HANDBOOK OF

Pain Management

A Clinical Companion to
Wall and Melzack's TEXTBOOK OF PAIN

To our wives, Lucy Melzack and Mary Wall,
with love and gratitude for all their encouragement and support.

Commissioning Editor: Michael J Houston
Project Development Manager: Aoibhe O'Shea, Glenys Norquay
Project Manager: Camilla Rockwood
Illustration Manager: Mick Ruddy
Designer: Sarah Russell
Illustrator: Marion Tasker

HANDBOOK OF

Pain Management

A Clinical Companion to Wall and Melzack's TEXTBOOK OF PAIN

Edited by

Ronald Melzack OC FRSC PhD
Department of Psychology
McGill University
Montreal
Quebec
Canada

Patrick D Wall FRS DM FRCP
(deceased)
Division of Physiology
St Thomas' Hospital
London
UK

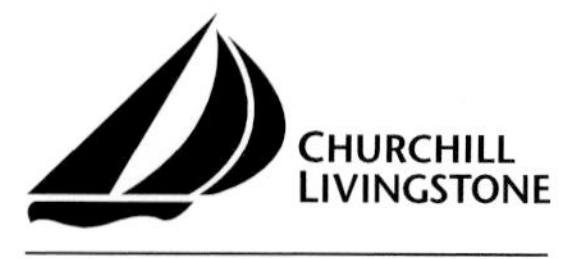

EDINBURGH LONDON NEW YORK OXFORD PHILADELPHIA ST LOUIS SYDNEY TORONTO 2003

CHURCHILL LIVINGSTONE
An imprint of Elsevier Limited

First published 2003

ISBN 0 443 017201 9

British Library Cataloguing in Publication Data
A catalogue record for this book is available from the British Library

Library of Congress Cataloging in Publication Data
A catalog record for this book is available from the Library of Congress

Notice
Medical knowledge is constantly changing. Standard safety precautions must be followed, but as new research and clinical experience broaden our knowledge, changes in treatment and drug therapy may become necessary or appropriate. Readers are advised to check the most current product information provided by the manufacturer of each drug to be administered to verify the recommended dose, the method and duration of administration, and contraindications. It is the responsibility of the practitioner, relying on experience and knowledge of the patient, to determine dosages and the best treatment for each individual patient. Neither the Publisher nor the editors assume any liability for any injury and/or damage to persons or property arising from this publication.
The Publisher

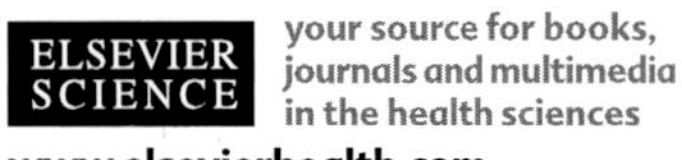

www.elsevierhealth.com

The Publisher's policy is to use **paper manufactured from sustainable forests**

Printed in China

Contents

Contributors List

Robert M Bennett MD
Department of Medicine
Oregon Health Sciences University
Portland, OR
USA

Charles B Berde MD PhD
Pain Treatment Service
Boston Children's Hospital
Boston, MA
USA

Aleksandar Berić MD DSc
Associate Professor of Neurology
Department of Neurology
Hospital for Joint Diseases
New York, NY
USA

Karen J Berkley PhD
Department of Psychology
Florida State University
Tallahassee, FL
USA

Laurence M Blendis MD FRCP FRCP(C)
Emeritus Professor of Medicine, University of Toronto
Visiting Professor, Sackler School of Medicine, Tel-Aviv University
Institute of Gastroenterology
Sourasky Tel-Aviv Medical Center
Tel-Aviv
Israel

Jörgen Boivie MD PhD
Department of Neurology
University Hospital
Linköping
Sweden

William Breitbart MD
Chief, Psychiatry Service
Department of Psychiatry and Behavioral Sciences
Memorial Sloan-Kettering Cancer Center
New York, NY
USA

Eduardo Bruera MD
Chair, Palliative Care and Rehabilitation Medicine
UT/MD Anderson Cancer Centre
Houston, TX
USA

Kay Brune MD PhD
Professor and Chairman
Department of Experimental and Clinical Pharmacology
University of Erlangen-Nürnberg
Erlangen
Germany

Arthur L Burnett MD
Department of Urology
Johns Hopkins University School of Medicine
Baltimore, MD
USA

Nathan I Cherny MB BS FRACD MD
Director, Cancer Pain and Palliative Care
Department of Medical Oncology
Shaare Zedek Medical Center
Jerusalem
Israel

Manon Choinière PhD
Institut de Cardiologie
de Montréal
Centre de Recherche
Montreal, Quebec
Canada

C A Chong MBBS FRCA
Pain Fellow
St Bartholomew's and
Whipps Cross University Hospitals
London
UK

John J Collins MB BS PhD FRACP
Head, Pain and Palliative Care Service
Children's Hospital at Westmead
Westmead, NSW
Australia

Michael Cousins AM MBBS MD
Pain Management and Research Centre
University of Sydney
St Leonards, NSW
Australia

Paul Creamer MD MRCP
Consultant Rheumatologist
Department of Rheumatology
Southmead Hospital
Bristol
UK

Shreelata Datta BSc
Cambridge
UK

Barbara de Lateur MD MS
Professor, Director and Lawrence Cardinal Shehan Chair
Department of Physical Medicine and Rehabilitation
Johns Hopkins University
Baltimore, MD
USA

David Dubuisson MD PhD
Clinical Associate Professor of Surgery,
University of South Carolina
Columbia, SC
USA

Howard L Fields MD PhD
Professor of Neurology and Physiology
Department of Neurology
University of California
San Francisco, CA
USA

Lucia Gagliese PhD
Assistant Professor
School of Kinesiology and Health Science, York University
Department of Anesthesia, University Health Network
Toronto, Ontario
Canada

Vivienne X Gallegos PhD
Registered Psychologist
West Vancouver, British Columbia
Canada

Ann Gamsa PhD
Director of Psychological Pain Services
McGill University Health Centre
Montreal General Hospital Pain Centre
Montreal, Quebec
Canada

Jan M Gybels MD PhD
Professor Emeritus of Neurosurgery
Department Neurosciences and Psychiatry
Belgium

Scott Haldeman DC MD PhD FRCPC
Clinical Professor, Department of Neurology
University of California, Irvine
Santa Ana, CA
USA

Per Hansson MD PhD DDS
Professor of Clinical Pain Research
Specialist in Neurology and Pain Medicine
Department of Surgical Sciences
Karolinska Hospital/Institute
Stockholm
Sweden

Raymond George Hill BPharm PhD
Executive Director of Pharmacology, The Neuroscience
Research Centre and Visiting Industrial Professor of Pharmacology,
University of Bristol.
Essex
UK

Anita Holdcroft MB ChB MD FRCA
Reader in Anaesthesia and Honorary Consultant Anaesthetist
Magill Department of Anesthesia
Imperial College London
Chelsea and Westminster Hospital
London
UK

Paul D Hooper DC MPH
Chair, Department of Principles and Practice
Southern California University of Health Sciences
Whittier, CA
USA

Malcolm IV Jayson MD FRCP
Emeritus Professor of Rheumatology
University of Manchester
Salford
UK

Troels Staehelin Jensen MD PhD
Professor of Experimental and Clinical Pain Research
Danish Pain Research Center
Aarhus University Hospital
Denmark

Julie A Jolin MD
Department of Obstetrics & Gynecology
UCLA Medical Center
Los Angeles, CA
USA

Justus F Lehmann MD
Professor and Chair, Retired
Department of Rehabilitation Medicine
University of Washington School of Medicine
Seattle, WA
USA

Donlin M Long MD PhD
Distinguished Service Professor
Department of Neurosurgery
Johns Hopkins Hospital
Baltimore, MD
USA

Thomas Lundeberg MD PhD
Professor, Department of Physiology and Pharmacology
Karolinska Institute
Stockholm
Sweden

Marco Maresca MD
Researcher
Dipartimento di Area Critica Medico Chirurgica
Università di Firenze
Florence
Italy

Bruce Masek PhD
Associate Professor of Psychiatry
Division of Child Psychiatry
Massachusetts General Hospital
Boston, MA
USA

John S McDonald MD
Professor of Obstetrics and Gynaecology
Chair, Department of Anesthesiology
Harbor-UCLA Medical Center
Torrance, CA
USA

Robert F McLain MD
Director, Spine Surgery Fellowship
Director, Spine Research Laboratory
Associate Professor, Ohio State University School of Medicine
Department of Orthopaedic Surgery
The Cleveland Clinic
Cleveland, OH
USA

Henry McQuay DM FRCA FRCP(Ed)
Professor of Pain Relief and Research Director
Pain Relief Unit
Churchill Hospital
Oxford
UK

Ronald Melzack OC FRSC PhD
Department of Psychology
McGill University
Montreal, Quebec
Canada

Harold Merskey DM FRCP FRCPC FRCPsych
Professor Emeritus of Psychiatry
London, Ontario
Canada

Kerry R Mills PhD MB FRCP
Professor of Clinical Neurophysiology
Academic Neuroscience Centre
King's College Hospital
London
UK

Richard Monks MDCM FRCP(C)
Clinical Associate Professor
Department of Psychiatry
University of British Columbia
Canada

Andrew Moore DSc DPhil
Pain Relief Unit
Churchill Hospital
Oxford
UK

Rajesh Munglani MD
Dept of Anaesthetic & Pain Clinic
West Suffolk Hospital
Bury St Edmonds
Suffolk
UK

Dianne J Newham PhD MCSP
Professor of Physiotherapy
GKT School of Biomedical Sciences
King's College London
London
UK

Lone Nikolajsen MD PhD
Consultant, Derpartment of Anaesthesia
Viborg Sygehus
Viborg
Denmark

Carl R Noback MD
Los Angeles, CA
USA

Akiko Okifuji PhD
Associate Professor
Dept of Anesthesiology
Pain Research and Management Center
Salt Lake City, UT
USA

Stephen D Passik PhD
Director, Symptom Management and Palliative Care
Associate Professor of Medicine and Behavioral Sciences
University of Kentucky – Markey Cancer Center
Lexington, KY
USA

Michael Platt
Consultant Anaesthetist
St Mary's Hospital
London
UK

Ian Power MD FRCA FFPMANZCA, FANZCA
Professor of Anaesthesia, Critical Care & Pain Medicine
Royal Infirmary
Little France
Edinburgh
UK

Paolo Procacci MD
Professor of Internal Medicine
The Pain Centre
University of Florence
Firenze
Italy

Andrea J Rapkin MD
Professor of Obstetrics and Gynecology
University of California, Los Angeles
Los Angeles, CA
USA

Barry D Rosenfeld PhD
Associate Professor of Psychology, Fordham University
Clinical Associate Professor of Psychology,
New York University School of Medicine
New York, NY
USA

Bo Salén MD
Orthopaedic Surgeon and Physician
Northwest Orthopaedics
Åre
Sweden

Peter S Sándor MD
Neurology Department
University Hospital
Zürich
Switzerland

Cicely Saunders FRCP
Founder, St Christopher's Hospice
London
UK

John W Scadding MD FRCP
Consultant Neurologist
The National Hospital for Neurology and Neurosurgery
London
UK

Jean Schoenen MD PhD
Professor of Neuroanatomy and Consultant Neurologist
Headache Research Unit
Department of Neuroanatomy and Neurology
University of Liege
Belgium

Yair Sharav DMD MS
Professor of Oral Medicine
Hebrew University - Haddassah
Jerusalem
Israel

Anders E Sola MD MS
Seattle, WA
USA

Erik Spangfort MD PhD
(deceased)
Late Associate Professor of Orthopaedic Surgery
Former Chief Orthopaedic Surgeon and Head of Spinal Unit
Huddinge University Hospital
Karolinska Institute
Stockholm
Sweden

Catherine Sweeney MB BCh BAO
Research Officer
Marymount Hospice
St Patrick's Hospital
Cork
Ireland

Ron R Tasker MD MA FRCS(C)
Division of Neurosurgery
Toronto Western Hospital
Toronto, Ontario
Canada

Dennis C Turk PhD
John & Emma Bonica Professor of Anesthesiology & Pain Research
Department of Anesthesiology
University of Washington
Seattle, WA
USA

Patrick D Wall FRS DM FRCP
(deceased)
Division of Physiology
St Thomas' Hospital
London
UK

James N Weinstein DO MS
Dartmouth Hitchcock Medical Center
Lebanon, NH
USA

Ursula Wesselmann MD PhD
Associate Professor of Neurology, Neurological Surgery and Biomedical Engineering
Department of Neurology
Johns Hopkins University School of Medicine
Baltimore, MD
USA

Joanna Zakrzewska MD FDSRCS FFDRCSI
Senior Lecturer and Honorary Consultant
Department of Oral Medicine
St Bartholomew's and the Royal London School of Medicine and Dentistry
London
UK

Hanns Ulrich Zeilhofer MD
Professor of Pharmacology
University of Erlangen-Nürnberg
Erlangen
Germany

Massimo Zoppi MD
Professor of Rheumatology
Dipartimento di Medicina Interna
Università di Firenze
Florence
Italy

Introduction: the pain revolution

Ronald Melzack

The explosive growth of our knowledge of every aspect of pain in recent years has produced major advances in the classification and management of the varieties of pain. An indication of our progress is the steady increase in size of successive editions of handbooks and textbooks. For example, the 4th edition of the *Textbook of Pain* (Wall and Melzack 1999) exceeds 1500 pages. Although its contents are outstanding, its bulk makes it difficult to handle when it is urgently needed in a clinical setting. This handbook, therefore, is a 'clinical companion' to our *Textbook of Pain*—an accessible summary of our current knowledge of clinical pain states and their management.

To produce this *Handbook of Pain Management*, authors of chapters of the *Textbook of Pain*—who are acclaimed authorities on pain diagnosis and therapy—were invited to contribute a shorter, updated version of their chapters. Sadly, my long-time colleague and friend Patrick Wall died on August 8, 2001, a few months after we invited the contributors to take part in this project. Fortunately, the authors affirmed their enthusiasm for a shorter handbook and contributed outstanding chapters. This book fulfils two aims Pat and I have always shared: to advance the frontiers of knowledge about pain, and to make the new ideas and facts as widely available as possible.

The field of pain has undergone a major revolution and this volume reflects these exciting advances. We now possess new concepts of pain and an array of recently developed approaches to pain management. There are several overlapping facets to the pain revolution.

The revolution in pain theory: the dominant role of the brain

The revolution began with a radical change in theory. The traditional view of pain is that injury or other somatic pathology activates pain receptors and fibres that transmit their messages directly up the spinal cord to the brain where they are perceived (Fig. 1). This concept explicitly assumes that pain perception always has an underlying physical cause—injury, infection, or some disease process. Pain in the absence of such a cause is usually attributed to psychological illness or malingering.

To replace this traditional approach to pain, we proposed the gate control theory (Melzack and Wall 1965), which states that spinal transmission is continuously modulated by the relative activity in large and small fibres and by descending messages from the brain. The gate theory's emphasis on the dynamic role of the brain in pain processes had a

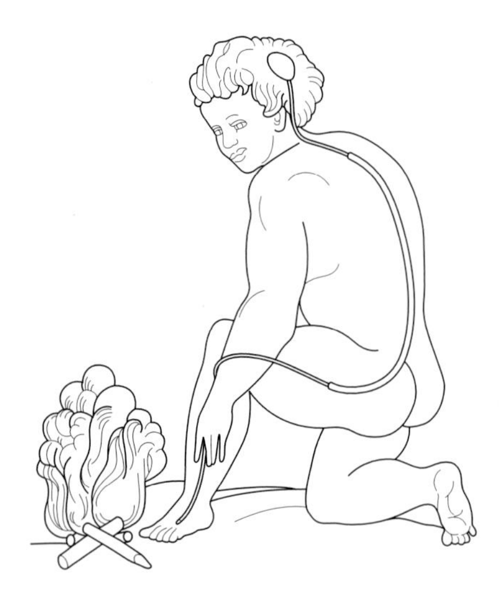

Fig. 1 Descartes' concept of the pain pathway. He writes: 'If for example fire (A) comes near the foot (B), the minute particles of this fire, which as you know move with great velocity, have the power to set in motion the spot of the skin of the foot which they touch, and by this means pulling upon the delicate thread (cc) which is attached to the spot of the skin, they open up at the same instant the pore (d e) against which the delicate thread ends, just as by pulling at one end of a rope one makes to strike at the same instant a bell which hangs at the other end.'

powerful scientific and clinical impact (Melzack and Wall 1996). Psychological factors, which were previously dismissed as 'reactions to pain', are now seen to be an integral part of pain processing, thereby opening new avenues for pain management by psychological therapies. Similarly, the concept of spinal sensory modulation provides a physiological rationale for physical therapists and other health-care professionals who use transcutaneous electrical nerve stimulation (TENS) and other stimulation techniques to treat pain.

The frontiers of pain theory have advanced still further into the brain. We now know that specialized parallel processing systems in the brain are selectively associated with the sensory-discriminative, affective-motivational, and cognitive-evaluative dimensions of subjective pain experience (Melzack and Casey 1968, Melzack and Wall 1996). The brain structures involved in pain include somatosensory projection areas, the anterior cingulate cortex and other limbic system structures, the prefrontal and posterior parietal cortex, the insula, hypothalamus and midbrain periaquaductal grey area, portions of the thalamus, and extensive interconnecting pathways (Ingvar and Hsieh 1999, Bushnell et al 2000). These brain areas compose a 'central pain matrix' (Ingvar and Hsieh 1999).

The impact of phantom limb pain

A major discovery that forces us to recognize the powerful role of the brain in pain perception is the evidence that a cordectomy—total removal of several segments of spinal cord so that there is no possible route for peripheral sensory information from the legs to arrive at the brain—does not stop intense pain in the phantom half of the body (Melzack and Loeser 1978, Gybels and Sweet 1989). Terrible pain is perceived in the phantom legs despite the obliteration of sensory input. The dominant role of the brain in our perception of the body is further supported by strong evidence that vivid phantom limbs are felt by people born without one or more limbs (Melzack et al 1997, Brugger et al 2000), indicating that the neural networks for perception of the body as well as the qualities of pain we feel in it are genetically built into the brain. Another built-in quality is the sense of 'self'; people with lesions of the posterior parietal cortex often deny that the contralateral half of their body is their own even when it is painfully stimulated (Sandifer 1946, Melzack 1989).

These remarkable observations refute the classical theory that attributes the qualities of experience to specific peripheral receptors and nerve fibres. It seems common sense to talk about 'pain pathways' to the brain. However, pain is not injury; the qualities of pain experience must not be confused with the physical event of injuring skin or bone. There are no receptor equivalents to stinging, smarting, rasping, and itchy. The perceptual qualities are produced by built-in neural networks in the brain—in the 'central pain matrix' described above—which compose what I have called the 'body-self neuromatrix' (Melzack 1990, 1995). We tend to assume that sensations are always produced by stimuli and that perceptions in the absence of stimuli are psychologically abnormal. Yet the extraordinary reality of painful phantom limbs indicates that this notion is wrong. The brain does more than detect and analyse sensory inputs; it creates perceptual experience even in the absence of external inputs. We do not need a body to feel a body or a physical injury to feel pain.

Descartes' depiction of pain as a simple, straight-through neural transmission system, shown in Fig. 1, requires further consideration (Lott 1986). These early events after injury, in fact, represent only Stage 1—the transmission of messages to the brain—of Descartes' larger conceptual scheme for pain. Stage 2 is the much more extraordinary transformation of the nerve messages into conscious experience within the brain. Descartes, in the 1600s, ascribed the transformation to a non-physical mind (or soul) that resides in the central part of the brain. In the twenty-first century, the challenge to scientists is to discover what happens in the brain during Stage 2. *How* are nerve impulses transformed into the conscious experience of pain? The pain revolution has advanced from Stage 1 skin-to-brain transmission mechanisms to Stage 2: the creative transformation by the brain of patterns of nerve impulses into the perceptual qualities, emotions, and meanings that compose the stream of subjective experience.

The role of stress

By recognizing the dominant role of the brain, which generates our subjective experiences and activates our defense systems, we are now able to appreciate the intimate relationship between pain and stress. We are so accustomed to considering pain as a sensory phenomenon that we have long ignored the fact that injury does more than produce pain; it also disrupts the brain's homeostatic regulation systems, thereby producing 'stress' and initiating complex programs to reinstate homeostasis. The stress system vastly expands the puzzle of pain and provides valuable clues in our quest to understand chronic pain (Melzack 1998, 1999).

Hans Selye (1956), who founded the field of stress research, observed that stress is produced by psychological threat and insult to the body-self as well as by physical injury and disease. The disruption of homeostasis by psychological and physical stress activates programmes of neural, hormonal, immunological, and behavioural activity selected from a genetically determined repertoire (Chrousos and Gold 1992, Sapolsky 1994). The release of cortisol and noradrenaline (norepinephrine) set the stage for the body's response to injury or other threats. Cortisol is an essential hormone for survival because it is responsible for producing and maintaining high levels of glucose necessary for the response to stress. However, it is potentially destructive because, to ensure a high level of glucose, it breaks down the protein in muscle and inhibits the ongoing replacement of calcium in bone. Sustained stress and cortisol release, therefore, can produce myopathy, weakness, fatigue, and decalcification of bone (Sapolsky 1994) and thereby contribute to the development of fibromyalgia, rheumatoid arthritis, and chronic fatigue syndrome (Chrousos and Gold 1992).

Prolonged cortisol release, moreover, also suppresses the immune system, providing a link between pain and some of the autoimmune diseases (Melzack 1999). Many autoimmune diseases such as rheumatoid arthritis, lupus, and scleroderma are also pain syndromes. Furthermore, more women than men suffer from autoimmune diseases as well as from chronic pain syndromes (Chap. 39). These relationships among stress, gender, the immune system, and chronic pain syndromes reveal the need to study pain in a biological context far broader than a 'pain pathway'.

The revolution in defining pain: from reflexes to subjective experience

The focus on reflexes in twentieth-century physiology and psychology led to definitions of pain in terms of innate and conditioned reflex responses to noxious stimulation: escape, avoidance, and other 'aversive behaviours'. Subjective experience was deemed to be unscientific. In the 1940s, however, WK Livingston (1943, 1998) argued that 'nothing can properly be called pain unless it is consciously perceived as such'. In short, pain is not a form of behaviour; it is what we feel. The definition of pain as a subjective experience—and only that—was finally established by Harold Merskey and his colleagues. Merskey (1979) presided over a Committee of the International Association for the Study of Pain that provided a definition now widely accepted: 'Pain is an unpleasant sensory and emotional experience associated with actual or potential tissue damage, or described in terms of such damage.' Merskey's report goes on to say:

> Pain is always subjective. Each individual learns the application of the word through experience related to injury in early life. . . . It is unquestionably a sensation in a part of the body but it is also always unpleasant and therefore also an emotional experience. . . . Many people report pain in the absence of tissue damage or any likely pathophysiological cause . . . If they regard their experience as pain and if they report it in the same ways as pain caused by tissue damage, it should be accepted as pain. This definition avoids tying pain to the stimulus.

Scientific research on pain experience requires measurement instruments, and several valid, reliable instruments are available (Melzack and Katz 1999). The most widely used is the McGill Pain Questionnaire (MPQ; Melzack 1975), which comprises 20 sets of verbal descriptors to measure the sensory, affective (emotional), and cognitive dimensions

SHORT FORM McGILL PAIN QUESTIONAIRE
Ronald Melzack

PATIENTS NAME: .... DATE: ....

	NONE		MILD		MODERATE		SEVERE	
THROBBING	0)	______	1)	______	2)	______	3)	______
SHOOTING	0)	______	1)	______	2)	______	3)	______
STABBING	0)	______	1)	______	2)	______	3)	______
SHARP	0)	______	1)	______	2)	______	3)	______
CRAMPING	0)	______	1)	______	2)	______	3)	______
GNAWING	0)	______	1)	______	2)	______	3)	______
HOT-BURNING	0)	______	1)	______	2)	______	3)	______
ACHING	0)	______	1)	______	2)	______	3)	______
HEAVY	0)	______	1)	______	2)	______	3)	______
TENDER	0)	______	1)	______	2)	______	3)	______
SPLITTING	0)	______	1)	______	2)	______	3)	______
TIRING-EXHAUSTING	0)	______	1)	______	2)	______	3)	______
SICKENING	0)	______	1)	______	2)	______	3)	______
FEARFUL	0)	______	1)	______	2)	______	3)	______
PUNISHING-CRUEL	0)	______	1)	______	2)	______	3)	______

NO PAIN |—|—|—|—|—|—|—|—|—|—| WORST POSSIBLE PAIN

0 1 2 3 4 5 6 7 8 9 10

P P I

0 NO PAIN ____
1 MILD ____
2 DISCOMFORTING ____
3 DISTRESSING ____
4 HORRIBLE ____
5 EXCRUCIATING ____

Fig. 2 The short-form McGill Pain Questionnaire. Descriptors 1–11 represent the sensory dimension of pain experience and 12–15 represent the affective dimension. Each descriptor is ranked on an intensity scale of 0 = none, 1 = mild, 2 = moderate, 3 = severe. The Present Pain Intensity (PPI) of the standard long-form McGill Pain Questionnaire and the visual analogue numerical scale (VANS) are also included to provide overall pain intensity scores.

of pain experience. The questionnaire provides numerical scores for each subjective quality of experience. A short-form MPQ is now used frequently for clinical practice and research trials (Melzack 1987; Fig. 2).

The change in the definition of pain from an injury-produced response to a multidimensional subjective experience opens the door to new forms of pain management. Peripheral and spinal mechanisms are obviously important and need to be fully investigated, but they are only part of the story of pain. Many people suffer severe chronic pain in the absence of discernible physical causes. Our ignorance of the causes of many pain states forces us toward the brain, where subjective experience occurs.

The revolution in pain management: from blocking a 'pain pathway' to multiple interacting approaches

The revolution in pain theory and definition has taken us from the concept of a specific, dedicated pathway as the exclusive source of pain to brain mechanisms that integrate inputs from parallel sensory, emotional, and cognitive systems. These systems generate output patterns that are transformed into the subjective experience of pain as well as strategies of homeostatic and behavioural responses to stop the pain and return to optimal health. The concept of a body-self neuromatrix provides us with a model to describe the inputs that impinge on the widespread integrative neural network (Fig. 3) and also provides guidelines for ways to modulate the network's output patterns to diminish or abolish pain. Implicit in this concept is the assumption that, in addition to sensory influences on the synaptic architecture of the neuromatrix, genetic determinants may predispose toward the development of chronic pain syndromes.

The management of pain depends, of course, on the kind of pain. Brief, acute pains, usually after an injury or infection, have genuine survival value. They may prevent or minimize serious damage to the body and are important for learning to avoid future encounters. Continuing pain during healing may also prevent reinjury (Chap. 1).

In contrast, chronic pain is destructive and serves no useful purpose. One form of chronic pain is associated with unremitting diseases such as cancer (Chaps. 42–45) and arthritis (Chaps. 2, 3) that destroy body tissue. Chronic pain may also be caused by protruding discs in the spine (Chaps. 5, 19), insufficient blood supply to heart tissue (Chap. 9), severe burns (Chap. 41), and a variety of other pathologies of the body's functions. Attempts to relieve these pains often work. Cancer pain, for example, can be greatly diminished, sometimes abolished entirely, by appropriate doses of morphine or other opioid drugs (Chaps. 24, 42–45). Yet despite the best efforts in hospitals with outstanding facilities, 5–10% of patients with cancer continue to have moderate to high levels of pain.

The second type of chronic pain is usually out of proportion to an injury or other pathology and may persist long after healing is complete, its causes often being a mystery. Trigeminal and postherpetic neuralgia (Chaps. 14, 17), pelvic and urogenital pain (Chaps. 10, 12), most back pains and headaches (Chaps. 5, 15), and 'myofascial pains' (Chaps. 6, 7) are some of the kinds of chronic pain that are difficult to control. In recent years, however, major advances have been made in our understanding and management of almost all of these pain states (Chaps. 5–18).

The new pharmacology of pain

Impressive advances have been made in pharmacology. New antipyretic (non-narcotic) analgesics (Chap. 22) and recently developed opioids and novel delivery systems (Chap. 24) have helped countless people. So too, advances in the use of local anaesthetics and epidurals (Chap. 25) and atypical analgesic drugs and sympathetic blockers (Chap. 26) have brought relief to many patients.

The most extraordinary drugs, however, are the new arrivals often labelled as 'adjuncts'. Developed originally to combat depression and epilepsy, they are unexpected sources of major relief for many severe, previously intractable, chronic pains (Chap. 23). These drugs are now the first line of attack against a wide variety of chronic pains. In addition to antidepressant and antiepilepsy drugs, neuroleptics and possibly lithium are effective for some kinds of pain (Chap. 24). Furthermore, clonidine, tramadol, mexiletine, and possibly cannabinoids relieve some types of pain in some people (Chaps. 22–26). These drugs, which relieve some of the most terrible, debilitating pains, are not mere 'adjuncts'; they are the 'new generation analgesics'. We need a new classification system and a new nomenclature for antipain drugs.

These advances in the pharmacology of pain did not come from Stage 1 research on the pain transmission pathways. They came instead from hunches and fortuitous discoveries made by observant clinicians who had the courage to publish articles and letters in medical journals to propose that antiepilepsy, antidepressant, antipsychotic, and other drugs that act on brain functions are also antipain drugs.

Stress presents a wide-open field for pharmacology. Stress reactions are part-and-parcel of pain-producing events—accidents, disease, day-to-day threats and challenges, childhood or marital physical abuse. These stresses trigger programmes of brain activities to correct the disruptions by activating the endocrine, sympathetic, immune, and behavioural systems. Sometimes these 'good programmes' may run amok and create conditions that produce pain rather than ameliorate it. Steroids are sometimes used effectively for these pain problems, but they must be used cautiously. Pharmacological research is urgently needed to find new, safe steroids or other stress-related compounds.

Despite the impressive advances and optimistic outlook, many chronic pains remain intractable. Consider phantom limb pain (Chap. 16). About 60–70% of amputees suffer terrible pain. The pain may be relieved in some patients by local anaesthetic injections or some combination of drugs. However, tragically, the cause of the pain is poorly understood and no widely effective treatment has yet been found. Similarly many people who suffer headaches, backaches, and other forms of chronic pain are helped by several therapies now available, but many are not. For example, we have excellent new drugs for some kinds of headache, but not for all (Chap. 15). Our understanding of headache has advanced substantially in recent years, but the continued suffering by countless people indicates we still have a long way to go.

Multidisciplinary pain clinics; hospice and palliative care services

Another major feature of the revolution is the development by John Bonica of the concept of the multidisciplinary pain clinic (see Bonica 1990), and the establishment by Cicely Saunders of St. Christopher's Hospice and associated palliative care services (Saunders 1976, Mount 1984). These events in the 1950s and 1960s mark an extraordinary breakthrough in the field of pain.

Pain, classically a symptom of injury, is now recognized as a major problem of challenging complexity. No longer merely a symptom, chronic pain states now often require several specialized therapists to examine, classify, and attempt to treat the pain. So too, terminally ill people with intense pain need more than aspirin or acetaminophen. Every bit of the armamentarium must be used to battle against pain—especially the opiates in the doses needed, on a fixed schedule to prevent the return of pain, and as long as needed. A wide range of therapists and other caregivers are enlisted to provide palliative care. Patient-controlled analgesia (PCA) and transdermal patches are reliable delivery systems for people in severe pain (Chaps. 24, 41–45). Pain is an evil to be abolished by every available means. We owe a tremendous debt to John Bonica and Cicely Saunders for fighting against the pressures to maintain the status quo. They instituted a profound sense of caring for the individual human's welfare. The challenge ahead is to extend this revolution to the poor in Western countries and the 80% of humanity who live in the third-world countries in Africa, Asia, and South America.

The rapid rise of non-drug therapies

The pain revolution has had a tremendous impact on the development of new non-drug therapies. Psychological therapies, which were generally used as a last resort when drugs or neurosurgery failed, are now an integral part of pain management strategies. The recognition that pain is the result of multiple contributions (Fig. 3) gave rise to a rich variety of psychological approaches: relaxation techniques, hypnotic suggestion, and ingenious methods of cognitive and behavioural therapy (Chaps. 33–36). So too, TENS and physical therapy procedures have evolved rapidly, bringing striking pain relief to large numbers of people (Chaps. 30–32). At the same time, techniques for electrical stimulation of the spinal cord and brain have been evolving and show promise for the relief of selective kinds of pain (Simpson 1999, and see Chap. 20). An important feature of the development of these psychological and physical procedures was the careful assessment and evaluation of all the variables relevant to pain (Turk and Melzack 2001).

The revolution in science: from a closed pain pathway to an open biological system

The pain revolution has taken us from a specific pain pathway to an open biological system that comprises multiple sensory inputs, memories of past experiences, personal and social expectations, genetic contributions, gender, ageing, and stress patterns involving the endocrine, autonomic, and immune systems. Pain has become a major challenge to medicine, psychology, and all the other health sciences and professions. Every aspect of life, from birth to dying, has characteristic pain problems. Genetics, until recently, was rarely considered relevant to understanding pain; yet sophisticated laboratory studies (Mogil et al 2000) and clinical observations (see Melzack 1999) have established genetic predispositions related to pain as an essential component of the field. The study of pain, therefore, now incorporates research in epidemiology and medical genetics as well as sociological and cultural studies. The field of pain has broadened in other exciting ways. Dworkin (1997) and Linton (2002) have searched for and found significant relationships between some chronic pain states and several features of prior acute pain or physical and sexual abuse. The elucidation of these relationships could lead to the prevention of serious pain syndromes.

The basic sciences are also pushing into exciting new territory. At the forefront of basic research in pain is the discovery that glial cells in the spinal cord—traditionally thought to simply maintain the metabolism of neurons—release immune products (cytokines) after peripheral nerve or spinal root injury (Colburn and DeLeo 1999, Watkins et al 2001). Cytokines produce spinal inflammation, which could contribute to spinal and neuropathic pains. If glial cells in selected regions of the brain have the same immune-inflammatory effects as in the cord, the implications for understanding pain could be enormous.

The impact of the pain revolution is revealed by the contents of this handbook. The further we move from a stimulus-driven concept of pain, the better we recognize the validity of baffling pain syndromes that often have no obvious pathology to explain the presence of pain or its terrible intensity. They include neuropathic pains, backache, fibromyalgia, pelvic, urogenital, and other pains (Chaps. 5–18), which become increasingly comprehensible when we extend our diagnostic search to consider multiple causal mechanisms.

A new historical perspective and some predictions

Two streams of research have evolved since Descartes' concept of pain (Fig. 1). The first stream derives from Descartes' mechanistic Stage 1 transmission system from skin to brain. Stream 1 research begins with the stimulation of sensory receptors and follows inputs up to the brain, but shows little interest in subjective perception: the brain simply produces sensation that passively reflects the sensory input. This 'bottom-up' approach to pain physiology continues to be the defining feature of Stream 1 research.

The second stream of research begins with people's descriptions of their pain, followed by a search for mechanisms. This 'top-down' approach to pain has its origins in S. Weir Mitchell's studies of nerve-injury pain during the American Civil War. Mitchell (1872) investigated phantom limb pain and causalgia, and recognized that both kinds of pain are strikingly out of proportion to injury. Excruciating phantom limb pains are reported by people whose stump and surrounding tissues have healed perfectly. Similarly, the horrible burning pain of causalgia is often associated with minor nerve injuries. Livingston (1943), after confirming Mitchell's observations in a civilian population, then searched for the causes of such intense, prolonged pain and was forced to shift his search for abnormal mechanisms from peripheral nerves to the spinal cord. This 'top-down' stream in the history of pain continued to evolve with the reports by Beecher (1959) of high levels of pain relief by placebos (Chap. 33), and the astonishing fact that little or no pain is felt by soldiers after major injuries at the battlefront—a fact confirmed in a civilian population (Melzack et al 1982). These observations are a convincing refutation of the concept that pain is a specific sensation produced by injury (see Melzack and Wall 1996).

By 1965 both streams were powerful but different from each other. One started with the stimulation of peripheral tissues and searched for the routes upward; the other started with subjective reports and explored downward. The power of the gate control theory, I believe, is that it brought both streams together by adding 'central control'—that is, psychological processes in the brain such as past experience, suggestion, and attention that act down on spinal gates and modulate pain-signalling transmission. The 'hybrid vigour' of the conjoined conceptual streams produced the revolution that ensued and the explosion in research.

Fortunately, a remarkable technology that holds great promise for a new creative period in pain research and therapy has evolved. PET and fMRI imaging techniques are being used increasingly to study pain-associated physiological events in the brains of human beings who can simultaneously report their subjective experiences (Bushnell et al 2000, Ingvar and Hsieh 1999). These techniques have confirmed pain-related activity in somatosensory projection areas, limbic structures, frontal and posterior parietal cortex, and related integrative structures. Lesions of these areas in humans also reveal selective disruption of the sensory, affective, and cognitive dimensions of pain experience (Bouckoms 1994, Melzack and Wall 1996, Ingvar and Hsieh 1999). These widely distributed, highly interconnected areas provide powerful supporting evidence for the concept of a body-self neuromatrix with multiple inputs and outputs as shown in Fig. 3.

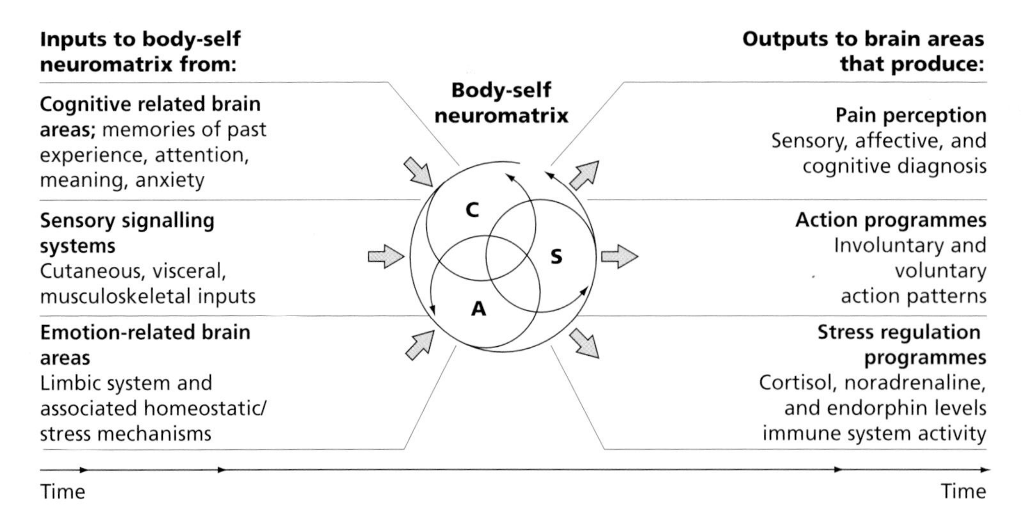

Fig. 3 Factors that contribute to the patterns of activity generated by the body-self neuromatrix, which comprises parallel, interacting sensory (S), affective (A), and cognitive (C) neuromodules. The output patterns from the neuromatrix project to other brain areas that produce the multiple dimensions of pain experience as well as concurrent homeostatic and behavioural responses.

I believe that this rapidly growing focus on the brain together with the exciting developments in imaging and other neuroscience techniques will again produce the hybrid vigour that characterized the impact of the gate control theory. Hopefully, animal models of human chronic pain syndromes, particularly neuropathic pain (Mao 2002), will allow parallel imaging studies of human brain activity during pain experience and microelectrode studies of brain activity in animals. Parallel studies such as these will provide essential information about brain function.

By using these parallel methods to study drug effects on brain activity, the new pharmacology will continue to flourish. Still more, the use of computer modelling and systems analysis as guides to explore the brain should reveal how multiple inputs are integrated in parallel, widely distributed networks, how the 'language' of the brain—temporal and spatial patterns of nerve impulses—produces output patterns that contain information about sensory, emotional, and cognitive dimensions, and how the continuous stream of that language is transformed into the pains we feel. This knowledge, together with the study of psychological procedures, such as relaxation (Chap. 34) and hypnosis (Chap. 35), whose effects on the brain can be followed in real time (Bushnell et al 2000), will contribute to the control of chronic pain.

The pain mission of the health professions

This volume is testimony to the recent advances in diagnosing and managing clinical pain states. The contributors describe procedures and strategies to combat a wide range of acute and chronic pains. Unfortunately, many people suffering various forms of pain are not helped because we lack the necessary knowledge. Still worse, many people suffer even though we have the knowledge but our educational, health care, or other social systems have failed.

We have a mission—all of us—to rectify the existing situation, for cancer pain as well as post-surgical pain, for pain in adults and in children, and for any kind of severe pain that can be helped by sensible administration of drugs and other pain therapies. In addition to educating one another in current pain research and therapy, as we do in journals and congresses, we must promote education on the management of pain for medical students and all health professionals. We must also teach patients to communicate better about their pain, and inform them that they have a right to freedom from pain, that each suffering human being deserves the best that the health professions have to offer. We must also get our message to those in government that pain is a major plague that saps the strength of society, that funds for research and therapy are urgently needed, that regulations regarding the supply of drugs must be modified to reflect the needs of people in pain, not just the misdeeds of street addicts. If we can pursue these goals together—as scientists and therapists, as members of the full range of scientific and health professions—we can hope to meet the goal we all strive for: to help our fellow human beings who suffer pain.

References

Beecher HK 1959 Measurement of subjective response. Oxford University Press, New York

Bonica JJ (ed) 1990 The management of pain, 2nd edn. Lea and Febiger, Philadelphia

Bouckoms AJ 1994 Limbic surgery for pain. In: Wall PD, Melzack R (eds) Textbook of pain, 3rd edn. Churchill Livingstone, Edinburgh, pp 1171–1187

Brugger P, Kollias SS, Müri RM, Crelier G, Hepp-Reymond MC, Regard M 2000 Beyond re-membering: phantom sensations of congenitally absent limbs. Proceedings of the National Academy of Sciences 97: 6167–6172

Bushnell MC, Duncan GH, Ha B, Chen J-I, Olausson H 2000 Non-invasive brain imaging during experimental and clinical pain. In: Eevor M, Rowbotham MC, Weisenfeld-Hallin Z (eds) Progress in pain research and management, vol 16. IASP Press, Seattle, pp 485–495

Chrousos GP, Gold PW 1992 The concept of stress and stress system disorders. Journal of the American Medical Association 267: 1244–1252

Colburn RW, DeLeo JA 1999 The effect of perineural colchicine on nerve injury-induced spinal glial activation and neuropathic pain behavior. Brain Research Bulletin 49: 419–427

Dworkin RH 1997 Which individuals with acute pain are most likely to develop a chronic pain syndrome? Pain Forum 6: 127–136

Gybels JM, Sweet WH 1989 Neurosurgical treatment of persistent pain. Karger, Basel

Ingvar M, Hsieh J-C 1999 The image of pain. In: Wall PD, Melzack R (eds) Textbook of pain, 4th edn. Churchill Livingston, Edinburgh, pp 215–233

Linton SJ 2002 A prospective study of the effects of sexual or physical abuse on back pain. Pain 96: 347–351

Livingston WK 1943 Pain mechanisms. Macmillan, New York

Livingston WK 1998 Pain and suffering. IASP Press, Seattle

Lott TL 1986 Descartes on phantom limbs. Mind & Language 1: 243–271

Mao J 2002 Translational pain research: bridging the gap between basic and clinical research. Pain 97: 183–187

Melzack R 1975 The McGill Pain Questionnaire: major properties and scoring methods. Pain 1: 277–299

Melzack R 1987 The Short Form McGill Pain Questionnaire. Pain 30: 191–197

Melzack R 1989 Phantom limbs, the self and the brain. Canadian Psychology 30: 1–16

Melzack R 1990 Phantom limbs and the concept of a neuromatrix. Trends in Neurosciences 13: 88–92

Melzack R 1995 Phantom limb pain and the brain. In: Bromm B, Desmedt JE (eds) Pain and the brain. Raven Press, New York, pp 73–82

Melzack R 1998 Pain and stress: clues toward understanding chronic pain. In: Sabourin M, Craik F, Robert M (eds) Advances in psychological science, vol 2, Biological and cognitive aspects. Psychology Press, Hove, pp 63–85

Melzack R 1999 Pain and stress: a new perspective. In: Gatchel RJ, Turk DC (eds) Psychosocial factors in pain. Guilford Press, New York, pp 89–106

Melzack R, Casey KL 1968 Sensory, motivational, and central control determinants. In: Kenshalo D (ed) The skin senses. Thomas, Springield IL, pp 423–443

Melzack R, Katz J 1999 Pain measurement in persons in pain. In: Wall PD, Melzack R (eds) Textbook of pain, 4th edn. Churchill Livingston, Edinburgh, pp 409–426

Melzack R, Loeser JD 1978 Phantom body pain in paraplegics: evidence for a central pattern generating mechanism for pain. Pain 4: 195–210

Melzack R, Wall PD 1965 Pain mechanisms: a new theory. Science 150: 971–979

Melzack R, Wall PD 1996 Challenge of pain (updated 2nd edn): Penguin Books, London

Melzack R, Wall PD, Ty TC 1982 Acute pain in an emergency clinic: latency of onset and descriptor patterns related to different injuries. Pain 14: 33–43

Melzack R, Israel R, Lacroix R, Schultz G 1997 Phantom limbs in people with congenital limb deficiency or amputation in early childhood. Brain 120: 1603–1620

Merskey H, IASP Subcommittee on Taxonomy 1979 Pain terms: a list with definitions and notes on usage. Pain 6: 249–252

Mitchell SW 1872 Injuries of nerves and their consequences. Lippincott, Philadelphia

Mogil JS, Yu L, Basbaum AI 2000 Pain genes? Annual Review of Neuroscience 23: 777–811

Mount BM 1984 Psychological and social aspects of cancer pain. In: Wall PD, Melzack R (eds) Textbook of pain, 1st edn. Churchill Livingston, Edinburgh, pp 460–471

Sandifer PH 1946 Anosognosia and disorders of the body scheme. Brain 69: 122–137

Sapolsky RM 1994 Why zebras don't get ulcers: a guide to stress, stress-related diseases, and coping. WH Freeman, New York

Saunders C 1976 Care of the dying. Nursing Times 72: 3–24

Selye H 1956 The stress of life. McGraw-Hill, New York

Simpson BA 1999 Spinal cord and brain stimulation. In: Wall PD, Melzack R (eds) Textbook of pain, 4th edn. Churchill Livingston, Edinburgh, pp 1353–1381

Turk DC, Melzack R 2001 Handbook of pain assessment, 2nd edn. Guilford Press, New York

Wall PD, Melzack R (eds) 1999 Textbook of pain, 4th edn. Churchill Livingston, Edinburgh

Watkins LR, Milligan ED, Maier SF 2001 Glial activation: a driving force for pathological pain. Trends in Neuroscience 24: 450–455

Section 1

Clinical pain states

Chapter 1

Acute and postoperative pain

Michael Cousins and Ian Power

Introduction

Acute pain usually signals impending or actual tissue damage and thus permits the individual to avoid further injury. It may also prevent harmful movement, for example, in the case of a fracture. Reduced mobility associated with acute pain may therefore aid healing. However, the organism benefits only briefly from this effect and its prolongation results in an adverse outcome (Bonica 1985, Cousins and Phillips 1986, Kehlet 1988). Pain also initiates complex neurohumoral responses that help initially to maintain homeostasis in the face of an acute disease or injury; if these changes are excessive or unduly prolonged, they may cause morbidity or mortality (Cousins and Phillips 1986, Kehlet 1988). Psychological responses to acute pain may initially be helpful in coping with the physical insult; however, if excessively severe or prolonged, they may become deleterious. The complexity of acute pain requires an understanding of safe and effective principles to treat it (Box 1.1).

Acute pain mechanisms

The perception of acute pain is a complex interaction that involves sensory, emotional, and behavioural factors. The role of psychological factors, which include a person's emotional and behavioural responses, must always be considered to be an important component in the perception and expression of acute pain.

The biological processes involved in our perception of acute pain are no longer viewed as a simple 'hard-wired' system with a pure 'stimulus–response' relationship. Trauma to any part of the body, and nerve damage in particular, can lead to changes within other regions of the nervous system, which influence subsequent responses to sensory input. There is increasing recognition that long-term changes occur within the peripheral and central nervous system following noxious input. This 'plasticity' of the nervous system then alters the body's response to further peripheral sensory input.

Peripheral sensitization

Surgical trauma or other noxious stimuli associated with acute pain are associated with an injury response or 'inflammatory response'. Part of the inflammatory response is the release of intracellular contents from damaged cells and inflammatory cells such as macrophages, lymphocytes, and mast cells. Nociceptive stimulation also results in a neurogenic inflammatory response and the eventual release of chemicals that sensitize high-threshold

BOX 1.1
Principles of safe and effective acute pain management. (Adapted from NHMRC 1999)

- Adverse physiological and psychological effects result from unrelieved severe pain.
- Proper assessment and control of pain require patient involvement.
- Effective pain relief requires flexibility and tailoring of treatment to an individual rather than rigid application of formulae and prescriptions.
- Pain is best treated early, because established, severe pain is more difficult to treat (Bach et al 1988, Katz et al 1996).
- While it is not possible or always desirable to completely alleviate all pain in the postoperative period, it should be possible to reduce pain to a tolerable or comfortable level.
- Postoperative analgesia should be planned preoperatively, with consideration given to the type of surgery, medical condition of the patient, perioperative use of analgesics, and regional anaesthetic techniques.
- Ultimate responsibility for pain management should be assigned to those most experienced in its administration and not to the most junior staff members.

Safe and effective analgesia also depends on:

- Frequent assessment and reassessment of pain intensity and charting of analgesia.
- Adequate education of all involved in pain management, including the patient.
- Formal programmes, protocols, and guidelines covering acute pain management relevant to the institution.
- Formal quality assurance programmes to regularly evaluate the effectiveness of pain management.

nociceptors, resulting in the phenomenon of peripheral sensitization.

Following sensitization, low-intensity mechanical stimuli which would not normally cause pain are now perceived as painful. There is also an increased responsiveness to thermal stimuli at the site of injury. This zone of 'primary hyperalgesia' surrounding the site of injury is caused by peripheral changes and is a feature commonly observed following surgery and other forms of trauma (see Levine and Reichling 1999, Raja et al 1999).

NSAIDs

Non-steroidal anti-inflammatory drugs (NSAIDs) are commonly used for 'peripheral' analgesia and one of their actions is a reduction in the inflammatory response (Merry and Power 1995, Walker 1995). Agents such as aspirin and other NSAIDs provide their anti-inflammatory action by blocking the cyclooxygenase pathway. Cyclooxygenase exists in two forms, COX1 and COX2. While COX1 is always present in tissues, including the gastric mucosa, COX2 is induced by inflammation (Seibert et al 1994). This presents an opportunity for the development of agents that have a selective anti-inflammatory effect without gastric side effects. Selective COX2 inhibitor drugs (e.g. rofecoxib, celecoxib) that may offer analgesia with no antiplatelet effect and less gastrointestinal toxicity than NSAIDs have been developed; renal toxicity, effects in aspirin-sensitive asthmatic individuals, and long term cardiovascular effects are as yet unclear (Kam and Power 2000). Besides the peripheral action of NSAIDs, there is increasing evidence that they exert their analgesic effect through central mechanisms (Urquhart 1993, Walker 1995).

Peripheral action of opioids

Opioids have traditionally been viewed as centrally acting drugs. However, there is now evidence for the action of endogenous opioids on peripheral sites following tissue damage (Stein et al 1989, Stein 1993). Opioid receptors are manufactured in the cell body (dorsal root ganglion) and transported toward the central terminal in the dorsal horn and toward the periphery. These peripheral receptors then become active following local tissue damage. This occurs with unmasking of opioid receptors and the arrival of immunocompetent cells that possess opioid receptors and have the ability to synthesize opioid peptides. This has led to an interest in the peripheral administration of opioids, such as intra-articular administration following knee surgery or arthroscopy (Haynes et al 1994, Stein 1995) or topical administration of morphine (Tennant et al 1993). Despite initial enthusiasm with this technique, some workers have expressed doubt about the usefulness and cost-benefit of intra-articular morphine, particularly following arthroscopy or minor knee surgery (Aasbo et al 1996). However, opioids with physicochemical properties favouring peripheral action are under development and, if successful, such drugs may be useful for regional application (Binder et al 2001). Medium-sized peptides are under development with a view to a localized action, thus avoiding systemic uptake.

Peripheral nerve injury

Recent studies have demonstrated that section of, or damage to, a peripheral nerve results in a number of biochemical, physiological, and morphological changes that act as a focus of pain in themselves (see Ollat and Cesaro 1995, Devor and Seltzer 1999). Neuroplasticity changes that maintain sensory input may occur at peripheral and/or spinal levels. In the postsurgery or post-trauma patient, neuropathic pain may have an early onset within the first 24 hours; this is contrary to classic teaching. There may also be a delayed onset on the order of 10 days. Agents used for the management of peripheral neuropathic pain are described in Chaps. 22–26.

Sympathetic nervous system

The sympathetic nervous system also has an important role in the generation and maintenance of acute pain states (McMahon 1991, Jänig and McLachlan 1994, Jänig 1996). Inflammation can result in the sensitization of primary nociceptive afferent fibres by prostanoids that are released from sympathetic fibres (Levine et al 1993). Following nerve injury, sympathetic nerve stimulation or the administration of noradrenaline (norepinephrine) can excite primary afferent fibres via an action at α-adrenoceptors; also there is innervation of the dorsal root ganglion by sympathetic terminals (McLachlan et al 1993). This means that activity in sympathetic efferent fibres can lead to abnormal activity or responsiveness of the primary afferent fibre.

Dorsal horn mechanisms of importance to acute pain

The dorsal horn is the site of termination of primary afferents, and there is a complex interaction among afferent fibres, local intrinsic spinal neurons and the endings of descending fibres from the brain. Moreover, pharmacological studies have identified the many neurotransmitters and neuromodulators involved in pain processing in the dorsal horn (Wilcox 1991, Doubell et al 1999).

Central sensitization

The changes that occur in the periphery following trauma lead to the phenomenon of 'peripheral sensitization' and primary hyperalgesia. The sensitization that occurs, however, can only be partly explained by the changes in the periphery. Following injury, there is an increased responsiveness to normally innocuous mechanical stimuli (allodynia) in a zone of 'secondary hyperalgesia' in uninjured tissue surrounding the site of injury. In contrast to the zone of primary hyperalgesia, there is no change in the threshold to thermal stimuli. These changes are believed to be a result of processes that occur in the dorsal horn of the spinal cord following injury (Bennett et al 1989). This is the phenomenon of central sensitization (Doubell et al 1999).

Several changes have been noted to occur in the dorsal horn with central sensitization (Dubner and Ren 1994). Firstly, there is an expansion in receptive field size so that a spinal neuron will respond to stimuli that would normally be outside the region that responds to nociceptive stimuli. Secondly, there is an increase in the magnitude and duration of the response to stimuli that are above threshold in strength. Lastly, there is a reduction in threshold so that stimuli that are not normally noxious activate neurons that normally transmit nociceptive information. These changes may be important both in acute pain states such as postoperative pain and in the development of chronic pain (Wilcox 1991).

Modulation at a spinal level

Transmission of nociceptive information is subject to modulation at several levels of the neuraxis including the dorsal horn. Afferent impulses arriving in the dorsal horn initiate inhibitory mechanisms, which limit the effect of subsequent impulses. Inhibition occurs through the effect of local inhibitory interneurons and descending pathways from the brain. In the dorsal horn, incoming nociceptive messages are modulated by endogenous and exogenous agents that act on opioid, α-adreno-, GABA, and glycine receptors located at pre- and postsynaptic sites.

Opioids are widely used and generally efficacious in the management of pain. Opioid receptors are found both pre- and postsynaptically in the dorsal horn, although the majority (about 75%) are located presynaptically (Besse et al 1990). Activation of presynaptic opioid receptors results in a reduction in the release of neurotransmitters from the nociceptive primary afferent (Hori et al 1992). However, the changes that occur with inflammation and neuropathy can produce significant changes in opioid sensitivity that involve a number of mechanisms (see Yaksh 1999).

Activation of α-adrenoceptors in the spinal cord has an analgesic effect either by endogenous release of noradrenaline (norepinephrine) by descending pathways from the brainstem or by exogenous spinal administration of agents such as clonidine (Yaksh and Reddy 1981). Furthermore, α-adrenoceptor agonists appear to have a synergistic effect with opioid agonists (Meert and De Kock 1994). There are a number of α-adrenoceptor subtypes, and the development of selective α-adrenoceptor subtype agonists has the potential to provide effective new analgesic agents with reduced side effects.

Both GABA and glycine are involved in tonic inhibition of nociceptive input, and loss of their inhibitory action can result in features of neuropathic pain such as allodynia (Sivilotti and Woolf 1994).

Descending inhibition involves the action of endogenous opioid peptides as well as other neurotransmitters, including serotonin and noradrenaline (norepinephrine) and GABA (for review see Fields and Basbaum 1994). Many of the traditional strategies available in acute pain management such as the use of opioids act via these inhibitory mechanisms. The elucidation of inhibitory mechanisms has resulted in the use of new techniques that aim to stimulate these inhibitory pathways. It has also provided a clearer rationale for techniques already in use, such as transcutaneous electrical nerve stimulation, and epidural/intrathecal opioid and non-opioid drug administration.

Aetiology and features of acute pain

Acute pain may arise from cutaneous, deep somatic, or visceral structures. Careful mapping of the principal superficial dermatomes is important for the effective use of neural blockade techniques. Visceral pain is much more vaguely localized than somatic pain and has other unique features (Table 1.1). The convergence of visceral and somatic afferents has been proven and this helps to explain referred pain. Also important viscerosomatic reflexes have been identified.

The relief of visceral pain requires blockade of visceral nociceptive fibres that travel to the spinal cord by way of the sympathetic chain. The viscera and the spinal cord segments associated with their visceral nociceptor afferents are shown in Table 1.2. Visceral pain is 'referred' to the body surface areas, as shown in Fig. 1.1. It should be noted that there is considerable overlap for the various organs. Thus it is not surprising that there is a substantial error rate in the diagnosis of visceral pain. Also, there are important viscerosomatic and somaticovisceral reflexes that may make diagnosis and treatment difficult.

The temporary relief of visceral pain by blockade of the somatic referred area poses potential problems of interpretation of 'diagnostic' local anaesthetic nerve blocks. It appears that the processes of peripheral and central sensitization that have been described previously in this chapter may be shared by somatic and visceral structures. This may account for the heightened response of visceral structures to a relatively benign stimulus following inflammation or tissue damage ('visceral hyperalgesia').

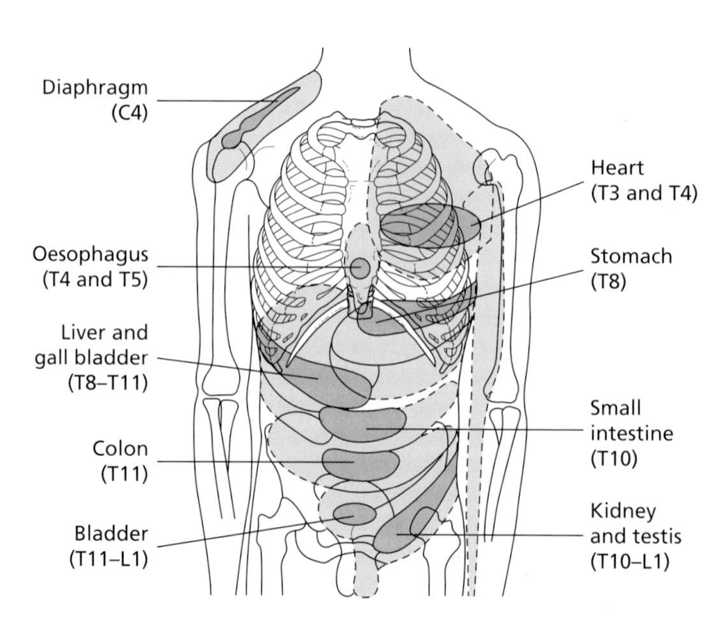

Fig. 1.1 Viscerotomes. Approximate superficial areas to which visceral pain is referred, with related dermatomes in brackets. The dark areas are those most commonly associated with pain in each viscus. The grey areas indicate approximately the larger area that may be associated with pain in that viscus. (Reproduced from Cousins 1987.)

Table 1.1 Visceral pain compared with somatic pain[a]

Factors	Somatic: well localized	Visceral: poorly localized
Radiation	May follow distribution of somatic nerve	Diffuse
Character	Sharp and definite	Dull and vague (may be colicky, cramping, squeezing, etc.)
Relation to stimulus	Hurts where the stimulus is associated with external factors	May be 'referred' to another area; associated with internal factors
Time relations	Often constant (sometimes periodic)	Often periodic and builds to peaks (sometimes constant)
Associated symptoms	Nausea usually only with deep somatic pain owing to bone involvement	Often nausea, vomiting, sickening feeling

[a]Reproduced from Cousins and Bridenbaugh (1998) with permission.

Table 1.2 Viscera and their segmental nociceptive nerve supply[a]

Viscus	Spinal segments of visceral nociceptive afferents[b]
Heart	T1–T5
Lungs	T2–T4
Oesophagus	T5–T6
Stomach	T6–T10
Liver and gallbladder	T6–T10
Pancreas and spleen	T6–T10
Small intestine	T9–T10
Large intestine	T11–T12
Kidney and ureter	T10–L2
Adrenal glands	T8–L1
Testis, ovary	T10–T11
Urinary bladder	T11–L2
Prostate gland	T11–L1
Uterus	T10–L1

[a]Reproduced from Cousins & Bridenbaugh (1998) with permission
[b]These travel with sympathetic fibres and pass by way of sympathetic ganglia to the spinal cord. However, they are *not* sympathetic (efferent) fibres. They are best referred to as visceral nociceptive afferents. *Note*: Parasympathetic afferent fibres may be important in upper abdominal pain (vagal fibres, coeliac plexus).

Features of acute pain

There are important differences between most types of acute pain and chronic pain. In acute pain the nervous system is usually intact; the pain is caused by trauma, surgery, acute 'medical' conditions, or a physiological process (e.g., labour). Facial grimaces and signs of increased autonomic activity and other potentially harmful effects may be evident: for example, hypertension, tachycardia, vasoconstriction, sweating, increased rate and decreased depth of respiration, skeletal muscle spasm, increased gastrointestinal secretions, decreased intestinal motility and increased sphincter tone, urinary retention, venous stasis and potential for thrombosis, and possible pulmonary embolism, anxiety, confusion, and delirium. Also, the pain usually ceases when the wound heals or the medical condition improves. Patients are usually aware that the pain will improve as they recover, and thus an end is in sight. This may not be so if patients are ill prepared and poorly informed.

Some patients with chronic pain may have superimposed acute pain (e.g., when they require further surgery or develop a bone fracture owing to metastatic cancer) (Foley 1985). Such patients may not have an intact nervous system and may have marked pre-existing psychological problems, opioid tolerance, and other problems.

Extensive somatic and sympathetic blockade may be required to relieve acute pain associated with some types of major surgery. For example, the following may be required for pain after thoracoabdominal oesophagogastrectomy with cervical anastomosis: C3–C4 and T2–T12 sensory nerves (somatic structures in neck, thorax, and abdomen); cervicothoracic sympathetic chain and coeliac plexus (intrathoracic and abdominal viscera); C3, C4 phrenic nerve sensory afferents (pain from incision in central diaphragm referred to shoulder tip).

Segmental and suprasegmental reflex responses to acute pain result in muscle spasm, immobility, vasospasm, and other adverse effects, as described above. This may intensify the pain by way of various vicious cycles, which include increased sensitivity of peripheral nociceptors. Acute pain that is unrelieved results in anxiety and sleeplessness, which in turn increase pain. Also anxiety and a feeling of helplessness, before as well as after surgery, increase pain. Their prevention and relief are valuable adjuncts to other treatments. Psychological journals contain much of relevance to acute pain. After major surgery, or severe trauma, or painful medical conditions (e.g., pancreatitis), acute pain may persist for more than 10 days (Bonica 1985). In such situations the pain and its sequelae become similar to chronic pain. It is not uncommon for such patients to show anger, depression, and other characteristics of chronic pain (Bonica 1985, Cousins and Phillips 1986). Thus one should be wary of drawing too sharp a distinction between acute and chronic pain: as acute pain persists, more emphasis may need to be placed on psychological in addition to physical and pharmacological approaches to treatment. An increasingly important role of acute pain services is to identify patients with emerging chronic pain problems. In many situations such patients can be identified by 2–3 weeks postsurgery or -trauma. However, a clear diagnosis may require assessment of the relative roles of physical, psychological, and environmental factors.

Pain management: clinical issues

Spinal administration of agents

The elucidation of the types of receptors present pre- and postsynaptically around nociceptive transmission neurons in the dorsal horn has led to the use of spinal drug administration as a pain management technique. The application of relatively low doses of agents acting at specific receptor types within the spinal cord with the relative avoidance of side effects has been a major advance in the management of some pain problems.

Pre-emptive analgesia

The discovery of the changes associated with the phenomenon of central sensitization has led to attempts to prevent these changes occurring. It has been demonstrated that early postoperative pain is a significant predictor of long-term pain (Katz et al 1996). It was hoped that steps that would reduce or abolish noxious input to the spinal cord during a painful event such as surgery would reduce or minimize spinal cord changes and thereby lead to reduced pain postoperatively and in the long term. However, it is still not known what duration or degree of noxious input is required before these long-term changes occur.

This concept has led to an increasing interest in the use of pre-emptive analgesia. Many trials have purported to show that pre-emptive analgesia results in reduced postoperative pain, decreased analgesic requirements, improved morbidity, and decreased hospital stay (for reviews see Dahl and Kehlet 1993, Woolf and Chong 1993). However, despite studies that appear to indicate the advantages of pre-emptive analgesia, Dahl and Kehlet (1993) and Woolf and Chong (1993) conclude that further trials are necessary before a definitive statement can be made for acute pain.

Acute pain and multimodal analgesia

There is excellent evidence that patients benefit from the use of multimodal, or balanced, analgesia after surgery (Table 1.3). NSAIDs, paracetamol, local anaesthetics, other non-opioid analgesics, and opioids are employed in combination to improve pain relief (Kehlet and Dahl 1993a, b). Multimodal analgesia employs a variety of drugs, given perhaps by different routes, to achieve analgesia, with a reduction in the incidence and severity of side effects (Kehlet 1989, 1997). For example, the addition of regular postoperative injections of the NSAID ketorolac to a regimen previously based on intercostal nerve blocks and patient-controlled (PCA) morphine significantly improved analgesia after thoracotomy (Power et al 1994). Non-opioid analgesics contribute significantly to multimodal analgesia and postoperative recovery of the patient by minimizing opioid side effects including the inevitable opioid-induced gastrointestinal stasis that delays the resumption of normal enteral nutrition after surgery. After bowel surgery multimodal analgesia comprising epidural analgesia using a mixture of local anaesthetics and low-dose opioids provides excellent analgesia and hastens the rate of recovery of gastrointestinal function after surgery of the colon, especially if systemic NSAIDs are used to avoid the need for opioid administration after the epidural has been ceased (Liu et al 1995a).

It is possible to eliminate pain after surgery using multimodal analgesia with a significant reduction in total opioid consumption (Schulze et al 1988, Dahl et al 1990). However, the effect on morbidity and mortality has been disappointing in

Table 1.3 Scientific evidence for pharmacological interventions to manage postoperative pain in adults[a]

Intervention	Level of evidence	Comments
NSAIDs		
Oral (alone)	I	Effective for mild to moderate pain. Relatively contraindicated in patients with renal disease and risk of or actual coagulopathy. Risk of coagulopathy, gastrointestinal bleeding, and other risk factors should be carefully sought.
Oral (adjunct to opioid)	I	Potentiating effect resulting in opioid sparing. Cautions as above.
Parenteral (ketorolac)	I	Effective for moderate to severe pain. Useful where opioids contraindicated or to produce 'opioid sparing', especially to minimize respiratory depression, sedation, and gastrointestinal stasis. Best used as part of a multimodal analgesia regimen.
Opioids		
Oral	IV	As effective as parenteral in appropriate doses. Use as soon as oral medication tolerated.
Route of choice.[b]		
Intramuscular	I	Has been the standard parenteral route, but injections painful and absorption unreliable. Hence, avoid this route when possible.[b]
Subcutaneous	I	Preferable to intramuscular because of patient comfort and a reduced risk of needlestick injury.[b]
Intravenous	I	Parenteral route of choice after major surgery. Suitable for titrated bolus or continuous administration. Significant risk of respiratory depression with inappropriate dosing.[b]
PCA (systemic)	I	Intravenous or subcutaneous routes recommended. Good steady level of analgesia. Popular with patients but requires special infusion pumps and staff education. See cautions about opioids above.[b]
Epidural and intrathecal	I	When suitable, provides good analgesia. Risk of respiratory depression (as with opioids by other routes), but sometimes delayed in onset. Requires careful monitoring. Use of infusion pumps requires additional equipment and staff education. Expensive if infusion pumps are employed.[b]
Local anaesthetics		
Epidural and intrathecal	I	Indications in particular settings. Effective regional analgesia. May blunt 'stress response' and aid recovery. Opioid sparing. Addition of opioid to local anaesthetic may improve analgesia. Risks of hypotension, weakness, numbness. Requires careful monitoring. Use of infusion pump requires additional equipment and staff education. Expensive if infusion pumps are employed.[b]
Peripheral nerve block	I	Plexus block, peripheral nerve block and infitration. Effective regional analgesia. Opioid sparing.

[a]Adapted from NHMRC (1999).
[b]The administration of opioids by any route requires monitoring.

some studies (Moiniche et al 1994a), demonstrating that very good pain control is not automatically associated with an improvement in outcome. Recent research has suggested, however, that the use of multimodal analgesia after major surgery may improve recovery and thus reduce costs (Brodner et al 1998). Kehlet has proposed that the 'pain-free state' should be employed as a fundamental component of an aggressive regimen of postoperative mobilization and early oral feeding in a process of acute rehabilitation after surgery (Kehlet and Dahl 1993a). Clearly, multimodal analgesia employing non-opioids to minimize opioid requirements has the particular advantage over unimodal systemic opioid administration of providing excellent pain relief upon movement, allowing early mobilization. In addition, by using non-opioids as part of a balanced analgesic plan, the patient can return to normal enteral nutrition much more quickly by avoiding the undesirable opioid problems of gastrointestinal stasis and nausea and vomiting (Moiniche et al 1994a, b; Bardram et al 1995).

Psychological factors and acute pain

Psychological response

Severe pain can cause a number of changes in an individual's behaviour, including increased self absorption and withdrawal from interpersonal contact. Fear and anxiety are the major emotional concomitants of acute pain and are especially pronounced when associated with fear of death. Severe acute pain that remains unrelieved for days on end may lead to depression and helplessness as a result of patients experiencing a loss of control over their environment. It is now generally agreed that unrelieved severe acute pain exacerbates premorbid tendencies for anxiety, hostility, depression, or preoccupation with health. In a few cases, the inability to cope with pain may create an acute psychotic reaction (Peck 1986). Acute pain is one of the important factors contributing to the development of delirium in intensive care units (Cousins and Phillips 1986).

Psychological factors affecting the acute pain response

Large individual differences in responsiveness to noxious stimuli are well documented. Clinical observations by Beecher (1946) of wounded soldiers were the first clear description of individual differences in pain response to acute injury. He reported that 65% of soldiers who were severely wounded in battle felt little or no pain. In a study of patients in an emergency unit, 30% did not feel pain at the time of injury and some experienced delays of up to 9 hours before the onset of pain. Melzack et al (1982) concluded 'Clearly the link between injury and pain is highly variable: injury may occur without pain and pain without injury'. Peck (1986) observes that anxiety is the psychological variable that is most reliably related to high levels of pain. Fear of death and general anxiety about bodily well-being are associated with acute postoperative pain, trauma pain, and other situations of acute pain.

Some important implications for treatment have arisen from knowledge of the psychological factors affecting the acute pain response:

1. Measures to reduce anxiety levels have an important bearing on the acute pain experienced by patients and their need for pain treatment (Egbert et al 1964, Fortin and Kirovac 1976, Chapman and Cox 1977, Peck 1986).
2. Approaches that give patients more control are likely to be successful in reducing anxiety and decreasing the requirement for pain and medication. Patient-controlled analgesia (PCA) is a highly successful example.
3. The relief of acute pain is likely to reduce the risks of unwanted psychological sequelae, such as depression, poor motivation to return to normal activities, antipathy towards further surgical procedures, and, in some situations, psychotic reactions.

Psychological methods for reducing pain are discussed in Chaps. 33–36.

Pathophysiology and complications of unrelieved acute pain

In general, severe acute pain results in abnormally enhanced versions of the physiological and psychological responses. Treatment should therefore be instituted before or during the period of functional impairment resulting from the pathophysiology of acute severe pain.

Respiratory system

After surgery or trauma to the chest or abdominal region, respiratory dysfunction is the most common and most important result of the pain associated with such situations. Involuntary spinal reflex responses to the noxious input from the injured area result in reflex muscle spasm in the immediate region of the tissue injury, as well as in muscle groups cephalad and caudad to the injury site. This is not surprising when one considers that nociceptive afferents commonly travel two to three segments above or below their site of entry into the dorsal horn. Pain may also result in voluntary reduction of muscle movement in the thorax and abdominal area. The end result is often described in the clinical setting as 'muscle splinting', which means muscle contraction on either side of the injured area in an attempt to 'splint' the area to prevent movement, comparable to the way one would apply an external splint to a fractured bone. This splinting is often associated with partial closure of the glottis, which produces a 'grunting' sound during breathing. The glottic closure is probably part of a primitive response that permits an increase in intra-abdominal and intrathoracic pressure, associated with muscle spasm, to brace the individual against an impending injury.

Such a response needs to be effectively treated. In addition to decreased tidal volume, there are decreases in vital capacity, functional residual capacity (FRC), and alveolar ventilation. FRC may become less than the volume at which small airway closure occurs. The potential for this problem is in elderly patients, smokers, and those with respiratory disease. This situation progresses to regional lung collapse (atelectasis), associated with considerable impairment of pulmonary gas exchange as a result of alteration of the relationship between ventilation and perfusion of the lung (V/Q inequality) leading to hypoxaemia. The low volume of ventilation also causes hypercarbia and contributes to the hypoxaemia. As a result of the muscle splinting, the patient is unable to cough and clear secretions, and this contributes to lobular or lobar collapse (Craig 1981). Infection often follows this situation, leading to pneumonia. Inability to co-operate with chest physiotherapy further complicates treatment and greatly prolongs the course of pulmonary complications and in turn prolongs hospital stay.

It is not commonly recognized that elderly patients and those in poor general condition may suffer pulmonary complications following lower abdominal and peripheral limb surgery, as a result of unrelieved severe pain that causes them to become immobile, resulting in a hypostatic pneumonia, initially at the base of the lung. This was demonstrated by Modig (1976), who reported on a group of elderly patients following total hip replacement. Those patients who were managed with routine intramuscular opioids had low tidal volumes and high respiratory rates associated with hypoxaemia. It seemed likely that the hypoxaemia was due to immobility and other adverse reflexes resulting from pain, because patients who were managed with epidural analgesia, and were completely pain free, did not show these abnormalities in pulmonary function.

Recent basic and clinical studies have demonstrated a 'viscerosomatic' reflex involving the diaphragm, with changes in amplitude and pattern of diaphragm activity in response to noxious visceral stimuli. This can be blocked by epidural bupivacaine (Mankikian et al 1988).

The classic clinical picture of the patient with unrelieved severe pain and impending respiratory failure is as follows: obvious splinting of abdominal and thoracic muscles; grunting on expiration, and small tidal volume and very rapid respiratory rate. Unfortunately, this is a very inefficient and energy-consuming method of respiration and may result in a high oxygen consumption that is not matched by an increase in cardiac output. This may cause excessive desaturation of mixed venous blood which will contribute to hypoxaemia (Bowler et al 1986). Impressive correction of the majority of these abnormalities in pulmonary function can be obtained with effective pain relief associated with epidural block (Bowler et al 1986, Scott 1988). The cumulative evidence of many clinical trials, when subjected to meta-analysis, has confirmed the superiority of epidural over systemic opioid administration in minimizing postoperative pulmonary morbidity.

Cardiovascular system

It is generally agreed that severe acute pain results in sympathetic overactivity with increases in heart rate, peripheral resistance, blood pressure, and cardiac output. The end result is an increase in cardiac work and myocardial oxygen consumption. Because heart rate is greatly increased, diastolic filling time is decreased and this may result in reduced oxygen delivery to the myocardium. Thus an imbalance results between myocardial oxygen demand and oxygen supply, with a resultant risk of hypoxaemia. Also, it is now known that α-receptors in the coronary vasculature may respond to intense sympathetic stimulation by producing coronary vasoconstriction. The end result of this pathophysiology may be myocardial ischaemia associated with anginal pain and even myocardial infarction. The potential for this situation is increased in patients with pre-existing coronary artery disease (Bowler et al 1986, Scott 1988). Anginal pain is associated with increased anxiety, further increases in circulating catecholamines, and further potential for coronary artery constriction.

The effects of postoperative pain on cardiovascular variables have been demonstrated by Sjögren and Wright (1972). That the cardiovascular changes were predominantly due to noxious stimuli is illustrated by the effect of epidural analgesia in preventing and reversing these abnormalities (Sjögren and Wright 1972, Hoar and Hickey 1976, Kumar and Hibbert 1984). There is impressive evidence from animal studies that noxious stimulation results in coronary artery vasoconstriction and potential for myocardial ischaemia.

Prevention of these noxious stimuli with thoracic epidural analgesia greatly improves the oxygen supply to the myocardium and reduces the myocardial ischaemic insult (Vik-Mo et al 1978, Klassen et al 1980). Epidural blocks also decrease the incidence of myocardial ischaemic episodes intraoperatively (Reiz et al 1982) and postoperatively (Yeager et al 1987). Yeager et al found an overall decrease in mortality associated with effective pain relief produced by epidural blockade compared with conventional and less effective methods of pain relief. A recent study has shown that there is an increase in myocardial ischaemia upon cessation of epidural analgesia in patients who have had aortic surgery (Garnett et al 1996). Acute anginal pain in non-surgical patients can be relieved with thoracic epidural block, and at the same time, blood flow in 'at risk' myocardium is improved by increasing the diameter of stenosed coronary artery segments (Blomberg et al 1990).

It is important to realize that there is evidence that other analgesics can reduce the incidence of myocardial ischaemia after surgery. In a recent study of patients having elective hip or knee arthroplasty, Beattie et al found that the addition of a continuous infusion of ketorolac (5 mg/h for 24 h) to a PCA morphine regimen reduced pain scores and arterial blood pressure, heart rate, and the duration of myocardial ischaemia (Beattie et al 1997). It is not clear whether this is a benefit of improved analgesia per se, a consequence of NSAID inhibition of thromboxane production, or an intrinsic effect on the heart.

In the peripheral circulation, acute pain is associated with decreased limb blood flow and this can be particularly serious in patients undergoing vascular grafting procedures. Relief of pain with epidural blockade results in a reversal of reductions in blood flow associated with surgical trauma and acute pain (Cousins and Wright 1971), and in an improved outcome (Tuman et al 1991). Severe postoperative pain and high levels of sympathetic activity may be associated with reduced arterial inflow and decreased venous emptying (Modig et al 1980). In association with changes in blood coagulability and immobility of patients, this may lead to venous thrombosis and pulmonary embolism (Modig et al 1983). Although increased sympathetic activity due to pain would be expected to reduce renal blood flow and also hepatic blood flow, data documenting such changes in patients with pain have not been obtained.

Musculoskeletal system

As noted above, segmental and suprasegmental motor activity in response to pain results in muscle spasm that may further increase pain, thus setting up a vicious circle. This vicious circle may also activate marked increases in sympathetic activity, which further increases the sensitivity of peripheral nociceptors. This situation can result in widespread disturbances, even in patients with relatively localized nociceptive foci in the long bones or other areas of the bony skeleton. Recent data indicate that persistent postoperative pain and limitation of movement may be associated with marked impairment of muscle metabolism, muscle atrophy, and significantly delayed normal muscle function. These changes appear to be due to pain and reflex vasoconstriction, and possibly reflex responses that can be at least partly reversed by the relief of pain with epidural analgesia. Patients managed in this manner appear to have a much quicker return to normal function (Bonica 1985).

Gastrointestinal and genitourinary systems

Increased sympathetic activity increases intestinal secretions and smooth muscle sphincter tone, whereas it decreases intestinal motility. Gastric stasis and even paralytic ileus may occur. These changes are at least partly related to severe pain and a resultant increase in sympathetic activity. However, the administration of opioid analgesic drugs may also make a significant contribution to delayed gastric emptying (Nimmo 1984). There is some evidence that pain relief with neural blockade may reduce the transit time of X-ray contrast media through the gut, from up to 150 h in a control group to 35 h in a group receiving epidural analgesia (Ahn et al 1988).

There is also evidence that the pain-related impairment of intestinal motility may be relieved by epidural local anaesthetic but not by epidural opioid (Scheinin et al 1987, Thoren et al 1989, Wattwil et al 1989, Thorn et al 1992, Liu et al 1995a, b). Furthermore, systemic, intravenous, administration of lidocaine (lignocaine) speeds the return of bowel function after radical prostatectomy, and reduces pain and shortens hospital stay (Groudine et al 1998).

Increased sympathetic activity postoperatively

also results in increased urinary sphincter activity that may result in urinary retention. However, the role of pain is difficult to assess, because opioid analgesic drugs may result in a significant incidence of urinary retention.

General stress response to acute injury

Surgery and other forms of trauma generate a catabolic state as a result of increased secretion of catabolic hormones and decreased secretion or action of anabolic hormones. The results for the patient include pain; nausea, vomiting, and intestinal stasis; alterations in blood flow, coagulation, and fibrinolysis; alterations in substrate metabolism; alterations in water and electrolyte handling by the body; increased demands on the cardiovascular and respiratory systems. This stress response to surgery and trauma, together with the modifying effects of analgesics, has been discussed recently by Liu et al (1995b) and Kehlet (1996, 1998).

The responses to surgical and other trauma may be divided into two phases. The initial acute 'ebb' or 'shock phase' is characterized by a hypodynamic state, a reduction in metabolic rate, and depression of most physiological processes. With surgical trauma this phase is either absent or very transient during the operative period.

The second phase is the hyperdynamic or 'flow phase', which may last for a few days or weeks, depending on the magnitude of the surgical or traumatic insult or on the occurrence of complications. Characteristically in this phase, metabolic rate and cardiac output are elevated (Kehlet 1998). There is some evidence that nociceptive impulses play an important part in the ebb phase and in the early part of the flow phase. However, there are a substantial number of other factors that contribute to initiation of the stress response, and it seems likely that these play an increasingly important part in the flow phase. This is an important area for investigation because the major benefits from the relief of severe postoperative pain with potent techniques may be obtained in the first 48 h following surgery (Cousins and Phillips 1986).

Major endocrine and metabolic changes are elicited by surgical trauma (Wilmore 1983; Liu et al 1995b; Kehlet 1996, 1998). However, there is powerful evidence that local anaesthetic and opioid neural blockade may produce a powerful modification of the responses to surgical injury (Kehlet 1989, 1996, 1998). Neural blockade with local anaesthetics may diminish a predominant part of the physiological response to surgical or other procedures in the lower abdomen or lower extremities. This usually occurs in situations where postoperative pain is completely alleviated. The inhibitory effect is much less pronounced during and following major abdominal and thoracic procedures, possibly because of the difficulty in obtaining sufficient afferent neural blockade. To obtain a pronounced reduction of the surgical stress response, it is necessary to maintain pain relief with continuous epidural analgesia for at least 48–72 h postoperatively (Kehlet 1989, 1996, 1998; Liu et al 1995b).

Current data indicate that pain relief by epidural or intrathecal administration of opioids is less efficient in reducing the stress response (Liu et al 1995b). However, studies of mixtures of local anaesthetics and opioids indicate that this combination may be capable of a more potent modification of the stress response. A convincing demonstration of the efficacy of pain relief with epidural blockade in modifying the stress response is the significant improvement in cumulative nitrogen balance obtained when pain relief is provided both intra- and postoperatively with continuous epidural neural blockade (Brandt et al 1978).

Changes in coagulation and fibrinolysis associated with major surgery may be partly modified by pain relief with neural blockade (Jorgensen et al 1991). However, interpretation of these results is complex, because factors other than pain may be involved. Also the absorption of local anaesthetics associated with neural blockade may result in an antithrombotic effect (Kehlet 1998). Encouragingly, a clinical study comparing the effects of epidural and general anaesthesia in peripheral vascular surgery has found that the epidural group needed fivefold fewer repeat operations for graft failure within 1 month (Christopherson et al 1993). Changes in immunocompetence and acute-phase proteins are well documented in association with surgical trauma. Pain relief with neural blockade has a mild influence on various aspects of the surgically induced impairment of immunocompetence. The mechanism has not been completely elucidated (Kehlet 1998).

Adverse effects of unrelieved pain are likely to manifest themselves in failure in more than one system, particularly in high-risk surgical patients. This question was examined by Yeager et al (1987) in a controlled study of high-risk patients undergoing major surgery. Patients were randomly assigned to receive general anaesthesia and epidural local anaesthetic during surgery followed by epidural opioid after surgery, or general anaesthesia alone during surgery followed by parenteral opioid postoperatively. The results showed a striking difference in morbidity in several systems and in mortality between the two groups. Of further interest was the substantial reduction in cost of treatment for the group receiving epidural analgesia. The precise role of pain relief in producing these more favourable results with epidural analgesia is not certain because intraoperative epidural local anaesthesia permitted a reduction in doses of anaesthetic agents and resulted in efferent sympathetic blockade in addition to blockade of nociceptive afferents. Postoperatively, however, it is likely that the effects of epidural opioids were predominantly due to pain relief. Unfortunately, corroborative evidence of reduced morbidity and mortality following potent methods of pain relief is hard to find (Scott and Kehlet 1988, Liu et al 1995b).

Other forms of acute pain

Tissue trauma usually, but not always, results in immediate sharp pain followed by neurochemical events associated with the inflammatory response. In the case of musculoskeletal pain, mechanical factors such as physical distension of joints or fascial compartments may contribute, as may ischaemia. In acute visceral trauma, distension, obstruction, ischaemia, chemical irritation from rupture of viscera into the peritoneal cavity, infection, and other factors may also play a part.

Patients with more localized and minor trauma were studied by Melzack et al (1982). The patients presented to an emergency department with simple fractures, dislocations, strains, sprains, lacerations, and bruises. Of the 138 patients studied, 37% did not feel pain at the time of injury; of 46 patients with injuries limited to the skin, 53% had a pain-free period, whereas of 86 patients with deep tissue injuries (e.g., fractures, sprains, amputation, bruises, stabs, and crushes) only 28% had a pain-free period. Delay periods varied from a few minutes up to several hours (Melzack et al 1982). Using the McGill Pain Questionnaire, it was found that the sensory scores were similar to those of patients with chronic pain, but the affective scores were lower. The descriptions used were very similar for the types of injury: 'hot' or 'burning' characterized fractures, cuts, and bruises; cuts and lacerations had a 'throbbing' or 'beating' quality; sprains or fractures and bruises had a 'sharp' quality (Melzack et al 1982).

In the case of pain following major trauma, it is likely that the pathophysiological response is almost identical to that of postoperative pain. However, because of the lack of preparation, suddenness of the injury, and associated severe psychological responses, anxiety levels are usually very high, and CNS responses initiate pronounced versions of the changes in various body systems that have been described above (Hume and Egdahl 1959, Wilmore et al 1976, Wilmore 1983). Acute pancreatitis is an example of an acute medical condition that may be accompanied by severe pain and pronounced abnormal reflex responses. The abdominal pain is usually accompanied by severe abdominal muscle spasm, with a resultant decrease in diaphragmatic movement, and progressive hypoventilation with a potential for hypoxaemia and hypercarbia. The release of pancreatic enzymes and other substances into the peritoneal cavity is associated with severe pain. It is also possible that depressant toxic substances that may result in cardiovascular depression and shock are released. Once again, the precise role of pain in contributing to these events is unclear. There are clinical reports of the relief of pain of acute pancreatitis with epidural local anaesthetics or opioids and an associated improvement in the overall condition of the patient (Cousins and Phillips 1986).

Myocardial infarction produces a disruption of the usual reciprocal relationship between sympathetic and parasympathetic control of cardiac function, frequently with overactivity of both systems. It is likely that these changes are substantially induced by haemodynamic alterations associated with myocardial infarction. However, it is possible that pain and associated increases in sympathetic activity, as well as increases in vagal activity, may contribute to the problem. Sudden changes in vagal activity may result in severe bradycardia, atrioventricular block, peripheral vasodilatation (faint response), and severe hypotension that may progress to cardiogenic shock. As indicated above, experimental evidence in animals (Vik-Mo et al 1978, Klassen et al 1980) and in man (Reiz et al 1982, Yeager et al 1987, Blomberg et al 1990) indicate that epidural neural blockade may substantially modify these adverse effects. It is not known how much of this effect is due to blockade of efferent sympathetic activity and how much is due to blockade of afferent nociceptive impulses from the myocardium.

The relief of pain in emergency departments need not be delayed by undue concerns that important symptoms may be masked as a consequence. Indeed the early administration of opioids in patients with an 'acute abdomen' does not impair the diagnosis of serious pathology, but may facilitate it. Therefore, appropriate analgesia must not be withheld from such patients (Zolte and Cust 1986, Attard et al 1992).

Clinical syndromes of acute pain: implications for diagnosis and treatment

A wide variety of situations may produce acute pain, including pathological events in patients with chronic pain. Prominent in this respect are patients with cancer who are subject to acute episodes of pain as a result of pathological fractures of long bones, acute intestinal obstructions, and other problems (see Chaps. 42, 44). Patients with chronic occlusive vascular disease may also suffer acute episodes of pain during an exacerbation of their condition in winter months. Another chronic condition that may present with acute episodes of pain is the acquired immune deficiency syndrome (AIDS). Acute pain may arise from cutaneous, deep somatic, or visceral structures. Careful mapping of the precise area of the pain is important. In the case of pain arising entirely from cutaneous structures, it is helpful to determine which dermatomes or superficial nerves are involved in the pain. In the case of deep somatic or visceral pain, some guidance as to the source of pain can be obtained by reference to classic viscerotome regions and also to superficial areas to which visceral pain is referred (Fig. 1.1). There is considerable overlap in the viscerotomes for various body organs, which undoubtedly results in a high error rate in the diagnosis of acute visceral pain. It is important to be aware of the spinal cord segments associated with nociceptive input from the various viscera (Table 1.2).

There are a number of general differences between visceral and somatic pain and these are summarized in Table 1.1 (Cousins 1987). Further complicating the differentiation of somatic and visceral pain are viscerosomatic and somatovisceral reflexes. A classic example of various neural pathways associated with acute pain is acute appendicitis. During the early phases of inflammation of the appendix, pain is conveyed by visceral nociceptive afferents arising from the appendix and conveyed to segment T10 of the spinal cord. As indicated in Fig. 1.1, this viscerotome is represented centrally around the umbilical area. The inflammation associated with the appendicitis spreads to the parietal peritoneum in the region of the right iliac fossa and pain becomes localized in this region, as somatic nociceptive afferents in the T10 and L1 region become involved. However, there may be wide variations in this pattern as the result of anatomical placement of the appendix, the initiation of viscerovisceral and viscerosomatic reflexes, and other factors.

In differentiating between the various causes of acute pain, the following are of particular importance: onset, time relations after onset, characteristics and intensity of pain, site and radiation, and symptoms associated with the pain. Usually, but not always, it is possible to determine whether the pain has a somatic or visceral origin by reference to the factors outlined in Table 1.1. In the case of visceral pain, a rapid onset suggests mechanisms such as rupture of an organ or arterial occlusion due to embolus. More gradual onset is suggestive of inflammation or infection. Constant pain may be associated with ischaemia or inflammation, whereas intermittent pain may be associated with periodically increased pressure in hollow organs due to obstruction.

An important example of referred pain is provided by the life-threatening situation of a torn spleen, with bleeding under the diaphragm which results in stimulation of phrenic afferent fibres (C3 and C4) and thus referral of pain to the shoulder tip region. In the thoracic region, pain due to acute trauma in the apical region of the lung may activate somatic afferents in the brachial plexus (C5–T1), resulting in pain on the outer aspect of the arm and shoulder and radiation into other regions of the arm. Pain emanating from trauma to the mediastinum may be diffusely located over the retrosternal area but may also radiate into the neck and abdomen. Because of the involvement of sympathetic afferent fibres that may involve segments from at least C8–T5, it is possible for pain to be referred into one or the other arm. The pain of acute gallbladder and bile duct disease is usually located either diffusely in the upper abdomen or the right upper quadrant and may radiate to the back near the right scapula. This is often a colicky pain related to eating and may be relieved by vomiting. Acute pain involving the liver is also located diffusely in epigastrium and right upper quadrant. It may be a constant dull pain and have a sickening component. Acute pancreatitis pain is usually located high in the upper abdomen or left upper quadrant and radiates directly through to the back in the region of the first lumbar vertebra to the left of this area or to the interscapular region. The pain is usually described as being very severe, constant, and dull.

Pain from the kidney usually radiates from the region of the loin to the groin and sometimes to the penis if the ureter is also involved, for example due to a stone in the ureter (renal colic). It seems likely that reflex increase in sympathetic activity associated with renal colic may intensify the pain and set up a vicious circle, which prevents the passage of the stone due to intense spasms of the ureter. Relief of such pain with continuous epidural block will sometimes not only result in highly effective pain relief, but also the passage of the stone (Scott 1988). The irritant presence of a stone in the ureter sets up a painful cycle of uncoordinated ureteric muscle contraction by stimulating local prostaglandin release and hence smooth muscle spasm. By inhibition of prostaglandin production, NSAIDs are more effective than opioids in relieving the pain of renal colic (Hetherington and Philp 1986).

Following surgery, the treatment of acute pain cannot be carried out without reference to the cause of the pain. This is so because of different requirements for drug treatment of somatic and visceral pain; also, as indicated above, the use of neural blockade techniques may be greatly influenced by neural pathways involved in the pain. 'Incident pain' is pain occurring other than at rest, such as during deep breathing and coughing or during ambulation. This pain usually, not unexpectedly, has a higher requirement for analgesia. Another cause of apparently increased levels of pain is opioid tolerance in patients treated with opioids for 7–10 days or more before surgery. Of particular importance, pain of certain patterns may be indicative of the development of postoperative complications that require surgical correction rather than pressing on blindly with the treatment of pain. A sudden increase in the requirements for intravenous opioid infusion, epidural administration of opioids, or local anaesthetics should be carefully examined, bearing in mind the possibility that a new event has occurred. A similar situation exists in patients treated in a critical care unit following trauma and who have been stabilized initially on an analgesic regimen. In the experience of one of these authors, the development of an important complication is frequently associated with pain that will break through an analgesic regimen that was previously successful (Cousins and Phillips 1986).

The possibility of the development of neuropathic pain should be borne in mind after surgery as it is often missed in patients with acute pain, and may require specific therapy (Hayes and Molloy 1997). The pain may be associated with injury, disease, or surgical section of the peripheral or central nervous system. One diagnostic clue after surgery or trauma is an unexpected increase in opioid consumption, as neuropathic pain may respond poorly to opioids.

Long-term effects of surgical incision and acute tissue trauma

It is usually assumed that surgical incision is followed by an orderly healing process with minimal residual potential for continuing pain. However, surgical incision is often complicated by the division of small peripheral nerves and sometimes larger nerves, in addition to a variable amount of tissue trauma, retraction, and compression of tissues, and other factors. Interestingly, there is no convincing evidence that pain problems are less frequent after elective surgical incision and associated tissue trauma compared to traumatic injuries.

The subject of continuing pain following traumatic injury is very large and is considered in many other chapters in this book. Important examples are the following: stump pain, phantom limb pain, complex regional pain syndrome (CRPS types I and II), trigeminal neuralgia secondary to trauma, occipital neuralgia due to trauma, cervical sprain or whiplash syndrome, acute postmastectomy pain, post-thoracotomy pain, abdominal cutaneous nerve entrapment syndrome, and a large variety of postoperative neuralgias involving peripheral nerves such as the iliohypogastric, ilioinguinal, genitofemoral, lateral femoral cutaneous, obturator, femoral, sciatic, and ulnar nerves (Merskey 1986, IASP Task Force on Taxonomy 1994).

The precise incidence of persistent pain following surgical incision and trauma is difficult to determine (Perkins and Kehlet 2000, Macrae 2001). However, in our experience, it is seen in at least 10% of surgical operations. There is strong evidence from animal studies that there is a genetic predisposition to the development of spontaneous activity in neuromas. This evidence is supported by observations that patients who develop neuromas and incisional pain frequently have similar problems if an attempt is made to remove the neuroma tissue surgically. Such patients tend to have similar problems when operations on other parts of the body are carried out. Thus, the preceding history of the patient is important and may point to the need for careful surveillance and the early use of appropriate treatment measures.

Surgical textbooks discuss factors in wound

healing such as gentleness of handling tissues, different methods of suturing, use of appropriate suture material, avoidance of haematoma and infection, and other factors (Sabiston 1982). However, there appears to have been only limited investigation of factors that have a significant influence on the development of various pain syndromes following surgical incision. It is generally held that incisions that cut across muscle fibres cause more postoperative pain than those that separate fibres. One of the few studies to test this hypothesis compared a dorsal approach to the kidney (muscle-separating) with the classic flank approach (muscle-cutting). The former was associated with a lesser requirement for postoperative analgesia and shorter hospital stay (Freiha and Zeineh 1983). Unfortunately patients were not followed up to determine the comparative incidence of postincisional pain.

Clinical observation suggests that the following operations are particularly prone to be associated with long-term pain in or near the surgical incision: lateral thoracotomy (50%); cholecystectomy; nephrectomy (flank incision); radical mastectomy (50%); vein-stripping (especially long saphenous because of proximity to saphenous nerve); inguinal herniorrhaphy; episiotomy; various operations on the arm and hand; facial surgery (Litwin 1962, White and Sweet 1962, Applegate 1972, Lindblom 1979, Tasker et al 1983, Kitzinger 1984). Perkins and Kehlet have surveyed surgical factors that may be involved (Perkins and Kehlet 2000). Nerve injury during surgery appears to play a key role. Patient factors such as genetic makeup (Inbal et al 1980), middle to old age (Tasker et al 1983), and the presence of unrelieved pain prior to surgery may be important (Melzack 1971). The latter is supported in animal studies, where injury prior to denervation of a limb by neurectomy resulted in increased self-mutilation (autotomy) compared to animals who were not injured prior to neurectomy (Coderre et al 1986). The study suggests that tissue damage and unrelieved pain prior to surgery may predispose to persistent pain problems following surgery. This is supported by the clinical observation that patients with pain due to occlusive vascular disease have a lower incidence of postamputation pain if their pain is relieved by neurolytic sympathectomy (Cousins et al 1979) or by epidural block (Bach et al 1988) prior to amputation.

The long-term effects of surgical incision can be considered in three broad categories: the postoperative neuralgias, complex regional pain syndromes (types I and II), and deafferentation syndromes. These are discussed in Chapter 17.

Conclusion

Acute pain has emerged as an important issue because of associated morbidity and mortality. The challenge is to employ multimodal analgesia, early nutrition, and rapid mobilization after surgery and trauma to aid acute rehabilitation to the benefit of the patient. The aim should be that the majority of patients have good relief of acute pain together with rapid functional recovery. To achieve this result requires a substantial educational and organizational effort to apply the knowledge and methodology now available, with close cooperation between anaesthetic, surgical, and nursing staff.

References

Aasbo V, Raeder JC, Grogaard B, Roise O 1996 No additional analgesic effect of intra-articular morphine or bupivacaine compared with placebo after elective knee arthroscopy. Acta Anaesthesiologica Scandinavica 40: 585–588

Ahn H, Andaker L, Bronge A et al 1988 Effect of continuous epidural analgesia on gastro-intestinal motility. British Journal of Surgery 75: 1176–1178

Applegate WV 1972 Abdominal cutaneous nerve entrapment syndrome. Surgery 71: 118

Attard AR, Corlett MJ, Kidner NJ et al 1992 Safety of early pain relief for acute abdominal pain. British Medical Journal 305: 554–556

Bach S, Noreng MF, Tjellden NU 1988 Phantom limb pain in amputees during the first 12 months following limb amputation, after preoperative lumbar epidural blockade. Pain 33: 297–301

Bardram L, Funch-Jensen P, Jensen P, Crawford ME, Kehlet H 1995 Recovery after laparoscopic colonic surgery with epidural analgesia, and early oral nutrition and mobilisation. Lancet 345: 763–764

Beattie WS, Warriner CB, Etches R et al 1997 The addition of continuous intravenous infusion of ketorolac to a patient-controlled analgesic morphine regime reduced postoperative myocardial ischemia in patients undergoing elective total hip or knee arthroplasty. Anesthesia and Analgesia 84: 715–722

Beecher H K 1946 Pain in men wounded in battle. Annals of Surgery 123: 96

Bennett GJ, Kajander KC, Sahara Y, Iadarola MJ, Sugimoto T 1989 Neurochemical and anatomical changes in the dorsal horn of rats with an experimental painful peripheral neuropathy. In: Cervero F, Bennett GJ, Headley PM (eds) Processing of sensory information in the superficial dorsal horn of the spinal cord. Plenum, Amsterdam, pp 463–471

Besse D, Lombard MC, Zakac JM, Roques BP, Besson J-M 1990 Pre- and postsynaptic distribution of mu, delta and kappa opioid receptors in the superficial layers of the cervical dorsal horn of the rat spinal cord. Brain Research 521: 15–22

Binder W, Machelska H, Mousa S, Schmitt T, Riviere PJM, Junien JL, Stein C, Schafer M 2001 Analgesic and antiinflammatory effects of two novel kappa-opioid peptides. Anesthesiology 94: 1034–1044

Blomberg S, Emanuelsson H, Kuist H, Lamm C et al 1990 Effects of thoracic epidural anaesthesia on coronary arteries and arterioles in patients with coronary artery disease. Anesthesiology 73(5): 840–847

Bonica JJ 1985 Biology, pathophysiology and treatment of acute pain. In: Lipton S, Miles J (eds) Persistent pain. Grune & Stratton, Orlando, pp 1–32

Bowler G, Wildsmith J, Scott DB 1986 Epidural administration of local anaesthetics. In: Cousins MJ, Phillips GD (eds) Acute pain management. Churchill Livingstone, New York, pp 187–236

Brandt MR, Fernandes A, Mordhorst R, Kehlet H 1978 Epidural analgesia improves postoperative nitrogen balance. British Medical Journal 1: 1106–1108

Brodner G, Pogatzki E, Van Aken H, Buerkle H, Goeters C, Schulzki C, Nottberg H, Mertes N 1998 A multimodal approach to control postoperative pathophysiology and rehabilitation in patients undergoing abdominothoracic esophagectomy. Anesthesia and Analgesia 86: 228–234

Chapman C R, Cox GB 1977 Anxiety, pain and depression surrounding elective surgery: a multivariate comparison of abdominal surgery patients with kidney donors and recipients. Journal of Pyschosomatic Research 21: 7

Christopherson R, Beattie C, Frank SM et al 1993 The perioperative ischemia randomized anesthesia trial study group: perioperative morbidity in patients randomized to epidural or general anesthesia for lower-extremity vascular surgery. Anesthesiology 79: 422–434

Coderre T, Grimes RW, Melzack R 1986 Autonomy after nerve section in the rat is influenced by tonic descending inhibition from locus coeruleus. Neuroscience Letters 67: 81–86

Cousins MJ 1987 Visceral pain. In: Andersson S, Bond M, Mehta M, Swerdlow M (eds) Chronic non-cancer pain: assessment and practical management. MTP Press, Lancaster 119–132

Cousins MJ, Bridenbaugh PO (eds) 1998 Neural blockade in clinical anaesthesia and management of pain, 3rd edn. Lippincott–Raven, Philadelphia

Cousins MJ, Phillips GD (eds) 1986 Acute pain management. Clinics in critical care medicine. Churchill Livingstone, Edinburgh

Cousins MJ, Wright CJ 1971 Graft, muscle and skin blood flow after epidural block in vascular surgical procedures. Surgery, Gynecology and Obstetrics 133: 59

Cousins MJ, Reeve TS, Glynn CJ, Walsh JA, Cherry DA 1979 Neurolytic lumbar sympathetic blockade: duration of denervation and relief of rest pain. Anaesthesia and Intensive Care 7: 121–135

Craig DB 1981 Postoperative recovery of pulmonary function. Anesthesia and Analgesia 60: 46

Dahl JB, Kehlet H 1993 The value of pre-emptive analgesia in the treatment of postoperative pain. British Journal of Anaesthesia 70: 434

Dahl JB, Rosenberg J, Dirkes WE, Morgensen T, Kehlet H 1990 Prevention of postoperative pain by balanced analgesia. British Journal of Anaesthesia 64: 518–520

Devor M, Seltzer Z 1999 Pathophysiology of damaged nerves in relation to chronic pain. In: Wall PD, Melzack R (eds) Textbook of Pain, 4th edn. Churchill Livingstone, Edinburgh, pp 129–164

Doubell TP, Mannion RJ, Woolf CJ 1999 The dorsal horn: state-dependent sensory processing, plasticity and the generation of pain. In: Wall PD, Melzack R (eds) Textbook of Pain, 4th edn. Churchill Livingstone, Edinburgh, pp 165–182

Dubner R, Ren K 1994 Central mechanisms of thermal and mechanical hyperalgesia following tissue inflammation. In: Boivie J, Hansson P, Lindblom U (eds) Touch, temperature, and pain in health and disease: mechanisms and assessments. IASP Press, Seattle, pp 267–277

Egbert LD, Battit GE, Welch CE et al 1964 Reduction of postoperative pain by encouragement and instruction of patients. New England Journal of Medicine 270: 825

Fields HL, Basbaum AI 1994 Central nervous system mechanisms of pain modulation. In: Wall PD, Melzack R (eds) Textbook of pain, 3rd edn. Churchill Livingstone, Edinburgh, pp 243–257

Foley KM 1985 The treatment of cancer pain. New England Journal of Medicine 313: 84

Fortin F, Kirovac S 1976 A randomized controlled trial of pre-operative patient education. Educational Journal of Nursing Studies 13: 11

Freiha F, Zeineh S 1983 Dorsal approach to upper urinary tract. Urology 21: 15–16

Garnett RL, MacIntyre A, Lindsay P 1996 Perioperative ischemia in aortic surgery: combined epidural/general anesthesia and epidural analgesia vs general anesthesia and IV analgesia. Canadian Journal of Anaesthesia 43: 769–778

Groudine SB, Fisher HAG, Kaufman RP et al 1998 Anesthesia and Analgesia 86: 235–239

Hayes C, Molloy AR 1997 Neuropathic pain in the perioperative period. In: Molloy AR, Power I (eds) International anesthesiology clinics. Acute and chronic pain. Lippincott–Raven, Philadelphia, pp 67–81

Haynes TK, Appadurai IR, Power I, Rosen M, Grant A 1994 Intra-articular morphine and bupivacaine analgesia after arthroscopic knee surgery. Anaesthesia 49: 54–56

Hetherington JW, Philp NH 1986 Diclofenac sodium versus pethidine in acute renal colic. British Medical Journal 292: 237–338

Hoar PF, Hickey RF 1976 Systemic hypertension following myocardial revascularization: a method of treatment using epidural anesthesia. Journal of Thoracic and Cardiovascular Surgery 71: 859

Hori Y, Endo K, Takahashi T 1992 Presynaptic inhibitory action of enkephalin on excitatory transmission in superficial dorsal horn of rat spinal cord. Journal of Physiology 450: 673–685

Hume DM, Egdahl RH 1959 The importance of the brain in the endocrine response to injury. Annals of Surgery 150: 697

IASP Task Force on Taxonomy 1994 Classification of chronic pain. IASP Press, Seattle

Inbal R, Devor M, Tuchendler O, Licblich L 1980 Autonomy following nerve injury: genetic factors in the development of chronic pain. Pain 9: 327–337

Jänig W 1996 The puzzle of 'reflex sympathetic dystrophy': mechanisms, hypotheses, open questions. In: Janig W, Stanton-Hicks M (eds) Reflex sympathetic dystrophy: a reappraisal. IASP Press, Seattle, pp 1–24

Jänig W, McLachlan EM 1994 The role of modifications in noradrenergic peripheral pathways after nerve lesions in the generation of pain. In: Fields HL, Liebeskind JC (eds) Progress in pain research and management. IASP Press, Seattle, pp 101–128

Jorgensen L, Rasmussen L, Nielsen A, Leffers A, Albrecht-Beste E 1991 Antithrombotic efficacy of continuous extradural analgesia after knee replacement. British Journal of Anaesthesia 66: 8–12

Kam PCA, Power I 2000 New selective Cox-2 inhibitors. Pain Reviews 7: 3–13

Katz J, Jackson M, Kavanagh BP, Sandler AN 1996 Acute pain after thoracic surgery predicts long-term post-thoracotomy pain. Clinical Journal of Pain 12: 50–55

Kehlet H 1988 Modification of responses to surgery by neural blockade: clinical implications. In: Cousins MJ, Bridenbaugh PO (eds) Neural blockade in clinical anesthesia and management of pain, 2nd edn. Lippincott, Philadelphia, pp 145–188

Kehlet H 1989 Surgical stress: the role of pain and analgesia. British Journal of Anaesthesia 63: 189–195

Kehlet H 1996 Effect of pain relief on the surgical stress response. Regional Anesthesia 21(6S): 35–37

Kehlet H 1997 Multimodal approach to control postoperative pathophysiology and rehabilitation. British Journal of Anaesthesia 78: 606–617

Kehlet H 1998 Modification of responses to surgery by neural blockade: clinical implications. In: Cousins MJ, Bridenbaugh PO (eds) Neural blockade in clinical anesthesia and management of pain, 3rd edn. Lippincott-Raven, Philadelphia, pp 129–178

Kehlet H, Dahl JB 1993a The value of 'multimodal' or 'balanced

analgesia' in postoperative pain treatment. Anesthesia and Analgesia 77: 1048–1056
Kehlet H, Dahl JB 1993b Postoperative pain [Review]. World Journal of Surgery 17: 215–219
Kitzinger S 1984 Episiotomy pain. In: Wall PD, Melzack R (eds) Textbook of pain, 1st edn. Churchill Livingstone, Edinburgh, pp 293–303
Klassen GA, Bramwell PR, Bromage RS, Zborawska-Sluis DT 1980 Effect of acute sympathectomy by epidural anesthesia on the canine coronary circulation. Anesthesiology 52: 8–15
Kumar B, Hibbert GR 1984 Control of hypertension during aortic surgery using lumbar extradural blockade. British Journal of Anesthesia 56: 797
Levine JD, Reichling DB 1999 Peripheral mechanisms of inflammatory pain. In: Wall PD, Melzack R (eds) Textbook of Pain, 4th edn. Churchill Livingstone, Edinburgh, pp 59–84
Levine JD, Fields HL, Basbaum AI 1993 Peptides and the primary afferent nociceptor. Journal of Neurosciences 13: 2273–2286
Lindblom U 1979 Sensory abnormalities in neuralgia. In: Bonica JJ, Liebeskind JC, Albe-Fessard DL (eds) Advances in pain research and therapy, vol 3. Raven Press, New York, pp 111–120
Litwin MS 1962 Postsympathectomy neuralgia. Archives of Surgery 84: 591–595
Liu SS, Carpenter RL, Mackey DC et al 1995a Effects of perioperative analgesic technique on rate of recovery after colon surgery. Anesthesiology 83: 757–765
Liu SS, Carpenter RL, Neal JM 1995b Epidural anesthesia and analgesia. Their role in postoperative outcome. Anesthesiology 82: 1474–1506
Macrae WA 2001 Chronic pain after surgery. British Journal of Anaesthesia 87: 88–98.
Mankikian B, Cantineau JP, Bertrand M et al 1988 Improvement of diaphragmatic dysfunction by extradural block after upper abdominal surgery. Anesthesiology 68: 379–386
McLachlan EM, Jänig W, Devor M, Michaelis M 1993 Peripheral nerve injury triggers noradrenergic sprouting within dorsal root ganglia. Nature 363: 543–546
McMahon SB 1991 Mechanisms of sympathetic pain. British Medical Bulletin 47: 584–600
Meert TF, De Kock M 1994 Potentiation of the analgesic properties of fentanyl-like opioids with α_2-adrenoceptor agonists in rats. Anesthesiology 81: 677–688
Melzack R 1971 Phantom limb pain. Anesthesiology 35: 409
Melzack R, Wall PD, Ty TC 1982 Acute pain in an emergency clinic: latency of onset and description patterns. Pain 14: 33
Merry A, Power I 1995 Perioperative NSAIDs: towards greater safety. Pain Reviews 2: 268–291
Merskey H 1986 Classification of chronic pain. Descriptions of chronic pain syndromes and definition of pain terms. Pain 3(suppl): S1–S225
Modig J 1976 Respiration and circulation after total hip replacement surgery: a comparison between parenteral analgesics and continuous lumbar epidural block. Acta Anaesthesiologica Scandinavica 20: 225–236
Modig J, Malmberg P, Karlstom G 1980 Effect of epidural versus general anesthesia on calf blood flow. Acta Anaesthesiologica Scandinavica 24: 305
Modig J, Borg T, Karlstom G, Maripuu E, Sahlstedt B 1983 Thromboembolism after hip replacement: role of epidural and general anesthesia. Anesthesia and Analgesia 62: 174–180
Moiniche S, Hjortso NC, Hansen BL et al 1994a The effect of balanced analgesia on early convalescence after major orthopaedic surgery. Acta Anaesthesiologica Scandinavica 38: 328–335
Moiniche S, Dahl JB, Rosenberg J, Kehlet H 1994b Colonic resection with early discharge after combined subarachnoid-epidural analgesia, preoperative glucocorticoids, and early postoperative mobilization and feeding in a pulmonary high-risk patient. Regional Anesthesia 19: 352–356
NHMRC 1999 Acute pain management: Scientific evidence. National Health and Medical Research Council of Australia, Canberra
Nimmo WS 1984 Effect of anaesthesia on gastric motility and emptying. British Journal of Anaesthesia 56: 29–37
Ollat H, Cesaro P 1995 Pharmacology of neuropathic pain. Clinical Neuropharmacology 18: 391–404
Peck C 1986 Psychological factors in acute pain management. In: Cousins M J, Phillips G D (eds) Acute pain management. Churchill Livingstone, Edinburgh, pp 251–274
Perkins FM, Kehlet H 2000 Chronic pain as an outcome of surgery—a review of predictive factors. Anesthesiology 93: 1123–1133.
Power I, Bowler GMR, Pugh GC, Chambers WA 1994 Ketorolac as a component of balanced analgesia after thoracotomy. British Journal of Anaesthesia 72: 224–226
Raja SN, Meyer RA, Ringkamp M, Campbell JN 1999 Peripheral neural mechanisms of nociception. In: Wall PD, Melzack R (eds) Textbook of Pain, 4th edn. Churchill Livingstone, Edinburgh, pp 11–58
Reiz S, Balfors E, Sorensen MR et al 1982 Coronary hemodynamic effects of general anesthesia and surgery. Regional Anesthesia 7(suppl): S8–S18
Sabiston DC 1982 Davis Christopher textbook of surgery: the biological basis of modern surgical practice, 2nd edn. Saunders, Philadelphia, pp 265–286
Scheinin B et al 1987 The effect of bupivacaine and morphine on pain and bowel function after colonic surgery. Acta Anaesthesiologica Scandinavica 31: 161–164
Schulze S, Roikjaer O, Hasseistrom L, Jensen NH, Kehlet H 1988 Epidural bupivacaine and morphine plus systemic indomethacin eliminates pain but not systemic response and convalescence after cholecystectomy. Surgery 103: 321–327
Scott DB 1988 Acute pain management. In: Cousins MJ, Bridenbaugh PO (eds) Neural blockade in clinical anesthesia and management of pain, 2nd edn. Lippincott, Philadelphia, pp 861–864
Scott N, Kehlet H 1988 Regional anaesthesia and surgical morbidity. British Journal of Surgery 75: 199–204
Seibert K, Zhang Y, Leahy K 1994 Pharmacological and biochemical demonstration of the role of cyclooxygenase 2 in inflammation and pain. Proceedings of the National Academy of Science of USA 91: 12013–12017
Sivilotti L, Woolf CJ 1994 The contribution of $GABA_A$ and glycine receptors to central sensitization: disinhibition and touch-evoked allodynia in the spinal cord. Journal of Neurophysiology 72: 169–179
Sjogren S, Wright B 1972 Circulatory changes during continuous epidural blockade. Acta Anaesthesiologica Scandinavica 46(suppl): 5
Stein C 1993 Peripheral mechanisms of opioid analgesia. Anesthesia and Analgesia 76: 182–191
Stein C 1995 Morphine—a local 'analgesic'. Pain: Clinical Updates 3: 1–4
Stein C, Millan MJ, Shippenberg TS 1989 Peripheral opioid receptors mediating antinociception in inflammation: evidence for involvement of mu, delta, and kappa receptors. Journal of Pharmacology and Experimental Therapeutics 248: 1269–1275
Tasker RR, Tsuda T, Hawrylyshyn P 1983 Clinical neurophysiological investigation of deafferentation pain. In: Bonica JJ, Lindblom U, Iggo A (eds) Advances in pain research and therapy, vol 5. Raven, New York, pp 713–738
Tennant F, Moll D, Depaulo V 1993 Topical morphine for peripheral pain. Lancet 342: 1047–1048
Thoren T, Sundberg A, Wattwil M, Garvill JE et al 1989 Effects of epidural bupivacaine and epidural morphine on bowel

function and pain after hysterectomy. Acta Anaesthesiologica Scandinavica 33: 181–195
Thorn SE, Wattwil M, Naslund I et al 1992 Post-operative epidural morphine but not epidural bupivacaine, delays gastric emptying on the first day after cholecystectomy. Regional Anesthesia 17(2): 91–94
Tuman KJ, McCarthy RJ, March RJ et al 1991 Effects of epidural anesthesia and analgesia on coagulation and outcome after major vascular surgery. Anesthesia and Analgesia 73: 696–704
Urquhart E 1993 Central analgesic activity of nonsteroidal antiinflammatory drugs in animal and human pain models. Seminars in Arthritis and Rheumatism 23: 198–205
Vik-Mo H, Ottsen S, Renck H 1978 Cardiac effects of thoracic epidural analgesia before and during acute coronary artery occlusion in open-chest dogs. Scandinavian Journal of Clinical and Laboratory Investigation 38: 737–746
Walker JS 1995 NSAID: an update on their analgesic effects. Clinical and Experimental Pharmacology and Physiology 22: 855–860
Wattwil M, Thoren T, Hennerdal S, Garvill JE et al 1989 Epidural analgesia with bupivacaine reduces postoperative paralytic ileus after hysterectomy. Anesthesia and Analgesia 68: 353–358
White JC, Sweet WH 1962 Pain and the neurosurgeon. Thomas, Springfield, IL, pp 11–49
Wilcox GL 1991 Excitatory neurotransmitters and pain. In: Bond MR, Charlton JE, Woolf CJ (eds) Proceedings of the VIth World Congress on Pain. Elsevier, Amsterdam, pp 97–117
Wilmore DW 1983 Alterations in protein, carbohydrate and fat metabolism in injured and septic patients. Journal of the American College of Nutrition 2: 3
Wilmore DW, Long JM, Mason AD, Pruitt BA 1976 Stress in surgical patients as a neurophysiologic reflex response. Surgery, Gynecology and Obstetrics 142: 257
Woolf CJ, Chong MS 1993 Preemptive analgesia—treating postoperative pain by preventing the establishment of central sensitization. Anesthesia and Analgesia 77: 362–379
Yaksh TL 1999 Central pharmacology of nociceptive transmission. In: Wall PD, Melzack R (eds) Textbook of Pain, 4th edn. Churchill Livingstone, Edinburgh, pp 253–308
Yaksh TL, Reddy SVR 1981 Studies in the primate on the analgesic effects associated with intrathecal actions of opiates, alpha-adrenergic agonists and baclofen. Anesthesiology 54: 451–467
Yeager MP, Glass DD, Neff RK, Brinck-Johnson T 1987 Epidural anesthesia and analgesia in high risk surgical patients. Anesthesiology 66: 729–736
Zolte N, Cust MD 1986 Analgesia in the acute abdomen. Annals of the Royal College of Surgeons of England 68: 209–2100

Chapter 2

Osteoarthritis

Paul Creamer

Introduction

Osteoarthritis (OA) is the most common form of arthritis, and is a major cause of morbidity, limitation of activity, and health care utilization (Lawrence et al 1990). Pain is the major symptom of OA and the main reason why affected individuals elect to seek medical care. Pain is also a major determinant of functional loss. Despite its importance, there is much about OA pain that remains unclear including, for example, the anatomical cause of pain and the reason for the poor correlation between pain and radiographic change. This chapter provides a brief overview of OA followed by a more detailed description of the nature, causes, and treatment of pain. Back pain is dealt with elsewhere: this chapter will concentrate on peripheral joint OA with particular emphasis on the knee.

Aetiopathogenesis of osteoarthritis

Osteoarthritis is a disorder of synovial joints characterized by destruction of articular cartilage and remodelling of subchondral bone. The traditional concept of OA as 'wear and tear' has been replaced by a model in which OA is seen as an active process resulting in breakdown of the balance between cartilage formation and catabolism. Thickening of subchondral bone, detectable by an increase in activity on bone scan, is also an early feature and may predict the future development of OA in the hand (Fig. 2.1) (Hutton et al 1986) and the knee (Dieppe et al 1993). It is unclear whether bone or cartilage represent the primary lesion in OA but clearly both are potential areas for therapeutic intervention.

Macroscopically, these changes result in focal cartilage loss with sclerosis and osteophyte formation at the joint margins. Some of these features correspond to radiographic changes on which the diagnosis of OA is usually made (Fig. 2.2, Table 2.1).

Rather than being a single pathology, the 'osteoarthritic disorders' are a group of overlapping distinct diseases varying in risk factors, clinical features, radiographic features, and outcomes. Factors increasing systemic vulnerability to OA include genes, age, gender, race, and nutrition. Local biomechanical factors include malalignment, previous damage, muscle weakness, joint laxity, and proprioceptive defects. Local factors, together with extrinsic factors acting on the joint such as obesity, physical activity, occupational overuse, and trauma, probably determine which joints get OA in a susceptible individual.

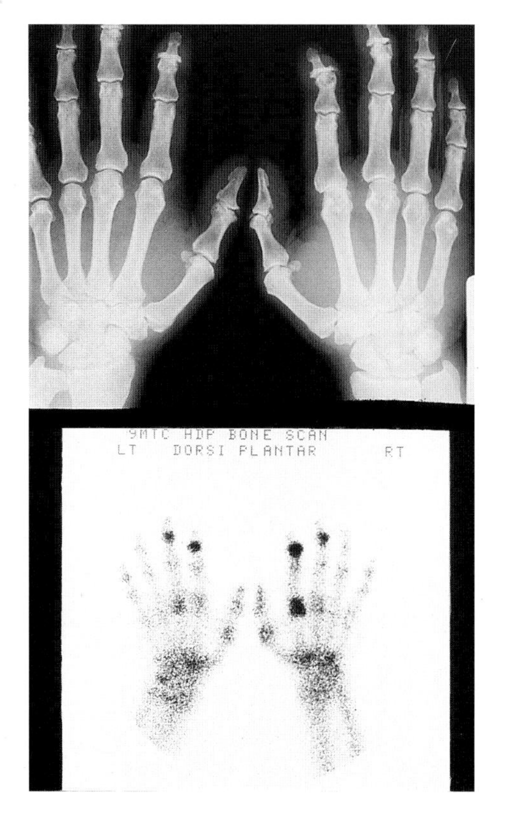

Fig. 2.1 Plain radiograph (top) and Tc^{99} scintigraphy (bottom) of a patient with hand OA. Note the 'hot' joints on scan, corresponding to sites of radiographic change.

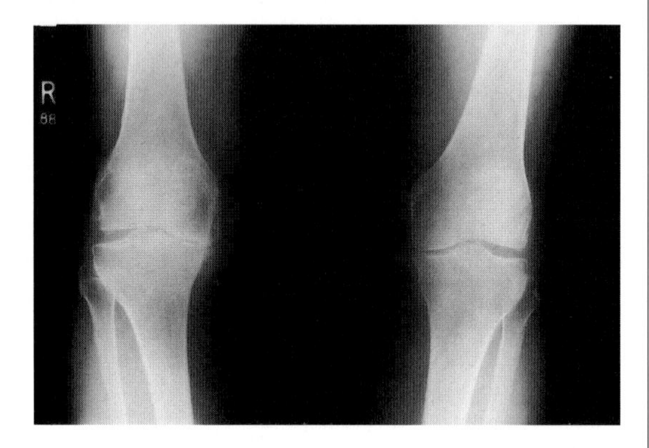

Fig. 2.2 Radiograph of tibiofemoral OA, showing joint space narrowing, sclerosis, and osteophyte formation.

Clinical features of osteoarthritis

Commonest sites for OA include the interphalangeal joints of the hand (Fig. 2.3), thumb base, knees, hips, and facet joints of the cervical and lumbar spine. Much OA appears to be asymptomatic: when it does cause problems these include pain, stiffness after inactivity, deformity, swelling, and loss of function.

Table 2.1 Relationship between pathological and radiographic features of osteoarthritis

Pathological features	Radiographic features
Focal areas of loss of articular cartilage	Asymmetric loss of interbone distance ('joint space narrowing')
Marginal lipping and overgrowth	Osteophytosis of bone
Remodelling of subchondral bone	Sclerosis and cysts in subchondral bone, altered bony contour
Capsular thickening and mild chronic synovitis	

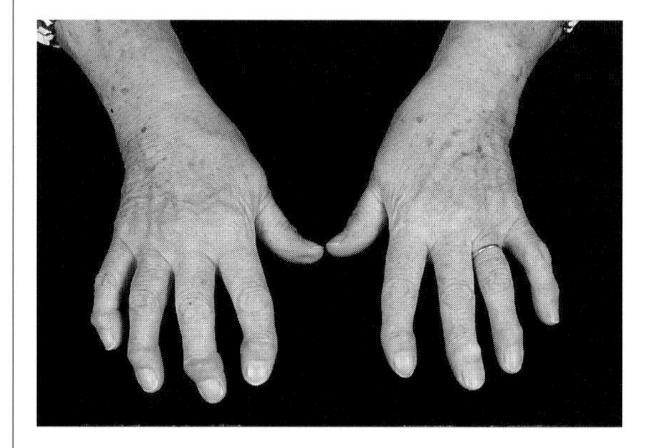

Fig. 2.3 Interphalangeal OA.

The diagnosis of OA still relies on radiographic features including osteophyte, joint space narrowing, and bony sclerosis. It is clear that considerable pathological change may occur before radiographs become abnormal (Fife et al 1991). Arthroscopy allows direct visualization of cartilage; scoring systems to standardize recording of cartilage damage are now available (Ayral et al 1996). Magnetic resonance imaging (MRI) has the advantage of being non-invasive and allowing assessment of non-bony structures; however, the cost and expertise required for interpretation makes it impractical for routine use.

Pathophysiology of joint pain

Most afferent fibres in articular nerves are unmyelinated, comprising C (group IV) fibres and postganglionic sympathetic fibres. Heavily myelinated Aβ (group II) fibres and thinly myelinated Aδ (group III) fibres comprise about 20% of the total fibres (Kidd 1996). There is rich innervation to articular capsule, tendons, ligaments, synovium, and periosteum via a mixture of free nerve endings and receptors. These sensory nerves respond to mechanical stimuli such as stretching of the joint capsule but also to chemical mediators such as lactic acid, histamine, kinins, and substance P. Such inflammatory mediators may stimulate pain fibres directly but may also sensitize fibres to mechanical stimuli. There is therefore potential for acute injury or inflammation to sensitize nerves such that they respond even when the original stimuli is removed. This 'neurogenic plasticity' may operate at both peripheral and spinal levels and is likely to be mediated by upregulation of specific receptors such as those for *N*-methyl-D aspartate (NMDA). Clearly these represent potential targets for therapeutic intervention. Although there is evidence for a central role for pain production in some patients, peripheral mechanisms are probably more important; for example, intra-articular local anaesthetic effectively abolishes pain temporarily in many patients with knee OA (Creamer et al 1996).

Measurement of pain in osteoarthritis

In community studies, the presence of knee pain is usually ascertained by a question such as: 'Have you ever had pain in or around the knee on most days for at least a month?' (Lawrence et al 1990). Subjective pain severity may be graded using a simple Likert scale (none, mild, moderate, severe, very severe) or a visual analogue scale. The stem question may be a simple 'how bad is your (knee, hip, hand) pain?' but additional valuable information can be obtained by asking about pain with different activities: stairs, walking, rest, and so on. Such information is obtained in questionnaires specifically designed to assess lower limb OA: examples include the WOMAC (Bellamy et al 1988) and Lequesne (1991) indices.

An attempt is sometimes made to assess the quality of pain in OA, using the McGill Pain Questionnaire (MPQ; Melzack 1975). This instrument allows subjects to select words (total = 76) that describe their pain. The MPQ was not specifically designed for arthritis pain, and some of the descriptors used may reflect mood disturbance rather than pure pain.

Finally, the effect of pain on observed behaviour in OA can be assessed, by videotaping patients while they undergo a standard activity programme (Keefe et al 1987a). Behaviours such as guarding, active rubbing, unloading the joint, rigidity, and joint flexing can be scored by independent observers.

Epidemiology of osteoarthritic pain

Most studies of pain in OA have looked at the knee. The prevalence of knee pain in 40- to 79-year-old community dwellers in the UK is about 25.3% (O'Reilly et al 1996). Radiographic knee OA was reported in 76% of those with pain. Less data are available on other joints. Using a definition of 'mild to severe pain during the last month', Carman (1989) reported a prevalence of hand pain of 37% in 50–74 year olds, of whom 45% had definite OA.

The chances of reporting the presence of pain rise with increasing radiographic severity but in general there is only a weak association between pain and structural damage. Community studies confirm that about 7–14% of the subjects with normal knee X-rays report knee pain: potential explanations include sources of pain not visible on an X-ray, insensitivity of radiographs, or inadequate views being taken (e.g., failure to assess the patellofemoral joint at the knee). Moreover, only 40–80% of the subjects with unequivocal radiographic knee OA report pain: perhaps due to inadequacies of the question being asked, or because pain may be a phasic process. Pain severity (as opposed to presence) in outpatients bears no relationship to X-ray change, but is more determined by factors such as obesity and coping strategies (Creamer et al 1999).

Pain in OA is not simply the result of structural changes but, rather, the outcome of a complex interplay between structural change, peripheral and central pain processing mechanisms, and subjective differences in what constitutes pain, in turn influenced by cultural, gender, and psychosocial factors. It is perhaps more helpful to regard knee pain and radiographic knee OA as separate problems: certainly they appear to differ in their risk factors (Davis et al 1992).

Subjects with clinical features such as crepitus and morning stiffness are more likely to report pain. For a given degree of radiographic severity, women tend to report pain more often than men. Age does not appear to be related to pain reporting. Increasing body mass index has been found to be a risk factor for pain in knee OA in some studies. Quadriceps weakness is a major risk factor for knee pain and subsequent disability (McAlindan et al 1993, Slemenda et al 1997).

Anatomical causes of pain in osteoarthritis

The anatomical source of pain in OA remains unclear. Any theory must take account of the fact that the principal structure involved (articular cartilage) possesses few pain-sensitive fibres: pain must therefore be arising from other tissues. Structures with the potential to cause pain in OA are listed in Table 2.2.

Psychosocial factors are important in OA, as in any chronic pain. Rates of depression and anxiety are increased in community subjects with knee pain compared to healthy controls (Dexter and Brandt 1994). Prevalence in hospital outpatients is even higher: 33% of patients with hip/knee OA had 'possible' depression compared to 19% healthy population (Hawley and Wolfe 1993). Differences between hospital and community subjects may reflect severity of disease, but depression may also play a role in the decision by patients to seek medical care.

Using the MPQ as a measure of pain severity, significant correlations between anxiety and depression and knee pain severity in hospital patients have been reported (Summers et al 1988). A community survey of elderly subjects reporting sporadic, episodic, or chronic knee pain (Hopman-Rock et al 1996) also found that chronicity and severity of pain were associated with higher psychosocial disability when compared with age-matched pain-free controls from the same community.

Personality traits such as hypochondriasis have been shown to be associated with greater pain severity in OA of the hip (Lunghi et al 1978) and knee (Lichtenberg et al 1986) as have 'life stress' and 'daily hassles'. Lower formal education level has been reported to be a risk factor for both radiographic and symptomatic knee OA (Hannan et al 1992).

Table 2.2 Potential sources of pain in OA

Bone:	Raised intra-osseous pressure
	Growing osteophyte
	Subchondral fractures
Inflammation	
Soft tissue:	Capsule
	Ligament
	Menisci
Central/psychosocial	

The mechanisms by which psychosocial factors are related to knee pain are unclear, and cross-sectional studies do not allow us to make inferences about cause and effect. Pathophysiological effects of anxiety or depression include increased muscle tension, which may be painful. Anxiety, manifested by persistent attempts to avoid knee pain, may lead to loss of muscle bulk and generalized deconditioning and loss of confidence. It is possible that overavoidance of movement in knee pain leads to a chronic cycle of inactivity, muscle wasting and weakness, and further pain and inactivity (Dekker et al 1993). Depression may also result in maladapted 'coping strategies' or affect the patient's belief about their ability to cope with pain, which in itself results in higher reported pain severity (Keefe et al 1987b).

Psychological factors may also be important in predicting response to therapies and determining patients' adherence to treatment. In a study of exercise for patients with knee arthritis, for example, the most powerful predictors of maintaining exercise at 3 months were baseline anxiety and depression (Minor and Brown 1993).

The nature of osteoarthritic pain

Pain due to OA is generally 'aching' or 'throbbing', insidious in onset, localized, and not associated with any systemic disturbance. The severity of OA pain is comparable to that of RA.

Characteristically, pain is worse on use of the affected joint (e.g., going up or down stairs for knee OA), worse in the evenings, and eased by rest. A significant proportion of subjects, however, do complain of pain at night: such patients have generally had symptoms for longer than those without night pain and may have more severe disease. In addition to diurnal variation, some patients show a day-to-day variation, with symptoms being worse at the weekends (Bellamy et al 1990).

The location of pain in OA generally corresponds to the affected joint but referred pain may be seen: for example, pain from hip OA may be felt in the knee and pain from spinal OA may be felt in the hip or buttock. At the knee, most pain either is diffusely felt anteriorly over the surface of the patella or is localized to the inferomedial aspect of the joint.

Management of pain in osteoarthritis

Pain is the most frequent symptom of OA and, in the absence of therapies that may modify the underlying disease process, treatments for OA are primarily assessed by their ability to reduce pain. Ideally, treatments would be based on knowledge of pathogenesis: however, because we do not know the cause of pain in OA, treatment is to some extent empirical. Nevertheless, four areas may be identified: correction of abnormal mechanical stress, modulation of central perception of pain, drug therapy, and surgery.

Correction of abnormal biomechanics

Knee OA is largely a biomechanical disorder. The aim of biomechanical intervention is to reduce pain and improve function by altering weight distribution through the joint, re-aligning to correct deformities, and improving stability and patient confidence.

Weight reduction

Obesity is a risk factor for OA, particularly at the knee and in women. Weight loss is associated with a lower chance of developing symptomatic OA and incident radiographic OA (Felson et al 1997) and probably reduces symptoms. In a study of overweight postmenopausal women with symptomatic knee OA (Martin et al 1996), weight loss during a 6-month programme of dietary counselling and exercise was associated with a reduction in both pain and disability. The paucity of other data may reflect that losing weight by diet alone is clearly not easy, particularly in the elderly who may be relatively immobile.

Orthotics

A walking stick and shock-absorbing footwear can reduce load bearing in the affected joint by 20–30% with a consequent reduction in symptoms. Lateral heel wedges are a method of decreasing the lateral thrust found in medial compartment OA with varus deformity and can also reduce pain (Ogata et al 1997). Soft neoprene sleeves with additional patellar padding may improve patellar tracking and may also act by improving proprioception. Other orthotic devices, such as splints, braces, and neck collars, aim to correct deformity and instability. Patients with knee OA who have patellofemoral joint disease have been shown to benefit from medial taping of the patella (Cushnaghan et al 1994). Modification of the patient's environment (raised chairs, toilet seats, dressing aids) should be considered.

Quadriceps strengthening

Quadriceps weakness may be a risk factor for radiographic OA (Slemenda et al 1997) and is clearly an important determinant of function and pain (Dekker et al 1993, McAlindon et al 1993). Several studies, of 3–6 months in duration, have documented that quadriceps strengthening exercises are effective in reducing pain and improving function in patients with knee OA (Fisher et al 1993) and can be taught to subjects in their own home (O'Reilly 1999). Quadriceps strengthening can be accomplished by both isometric and isotonic resistive exercise. Suitable exercises for patients with knee OA are given in Table 2.3.

Aerobic exercise

Aerobic conditioning exercise, either supervised fitness walking or aquatics, has been shown to be well tolerated and more effective than conventional physical therapy or standard medical care in patients with OA of the hip and/or knee. Home exercises are as effective as outpatient hydrotherapy in hip OA. A multicentre study (Ettinger et al 1997) on community-dwelling adults with knee OA and self-reported physical disability aged 60 and above demonstrated that participation in either aerobic or resistive exercise was superior to patient education alone.

Central pain modification

Cognitive behavioural approaches, designed to improve self-efficacy and coping strategies, are also beneficial. These interventions emphasize the control of pain by understanding the interaction of emotions and cognition with the physical and behavioural aspects of pain. In one study (Keefe et al 1996), patients with knee OA who participated in a programme that involved their spouse had

Table 2.3 Exercises suitable for home treatment of knee OA[a]

Exercise
1. Isometric quads contraction in extension for 5 seconds (subject sits on floor against wall, legs extended, towel under knee, pushes knee into floor against towel)
2. Isotonic quads contraction held in mid flexion for 5 seconds (subject in chair, partially extends lower leg and holds)
3. Isotonic hamstring contraction (lies on front and bends knee bringing foot towards body)
4. Isotonic quads with resistance band held for 5 seconds (as 2)
5. Dynamic stepping: walking up and down 1 step
Increased to maximum of 20 reps on each leg

[a]Modified from O'Reilly et al (1999).

greater improvement in pain, psychological disability, self-efficacy, and pain behaviours, as well as better marital adjustment and coping skills, compared to patients who participated in a traditional programme without their spouse.

Education is also an effective treatment. The Arthritis Self-Help Course has been shown to be effective. This course consists of six weekly education sessions focusing on exercise, relaxation techniques, joint protection techniques, and a description of the various medications used in treating patients with arthritis. Studies by Lorig and colleagues (Lorig and Holman 1993) have shown that patients with OA who participate in this programme have significant improvement in knowledge, pain, and quality of life, and a decreased frequency of physician visits and lower health care costs.

Finally, provision of social support through simple telephone contact can improve functional status and pain in patients with OA (Weinberger et al 1993). The content of the telephone calls seems to be important: symptom monitoring is not as effective as specific advice and counselling (Maisiak et al 1996).

Drug therapy

First-line drug therapy in OA should be a trial of simple analgesics such as paracetamol, coproxamol, or tramadol. These drugs are safe, effective, and well tolerated. Only when analgesia and non-pharmacological therapy have been fully tested should non-steroidal anti-inflammatory drugs (NSAIDs) be given.

Evidence for the superiority of NSAIDs over paracetamol is largely lacking and, at least under trial conditions, many patients on chronic NSAID therapy for knee OA can cease this medication without apparent deterioration in symptoms. A small proportion of patients with OA do seem to derive sustained benefit from NSAIDs: it is tempting to suggest that these patients have a more 'inflammatory' type of OA, but it is not possible from clinical examination to predict those patients who will respond (Bradley et al 1992). The use of NSAIDs is associated with appreciable morbidity, particularly in the elderly (the group most likely to have OA): this can be minimized by using the smallest effective dose and a co-prescription of gastroprotective agents and by encouraging 'intelligent non-compliance' (i.e., only take the tablets if you have pain). Novel highly selective COX2 inhibitors (rofecoxib, celecoxib) are no more effective than traditional NSAIDs but probably have a lower risk of serious gastrointestinal complications. NSAIDs may also be given as topical creams or gels, which are safe, popular with patients, and effective—perhaps because they give the patient a degree of control over their symptoms. Topical capsaicin, a specific substance P depletor derived from the pepper plant, can also be of value especially in hand OA.

IA steroid injections are widely used. Controlled trials, confined to the knee, provide some evidence supporting their efficacy over placebo, but only for up to 4 weeks (Creamer 1997). This contrasts with clinical practice that suggests that some patients have a sustained response lasting up to 6 months. Efforts to identify predictors of response have proved largely unsuccessful, although some studies have reported that the presence of effusion (Gaffney et al 1995) or local tenderness (Jones and Doherty 1996) may be associated with a better response. A recent report (Griffith et al 1997) found significant improvement in pain, stiffness, and range of movement after steroid or anaesthetic injection at the hip but both injections were equally effective. Anecdotally, injection of the carpometacarpal joint can be very helpful in thumb-base OA. Steroid injections are remarkably safe and well tolerated.

Hyaluronic acid (HA) forms the backbone of the proteoglycan molecule and is the major constituent of synovial fluid. In addition to its mechanical role as a lubricant, shock absorber, and buffer between articular cartilage surfaces, it also may have a role in binding inflammatory mediators and neuropeptides associated with pain production. Preparations of HA are available for use by intra-articular injection in knee OA. Several studies suggest a modest benefit when compared to placebo injections (Dougados et al 1993, Lohmander et al 1996) or intra-articular steroids (Jones et al 1995). Given the reluctance to use NSAIDs in the elderly, there may be a role for intra-articular hyaluronic acid in the treatment of selected elderly patients with knee OA: for example, in those in whom surgery is contraindicated and whose pain is not controlled by simple oral and/or topical analgesics.

Glucosamine is an aminomonosaccaride, which is essential for the formation of the glycosaminoglycans in articular cartilage. Doses of 1500 mg daily produce greater improvement in pain than placebo and are as effective as ibuprofen 1200 mg daily (Muller-Fassbender et al 1994) with fewer gastrointestinal adverse reactions. A longer study (Reginster et al 2001) has confirmed a clinical benefit though a reported disease-modifying action remains controversial.

Finally low doses of tricyclics at night may improve sleep quality and pain.

Surgical procedures

Tidal lavage (the instillation and drainage of 500 ml–2 L of saline) is effective in some patients with knee OA that has not responded to standard medical therapy, and is particularly useful in those for whom surgery is contraindicated or refused (Ravaud et al 1999). Traditionally, lavage has been performed at the same time as arthroscopy but can also be achieved using a 'needle' arthroscope or even a sterile disposable 14-gauge cannula, thereby avoiding the need for an operating room and anaesthesia. The mechanism of action of lavage is unknown: reduction of secondary synovitis induced by crystals or joint debris, removal of inflammatory mediators, and stretching of joint capsule have all been suggested. An improvement in quadriceps muscle function after lavage has been demonstrated (Gibson et al 1992).

Finally, total joint replacement (TJR) (Dieppe et al 1999) is an excellent treatment for OA and has been responsible for a dramatic improvement in the quality of life of individuals with severe symptomatic lower limb OA who have failed to respond to medical management. Highly significant changes in pain, mobility, social function, and global health status are detectable at 3 months; improvement may continue for up to a year (Hawker et al 1998).

Future developments in osteoarthritis

The development of better methods of understanding OA, such as MRI scanning or use of biochemical markers, will allow rational assessment of interventions designed both to modify disease and to reduce symptoms. Disease modification may be possible by targeting the enzymes that promote inflammation and break down cartilage, including chemically modified tetracyclines and other metalloproteinase inhibitors (Ryan et al 1996) and interleukin-1 receptor antagonist (Caron et al 1996), or by reducing bone turnover perhaps using bisphosphonates. Autologous cartilage transplantation may be useful in patients with early disease and focal cartilage defects (Brittberg et al 1994). Mechanical factors and injury also represent targets for prevention, for example by modifying work practices in high-risk groups. The proven disease-modifying effect of simple interventions such as weight reduction should not be underestimated. Symptom reduction may come with better analgesics acting centrally or locally and with the refinement of interventions designed to tackle the patient's emotional and attitudinal response to disease.

References

Ayral X, Dougados M, Listrat V et al 1996 Arthroscopic evaluation of chondropathy in osteoarthritis of the knee. Journal of Rheumatology 23: 698–706

Bellamy N, Buchanan WW, Goldsmith CH et al 1988 Validation study of WOMAC: a health status instrument for measuring clinically important patient relevant outcomes to antirheumatic drug therapy in patients with osteoarthritis of the hip or knee. Journal of Rheumatology 15: 1833–1840

Bellamy N, Sothern R, Campbell J 1990 Rhythmic variations in pain perception in osteoarthritis of the knee. Journal of Rheumatology 17: 364–372

Bradley JD, Brandt KD, Katz BP et al 1992 Treatment of knee osteoarthritis: relationship of clinical features of joint inflammation to the response to a nonsteroidal antiinflammatory drug or pure analgesic. Journal of Rheumatology 19: 1950–1954

Brittberg M, Lindahl A, Nilsson A et al 1994 Treatment of deep cartilage defects in the knee with autologous chondrocyte transplantation. New England Journal of Medicine 331: 889–895

Carman WJ 1989 Factors associated with pain and osteoarthritis in the Tecumseh Community Health Study. Seminars in Arthritis and Rheumatism 18: 10–13

Caron JP, Fernandes JC, Martel-Pelletier J et al 1996 Chondroprotective effect of intraarticular injections of interleukin-1 receptor antagonist in experimental osteoarthritis. Suppression of collagenase-1 expression. Arthritis and Rheumatism 39: 1535–1544

Creamer P 1997 Intra-articular steroid injections in osteoarthritis: do they work and if so how? (Editorial). Annals of the Rheumatic Diseases 56: 634–635

Creamer P, Hunt M, Dieppe PA 1996 Pain mechanisms in osteoarthritis of the knee: effect of intraarticular anesthetic. Journal of Rheumatology 23: 1031–1036

Creamer P, Lethbridge-Cejku M, Hochberg M 1999 Determinants of pain severity in knee osteoarthritis: effect of demographic and psychosocial variables using three pain measures. Journal of Rheumatology 26: 1785–1792

Cushnaghan J, McCarthy C, Dieppe P 1994 Taping the patella medially: a new treatment for osteoarthritis of the knee joint? British Medical Journal 308: 753–755

Davis M, Ettinger W, Neuhaus J et al 1992 Correlates of knee pain among US adults with and without radiographic knee osteoarthritis. Journal of Rheumatology 19: 1943–1949

Dekker J, Tola P, Aufdemkampe G, Winckers M 1993 Negative affect, pain and disability in osteoarthritis patients: the mediating role of muscle weakness. Behaviour Research and Therapy 31: 203–206

Dexter P, Brandt K 1994 Distribution and predictors of depressive symptoms in osteoarthritis. Journal of Rheumatology 21: 279–286

Dieppe PA, Cushnaghan J, Young P, Kirwan J 1993 Prediction of the progression of joint space narrowing in osteoarthritis of the knee by scintigraphy. Annals of the Rheumatic Diseases 52: 557–563

Dieppe P, Basler HD, Chard J, Croft P, Dixon J, Hurley M, Lohmander S, Raspe H 1999 Knee replacement surgery for osteoarthritis: effectiveness, practice variations, indications and possible determinants of utilization. Rheumatology 38: 73–83

Dougados M, Nguyen M, Listrat V, Amor B 1993 High molecular weight sodium hyaluronate (hyalectin) in osteoarthritis of the knee: a 1 year placebo-controlled trial. Osteoarthritis and Cartilage 1: 97–103

Ettinger WH, Burns R, Messier SP et al 1997 A randomized trial comparing aerobic exercise and resistance exercise with a health education program in older adults with knee

osteoarthritis. Journal of the American Medical Association 277: 25–31
Felson DT, Zhang Y, Hannan MT et al 1997 Risk factors for incident radiographic knee osteoarthritis in the elderly. Arthritis and Rheumatism 40: 728–733
Fife RS, Brandt K, Braunstein E et al 1991 Relationship between arthroscopic evidence of cartilage damage and radiographic evidence of joint space narrowing in early osteoarthritis of the knee. Arthritis and Rheumatism 34: 377–382
Fisher NM, Gresham GE, Abrams M et al 1993 Quantitative effects of physical therapy on muscular and functional performance in subjects with osteoarthritis of the knees. Archives of Physical Medicine and Rehabilitation 74: 840–847
Gaffney K, Ledingham J, Perry JD 1995 Intra-articular triamcinolone hexacetonide in knee osteoarthritis: factors influencing the clinical response. Annals of the Rheumatic Diseases 54: 379–381
Gibson JN, White MD, Chapman VM, Strachan RK 1992 Arthroscopic lavage and debridement for osteoarthritis of the knee. Journal of Bone and Joint Surgery 74B: 534–537
Griffith SM, Dziedzic K, Cheung NT et al 1997 Clinical outcomes: a double blind randomised controlled trial to compare the effect of intra-articular local anaesthetic and local anaesthetic plus steroid in hip arthritis. British Journal of Rheumatology 36(suppl 2): 21
Hannan MT, Anderson JJ, Pincus T, Felson DT 1992 Educational attainment and osteoarthritis: differential associations with radiographic changes and symptom reporting. Journal of Clinical Epidemiology 45: 139–147
Hawker G, Wright J, Coyte P, Paul J, Dittus R, Croxford R, Katz B 1998 Health-related quality of life after knee replacement. Journal of Bone and Joint Surgery 80: 163–173
Hawley DJ, Wolfe F 1993 Depression is not more common in RA: a 10 year longitudinal study of 6153 patients with rheumatic disease. Journal of Rheumatology 20: 2025–2031
Hopman-Rock M, Odding E, Hofman A et al 1996 Physical and psychosocial disability in elderly subjects in relation to pain in the hip and/or knee. Journal of Rheumatology 23: 1037–1044
Hutton CW, Higgs ER, Jackson PC et al 1986 99mTc HMDP bone scanning in generalised nodal osteoarthritis. II The four hour bone scan predicts radiographic change. Annals of the Rheumatic Diseases 45: 622–626
Jones A, Doherty M 1996 Intra-articular corticosteroids are effective in osteoarthritis but there are no clinical predictors of response. Annals of the Rheumatic Diseases 55: 829–832
Jones AC, Pattrick M, Doherty S, Doherty M 1995 Intra-articular hyaluronic acid compared to intra-articular triamcinolone hexacetonide in inflammatory knee osteoarthritis. Osteoarthritis and Cartilage 3: 269–273
Keefe FJ, Caldwell DS, Queen K et al 1987a Osteoarthritis knee pain: a behavioral analysis. Pain 28: 309–321
Keefe FJ, Caldwell DS, Queen KT et al 1987b Pain coping strategies in osteoarthritis patients. Journal of Consulting and Clinical Psychology 55: 208–212
Keefe FJ, Caldwell DS, Baucom D et al 1996 Spouse-assisted coping skills training in the management of osteoarthritic knee pain. Arthritis Care and Research 9: 279–291
Kidd B 1996 Problems with pain—is the messenger to blame? Annals of the Rheumatic Diseases 55: 276–283
Lawrence RC, Everett DF, Hochberg MC 1990 Arthritis. In: Huntley R, Cornoni-Huntley J (eds) Health status and well being of the elderly: National Health and Nutrition Examination I epidemiologic follow-up study. Oxford University Press, New York, pp 133–151
Lequesne M 1991 Indices of severity and disease activity for osteoarthritis. Seminars in Arthritis and Rheumatism 20(suppl 2): 48–54
Lichtenberg PA, Swensen CH, Skehan MW 1986 Further investigation of the role of personality, lifestyle and arthritic severity in predicting pain. Journal of Psychosomatic Research 30: 327–337
Lohmander LS, Dalen N, Englund G et al 1996 Intra-articular hyaluronan injections in the treatment of osteoarthritis of the knee: a randomized, double blind, placebo controlled trial. Annals of the Rheumatic Diseases 55: 424–431
Lorig KR, Holman HR 1993 Arthritis self management studies: a 12 year review. Health Education Quarterly 20: 17–28
Lunghi M, Miller P, McQuillan W 1978 Psychosocial factors in osteoarthritis of the hip. Journal of Psychosomatic Research 22: 57–63
McAlindon T, Cooper C, Kirwan JR, Dieppe PA 1993 Determinants of disability in osteoarthritis of the knee. Annals of the Rheumatic Diseases 52: 258–262
Maisiak R, Austin J, Heck L 1996 Health outcomes of two telephone interventions for patients with rheumatoid arthritis or osteoarthritis. Arthritis and Rheumatism 39: 1391–1399
Martin K, Nicklas BJ, Bunyard LB et al 1996 Weight loss and walking improve symptoms of knee osteoarthritis. Arthritis and Rheumatism 39(suppl): S225
Melzack R 1975 The McGill pain questionnaire: major properties and scoring methods. Pain 1: 277–299
Minor MA, Brown JD 1993 Exercise maintenance of persons with arthritis after participation in a class experience. Health Education Quarterly 20: 83–95
Muller-Fassbender H, Bach GL, Haase W et al 1994 Glucosamine sulfate compared to ibuprofen in osteoarthritis of the knee. Osteoarthritis and Cartilage 2: 61–69
Ogata K, Yasunaga M, Nomiyama H 1997 The effect of wedged insoles on the thrust of osteoarthritic knees. International Orthopaedics 21: 308–312
O'Reilly S, Muir KR, Doherty M 1996 Screening for pain in knee osteoarthritis: which question? Annals of the Rheumatic Diseases 55: 931–933
O'Reilly SC, Muir KR, Doherty M 1999 Effectiveness of home exercise on pain and disability from osteoarthritis of the knee: a randomised controlled study. Annals of the Rheumatic Diseases 58: 15–19
Ravaud P, Moulinier L, Giraudeau B, Ayral X, Guerin C, Noel E, Thomas P, Fautrel B, Mazieres B, Dougados M 1999 Effects of joint lavage and steroid injection in patients with osteoarthritis of the knee: results of a multicenter, randomized, controlled trial. Arthritis and Rheumatism 42: 475–482
Reginster JY et al 2001 Long term effects of glucosamine sulphate on osteoarthritis progression: a randomised placebo controlled clinical trial. Lancet 357: 251–256
Ryan ME, Greenwald RA, Golub LM 1996 Potential of tetracyclines to modify cartilage breakdown in osteoarthritis. Current Opinions in Rheumatology 8: 238–247
Slemenda C, Brandt KD, Heilman DK et al 1997 Quadriceps weakness and osteoarthritis of the knee. Annals of Internal Medicine 127: 97–104
Summers MN, Haley WE, Reveille JO, Alarcon GS 1988 Radiographic assessment and psychological variables as predictors of pain and functional impairment in osteoarthritis of the knee or hip. Arthritis and Rheumatism 31: 204–209
Weinberger M, Tierney WM, Cowper PA et al 1993 Cost-effectiveness of increased telephone contact for patients with osteoarthritis. A randomized, controlled trial. Arthritis and Rheumatism 36: 243–246

Chapter 3

Rheumatoid arthritis

Malcolm I V Jayson

Introduction

Rheumatoid arthritis (RA) is a complex multi-system inflammatory disorder in which the principle problems affect the synovial linings of the joints and tendons. In acute disease many patients develop generalized malaise and weight loss, and specific complications may affect other organ systems. Occasionally these features predominate.

The cause of RA is unknown but the prevailing view is that both inherited and environmental factors are important, with systemic autoimmune reactions precipitating a cascade of inflammatory changes.

There is an increased familial aggregation of the disease and, in particular, greater concordance in monozygotic than dizygotic twins. The best documented genetic marker for RA is the class II major histocompatibility complex (MHC) antigen HLA DR4. The presence of this inherited HLA marker conveys a sixfold increase in the relative risk of developing this disease. Some 50% of patients with RA carry the DR4 antigen. In particular it is associated with more severe disease and systemic complications (Westedt et al 1986). The presence of this tissue type acts as a susceptibility factor for autoimmune events but the mechanism for this remains to be determined.

Against this background environmental factors are believed to precipitate the development of this problem. Much effort has gone into identifying a possible infective basis for the development of RA in genetically predisposed individuals. A wide variety of organisms have been implicated, but in contrast to reactive arthritis and other forms of chronic inflammatory disease, no definitive evidence of a specific causative microorganism has been identified.

Many patients blame the onset of RA on a stressful event. The evidence for this is weak but undoubtedly psychological distress exacerbates patients' perception of severity of the disease.

Despite many claims, diet plays little role in RA. Some patients have individual allergies and may develop acute synovitis on exposure to specific types of food but this is very different from the rheumatoid process. Numerous studies on the effects of diet on arthritis have been undertaken but with little positive results. A very high intake of fish oil may lead to a decrease in the ability to generate certain inflammatory cytokines and have a limited anti-inflammatory effect.

The prevalence of the disease varies considerably between different populations. In part this is due to different genetic make-ups but environmental factors also play their part. For example, in

Africa there is a considerably lower prevalence in rural black groups than in urbanized populations (Beighton et al 1975).

Pathology

The normal synovial lining of diarthrodial joints is a delicate tissue layer up to three cells thick and a loosely arranged stroma with connective tissue, microvasculature, and lymphatics. In early active disease the synovium becomes swollen, hypertrophic, and inflamed. Microscopically the stroma is invaded by lymphocytes and plasma cells. Fibrin deposition may occur on the surface of the hypertrophic synovium. The synovial stroma is replaced by proliferation of local connective tissue cells by the process of mesenchymoid transformation. Excess production of synovial fluid leads to joint swelling and clinically detectable effusions. The cellular content of rheumatoid synovial fluid consists principally of polymorphonuclear leucocytes. The destructive phase of the disease is associated with the production of chronic granulation tissue or pannus, which spreads over the articular cartilage surface. Cartilage destruction appears on the deep surface of the pannus and is seen as loss of joint space on X-ray. Bone erosions usually appear first at the joint margins at the point of normal synovial reflection and where bone is relatively unprotected by cartilage. Neutral proteolytic enzymes (Barrett and Saklatvala 1981) secreted by macrophages in the pannus and acidic lysosomal enzymes secreted by polymorphonuclear leucocytes in the synovial fluid both play a part in bone and cartilage destruction. In severe forms of the disease continued bone and cartilage destruction is associated with irreversible deformity and, particularly in weight-bearing joints, secondary osteoarthritis may occur.

Clinical features

RA occurs in both sexes but is two or three times more common in females than males. It may start at any age but with an increasing incidence in older people. The overall prevalence is about 1% of the population. In recent years the incidence of the disease appears to be decreasing with its effects being less severe.

RA is a generalized disease with the most obvious problems affecting the joints. Severe forms of the disease may be associated with both articular and extra-articular features and the symptoms and signs of a systemic disease process. These include general malaise and lassitude, weight loss, and low-grade pyrexia. The disease onset is insidious in up to 70% of patients but may be acute and associated with systemic upset and fever.

Articular clinical features

Established rheumatoid disease is typically a symmetrical peripheral inflammatory polyarthritis that most often involves the small joints of the hands and feet, the wrists, ankles, knees, and cervical spine. The shoulders and elbows may be involved and the hips and lumbar spine less frequently. In severe forms of the disease any synovial joint may be affected.

In early active rheumatoid disease there is pain, soft-tissue swelling, and stiffness. The pain and stiffness of active inflammation are typically worse in the early morning and improve with activity during the day, although many patients develop further symptoms when they become tired in the early evening. Gelling or stiffening of the joints with rest or inactivity are also typical of inflammatory disease. On examination the soft-tissue joint swelling of active RA is due to synovial hypertrophy and effusion and is warm and tender. Muscle wasting appears rapidly around painful swollen joints, and there is sometimes periarticular inflammatory oedema.

In late-stage destructive RA problems of deformity and loss of function predominate with relatively little active inflammation.

The pattern of changes is similar in various joints and is exemplified by the patterns seen in the hands. In early disease there is inflammation of the metacarpophalangeal and proximal interphalangeal joints (Fig. 3.1) with pain and swelling. The

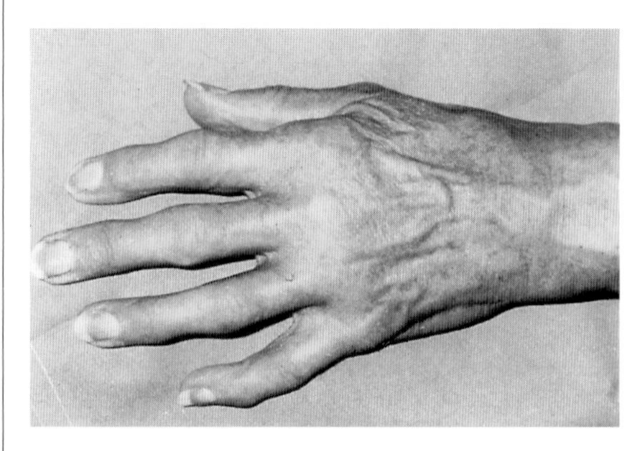

Fig. 3.1 Early rheumatoid inflammation of the proximal interphalangeal and metacarpophalangeal joints of the hand.

inflammation may also affect the tendon sheaths, contributing to impaired finger movement and poor grip. Synovitis of the wrists and of the flexor tendon sheaths may lead to compression of the median nerve and produce features of the carpal tunnel syndrome. As the disease advances a variety of deformities may develop due to combinations of synovitis, joint erosion and instability, tendon sheath synovitis and rupture, and progressive deformities (Figs. 3.2, 3.3, 3.4). Analogous progressive changes may affect any synovial joints and in particular the feet, ankles, knees, elbows, shoulders, and neck.

Extra-articular clinical features

Extra-articular features are found particularly in patients with the most severe forms of articular disease.

The pathogenesis of many of the systemic features, such as vasculitis and nodules, are thought to be related to the local deposition of circulating immune complexes containing IgM and possibly IgG rheumatoid factors.

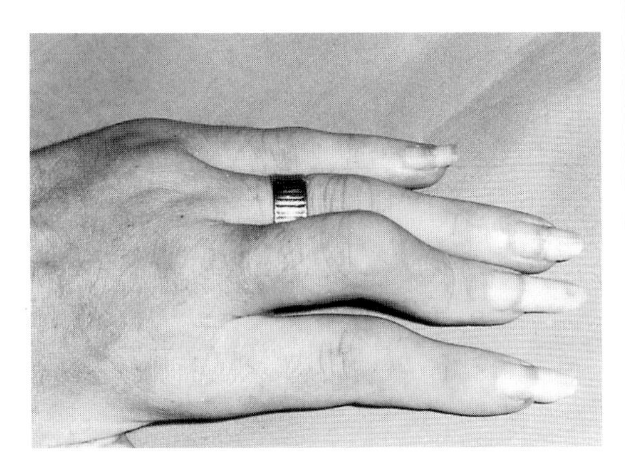

Fig. 3.2 The boutonnière, or buttonhole, deformity of the middle finger.

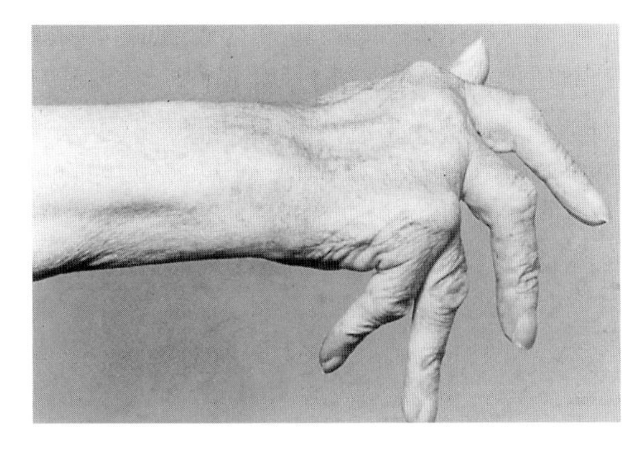

Fig. 3.3 Ulnar deviation of the fingers.

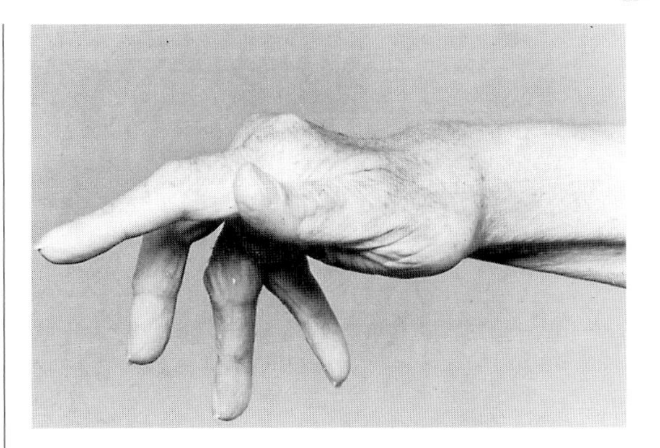

Fig. 3.4 Rupture of extensor tendons with 'dropped fingers'.

Nodules

Rheumatoid nodules are found most frequently in subcutaneous regions subject to recurrent mechanical stress. Common sites include the subcutaneous borders of the forearms, the olecranon, often in association with an olecranon bursa, and also over sites such as the tips of the fingers and sacrum. Rheumatoid nodules in these sites are firm, non-tender, and larger and less transient than the small nodules of rheumatic fever. In certain areas, such as over the sacrum, nodules may ulcerate and become infected bedsores. They can form a potential focus for systemic infections. Although most frequently found in the subcutaneous regions, these nodules may also occur as intracutaneous nodules and within other tissues such as the sclera, lung, pleura, and myocardium.

The histology of the rheumatoid nodule is almost specific for RA and consists of a central area of fibrinoid necrosis surrounded by a palisade layer of histiocytes and peripherally by a zone of loose connective tissue (Gardner 1992). The presence of rheumatoid nodules may be helpful for clinical diagnosis, and their presence indicates an adverse prognosis.

Vasculitis

This is an uncommon but potentially fatal complication found in the most severe forms of the disease. All sizes of blood vessels may become affected. Cutaneous vasculitis is most often seen as nailfold haemorrhages in the fingers. Patients with these lesions do not always develop the more serious forms of vasculitis although they are at increased risk of doing so. More serious forms of cutaneous vasculitis may be associated with persistent cutaneous ulceration which often appears in the lower leg and may prove resistant to treatment. Medium or large blood vessels may become involved and present clinically with gangrene of the fingers, small bowel infarction or perforation, and pulmonary hypertension. Small-vessel vasculitis is thought to underline many of the other extra-articular disease features such as peripheral neuropathy and probably nodule formation.

The histological changes found in rheumatoid vasculitis range from intimal hyperplasia to an inflammatory reaction affecting all layers of the vessel wall and are sometimes associated with necrosis (Fassbender 1975). Immunological tests often show high titres of circulating IgM rheumatoid factors, antinuclear antibodies, and evidence of circulating immune complex activity, such as reduced serum complement levels and sometimes circulating cryoglobulins.

Patients with severe forms of vasculitis are medical emergencies and often require aggressive treatment with corticosteroids and immunosuppressive drugs.

Haematology

The anaemia of RA is similar to that found in other chronic disorders such as malignancy, chronic infections, and uraemia. This anaemia is usually normocytic normochromic, but may be hypochromic and, less commonly, macrocytic. The degree of anaemia in rheumatoid disease roughly correlates with the erythrocyte sedimentation rate (ESR). Typically the serum iron and total iron binding capacity are reduced and serum ferritin is elevated. The anaemia is associated with an increased affinity of the reticuloendothelial system for iron, and bone marrow iron stores are plentiful. The anaemia of rheumatoid disease is to be distinguished from that of iron deficiency; the latter commonly results from gastrointestinal blood loss, which is frequently a side effect of non-steroidal anti-inflammatory drug (NSAID) therapy. In an iron deficiency anaemia serum iron is low but the total iron binding capacity is elevated and the bone marrow iron stores are reduced. Two types of anaemia may coexist, and factors that might suggest that iron deficiency is contributing to anaemia include a history of melaena or recent dyspepsia, a sudden drop in haemoglobin, or a haemoglobin value much lower than 9 g/dl. Unless there is coincidental iron deficiency, oral iron therapy does not improve the anaemia of RA. Parenteral iron is occasionally used, but the main treatment of this anaemia consists of measures directed at suppressing the underlying disease process.

Felty's syndrome is the association of RA with splenomegaly and leucopenia. Other features of the syndrome may include normocytic normochromic anaemia, thrombocytopenia, lymphadenopathy, cutaneous ulceration, and pigmentation. The major hazard of the condition is recurrent major or minor infection. Patients with Felty's syndrome tend to have more severe forms of articular disease and on serological testing usually have high titres of IgM rheumatoid factor and antinuclear factors.

The leucopenia of Felty's syndrome usually lies between 800 and 2500 cells/mm^3 and is associated with a fall in granulocyte number. Occasionally a leucopenia of less than 800 cells/mm^3 is seen. The most frequent bone marrow abnormality found is granulocyte maturation arrest. The pathogenesis of Felty's syndrome is multifactorial and includes both an increased peripheral destruction partly attributable to circulating immune complexes and depression of granulopoiesis by a splenic humoral factor. Excessive margination of leucocytes in the peripheral circulation may account for some of the apparent fall in circulating cell counts.

The treatment of Felty's syndrome is only indicated if the leucopenia is associated with significant recurrent infection. Although corticosteroid therapy may increase the peripheral white cell count, it also increases the susceptibility to infection and is of uncertain value in the treatment of Felty's syndrome. Gold or penicillamine therapy can be very effective but these drugs must be used carefully because of their potential toxic effects on the bone marrow. A proportion of patients with this condition respond to splenectomy, although the operation itself is associated with significant postoperative mortality. Rarely, despite a rise in the peripheral white cell count after splenectomy, susceptibility to infection does not improve and patients die of fulminating septicaemia. The removal of splenic factors normally helpful in the defence against infection may be responsible. Immunization against disease and prompt aggressive treatment of any infections becomes essential.

Thrombocytosis or an increase in the circulating platelet count may be seen in active rheumatoid disease and probably represents a non-specific effect of inflammation. This thrombocytosis is not usually clinically significant.

Sjögren's syndrome

Sjögren's syndrome is the association of keratoconjunctivitis sicca (KCS) and/or xerostomia with RA or other connective tissue disorders. Dysfunction of lacrimal and salivary glands is associated with lymphocytic infiltration, which may progress to fibrosis and complete loss of acinar tissue. This is distinguished from the gland dysfunction due to simple atrophy in old age. Estimates of the prevalence of Sjögren's syndrome vary between 13 and 58% of rheumatoid patients (Benedek 1993).

The symptoms of KCS are a gritty feeling or irritation of the eyes. This is often worse first thing in the morning when patients find it difficult to open their eyes. The lysozyme content of tears is reduced and the eyes may be subject to recurrent infection. The diagnosis of KCS is best confirmed with a slit lamp, when absence of the normal tear film will be noted. In addition, thick strands of mucus may be seen sticking to the conjunctiva and cornea. Two drops of 1% rose bengal instilled into the eye can be used to show up the mucus strands and abnormal epithelium of the dry conjunctiva. In the absence of a slit lamp the reduction in tear secretion may be demonstrated by the Schirmer tear test. A strip of filter paper is hooked over the lower lid at the junction of the middle and outer thirds and wetting of less than 10 mm of the paper over a 5-min period is considered abnormal. The symptoms of KCS are usually relieved by the regular instillation of artificial tear drops into the affected eyes. Occasionally, tarsorrhaphy or lacrimal canal ablation is indicated.

The xerostomia may be associated with recurrent salivary gland swelling. A clinical diagnosis of xerostomia may be made if the patient complains of a dry mouth and on examination there is no salivary pool in the floor of the mouth. Again it is advisable to consider other non-specific factors such as drug therapy and anxiety before attributing all complaints of mouth dryness to this condition. Biopsy of minor salivary glands from the lip may be used to confirm the diagnosis. Other investigations that have been used in the formal assessment of xerostomia include measurement of salivary flow rate following cannulation of the parotid duct, sialography, and radioisotope imaging of the salivary glands. Treatment of the xerostomia of Sjögren's syndrome is unsatisfactory.

Artificial saliva is available and may prove helpful. Dental hygiene is important, as patients with the condition are susceptible to dental caries. Local radiotherapy to the involved glands is not helpful and increases the risk of these patients developing lymphoma to which they already have an increased susceptibility.

Secretions from other endothelial surfaces may also be affected, so that other features of the condition may include dysphagia, dyspareunia, and dryness of the skin. Sjögren's syndrome may be associated with a number of immunological symptoms, including renal tubular acidosis and autoimmune thyroid disease.

Ophthalmic

Keratoconjunctivitis sicca is the most frequent eye feature of rheumatoid disease. Scleritis (Jayson and Jones 1971) is less common but is potentially more serious. It may occur in diffuse or nodular forms. Rarely, a severe necrotizing form of scleritis is seen. The complications of untreated scleritis include perforation of the sclera, glaucoma, and cataract. Systemic steroids in dosages of around 60 mg daily, local steroid drops, and sometimes immunosuppressive drugs may be required for the treatment of this condition. Milder attacks may respond to NSAIDs.

Respiratory

Pleurisy and pleural effusions are the most common forms of pulmonary involvement by the disease. Rheumatoid pleural effusions show lymphocytosis and reduced glucose content in the absence of infection. Sometimes macrophages containing IgM inclusions (ragocytes) are present, and immunological tests for antinuclear antibodies and IgM rheumatoid factor may be positive. The histology of the underlying pleura often shows non-specific changes of chronic inflammation, but occasionally rheumatoid nodule formation is seen.

Interstitial fibrosis (fibrosing alveolitis) may occur uncommonly as the cause of progressive breathlessness in seropositive, nodular rheumatoid disease, particularly in smokers (Hyland et al 1983). The associated features found in the idiopathic condition are also found in the form associated with rheumatoid disease and include finger clubbing, coarse pleural crepitations, and widespread pulmonary shadows on chest X-ray. Treatment with corticosteroid drugs is usually disappointing but occasionally immunosuppressive drugs appear to help. Asymptomatic impairment of carbon monoxide diffusion capacity in the absence of radiological change is common in rheumatoid disease, as in other forms of connective tissue disease, and usually does not progress to symptomatic interstitial fibrosis.

Rheumatoid nodules may appear in the lungs as nodules of varying size and need to be differentiated from other causes of pulmonary shadowing such as neoplasms and tuberculosis.

Seropositive rheumatoid arthritics who are coal miners or are exposed to industrial dusts may develop gross forms of pulmonary fibrosis and nodules. Caplan (1953) originally described such lesions in coal miners.

Destructive airways disease has been shown to be more frequent in RA patients than in controls matched for smoking habits. A rare and progressively fatal form of obstructive bronchiolitis has also been described in a group of rheumatoid patients.

Cardiovascular

Pericardial effusions may be detected by echocardiography. They are frequently asymptomatic. Rarely, cardiac tamponade may result from massive effusions (Hara et al 1990).

Clinical forms of rheumatoid disease affecting the myocardium or cardiac valve structures are rare. However, postmortem studies have shown non-specific valvulitis in up to 30% of rheumatoid patients. Rheumatoid granulomas of the myocardium have also been noted in postmortem studies. Rheumatoid disease is an uncommon cause of chronic valve malfunction, but granulomas have been frequently noted in the aortic and mitral valves in patients receiving cardiac valve surgery.

Neurological

Peripheral nerve symptoms in rheumatoid patients may arise from entrapment neuropathies and cervical myelopathy. Symptoms of entrapment neuropathy can usually be relieved by appropriate decompression. The sites of entrapment include compression of the median nerve at the wrist (carpal tunnel syndrome), compression of the posterior tibial nerve at the ankle (tarsal tunnel syndrome), and ulnar nerve compression at the elbow (ulnar neuritis).

Rheumatoid peripheral neuropathies fall into two pain groups—severe sensorimotor neuropathy and milder sensory neuropathy (Chamberlain and Bruckner 1970). The former is associated with a sudden loss of motor and sensory function and often picks out isolated nerves in a mononeuritis multiplex pattern. It is associated with the more severe forms of seropositive nodular disease and there is often evidence of vasculitis elsewhere. Nerve conduction tests usually show features of muscle denervation and the condition is thought to be produced by vasculitis of the vasa nervorum. The sensory type of neuropathy usually occurs as a glove-and-stocking pattern of sensory loss, and if motor signs occur they are usually minor. Nerve conduction tests may be normal or may show slowing of motor and sensory conduction.

Cervical myelopathy from atlantoaxial or subaxial subluxation of the cervical spine can be confused with a peripheral neuropathy and has been discussed earlier.

Renal and hepatic

Slight impairment of renal function is common in rheumatoid patients (Wish and Kammer 1993), and liver enlargement is found clinically in about 11% of rheumatoid patients (Whaley and Webb 1977). These problems are discussed by Jayson (1999).

Septic arthritis

This severe and potentially fatal complication is found particularly in patients with the most severe forms of rheumatoid disease. Presentation may be acute, with one disproportionately painful and inflamed joint and pyrexia. At other times septic arthritis may present in a more obscure fashion such as feeling unwell or even with an apparent flare of the disease. Fever and leucocytosis may be absent in elderly debilitated and steroid-treated patients most prone to develop this condition (Ostensson and Geborek 1991). *Staphylococcus aureus* is the organism most frequently isolated. Prompt diagnosis and treatment are essential in order to minimize joint damage and to preserve life.

Laboratory findings

The diagnosis of RA is made mainly on clinical grounds but laboratory investigations may help. They provide objective measurements of disease activity and sometimes have prognostic value. The anaemia of rheumatoid disease has been discussed. In active disease the ESR, plasma viscosity, and acute-phase reactants such as C-reactive protein are elevated and provide a rough guide to disease activity. As a non-specific feature of chronic inflammation, serum albumin may be reduced and alpha and gamma globulin elevated on protein electrophoresis. All the immunoglobulin components (IgG, IgA, and IgM) may be elevated or sometimes just IgG is increased. The serological tests for IgM rheumatoid factor become positive in 75% of patients with RA.

Prognosis

The natural history of RA is variable. A high proportion of patients with the disease have a mild illness with a good prognosis. In a 10-year follow-up of a group of rheumatoid patients who were treated fairly conservatively by present-day practices, Duthie and colleagues found that over 50% had an eventual satisfactory outcome while only 11% became completely disabled (Duthie et al 1955). The following are adverse prognostic factors: development of erosions within 1 year of onset, poor functional capacity early in the disease course, the presence of extra-articular disease features, a persistently high ESR, and failure to respond to NSAIDs. Some studies also suggest that the histocompatibility antigen DR4 may be associated with severe disease (Westedt et al 1986).

Therapy

Decisions on effective treatment depend on the stage and activity of the disease. When there is early active inflammation the emphasis is on suppression of inflammation by general measures and antirheumatic drugs. In the late stages when destructive disease and secondary osteoarthritis predominate, the emphasis of management shifts towards relief of pain by provision of simple analgesics, improving joint function, and reconstructive surgery. The prognosis in the majority of patients is reasonable and the aim of treatment is to suppress the disease process to prevent and limit the onset of erosions and the development of deformities and disabilities.

Principles of management

The pattern of rheumatoid disease becomes established very quickly after onset. Indeed joint erosions develop within the first few months. In consequence aggressive treatment at an early stage appears effective, preventing the establishment of permanent changes and deformity. In many rheumatological centres early arthritis clinics have been instituted with the result that patients receive active aggressive treatment at an early stage. This appears effective in preventing damage and long-term disability.

General measures

The long-term management of patients with RA is undertaken by a management team that includes not only rheumatologists but also orthopaedic surgeons, physiotherapists, occupational therapists, chiropodists/podiatrists, social workers, disablement resettlement officers, and nurses. The programme includes advice and education about the nature of the disease and the aims and limitations of treatment. During phases of active disease many patients require an extra rest period during the day. Physiotherapists and occupational therapists help by prescribing exercises designed to maintain and restore muscle function and ranges of joint movements, providing splints to prevent or reduce deformities, and providing aids to improve function. During major disease exacerbations short periods in bed, together with splinting of particularly inflamed joints, are helpful. Individual inflamed joints may be controlled by aspirating synovial effusions and injection of slow-release corticosteroids under strict aseptic conditions.

Drug therapy

The drugs used in the treatment of RA can be considered under the following headings:

1. simple analgesics
2. NSAIDs
3. second-line antirheumatic drugs
4. immunosuppressives and corticosteroids
5. TNF-α inhibitors

Simple analgesics

These include paracetamol, often in mixtures with codeine, dextropropoxyphene, and others, which act on the central nervous system. They are not very effective in relieving the pain of acute inflammation and are of more use for the pain of secondary osteoarthritis and for a top-up effect in patients in whom the NSAIDs prove inadequate. These drugs do not have the gastrointestinal effects of the non-steroidal anti-inflammatory agents discussed in detail in Chap. 22. Narcotic analgesics are virtually never required for RA.

Non-steroidal anti-inflammatory drugs

Drugs in this group provide symptomatic relief of pain and stiffness. However, they do not alter the natural history of the disease and on their own do not prevent the development of progressive joint damage. These agents may be adequate for many rheumatoid patients but now we believe that second-line antirheumatic agents should be the initial treatment at an early stage.

Soluble aspirin was the prototype of this type of drug but is now largely replaced by newer agents such as the propionic acid derivatives. These are better tolerated but are not significantly more effective.

There is some evidence from studies of osteoarthritis that some anti-inflammatory drugs such as indomethacin may actually exacerbate damage to articular cartilage. All these drugs may cause gastrointestinal ulceration and bleeding in susceptible patients. If a patient suffers from dyspepsia it may be possible to administer the drug successfully as a suppository, as it is then absorbed more slowly and lower peak levels occur in the peripheral blood. Other alternatives include the prophylactic use of antiulcer drugs or the use of prodrugs, such as benoxaprofen, in which the agent is taken in an inactive form and only activated after absorption through the intestinal muscosa. Both the anti-inflammatory properties and the gastrointestinal adverse toxicity of these agents are in part due to their abilities to inhibit the cyclo-oxygenase enzymes involved in prostaglandin synthesis.

We now know that there are two forms of cyclo-oxygenase enzymes (COX1 and COX2). Inhibition of COX1 is more likely to lead to gastrointestinal toxicity, whereas the anti-inflammatory effects are mediated by inhibition of COX2. We now have a new generation of anti-inflammatory drugs specifically targeted at COX2. These have anti-inflammatory effects similar to those of standard anti-inflammatory agents but seem less likely to cause dyspepsia and gastrointestinal problems (Emery et al 1999). Various strategies are now available to reduce the risks of gastrointestinal toxicity (Wolfe et al 1999).

Second-line antirheumatic drugs

Active RA is now treated aggressively in most units and the second-line antirheumatic drugs are instituted rapidly if there is evidence of active inflammation. These drugs are given on a long-term basis, and all have a delay from the start of treatment until the onset of action of commonly 2 or 3 months.

Sulfasalazine This agent is effective in causing remission of RA. The usual regimen is to start with 0.5–1.0 g of the enteric-coated form daily and increase by weekly increments to a maximum of 1 g three times per day. Gastrointestinal side effects such as nausea may occur but more serious problems such as blood dyscrasias are rare. Sulfasalazine may uncommonly cause hepatotoxicity and in males a fall in sperm count. Regular monitoring of the blood count, urea, creatinine, and liver function is required.

Antimalarials Chloroquine and hydroxychloroquine have definite disease-suppressing properties. There is a small risk of producing retinopathy and visual impairment but this is minimized if the daily dosage is kept as low as possible and the eyes are monitored by an ophthalmologist. Gastrointestinal problems are uncommon, and these agents lack the haematological and renal side effects found in many more potent antirheumatic drugs.

Gold therapy Gold salts have been used in the treatment of RA since the 1930s. Intramuscular sodium aurothiomalate (Myocrisin) is the gold salt most commonly used in the UK, although an oral preparation has also been introduced. In a commonly used regimen, after incremental test doses, the drug is given as 50 mg weekly by intramuscular injections to a maximum of 1 g or until there is disease remission or toxicity. Once remission has occurred and maximum benefit appears to have been achieved, it is usual to lengthen the intervals between injections and reduce the dose to a monthly maintenance regimen. If there has been no response to the gold after a cumulative dose of 1 g has been given, most physicians withdraw the drug, but it is possible to try increasing the weekly injection dose (Rothermick et al 1976).

Possible side effects of gold therapy include minor skin rashes, itching, exfoliative dermatitis, stomatitis, renal problems, blood dyscrasias, hepatotoxicity, and penumonitis. All patients receiving gold therapy will require regular monitoring of the skin, blood, and urine.

D-Penicillamine This drug was initially used as a chelating agent in the treatment of Wilson's disease. It is given orally but otherwise has indications and side effects similar to those of gold salts. The usual starting dose is 125 or 250 mg daily, and it is important to take this drug well away from food as it can combine with food nutrients. Some patients respond to doses as low as this but if there is no improvement the dosage is slowly increased by similar amounts, at intervals, to a maximum of 750 mg daily. Most commonly the final dose is around 375 mg per day. Adverse effects include skin rashes, blood dyscrasias, and renal problems. Rare side effects include immunological syndromes such as myasthenia gravis and drug-induced systemic lupus erythematosus. Regular monitoring of the skin, blood, and urine for toxicity is essential.

Levamisole This is a second-line antirheumatic agent that appears effective in long-term disease control. Careful monitoring of the blood count, urea, creatinine, and liver function is essential (Smolen et al 1999).

Immunosuppressives and corticosteroids

Immunosuppressive agents, and in particular methotrexate, are frequently used for patients with severe persistent disease not controlled by more conservative measures. Methotrexate is a folic acid antagonist with immunosuppressive properties. It is given in a weekly dose, starting at 5 mg, and then increasing usually to a maximum of 15 mg per week but occasionally more. It appears much more effective than the second-line antirheumatic agents (Ward 1985). The onset of benefit commonly does not start for at least a month after initiating treatment. Adverse effects are uncommon but may affect blood, liver, and lungs, and the drug is contraindicated in patients with a high alcohol intake. Careful monitoring of the blood and liver function is essential. Co-prescription of folic acid, usually on the third day after the methotrexate, may reduce the risk of gastrointestinal problems.

Alternative immunosuppressive agents such as cyclophosphamide are used for very severe individual cases and are sometimes given as bolus infusions. They are usually reserved for patients with complications such as severe forms of vasculitis and for patients who have failed to respond to more conservative therapy.

Cyclosporin is an immunosuppressive agent used following transplantation surgery. It is effective in severe and resistant forms of RA. Common problems of treatment include some impairment of renal function and the development of hypertension. Careful monitoring is essential.

Oral corticosteroids such as prednisolone have dramatic effects in relieving symptoms. Unfortunately, once patients have started on steroids it is commonly very difficult, if not impossible, to withdraw them. Patients receiving steroid therapy over a number of years frequently develop severe adverse effects such as osteoporosis, hypertension, and dermal atrophy, and in the long run these may outweigh the benefits in relieving the arthritis symptoms. The decision to start corticosteroids is a major one and should only be taken after careful consideration. The bone mineral density should be checked in patients maintained on steroids. If necessary, bone-strengthening measures such as calcium and vitamin D, oestrogens, or biophosphates are added.

Local steroid injections are helpful when one or two joints or tendon sheaths show continued inflammation. If there is any suspicion of infection, the synovial fluid should be aspirated and cultured and the steroid injection given later. Slow-acting steroid preparations are usually used. Fluorinated steroids should be avoided for very superficial injections, as they are more likely than other steroid preparations to cause dermal atrophy.

TNF-a inhibitors

Research has focused on the molecular mechanisms underlying chronic inflammation. In particular tumour necrosis factor-α (TNF-α) has been shown to play a key role in the inflammatory process. Specific inhibition of TNF-α has proved effective in treating rheumatoid arthritis (Moreland et al 1999). The two drugs currently available are etanercept and inflixamab. The former is given by subcutaneous injection twice a week, the latter by intravenous infusion. Etanercept can be used on its own or in combination with immunosuppressive agents, whereas the latter is necessary for inflixamab. These drugs have proved very effective for patients with severe disease, and indeed there is now evidence that they will prevent the development and progress (Bathon et al 2000) of joint erosion and damage.

The principal concern is that resistance to infection is reduced and these drugs are contraindicated in the presence of infection. There is some concern about long-term use and possible predisposition towards malignancy. Etanercept may also give rise to local skin reactions.

These drugs are proving very effective and helpful, but are extremely expensive with resulting difficulties in access. They are gradually becoming more freely available.

Surgery

Surgery is indicated for the relief of pain and prevention of loss of function when medical measures prove inadequate. The programme is best planned in a combined clinic held jointly by the rheumatologist and the orthopaedic surgeon.

In early disease synovectomy may be helpful symptomatically when synovial swelling is localized to one or two joints and significant erosions have not appeared. Tenosynovectomy may help when synovial hypertrophy has involved tendon sheaths and is affecting hand function or threatening tendon rupture. Decompression may be required for the relief of nerve entrapment syndromes.

In advanced cases, joint replacements are now available for a variety of joints and are continually being improved. Hip and knee replacements are commonplace and are the most successful. Replacements are available for the shoulder, elbow, and ankle.

Other surgical procedures sometimes used include excision arthroplasty, fusion, and repair of ruptured tendons.

References

Barrett AJ, Saklatvala H 1981 Proteinases in joint disease. In: Kelley WN, Harris ED, Ruddy SF, Sledge CB (eds) Textbook of rheumatology. Saunders, Philadelphia, pp 195–209

Bathon JM, Martin RW, Fleischmann RM et al 2000 A comparison of etanercept and methotrexate in patients with early rheumatoid arthritis. New England Journal of Medicine 343: 1586–1602

Beighton P, Soloman L, Valkenburgh HA 1975 Rheumatoid arthritis in a rural South African population. Annals of Rheumatic Disease 34: 136–141

Benedek TG 1993 Association between rheumatic diseases and neoplasia. In: Maddison PH et al (eds) Oxford textbook of rheumatology. Oxford University Press, Oxford, pp 1070–1082

Caplan A 1953 Certain unusual radiological appearances in the chest of coalminers suffering from rheumatoid arthritis. Thorax 8: 29–37

Chamberlain MA, Bruckner FE 1970 Rheumatoid neuropathy. Clinical and electrophysiological features. Annals of the Rheumatic Diseases 29: 609–616

Duthie JR, Thompson M, Wier MM, Fletcher WB 1955 Medical and social aspects of the treatment of rheumatoid arthritis with special reference to factors affecting prognosis. Annals of the Rheumatic Diseases 14: 133–149

Emery P, Zeidler H, Kvien TK et al 1999 Celecoxib versus diclofenar in long-term management of rheumatoid arthritis: randomised double-blind comparison. The Lancet 354: 2106–2111

Fassbender HG 1975 Rheumatoid arthritis in pathology of rheumatic diseases. Springer-Verlag, Berlin, pp 70–210

Gardner DL 1992 Pathological basis of the connective tissue disease. Edward Arnold, London, pp 485–487

Hara KS et al 1990 Rheumatoid pericarditis: clinical features and survival. Medicine 69: 81–91

Hyland RH, Gordon DA, Broder I, Davies GM et al 1983 A systemic controlled study of pulmonary abnormalities in rheumatoid arthritis. Journal of Rheumatology 10: 395–405

Jayson MIV 1999. Rheumatoid arthritis. In: Wall PD, Melzack R (eds) Textbook of Pain, 4th edn. Churchill Livingstone, Edinburgh, pp 505–516

Jayson MIV, Jones DEP 1971 Scleritis and rheumatoid arthritis. Annals of the Rheumatic Diseases 30: 343–347

Moreland LW, Schiff MH et al 1999 Etanercept therapy in rheumatoid arthritis. Annals of Inernal Medicine 130: 478–486

Ostensson A, Geborek P 1991 Septic arthritis as a non-surgical complication in rheumatoid arthritis and relation to disease severity and therapy. British Journal of Rheumatology 30: 35–38

Rothermick NO, Philips VK, Bergen W, Rhomas MH 1976 Chrysotherapy. A prospective study. Arthritis and Rheumatism 19: 1321–1327

Smolen JS, Kalden JR et al 1999 Efficacy and safety of leflunamide compared with placebo and sulphasalazine in active rheumatoid arthritis: a double-blind, randomised, multi-centre trial. Lancet 353: 259–266

Ward T 1985 Historical perspective on the use of methotrexate for the treatment of rheumatoid arthritis. Journal of Rheumatology (suppl i): 3–6

Westedt ML, Breedveld FC, Schrevder GM Th, d'Amato J, Cats N, de Vries RRP 1986 Immunogenetic heterogeneity of rheumatoid arthritis. Annals of the Rheumatic Diseases 45: 534–538

Whaley K, Webb J 1977 Liver and kidney disease in rheumatoid arthritis. Clinics in Rheumatic Diseases 3: 527–547

Wish JB, Kammer GM 1993 Nephrological aspects of management in the rheumatic diseases. In: Maddison PH et al (eds) Oxford text book of rheumatology. Oxford University Press, Oxford, pp 179–187

Wolfe MM, Lichtenstein DR, Singh G 1999 Gastrointestinal toxicity of nonsteroidal anti-inflammatory drugs. New England Journal of Medicine 340: 1888–1899

Chapter 4

Muscles, tendons, and ligaments

Dianne J Newham and Kerry R Mills

Introduction

Musculoskeletal soft tissue is composed of muscle, tendon, and ligament, and it is often difficult for both patient and clinician to distinguish which are the source of pain, and more than one is often affected at the same time. The cardinal signs of damage to the non-contractile soft tissues are pain, tenderness, swelling and loss of function. Usually musculoskeletal pain is clearly associated with trauma or exercise and is self-resolving but a variety of pathological conditions may give rise to myalgia. Diseases of collagen and connective tissue are relatively rare, but often have a devastating effect (Pope 1998).

Muscle pain

Association with exercise

There is usually a clear association between muscle pain and exercise but two very different time courses may occur. In one case, often called ischaemic pain, it occurs during exercise and rapidly increases in intensity until contractions stop and blood flow is restored, whereupon it disappears rapidly. Alternatively, pain may not occur until hours later and persist for days.

Ischaemic muscle pain

Intermittent claudication and angina pectoris are two well-known examples of this type of pain that occurs in muscles whose blood supply is unduly compromised. In normal subjects it disappears rapidly after contractions stop, leaving no residual effects. Accumulation of metabolites is responsible although the stimulus, or combination of stimuli, is not clear. Lactic acid is not the prime algesic substance as patients with myophosphorylase deficiency (McArdle's syndrome) experience particularly severe pain during exercise, despite an inability to produce lactic acid (Schmid and Hammaker 1961, Cady et al 1989). Furthermore, clearance of intramuscular lactic acid is slower than the disappearance of pain. Possible agents, acting alone or in combination, are thought to include histamine, acetylcholine, serotonin, and bradykinin. Potassium (Lendinger and Sjogaard 1991) and adenosine (Sylven et al 1988) are currently receiving considerable attention in this respect.

Delayed-onset muscle pain

Heavy or unaccustomed exercise may be associated with muscle pain that occurs about 8 h later and persists for days. It is particularly associated with unaccustomed eccentric contractions (Newham et al 1983c, 1988; Stauber 1989; Clarkson and Newham 1995). These generate the highest force per active fibre (Katz 1939, Abbott et al 1952) and have the lowest metabolic cost per unit force (Curtin and Davies 1973, Menard et al 1991). Thus it is likely to be caused by mechanical rather than metabolic factors. It is associated with considerable muscle damage, shown by structural (Newham et al 1983b, Friden 1984, Jones et al 1986, Newham 1988), biochemical (Newham et al 1983a, 1986a,b; Stauber 1989), and radioisotopic changes (reviewed by Clarkson and Newham 1995). However, none of these damage markers follow the same time course as the pain (Jones et al 1986, Newham et al 1986b). Evidence increasingly indicates connective tissue damage (Brown et al 1997) along with inflammatory processes. The affected muscles are tender and often feel swollen. Increased intramuscular pressures have been reported in muscles in non-compliant compartments (Friden et al 1986), but not in others (Newham and Jones 1985).

There is conflicting evidence about the effect of steroidal and non-steroidal anti-inflammatory agents on delayed-onset pain (Janssen et al 1983, Kuipers et al 1983, Headley et al 1986).

Clinical myalgia

Signs and symptoms

The vocabulary of patients presenting with myalgia is relatively restricted. Common terms are stiffness, soreness, aching, spasms or cramps, and tenderness. The symptom of stiffness usually means discomfort on muscle movement, rather than increased compliance. Muscle pain is most often reported as having a dull, aching quality. Sharp, lancinating pain is relatively rare, although acute tenderness from a 'trigger point' (Travell and Simons 1998) may occur. Muscle pain is usually exacerbated by voluntary contraction, although rarely the opposite may be the case.

The terms cramp, contracture, spasm, and tetanus or tetany have precise definitions but are often used inaccurately (Simons and Mense 1998). Cramps are strong, involuntary contractions of rapid onset that are extremely painful and associated with electromyographic signals similar to those of a normal voluntary contraction (Mills et al 1982b). A contracture is an extremely rare form of involuntary contraction due to depletion of muscle adenosine triphosphate (ATP) and is electrically silent. It is a sign of rare metabolic disorders (e.g., myophosphorylase deficiency). Spasm usually implies a reflex contraction of the muscles surrounding an injured or inflamed structure. Tetany is an involuntary contraction, often in carpopedal muscles, and is usually associated with hypocalcaemia or hypocapnia (Layzer and Rowland 1971). Less common are myotonia and dystonia.

Associated signs and symptoms

Patients with myalgia often complain of weakness, fatigability, or exercise intolerance (discussed under 'Investigation of muscle pain' below). Swelling of painful muscles is often reported, but rarely substantiated. If it is, it almost always implies serious underlying pathology and occurs in polymyositis, dermatomyositis, myophosphorylase and phosphofructokinase deficiencies, and acute alcoholic myopathy. Enquiry should be made about alcohol, diet, and fasting. A drinking bout in an alcoholic may precipitate acute alcoholic myopathy and even myoglobinuria. A diet deficient in vitamin D is associated with osteomalacia, causing bone and muscle pain (Smith and Stern 1967). Attacks of pain and weakness occur in carnitine palmityltransferase deficiency, particularly during prolonged exercise after fasting or after a high-fat, low-carbohydrate diet or meal (Di Mauro and Di Mauro 1973, Bank et al 1975). Fasting may be used as a provocative test for this condition (Carroll et al 1979).

Differentiation of muscle pain from pain in other tissues

Pain localization is poor in skeletal muscle, and patients may also be unable to differentiate it from pain arising from local noncontractile tissues. It is important to identify the painful tissue but this may be very difficult due to poor localization and referred pain; pain from an arthritic hip may be referred to the thigh muscles or knee joint, from a carpal tunnel syndrome to the forearm muscles, or from cervical spondylosis to the arm muscles.

Pain from joints and their capsules tends to be more localized than myalgia, and arthralgia is often worsened by passive joint movement. Capsular pain may be present only in specific joint positions (e.g., painful arc syndrome in the shoulder). Bone pain also tends to be poorly localized but, unlike myalgia, usually has a deep, boring quality. It is usually worse at night and tends to be unaffected by either movement or muscle activity.

Myalgia, exercise, and rest

Many patients presenting with myalgia describe a relationship with exercise. Others find no relationship or even that their pain is relieved by moderate exercise.

The paradigm of exercise-related muscle pain is intermittent claudication, in which pain occurs in the calf muscles during exercise then disappears after a period of rest. This is a pathological form of ischaemic muscle pain caused by stenosis of the feeding artery and is experienced distal to the stenosis. Thus thrombosis of the terminal aorta leads to pain in the buttocks (Leriche's syndrome), narrowing of the axillary artery by a cervical rib gives rise to forearm pain, and arteritis of cranial arteries may result in pain in the muscles of mastication during chewing. Reduced blood supply can also occur due to increased blood viscosity (e.g., Waldenström's macroglobulinaemia).

Other conditions in which myalgia is clearly related to exercise involve an impaired energy supply to a contracting muscle; the mechanism is presumably the same as ischaemic muscle pain. Myophosphorylase deficiency (Schmid and Mahler 1959), glycolytic disorders of muscle (McArdle 1951), and phosphofructokinase deficiency (Tarui et al 1965) all present as exercise-related myalgia with cramps and contracture. Contracture is a potentially serious event, because it leads to irreversible muscle breakdown and the release of large amounts of myoglobin may lead to renal cast formation and failure. A clear association between exercise and myalgia is also found in several of the mitochondrial myopathies (Land and Clark 1979) and in carnitine palmityltransferase deficiency (Bank et al 1975).

In those individuals where failure of energy or blood supply has been eliminated, the relationship of pain to exercise or rest appears to have no diagnostic or prognostic value (Mills and Edwards 1983).

Table 4.1 Principal medical conditions associated with myalgia

Trauma and sports injuries
Primary infective myositis
Inflammatory myopathies
Polymyositis
Dermatomyositis
Polymyositis or dermatomyositis in association with connective tissue disease
Viral myositis
Polymyalgia rheumatica
Myalgia of neurogenic origin
Muscle cramp
Impaired muscle energy metabolism
Cytosolic enzyme defects
Lipid storage myopathies
Mitochondrial myopathies
Drug-induced myalgia
Myalgic encephalomyelitis
Muscle pain of uncertain cause

Aetiology (Table 4.1)

Primary infective myositis

Direct infection of muscle with bacteria is uncommon. Tropical myositis (Taylor et al 1976) is an infection with *Staphylococcus aureus*, probably secondary to a viral myositis. It affects children and young adults in the tropics and is characterized by fever, muscle pains (often severe and localized to a single limb), and deep intramuscular abscesses. It usually responds to antibiotics and surgical drainage.

Parasitic infections of muscle that cause muscle pain and tenderness include trichinosis (Gould 1970), sparganonosis (Wirth and Farrow 1961), sarcosporidosis (Jeffrey 1974), and cysticercosis. Infection with *Trichinella spiralis*, usually by eating undercooked pork, is common in many parts of the world, especially the USA, but many cases are asymptomatic. The disease is ushered in with fever and periorbital oedema. Later myalgia and muscle weakness develop to reach a peak at 3 weeks. The prognosis depends on the heaviness of the infection; 2–10% of cases are fatal. Treatment with thiabendazole and steroids has been successful.

Inflammatory myopathies

Polymyositis and dermatomyositis (Pachman 1998, Targoff 1998) The idiopathic inflammatory myopathies, polymyositis and dermatomyositis, classified by Bohan and Peter (1975a,b) and Carpenter and Karpati (1981), have been reviewed extensively (Currie 1981, Mastaglia 1988, Dalakas 1988, Pachman 1998, Targoff 1998). In a few cases muscle pain may be a prominent feature but usually the presentation is of muscle weakness. Dermatomyositis presents more commonly in the female with acute or subacute onset of limb girdle weakness, dysphagia, muscle tenderness, and skin involvement. There is often involvement of other systems, such as the lungs and heart, and in 20% of cases there may be an associated carcinoma. Pathologically in dermatomyositis, there is evidence of a microangiopathy with immunoglobulin deposits on vessel walls that lead to microinfarcts. On muscle biopsy there may be striking perivascular atrophy. Polymyositis, on the other hand, presents equally in males and females and has a chronic course, respiratory muscle involvement is unusual, and muscle tenderness is infrequent. There is no skin involvement or involvement of other systems. Pathologically, muscle biopsy shows endomysial lymphocyte infiltration and cytotoxic T cells predominate.

Diagnosis rests on the findings of:

1. A muscle biopsy showing muscle cell necrosis, lymphocyte infiltration, phagocytosis, variation in size of both fibre types and basophilic fibres reflecting regeneration.
2. Electromyography (EMG) showing brief, small-amplitude polyphasic potentials and fibrillations (Marinacci 1965).
3. Plasma creatine kinase (CK), which is raised in the acute phase but may be normal in 30% of cases.
4. Raised inflammatory markers.

The clinical usefulness of steroid therapy is a widely held view, and the complications of long-term steroid therapy are said to be uncommon (Riddoch and Morgan-Hughes 1975, Bunch et al 1980, Currie 1981), although they must always be borne in mind (Carpenter et al 1977, Edwards et al 1981). Other immunosuppressive drugs such as azathioprine, cyclophosphamide, methotrexate, and cyclosporin, immunoglobulin infusions, whole-body irradiation, and plasmapheresis have all been tried but the results and the benefits are not clear cut.

Polymyositis in association with connective tissue disease Polymyositis may be seen in association with systemic lupus erythematosus (Tsokos et al 1981), progressive systemic sclerosis, mixed connective tissue disease, rheumatoid disease (Haslock et al 1970), Sjögren's syndrome, polyarteritis nodosa, and occasionally, myasthenia gravis. In polyarteritis nodosa muscle changes are probably due to infarction, but in the other conditions findings are similar to those in idiopathic polymyositis, although the changes of steroid myopathy are often superimposed.

Viral polymyositis Myalgia is a feature of most acute viral infections; in the vast majority of cases, influenza virus A or B or coxsackie virus A or B are the agents involved. Coxsackie B virus is the agent responsible for epidemic myalgia (Bornholm disease) in which there is fever, headache, and muscle pain in the chest and abdomen. The disease is rapidly self limiting, as is benign acute childhood myositis, which can follow influenza A or B virus infection.

Polymyalgia rheumatica This condition affects patients over the age of 55 and is characterized by pain and stiffness of the proximal muscles especially the shoulder girdle (Hamrin 1972). There may be mild anaemia, weight loss, and malaise. The erythrocyte sedimentation rate is typically over 50 mm in the first hour, but creatinine kinase (CK), muscle biopsy, and electromyography (EMG) are normal. There appears to be a close relationship between this condition and temporal, cranial, or giant cell arteritis. The response to steroids is usually immediate and dramatic (Bird et al 1979), most authorities advising a high initial dose of 40–60 mg per day.

Myalgia of neurogenic origin

Pain that appears to be localized to muscle may be a predominant feature in a number of neurogenic diseases. Cervical radiculopathy with pain radiating into the myotomal distribution of the roots, or nerve compression (e.g., carpel tunnel syndrome), may produce pain radiating into the arm muscles. Peripheral neuropathies may produce pain especially when they affect small fibres. Spasticity of any origin can give rise to flexor 'spasms' which can be very distressing. Treatment is difficult but diazepam and baclofen can be tried.

Muscle cramps

Apart from the benign 'ordinary' muscle cramps experienced by most individuals, cramps are also seen in glycolytic disorders (see below), in dehydration, in uraemia, with certain drugs such as salbutamol, phenothiazine, vincristine, lithium, cimetidine, and bumetanide (Lane and Mastaglia 1978), after haemodialysis, and in tetanus (Layzer 1994).

The 'stiff man' syndrome, first described by Moersch and Woltman (1956) and reviewed by Gordon et al (1967) and Layzer (1994), is characterized by continuous board-like stiffness of muscles, paroxysms of intense cramp, abolition of muscle stiffness during sleep, and a normal motor and sensory examination. Stiffness treatment with diazepam, often in very large doses, has been reported.

Neuromyotonia (Isaacs' syndrome) features widespread fasciculation, generalized stiffness, excessive sweating, and continuous motor unit activity, which persist during sleep and anaesthesia (Isaacs 1961, Newsom-Davis and Mills 1992). In all the above conditions the defect is thought to be in the spinal cord or motor axons.

Impaired muscle energy metabolism

Cytosolic enzyme defects

Myophosphorylase deficiency (McArdle's disease) In 1951 McArdle first described a patient with exercise-induced muscle pain and contractures, and postulated a defect in muscle glycolysis. Myophosphorylase deficiency was demonstrated by Mommaerts et al (1959) and Schmid and Mahler (1959) in further cases. The symptoms usually begin in early adolescence with painful muscle stiffness, cramps, contractures, and muscle weakness induced by vigorous exercise. The symptoms disappear after a period of rest but contractures may persist for several hours. Moderate exercise may be performed for long periods without symptoms developing, but if they do, further exercise may result in resolution of the pain. This is the 'second wind' phenomenon (Pernow et al 1967), thought to be due to a combination of increased muscle blood flow and the mobilization of free fatty acids and glucose from the liver. The condition has a relatively benign course, symptoms becoming less troublesome after the age of 40 years. Patients often have no physical signs at rest, although quadriceps weakness may be demonstrated by quantitative testing. CK is elevated at rest and reaches very high values as contractures resolve. EMG may be normal or show myopathic changes, but the definitive investigation is muscle biopsy showing excessive glycogen deposition and a reduction or absence of myophosphorylase. Biopsy in an acute attack may, in addition, show muscle cell necrosis.

Phosphofructokinase deficiency (Tarui et al 1965) The symptoms of this condition are very similar to those of McArdle's disease but may begin early in childhood and contractures are less frequent. Diagnosis is achieved by the demonstration of the absence of phosphofructokinase (PFK) activity and of glycogen accumulation in muscle.

Other enzyme deficiencies A number of other enzyme deficiencies that cause exercise intolerance, exercise-induced muscle pains, and muscle fatigue have been reported. Phosphoglycerate kinase deficiency (type 9 glycogenesis) (Di Mauro et al 1983), phosphoglycerate mutase deficiency (type 10 glycogenesis) (Di Mauro et al 1982), and lactate dehydrogenase deficiency (Kanno et al 1980) have been reported in only a few cases.

Lipid storage myopathies Transport of long-chain fatty acids to the interior of the mitochondrion depends on the enzyme carnitine palmityltransferase (CPT) located on the inner membrane and the carrier molecule carnitine. Deficiency of either would be expected to lead to a block in energy supply once intramuscular glycogen stores were depleted.

Systemic carnitine deficiency, in which both muscle and plasma carnitine are low, presents in childhood with episodes of nausea, vomiting, encephalopathy, and muscle weakness (Karpati et al 1975). Muscle carnitine deficiency (Willner et al 1979), in which plasma carnitine is normal, presents in young adults with proximal muscle weakness and pain. CK is usually raised and the EMG myopathic. Muscle biopsy shows lipid accumulation beneath the plasma membrane and between myofibrils, and low levels of carnitine.

CPT deficiency usually presents in adolescence with attacks of muscle pain, weakness, and myoglobinuria precipitated by prolonged exercise, especially after fasting or after a low-carbohydrate, high-fat diet (Bertorini et al 1980). CK is usually normal between attacks but rises markedly during and after attacks of pain. Muscle biopsy at the height of an attack may show lipid accumulation and/or muscle cell necrosis, and assay for CPT shows very low levels.

Mitochondrial myopathies This is a heterogeneous group of conditions, often presenting with muscle weakness and/or exercise-induced pain, and distinguished by the finding, usually on electron microscopy, of mitochondria of abnormal size, shape, or numbers, often with crystalline inclusions. Many patients may have 'ragged red fibres' on the modified Gomori trichrome stain. With increasingly sophisticated biochemical investigations, metabolic abnormalities isolated to particular segments of the cytochrome chain can now be distinguished (Petty et al 1986, Morgan-Hughes et al 1987, Holt et al 1989). Several other mitochondrial cytopathies have been associated with a bewildering number of other abnormalities: deafness, myoclonus, encephalopathy, ophthalmoplegia, growth retardation, and retinitis pigmentosa (Kearns–Sayre syndrome), as reviewed by Petty et al (1986).

Drug-induced myalgia

A large number of agents have now been catalogued as the cause of muscle pain (Lane and Mastaglia 1978). A polymyositis can be produced by D-penicillamine, with myopathic features on EMG, muscle cell necrosis, and an inflammatory infiltrate on muscle biopsy samples. A severe acute rhabdomyolysis with myoglobinuria and the threat of renal failure can be induced by diamorphine, amphetamine, phencyclidine, and alcohol.

Myalgic encephalomyelitis/chronic fatigue syndrome

The well-publicized syndrome of myalgic encephalomyelitis (ME) commonly presents with diffuse muscle pain, which is exacerbated by muscle activity, marked exercise intolerance, weakness, and fatigability. Other symptoms include loss of concentration and sleep disturbance. A proportion of cases relate the onset of symptoms to a viral illness, giving rise to the term postviral (fatigue) syndrome. The multiplicity of possible symptoms often makes diagnosis difficult and a consensus on diagnostic criteria has been agreed (Dawson 1990). It may occur sporadically or in epidemics and is most common in young and middle-aged women (Behan and Bakheit 1991). Currently there is much debate about whether the aetiology is physical or psychological (Wessely 1990). Irrespective of the underlying mechanisms, the symptoms affect a large number of individuals, some of whom will recover over a few months or years, while others are transformed into chronic invalids (Wessely and Newham 1993). Behan et al (1991) presented a series of expert reviews on the diagnosis, aetiology, clinical findings, and management of the syndrome.

There is a lack of agreement about whether the patients show immunological indications of chronic viral infections. Hyperventilation is reported as being a common finding, which when treated brings symptomatic improvement. There is neurophysiological evidence of attentional deficits and slowed information processing (Prasher et al 1990). There appears to be an increased incidence of psychiatric disorder in these patients, compared to normal individuals and those with muscle disease (Wessely and Powell 1989, Wood et al 1991).

On objective muscle testing there is no evidence of muscle wasting, weakness, or abnormal fatigability, due to either central or peripheral mechanisms (Stokes et al 1988, Edwards et al 1991, Lloyd et al 1991, Rutherford and White 1991). Neither are there consistent histochemical or metabolic changes, other than the non-specific changes associated with immobility. Blood levels of skeletal muscle cytoplasmic enzymes (e.g., CK), usually raised with muscle damage, are normal.

Muscle pain of uncertain cause

Vague muscle aches and pains commonly form part of the symptomatology in depressive illness and in individuals with a neurotic or obsessive personality disorder. However, care must be taken not to dismiss these symptoms; the depression may be secondary to an organic muscle abnormality.

In large studies a group of patients always appear who complain of muscle pain, in whom no abnormality can be found despite exhaustive investigation (Serratrice et al 1980, Mills and Edwards 1983, Simons and Mense 1998). Rational criteria to filter out those patients with organic abnormalities appear to be the measurement of ESR and CK. If either of these is abnormal, then muscle biopsy, EMG, exercise, and strength testing should be performed. However, there exists a considerable group of patients with muscle pain in whom no definite muscle abnormality can be found. Undoubtedly, a number of specific muscle abnormalities remain to be characterized.

The term 'repetitive strain injury' has recently gained popularity as a catch-all term for pain developing as the consequence of some repetitive occupation. Although changes in muscle biopsy specimens have been reported (Fry 1986), there has been no firm confirmation of any neurological or rheumatological abnormality (Barton et al 1992).

Primary fibromyalgia (Bengtsson 1986) or 'fibrositis' (Bennett 1981) is a disorder in which histological abnormalities have been detected (Bartels and Danneskiold-Samsoe 1986, Bengtsson et al 1986a), as have reduced high-energy phosphate levels (Bengtsson et al 1986b), although the clear definition of the syndrome remains controversial (Hazleman 1998).

Investigation of muscle pain

Muscle biopsy

This is often the definitive investigation in the management of myalgia. Percutaneous muscle biopsy is suitable for histological, histochemical, electron microscopic, and metabolic characterization. Needle biopsies (Edwards et al 1980) are suitable for all these procedures, and the conchotome modification allows the removal of larger samples (Dietrichson et al 1987). These procedures are relatively atraumatic and can be used serially for following progress. Open biopsy is still practised and may have advantages in 'patchy' diseases such as focal polymyositis or in arthritic diseases (e.g., polyarteritis nodosa); however, in the majority of primary investigations of myalgia it is unnecessary and unethical.

Muscle biopsy is useful in the diagnosis of inflammatory myopathies by demonstrating muscle cell necrosis and inflammatory cell infiltrate, although there is poor correlation between morphology and myalgia. With neurogenic pain, fibre-type grouping may be found. In metabolic disorders, histochemistry reveals the absence or reduction of enzymes such as myophosphorylase. Direct measurement can be made of enzymes such as carnitine palmityltransferase and mitochondrial activity. It is essential in the analysis of mitochondrial myopathies where there is a defect either in mitochondrial substrate transport or in electron transport (Gohil et al 1981).

Biochemical markers of muscle damage

Myoglobinuria and myoglobinaemia Myoglobinuria is an important sign of muscle disease (Rowland et al 1964). It may be the presenting complaint in a number of conditions with exercise-induced pain or a concomitant of severe polymyositis, viral myositis, or alcoholic myopathy.

When muscle fibres degenerate, myoglobin leaks into the plasma and is sufficiently small to pass into the urine. This is important because of the potentially fatal complication of oliguric renal failure due to acute tubular necrosis (Paster et al 1975). Myoglobinuria can also occur in normal individuals after prolonged strenuous exercise, especially at high ambient temperatures (Demos et al 1974). It is seen in <74% of myositis cases and may precede CK elevation in relapses.

Creatine kinase CK exists as three isoenzymes, MM, MB, and BB, with MM predominating (95–99%) in normal skeletal muscle. All three isoenzymes may occasionally be seen, probably because of regeneration of immature fibres in various myopathies, but usually the MM isoenzyme is predominantly elevated. It has been suggested that the MB fraction emanating from heart muscle can be used as an indicator of cardiac involvement in polymyositis. However, it can be elevated in <28% of patients with polymyositis uncomplicated by cardiac disease.

Leakage of CK into plasma is usually taken as evidence of muscle damage, but is also caused by prolonged moderate exercise in normal individuals (Thomson et al 1975, Brooke et al 1979). Plasma CK is higher in outpatients with high levels of habitual activity than inpatients (Griffiths 1966). Intramuscular injections and electromyography also cause a rise in CK.

CK is grossly elevated in muscular dystrophies, especially Duchenne, and may be elevated in spinal muscular atrophy, motor neurone disease, post-poliomyelitis muscular atrophy, hypothyroidism, and toxic muscle damage. In acute rhabdomyolysis, CK can reach very high values and be associated with myoglobinuria. Nevertheless it can be used as a screening test in painful myopathies of less dramatic onset, because it may be elevated in asymptomatic periods between attacks; e.g., in McArdle's disease it is usually 5–15 times the upper limit of normal, but may rise to 100 times this level during and after a painful cramp or contracture. CK may be elevated in myoadenylate deaminase deficiency (Fishbein et al 1978), but is normal between attacks of muscle pain in carnitine palmityltransferase deficiency (Morgan-Hughes 1982). In polymyositis and dermatomyositis it is usually elevated, but even in acute myositis it may be normal. Only in 3% of patients does the CK remain normal throughout the entire clinical course of polymyositis. In polymyositis it may rise 5–6 weeks before a relapse and decrease 3–4 weeks before an improvement in muscle strength (Bohan and Peter 1975b). CK is usually normal in polymyalgia rheumatica.

3-Methylhistidine This amino acid is excreted unchanged in the urine and may be used as an indicator of muscle breakdown, if related to the total excretion of creatinine (McKeran et al 1977). However, other actin-containing tissues such as skin and gut may turn over 3-methylhistidine much faster, and there are uncertainties about interpretation.

Erythrocyte sedimentation rate Inflammatory myopathies, particularly polymyalgia rheumatica (Panayi 1998), cause a rise in the erythrocyte sedimentation rate (ESR). This simple investigation is useful as a screening test for active disease and in monitoring progress.

Magnetic resonance techniques

Spectroscopy Patients with the metabolic disorders of myophosphorylase deficiency (Ross et al 1981, Radda et al 1984) and phosphofructokinase deficiency (Chance et al 1982, Edwards et al 1982a, Cady et al 1985, 1989) usually have normal spectra at rest, as do patients with alcoholic myopathy (Bollaert et al 1989). Exercise causes unusually large metabolic changes, with the exception of the internal pH in myophosphorylase deficiency, which shows no or little change.

Mitochondrial myopathies are associated with excessive changes in pH, Pi, and PCr during exercise and sometimes in unexercised, resting muscle (Gadian et al 1981, Narayana et al 1989, Matthews et al 1991a,b) and in numerous neuromuscular diseases (Barany et al 1989). Patients with peripheral vascular disease (PVD) often show signs of excessive metabolism at rest (Hands et al 1986), as do those with hypothyroidism (Kaminsky et al 1992). In PVD the metabolic abnormalities are greater in those with rest pain (Hands et al 1990). Vascular surgery eliminates symptoms and abolishes the metabolic abnormalities (Hands et al 1986).

MRS has failed to detect metabolic abnormality in the tender points of patients with fibromyalgia (De Blecourt et al 1991).

Normal individuals with delayed-onset muscle pain have an unusually high Pi concentration in resting muscle (Aldridge et al 1986, McCully et al 1988) before the onset of pain. It is also found in some patients with primary muscle diseases (Barany et al 1989) that are usually pain free. This may be a non-specific finding unrelated to myalgia (Newham and Cady 1990).

Imaging Individual muscle groups and also their relative composition of fat and water can be seen, enabling sensitive monitoring of therapies (Fleckenstein et al 1991b). In patients presenting with muscle pain, intramuscular masses (Turner et al 1991), abscesses (Stephenson et al 1991), and anomalous muscles (Paul et al 1991, Sanger et al 1991) have been identified.

Valuable information can be obtained for differential diagnosis and also in cases of referred pain (Chevalier et al 1991, Halpern et al 1997, Stoller 1997). MRI can determine the aetiology of shoulder (Fritz et al 1992) and foot pain (Kier et al 1991) with greater accuracy than other imaging techniques (Nelson et al 1991, Kier et al 1991). Myositis ossificans circumspecta (pseudomalignant osseous soft-tissue tumour) may be differentiated from malignant neoplasms (Ehara et al 1991). Imaging techniques may be combined with spectroscopy to study tumour site, size, and metabolic characteristics (Zlatkin et al 1990).

The distribution and severity of individual muscle involvement can be determined (Lamminen 1990, Fleckenstein et al 1991b). Exercise testing may reveal further abnormalities (Amendola et al 1990, Fleckenstein et al 1991a).

Traumatic and sports injuries are readily visualized (Fleckenstein et al 1989, Greco et al 1991, Farley et al 1992), although the actual level and extent of damage is not always clear. They may be accompanied by haemorrhage (De Smet et al 1990).

As with other investigations, the technique to be used should be chosen with care (Erlemann et al 1990, Greco et al 1991), and both operator and obesity of the subject may affect accuracy (Nelson et al 1991).

Radioisotope scanning

An excessive uptake of radioisotope-labelled complexes into muscle occurs in a variety of muscle diseases, most being pain free (Bellina et al 1978, Giraldi et al 1979). The extent of uptake in patients with polymyositis and dermatomyositis may have prognostic value (Buchpiguel et al 1991).

Affected bone and soft tissues can be identified in trauma and sports injuries (Elgazzar et al 1989, Rockett and Freeman 1990, Halpern et al 1997). Muscular involvement may be identified in cases of ischaemic damage (Yip et al 1990, Rivera-Luna and Spiegler 1991) and PVD (Sayman and Urgancioglu 1991).

Increased muscle uptake of isotope has been observed after exercise in normal, pain-free individuals (Matin et al 1983, Valk 1984). When pectoral muscles are involved there is the possibility of a false diagnosis of exercise-induced left ventricular dysfunction (Campeau et al 1990). Similar findings occur with delayed-onset muscle pain (Jones et al 1986, Newham et al 1986b). The time course of muscle uptake parallels the changes in blood CK levels (Jones et al 1986, Newham et al 1986b), and both presumably reflect sarcolemmal changes. The mechanism of increased isotope uptake is unclear (for a review see Brill 1981), and different mechanisms may be involved in different situations.

Exercise testing

The energy supply for muscle contraction is held in essentially three pools:

- Creatine phosphate and ADP reform ATP, forming an instantly available energy buffer which lasts only a very short time.
- Glycogen stores within muscle provide an intermediate energy supply system.
- Long-term energy supply is provided by carbohydrate and fat in endurance exercise.

Exercise testing needs to be tailored to test specific aspects of the system. There is a large literature on the response to exercise of normal individuals, and in many disease categories exercise testing may be revealing (Jones et al 1975). The performance of whole-body exercise, such as cycle ergonometry, stresses not only the neuromuscular system but also the cardiovascular and respiratory systems and is dependent on motivation. The technique may be useful not only for assessing overall work fitness, but can also provoke symptoms that can then be analysed further. It can also be useful in clinical management as patients can be reassured that they can exercise without producing excessive pain.

Many protocols for progressive exercise tests on a cycle ergometer are available (Jones et al 1975, McArdle et al 1991). Submaximal tests are usually performed at a work rate that is a fixed proportion of the previously determined maximal rate and continue for a fixed time with regular and frequent monitoring. Exercise testing is useful in myalgia when a metabolic muscle disease is suspected. In many mitochondrial myopathies (see below) there is a raised resting lactate that rises markedly after moderate exercise.

The prolonged exercise test (Brooke et al 1979) attempts to measure the individual's ability to switch to fatty acid oxidation once glycogen in muscle has been depleted.

Ischaemic forearm exercise tests (McArdle 1951, Munsat 1970, Sinkeler et al 1986) are designed to test the phosphorylase system in muscle. In normal subjects, lactate rises to between three and five times the resting level at 3 min. In McArdle's disease and phosphofructokinase deficiency, there is no rise in lactate. They should be performed with care because they may produce contractures in myophosphorylase-deficient patients.

Electromyography

Electrical activity can be recorded from muscles, either with surface electrodes or with intramuscular recording needles. With the former, activity from a large volume of tissue can be recorded, and this is useful in the study of abnormalities in the gross pattern of muscle activation (e.g., kinaesiological studies) and in the study of fatigue. The electrical properties of the skin, however, effectively filter out diagnostic information from the muscle signal. For diagnostic purposes, needle electromyography (EMG) is required (Hayward and Willison 1973, Daube 1983, Desmedt 1983). EMG is useful in distinguishing primary muscle diseases from those conditions associated with abnormalities of the anterior horn cell or motor axons. In primary muscle disease, motor unit potentials recorded with a conventional concentric needle electrode consist of brief, small-amplitude potentials. These summate to form a crowded recruitment pattern when the muscle is moderately activated. By contrast, in muscle that has undergone denervation followed by reinnervation, motor unit potentials of high amplitude and broad simple waveform are seen and, even when the muscle is producing its maximal force, they occur as discrete potentials repeating at high rates. In primary muscle disease, motor unit potentials may have maximal amplitude of 0.5–1 mV, whereas in chronic reinnervation due to a neurogenic process, motor unit potentials may be up to 20 mV in amplitude (Mills and Willison 1987).

Healthy muscle at rest is electrically silent. Spontaneous muscle fibre potentials (fibrillations) are most characteristically seen in acute denervating processes, but may also be seen in muscular dystrophies and inflammatory muscle diseases.

Apart from this major function in distinguishing primary muscle and neurogenic diseases, EMG may also be useful in other investigations of muscle pain. It can detect myotonia when clinical myotonia is absent, and can distinguish the electrically silent contracture of McArdle's disease from the excessive motor unit activity of a muscle cramp. Combined with nerve conduction studies, EMG can be used to assess the distribution of muscles affected by denervation, and may help to provide information about which nerve or nerve roots are involved.

Measurements of muscle force

The two most common force-related symptoms are weakness and excessive fatigability. They should be differentiated; weakness is a failure to achieve the expected force, while fatigue is an excessive loss of force generation during or after activity. Measurements of maximal voluntary force generation provide information about the presence and distribution of weakness, as well as about longitudinal changes in strength (Edwards 1982, Edwards et al 1980, 1983). Percutaneous electrical stimulation, through either the motor nerve or its intramuscular nerves, provides useful information about abnormalities in muscle contractile properties (Edwards et al 1977). Patients with both myalgia and weakness are likely to have a specific muscle problem. The distribution may be informative; for example, pain and weakness in the forearm and fingers may simply be a nerve entrapment syndrome, whereas proximal muscle weakness is often associated with primary muscle disease.

Muscle weakness and wasting are associated with, and may be the main presenting symptom of, both neuropathic and myopathic conditions, the former usually being pain free. Electromyographic studies and clinical examination enable the two to be distinguished. Myopathies are subdivided into atrophic and destructive forms. Atrophic myopathies may cause muscle pain (hypothyroid, osteomalacia) but others do not (steroid, Cushing's). Destructive myopathies are further subdivided into those of a destructive nature (muscular dystrophies) and inflammatory (polymyositis and dermatomyositis). In both categories the relationship with pain is very variable and does not appear to correlate well with any other findings. Pain is usually described as aching—especially on activity but sometimes at rest—and also as muscle tenderness. Muscle weakness and pain are reported by some, but not all, former victims of poliomyelitis for unknown reasons (Agre et al 1991).

There is always the possibility that poor motivation or central fatigue is preventing the generation of the maximal voluntary force. The superimposition of electrical or magnetic stimulation on a voluntary contraction determines whether it is maximal (Belanger and McComas 1981, Rutherford et al 1986, Gandevia et al 1995), because additional force is generated only if the voluntary contraction is submaximal and the true strength of the muscle can be estimated from submaximal efforts (Bigland-Ritchie et al 1986). Interestingly, patients with primary myopathy and myalgia rarely show activation failure (Rutherford et al 1986). By contrast, mechanical joint damage, which may be completely pain free, is strongly associated with incomplete voluntary activation (Newham et al 1989).

Peripheral fatigue is a failure of force generation despite the muscle being fully activated. Undue fatigability of this type is seen without pain in myasthenia gravis and myotonic disorders (Wiles and Edwards 1977, Ricker et al 1978). Fatigability and pain are found in mitochondrial myopathies (De Jesus 1974, Edwards et al 1982b). Using motor nerve stimulation, simultaneous measurements of force, and the compound muscle action potential allow the investigation of excitation and activation. These techniques have revealed that the excessive peripheral fatigue in myophosphorylase deficiency is mainly due to a failure of muscle membrane excitation (Wiles et al 1981, Linssen et al 1990).

Treatment

A number of drugs are available for myalgia. Aspirin and many other steroidal and non-steroidal anti-inflammatory drugs (e.g., ibuprofen, flurbiprofen, naproxen, indomethacin) may be used, but no single preparation has been shown to be superior. Diazepam and other benzodiazepines may be effective for muscle 'spasm', as may baclofen or dantrolene sodium, although the latter may impair force generation.

Quinine sulphate has long been used to treat night cramps and those associated with haemodialysis. In the latter case the drug appears to reduce the frequency but not the severity (Kaji et al 1976). Verapamil has helped some patients with exertional muscle pain (Lane et al 1986). A wide range of physical therapies is used, particularly in the case of trauma and sport injuries. The repertoire includes ice, transcutaneous nerve stimulation, and a variety of electrical treatments. Both immobilization and mobilization are considered important at different stages (Lehto and Jarvinen 1991, Renstrom 1991). Immobilization results in marked muscle atrophy, which, although reversible, may delay full rehabilitation (Appell 1990).

Surgical intervention is indicated in cases of severe or complete muscle tears, severe haematomas, and compartment syndromes.

Patients with myalgia of unknown aetiology may be offered a variety of treatments as part of behavioural therapy. Those with diffuse myalgia may be profoundly unfit as a result of inactivity, and some may have a degree of postural hypotension (Newham and Edwards 1979). A logical approach is to provide a well-supervised exercise programme (Edwards 1986), although the individual response to this is very variable. Most patients with ME report their symptoms to be increased by excessive exercise, although a carefully graded programme may be beneficial.

Dietary supplementation of essential fatty acids in ME (Behan et al 1990) and protein in McArdle's syndrome (Jensen et al 1990) has been reported to improve symptoms.

Occasionally, patients with mitochondrial cytopathies have been reported to respond to vitamins. The best-documented example (Eleff et al 1984) is a patient with complex III deficiency in whom vitamins K3 and C (which might be expected to bypass the metabolic defect) resulted in rapid clinical improvement.

Trauma and sports injuries

Direct trauma from many causes, ranging from intramuscular injections to sports and severe crush injuries, is an obvious cause of muscle pain. If sufficient muscle tissue is damaged, life is threatened by hypercalcaemia and acute renal failure from myoglobinuria. Sports injuries, from minor muscle sprains to complete rupture (e.g., hamstring rupture), may include direct trauma and are increasingly common in exercise-conscious cultures (Renstrom 1991, Harries et al 1994, de Lee and Prez 1994).

Muscle

Traumatic muscular damage is invariably associated with pain, which may have a gradual or immediate onset. It may be detected by imaging techniques, blood biochemistry, and the immunohistochemical (Fechner et al 1991) and routine histochemical examination of biopsy samples as described above. The combination of damage and immobilization (Appell 1990) results in considerable weakness and wasting, which may only be reversed by relatively long periods of rehabilitation.

In many cases the cause of injury is obvious and associated with forced lengthening of active muscle, but spontaneous ruptures, particularly of the hamstrings and pectoralis major (Kretzler and Richardson 1989), occur frequently. Ruptures and tears of limb muscles may mimic a compartment syndrome, while those in the abdominal musculature may cause groin pain. They are commonly associated with muscle spasms, which cause additional pain. Myositis ossificans is a potentially disabling complication that may be confused with a sarcoma (Booth and Westers 1989).

Activity-related compartment syndromes occur in muscle groups within a relatively inextensible fascial sheath, such as the anterior tibial muscles (Vincent 1994). Pain occurs during exercise and increases as it continues. Symptoms include pain and cramp-like sensations, very similar to those of intermittent claudication. They usually disappear at rest but tenderness may persist. Weakness, paralysis, and numbness may occur in acute cases, which tend to result in continued symptoms and raised intramuscular pressures at rest (Martens and Moeyersoons 1990).

Ligaments and tendons

There are only subtle morphological differences between these two structures (Oakes 1994). Tendons require greater flexibility and the ability to resist high forces. Ligaments are passive structures that are superior to tendons in their ability to sustain constant tension. Healthy structures are extremely strong, strength being related to cross-sectional area; forces <4000 N have been recorded in the Achilles tendon (Komi 1992). Injuries are thought to be caused by both overt trauma and also repeated, cumulative microtrauma associated with intense functional use, particularly in structures with a small cross-sectional area. Conversely, immobilization also weakens ligamentous collagen (Amiel et al 1983) as well as bone.

Injuries range from microscopic damage through partial tears to complete ruptures. The high forces involved may detach some bone that remains attached to the tendon or ligament. Muscles acting over two joints, such as the hamstrings and rectus femoris, appear to be particularly susceptible. This may be due to the complex neuromuscular control needed for co-contraction and relaxation in muscle groups with opposing actions.

Clinically it is extremely difficult to determine the exact location and extent of damage. Pain and tenderness usually accompany such lesions, but localization can be difficult. Palpation always involves the tendon as well as its sheath, and muscle contraction will apply force to both. Imaging techniques tend to overestimate the size of a lesion. Depending on the extent of damage, pain may be absent, may occur only on activity, or be constant and severe.

Tendon injuries

Many sporting activities stress tendons to a high proportion of their theoretical maximum (Alexander and Vernon 1975). The incidence of tendinitis and rupture may be associated with changes in the nature or intensity of activity.

The musculo-tendinous junction is a common site of failure (Curwin 1994). The last sarcomere of a muscle fibre shows increased folds which are thought to increase surface area and reduce stress at the junction (Oakes 1994). These are probably not reproduced during repair and may explain the frequent occurrence of repeat injuries. Intrinsic causes of the injury remain unknown, but may include inadequate muscle/tendon length, muscle weakness, or fatigue.

Repetitive use, combined with overuse and microtrauma, may cause a progressive attrition of tendon. Spontaneous tendon rupture is uncommon in young people and usually occurs with age-related degeneration. It is also rare under normal loading in the absence of previous injury or disease (Barfred 1971).

Compressive forces, such as those from the individual's own anatomy or tight shoes, may be an external cause.

Ligament injuries

These have a high incidence, particularly in association with sporting injuries. Ankle ligament sprains, possibly with bone avulsion, are the most common specific injury (McBride 1994). They may be acute or have gradual onset. Mechanical joint damage, including ligament injury, is associated with voluntary activation failure in related muscles (Hurley et al 1994).

Acute knee injuries are one of the most common career-ending events for competitive athletes

(Johnson 1994) and may involve one or more of the ligaments and menisci. Meniscal damage inevitably results in pain and functional impairment, but a damaged anterior cruciate ligament may mean either normal function or significant symptoms and substantial functional disability.

Injuries to the rotator cuff occur particularly in sports such as swimming, tennis, and baseball (Bowen and Warren 1994). Structures involved could include the supra- and infraspinati, teres major, and subscapularis muscles and their tendons and joint capsule as well as ligaments (Itio and Tabata 1992). The supraspinatus appears to be highly susceptible to injury, perhaps due to a relatively poor vasculature. There is frequently some degree of glenohumeral instability. Pain is poorly localized and may radiate down the affected arm. Night pain is common.

The prognosis for function is poor unless effective treatment is instigated early.

Treatment

Ligaments and tendons are poorly vascularized and heal slowly. Soft-tissue injuries present a challenge due to the conflicting demands of maintaining or increasing mobility and the requirement of injured tissues for low stress for healing (Curwin 1994). However, effective treatment is essential because many injuries will fail to heal spontaneously and chronic conditions tend to develop.

Remodelling and mobilization of connective tissue can continue for up to a year (Oakes 1994). Local collagen matrices may shorten the affected region and smaller diameter fibrils are retained, rendering the area weaker and susceptible to repeated injury. Reduced activity leads to atrophy in collagen as well as muscle tissue; however, regenerating fibres cannot tolerate high forces. Once fibrils are strong enough, application of load causes them to become larger and stronger (Butler et al 1978). Muscle hypertrophy probably also involves connective tissue changes.

Trauma frequently results in extravascular bleeding that needs to be removed. Extravascular blood in itself may increase tissue pressure to the point of pain and also acts as an irritant, leading to further pressure increases and possibly tissue necrosis.

The basic issue is whether initial treatment should be conservative or surgical. Improved imaging techniques have increased the ability to determine the location and extent of injury (Stoller 1997, Halpern et al 1997). The criteria are usually on symptoms and functional loss. Ruptures involving more than a small proportion of the structure are unlikely to spontaneously reunite with any degree of functional improvement and often lead to chronic conditions.

The approach for the first few days after surgery or injury is generally ice, rest, and anti-inflammatory agents. Applied forces are kept to a minimum to avoid further collagen damage, including that to regenerating fibrils. From about 5 days gentle movement and stress is introduced to increase collagen regeneration, fibril size, and cross-sectional area and to prevent the adverse consequences of immobilization and disuse atrophy. From 3 weeks onwards progressive stresses are placed on the tissue to increase cross-linking, size, and strength. Physical therapy is widely and intensively used and is thought to be essential for optimal healing and rehabilitation outcome (De Lee and Prez 1994, Harries et al 1994, Sallis and Massimo 1997). A prime goal is to prevent repeated injury, so attention must be paid to possible internal and external contributing factors.

Overuse

Great emphasis has been placed on the ability of training to protect against injury in sports (Safran et al 1989). Nevertheless, it is currently accepted that for many athletes overtraining in itself can produce a wide variety of symptoms, both physical and psychological (Fry et al 1991). Depression of the immune system is associated with overuse (Shepherd 1998).

There seems to be considerable individual variation in the susceptibility to sports-related injuries, which is little understood (Taimela et al 1990). The syndrome also involves tendons and ligaments (Renstrom 1994). It is wide ranging, involving both elite athletes and sedentary individuals involved in low-intensity, highly repetitive occupations (Simons and Mense 1998). Predisposing factors are classified as external (intensity, repetition, duration, environmental, clothing, footware, etc.) and internal (anatomical or postural abnormalities, muscle weakness, decreased flexibility and previous disorders).

In the past decade there has been a virtual epidemic of these syndromes but optimal treatment or prevention regimens remain unclear. However, these are important issues due to the high incidence and the fact that unresolved acute pain tends to become chronic and processed differently in the brain (Hsieh et al 1995).

References

Abbott BC, Bigland B, Ritchie JM 1952 The physiological cost of negative work. Journal of Physiology 117: 380–390

Agre JC, Rodriquez AA, Tafel JA 1991 Late effects of polio: a critical review of the literature on neuromuscular function. Archives of Physical Medicine and Rehabilitation 72: 923–931

Aldridge R, Cady EB, Jones DA, Obletter G 1986 Muscle pain after exercise is linked with an inorganic phosphate increase as shown by 31P NMR. Bioscience Reports 6: 663–667

Alexander DS, Vernon P 1975 The dimensions of knee and ankle muscles and the force they exert. Journal of Human Movement Studies 41: 115–123

Amendola A, Rorabeck CH, Vellett D, Vezina W, Rutt B, Nott L 1990 The use of magnetic resonance imaging in exertional compartment syndromes. American Journal of Sports Medicine 18: 29–34

Amiel D, Akesan WH, Harwood FL, Frank CB 1983 Stress deprivation effect on metabolic turnover of medial collateral ligament collagen; a comparison between 9 and 12 week immobilisation. Clinical Orthopaedics and Related Research 172: 265–270

Appell HJ 1990 Muscular atrophy following immobilisation. A review. Sports Medicine 10: 42–58

Bank WJ, Di Mauro S, Bonilla E, Capuzzi DM, Rowland LP 1975 A disorder of muscle lipid metabolism and myoglobinuria. Absence of carnitine palmityl transferase. New England Journal of Medicine 292: 443–449

Barany M, Siegel IM, Venkatasubrananian PN, Mok E, Wilbur AC 1989 Human leg neuromuscular diseases: P-31 MR spectroscopy. Radiology 172: 503–508

Barfred T 1971 Experimental rupture of Achilles tendon: comparison of various types of experimental rupture in rats. Acta Orthopaedica Scandinavica 42: 528–543

Bartels EM, Danneskiold-Samsoe B 1986 Histological abnormalities in muscle from patients with certain types of fibrositis. Lancet 7: 755–757

Barton NJ, Hooper G, Noble J, Steel WM 1992 Occupational causes of disorders in the upper limb. British Medical Journal 304: 309–311

Behan PO, Bakheit AMO 1991 Clinical spectrum of postviral fatigue syndrome. In: Behan PO, Goldberg DP, Mowbray JF (eds) Postviral fatigue syndrome. British Medical Bulletin 47: 793–809

Behan PO, Behan WM, Horrobin D 1990 Effects of high doses of essential fatty acids on the postviral fatigue syndrome. Acta Neurologica Scandinavica 82: 209–216

Behan PO, Goldberg DP, Mowbray JF (eds) 1991 Postviral fatigue syndrome. British Medical Bulletin 47

Belanger AY, McComas AJ 1981 Extent of voluntary unit activation during effort. Journal of Applied Physiology 51: 1131–1135

Bellina CR, Biachi R, Bombardini S et al 1978 Quantitative evaluation of ^{99m}Tc pyrophosphate muscle uptake in patients with inflammatory and non-inflammatory muscle diseases. Journal of Nuclear Medicine 22: 89–96

Bengtsson A 1986 Primary fibromyalgia. A clinical and laboratory study. Linkoping University, Dissertation 224

Bengtsson A, Henriksson K-G, Jarson J 1986a Muscle biopsy in primary fibromyalgia. Light microscopical and histochemical findings. Scandinavian Journal of Rheumatology 15: 1–6

Bengtsson A, Henriksson K-G, Jarson J 1986b Reduced high energy phosphate levels in painful muscle in patients with primary fibromyalgia. Arthritis and Rheumatism 29: 817–821

Bennett RM 1981 Fibrositis: misnomer for a common rheumatic disorder. Western Journal of Medicine 134: 405–413

Bertorini T, Yeh YY, Trevisan C, Standlan E, Sabesin S, Di Mauro S 1980 Carnitine palmityltransferase deficiency: myoglobinuria and respiratory failure. Neurology 30: 263–271

Bigland-Ritchie B, Furbush F, Woods JJ 1986 Neuromuscular transmission and muscular activation in human post-fatigue ischaemia. Journal of Physiology 337: 76P

Bird HA, Esselinck W, Dixon A St J, Mowat AG, Wood PHN 1979 An evaluation of the criteria for polymyalgia rheumatica. Annals of the Rheumatic Diseases 38: 424–439

Bohan A, Peter JB 1975a Polymyositis and dermatomyositis: part 1. New England Journal of Medicine 292: 344–347

Bohan A, Peter JB 1975b Polymyositis and dermatomyositis: part 2. New England Journal of Medicine 292: 402–407

Bollaert PE, Robin-Lherbier B, Escanye JM et al 1989 Phosphorus nuclear magnetic resonance evidence of abnormal skeletal muscle metabolism in chronic alcoholics. Neurology 39: 821–824

Booth DW, Westers BM 1989 The management of athletes with myositis ossificans traumatica. Canadian Journal of Sport Science 14: 10–16

Bowen MK, Warren RF 1994 Injuries of the rotator cuff. In: Harries M, Williams C, Stanish WD, Micheli LJ (eds) Oxford textbook of sports medicine. Oxford Medical Press, Oxford, pp 442–452

Brill DR 1981 Radionuclide imaging of non-neoplastic soft tissue disorders. Seminars in Nuclear Medicine 11: 277–288

Brooke MH, Carroll JE, Hagberg JM 1979 The prolonged exercise test. Neurology 29: 636–643

Brown SJ, Child RB, Day SH, Donnelly A 1997 Indices of skeletal muscle damage and connective tissue breakdown following eccentric muscle contractions. European Journal of Applied Physiology 75: 369–374

Buchpiguel CA, Roizenblatt S, Lucena-Fernandes MF et al 1991 Radioisotopic assessment of peripheral and cardiac muscle involvement and dysfunction in polymyositis/ dermatomyositis. Journal of Rheumatology 18: 1359–1363

Bunch TW, Worthington JW, Combs JJ, Ilstrup DM, Engel AG 1980 Azathioprine with prednisone for polymyositis. Annals of Internal Medicine 92: 365–369

Butler DL, Grood ES, Noyes FR, Zernicke RG 1978 Biomechanics of ligaments and tendons. Exercise and Sports Science Reviews 6: 125–182

Cady EB, Griffiths RD, Edwards RHT 1985 The clinical use of nuclear magnetic resonance spectroscopy for studying human muscle metabolism. International Journal of Technological Assessment in Health Care 1: 631–645

Cady EB, Jones DA, Lynn J, Newham DJ 1989 Changes in force and intracellular metabolites during fatigue of human skeletal muscle. Journal of Physiology 418: 311–325

Campeau RJ, Garcia OM, Correa OA, Mace JE 1990 Pectoralis muscle uptake of thallium-201 after arm exercise ergometry. Possible confusion with lung thallium-201 activity. Clinical Nuclear Medicine 15: 303–306

Carpenter JR, Bunch TW, Angel AG, O'Brien PC 1977 Survival in polymyositis: corticosteroids and risk factors. Journal of Rheumatology 4: 207–214

Carpenter S, Karpati G 1981 The major inflammatory myopathies of unknown cause. Pathological Annual 16: 205–237

Carroll JE, De Vivo DC, Brooke MH, Planner GJ, Hagberg JH 1979 Fasting as a provocative test in neuromuscular diseases. Metabolism 28: 683–687

Chance B, Eleff S, Bank W, Leigh JR, Warnell R 1982 ^{31}P NMR studies of control of mitochondrial function in phosphofructokinase deficient human skeletal muscle. Proceedings of the National Academy of Sciences USA 79: 7714–7718

Chevalier X, Wrona N, Avouac B, Larget B 1991 Thigh pain and multiple osteonecrosis: value of magnetic resonance imaging. Journal of Rheumatology 18: 1627–1630

Clarkson PM, Newham DJ 1995 Associations between muscle soreness, damage and fatigue. In: Gandevia SC et al (eds)

Fatigue: neural and muscular mechanisms. Advances in Experimental medicine and biology, vol 384. Plenum Press, New York, pp 457–470
Currie S 1981 Inflammatory mypathies. Polymyositis and related disorders. In: Walton JN (ed) Disorders of voluntary muscle, 4th edn. Churchill Livingstone, Edinburgh, pp 525–568
Curtin NA, Davies RE 1973 Chemical and mechanical changes during stretching of activated frog muscle. Cold Spring Harbor Symposia on Quantitative Biology 37: 619–626
Curwin SL 1994 The aetiology and treatment of tendinitis. In: Harries M, Williams C, Stanish W D, Micheli LJ (eds) Oxford textbook of sports medicine. Oxford Medical Press, Oxford, pp 512–528
Dalakas MC (ed) 1988 Polyositis and dermatomyositis, 1st edn. Butterworths, Boston
Daube JR 1983 Disorders of neuromuscular transmission: a review. Archives of Physical Medicine and Rehabilitation 64: 195–200
Dawson J 1990 Consensus on research into fatigue syndrome. British Medical Journal 300: 832
De Blecourt AC, Wolf RF, van Rijswijk MH et al 1991 In vivo ^{31}P magnetic resonance spectroscopy (MRS) of tender points in patients with primary fibromyalgia syndrome. Rheumatology International 1: 51–54
De Jesus PV 1974 Neuromuscular physiology in Luft's syndrome. Electroencephalography and Clinical Neurophysiology 14: 17–27
de Lee JC, Prez D 1994 Orthopaedic sports medicine, vol 11. Saunders, Philadelphia
Demos MA, Gitlin EL, Kagen L 1974 Exercise myoglobinuria and acute exertional rhabdomyolysis. Archives of Internal Medicine 134: 669–673
De Smet AA, Fischer DR, Heiner JP, Keene JS 1990 Magnetic resonance imaging of muscle tears. Skeletal Radiology 19: 283–286
Desmedt JE (ed) 1983 Computer aided electromyography. Progress in clinical neurophysiology, vol 10. Karger, Basel
Dietrichson P, Oakley J, Smith PEM, Griffiths RD, Helliwell TR, Edwards RHT 1987 Conchotome and needle percutaneous biopsy of skeletal muscle. Journal of Neurology, Neurosurgery and Psychiatry 50: 1461–1476
Di Mauro S, Di Mauro PM 1973 Muscle carnitine palmityltransferase deficiency and myoglobinuria. Science 182: 929–931
Di Mauro S, Miranda AF, Olarte M, Friedman R, Hays AP 1982 Muscle phosphoglycerate mutase (GAM) deficiency: a new metabolic myopathy. Neurology 32: 584–591
Di Mauro S, Dalakas M, Miranda AF 1983 Phosphoglycerate kinase deficiency: another cause of recurrent myoglobinuria. Annals of Neurology 13: 11–19
Douglas JG, Ford MJ, Innes JA, Munro JF 1979 Polymyalgia arteritica: a clinical review. European Journal of Clinical Investigation 9: 137–140
Edwards RHT 1982 Weakness and fatigue of skeletal muscles. In: Sarner M (ed) Advanced medicine, vol 18. Pitman Medical, London, pp 100–119
Edwards RHT 1986 Muscle fatigue and pain. Acta Medica Scandinavica (suppl) 711: 179–188
Edwards RHT, Young A, Hosking GP, Jones DA 1977 Human skeletal muscle function: description of tests and normal values. Clinical Science and Molecular Medicine 52: 283–290
Edwards RHT, Young A, Wiles CM 1980 Needle biopsy of skeletal muscle in diagnosis of myopathy and the clinical study of muscle function and repair. New England Journal of Medicine 302: 261–271
Edwards RHT, Isenberg DA, Wiles CM, Young A, Snaith ML 1981 The investigation of inflammatory myopathy. Journal of the Royal College of Physicians 15: 19–24
Edwards RHT, Dawson MJ, Wilkie DR, Gordon RE, Shaw D 1982a Clinical use of nuclear magnetic resonance in the investigation of myopathy. Lancet i: 725–731
Edwards RHT, Wiles CM, Gohil K, Krywawych S, Jones DA 1982b Energy metabolism in human myopathy. In: Schotland DC (ed) Disorders of the motor unit. Wiley, London, pp 715–728
Edwards RHT, Wiles CM, Mills KR 1983 Quantitation of human muscle function. In: Dyck P, Thomas PK, Lambert EH (eds) Peripheral neuropathy. Saunders, Philadelphia, pp 1093–1102
Edwards RHT, Newham DJ, Peters TJ 1991 Muscle biochemistry and pathophysiology in postviral fatigue syndrome. In: Behan PO, Goldberg DP, Mowbray JF (eds) Postviral fatigue syndrome. British Medical Bulletin 47: 826–837
Ehara S, Nakasato T, Tamakawa Y et al 1991 MRI of myositis ossificans circumscripta. Clinical Imaging 15: 130–134
Eleff S, Kennaway NG, Buist NRM et al 1984 ^{31}P-NMR studies of improvement of oxidative phosphorylation by vitamins K3 and C in a patient with a defect in electron transport and complex III in skeletal muscle. Proceedings of the National Academy of Sciences USA 81: 3529–3533
Elgazzar AH, Malki AA, Abdel-Dayem HM et al 1989 Indium-111 monoclonal anti-myosin antibody in assessing skeletal muscle damage in trauma. Nuclear Medicine Communications 10: 661–667
Erlemann R, Vassallo P, Bongartz G et al 1990 Musculoskeletal neoplasm: fast low-angle shot MR imaging with and without Gd-DTPA. Radiology 176: 489–495
Farley TE, Neumann CH, Steinbach LS, Jahnke AJ, Petersen SS 1992 Full-thickness tears of the rotator cuff of the shoulder: diagnosis with MR imaging. American Journal of Roentgenology 158: 347–351
Fechner G, Hauser R, Sepulchre MA, Brinkman B 1991 Immunohistochemical investigations to demonstrate vital direct damage of skeletal muscle. International Journal of Legal Medicine 104: 215–219
Fishbein WN, Armbrustmacher KW, Griffin JL 1978 Myoadenylate deaminase deficiency: a new disease of muscle. Science 200: 545–548
Fleckenstein JL, Weatherall PT, Parkey RW, Payne JA, Peshock RM 1989 Sports-related muscle injuries: evaluation with MR imaging. Radiology 172: 793–798
Fleckenstein JL, Haller RG, Lewis SF et al 1991a Absence of exercise-induced MRI enhancement of skeletal muscle in McArdle's disease. Journal of Applied Physiology 71: 961–969
Fleckenstein JL, Weatherall PT, Bertocci LA et al 1991b Locomotor system assessment by muscle magnetic resonance imaging. Magnetic Resonance Quarterly 7: 79–103
Friden J 1984 Muscle soreness after exercise: implications of morphological changes. International Journal of Sports Medicine 5: 57–66
Friden J, Sfakianos PN, Hargens AR 1986 Delayed muscle soreness and intramuscular fluid pressure: comparison between eccentric and concentric load. Journal of Applied Physiology 61: 2175–2179
Fritz RC, Helms CA, Steinbach LS, Genant KK 1992 Suprascapular nerve entrapment: evaluation with MR imaging. Radiology 182: 437–444
Fry HJH 1986 Overuse syndrome of the upper limb in musicians. Medical Journal of Australia 144: 182–185
Fry RW, Morton AR, Keast D 1991 Overtraining in athletes. An update. Sports Medicine 12: 32–65
Gadian DG, Radda GK, Ross BD et al 1981 Examinations of a myopathy by phosphorus nuclear magnetic resonance. Lancet ii: 774–775
Gandevia SC, Allen GM, McKenzie DK 1995 Central fatigue: critical issues, quantification and practical issues. In: Gandevia SC et al (eds) Fatigue: neural and muscular mechanisms. Advances in

experimental medicine and biology, vol 384. Plenum Press, New York, pp 281–294

Giraldi C, Marciani G, Molla N, Rossi B 1979 ^{99m}Tc-pyrophosphate muscle uptake in four subjects with Becker's disease. Journal of Nuclear Medicine 23: 45–47

Gohil K, Jones DA, Edwards RHT 1981 Analysis of muscle mitochondrial function with techniques applicable to needle biopsy samples. Clinical Physiology 1: 195–207

Gordon EE, Januszko DM, Kaufman L 1967 A critical survey of stiff-man syndrome. American Journal of Medicine 42: 582–599

Gould SE (ed) 1970 Trichinosis in man and animals. Thomas, Springfield, IL, pp 147–189

Greco A, McNamara MT, Escher RM, Trifilio G, Parienti J 1991 Spin-echo and STIR imaging of sports related injuries at 1.5 T. Journal of Computer Assisted Tomography 15: 994–999

Griffiths PD 1966 Serum levels of ATP and creatine phosphotransferase (creatine kinase). The normal range and effect of muscular activity. Clinica Chimica Acta 13: 413–420

Halpern B, Herring SA, Altchelk D, Herzog R (eds) 1997 Imaging in muscle and sports medicine. Blackwell Science, Malden, MA

Hamrin B 1972 Polymyalgia rheumatica. Acta Medica Scandinavica (suppl) 553: 1–131

Hands CJ, Bone PJ, Galloway G, Morris PJ, Radda GK 1986 Muscle metabolism in patients with peripheral vascular disease investigated by ^{31}P nuclear magnetic resonance spectroscopy. Clinical Science 71: 283–290

Hands LJ, Sharif MH, Payne GS, Morris PJ, Radda GK 1990 Muscle ischaemia in peripheral vascular disease studied by ^{31}P-magnetic resonance spectroscopy. European Journal of Vascular Surgery 4: 637–642

Harries M, Williams C, Stanish WD, Micheli LJ (eds) 1994 Oxford textbook of sports medicine. Oxford Medical Press, Oxford

Haslock DI, Wright V, Harriman DGF 1970 Neuromuscular disorders in rheumatoid arthritis. A motor-point muscle biopsy study. Quarterly Journal of Medicine 39: 335–358

Hayward M, Willison RG 1973 The recognition of myogenic and neurogenic lesions by quantitative EMG. In: Desmedt JE (ed) New developments in electromyography and clinical neurophysiology, vol 2. Karger, Basel, pp 448–453

Hazleman B 1998 Soft tissue rheumatology. In: Maddison PJ, Isenberg DA, Woo P, Glass D (eds) The Oxford textbook of rheumatology, 2nd edn. Oxford Medical Press, Oxford, pp 1489–1514

Headley SA, Newham DJ, Jones DA 1986 The effect of prednisolone on exercise induced muscle pain and damage. Clinical Science 70: 85P

Holt IJ, Harding AE, Cooper JM et al 1989 Mitochrondrial myopathies: clinical and biochemical features of 30 patients with major deletions of muscle mitochondrial DNA. Annals of Neurology 29: 600–608

Hsieh JC, Beifrage M, Stone-Elander P, Hansson P, Ingvar M 1995 Central representation of chronic ongoing neuropathic pain studied by positron emission tomography. Pain 63: 224–236

Hurley MV, Jones DW, Newham DJ 1994 Arthrogenic quadriceps inhibition and rehabilitation of patients with traumatic knee injury. Clinical Science 86: 305–310

Isaacs H 1961 A syndrome of continuous muscle fibre activity. Journal of Neurology, Neurosurgery and Psychiatry 24: 319–325

Itoi E, Tabata S 1992 Conservative treatment of rotator cuff tears. Clinical Orthopaedics 275: 165–173

Janssen E, Kuipers H, Venstrappen FTJ, Costill DL 1983 Influence of an anti-inflammatory drug on muscle soreness. Medicine and Science in Sports and Exercise 15: 165

Jeffrey HC 1974 Sarcosporidosis in man. Transactions of the Royal Society of Tropical Medicine and Hygiene 68: 17–29

Jensen KE, Jakobsen J, Thomsen C, Henriksen O 1990 Improved energy kinetics following high protein diet in McArdle's syndrome. A ^{31}P magnetic resonance spectroscopy study. Acta Neurologica Scandinavica 81: 499–503

Johnson RL 1994 Acute knee injuries. In: Harries M, Williams C, Stanish WD, Micheli LJ (eds) Oxford textbook of sports medicine. Oxford Medical Press, Oxford, pp 350–363

Jones DA, Newham DJ, Round JM, Tolfree SEJ 1986 Experimental human muscle damage: morphological changes in relation to other indices of damage. Journal of Physiology 375: 435–448

Jones NL, Campbell EJM, Edwards RHT, Robertson DG 1975 Clinical exercise testing. Saunders, Philadelphia

Kaji DM, Ackad A, Nottage WG, Stein RM 1976 Prevention of muscle cramps on haemodialysis patients by quinine sulphate. Lancet ii: 66–67

Kaminsky P, Robin Lherbier B, Brunotte F, Escanye JM, Walker P 1992 Energetic metabolism in hypothyroid skeletal muscle, as studied by phosphorus magnetic resonance spectroscopy. Journal of Clinical Endocrinology and Metabolism 74: 124–129

Kanno T, Sudo K, Takeuchi I et al 1980 Hereditary deficiency of lactate dehydrogenase M subunit. Clinica Chimica Acta 108: 267–276

Karpati G, Carpenter S, Engel A et al 1975 The syndrome of systemic carnitine deficiency. Neurology 25: 16–24

Katz B 1939 The relation between force and speed in muscular contraction. Journal of Physiology 96: 46–64

Kier R, McCarthy S, Dietz MJ, Rudicel S 1991 MR appearance of painful conditions of the ankle. Radiographics 11: 401–414

Komi PV 1992 Strength-shortening cycle. In: Komi PV (ed) Strength and power in sport. Blackwell Scientific, Oxford, pp 169–179

Kretzler HH Jr, Richardson AB 1989 Rupture of the pectoralis major muscle. American Journal of Sports Medicine 17: 453–458

Kuipers H, Kieren HA, Venstrappen FTJ, Costill DL 1983 Influence of a prostaglandin inhibiting drug on muscle soreness after eccentric work. Journal of Sports Medicine 6: 336–339

Lamminen AE 1990 Magnetic resonance imaging of primary skeletal diseases: patterns of distribution and severity of involvement. British Journal of Radiology 63: 946–950

Land JM, Clark JB 1979 Mitochondrial myopathies. Biochemical Society Transactions 7: 231–245

Lane RJM, Mastaglia FL 1978 Drug-induced myopathies in man. Lancet ii: 562–566

Lane RJM, Turnbull DM, Welch JL, Walton J 1986 A double blind placebo controlled cross-over study of verapamil on exertional muscle pain. Muscle and Nerve 9: 635–641

Layzer RB 1994 Muscle pain, cramps and fatigue. In: Engel AG, Franzini-Armstrong C (eds) Myology, vol 2, 2nd edn. McGraw-Hill, New York, pp 1754–1768

Layzer RB, Rowland LP 1971 Cramps. New England Journal of Medicine 285: 31–40

Lehto MU, Jarvinen MJ 1991 Muscle injuries, their healing processes and treatment. Annales Chirurgiae et Gynaecologiae 80: 102–108

Lendinger MI, Sjogaard G 1991 Potassium regulation during exercise and recovery. Sports Medicine 11: 382–401

Linssen WH, Jacobs M, Stegman DF, Joosten EM, Moleman J 1990 Muscle fatigue in McArdle's disease. Muscle fibre conduction velocity and surface EMG frequency spectrum during ischaemic exercise. Brain 113: 1779–1793

Lloyd AR, Gandevia SC, Hales JP 1991 Muscle performance, voluntary activation, twitch properties and perceived effort in normal subjects and patients with the chronic fatigue syndrome. Brain 114: 85–98

Marinacci AA 1965 Electromyography in the diagnosis of polymyositis. Electromyography 5: 255–268

Martens MA, Moeyerssoons JP 1990 Acute and recurrent effort-related compartment syndrome in sports. Sports Medicine 9: 62–68

Mastaglia FL (ed) 1988 Inflammatory diseases of muscle, 1st edn. Blackwell Science, Oxford
Matin P, Lang G, Ganetta R, Simon G 1983 Scintiographic evaluation of muscle damage following extreme exercise. Journal of Nuclear Medicine 24: 308–311
Matthews PM, Allaire C, Shoubridge EA, Karpati G, Carpenter S, Arnold DL 1991a In vivo muscle magnetic resonance spectroscopy in the clinical investigation of mitochondrial disease. Neurology 41: 114–120
Matthews PM, Berkovic SF, Shoubridge EA et al 1991b In vivo magnetic resonance spectroscopy of brain and muscle in a type of mitochondrial encephalomyopathy (MERRF). Annals of Neurology 29: 435–438
McArdle B 1951 Myopathy due to a defect in muscle glycogen breakdown. Clinical Science 10: 13–33
McArdle WD, Katch FI, Katch VL 1991 Exercise physiology: Energy, nutrition and human performance. Lea and Febiger, Philadelphia
McBride AM 1994 The acute ankle sprain. In: Harries M, Williams C, Stanish WD, Micheli LJ (eds) Oxford textbook of sports medicine. Oxford Medical Press, Oxford, pp 471–482
McCully KK, Argov Z, Boden BA, Brown RL, Blank WJ, Chance B 1988 Detection of muscle injury in humans with ^{31}P magnetic resonance spectroscopy. Muscle and Nerve 11: 212–216
McKeran RO, Halliday D, Purkiss D 1977 Increased myofibrillar protein catabolism in Duchenne muscular dystrophy measured by 3-methylhistidine excretion in the urine. Journal of Neurology, Neurosurgery and Psychiatry 40: 979–981
Menard MR, Penn AM, Lee JE, Dusik LA, Hall LD 1991 Relative metabolic efficiency of concentric and eccentric exercise determined by ^{31}P magnetic resonance spectroscopy. Archives of Physical Medicine and Rehabilitation 72: 976–983
Mills KR, Edwards RHT 1983 Investigative strategies for muscle pain. Journal of the Neurological Sciences 58: 73–88
Mills KR, Willison RG 1987 Quantification of EMG on volition. In: The London Symposia (electroencephalography and clinical neurophysiology, suppl 39). Elsevier, Amsterdam, pp 27–32
Mills KR, Newham DJ, Edwards RHT 1982 Severe muscle cramps relieved by transcutaneous nerve stimulation. Journal of Neurology, Neurosurgery and Psychiatry 45: 539–542
Moersch FP, Woltman HW 1956 Progressive fluctuating muscular rigidity and spasm ('stiff man' syndrome): report of a case and some observations in 13 other cases. Proceedings of the Staff Meetings of the Mayo Clinic 31: 421–427
Mommaerts WFHM, Illingworth B, Pearson CM, Guillory RJ, Seraydarian K 1959 A functional disorder of phosphorylase. Proceedings of the National Academy of Sciences of the USA 45: 791–797
Morgan-Hughes JA 1982 Defects of the energy pathways of skeletal muscle. In: Matthews WB, Glaser GH (eds) Recent advances in clinical neurology, vol 3. Churchill Livingstone, Edinburgh, pp 1–46
Morgan-Hughes JM, Cooper JM, Schapira AHV, Hayes DJ, Clark JB 1987 The mitochondrial myopathies. Defects of the mitochondrial respiratory chain and oxidative phosphorylation system. In: Ellingson JR, Murray NMF, Halliday AM (eds) The London Symposia (electroencephalography and clinical neurophysiology, suppl 39). Elsevier, Amsterdam, pp 103–114
Munsat TL 1970 A standardised forearm ischaemic test. Neurology 20: 1171–1178
Narayana PA, Slopis JM, Jackson EF, Jazle JD, Kulkarni MV, Butler IJ 1989 In vivo muscle magnetic resonance spectroscopy in a family with mitochondrial cytopathy. A defect in fat metabolism. Magnetic Resonance Imaging 7: 33–39
Nelson MC, Leather GP, Nirschl RP, Pettrone FA, Freedman MT 1991 Evaluation of the painful shoulder. A prospective comparison of magnetic resonance imaging, computerized tomographic arthrography, ultrasonography and operative findings. Journal of Bone and Joint Surgery 73A: 707–716
Newham DJ 1988 The consequences of eccentric contractions and their relation to delayed onset muscle pain. European Journal of Applied Physiology 57: 353–359
Newham DJ, Cady EB 1990 A ^{31}P study of fatigue and metabolism in human skeletal muscle with voluntary, intermittent contractions at different forces. NMR in Biomedicine 3: 211–219
Newham DJ, Edwards RHT 1979 Effort syndromes. Physiotherapy 65: 52–56
Newham DJ, Jones DA 1985 Intramuscular pressure in the painful human biceps. Clinical Science 69: 27P
Newham DJ, Jones DA, Edwards RHT 1983a Large and delayed plasma creatine kinase changes after stepping exercise. Muscle and Nerve 6: 36–41
Newham DJ, McPhail G, Mills KR, Edwards RHT 1983b Ultrastructural changes after concentric and eccentric contractions. Journal of Neurological Science 61: 109–122
Newham DJ, Mills KR, Quigley BM, Edwards RHT 1983c Pain and fatigue after eccentric contractions. Clinical Science 64: 55–62
Newham DJ, Jones DA, Edwards 1986a Plasma creatine changes after eccentric and concentric contractions. Muscle and Nerve 9: 59–63
Newham DJ, Jones DA, Tolfree SEJ, Edwards RHT 1986b Skeletal muscle damage: a study of isotope uptake enzyme efflux and pain after stepping exercise. European Journal of Applied Physiology 55: 106–112
Newham DJ, Hurley MV, Jones DW 1989 Ligamentous knee injuries and muscle inhibition. Journal of Orthopaedic Rheumatology 2: 163–173
Newsom-Davis JM, Mills KR 1992 Immunological associations in acquired neuromyotonia (Isaacs' syndrome): report of 5 cases and literature review. Brain 116: 453–469
Oakes B 1994 Tendons and ligaments—basic science. In: Harries M, Williams C, Stanish WD, Micheli LJ (eds) Oxford textbook of sports medicine. Oxford Medical Press, Oxford, pp 493–511
Pachman LM 1998 Polymyositis and dermatomyositis in children. In: Maddison PJ, Isenberg DA, Woo P, Glass D (eds) The Oxford textbook of rheumatology, 2nd edn. Oxford Medical Press, Oxford, pp 1287–1300
Panayi GS 1998 Polymyalgia rheumatica. In: Maddison PJ, Isenberg DA, Woo P, Glass D (eds) The Oxford textbook of rheumatology, 2nd edn. Oxford Medical Press, Oxford, pp 1373–1381
Paster SB, Adams DI, Hollenberg NK 1975 Acute renal failure in McArdle's disease and myoglobinuric states. Radiology 114: 567–570
Paul MA, Imanse J, Golding RP, Koomen AR, Meijer S 1991 Accessory soleus muscle mimicking a soft tissue tumour. Acta Orthopaedica Scandinavica 62: 609–611
Pernow BB, Havel RJ, Jennings DB 1967 The second wind phenomenon in McArdle's syndrome. Acta Medica Scandinavica (suppl) 472: 294–307
Petty RKH, Harding AE, Morgan-Hughes JA 1986 The clinical features of mitochondrial myopathy. Brain 109: 915–938
Pope FM 1998 Molecular abnormalities of collagen and connective tissue. In: Maddison PJ, Isenberg DA, Woo P, Glass D (eds) The Oxford textbook of rheumatology, 2nd edn. Oxford Medical Press, Oxford, pp 353–404
Prasher D, Smith A, Findley L 1990 Sensory and cognitive event-related potentials in myalgic encephalomyelitis. Journal of Neurology, Neurosurgery and Psychiatry 53: 247–253
Radda GK, Bone PJ, Rajagoplan B 1984 Clinical aspects of ^{31}P NMR spectroscopy. British Medical Bulletin 40: 155–159
Renstrom P 1991 Sports traumatology today. A review of common sports injury problems. Annales Chirugiae et Gynaecologiae 80: 81–93

Renstrom PAFH 1994 Introduction to chronic overuse injuries. In: Harries M, Williams C, Stanish WD, Micheli LJ (eds) Oxford textbook of sports medicine. Oxford Medical Press, Oxford, pp 531–545
Ricker K, Haass A, Hertel G, Mertens HG 1978 Transient muscular weakness in severe recessive myotonia congenita. Journal of Neurology 218: 253–262
Riddoch J, Morgan-Hughes JA 1975 Prognosis in adult polymyositis. Journal of the Neurological Sciences 26: 71–80
Rivera-Luna H, Spiegler EJ 1991 Incidental rectus abdominis muscle visualization during bone scanning. Clinical Nuclear Medicine 16: 523–527
Rockett JF, Freeman BL 1990 3D scintigraphic demonstration of pectineus muscle avulsion injury. Clinical Nuclear Medicine 15: 800–803
Ross BD, Radda GK, Gadian DG, Rolker G, Esiri M, Falloner-Smith J 1981 Examination of a case of suspected McArdle's syndrome with ^{31}P nuclear magnetic resonance. New England Journal of Medicine 304: 1338–1342
Rowland LP, Tahn S, Hirschberg E, Harter DH 1964 Myoglobinuria. Archives of Neurology 10: 537–562
Rutherford OM, White J 1991 Human quadriceps strength and fatigability in patients with post-viral syndrome. Journal of Neurology, Neurosurgery and Psychiatry 54: 961–964
Rutherford OM, Jones DA, Newham DJ 1986 Clinical and experimental application of the switch superimposition technique for the study of human muscle activation. Journal of Neurology, Neurosurgery and Psychiatry 49: 1288–1291
Safran MR, Seaber AV, Garrett WE Jr 1989 Warm-up and muscular injury prevention. An update. Sports Medicine 8: 239–249
Sallis RE, Massimo F (eds) 1997 ACSM's essentials of sports medicine. Mosby, London
Sanger JR, Krasniak CL, Matloub HS, Yousif NJ, Kneeland JB 1991 Diagnosis of an anomalous superficialis muscle in the palm by magnetic resonance imaging. Journal of Hand Surgery (America) 16: 98–101
Sayman HB, Urgancioglu I 1991 Muscle perfusion with technetium-MIBI in lower extremity peripheral arterial diseases. Journal of Nuclear Medicine 32: 1700–1703
Schmid R, Mahler R 1959 Chronic progressive myopathy with myoglobinuria: demonstration of a glycogenolytic defect in muscle. Journal of Clinical Investigation 38: 2044–2058
Schmid R, Hammaker L, 1961 Hereditary absence of muscle phosphorylase (McArdle's syndrome). New England Journal of Medicine 264: 223–225
Serratrice G, Gastaut JL, Schiand A, Pellissier JF, Carrelet P 1980 A propos de 210 cas de myalgies diffuses. Semaine des Hopitaux de Paris 56: 1241–1244
Shepherd JRL 1998 Acute and chronic over exercise: do depressed immune responses provide useful markers? International Journal of Sports Medicine 19: 59–171
Simons DG, Mense S 1998 Understanding of muscle tone as related to clinical muscle pain. Pain 75: 1–17
Sinkeler SP, Wevers RA, Joosten EM et al 1986 Improvement of screening of exertional myalgia with a standardised ischaemic forearm test. Muscle and Nerve 9: 731–737
Smith R, Stern G 1967 Myopathy, osteomalacia and hyperparathyroidism. Brain 90: 593–602
Stauber W 1989 Eccentric action of muscles: physiology, injury and adaptation. In: Pandolf KB (ed) Exercise and sports sciences reviews, vol 17. Williams & Wilkins, Baltimore, pp 157–186
Stephenson CA, Seibert JJ, Golladay ES et al 1991 Abscess of the iliopsoas muscle diagnosed by magnetic resonance imaging and ultrasonography. Southern Medical Journal 84: 509–511
Stokes M, Cooper R, Edwards RHT 1988 Normal strength and fatigability in patients with effort syndrome. British Medical Journal 297: 1014–1018
Stoller DW 1997 Magnetic resonance in orthopaedic and sports medicine. Lippincott, Philadelphia
Sylven C, Jonzon B, Fredholm BB, Kaijser L 1988 Adenosine injection into the brachial artery produces ischaemia-like pain or discomfort in the forearm. Cardiovascular Research 22: 674–678
Taimela S, Kujala UM, Osterman K 1990 Intrinsic risk factors and athletic injuries. Sports Medicine 9: 205–215
Targoff IN 1998 Polymyositis and dermatomyositis in adults. In: Maddison PJ, Isenberg DA, Woo P, Glass D (eds) The Oxford textbook of rheumatology, 2nd edn. Oxford Medical Press, Oxford, pp 1249–1286
Tarui S, Okuno G, Ikura Y, Tanaka T, Suda M, Nishikawa M 1965 Phosphofructokinase deficiency in skeletal muscle: a new type of glycogenosis. Biochemical and Biophysical Research Communications 19: 517–523
Taylor JF, Fluck D, Fluck D 1976 Tropical myositis: ultrastructural studies. Journal of Clinical Pathology 29: 1081–1084
Thomson WHS, Sweetin JC, Hamilton IJD 1975 ATP and muscle enzyme efflux after physical exertion. Clinica Chimica Acta 59: 241–245
Travell JG, Simons DG 1998 Myofascial pain and dysfunction. The Trigger Point Manual, 2nd edn. Williams & Wilkins, Baltimore, MD
Tsokos GC, Moutsopoulos HM, Steinberg AD 1981 Muscle involvement in systemic lupus erythematosus. Journal of the American Medical Association 246: 766–768
Turner RM, Peck WW, Prietto C 1991 MR of soft tissue chloroma in a patient presenting with left pubic and hip pain. Journal of Computer Assisted Tomography 15: 700–702
Valk P 1984 Muscle localisation of Tc 99m MDP after exertion. Clinics in Nuclear Medicine 9: 492–494
Vincent NE 1994 Compartment syndromes. In: Harries M, Williams C, Stanish WD, Micheli LJ (eds) Oxford textbook of sports medicine. Oxford Medical Press, Oxford, pp 564–568
Wessely S 1990 Old wine in new bottles: neurasthenia and ME. Psychological Medicine 20: 35–53
Wessely S, Newham DJ 1993 Virus syndromes and chronic fatigue. In: Vaeroy H, Merskey H (eds) Pain research and clinical management, vol 6. Progress in fibromyalgia and myofascial pain. Elsevier, Amsterdam, pp 349–360
Wessely S, Powell R 1989 Fatigue syndromes: a comparison of postviral fatigue with neuromuscular and affective disorders. Journal of Neurology, Neurosurgery and Psychiatry 52: 940–948
Wiles CM, Edwards RHT 1977 Weakness in myotonic syndromes. Lancet ii: 598–601
Wiles CM, Jones DA, Edwards RHT 1981 Fatigue in human metabolic myopathy. In: Porter R, Whelan J (eds) Human muscle fatigue: physiological mechanisms. Ciba Foundation Symposium 82. Pitman, London, pp 264–282
Willner J, Di Mauro S, Eastwood A, Hays A, Roohi R, Lovelace R 1979 Muscle carnitine deficiency: genetic heterogeneity. Journal of the Neurological Sciences 41: 235–246
Wirth WA, Farrow CC 1961 Human sparganosis. Case report and review of the subject. Journal of the American Medical Association 177: 6–9
Wood GC, Bentall RP, Gopfert M, Edwards RHT 1991 A comparative psychiatric assessment of patients with chronic fatigue syndrome and muscle disease. Psychological Medicine 21: 619–628
Yip TC, Houle S, Hayes G, Forrest I, Nelson L, Walker PM 1990 Quantitation of skeletal muscle necrosis using ^{99}Tc pyrophosphate with SPECT in a canine model. Nuclear Medicine Communications 11: 143–149
Zlatkin MB, Leninski RE, Shinkwin M et al 1990 Combined MR imaging and spectroscopy of bone and soft tissue tumours. Journal of Computer Assisted Tomography 14: 1–10

Chapter 5

Chronic back pain

Donlin M Long

Introduction

Back pain is one of the most common reasons why patients see physicians and ranks high in terms of total expenditures of health care dollars in the United States (Kelsey 1982, Frymoyer and Cats-Baril 1991, Anderson 1996). However, the problem is poorly understood and few treatments have been validated (Wiesel et al 1980, Weber 1983). One of the major issues is the lack of an appropriate classification system. Back pain is simply a complaint that originates in a large heterogeneous spectrum of diseases. Another major issue is that the actual pathophysiological causes of complaints are unknown (Long et al 1996). Even when the complaints can be associated with definable diseases, what is causing the back pain is unclear (Bogduk and Long 1980, Schwarzer et al 1995). There is reasonable evidence that overt instability causes pain and elimination of that instability will reduce pain. The strongest evidence is that root compression is associated with pain and neurological deficit (Kelsey 1975, 1982; Jonsson and Stromqvist 1993). Decompression is satisfactory treatment for a majority of patients (O'Connell 1951, Spangfort 1972). However, these two conditions are relatively rare in the spectrum of patients with back and/or leg pain complaints, and for the majority, the association of complaints with demonstrated structural abnormalities is tenuous at best (Hurme and Alaranta 1987, Weber 1994).

It is not surprising that therapies are problematical in a condition without known causes of pain (Boden et al 1990, Bigos et al 1994). Until there is a better scientific basis for understanding back pain and its treatment, we must use what is known to decide upon best current therapy for these patients (Bush et al 1992). The goal of this chapter is to provide the framework for the evaluation, diagnosis, treatment, choice, and assessment of treatment outcome for patients complaining of chronic low back pain with or without sciatica.

Classification of the complaint of low back pain

The most practical classification yet devised describes low back pain in terms of temporal characteristics. While incomplete, this classification is useful because so much of low back pain is still idiopathic (BenDebba et al 1997). *Transient low back pain* typically lasts a very short period of time and does not come to medical attention, except by history later. Treatment is usually symptomatic and instituted by the patient. Causes are virtually never known and the problem does not have great significance for practice or disability.

Acute low back pain is generally defined as pain that lasts from a few days to a few months. Back pain with or without leg radiation is common. Experience and some evidence says that the majority of these problems are self-limited and resolve spontaneously. Standard treatments have little influence upon the natural history (Long and Zeidman 1994). Typical treatment algorithms include short periods of bed rest, adequate analgesia, local physical measures, and watchful waiting. Some patients, particularly those with acute disc herniation, have intractable pain which cannot be allowed to resolve spontaneously because of its severity (Bigos et al 1994). Rarely, a significant neurological deficit may accompany pain. Both situations usually lead to prompt surgical intervention (Bell and Rothman 1984).

Persistent low back pain

In the most common schema, it is assumed that pain that persists for six months progressively leads to the chronic state defined by preoccupation with pain, depression, anxiety, and disability (Long et al 1988). In the recent past, we have identified a large group of patients in whom pain persists for more than six months without any concomitants of the chronic pain syndrome (BenDebba et al 1997). Ninety-five percent of patients seen demonstrated complaints of pain and dysfunction that reduced, but did not seriously affect, all activities otherwise. Psychological testing in them revealed patterns similar to those expected in any ill normal population. There was a 5% incidence of psychological dysfunction in the overall group. We have termed this constellation the *persistent low back pain syndrome* to differentiate it from the implications of the word chronic in the pain field. The majority of these patients suffered from spondylotic disease. There was no significant worsening or improvement with longitudinal evaluation, and these patients did not respond to typical modalities of therapy employed for them (Long et al 1996).

The chronic pain syndrome

For the past twenty years, there has been general agreement about the symptoms and signs that define a group of patients who chronically complain of pain (Long et al 1988, Long 1991). Virtually irrespective of the cause of the pain, these patients present with similar complaints and findings (Waddell et al 1980). They are preoccupied with pain and pain is the cause of their impairment. A very high percentage are depressed and anxious. There is an unusually high incidence of psychiatric diagnoses among them. An even larger number have features consistent with personality disorder. Drug misuse is common, although addictive behavior is relatively rare. These patients use medical resources heavily and are consistently disabled from pain. Specialized treatment facilities to deal with them have been developed throughout the world.

Evaluation of back and leg pain

The evaluation should begin with a careful history that describes the pain severity, location, and influences (Deyo et al 1992). Physical examination is unlikely to be diagnostic but will assess neurological and musculoskeletal abnormalities (McCombe et al 1989, Jonsson and Stromqvist 1993). During these examinations, listen for the danger signals such as night pain (intraspinal tumour), constant pain (cancer or infection), systemic symptoms (cancer or infection), and symptoms of other organ or systemic disease. Also, observe the patient's behaviour during the examination. Is there much pain behaviour? Are actions consistent with complaints? Is motor examination reliable (Waddell et al 1980)?

Unlike the acute pain problems, imaging is important in the chronic patients. Plain films with flexion/extension are important. MRI is best for most screening. CT can be used if bony pathology is suspected: with 2–3D reconstructions fixator artefacts can be reduced. CT myelogram is needed rarely, most commonly in patients with previous surgery (Wiesel et al 1984, Boden et al 1990, Cavanagh et al 1993, Ackerman et al 1997).

Back and leg pain as a manifestation of unexpected or intercurrent disease

In our own series of patients, an unexpected systemic disease was found in only 3% of patients (Long et al 1996). All had symptoms or signs that suggested something other than common spondylotic disease. Osseous metastases are the most common. Retroperitoneal inflammatory processes, sometimes associated with chronic gastrointestinal disease, pancreatitis, and chronic and acute renal disease all may cause back pain rarely. The clues that these do not represent spondylotic disease are usually obvious, although differentiation may occasionally be obscure. The pain from any of these processes is usually local. Leg radiation may occur secondary to lumbosacral plexus involvement, but is rarely typically sciatic. These pains are constant, tend not to be exacerbated by activity or relieved by rest, and are often associated with other signs or symptoms of systemic disease. Leg pain is non-radicular, as are the physical findings associated with infiltration of the plexus. Signs and symptoms that suggest intercurrent disease are intractable pain, unremitting pain, neurological deficit suggestive of lumbosacral plexus involvement, a history of cancer or inflammatory disease, a history of any disease likely to be complicated by infection, and a history of significant trauma. Evaluation of patients with any of these should include plain spine films and MRI for diagnosis. Treatment will depend upon the cause of presenting symptoms.

Osteoporosis

There is still an argument about whether osteoporosis alone can cause back pain. Many experts in spinal pain believe it can. However, the most common cause of intractable pain with osteoporosis is compression fracture. Pain with compression fracture is local and extremely severe. If the collapse is great enough, then individual nerve root compression signs and symptoms may occur. However, typically the pain does not radiate, it is focal in the back, and can be localized with great accuracy over the collapsed segment. Those at risk include post-menopausal women, and anyone with other disorders of calcium and estrogen metabolism, heavy smokers, prolonged steroid users, and any patient with prolonged immunosuppression. The diagnosis is made by plain X-ray. Treatment usually consists of rest, external support, limitation of activity, and time with therapy for the underlying problem. The pain often persists for six months or more following compression fracture.

Recently, vertebroplasty has been introduced. In this procedure, the acutely compressed segment is visualized with fluoroscopy. A needle is placed through the pedicle into the vertebral body and methyl methacrylate is injected to reinforce the collapse. Pain relief is usually immediate and may be very gratifying.

Spondylitis

The most common inflammatory condition to be associated with chronic back pain is *rheumatoid arthritis*. Back pain is usually not an early characteristic of the disease, so the diagnosis is known when back pain occurs. If systemic manifestations are not prominent, it can be difficult to be certain about the diagnosis on clinical grounds. Plain films, CT, and MR all suggest inflammatory spondylotic disease. The diagnosis is confirmed by serological testing. Treatment consists of three phases. The first is treatment of the underlying disease. The second is an exercise programme for lifelong maintenance of axial muscle strength. The third is surgical therapy for spinal instability or root compression syndromes. The majority of rheumatoid spinal problems requiring surgery are cervical, but spinal stenosis in the lumbar region does occur. The syndrome is typical neurogenic claudication. Surgery requires decompression and frequently fusion.

The second common problem is *ankylosing spondylitis*. This is a disease of males predominantly. Symptoms usually begin with back pain early in life and a progressive history of constant back pain is typical. Radicular or cord compression symptoms are uncommon. The diagnosis is made by the typical 'bamboo spine' appearance on plain X-ray or MRI. Treatment is typically symptomatic. As spontaneous fusion progresses up the spine, pain relents in the lumbar region, only to reappear at higher levels progressively.

Psoriatic arthritis is a rare similar disease. The problem is more facet arthropathy with synovial proliferation (Liu et al 1990). Thus in psoriatic arthritis, root compression syndromes are common and spinal stenosis is typical. Back pain alone is best treated symptomatically. Surgical decompression and occasional stabilization is required for root compression syndromes.

Acromegalic spondylitis is common in untreated patients. Fortunately, with the quality of therapy now available for these pituitary tumours, this problem has become very rare. The syndrome is similar to ankylosing spondylitis with progressive pain usually beginning in the lumbar region and which ceases with spontaneous fusion. Treatment is symptomatic.

Musculoskeletal pain syndromes

There are a group of people with idiopathic back and leg pain for whom no correlated underlying abnormality can be found (Panjabi et al 1982). Most complain of muscular tenderness and pain. Most have associated spasm and focal tenderness, with loss of range of motion (Pope et al 1994). There are no associated neurological signs. The back pain is typically local, but radiates diffusely upward and diffusely into hips and upper thighs (Mense 1991). The problem may be isolated to the lumbar spine or be a part of the larger syndrome called *myofascial pain*. Diagnosis is made by history and through the non-specific physical findings that typically are loss of range of motion, local pain and tenderness in muscles or at muscular insertions, and the presence of focal areas of myositis. Imaging studies typically are normal or have non-diagnostic spondylotic abnormalities. Treatment consists of anti-inflammatories, local passive therapy measures for focal areas of abnormality, and a long-term exercise program.

Abdominal and pelvic disease causing low back pain

It is rare for abdominal pelvic or hip disease to mimic spondylotic or idopathic low back pain, but a few specific diseases are important. The most common is likely to be metastatic disease to the lumbar spine, which can be diagnosed with appropriate imaging. Retroperitoneal inflammatory disease and cancer are other definable causes. Both chronic pelvic inflammatory disease and endometriosis produce low back pain and leg pain. Aortic aneurysm may produce chronic back pain associated with vascular claudication, although dissection is usually an acutely painful event. Intra-abdominal disease of other organs is so rarely confused with idiopathic chronic back pain that any are unlikely to be important in diagnosis. Renal, gallbladder, and bowel disease are so commonly associated with other symptoms that confusion in diagnosis is unlikely to occur.

Back pain as a manifestation of psychiatric disease

There is a strong tendency among physicians, and many others involved in treatment of chronic pain, to assume that all pain for which no diagnosable cause can be found is psychosomatic. Nowhere is this more true then with chronic back pain. The National Low Back Pain Study data indicate that the incidence of psychopathology is no greater in back pain patients than would be expected in any ill population. Three percent of patients in that study had a psychiatric diagnosis that was thought by the examiners to be the primary cause of the complaint (BenDebba et al 1997). However, in a population of more than 2000 patients admitted to a pain treatment programme for manifestations of the chronic pain syndrome, the incidence of psychopathology was much higher. Between 15 and 20% of these patients had a primary psychiatric diagnosis that was thought to be the origin of the pain complaint or at least an important mediator (Long et al 1988, Long 1991).

Endogeneous depression was the most common diagnosis. The psychiatrists involved with these patients separated this diagnosis from the reactive depression seen much more commonly. Somatiform disorder was the next most common diagnosis made, followed by schizophrenia. There is an important difference of opinion among pain specialists about what is the most common diagnosis. In some experiences, it is personality disorders. This chapter is not the place for an exhaustive review of these psychological factors. In this context, it is only important to emphasize that psychiatric disease may have pain as an important symptom. The presence of psychiatric disease does not eliminate the probability that the patient has a diagnosable separate cause.

It is much more likely that symptoms in patients with idiopathic low back pain are ascribed to psychosomatic causes than for patients with symptoms secondary to psychiatric disease to be misdiagnosed as organic problems.

Spondylotic low back pain (idiopathic)

The majority of patients who present complaining of low back pain with or without leg pain have associated spondylotic spinal disease. The presence of spondylosis and the complaints are at least correlated, but the correlation is far from certain (Boden et al 1990, Wiesel et al 1984). Even if the relationship is causative, the mechanisms by which the pain is produced are largely unknown. The diagnostic problem is that a substantial number of patients have spondylotic changes without any apparent related symptoms. Yet, in a sizeable majority of patients with chronic back pain complaints, spondylotic changes are present and are the only abnormalities that seem to explain the pain.

The history of the problem is the most important diagnostic tool. Patients with pain of apparent spondylitic origin characteristically have more pain when standing or load bearing. Most are improved by rest. A minority are worsened by reclining, although this is usually limited to reclining in extension. Non-steroidal analgesics are of limited use, and pain is temporarily relieved by simple local modalities such as heat and massage. The pain is local in the lumbar region and the patient often can precisely identify an origin with a fingertip. Severe back pain is often associated with non-radicular leg pain, usually diffuse and aching in anterior or posterior thighs. Associated true radicular pain is common, as is neurogenic claudication.

Diagnosis

Diagnosis is made with plain X-ray, CT, or MRI, all of which demonstrate different characteristics of the disease (Ackerman et al 1997). The earliest changes are dissication of the disc. The nucleus loses its definitive character and the disc narrows, becomes irregular, and loses water. First acute and then chronic inflammatory changes occur in the surrounding bone of the end plate and beyond. Discs erode the end plates and interosseous herniation occurs. There is associated ligamentous thickening, anterior and posterior disc bulges occur, and traction spurs appear anteriorly or posteriorly. The canal may narrow and degenerative changes in facets are typical. Canal narrowing is a combination of facet overgrowth, synovial hypertrophy, ligamentous thickening, and bony enlargement.

Treatment of spondylitic back pain

Surgical procedures are of value only for the relief of demonstrated nerve root compression, correction of a fixed deformity, or stabilizing an unstable segment (O'Connell 1951, Hanley et al 1991, Zdeblick 1993). Pain associated with spondylosis alone does not constitute a reason for surgery. For the majority of patients, no direct intervention is likely to be of value. Therapy is symptomatic (Waddell 1987a). For patients whose symptoms have been present six months or longer, there is strong new evidence that spontaneous improvement will not occur. The evidence is equally good that the usual conservative measures, as they are applied in a typical practice, are not useful and cannot be differentiated from no treatment. Our studies have examined many forms of standard physical therapy, manipulation therapy, and a wide variety of other treatments, including acupuncture, back schools, nutritional therapies, pain treatment centres, and cognitive therapies. We were unable to determine any effect of any of these treatments as currently applied in practice. Therefore, it will not suffice to simply refer patients for any of these treatments. A programme based upon the best available data should be individualized for each patient (Hsieh et al 1992, Koes et al 1992, Meade et al 1995).

Adequate analgesia is a first choice. Nonsteroidal anti-inflammatory analgesics are standard (Bigos et al 1994). Some investigators are examining the use of long-acting narcotics for the relief of pain of benign origin. Some patients will be benefited by short-term bracing, especially when active; so a trial lumbosacral support is worthwhile. There is reasonable evidence that an individualized exercise programme to strengthen the paravertebral and abdominal muscles, combined with local measures to restore painless range of motion, will benefit many patients. Weight loss has not been proven to be beneficial, but reduction in weight makes intuitive sense and is included in most vigorous rehabilitation efforts (Heliovaara 1987). These vigorous physical therapy programmes require real commitment from patient and physician, if they are to be successful. Serious osteoporosis should be treated, as well.

The facet syndrome

A small subset of patients have pain which apparently is generated from lumbar zygapophyseal joints (Bogduk and Long 1980, Moran et al 1988). Typically, these patients complain of local pain and often can point to the involved joint. Movement is painful. Rest is helpful, and axial loading particularly produces pain.

Imaging studies demonstrate arthropathy. Joints are hypertrophied. Synovial cysts are common. The cartilage end plates are eroded, and both acute and chronic inflammatory changes occur around the articular surfaces. Subluxations are common.

A diagnosis is validated when injection of local anaesthetic into the joint or its innervation produces pain relief. Radiofrequency destruction of the innervation has proven to be useful, providing lasting relief for the majority of patients who fit the diagnostic criteria. In our experience, this is a very small percentage, being no more than 1 to 2% of patients presenting with back pain (Bogduk and Long 1980).

Spinal stenosis

The syndrome of spinal stenosis is signified by back pain and leg pain with claudication. Patients typically present first with simple gait disturbance. That is, they have trouble walking well after ambulating for more than a short time. Then pain occurs and the hallmark of the diagnosis is painful weakness in both legs brought on by walking. Typically, these patients are relieved upon cessation of walking and often assume a flexed sitting position to speed resolution of symptoms. These features differentiate it from vascular claudication whose symptoms resolve immediately after cessation of activity. Sensory complaints are usually stocking-like and suggestive of metabolic peripheral neuropathy with which the problem is often confused. The neurological examination may be entirely normal at rest, but both motor and sensory loss can appear after activity.

The diagnosis is made with imaging studies. Either MRI or CT will make the diagnosis.

The treatment for spinal stenosis when symptoms are severe is surgical decompression. Outcomes are excellent. The issue is when are symptoms serious enough to warrant operation. The majority of patients have mild to moderate incapacity and do not necessarily require surgery. When symptoms become significantly incapacitating or when progressive important neurological deficits occur, then surgery is indicated.

Foraminal root compression syndrome

A variation of the spinal stenosis problem occurs when there is compression of an isolated root in a spondylotic foramen. Patients present with the acute disc herniation in terms of complaints, but the time course is protracted and onset has usually been gradual. Patients complain of sciatica or femoral pain in the accepted distribution of a single root. Sometimes root involvement is bilateral and occasionally more than one root on one side is affected. However, the syndrome is not of claudication. It is one of ongoing root compression. That is, the pain tends to be constant, although it is often exacerbated by activity, being upright, and axial loading. The associated reflex, motor, and sensory changes relate to the individual root. A positive straight leg raising is unusual, which is different than the tension sign of the acute disc herniation. Diagnosis is made by MR and CT, which visualize the neural foramina and the compression of the nerve root.

If the pain is tolerable and there is no major neurological deficit, then a thorough trial of an individualized exercise activity programme is indicated (Saal and Saal 1989). If the rehabilitation programme is not effective and pain is intractable, or if there are associated neurological deficits, then surgery should proceed (Saal et al 1990). The outcome of surgery should be as good as that enjoyed for acute disc herniation.

Spinal instability and progressive deformity syndromes

A significant number of patients with spondylotic disease will develop progressive spinal deformities. These are degenerative in nature for the majority, although congenital and traumatic instability certainly can occur and will be similar in presentation. Fortunately, the treatment is very much the same, so it makes very little difference about aetiology (Cholewicki and McGill 1996).

Degenerative spondylolisthesis

This is the most common of the problems encountered. The slip may occur in either anterior or posterior direction. It may be actively moving and demonstrable on dynamic films. It may be slowly progressive and occasionally may be fixed. Patients typically complain of back pain in the lumbar area with or without associated root signs. Diagnosis is made by plain X-rays, which should include dynamic films to be certain whether the spine is moving actively.

Treatment should be symptomatic, unless pain is intractable or significant nerve root compression with neurological deficit is occurring. Symptomatic therapies include bracing, modification of lifestyle, and individualized active exercise for axial muscle strengthening, range of motion, and leg strength. Surgery should be considered when axial back pain, radicular pain, or both are severe and disabling. Most patients with progressive listhesis or slowly progressive scoliotic deformities of any kind will require fixator use for stabilization and fusion. It is best to proceed when it is apparent that symptoms are serious enough to warrant surgery, but before extremely severe deformities occur (Raugstad et al 1982, Zdeblick 1993).

The failed back syndrome

The failed back syndrome is an imprecise term usually used to categorize a large group of patients who have undergone one or more operations on the lumbar spine without benefit (Waddell 1987b, Long 1991). The patient who has not benefited from one or more operations needs an evaluation that, if anything, is more complex than that for the patient who has not undergone surgery (Fager and Freidberg 1980). The goal of the evaluation should be the most precise definition of abnormalities possible, so that an individualized treatment plan can be prescribed. Patients fall into broad categories within this heterogeneous group that are useful for guiding the evaluation and the therapeutic plans (Long et al 1988). The first of these broad categories is a group of patients for whom *surgery was probably not indicated in the first place*. The second group of patients is those with clear indications for surgery, but in whom *surgery did not correct the original abnormality*. A third category of patients is those in whom some *significant complication of surgery* occurred and is now the pain generator. There is another very small group of patients in whom an *intercurrent diagnosis has been missed.*

Whatever the proposed treatment plan, precise definition of the abnormalities likely to be generating the pain and that must be treated is imperative (Frymoyer et al 1978). Specifically, if any reoperative surgery is to be done, it should be planned for abnormalities that are as well defined as those for first surgery (Finnegan et al 1979). It is still true in these patients that surgery will only benefit individuals who have nerve root compression or clearly demonstrable instability (Turner et al 1992).

Common post-operative pain syndromes

Inappropriate patient selection

Analysis of patients who present with failure of pain relief after first-time lumbar surgery often suggests that the majority have not met accepted criteria before operation and were lacking symptoms, signs, and imaging demonstration of either root compression or instability syndromes. When previous studies and records are available, they will validate or refute the original indications for surgery. The fact that the original surgery was not obviously indicated does not imply the patient does not now have a correctable problem. Re-evaluation is warranted. It is important to remember that failure of first surgery with residual pain is not an indication for a second surgery. Indications for surgery in reoperation should be as stringent as those applied for first (Spengler and Freeman 1979). Stereotyped addition of fusion because of a failed first procedure is unwarranted.

Failure to correct the initial pathology

Another common problem is that the original surgeon simply did not do an operation designed to completely correct the original disease. Common examples are failure to decompress a nerve root or roots through foraminotomy, failure to decompress the spinal canal, wrong level, failure to remove a disc entirely, and failure to recognize and stabilize unstable segments. Repeat of the imaging studies will usually demonstrate the residual abnormality. When these abnormalities are concordant with the patient's complaints, surgical repair is virtually as successful as first-time operation.

Surgical complications

There are a large number of complications that can occur. These include nerve root injury, pseudomeningocele, surgically induced instability, infection, and excessive scar formation.

Fixators have their own set of problems. Fusions may fail (pseudarthrosis) (Steinman and Herkowitz 1992). Hardware may loosen and even extrude. Sometimes hardward is inappropriately placed. It is important to examine all patients who have undergone fusion to assess the competency of bony fusion, location of fixators and their stability, and the appropriateness of fixator placement (Kozak and O'Brien 1990).

There are other problems related to surgery that are not direct or even immediate complications. Fixation of one or more spinal segments may lead to degeneration of the segment above. Sometimes this is acute, but more typically it is a chronic problem. The symptoms are those of instability and stenosis above the fusion.

A large number of patients have obviously thick scar, which may deform the thecal sac following surgery. The significance of these scars is uncertain. There is no evidence that operating upon those that are not compressive will benefit the patient (Bandschuh et al 1990).

Arachnoiditis

This is an unusual problem, if viewed as a clinical syndrome and not as a radiological finding. Many patients who have undergone spinal surgery with or without myelography demonstrate root adhesions and adherence of nerve roots to dural sac. Most of these findings have no obvious clinical significance, but some do seem to be associated with symptoms. However, chronic adhesive arachnoiditis is rarely progressive and needs to be considered with some patients. Symptoms of this rare syndrome are diffuse lower extremity pain, often burning in character, with slowly progressive loss of function. MRI may suggest arachnoiditis, but myelography is required to really be certain of the degree of arachnoiditis, particularly when spinal stenosis is present. Arachnoiditis was most commonly associated with infection when first described and then was described as a complication of myelography and surgery. Arachnoiditis is now seen in patients who have not had myelography, as a complication of surgery alone. When the rare progressive problem is present, there is little question of the relationship between the myelographic findings of arachnoiditis and the symptomatology. However, for the majority of patients, the relationship between arachnoiditis and symptoms is still uncertain. Simply finding arachnoiditis does not imply that this pathological process is the cause of the patient's complaints. Pain is usually treated by spinal cord stimulation (Long et al 1981).

Theoretical causes of low back pain

Because back and leg pain often are unaccompanied by obvious diagnosable instability or clearly defined nerve root compression, there have been extensive investigations into possible causes of the pain. In some patients, it appears that the pain arises mostly from ligaments and muscles (Panjabi et al 1982). At least, no other causes have been defined. Three other lines of investigation are being followed. The first of these suggests that the pain may be neuropathic in type and may originate from minor degrees of demyelinization and sensitization, probably accompanied by central receptor changes (Wall and Gutnick 1974, Calvin et al 1982, Devor et al 1991). A variety of factors and possible mechanisms are being examined. None of these are clearly applicable to typical patients with chronic back and leg pain, as yet.

A second important line of inquiry suggests that the nerve activation and sensitization is secondary to the release of inflammatory products secondary to degeneration, spondylotic changes, and/or surgical trauma (Schwarzer et al 1995).

A third general category is termed by its originators' micromovement. In this concept, the noxious stimuli come from small but abnormal degrees of movement in zygapophyseal joints and in and around the disc. These movements presumably would activate nociceptors in ligaments, periosteum, and muscles (Kuslich et al 1991, Gracely et al 1992).

Further evaluation of the patient without an apparent cause of pain

After all these specific abnormalities have been diagnosed or excluded there remains a majority of patients for whom no currently definable cause of pain has been found. Some of them respond well to non-specific conservative measures, but many do not. Many spinal experts have continued to examine these patients with physiologic techniques to try to add information to the anatomical data available from imaging studies.

The hypothesis that underlies the use of *temporary diagnostic blockade* to augment clinical decision making is straightforward; that is, anaesthetization of a pain generator should produce relief of the pain being produced. Additions include production of pain by mechanical irritation of the generator and control by placebo injections (Bogduk et al 1995a).

There is probably no current area in the field of spinal disease more misunderstood than is the use of diagnostic blocks to aid the clinician in identifying painful segments or structures in the lumbar spine. A few principles must be understood if blocks are to be applied appropriately. Current evidence indicates that these blocks are effective in identifying painful segments, but are not necessarily specific for individual structures blocked, since there appears to be much overlap in multiple blocks of different types in the same segment (Knox and Chapman 1993). Placebo-controlled blocks are more accurate than others. Blocks without a negative control are suspect (Bogduk et al 1995b).

Blocks in current use include blockade of zygapophyseal joints, individual root blocks, block of donor site and pseudarthroses, and provocative disc blockade. The current use of these blocks is to support a clinical impression of the origin of the complaint of pain. As yet, the next major step has not been taken. That is, there is no study available that clearly demonstrates the predictive power of any of these blocks to estimate the chance of a good result from a rationally chosen interventional procedure. Nevertheless, they are useful in the hands of an expert clinician who performs them well and interprets them without bias.

Alternatives for care of chronic low back pain

It is not surprising that a clinical problem as poorly understood as low back pain should generate a huge number of therapies devised to be helpful. Most are as yet unproven, although many are supported by long-standing practice.

The first general category comprises all those adjuncts that claim to make people more comfortable. The list is long: adjustable beds, firm mattresses, chairs, pillows, supports, and whirlpools to name a few. Patients may try those that seem attractive to them, and use those that are comfortable. I tend to discourage use of those that are excessively expensive and will not prescribe any.

Many patients are in long-term programmes of passive therapy measures such as heat, massage, and electrical stimulation, or active programmes of massage and manipulation. The value of any of these is not supported by strong evidence in chronic back pain. I tell patients to continue if they are convinced they are symptomatically better (O'Connell 1951).

Patients also seek acupuncture, and a variety of related and unrelated therapies such as are available from mail-order catalogues. None are supported by scientific data in chronic back pain, and I do not recommend any. This is also true of the many herbal remedies patients buy.

There are a large number of books, tapes, and videos available on the topic of back pain. Most are helpful; a few could be dangerous. It's best to find some you like and recommend them, rather than allowing the patient to choose indiscriminately. Many minimally invasive techniques that promise patients no-risk relief have appeared. Some of the most popular were and are chymopapain intradiscal injection (Martins et al 1978), steroid in epidural or intradiscal spaces (Heyse-Moore 1978, Berman et al 1984, Bowman et al 1993), percutaneous discectomy (Choy et al 1987, Kambin 1988, Onik et al 1990, Revel et al 1993), endoscopic laser discectomy, endoscopic discectomy, endoscopic fusion, and microdiscectomy. All are techniques for experts. Some have come and gone. Some are being evaluated. None are clearly established to have an important role in chronic low back and leg pain.

References

Ackerman SJ, Steinberg EP, Bryan RN, BenDebba M, Long DM 1997 Persistent low back pain in patients suspected of having herniated nucleus pulposus: radiologic predictors of functional outcome—implications for treatment selection. Radiology 203(3): 815–822

Anderson GBJ 1996 The epidemiology of spinal disorders. In: Frymoyer JW (ed) The adult spine, principles and practice, 2nd edn. Lippincott, Philadelphia

Bandschuh CV, Stein L, Slusser JH et al 1990 Distinguishing between scar and recurrent herniated disk in postoperative patients: Value of contrast-enhanced and MR imaging. American Journal of Neuroradiology 11: 949–958

Bell GR, Rothman RH 1984 The conservative treatment of sciatica. Spine 9: 54–56

BenDebba M, Torgerson WS, Long DM 1997 Personality traits, pain duration and severity, functional impairment, and psychological distress in patients with persistent low back pain. Pain 72: 115–125

Berman AT, Garbarino JL Jr, Fisher SM et al 1984 The effects of epidural injection of local anesthetics and corticosteroids on patients with lumbosciatic pain. Clinical Orthopaedics 188: 144–151

Bigos SJ, Bowyer O, Braen G et al 1994 Acute low back problems in adults. In: Clinical Practice Guideline No 14 (AHCPR Publication No 95-0642). US Department of Health and Human Services, Rockville, MD

Boden SD, Davis DO, Dina TS et al 1990 Abnormal magnetic-resonance scans of the lumbar spine in asymptomatic subjects: a prospective investigation. Journal of Bone and Joint Surgery 72A: 403–408

Bogduk N 1991 The lumbar disc and low back pain. Neurosurgery Clinics of North America 2: 791–806

Bogduk N, Long DM 1980 Percutaneous lumbar medial branch neurotomy. A modification of facet denervation. Spine 5(2): 193–200

Bogduk N, Aprill C, Derby R 1995a Discography. In: White AH (ed) Spine care: diagnosis and conservative treatment. CV Mosby, St. Louis, MO, pp 219–238

Bogduk N, Aprill C, Derby R 1995b Selective nerve root blocks. In: Wilson DJ (ed) Interventional radiology of the musculoskeletal system. Edward Arnold, London, pp 121–132

Bowman SJ, Wedderburn L, Whaley A et al 1993 Outcome assessment after epidural corticosteroid injection for low back pain and sciatica. Spine 18: 1345–1350

Bush K, Cowan N, Katz DE et al 1992 The natural history of sciatica associated with disc pathology: a prospective study with clinical and independent radiologic follow-up. Spine 17: 1205–1212

Calvin WH, Devor M, Howe JF 1982 Can neuralgias arise from minor demyelination? Spontaneous firing, mechanosensitivity and after-discharge from conducting axons. Experimental Neurology 75: 755–763

Cavanagh S, Stevens J, Johnson JR 1993 High-resolution MRI in the investigation of recurrent pain after lumbar discectomy. Journal of Bone and Joint Surgery 75B: 524–528

Cholewicki J, McGill SM 1996 Mechanical stability of the in vivo lumbar spine: implications for injury and chronic low back pain. Clinical Biomechanics 11: 1–15

Choy DS, Case RB, Field W et al 1987 Letter: Percutaneous laser nucleolysis of lumbar disks. New England Journal of Medicine 317: 771–772

Devor M, Basbaum AI, Bennett GJ et al 1991 Mechanisms of neuropathic pain following peripheral injury. In Basbaum AI, Besson JMR (eds) Towards a new pharmacotherapy of pain. Wiley, Chichester, pp 417–440

Deyo RA, Rainville J, Kent DL 1992 What can the history and physical examination tell us about low back pain? Journal of American Medical Association 268: 760–765

Fager CA, Freidberg SR 1980 Analysis of failures and poor results of lumbar spine surgery. Spine 5: 87–94

Finnegan WJ, Fenlin JM, Marvel JP et al 1979 Results of surgical intervention in the symptomatic multiply-operated back patient: Analysis of sixty-seven cases followed for three to seven years. Journal of Bone and Joint Surgery 61A: 1077–1082

Frymoyer JW, Cats-Baril WL 1991 An overview of the incidences and costs of low back pain. Orthopaedic Clinics of North America 22: 263–271

Frymoyer JW, Matteri RE, Hanley EN et al 1978 Failed lumbar disc surgery requiring second operation: a long-term follow-up study. Spine 3: 7–11

Gracely RH, Lynch SA, Bennett GJ 1992 Painful neuropathy: Altered central processing maintained dynamically by peripheral input. Pain 51: 175–194

Hanley EN Jr, Phillips ED, Kostuik JP 1991 Who should be fused? In: Frymoyer JW, Ducker TB, Hadler NM et al (eds) The adult spine: principles and practice, vol 2. Raven Press, New York, pp 1893–1917

Heliovaara M 1987 Body height, obesity, and risk of herniated lumbar intervertebral disc. Spine 12: 469–472

Heyse-Moore GH 1978 A rational approach to the use of epidural medication in the treatment of sciatic pain. Acta Orthopaedica Scandinavica 49: 366–370

Hsieh CY, Phillips RB, Adams AH et al 1992 Functional outcomes of low back pain: Comparison of four treatment groups in a

randomized controlled trial. Journal of Manipulative Physiological Therapeutics 15: 4–9
Hurme M, Alaranta H 1987 Factors predicting the result of surgery for lumbar intervertebral disc herniation. Spine 12: 933–938
Jonsson B, Stromqvist B 1993 Symptoms and signs in degeneration of the lumbar spine: a prospective, consecutive study of 300 operated patients. Journal of Bone and Joint Surgery 75B: 381–385
Kambin P 1988 Percutaneous lumbar discectomy: current practice. Surgical Rounds of Orthopaedics 2: 31–35
Kelsey JL 1975 An epidemiological study of acute herniated lumbar intervertebral discs. Rheumatological Rehabilitation 14: 144–159
Kelsey JL 1982 Idiopathic low back pain: Magnitude of the problem. In: White AA III, Gordon SL (eds) American Academy of Orthopaedic Surgeons Symposium on Idiopathic Low Back Pain. CV Mosby, St. Louis, MO, pp 5–8
Knox BD, Chapman TM 1993 Anterior lumbar interbody fusion for discogram concordant pain. Journal of Spinal Disorders 6: 242–244
Koes BW, Bouter LM, van Mameren H et al 1992 The effectiveness of manual therapy, physiotherapy, and treatment by the general practitioner for nonspecific back and neck complaints: a randomized clinical trial. Spine 17: 28–35
Kozak JA, O'Brien JP 1990 Simultaneous combined anterior and posterior fusion: An independent analysis of a treatment for the disabled low-back pain patient. Spine 15: 322–328
Kuslich SD, Ulstrom CL, Michael CJ 1991 The tissue origin of low back pain and sciatica: A report of pain response to tissue stimulation during operations on the lumbar spine using local anesthesia. Orthopedic Clinics of North America 22: 181–187
Liu SS, Williams KD, Drayer BP et al 1990 Synovial cysts of the lumbosacral spine: diagnosis by MR imaging. American Journal of Roentgenology 154: 163–166
Long DM 1991 Failed back surgery syndrome. Neurosurgery Clinics of North America 2(4): 899–919
Long DM, Zeidman SM 1994 Outcome of low back pain therapy. In: Hadley MN (ed) Perspectives in neurological surgery, vol 5, no 1. Quality Medical, St. Louis, pp 41–51
Long DM, Erickson D, Campbell J, North R 1981 Electrical stimulation of the spinal cord and peripheral nerves for pain control. A 10-year experience. Applied Neurophysiology 44: 207–217
Long DM, Filtzer DL, BenDebba M, Hendler NH 1988 Clinical features of the failed-back syndrome. Journal of Neurosurgery 69: 61–71
Long DM, BenDebba M, Torgerson WS et al 1996 Persistent back pain and sciatica in the United States: patient characteristics. Journal of Spinal Disorders 9(1): 40–58
Martins AN, Ramirez A, Johnston J et al 1978 Double-blind evaluation of chemonucleolysis for herniated lumbar discs: late results. Journal of Neurosurgery 49: 816–827
McCombe PF, Fairbank JC, Cockersole BC et al 1989 Reproducibility of physical signs in low-back pain. Spine 14: 908–918
Meade TW, Dyer S, Browne W et al 1995 Randomised comparison of chiropractic and hospital outpatient management for low back pain: results from extended follow up. British Medical Journal 311: 349–351
Mense S 1991 Considerations concerning the neurobiological basis of muscle pain. Canadian Journal of Physiological Pharmacology 69: 610–616
Moran R, O'Connell D, Walsh MG 1988 The diagnostic value of facet joint injections. Spine 13: 1407–1410
O'Connell JEA 1951 Protrusions of the lumbar intervertebral discs: a clinical review based on five hundred cases treated by excision of the protrusion. Journal of Bone and Joint Surgery 33B: 8–30
Onik G, Mooney V, Maroon JC et al 1990 Automated percutaneous discectomy: a prospective multi-institutional study. Neurosurgery 26: 228–233
Panjabi MM, Goel VK, Takata K 1982 Physiologic strains in lumbar spinal ligaments: an in vitro biomechanical study. Spine 7: 192–203
Pope MH, Phillips RB, Haugh LD et al 1994 A prospective randomized three-week trial of spinal manipulation, transcutaneous muscle stimulation, massage and corset in the treatment of subacute low back pain. Spine 19: 2571–2577
Raugstad TS, Harbo K, Oogberg A et al 1982 Anterior interbody fusion of the lumbar spine. Acta Orthopaedica Scandinavica 53: 561–565
Revel M, Payan C, Vallee C et al 1993 Automated percutaneous lumbar discectomy versus chemonucleolysis in the treatment of sciatica: A randomized multicenter trial. Spine 18: 1–7
Saal JA, Saal JS 1989 Nonoperative treatment of herniated lumbar intervertebral disc with radiculopathy: an outcome study. Spine 14: 431–437
Saal JA, Saal JS, Herzog RJ 1990 The natural history of lumbar intervertebral disc extrusions treated nonoperatively. Spine 15: 683–686
Schwarzer AC, Aprill CN, Derby R et al 1995 The prevalence and clinical features of internal disc disruption in patients with chronic low back pain. Spine 20: 1878–1883
Spangfort EV 1972 The lumbar disc herniation: A computer-aided analysis of 2,504 operations. Acta Orthopaedica Scandinavica 142(suppl): 1–95
Spengler DM, Freeman CW 1979 Patient selection for lumbar discectomy: an objective approach. Spine 4: 129–134
Steinmann JC, Herkowitz HN 1982 Pseudarthrosis of the spine. Clinical Orthopaedics 284: 80–90
Turner JA, Ersek M, Herron L et al 1992 Patient outcomes after lumbar spinal fusions. Journal of American Medical Association 268: 907–911
Waddell G 1987a A new clinical model for the treatment of low-back pain. Spine 12: 632–644
Waddell G 1987b Failures of disc surgery and repeat surgery. Acta Orthopaedica Belgica 53: 300–302
Waddell G, McCulloch JA, Kummel E et al 1980 Nonorganic physical signs in low back pain. Spine 5: 117–125
Wall PD, Gutnick M 1974 Ongoing activity in peripheral nerves: The physiology and pharmacology of impulses originating from a neuroma. Experimental Neurology 43: 580–593
Weber H 1983 Lumbar disc herniation: A controlled, prospective study with ten years of observation. Spine 8: 131–140
Weber H 1994 The natural history of disc herniation and the influence of intervention. Spine 19: 2234–2238
Wiesel SW, Cuckler JM, Deluca F et al 1980 Acute low-back pain: an objective analysis of conservative therapy. Spine 5: 324–330
Wiesel SW, Tsourmas N, Feffer HL et al 1984 A study of computer-assisted tomography: I. The incidence of positive CAT scans in an asymptomatic group of patients. Spine 9: 549–551
Zdeblick TA 1993 A prospective, randomized study of lumbar fusion: preliminary results. Spine 18: 983–991

Chapter 6

Upper extremity pain

Anders E Sola

Introduction

Upper extremity pain can be an enigma to physicians because it may be related to many different conditions: degeneration of cervical spine processes, degeneration of the affected joint, trauma to the cervical spine or affected joint, vascular compromise, nerve impingement, thoracic or abdominal pathology, or any combination of these elements. Further, pain that emanates from a joint area may involve muscle, ligaments, tendons, or the capsule. Therefore unless the aetiology of pain is obvious, the clinical management of upper extremity pain begins with a determination, through history and examination, of whether the pain is intrinsic to the shoulder area, extrinsic, or of combined aetiologies (Table 6.1) (DePalma 1973, Bateman 1978, Calliet 1981).

Intrinsic shoulder pain

Intrinsic pain is most often caused by acute trauma, minor chronic trauma (overuse or strain), arthritides (osteoarthritis is fairly common, rheumatoid arthritis less so), local infection or tumour, infectious arthritis, and capsulitis in association with any condition that causes splinting. When the supraspinatus tendon, acromioclavicular joint, sternoclavicular joint, or anterior subacromial area is implicated as the source of pain, the specific structure will be exquisitely sensitive to touch (Steindler 1959, DePalma 1973). Examination for trigger points requires more diligence and pressure to identify the cause of pain referral (Travell and Simons 1983).

Extrinsic shoulder pain

Cervical radiculopathy affecting the C5–T1 roots is a common neurological cause of shoulder pain; however, cervical lesions may cause multilevel nerve root irritation without radiculitis (Bateman 1978). Other neurological disorders affecting the shoulder are pathology in the cervical roots, the brachial plexus and the axillary, suprascapular, or other peripheral nerves (Gerhart et al 1985).

Additional causes of extrinsic pain are myofascial trigger points in the muscles of the neck and shoulder, severe temporomandibular joint disease, cervicodorsal ligamental sprains, thoracic outlet syndromes, injuries to the brachial plexus, and referred pain from visceral disorders, such as gallstones, cholecystitis, hepatitis, myocardial infarction, pneumonitis, or tumours of the lung or spinal cord (Bonica 1990). When pain is referred to the shoulder, a common site of pain is the anterior-

Table 6.1 Causes of shoulder pain

Intrinsic causes
The joint
Acromioclavicular separation
Acute with instability
Chronic with degenerative joint disease
Adhesive capsulitis (idiopathic, secondary)
Glenohumeral instability (capsular laxity, labrum tear)
Periarticular
Myofascial syndromes
Bursitis, tendinitis (supraspinatus, infraspinatus, bicipital)
Impingement (subacromial)
Rotator cuff tear
Other
Fracture (proximal humerus, scapula, clavicle)
Myofascial trigger points in interscapular, periscapular muscles
Tumour (metastatic, primary)
Extrinsic causes of shoulder pain
Elbow or wrist pathology (carpal tunnel syndrome)
Cervical or thoracic nerve root irritation; spondylosis; herniated disc
Injuries to the brachial plexus
Myofascial trigger points in the trapezii, levator scapulae, scalenae, pectoralis muscles
Thoracic outlet syndrome (cervical rib, scalenus anticus)
Somatic disorders (free air under diaphragm)
Visceral disorders (gallstones, cholecystitis, hepatitis, myocardial infarction, pneumonitis or tumours of lung/spinal cord)

Adapted from Gerhart et al (1985).

superior portion of the shoulder. Three clues suggest exclusively extrinsic causes:

1. virtual absence of objective findings in the shoulder joint
2. normal active and passive range of movement (ROM) without pain
3. absence of point tenderness with direct pressure on the bicipital tendon, supraspinatus tendon, and the clavicular joints.

Pain referred from the shoulder is rarely felt beyond the insertion of the deltoid; therefore a primary or secondary extrinsic cause is suggested when the extremities are affected. Pain of combined intrinsic and extrinsic aetiology increases with ageing; i.e., in older patients shoulder pain is more likely to be complicated by spondylosis or multiple involvement of nerve root and degeneration of the joint, particularly of muscles of the rotator cuff. Myofascial disorders are often present as a secondary disorder in conjunction with acute or non-acute trauma and degenerative conditions.

Finally, there are a number of factors that may contribute to the aetiology and intensity of a painful event. These include stressors, either physical or psychological, latent trigger points from previous injuries, and the patient's physical and psychological 'interpretation' of the pain and its importance.

Important elements of the history

The first purpose of the history is to determine whether the pain experienced in the upper extremity actually originates in the structures of the neck, shoulder, forearm, or wrist. Observation of the total patient is important. Does the patient appear ill? Is he or she feverish or reporting recent illness? What is the patient's age and general health status? Does the patient appear tense or report unusual stresses?

Pertinent data can usually be elicited by asking what the patient thinks the problem is. If it is necessary to lead the patient, the examiner should ask what has happened recently, whether the patient has been involved in a motor vehicle accident in the past, or whether there has been any change in work or recreational activities.

Always using the vocabulary of the patient, the history taker should question him or her closely about the chronological development of the symptoms and the onset and nature of the pain. Where is it felt? Does it feel superficial or deep, such as bone pain? What does it feel like? 'Pins and needles', 'burning sensations', and 'shooting pains' are terms easily understood. Does the patient experience a 'grating feeling' when turning the head or neck? Does he or she experience electric-like pain on flexion or extension of the neck? Has the patient experienced any arthritis/gout/rheumatic problems? Does the patient have other aches and pains? Difficulty in swallowing? Does the patient have unusual sensations into the hand or fingers? Has the patient had the same problem before? If so, what was the diagnosis and treatment?

It is wise also to question the effects of the pain. Is there anything the patient normally does that he or she cannot do because of pain? Does riding in a car aggravate the condition? Does pain result in limitation of movements or weakness? Is it worse at night? Does it interfere with sleep or result in the patient's assuming different sleeping positions?

The history should also include recent medical care and medication or drug use. Has the patient been treated recently by another physician? Were any X-rays taken? Has the patient been hospitalized, particularly because of injury to the back or upper extremity? Is the patient taking any drugs, antibiotics? Heavy alcohol consumption may be a significant clue and exposure to industrial chemicals may play a part in upper extremity pain. (See also Chap. 17 for a discussion of peripheral neuropathies caused by diabetes or thyroid disease, nutritional deficiencies, metabolic disorders, infections, and other entities.)

Examination

Head, neck, and cervical spine

A thorough screening to determine the probable aetiology of upper extremity pain usually begins with at least a routine evaluation of head, neck, and cervical spine. The few procedures outlined below are adequate to eliminate these structures as the probable source of pain in the initial assessment.

1. Visual inspection, looking for deformities, atrophy, loss of normal contour
2. Palpation of spinous and transverse processes, thyroid gland, and carotid pulse
3. Range of movement of head and neck, with rotation right to left, flexion/extension, and lateral bending
4. Distraction or evaluation of the effect of cervical traction by placing hands on occiput and under chin
5. Compression: if neural foramina are compromised, this may produce or intensify pain
6. Valsalva manoeuvre to determine whether straining with breath holding reproduces pain
7. Lhermitte's sign: flexion or extension of the head and neck causes lancinating or 'electric' shock radiating from neck into hands (Brody and Wilkins 1969)
8. Adson's test: in the modified Adson's test, the patient's arm is abducted to 90° and externally rotated with the elbow flexed. The patient turns the head towards the abducted arm, takes a deep breath, and coughs. The test is positive if the radial pulse is reduced or absent. This may indicate compression of the subclavian artery (Adson 1951).

Testing for radiculitis is based on radiation of symptoms such as sensory changes, weakness, and loss of reflexes. If the symptoms are aggravated by cervical tests that stretch the nerve roots, increase intraspinal pressure (Valsalva manoeuvre), or decrease the spinal foramina (head compression), the diagnosis is implied.

Cervical spondylosis, which results in gradually increasing clinical signs, may present multiple levels of nerve root irritation and contribute to confusion of diagnosis, particularly in patients over 55 years of age. In younger age groups, single nerve root involvement due to cervical herniation is more common (see Chap. 19).

A summary of neurological levels relating to the upper extremity is shown in Table 6.2. Weakness in any of these extremity structures calls for further evaluation of the cervical spine in addition to assessment of the extremity itself.

Local structures

The shoulder joint has the most complex motions of the body (Saha 1961, Post 1987). They are possible because the shoulder girdle is composed of three joints (the sternoclavicular, acromioclavicular, and glenohumeral) that work with the scapulothoracic

Table 6.2 Summary of neurological levels relating to upper extremity pain and/or dysfunction

	Motor	Sensory	Reflex
C5	Shoulder abduction, deltoids, biceps	Lateral aspect, arm (C5 axillary, nerve)	Biceps
C6	Wrist extension	Lateral forearm, musculocutaneous	Brachioradialis
C7	Wrist flexion	Middle finger	Triceps
	Finger extension		
C8	Finger flexion	Medial forearm	Finger flexion
			Hand intrinsics
T1	Finger abduction	Medial arm	Hand intrinsics

articulation in a synchronized pattern to provide extension, flexion, abduction, adduction, and internal and external rotation. ROM in any of the three joints may be inhibited because of pain, neurological deficit, or skeletal or soft tissue pathology. Both extremities should be tested for active and passive ROM to characterize the pain pattern and compared. ROM should also be tested against resistance. If any weakness is noted, a thorough muscle test and grading should be done.

Pain upon abduction between 60° and 120° suggests supraspinatus tendinitis; pain with forward flexion up to 90° with internal rotation suggests rotator cuff involvement due to impingement; pain at 140°–180° of abduction suggests acromioclavicular joint pain. In testing ROM, the first 30°–40° involve only glenohumeral motion and patients may compensate for restriction in this area with scapulothoracic motion.

Observations of joint noises, crepitation, or loss of normal gliding motion suggest that degenerative changes and intrinsic injury must be ruled out. A not uncommon condition is friction rub secondary to exostoses on either the scapula or rib, causing pain, although ROM may be normal. When this is suspected, special thoracic and scapular X-ray views are required.

Point tenderness examination of the two clavicular joints, supraspinatus tendon, bicipital tendon, and anterior subacromial region (for impingement syndrome) will usually be sufficient to identify local pathology. Figure 6.1 provides a review of shoulder structures with common points of tenderness. Palpation must be done gently, as excessive pressure will be painful and may irritate sensitive tissues. To palpate the bicipital groove, the arm is rotated externally (Yergason's test). The groove lies between the medial lesser tuberosity and the more lateral greater tuberosity. Passive extension of the shoulder will allow examination of the bursa and the cuff as it moves these structures forward; the insertion of the subscapularis is not palpable. Swelling and unusual warmth should be noted. Careful examination may reveal abnormal masses or thickening. Fluid can never be palpated in a normal synovial joint and its presence is a sign of joint pathology. If a ligament is tender or painful on palpation, the ligament has been injured or there is pathology at the joint. Palpation of muscle will identify sensitive trigger points that may be the primary or secondary cause of pain.

Supporting diagnostic procedures

Often careful history taking, palpation, and range of motion will establish a clear aetiology for upper extremity pain on the initial visit. However, with more complex problems or combined aetiologies,

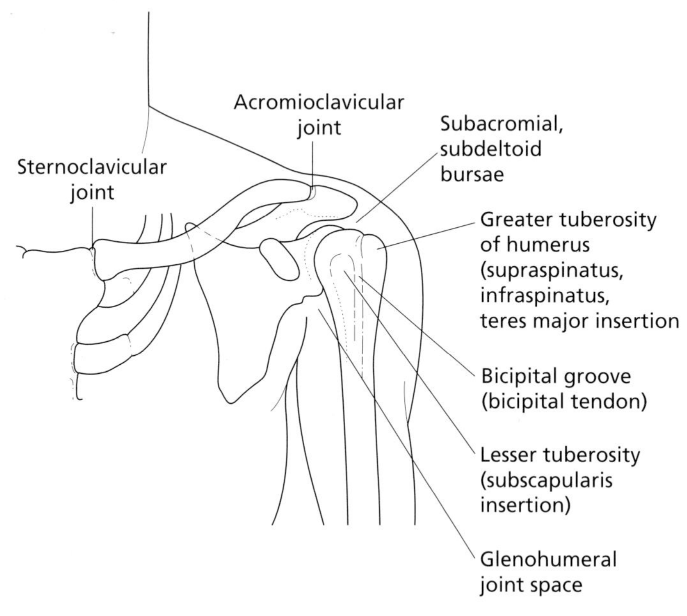

Fig. 6.1 Shoulder joint pain can arise from the greater tuberosity, the lesser tuberosity, the subacromial bursa, the subdeltoid bursa, bicipital groove and the long head of the biceps, the glenohumeral joint, and the acromioclavicular joint. When degenerative changes interact with clinical findings, severe pain, dysfunction, or loss of range of movement may result. Poor muscle tone, often associated with ageing, tends to exacerbate shoulder lesions.

two or three evaluation visits may be necessary, and it may be helpful to utilize supporting diagnostic procedures such as special roentgenographs or electromyograms (EMG) with peripheral nerve conduction studies.

Diagnostic radiographic studies

Radiographic studies are done on joints as indicated by the initial work-up. In any situation where diagnosis is difficult, these studies should include anterior/posterior and lateral views of the neck in extended, neutral, and flexed positions and also oblique views to visualize the neuroforamina. Routine shoulder films include anterior and posterior views and abduction, axillary, and bicipital groove views. Note that negative findings do not rule out pathology. Even positive findings do not necessarily explain the cause of pain or other symptoms.

High-resolution ultrasonography is particularly helpful as a non-invasive procedure to rule out rotator cuff tears. If there is any question or a tear is suspected, it is most easily confirmed by arthrography and magnetic resonance imaging (MRI). MRI holds great promise for evaluation and diagnosis of soft tissue injuries. MRI technology is particularly valuable in diagnosing damage to tendons, ligaments, and fibrocartilage and tears in the rotator cuff or glenoid labrum.

EMG and peripheral nerve conduction studies

EMG is particularly valuable for identifying peripheral neuropathies and for eliminating cervical lesions, discogenic disease, and nerve root entrapment as probable contributors to pain and dysfunction in the upper extremity. It is the only reliable tool for identifying peripheral neurocervical radiculitis.

Rotator cuff injuries

Tendinitis

Tendinitis is generally a non-traumatic lesion that occurs as the result of gradual degenerative changes in the rotator cuff. These changes may or may not be accompanied by calcium deposits in the tendon. A mild ache or discomfort may be present for months. In calcific tendinitis the ache may suddenly develop into an intolerable, unremitting pain, usually referred to the top or lateral aspect of the shoulder. The patient will usually hold the arm immobile against the body. Deep breathing may increase the pain. This acute episode may be associated with acute bursitis as a result of calcium, which may form in the tendon in response to injury, penetrating into the bursal sac. Since the condition is related to degenerative changes, it is more common after the fifth decade of life (Calliet 1981).

Signs and symptoms

It is usually possible to arrive at a working diagnosis of shoulder tendinitis through physical examination, including resisted range of motion. With involvement of the supraspinatus tendon, pain is often localized at the greater tuberosity of the humerus. The patient may be unable or unwilling to move the arm but full passive range of motion is possible. Pain upon resisted abduction is an indication of supraspinatus tendinitis. Infraspinatus involvement is also associated with pain localized at the greater tuberosity, but it is resisted external rotation that exacerbates the pain. Tendinitis of teres minor results in pain at the greater tuberosity, which is aggravated by resisted external rotation. Pain experienced locally at the lesser tuberosity may be tendinitis of the subscapularis. This will be further confirmed if the pain is associated with resisted medial rotation. Bicipital tendinitis most frequently involves the long head of the biceps muscle. Pain is experienced locally in the bicipital groove and at its attachment at the superior rim of the glenoid fossa.

Treatment course and prognosis

Calcific tendinitis in the acute stage may require immobilization of the arm in a sling, the use of cold packs, medication with oral anti-inflammatory and non-steroidal anti-inflammatory products, local anaesthetic, and steroid injections. Some patients may require the use of a narcotic for several days. If this treatment course is not successful, some physicians prefer to aspirate the joint. Milder cases usually respond to conservative treatment. The most important aspect of treatment is early mobilization of the shoulder starting with passive pendular exercises. These are followed by active pendular exercises as soon as tolerated.

Bursitis

Unfortunately, the term 'bursitis' is often used inappropriately for any painful shoulder. Specifically, bursitis is an acute inflammatory response usually associated with the deposition of calcific material. The bursa swells and impinges upon surrounding structures, causing excruciating pain. Primary bursitis is an uncommon entity, but it does occur. Inflammation of the bursa is more likely to occur secondarily to a tear or inflammation of adjacent tendon or muscle or to direct trauma. It is essentially a disease of middle age, being associated with degenerative changes of tendon, muscle, or the rotator cuff, although it is occasionally seen in a young patient.

Signs and symptoms

Subdeltoid bursitis is characterized by painful passive arc. Passive abduction is limited by pain at approximately 70° through 110°–115°, after which point the pain disappears. The pain is usually sharp and localized. Abduction and external rotation increase the pain dramatically, although any motion can cause pain. Pain seems to be aggravated at night. Roentgenograms may confirm the presence of calcific deposits. It is important to note, however, that only 35% of patients with X-ray evidence of calcium develop symptoms. Symptoms usually accompany calcium deposits greater than 1.5 cm.

Treatment course and prognosis

Treatment for bursitis is much the same as for calcific tendinitis. An unfortunate sequela of bursitis is adhesive capsulitis, particularly without proper treatment to ensure range of motion.

Bicipital tendinitis

The long head of the big tendon passes through the bicipital groove across the shoulder joint and is attached to the superior rim of the glenoid cavity. As a result of degenerative changes, chronic irritation may occur over the anterior aspect of the shoulder. This is often related to repetitious movement. This condition is frequently misdiagnosed as bursitis because of the similarity of location of pain.

Signs and symptoms

Bicipital tendinitis should be suspected if there is pain and tenderness to pressure over the bicipital groove. Yergason's sign (increased pain on resistance to supination) is a positive indicator, as is a palpable, swollen tendon. The pain of bicipital tendinitis may occur after heavy lifting and is associated with unusual athletic activity in young adults.

Treatment course and prognosis

Most of these patients respond to conservative treatment of resting the arm in a sling and providing analgesics for pain. Some clinicians advise local injections of steroids, but this writer has seen several cases in which this treatment has resulted in rupture of the tendon. Range of motion must be maintained during treatment to prevent 'frozen shoulder' or adhesive capsulitis. This is usually done passively until pain is adequately controlled, at which time active exercises are introduced.

Rotator cuff tears

The rotator cuff is a band of tendinous-fibrous tissue composed of the tendons of the subscapularis, supraspinatus, infraspinatus, and teres minor muscles, which fuse around the anatomic neck of the humerus where it inserts with the joint capsule. This part of the cuff is characterized by a marginal blood supply, which contributes to early degeneration, which in turn is associated with minor tears from normal activities.

Tears of the rotator cuff should be considered in conjunction with injuries sustained while working with arms overhead, with falls involving striking the shoulder or breaking the force of the fall with an outstretched hand, and with fractures or dislocations of the shoulder and greater tuberosity of the humerus. Residual pain subsequent to an earlier injury with loss of range of motion should also suggest rotator cuff tear. Degenerative cervical disease is a predisposing factor. Small tears may not require treatment. It has been reported that 30% of cadavers have rotator cuff tears.

Signs and symptoms

Rotator cuff tears are associated with pain at the anterolateral margin of the acromion. They are rare in patients under 40 years with the exception of those using the joint heavily. The patient, most often a labourer between the ages of 40 and 65, reports feeling a tear or snap in the shoulder, followed by severe pain if the tear is extensive. With less severe tears, the pain may increase in intensity, reaching a peak after 48 h and remaining in an acute stage for several days. Shoulder motion increases the pain, which is usually felt first in the shoulder joint but may spread to the posterior scapular area and to the deltoid and forearm. Frequently the pain is described as a deep, throbbing sensation and it may interfere with sleep.

Physical findings may include exquisite tenderness on pressure over the greater tuberosity, reduced abduction or pain on resisted abduction, and weakness on forward flexion or pain on internal rotation. Scapulohumeral dysrhythm may be present. The patient may be unable to control lowering of the arm to his side and it may drop freely. This is a useful guide for rotator cuff tears, but it should be noted that injuries to the suprascapular and axillary nerves, as well as fifth cervical root lesions, produce the same clinical sign. Atrophy of the rotator cuff suggests an injury several weeks old that involves the supraspinatus or infraspinatus muscles.

To rule out a diagnosis of rotator cuff impingement, 5 ml of local anaesthetic is injected laterally into the subacromial bursa just underneath the acromial arch. Relief of pain and improved strength around the shoulder joint following injection confirm rotator cuff impingement syndrome.

Treatment course and prognosis

Suspected lesions must be confirmed by contrast radiography, ultrasonography, or MRI. Minor tears respond to non-surgical treatment and usually heal within 2 months. Since tears are often associated with some degree of degenerative process, they tend to be a chronic problem. Severe tears should be evaluated by an orthopaedic surgeon for possible repair (Neviaser 1975, Post 1987) (Table 6.3).

Adhesive capsulitis

Adhesive capsulitis affects the glenohumeral joint. Adhesions form as a result of an inflammatory response, which produces saturation with a serofibrinous exudate. It is a common finding secondary to heavy use, immobilization, injury, tendonitis, fractures about the shoulder, infections, neoplasms, general surgery, and heart attacks. Bicipital tenosynovitis is also reported as a frequent cause. McLaughlin (1961) maintains that a shoulder that is put through the full range of movement a few times daily will not develop adhesive capsulitis, indicating that prolonged dependency is the initiating factor. The condition is unusual in patients under 40 years of age.

Signs and symptoms

The patient may report pain with a gradual onset without any known injury. It is often seen in sedentary persons who have recently begun to participate in an activity involving the upper extremities, such as golf, tennis, or bowling (Neer and Welsh 1977). The patient will have difficulty putting on a shirt, combing hair, or placing the hand in a back pocket. There may be little pain on palpation, but it will be aggravated by both external and internal rotation. Pain may seem to localize in the deltoid, particularly at its insertion, and frequently causes suffering at night.

A tentative diagnosis of adhesive capsulitis must be confirmed with arthrography to differentiate a simple stiff shoulder from the inflammatory condi-

Table 6.3 Shoulder pain: clinical findings and treatment

Differential diagnosis	Key findings	Key tests	Treatment
Impingement syndrome	Acromial pain on humeral forward flexion beyond 90°, tenderness on anterior insertion supraspinatus tendon	Reduced pain with subacromial lidocaine	NSAID; subacromial steroid injection (×3 max); cuff-strengthening exercises; acromioplasty
Rotator cuff tears	Weak external rotation; supraspinatus atrophy; painful arc 60°–120°; difficulty initiating abduction; usually more painful at night; uncommon in patients under 40 years	Drop-arm test positive; subacromial dye extravasation on arthrogram	Cuff-strengthening exercises for small tears; surgery large tears
Supraspinatus tendinitis	Pain tenderness; pain with external rotation	Calcification on X-ray	NSAID; acromioplasty
Biceps tendinitis	Positive Yergason's test; tender bicipital groove; anterior shoulder pain	None	NSAID; restricted-activity; surgery
Frozen shoulder	Diffuse pain and tenderness; decreased passive glenohumeral motion	Reduced capsular space on arthrogram	Range of movement exercises
Glenohumeral arthritis	Increased pain with activity; barometric sensitivity	X-rays	NSAID; arthroplasty
AC joint arthritis	AC; joint tenderness and pain with adduction 140°–180°	X-ray, injections of lidocaine into AC joint decreases pain	NSAID; AC joint steroid injection (×3 max); distal clavicle resection

Adapted from Lippert and Teitz (1987). AC = acromioclavicular; NSAID = nonsteroidal antiinflammatory drug.

tion. Neviaser (1975) classifies patients according to how much of the injected dye is accepted into the capsule and what the patient's range of passive abduction indicates. Abduction to more than 90° and dye acceptance of more than 10 ml indicates a mild form. Moderate involvement includes patients who cannot abduct over 90° and whose capsular joint space measures from 5 to 10 ml. A third classification is severe capsulitis, which is usually seen only after proximal humerus fracture in patients with osteoporosis or following severe shoulder dislocation.

Treatment course and prognosis

The best treatment for adhesive capsulitis is prevention with regular, daily range of movement exercises. Fortunately, many cases respond to a conservative treatment programme consisting mainly of steroid therapy and pain management in conjunction with an aggressive physical therapy programme carried out by a qualified physical therapist. The judicious use of steroids injected into the rotator cuff and intra-articular space may be helpful when applied in combination with intensive physical therapy (Sheon et al 1987).

Local anaesthetics may be adequate to facilitate therapy but local nerve block, particularly of the suprascapular nerve, may be indicated. Muscle relaxants are sometimes helpful. Trigger points can be injected with either lidocaine or procaine to reduce the possibility of a pain cycle. Manipulation is frequently used. When the degree of involvement is greater, manipulation may require anaesthesia. The arm may be positioned in 90° abduction during a period of 2 weeks bedrest, followed by a 3- to 6-month therapy programme usually leading to full recovery. The use of narcotics is not recommended over an extended period of time. Depression is not uncommon in these patients, and it should be recognized and treated as necessary.

Bicipital lesions

Bicipital subluxation

The same type of degenerative process that precipitates tendonitis can predispose older patients towards subluxation of the tendon. In younger individuals this condition may be associated with sports activities.

Signs and symptoms

When the transverse ligament is torn, local tenderness is normally experienced. The clinician may be able to feel the muscle 'snap' in and out of the groove upon passive rotation of the arm in the abducted position.

Treatment course and prognosis

When subluxation occurs in a young active person, surgery is indicated. Bicipital subluxation can lead to chronic tenosynovitis. In the older individual, restriction of activity may be the preferable course unless the patient is experiencing severe pain.

Bicipital rupture

Bicipital rupture is another condition that is usually related to degenerative changes in the biceps tendon or muscle. It may be a painless condition in which the biceps has completely separated between the muscle belly and the tendon or away from the supraglenoid fossa.

Signs and symptoms

Complete separation can usually be visualized. The flaccid biceps muscle bulges.

Treatment course and prognosis

In younger patients surgical repair is indicated. In older patients, if decrease of upper extremity strength would not impair lifestyle, no treatment is required although it may be desirable for cosmetic reasons.

Acromioclavicular joint lesions

Lesions of the acromioclavicular joint are one of the most overlooked causes of shoulder and arm pain. The joint is subject to arthritic involvement, to various injuries including sprains, contusions, and separations, and to tumours, although these are rare (DePalma 1957).

Signs and symptoms

Pain associated with the acromioclavicular joint is usually local without referral. It is aggravated by shrugging the shoulder and by full passive adduction of the arm across the chest. X-rays are not particularly useful for diagnostic purposes if the aetiology is an arthritic process, but they will rule out separation of the joint. Separation usually involves pain over the entire shoulder, often accompanied by weakness of all shoulder movements and loss of function. Palpation of the clavicular attachment may reveal subluxation, in which the clavicle usually displaces upward.

The symptoms of degenerative arthritis include tenderness, swelling, and/or warmth over the joint.

Treatment course and prognosis

In the case of mild injury of the joint, a shoulder elbow strap is used for immobilization for 1–2 weeks as needed. If the injury is more severe (subluxation) the strap is worn for up to 5–6 weeks. Surgery may be necessary if immobilization is not successful. The shoulder joint must be passively put through the range of movement as tolerated by pain. In addition, appropriate measures to prevent disabilities to the hand, wrist, and elbow must be taken.

Arthritis

The shoulder joint has only minimal susceptibility to arthritis, probably because it is not a weight-bearing joint and only under certain conditions is it a power-bearing joint. To a great extent it escapes the destructive degenerative changes of repeated pressure and trauma. The major exception to this is athletes, particularly those who load the joint in 'bursts'. Osteoarthritis is moderately common among persons who play baseball and overhead racquet sports, skiers, and musicians, being activity related rather than disease related. However, osteoarthritis and traumatic arthritis do occur in other patients and symptoms of painful, swollen, warm joints should suggest a systematic work-up for arthritic involvement. Other arthritides, including rheumatoid arthritis, are discussed elsewhere in this book.

Hemiplegia

Shoulder pain is a common complaint of people with hemiplegia. It can be so severe that it interferes with the rehabilitation programme that is so crucial immediately after 'stroke'. Appropriate splinting to prevent capsular stretching and resultant subluxation of the glenohumeral joint is necessary early in therapy and should help to prevent the complication of pain.

Treatment of the pain is comparable to that used in other painful shoulder conditions: injections of steroids, local anaesthetics, suprascapular nerve block, and oral medications consistent with the medical status of the patient. These patients should be managed by medical personnel trained in rehabilitation or by a health care team that includes a physical therapist.

Pain of combined aetiologies

Myofascial disorders

An understanding of myofascial disorders, their pain patterns, incidence, origins, and proper treatment is absolutely essential in treatment of upper extremity pain (Travell and Rinzler 1952; Sola and Kuitert 1955; Sola et al 1955; Sola and Williams 1956; Kraft et al 1968; Kraus 1970; Simons 1975, 1976; Travell 1976; Melzack et al 1977; Sola 1981, 1984; Bonica 1990, Roberts and Hedges 1991; Travell and Simons 1983).

Like the lower back, the shoulder and neck region are commonly the 'storehouse' of numerous latent points that, when challenged by physical (and, to some degree, emotional) stressors, can cause pain. The mechanism of pain can be described as follows: from an initiating stimulus such as trauma, fatigue, or stress, a physiological response is generated and a particular trigger point (TP) begins to send distress signals to the central nervous system. Muscles associated with the trigger point become tense and soon muscle fatigue is experienced. Local ischaemia occurs, leading to change in the extracellular environment of the affected cells, including release of algesic agents. These feed into a cycle of increasing motor and sympathetic activity, and other trigger points 'flare up', contributing to the cycle (Zimmerman 1979). These interactions may magnify a painful event far out of proportion to its precipitating challenge. Furthermore, once established as a cycle, a painful event may sustain itself despite control of the stimulus that originally initiated the cycle. Thus, proper and adequate treatment of a local injury may not provide alleviation of pain. Figure 6.2 graphically describes the process and interacting elements.

Trigger-point syndromes affect virtually everyone, either in a primary role of translating stress responses into pain or in a secondary role in which activation intensifies or prolongs pain from another stimulus. Trigger-point pain varies from slight discomfort to severe unrelenting pain and is described as either sharp or dull. It can also simulate the pain of visceral disorders that are referred to the shoulder area.

It is important to note that although trigger-point pain can affect both sides of the body, it is commonly confined to one side and is often associated with ipsilateral hypersensitivity in muscles seemingly quite removed from the reported problem. For example, pain in the neck and shoulder is commonly associated with gluteal TPs that are exquisitely sensitive to pressure even though the patient may not report overt pain in these muscles. In such cases treatment must involve the remote ipsilateral TPs as well as those in the painful area (see Fig. 6.3).

Treatment course and prognosis

An injection of local anaesthetic or physiological saline into the TPs is often adequate to break the

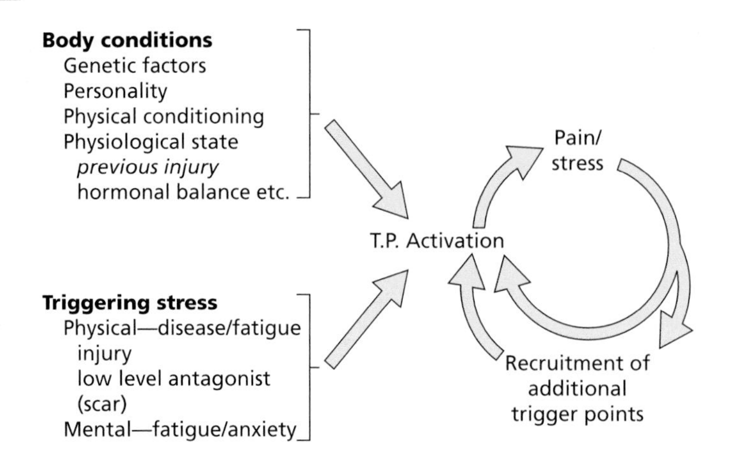

Fig. 6.2 A variety of stress-inducing stimuli may be implicated in the onset of myofascial pain. The power of these stimuli to induce pain is moderated by the genetics, personality, conditioning, and physiological state of a particular individual. Once established, however, a painful event may sustain itself despite control or elimination of the initiating stimuli.

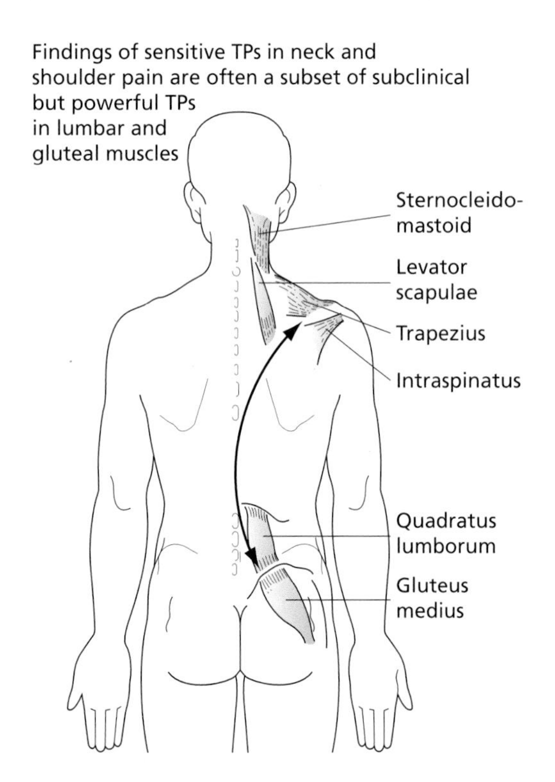

Fig. 6.3 An ipsilateral pattern of pain is very common, with simultaneously active painful trigger points in the neck and shoulder, quadratus lumborum, and gluteal muscles. Hyperactive trigger points (TPs) in the lumbar gluteal muscles must be treated before positive results can be expected from treatment of TPs in head, neck, or extremities.

pain cycle (Bray and Sigmond 1941, Frost et al 1980, Tfelt-Hansen et al 1980). The use of vasocoolants, such as fluoromethane spray, has been shown to be a helpful technique by Travell and Daitz (1990). The insertion of thin solid needles alone (dry needling as described by Gunn 1989) has often been found to be as effective as injection without subjecting the patient to the added tissue disruption caused by edged hypodermic needles. When dry needling, local anaesthetic, or saline injection proves inadequate, injection of a weak solution of dexamethasone (1 cc diluted in 100 cc of normal saline) is a useful procedure (Edagawa 1994). This treatment presumes that there are no contraindications to steroid use such as diabetes or clotting disorders. When the pain is secondary to another stimulus, particularly nerve root lesions or nerve compression, the treatment is never more than moderately successful in relieving pain. Therefore this procedure is useful as a differential diagnostic tool, as it interrupts the pain cycle and allows exposure of the underlying disorder. Other treatments are being explored. Periosteal stimulation reportedly enhances the effectiveness of TP injection, reducing myofascial pain (Lawrence 1978). There is also new work in the use of laser therapy and interesting work in progress on electromagnetic fields to relieve pain.

Reflex dystrophy-like syndromes

Reflex dystrophies are part of the group of sympathetic disorders whose features may include throbbing, burning or aching pain, hyperaesthesia, hyperalgesia, and oedema and/or erythema. These are serious, painful, and disabling disorders. Onset may be triggered by coronary ischaemia, hemiplegia, adhesive capsulitis, bicipital tendinitis, trauma, or even simple bruises or sprains. In a study of 140 patients with reflex dystrophy, 40% of the cases occurred following soft tissue injury, 25% following fractures, 20% were postoperative, 12% followed myocardial infarction, and 3% followed CVA. It was also noted that 37% of these patients had significant emotional disturbances at the time of onset. Thus elements of the process include CNS involvement and the entire myofascial pain cycle of stressors, trigger-point activation, pain, and sympathetic involvement (Pak et al 1970). Treatment must be instituted immediately and includes injection of the affected trigger points with an anaesthetic–corticosteroid mixture by a specialist and physical therapy. If this provides no relief, one must resort to sympathetic blocks, oral corticosteroids, and, finally, sympathectomy. Early treatment of the affected TPs has shown great promise in breaking this cycle.

Shoulder–hand syndrome

Signs and symptoms

The disease has several stages. Onset is usually insidious. The patient may present with a burning pain involving the shoulder and vasomotor changes in the hand and fingers. This phase may last several months. After this initial phase, shoulder pain may ease but trophic changes appear: atrophy of the muscles in the affected extremity, thickening of palmar fascia, demineralization, and atrophy of the nails. By the time these trophic changes have occurred, it is extremely difficult to reverse the disease process despite aggressive treatment and the end result is flexion deformities of the fingers. At this stage vasomotor changes are absent.

Treatment course and prognosis

This condition requires aggressive treatment. Residual damage is usually irreversible; surgery has not proven successful in restoring function. The pain associated with shoulder–hand syndrome can be excruciating and the patient will normally require narcotics for pain management. Phenobarbital should not be given but other sedatives may be used. Sympathetic blocks done early in the course of the disease may be helpful, as well as corticosteroid therapy. Injection of local anaesthetics into hypersensitive areas of the shoulder or the suprascapular nerve may also be helpful. From the outset, treatment must be accompanied by an intensive physical therapy programme to maintain function.

Overuse syndromes

Although a given action or set of actions may be well within the body's capabilities, excessive repetition may, through interference with circulation, repeated microinjury, buildup of waste products, or any of these and other factors, stress a tissue beyond its anatomical or physiological limits. The stressor may be either dynamic, as in the case of repetitive movement, or static, as in the case of prolonged bracing or maintenance of a particular posture.

One should suspect an overuse syndrome when a patient reports that he or she:

1. performs a repetitive task
2. maintains a fixed posture for long periods of time
3. lifts above or below a mechanically strainful height
4. performs a tedious or monotonous task.

Furthermore, it should be suspected when numerous other workers or participants have been disabled performing the same tasks. Such a finding would suggest that an evaluation of the ergonomics of the workplace would be in order (Sheon et al 1987, Khalil et al 1994).

The repeated movements of certain sports such as tennis, swimming and baseball, and extended periods of wrist pressure involved in cycling are well-documented sources of overuse injury. So too are certain occupations. Inflammation is rarely apparent on physical examination in patients with overuse syndrome, and it is often not clear whether the injured structure is tendon, muscle, ligament, joint capsule, or a combination of these (Sataloff et al 1990).

Carpal tunnel syndrome

Carpal tunnel syndrome is the second most common industrial injury in the United States, surpassed only by low back pain. Workers in occupations that require heavy wrist activity, such as data entry operators, grocery checkers, pipefitters, tool workers, carpenters, secretaries, and pianists, are considered most at risk for this syndrome. Recent findings suggest that the condition is exacerbated by psychological stressors such as boredom, insecurity, or the stress of other painful processes.

Carpal tunnel syndrome is caused by pressure on the median nerve; this may be due to increased synovial hypertrophy, as it occurs in rheumatoid arthritis, gout, hypothyroidism, diabetes, ganglion tumours or lipomas, pregnancy, and trauma. Biomechanical studies have shown that intracarpal pressure is particularly increased with flexor and ulnar deviation. Rosenbaum and Ochoa (1993) suggest that Phalen's wrist flexion test is more reliable than Tinel's nerve stimulation of the median nerve at the wrist in diagnosis of carpal tunnel syndrome.

Signs and symptoms

This syndrome causes paraesthesias and dysthaesias along the median nerve into the hand and wrist. The pain may be localized at the wrist, but may also show retrograde spread to the elbow or shoulder. Shaking or moving the hand may relieve symptoms, suggesting a pressure gradient involving the lymphatic or circulatory system. However, if such shaking causes increased pain, cervical radiculitis should be suspected. Thenar atrophy may be present.

Treatment course and prognosis

Conservative treatment measures include splinting, cortisone injections, rest, and/or change in activities. Treatment of trigger points in the forearm, shoulder, neck, and, often, gluteal region may help relieve both the pain and dystrophy-like syndromes. In difficult cumulative disorders the patient should ideally begin a 'work-hardening' programme under the supervision of trained hand, occupational, or physical therapists to develop strength and endurance. Ergonomic improvements in the workplace may also be required. When other treatments are not effective, surgical release is recommended. Although Silverstein et al (1987) have reported that 58% of surgically treated patients return to their former job, none of these returned to jobs that required forceful repetitive motion.

Other peripheral entrapment syndromes

Among the most puzzling pains of the extremity are the peripheral neuropathies. The causes are obscure and differential diagnosis is not easy, especially since cervical nerve root irritation must be considered (Kopell and Thompson 1973, Dyck et al 1976). There is evidence that radiculitis increases the susceptibility to nerve entrapment (Upton and McComas 1973, Bland 1987). Table 6.4 gives some

Table 6.4 Differentiating between radiculopathy and entrapment syndromes

Radiculopathy	Entrapment
Involves posterior division of cervical root; radiation along medial border of scapula.	Signs uncommon with entrapment.
Pain with coughing, sneezing, Valsalva manoeuvre, highly specific for radiculopathy when present.	Signs not associated with entrapment.
Pain increases with use of hand.	Carpal tunnel syndrome pain is relieved by massage, shaking hand, immersion of hand in water, changing positions.
Muscle weakness rarely severe. Most easily identified; deltoid, infraspinatus (C5); biceps, wrist extensors (C6); triceps, long finger flexors, finger extensors (C7); intrinsic muscles of hand and wrist flexors (C8); arm and when testing muscle.	Not a diagnostic feature.
Electrophysiological studies	**Electrophysiological studies**
Nerve conduction studies almost always normal with uncomplicated radiculopathy. EMGs done on a number of arm muscles may show changes in a radicular pattern. Paraspinus muscles may be denervated, confirming nerve root damage. Myelography/computerized tomography delineates lateral disc protrusion.	Local changes may be present.
Treatment	**Treatment**
Successful response to several weeks of conservative treatment (traction, cervical collar, local massage and analgesics) confirms diagnosis.	In early stages is likely to respond to conservative treatment; splinting, cortisone, rest. More advanced may require surgical release.

guidelines to differentiate between entrapment and peripheral radiculopathy (Dawson et al 1983, 1990). Peripheral radiculopathy must also be differentiated from cervical spondylosis and other less common entities that cause cervical root irritation, such as tumours, infection, osteophytes, prolapsed disc, fractures, and epidural abscess (see Chaps. 17 and 19). Note that patients can usually distinguish between pain that radiates from the hand to the shoulder and pain that originates in the neck or shoulder and spreads to the hand. The only definitive way to diagnose peripheral neuropathy is by electromyography and nerve conduction studies in addition to routine radiological studies.

Any one of the entrapment syndromes can cause hand, forearm, and shoulder pain which is not consistent in character. Generally, there is some local pain at the area of entrapment, but muscles distal to the entrapment may or may not have pain involvement. Frequently the pain experienced is intermittent, low grade, and worse at night. Scapulocostal irritation and myofascial disturbances tend to distort the pain patterns to peripheral nerve compression. Carpal tunnel syndrome is the most common of the nerve compression syndromes affecting the median nerve. Two other conditions related primarily to median nerve compression are pronator teres syndrome and anterior interosseous nerve syndrome. Conditions affecting the radial nerve are radial palsy and posterior interosseous syndrome. Ulnar nerve compression is associated with cubital tunnel syndrome and Guyon's canal compression. In addition to the conditions described in Table 6.5, compression of the suprascapular nerve can cause dull, deep pain in the rhomboid area, and dorsal scapular nerve syndrome can cause pain particularly in the posterolateral aspect of the shoulder.

Treatment course and prognosis

Treatment for these syndromes follows much the same pattern as treatment for carpal tunnel syndrome and includes splinting, cortisone injections, rest, and/or change in activities, as well as treatment of trigger points in the affected and related areas to help relieve both the pain and dystrophy-like syndromes.

Tennis elbow or epicondylitis

Signs and symptoms

The patient complains of severe pain in the elbow, frequently radiating to wrist or shoulder. Any grasping movements are painful and the patient may drop things from the hand. The pain is usually described as 'deep'. Pressure applied over the lateral condyles causes extreme pain. Dorsiflexion of the wrist may be painful. This clinical picture of pain is usually accompanied by a history of overuse of the extensors and supinators of the wrist in sports such as tennis and golf and in occupations requiring similar motions such as hammering. In older patients, this lesion is more likely to be a chronic condition unrelated to a specific activity and much less amenable to treatment.

Table 6.5

Nerve	Syndrome	Signs/symptoms
Median nerve	Pronator teres	Pain, paraesthesias and associated weakness in flexor muscles of the forearm and thenar muscles.
	Anterior interosseous	Weakness or paralysis in the index and middle fingers. Pronator teres weak when elbow flexed. Pronator quadratus weak in pronation.
Radial nerve	Radial palsy	Affects all muscles of the forearm supplied by the radial nerve. Usually painless, frequent hyperparaesthesia.
	Posterior interosseous	The patient is able to extend the wrist but unable to extend metacarpophalangeal joints of the fingers, unable to abduct the thumb, and unable to extend the distal joint of the thumb.
Ulnar nerve	Cubital tunnel	May experience pain along the ulnar border of the forearm, weakness of intrinsic muscles of the hand and hyperaesthesias.
	Guyon's canal compression	Associated with fractures or aneurysm of the small artery. The patient may experience local pain and numbness in the ulnar distribution of the fourth and fifth fingers.

Treatment course and prognosis

Treatment depends on the structures involved. Common extensor and flexor tendons will usually respond to steroids and local anaesthetic. When the extensor carpi radialis tendon is involved, the pain may originate with muscle rather than on the epicondyle and a local anaesthetic may be indicated. Muscle involvement is uncommon at the supracondylar ridge. Joint dysfunction at any of the three elbow joints can cause pain simulating tennis elbow. These are treated by manipulation. Refractory cases of tennis elbow are frequently treated by surgery. Trigger points may occur in any of the muscles around the elbow joint and these frequently respond to injection therapy. Trigger points in the scalenus anticus muscle can frequently refer pain to this area (Zohn and Mennell 1976).

Olecranon bursa

Signs and symptoms

The olecranon bursa, which lies over the bony olecranon process, is frequently injured by constant mechanical pressure. Clinically, the bursa sac area becomes red and swollen, warm to the touch, and tender on palpation. Occasionally it may become infected. Patients who have gout and rheumatoid arthritis are prone to this disorder.

Treatment course and prognosis

Pain and swelling usually subside if a cushioning ring is used around the area of irritation to prevent further mechanical pressure. If pain persists, fluid can be aspirated from the bursal sac and examined for evidence of infection and/or to differentiate between aetiologies. If the condition is persistent or recurrent, surgical excision may be the treatment of choice.

Ligamental injuries

Ligamental injuries are common at the wrist. Diagnosis is made on the basis of local pain and tenderness. The most frequent of these injuries is sprain of the ulnar collateral ligament, which is characterized by pain on radial deviation. When the radial ligament is sprained or torn, pain is present on ulnar deviation. The ulnar-capitate sprain is also quite common. With flexion of the wrist, pain is felt at the dorsal aspect.

Treatment course and prognosis

Local management with steroid injection treatment is usually effective for ligamental injuries. Ruptures may require surgical intervention.

De Quervain's disease (constrictive tenosynovitis)

Signs and symptoms

The patient will present with pain in the wrist and thumb area and weakness of grip. In the acute state, there may be local swelling with symptoms similar to wrist sprain. Examination will reveal marked tenderness to pressure over the styloid process and over the tendons, abductor pollicis longus, and extensor pollicis brevis.

The pain is related to thickening and stenosis of the sheath surrounding the tendons. Diagnosis of De Quervain's disease is affirmed by holding the patient's thumb in flexion and abducting the wrist. This will elicit a pain response.

Treatment course and prognosis

Immobilization is recommended and the area is injected with long-acting anaesthetic. Injectable steroid therapy is also appropriate.

Trigger finger

Small tears in the flexor tendon may form a nodule that interferes with normal gliding motion through the tendon sheath, causing the finger to snap in extension. Palpation of the tendon sheath will usually be painful.

Treatment is the same as for De Quervain's disease: immobilization, steroid injection, and surgical release if necessary.

Impingement syndromes

Impingement syndromes are common in athletes and persons doing heavy physical labour. Impingement is diagnosed by point tenderness over the anterior insertion of the supraspinatus tendon and positive findings on forward flexion with internal rotation. The critical test is relief of symptoms with use of local anaesthetic injected into the anterior acromial process (coracoid acromial ligament).

Tendinitis, rotator cuff tears, and adhesive capsulitis may all be components of a degenerative process beginning with impingement. When impingement syndromes are present in young persons, they are almost always associated with racquet sports, swimming, baseball, football, and repetitive overhead motions (Moseley 1969, Post 1987, Nichols and Hershman 1990).

Neer and Welsh (1977) have suggested three stages:

- Stage I is characterized by oedema and/or inflammation and usually occurs in patients between the ages of 15 and 30 years. Treatment at this stage is conservative; restriction of shoulder movement, anti-inflammatory medications, and ice packs. Occasionally steroid injections are given if these measures do not provide relief.
- Stage II is characterized by fibrosis and thickening of the rotator cuff, which further compromises subacromial mechanisms. If the patient does not respond to conservative treatment and cuff tear has been ruled out, a partial anterior acromioplasty and sectioning of the coracoid acromial ligament may be necessary.
- Stage III is usually associated with patients over the age of 40 years, when further degeneration has taken place, and it may include partial tears of the rotator cuff and bony changes. Surgery may be necessary to correct the condition, particularly if tears are involved (Post 1987). The diagnosis can be confirmed by an arthrogram (see Table 6.3).

Thoracic outlet syndrome

Thoracic outlet syndrome is most commonly caused by compression or irritation of the inferior portion of the brachial plexus by the scalene muscles, rib, clavicle, or pectoralis minor muscle. This affects the ulnar and, sometimes, the medial nerves. In a small percentage of cases the subclavian vein may also be compressed.

Signs and symptoms

There is often a gradual increase in discomfort culminating in pain involving the upper extremity, lower neck region, shoulder, and arm. The pain tends to be intermittent and is associated with movement, particularly with lifting objects overhead. The patient may describe a 'pins and needles' sensation in the forearm and wrist and may experience weakness or numbness in the fourth or fifth finger. Symptoms are usually worse in the morning than later in the day. The condition is seen most often in young adult patients with poor posture and is reported more frequently in women.

Palpation or percussion during examination may indicate tenderness of the brachial plexus. A confirming test is to have the patient assume a sitting position with both arms elevated to 90° abduction with external rotation. The elbows are maintained somewhat behind the frontal plane. The position is held for 3 min while slowly opening and closing the hands. If radial pulses remain strong but the patient experiences the usual symptoms, the test is positive.

Treatment course and prognosis

A conservative treatment approach is to recommend posture-related therapy and mild exercise to strengthen shoulder muscles. If the problem can be associated with a particular type of activity or position during sleeping, these should be modified. Medication for muscle relaxation may be indicated. However, all these measures are limited if the condition has progressed to the extent that only surgical procedures can provide decompression.

Cervical sprain

Cervical sprain or 'whiplash' injury is associated with the rapid acceleration of the neck into hyperextension and/or flexion with subsequent rebound and reflex splinting. Although whiplash can cause cord damage it is most commonly associated with some trauma to the supporting muscles, tendons, and ligaments. It may also be associated with damage or functional compromise of the cervical nerve roots either directly or through the pressures of subsequent muscle spasm (Bland 1987, Bonica 1990, Johnson 1996).

The short-term signs of cervical sprain include stiffness and pain in the neck and shoulder girdle, hoarseness or dysphagia (in anterior damage), headache, and various sympathetic dystrophy-like symptoms. A normal neurological examination with no swelling or apparent trauma to the neck may be taken as a good indication that there is no spinal or cord damage. Even if the injury appears minimal, the patient must be carefully followed for several days following the incident (Borchgrevink et al 1998). Muscles and ligaments heal within 4–6 weeks, whereas intervertebral discs heal slowly because they have no blood supply. If there is any suspicion of damage to the cervical spine or cord, one must obtain a transtable lateral view of the entire cervical spine.

If spinal injury has been ruled out, immediate treatment includes applying mild cervical traction and physical therapy and administration of non-steroidal anti-inflammatory medications. A soft cervical collar may be indicated for a short time although these have not generally been found to be effective. Spasm and TPs in the involved muscles may affect nerve roots as low as T7 (see Fig. 6.4). Muscles of the lower back are also commonly involved. Thus one must carefully examine the lower torso for painful foci and trigger points with

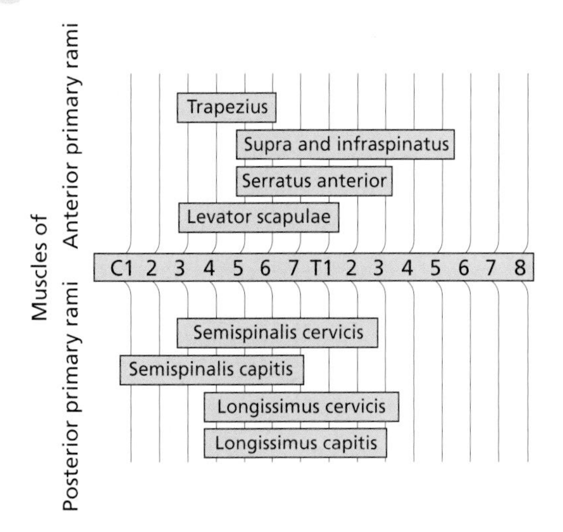

Fig. 6.4 This schematic illustration gives examples of upper extremity muscles supplied by the anterior primary rami of the cervical spine. Note the length of the muscles supplied by the posterior rami shown for the same cervical region. Activation of trigger points (TPs) that exist along the entire length of a muscle can cause or intensify pain felt in muscles supplied by any common nerve segment. Therefore, pain experienced along a muscle such as the semispinalis capitis can contribute to shoulder pain. Injection treatment of posterior primary rami muscles beginning at T6 is indicated if hypersensitive TPs are found in the muscles.

particular attention to the paraspinal muscles and the gluteal muscle group. Trigger points in these muscles are not only sources of localized pain but may exacerbate problems in the neck and shoulders, making treatment in those areas less effective if left untreated (see Fig. 6.3).

Multiple upper extremity lesions

One of the problems in managing upper extremity pain is that several lesions may be contributing to it. This is particularly true in the case of a middle-aged or older patient who sustains an injury. Unrelieved or persistent pain following seemingly satisfactory healing of the point of injury should always suggest further evaluation for potential cervical problems. Further assessment should also include examination of the shoulder, elbow, and wrist for joint dysfunction and hypersensitive TPs and tendons, bursae, rotator cuff, and joint capsule for undiagnosed injuries along the path of shock absorption. Any injury site has the potential for setting up a dystrophy-like syndrome. It is unfortunate for the patient if the clinician overlooks these sequelae, since they can usually be treated effectively and the pain eliminated.

References

Adson AW 1951 Cervical ribs: symptoms, differential diagnosis and indications for section of the insertion of the scalenus anticus muscle. Journal of the International College of Surgeons 16: 546–559

Bateman JE 1978 The shoulder and neck, 2nd edn. Saunders, Philadelphia

Bland JH 1987 Disorders ot the cervical spine: diagnosis and medical management. Saunders, Philadelphia, chaps 13, 20

Bonica JJ 1990 The management of pain, 2nd edn. Lea & Febiger, Philadelphia, chaps 21, 40, 47, 52

Borchgrevink GE, Kaasa A, McDonagh D, Stiles TC, Haraldseth O, Lereim I 1998 Acute treatment of whiplash neck sprain injuries. A randomized trial of treatment during the first 14 days after a car accident. Spine 23(1): 25–31

Bray EA, Sigmond H 1941 The local and regional injection treatment of low back pain and sciatica. Annals of Internal Medicine 15: 840–852

Brody IA, Wilkins RH 1969 Lhermitte's sign. Archives of Neurology 21: 338–340

Calliet R 1981 Shoulder pain, 2nd edn. Davis, Philadelphia

Dawson DM, Hallet M, Millender LH 1983 Entrapment neuropathies. Little, Brown, Boston

Dawson DM, Hallet ML, Millender LH 1990 Entrapment neuropathies, 2nd edn. Little, Brown, Boston

DePalma AF 1957 Degenerative changes in sternoclavicular and acromioclavicular joints in various decades. Thomas, Springfield, IL

DePalma AF 1973 Surgery of the shoulder, 2nd edn. Lippincott, Philadelphia

Dyck PJ, Lambert EH, O'Brien PC 1976 Pain in peripheral neuropathy related to rate and kind of nerve fiber degeneration. Neurology 26: 466–477

Edagawa N 1994 Body wall medicine. W4 Group, Mississauga, Ontario

Frost FA, Jeason B, Siggaard-Anderson JA 1980 A controlled, double-blind comparison of mepivacaine injection versus saline injection for myofascial pain. Lancet 1: 499–501

Gerhart TN, Dohlman LE, Warfield CA 1985 Clinical diagnosis of shoulder pain. Hospital Practice 20(9): 134–141

Gunn CC 1989 Treating myofascial pain: intramuscular stimulation (IMS) for myofascial pain syndromes of neuropathic origin. Health Sciences Center for Educational Resources, University of Washington, Seattle

Johnson G 1996 Hyperextension soft tissue injuries of the cervical spine—a review. Journal of Accident and Emergency Medicine 13(1): 3–8

Khalil T, Abdel-Moty E, Steele-Rosomoff R, Rosomoff H 1994 The role of ergonomics in the prevention and treatment of myofascial pain. In: Rachlin ES (ed) Myofascial pain and fibromyalgia. Mosby, St Louis

Kopell HP, Thompson W 1973 Peripheral entrapment neuropathies. Williams & Wilkins, Baltimore

Kraft GH, Johnson EW, LaBan MM 1968 The fibrositis syndrome. Archives of Physiological Medicine and Rehabilitation 49: 155–162

Kraus H 1970 Clinical treatment of back and neck pain. McGraw-Hill, New York

Lawrence RM 1978 New approach to the treatment of chronic pain: combination therapy. American Journal of Acupuncture 6: 59–62

Lippert FG III, Teitz CC 1987 Diagnosing musculoskeletal problems—a practical guide. Williams & Wilkins, Baltimore

McLaughlin HL 1961 The 'frozen shoulder'. Clinical Orthopedics 20: 126–131

Melzack R, Stillwell DM, Fox EJ 1977 Trigger points and

acupuncture points for pain: correlations and implications. Pain 3: 3–23
Moseley HF 1969 Shoulder lesions, 3rd edn. E & S Livingstone, Edinburgh, pp 75–81, 243–292
Neer CS II, Welsh RP 1977 The shoulder in sports. Orthopedic Clinics of North America 8: 583–591
Neviaser JS 1975 Arthrography of the shoulder: the diagnosis and management of the lesions visualized. CC Thomas, Springfield, IL
Nichols JA, Hershman EB 1990 The upper extremity in sports medicine. Mosby, St Louis
Pak TJ, Martin GM, Magnes JL, Kavanaugh GJ 1970 Reflex sympathetic dystrophy. Minnesota Medicine 53: 507–512
Post M 1987 Physical examination of the musculoskeletal system. Year Book Medical Publishers, Chicago
Roberts JR, Hedges JR 1991 Clinical procedures in emergency medicine, 2nd ed. Saunders, Philadelphia, chap 64
Rosenbaum RB, Ochoa JL 1993 Carpal tunnel syndrome and other disorders of the median nerve. Butterworth-Heinemann, New York
Saha AK 1961 Theory of shoulder mechanism. Thomas, Springfield, IL
Sataloff RT, Brandfonbrenner AG, Lederman RJ 1990 Textbook of performing arts medicine. Raven Press, New York
Sheon RP, Moskowitz RW, Goldberg VM 1987 Soft tissue rheumatic pain, 2nd edn. Lea & Febiger, Philadelphia
Silverstein B, Fine L, Stetson D 1987 Hand–wrist disorders among investment casting plant workers. Journal of Hand Surgery 12A: 838–844
Simons DG 1975 Muscle pain syndromes. Part I. American Journal of Physical Medicine 54: 289–311
Simons DG 1976 Muscle pain syndromes. Part II. American Journal of Physical Medicine 55: 15–42
Sola AE 1981 Myofascial trigger point therapy. Resident Staff Physicians 27: 38–48
Sola AE 1984 Treatment of myofascial pain syndromes. In: Benedetti C et al (eds) Advances in pain research and therapy. Raven Press, New York, p 13
Sola AE, Kuitert JH 1955 Myofascial trigger point pain in the neck and shoulder girdle: 100 cases treated by normal saline. Northwest Medicine 54: 980–984
Sola AE, Williams RL 1956 Myofascial pain syndromes. Neurology 6: 91–95
Sola AE, Rodenberg ML, Getty BB 1955 Incidence of hypersensitive areas in posterior shoulder muscles. American Journal of Physical Medicine 34: 585–590
Steindler A 1959 Lectures on the interpretation of pain in orthopedic practice. Thomas, Springfield, IL
Tfelt-Hansen P, Olesen J, Lous I et al 1980 Lignocaine versus saline in migraine pain. Lancet 1: 1140
Travell J 1976 Myofascial trigger points. In: Bonica JJ (ed) Advances in pain research and therapy. Raven Press, New York
Travell J, Daitz B 1990 Myofascial pain syndromes: the Travell trigger point tapes. Williams & Wilkins Electronic Media, Baltimore
Travell J, Rinzler SH 1952 The myofascial genesis of pain. Postgraduate Medicine 11: 425–434
Travell J, Simons DG 1983 Myofascial pain and dysfunction: the trigger point manual. Williams & Wilkins, Baltimore
Upton ARM, McComas AJ 1973 The double crush syndrome in nerve entrapment syndromes. Lancet 2: 359
Zimmermann M 1979 Peripheral and central nervous mechanisms of nociception, pain and pain therapy: facts and hypotheses. In: Bonica JJ, Liebeskind JC, Albe-Fessard DG (eds) Advances in pain research and therapy, vol 3. Lippincott–Raven, Philadelphia, pp 3–32
Zohn DA, Mennell JM 1976 Musculoskeletal pain: diagnosis and physical treatment. Little, Brown, Boston

Chapter 7

Fibromyalgia

Robert M Bennett

Introduction

Fibromyalgia is a multisymptomatic syndrome defined by the core feature of chronic widespread pain (Bennett 1981, Yunus et al 1981, Goldenberg 1987). Many of these patients also have severe fatigue and associated symptoms related to visceral hyperalgesia, such as irritable bowel and bladder. This population accounts for about 20% of patients consulting rheumatologists in North America (White et al 1995). Contemporary research implicates abnormalities of sensory processing and neuroendocrine dysfunction as being related to the symptomatology of these patients.

Historical perspective

The first use of the word 'fibrositis' is attributed to Sir William Gowers in a lecture on the subject of lumbago that was published in the *British Medical Journal* in 1904 (Gowers 1904). To quote from this lecture: 'I think we need a designation for inflammation of the fibrous tissue—we may conveniently follow the analogy of "cellulitis" and term it "fibrositis"'. Ralph Stockman, a Glasgow pathologist, described foci of inflammation in the interstitium of muscle bundles, the so-called 'myalgic nodules', that very same year (Stockman 1904). These histological findings were never verified and the diagnosis of 'fibrositis' became equated with the concept of 'psychogenic rheumatism' for much of the middle third of the twentieth century. The description of an objective sleep abnormality in these patients by Moldofsky in 1976 and the rediscovery of defined tender areas by Smyth in 1977 led to a re-evaluation of the 'fibrositis concept' in the 1980s. It became evident that these patients made up a substantial proportion of those seeing rheumatologists. This led the American College of Rheumatology (ACR) to commission a multicenter study to provide diagnostic guidelines. The results of this study were published in 1990 (Wolfe et al 1990) and are generally referred to as the 1990 ACR guidelines. They adopted the name of fibromyalgia as the old name of 'fibrositis' was considered to represent a pathological notion that was now discredited.

Diagnosis

The 1990 American College of Rheumatology's guidelines for making a diagnosis of fibromyalgia are the most widely used criteria in current use (Wolfe et al 1990). They comprise one historical feature and one physical finding. The historical feature is widespread pain of 3 months or more. Widespread is defined as pain in an axial distribution plus pain on both left and right sides of the body, and pain above and below the waist. The physical finding is the presence of 11 or more out of 18 specified tender points. A tender point is defined in terms of its location and the patient's experience of pain on digital palpation with an approximate force of 4 kg (the amount of pressure required to blanch a thumbnail). The locations of the 18 tender points are shown in Fig. 7.1.

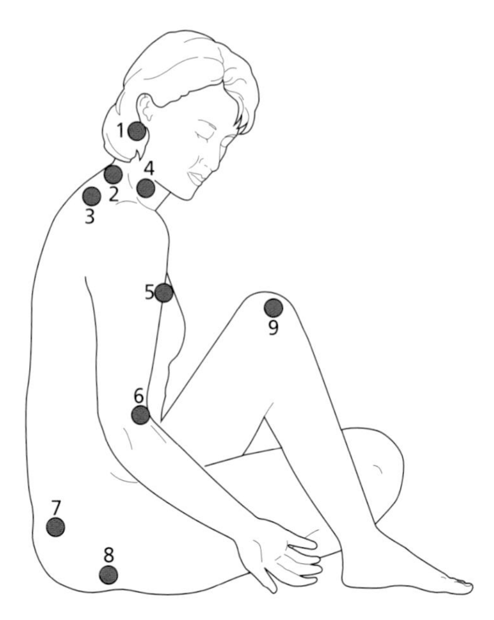

1. Insertion of nuchal muscles into occiput
2. Upper border of trapezius—mid-portion
3. Muscle attachments to upper medial border of scapular
4. Anterior aspects of the C5, C7 intertransverse spaces
5. 2nd rib space—about 3 cm lateral to the sternal border
6. Muscle attachments to lateral epicondyle
7. Upper outer quadrant of gluteal muscles
8. Muscle attachments just posterior to greater trochanter
9. Medial fat pad of knee proximal to joint line

Fig. 7.1 American College of Rheumatology 1990 criteria—recommended tender point locations: a total of 11 or more tender points in conjunction with a history of widespread pain is characteristic of the fibromyalgia syndrome.

Epidemiology

Chronic musculoskeletal pain is commonly encountered in the general population. In the north of England, prevalence rates of 11.2% for chronic widespread pain and 43% for regional pain were found (Croft et al 1993). In a Kansas study (Wolfe et al 1995) the prevalence of chronic widespread musculoskeletal pain was more common in women and increased progressively from ages 18 to 70—with a 23% prevalence in the seventh decade. There appears to be a tendency for some subjects with regional pain syndromes to develop the widespread pain of fibromyalgia (Forseth et al 1999a). The overall prevalence of fibromyalgia in the Kansas population was 2%, with a prevalence of 3.4% in women and 0.5% in men. All epidemiological studies have reported that chronic widespread pain is more prevalent than the ACR defined diagnosis of fibromyalgia, and it is conceptualized that fibromyalgia is at one end of a continuous spectrum of chronic pain (MacFarlane 1999).

Clinical features

Pain

The core *symptom* of the fibromyalgia (FM) syndrome is chronic widespread pain (Wolfe et al 1990). The pain is usually perceived as arising from muscle; however, many fibromyalgia patients also report joint pain (Reilly and Littlejohn 1992). Stiffness, worse in the early morning, is a prominent symptom of most FM patients; along with the perception of articular pain this may reinforce the impression of an arthritic condition. Fibromyalgia pain and stiffness typically have a diurnal variation, with a nadir during the hours of about 11.00 am to 3.00 pm (Moldofsky 1994).

Fatigue

Easy fatigability from physical exertion, mental exertion, and psychological stressors are typical of fibromyalgia (Yunus et al 1981). The etiology of fatigue in fibromyalgia is multifaceted and is thought to include non-restorative sleep, deconditioning, dysautonomia, depression, poor coping mechanisms, and secondary endocrine dysfunction involving the hypothalamic pituitary adrenal axis and growth hormone deficiency (Bennett et al 1997, Pillemer et al 1997). Patients with the chronic fatigue syndrome (CFS) have many similarities with FM patients (Aaron and Buchwald 2001). About 75% of patients meeting the diagnostic criteria of CFS also meet the criteria for diagnosis of FM (Goldenberg et al 1990).

Disordered sleep

Fibromyalgia patients usually report disturbed sleep (Moldofsky et al 1975). Even if they sleep continuously for 8 to 10 h they awake feeling tired. This is referred to as non-restorative sleep. Most relate to being light sleepers, being easily aroused by low-level noises or intrusive thoughts. Many exhibit an alpha–delta EEG pattern, which would explain their never getting into the restorative stages 3 and 4 of non-REM sleep (Moldofsky 1989). However an alpha intrusion rhythm in delta sleep is not invariable in fibromyalgia nor is it specific (Hauri and Hawkins 1973). The experimental induction of alpha–delta sleep in healthy individuals has been reported to induce musculoskeletal aching and/or stiffness as well as increased muscle tenderness (Moldofsky and Scarisbrick 1976). A poor night's sleep is often followed by a worsening of fibromyalgia symptoms the next day (Affleck et al 1996).

Cognitive dysfunction

Cognitive dysfunction is a major problem, according to self-reports, for many fibromyalgia patients (Park et al 2001). Patients commonly describe difficulties with short-term memory, concentration, logical analysis, and motivation. Problems with cognitive function are being increasingly recognized in fibromyalgia patients and are the subject of increasing research efforts (Glass and Park 2001). Currently, defects have been described in terms of working memory, episodic memory, and verbal fluency. These decreases in cognitive performance has been estimated to be equivalent to 20 years of aging (Glass and Park 2001).

Associated disorders

It is not unusual for fibromyalgia patients to have an array of somatic complaints other than musculoskeletal pain, such as irritable bowel syndrome, restless leg syndrome, dysautonomia, cognitive dysfunction, chemical hypersensitivity, and irritable bladder (Clauw 1995). It is now thought that these symptoms are in part a result of the abnormal sensory processing and the neuroendocrine effects of chronic stress.

Psychological distress

As in many chronic conditions there is an increased prevalence of psychological diagnoses in fibromyalgia patients. Depression is more common in fibromyalgia patients than in healthy controls (Burckhardt et al 1994, Yunus 1994). Importantly fibromyalgia is not common in patients with major depression, even those depressed individuals who complained of pain did not have multiple tender points (Fassbender et al 1997). Psychological distress in fibromyalgia may in part determine who becomes a patient (Aaron et al 1996). There is increasing acceptance that post-traumatic stress disorder may be associated with fibromyalgia (Amir et al 1997). Although psychiatric disorders are more prevalent in fibromyalgia patients than fibromyalgia non-patients, they do not seem to be intrinsically related to the pathophysiology of the fibromyalgia syndrome, but rather appear to be a result of symptom severity (Aaron et al 1996).

Initiation and maintenance of fibromyalgia

Fibromyalgia seldom emerges out of the blue. Most patients relate an acute injury, repetitive work related pain, athletic injuries, or another pain state. It is not uncommon for a regional pain syndrome to evolve into fibromyalgia (Forseth et al 1999b). Others attribute stress, infections, and toxins to its onset. Fibromyalgia is commonly found as an accompaniment of rheumatoid arthritis, low back pain, SLE, Sjogren's and inflammatory bowel disease, and osteoarthritis (Morand et al 1994, Urrows et al 1994, Lapossy et al 1995, Bennett 1997, Sperber et al 1999). There is a reported 22% prevalence of fibromyalgia one year after whiplash injuries (Buskila et al 1997). A striking familial prevalence of fibromyalgia has been reported by Buskila et al 1996). This suggests that subjects destined to develop fibromyalgia either are genetically predisposed (nature) or have past life events or experiences that favor its later development (nurture).

Prognosis and impact

Fibromyalgia symptomatology often persists over many years (Bengtsson et al 1994). Chronic musculoskeletal pain often severely impacts a patient's quality of life (Burckhardt et al 1993). An analysis of 1604 fibromyalgia patients followed in academic centres reported that pain, fatigue, sleep disturbance, functional status, anxiety, depression, and health status were essentially unchanged after 7 years of follow-up (Wolfe et al 1997a). There is some evidence that fibromyalgia patients seen in the community, rather than tertiary care centres, have a better prognosis (Granges et al 1994). The consequences of pain and fatigability influence motor performance; everyday activities take longer in fibromyalgia patients, they need more time to get started in the morning, and they often require extra rest periods during the day (Henriksson CM 1994). They have difficulty with repetitive sustained motor tasks, unless frequent time-outs are taken. Tasks may be well tolerated for short periods of time, but when carried out for prolonged periods become aggravating factors (Waylonis et al 1994). The adaptations that fibromyalgia patients have to make in order to minimize their pain experience often has a negative impact on both vocational and avocational activities.

Disability

Despite the superficial appearance of normality many fibromyalgia patients have difficulty with remaining competitive in the work force (Bennett 1996a). Most FM patients report that chronic pain and fatigue adversely affect the quality of their life and negatively impact their ability to be competitively employed (Henriksson 1995). The extent of reported disability in FM varies greatly from country to country—probably reflecting differences in political philosophies and socio-economic realities. A survey of fibromyalgia patients seen in academic centres reported that 70% perceived themselves as being disabled. Sixteen percent were receiving Social Security benefits (SSD); this compares to 2.2% of the US population (Wolfe et al 1997b).

Pathogenesis

The contemporary aetiological paradigm for fibromyalgia is that of a complex hyperalgesic pain syndrome, in which abnormalities of central sensory processing interact with peripheral pain generators and neuro-endocrine pathways to generate a wide spectrum of patient symptomatology and distress. It is now thought that both peripheral and central factors contribute in varying degrees to the expression of symptoms labelled as fibromyalgia.

For most of the twentieth century fibrositis/fibromyalgia was considered to be a muscle disease. It is now appreciated that there are no distinctive muscle changes that can define fibromyalgia in terms of a specific tissue pathology (Simms 1996). However, this does not mean that non-pathological muscle pain problems, such as exertional muscle microtrauma, are of no relevance to the pathogenesis. Indeed, it is hypothesized that any tissue-generated cause of pain (a peripheral pain generator) can accentuate and/or perpetuate central pain mechanisms.

Focal loci of muscle pain are referred to as myofascial trigger points. These are hyperalgesic zones in muscle that often feel indurated on palpation. Prolonged pressure over these areas may cause a pattern of pain that is referred distally—hence the name 'trigger points' (Travell and Simons 1992). Kellgren pioneered studies using hypertonic saline to evaluate the correlates of painful foci within muscle (Kellgren 1938). Graven-Nielsen has demonstrated that hypertonic saline-induced muscle pain demonstrates temporal and spatial summations influenced by central facilitatory and inhibitory mechanisms (Basbaum and Fields 1984, Graven-Nielsen et al 1997). These experiments highlight the importance of focal muscle pain in inducing a state of central sensitization and are postulated to be relevant to abnormal sensory processing in fibromyalgia patients (Henriksson KG 1994, Bennett 1996c).

Muscle microtrauma, a normal occurrence in healthy individuals, has been postulated to be one cause of peripheral nociceptive input in fibromyalgia patients (Bennett 1993). It is difficult to diagnose this phenomenon as the act of biopsying a muscle can cause trauma. However, NMR spectroscopy can evaluate living untraumatized muscle. Three NMR studies have reported an increase in phosphodiester peaks in fibromyalgia compared to controls (Jubrias et al 1994, Park et al 2000, Sprott et al 2000). Phosphodiester peaks occur in musculodystrophies (Younkin et al 1987) and also with increasing age (Satrustegui et al 1988). They are thought to result from the lipid peroxidation of sarcolemmal membrane proteins. This process occurs in calcium-activated muscle damage (muscle microtrauma) (Armstrong et al 1991).

There are several lines of evidence to suggest that the pain experience of fibromyalgia patients is in part the result of disordered sensory processing at a central level.

Qualitative differences in pain

An objective measure of applied force to a tender point can be obtained by dolorimetry (Campbell et al 1983). A study using an electronic dolorimeter recorded the subject's assessment of pain intensity on a 0- to 10-cm visual analogue scale (VAS) at varying levels of applied force (Bendtsen et al 1997). Distinctly different response curves were obtained for controls and fibromyalgia patients. Similar abnormalities of pain processing in fibromyalgia patients have also been reported for heat and cold (Kosek et al 1996).

Deficient pain modulation in response to repeated thermal stimuli

An up-regulation of pain threshold can be demonstrated in normal individuals by subjecting them to repeated non-noxious skin stimulation. This is the basis for the use of transcutaneous nerve stimulators (TENS) in the management of chronic pain states. The physiological basis for this effect is the inhibition of dorsal horn neuron excitability by persistent stimulation of type A myelinated axons (Wall and Cronly-Dillon 1960). This effect, known as diffuse noxious inhibitory control (DNIC), is defective in fibromyalgia subjects (Lautenbacher and Rollman 1997), thus supporting the notion that they have a defective descending inhibitory pain system (Mense 2000).

Hyper-responsive somatosensory induced potentials

Somatosensory-induced potentials refer to the electrophysiological activity in the brain that can be measured by skull electrodes in response to peripheral sensory stimulation. Gibson et al reported an increased late nociceptive (CO_2-laser stimulation of skin) evoked somatosensory response in 10 FM patients compared to 10 matched controls (Gibson et al 1994). Lorenz et al (1996) have reported increased amplitude of the N170 and P390 brain somatosensory potentials in fibromyalgia compared to controls evoked by laser stimulation of the skin. Furthermore they observed a response in both hemispheres, whereas in controls the response was localized to one side of the brain. These two studies provide objective evidence that fibromyalgia patients have an altered processing of nociceptive stimuli in comparison to pain-free controls.

Secondary hyperalgesia on electrocutaneous stmulation

Primary hyperalgesia is the normal perception of pain from nociceptor stimulation in an injured tissue. Secondary hyperalgesia refers to pain elicited from uninjured tissues (Magerl et al 1998). Arroyo and Cohen, while attempting to treat fibromyalgia patients with electrical nerve stimulation, reported sensory phenomena characteristic of secondary hyperalgesia (Arroyo and Cohen 1993).

Abnormalities on SPECT imaging

Pain-induced changes in brain blood flow or metabolism can now be visualized by several different imaging techniques (Bradley et al 2000). There are reports of reduced thalamic blood flow in fibromyalgia subjects (Mountz et al 1995, Kwiatek et al 2000). It is interesting that chronic pain states have been associated with thalamic blood flow, whereas acute pain *increases* thalamic blood flow. The reason for this difference is postulated to be a disinhibition of the medial thalamus, which results in activation of a limbic network (Craig 1998).

Elevated levels of substance P in the CSF

Substance P is an important nociceptive neurotransmitter. There are three definitive studies that have shown a threefold increase of substance P in the CSF of fibromyalgia patients compared to that in controls (Vaeroy et al 1988, Russell et al 1994, Liu et al 2000). Animal models of hyperalgesia and hypoalgesia have implicated substance P as a major aetiological factor in central sensitization and have highlighted the relevance of substance P in human pain states (Abbadie et al 1996).

Elevated levels of nerve growth factor

Nerve growth factor (NGF) is required for the normal development of sympathetic and sensory neurons. Giovengo et al have reported a fourfold elevation of NGF in the CSF of patients with primary fibromyalgia compared with that of healthy controls and other pain patients (Giovengo et al 1999). The intravenous administration of recombinant nerve growth factor in humans results in a muscle pain syndrome resembling fibromyalgia that lasts for up to a week after the initial injection. The mechanism whereby NGF causes hyperalgesia is hypothesized to be related to its stimulation of protein synthesis in the CNS (Bennett 2001).

Beneficial response to an NMDA receptor antagonist

The excitatory amino acid glutamine reacting with NMDA (*N*-methyl-D-aspartic acid) receptors plays a central role in the generation of non-nociceptive pain. Two studies have reported that intravenous ketamine (an NMDA receptor antagonist) attenuates pain and increases pain threshold, as well as improving muscle endurance in FM patients (Sorensen et al 1995). The experimental induction of pain summation and referral by intramuscular hypertonic saline in fibromyalgia is attenuated by the use of ketamine (Graven-Nielsen et al 2000).

Experimentally induced central hyperexcitability

Temporal summation of nociceptive impulses at the level of the spinal cord normally occurs when unmyelinated C fiber input exceeds a rate of one impulse every 2–3 s. There is good experimental evidence that this neurophysiological process is a critical event in the development of central sensitization (Koltzenburg et al 1994). An amplification of temporal summation has been demonstrated after repetitive thermal stimulation of the palmar skin in fibromyalgia patients (Staud et al 2001) and after intramuscular electrical stimulation of muscle (Sorensen et al 1998).

Management

The management of fibromyalgia patients is an exercise in symptom palliation and maintenance of physical and emotional functionality. The successful management of fibromyalgia patients requires a thorough analysis in terms of the bio-psycho-social model of disease. The major management issues that usually require attention are shown in Table 7.1.

Table 7.1 The components of a fibromyalgia treatment programme

1. Diagnosis and evaluation
2. Education
3. Pain
4. Fatigue
5. Sleep
6. Psychological disorders
7. Endocrine dysfunction
8. Dysautonomia
9. Deconditioning
10. Cognitive dysfunction
11. The existential crisis
12. Associated syndromes

Diagnosis and evaluation

The diagnosis of fibromyalgia is usually based on 1990 recommendations of the American College of Rheumatology classification criteria (Wolfe et al 1990). However, it is increasingly evident that many patients with widespread pain have less than the recommended 11 out of 18 tender points. If a patient has widespread pain and tenderness in many other areas, they are unlikely to have a different neuro-physiological basis for their pain than patients with strictly ACR-defined fibromyalgia. Thus it is important to look at other sites that commonly harbour myofascial trigger points. The reason for this more extensive evaluation is twofold: (1) to establish a probable diagnosis fibromyalgia in patients with less than 11 tender points, and (2) to find relevant myofascial pain generators that would benefit from trigger point therapy (Borg-Stein and Stein 1996).

Fibromyalgia is not a diagnosis of exclusion, and thus laboratory tests and imaging studies play no role in establishing the diagnosis according to the 1990 ACR criteria. However, fibromyalgia patients may have concomitant conditions that are relevant to overall management in terms of peripheral pain generators that can accentuate and maintain central sensitization. In many cases these concomitant problems investigational approach to diagnosis. A fibromyalgia-focused history and examination is an important requisite in obtaining data for an effective management programme. The history and examination will probably suggest certain problems that need further evaluation in terms of specialist referral or investigations.

Education

There is good evidence that higher educational attainments are associated with a better prognosis in many chronic diseases (Ramos-Remus et al 2000). There are several studies that support the value of education in fibromyalgia patients (Gowans et al 1999, Mannerkorpi et al 2000). Indeed, education has several components common to cognitive behavioural techniques, such as goal setting and reassessment of priorities. Important educational issues are shown in Table 7.2.

Table 7.2 The components of a fibromyalgia educational programme

1. Validate symptoms
2. Emphasize non-destructive (*not necessarily benign*) nature of FM
3. Focus on improving function, not complete eradication of symptoms—as in many other chronic diseases
4. Discuss importance of mind–body relationships—teach meditation and relaxation techniques
5. Discuss drug and non-drug therapy options
6. Discuss 'touted cures' for FM
7. Explain the importance of gentle life-long exercise
8. Inform about principles of sleep hygiene
9. Discuss pacing of activities, feelings of guilt and improved assertiveness
10. Emphasize patient's *active* role in any treatment plan

Table 7.3 Peripheral pain generators

Myofascial trigger points
Degenerative joint disease
Inflammatory joint disease
Bursitis
Tendinitis
Developmental defects (e.g., scoliosis)
Hypermobility syndrome
Neuropathic pain
Injuries/trauma
Repetitive strain
Visceral pain (e.g., IBS, endometriosis)
Herniated discs
Spinal stenosis/Chiari malformation
Recurrent headaches (e.g., migraine)

Pain

In considering the management of pain in FM it is logical to focus on the major sites of pain generation/processing, namely peripheral pain generation, dorsal horn sensitization, psychological influences, and the descending pain pathway.

There is no specific tissue pathology, at least in peripheral tissues, that can be said to be characteristic of fibromyalgia (Simms 1996). However, this fact should not be taken as negating the importance of peripheral nociceptive mechanisms. Once the CNS is sensitized, peripheral pain generators will not only be perceived as being more painful, but a persistent barrage of nociceptive impulses will prolong and amplify the biochemical machinery of central sensitization. Common peripheral pain generators are shown in Table 7.3. Although some peripheral pain generators, notably arthritic disorders, may be helped by NSAIDs, central pain is not usually very responsive to these agents. Thus the use of NSAIDs is usually adjunctive to the use of centrally acting analgesics. Specific treatments for other pain generators would include, for example, gabapentin in neuropathic pain and 5-HT_{1D} antagonists in vascular headaches. Some pain generators, such as osteoarthritis of the knees or bursitis, may be helped by local corticosteroid injections. In other instances surgery may be appropriate (e.g., severe osteoarthritis of the hips, Chiari malformation, endometriosis). As the commonest pain generators, in most fibromyalgia patients, are myofascial trigger points it is imperative that these be identified and effectively managed in terms of pacing, stretching, improved physical conditioning, self-help techniques such as acupressure and spray and stretch, and physician intervention in terms of procaine or botulinum toxin injections.

Most of the drugs used to treat pain act at the level of the dorsal horn. The modulation of the 'nociceptive amplification' that occurs at the first synapse is mainly pharmacological (Reveille 2000). The descending pain system originates in the midbrain and terminates at the level of dorsal horn neurons, thus influencing spinal cord sensitization (Willis and Westlund 1997). This descending system is responsible for such diverse events as the placebo effect, fear-induced hypoalgesia, anticipatory hyperalgesia, the benefits of cognitive behavioural therapy, the action of opioids, and inflammation-induced hyperalgesia. Thus cortical and subcortical circuits can modulate dorsal horn activity through emotional states related to attention, motivation, and cognition. Currently the only FDA-approved drugs that modulate dorsal horn cell reactivity are those that activate or amplify the *descending* pain system; these include opioids, tricyclic antidepressants, and alpha-2 adrenergic agonists.

Antidepressants such as amitriptyline have long been a mainstay in the treatment of chronic pain states (Fishbain 2000), including fibromyalgia

(Carette et al 1986). A meta-analysis of antidepressants, in the treatment of fibromyalgia, analysed 13 randomized, placebo-controlled trials (O'Malley et al 2000). The odds ratio for improvement with therapy was 4.2. Analysing the effect on specific symptoms indicated that antidepressants improved sleep, fatigue, pain, and well-being—in that order. Only one study found a correlation between symptom benefit and improvement in depression. Despite their widespread use, the long-term efficacy of antidepressants in managing fibromyalgia pain has not been well established (Carette et al 1994).

Opioids are effective in most acute and chronic pain states. Although opioids are fairly commonly used in the treatment of fibromyalgia (Wolfe et al 1997a), there have been no controlled clinical trials. The main problems related to long-term use of opioids are the effects on cognition, reduced motivation to pursue non-pharmacological treatment modalities, aggravation of depression, and negative stigmatization by the medical profession and society in general (Savage 1996). The usual cited concerns regarding addiction are now known to be unfounded—only occurring in about 0.5% of opioid-treated chronic pain patients (Portenoy 1996). All patients taking opioids can be expected to develop dependency; this, however, is not the same as addiction, but implies that this class of medications cannot be abruptly stopped without the patient experiencing withdrawal symptoms. Addiction is a dysfunctional state occurring as a result of the unrestrained use of a drug for its mind-altering properties; manipulation of the medical system and the acquisition of narcotics from non-medical sources are common accompaniments. Addiction should not be confused with 'pseudo-addiction'. This is a drug-seeking behaviour generated by attempts to obtain appropriate pain relief in the face of undertreatment of pain (Weissman and Haddox 1989). Opiates should not be the first choice of analgesia in fibromyalgia, but they should not be withheld if less powerful analgesics have failed.

Tramadol (Ultram) is proving to be a useful drug to treat pain in chronic conditions, including fibromyalgia (Roth 1998, Schnitzer et al 2000). Tramadol has a dual mechanism of acting both as a weak opioid agonist and as an inhibitor of the reuptake of serotonin and noradrenaline (norepinephrine) at the level of the dorsal horn (Lewis and Han 1997). A double-blinded study demonstrated its efficacy and tolerability in the management of fibromyalgia pain at an average dose of 200 mg/day (Russell et al 1997). A combination of tramadol and acetaminophen (Ultracet) has also been reported to benefit fibromyalgia pain and other symptoms (Bennett et al 2001).

Alpha-2 adrenergic agonists such as tizanidine (Zanaflex) have been used successfully in some chronic pain disorders (Fogelholm and Murros 1992). The experimental basis for this antinociceptive action is the observation that intrathecally administered alpha-2 adrenergic agonists, but not beta-adrenergic receptor agonists, produce a powerful analgesia in both experimental animals and man (Nabeshima et al 1987, Coward 1994). There have been no trials of these agents in fibromyalgia. There is anecdotal evidence for tizanidine being useful in FM-related pain, as not only is it antinociceptive but it is also an antispasmodic (Smith and Barton 2000), which cause drowsiness—a benefit in fibromyalgia patients if it is given in the evening.

5-HT3 antagonists have been the subject of several encouraging short-term trials in fibromyalgia patients (Farber et al 2000, Haus et al 2000). 5-HT3 receptors are found only in neuronal tissues, both central and peripheral (Tecott et al 1993). The complex biochemistry of 5-HT3 receptors suggests that antagonists would have nociceptive and antinociceptive actions in different circumstances. When activated the 5-HT3 receptor causes a rapid membrane depolarization with resultant rise in cytosolic Ca^{++}, which in turn modulates the release of neuro-active molecules such as substance P, serotonin, GABA, acetylcholine, cholecystokinin, and dopamine (Wolf 2000). Longer-term studies in fibromyalgia patients are needed before the efficacy of this class of drugs can be fully evaluated.

Drugs that modulate the *ascending* pain system are less commonly used. However, there is experimental evidence that blocking NMDA receptors with ketamine ameliorates pain in fibromyalgia subjects (Sorensen et al 1995). Dextromethorphan is a weak NMDA receptor antagonist that has been successfully used in neuropathic pain (McQuay et al 1994) and more recently as an adjunct to tramadol and treatment of fibromyalgia (Clark and Bennett 2000). Logically inhibiting the release of substance P or blocking its interaction with the NK-1 receptor should be beneficial. However, clinical trials of a first-generation substance P antagonist were disappointing in chronic pain states (Hill 2000). To date NGF antagonists have not been used in human clinical trials.

Fatigue

The common treatable causes of chronic fatigue in fibromyalgia patients are: (1) inappropriate dosing of medications (TCAs, drugs with antihistamine actions, benzodiazapines, etc.), (2) depression, (3) aerobic deconditioning, (3) a primary sleep disorder (e.g. sleep apnoea), (4) non-restorative sleep (see above), (5) neurally mediated hypotension, and (6) growth hormone deficiency (Bennett et al 1998). Many of these causative factors are most amenable to non-pharmacological interventions. However, sleep problems, depression and other psychological stressors, some features of dysautonomia, and endocrine dysfunction are appropriately treated with drugs. Recent studies using the 5-HT3 receptor antagonist tropisetron reported benefits both in fibromyalgia-related fatigue and in chronic fatigue syndrome (Spath et al 2000). There are anecdotal reports that modafinal (Provigil), a non-amphetamine drug used in narcolepsy and sleep deprivation situations, is of some benefit in improving non-specific fatigue (Lyons and French 1991).

Sleep

Most fibromyalgia patients relate to being light sleepers, being easily aroused by low-level noises or intrusive thoughts. Many exhibit an alpha–delta EEG pattern, which would explain their never getting into the restorative stages 3 and 4 of non-REM sleep (Drewes et al 1995). Important non-pharmacological aspects of sleep management include ensuring an adherence to the basic rules of sleep hygiene and regular low-grade exercise. The use of low-dose tricyclic antidepressants (amitriptyline, trazadone, doxepin, imipramine, etc.) has been the mainstay of sleep pharmacotherapy in FM patients (Goldenberg 1989, Carette et al 1994). Many fibromyalgia patients cannot tolerate TCAs due to unacceptable levels of daytime drowsiness or weight gain. In these patients, benzodiazapine-like medications such as aprazolam (Russell et al 1991), zolpidem (Moldofsky et al 1996), and zopiclone (Drewes et al 1991) have been shown to be beneficial in a few trials. A subset of fibromyalgia patients suffer from a primary sleep disorder, which requires specialized management. About 25% of male and 15% of female fibromyalgia patients have sleep apnoea, which usually requires treatment with positive airway pressure (CPAP) or surgery. By far the commonest sleep disorder in fibromyalgia patients is restless leg syndrome/periodic limb movement disorder. Treatment is usually with L-dopa/carbidopa (Sinemet 10/100 mg at suppertime) or clonazepam (Klonipin 0.5 or 1.0 mg at bedtime) (Montplaisir et al 1992). More recently other dopamine agonists such as pergolide, tolixepole, and pramixepole have been proven to be effective.

Psychological distress

Having a chronic painful disease for which there is currently no generally accepted cure often produces a cascade of emotional reactions that can be likened to an existential crisis (Chapman and Gavrin 1999). Approximately 30% of fibromyalgia patients have significant current depression and about 60% have a lifetime prevalence of depressive illness (Okifuji et al 2000). It is generally assumed that treating depression fibromyalgia patients is no different than treating primary depressive illness. There are no trials that have specifically addressed the issue of treating depression in FM patients; however, one article addressed this issue in a useful review (Gruber et al 1996). Although antidepressant medications are commonly used in the treatment of pain and sleep in fibromyalgia patients, the doses used are usually suboptimal for treating depressive illness. Further FM patients may be taking many other medications with the potential for adverse interactions and are more sensitive to medication side effects. In that FM patients often develop stressors related to psychosocial/economic issues, therapy focusing on problem-solving techniques and cognitive restructuring may be beneficial in addition to drug therapy. Patients with poor coping strategies often tend to catastrophize adverse life events—which they perceive as being helpless to influence. Psychological intervention in terms of improving the internal locus of control and more effective problem solving is important in such patients. Techniques of cognitive-behavioural therapy seem particularly well suited to effect these changes and may be enhanced when done as a part of group therapy (Goldenberg et al 1994).

Deconditioning

The notion that 'exercise is good for fibromyalgia patients' is an accepted contemporary truth (Clark et al 2001) supported by many studies. The benefits of exercise are based on reasonable scientific evidence, but exercise may also be deleterious (Mengshoel et al 1995). Whether it is good or bad for fibromyalgia patients probably depends upon many variables, such as age, current level of conditioning, rate of increase of exercise intensity, frequency of exercise, ratio of eccentric to concentric muscle use, hormonal anabolic status, and negative factors such as obesity, arthritis, and concomitant muscle disease. There are some similarities between fibromyalgia symptomatology and the overtraining syndrome. Overtraining results in a syndrome of chronic fatigue, reduced performance, depression, impaired hormonal stress responses, increased susceptibility to muscle damage, and infections (Urhausen et al 1998). A carefully planned individual exercise programme is always needed to optimize the benefits and minimize increased pain and fatigue (Clark 1994).

Endocrine dysfunction

There is no good evidence that fibromyalgia is primarily due to an endocrine disorder. However, common problems such as hypothyroidism and menopausal symptoms will often aggravate pain and fatigue, and appropriate replacement therapy is usually indicated. There has been much interest in abnormalities of the hypothalamic–pituitary–adrenal axis (HPA) in fibromyalgia patients (Crofford et al 1994, Pillemer et al 1997). The general impression is that fibromyalgia patients have a somewhat reduced HPA responsiveness. However, replacement therapy with Prednisone 15 mg/day was not shown to be therapeutically useful in fibromyalgia (Clark et al 1985). About one-third of fibromyalgia patients are growth hormone deficient (Bennett et al 1997), and replacement therapy has been reported to benefit such patients (Bennett et al 1998).

Associated disorders

Recognition and treatment of problems commonly associated with fibromyalgia are important in the overall management scheme.

Chronic fatigue

The common treatable causes of chronic fatigue in fibromyalgia patients are: (1) inappropriate dosing of medications (TCAs, drugs with antihistamine actions, benzodiazapines, etc.), (2) depression, (3) aerobic deconditioning, (3) a primary sleep disorder (e.g. sleep apnoea), (4) non-restorative sleep (see above), (5) neurally mediated hypotension, and (6) growth hormone deficiency (Bennett et al 1997, 1998).

Restless leg syndrome

Treatment is simple and very effective—L-dopa/levodopa (Sinemet) in an *early* evening dose of 10/100 mg (a minority require a higher dose or use of the long-acting preparations). Some patients respond to gabapentin. Recalcitrant cases are often helped by low-dose opioid therapy.

Irritable bowel syndrome

Treatment involves (1) elimination of foods that aggravate symptoms, (2) minimizing psychological distress, (3) adhering to basic rules for maintaining a regular bowel habit, and (4) prescribing medications for specific symptoms: constipation (stool softener, fibre supplementation, and gentle laxatives such as bisacodyl), diarrhoea (loperamide or diphenoxylate), and antispasmodics (dicycloverine (dicyclomine) or anticholinergic/sedative preparations such as Donnatal).

Irritable bladder syndrome

Treatment involves (1) increasing intake of water, (2) avoiding bladder irritants such as fruit juices (especially cranberry), (3) pelvic floor exercises (e.g. Kagel exercises), and (4) the prescription of antispasmodic medications (e.g. oxybutinin, flavoxate, hyoscamine).

Cognitive dysfunction

This is a common problem for many fibromyalgia patients. It adversely affects the ability to be competitively employed and may cause concern as to an early dementing type of neurodegenerative disease. In practice the latter concern has never been a problem and patients can be reassured. The cause of poor memory and problems with concentration is, in most patients, related to the distracting effects of chronic pain and mental fatigue. Thus the effective treatment of cognitive dysfunction in fibromyalgia is dependent on the successful management of the other symptoms.

Cold intolerance

Treatment involves: (1) keeping warm, (2) low-grade aerobic exercise (which improves peripheral circulation), (3) treatment of neurally mediated hypotension (see below), and (4) the prescription of vasodilators such as the calcium channel blockers (but these may aggravate the problem in patients with hypotension).

Multiple sensitivities

Treatment involves being aware that this is a fibromyalgia-related problem and employing avoidance tactics. Medications often need to be started at half the usual doses.

Dizziness

Treatable causes related to fibromyalgia include: (1) proprioceptive dysfunction secondary to muscle deconditioning, (2) proprioceptive dysfunction secondary to myofascial trigger points in the sterno-cleido-mastoids and other neck muscles, (3) neurally mediated hypotension (see below), and (4) medication side effects. Treatment is dependent upon making an accurate diagnosis.

Neurally mediated hypotension

Treatment involves: (1) education as to the triggering factors and their avoidance, (2) increasing plasma volume (increased salt intake, prescription of florinef), (3) avoidance of drugs that aggravate hypotension (e.g., TCAs, antihypertensives), (4) preventing reflex (β-adrenergic antagonists or disopyramide), and (5) minimizing the efferent limb of the reflex (α-adrenergic agonists or anticholinergic agents).

Multidisciplinary team therapy

Most of the recommendations for management assume a one-on-one doctor–patient encounter. In the era of cost-effective medicine it is often difficult to accommodate the demands of these patients. However, most of these same recommendations can be incorporated into a multidisciplinary treatment programme using a team of interested health professionals (nurse practitioners, clinical psychologists, exercise physiologists, mental health care workers, and social workers) (Goldenberg 1989, Bennett 1996b, Turk et al 1998). In this way groups of 5–15 patients can be seen in designated sessions several times a month. Patients are usually appreciative of meeting others who share similar problems, and the dynamics of group therapy is often a powerful aid to cognitive-behavioural modifications. Such groups can be encouraged to develop a sense of camaraderie in solving mutual problems. This form of therapy has proved beneficial in one 6-month programme, with continuing improvement out to 2 years after leaving the programme (Bennett et al 1996).

References

Aaron LA, Buchwald D 2001 A review of the evidence for overlap among unexplained clinical conditions. Annals of Internal Medicine 134: 868–881

Aaron LA et al 1996 Psychiatric diagnoses in patients with fibromyalgia are related to health care-seeking behavior rather than to illness. Arthritis and Rheumatism 39: 436–445

Abbadie C et al 1996 Spinal cord substance P receptor immunoreactivity increases in both inflammatory and nerve injury models of persistent pain. Neuroscience 70: 201–209

Affleck G et al 1996 Sequential daily relations of sleep, pain intensity, and attention to pain among women with fibromyalgia. Pain 68: 363–368

Amir M et al 1997 Posttraumatic stress disorder, tenderness and fibromyalgia. Journal of Psychosomatic Research 42: 607–613

Armstrong RB, Warren GL, Warren JA 1991 Mechanisms of exercise-induced muscle fibre injury. Sports Medicine 12: 184–207

Arroyo JF, Cohen ML 1993 Abnormal responses to electrocutaneous stimulation in fibromyalgia. Journal of Rheumatology 20: 1925–1931

Basbaum AI, Fields HL 1984 Endogenous pain control systems: brainstem spinal pathways and endorphin circuitry. Annual Review of Neuroscience 7: 309–338

Bendtsen L et al 1997 Evidence of qualitatively altered nociception in patients with fibromyalgia. Arthritis and Rheumatism 40: 98–102

Bengtsson A et al 1994 Long term follow-up of fibromyalgia patients: clinical symptoms, muscular function, laboratory tests—an eight year comparison study. Journal of Musculoskeletal Pain 2: 67–80

Bennett DL 2001 Neurotrophic factors: important regulators of nociceptive function. Neuroscientist 7: 13–17

Bennett R 1997 The concurrence of lupus and fibromyalgia: implications for diagnosis and management. Lupus 6: 494–499

Bennett RM 1981. Fibrositis: misnomer for a common rheumatic disorder. Western Journal of Medicine 134: 405–413

Bennett RM 1993 The origin of myopain: An integrated hypothesis of focal muscle changes and sleep disturbance in patients with the fibromyalgia syndrome. Journal of Musculoskeletal Pain 1: 95–112

Bennett RM 1996a Fibromyalgia and the disability dilemma. A new era in understanding a complex, multidimensional pain syndrome. Arthritis and Rheumatism 39: 1627–1634

Bennett RM 1996b Multidisciplinary group programs to treat fibromyalgia patients. Rheumatic Disease Clinics of North America 22: 351–367

Bennett RM 1996c The contribution of muscle to the generation of fibromyalgia symptomatology. Journal of Musculoskeletal Pain 4: 35–59

Bennett RM et al 1996 Group treatment of fibromyalgia: a 6 month outpatient program. Journal of Rheumatology 23: 521–528

Bennett RM et al 1997 Hypothalamic-pituitary-insulin-like growth factor-I axis dysfunction in patients with fibromyalgia. Journal of Rheumatology 24: 1384–1389

Bennett RM, Clark SR, Walczyk J 1998 A randomized, double-blind, placebo-controlled study of growth hormone in the treatment of fibromyalgia. American Journal of Medicine 104: 227–231

Bennett RM et al 2001 Efficacy and safety of a tramadol/acetaminophen combination (Ultracet) in the management of fibromyalgia-related pain: a multicenter, outpatient, randomized, double-blind, placebo controlled study.

Borg-Stein J, Stein J 1996 Trigger points and tender points: one and the same? Does injection treatment help? Rheumatic Disease Clinics of North America. 22: 305–322

Bradley LA et al 2000 Use of neuroimaging to understand abnormal pain sensitivity in fibromyalgia. Current Rheumatology Reports 2: 141–148

Burckhardt CS, Clark SR, Bennett RM 1993 Fibromyalgia and quality of life: a comparative analysis. Journal of Rheumatology 20: 475–479

Burckhardt CS et al 1994 Assessing depression in fibromyalgia patients. Arthritis Care Research 7: 35–39

Buskila D et al 1996 Familial aggregation in the fibromyalgia syndrome. Seminars in Arthritis and Rheumatism 26: 605–611

Buskil D et al 1997 Increased rates of fibromyalgia following cervical spine injury. A controlled study of 161 cases of traumatic injury. Arthritis and Rheumatism 40: 446–452

Campbell SM et al 1983 Clinical characteristics of fibrositis. I.A 'blinded' controlled study of symptoms and tender points. Arthritis and Rheumatism 26: 817–824

Carette S et al 1986 Evaluation of amitriptyline in primary fibrositis. A double-blind, placebo-controlled study. Arthritis and Rheumatism 29: 655–659

Carette S et al 1994 Comparison of amitriptyline, cyclobenzaprine,

and placebo in the treatment of fibromyalgia. Arthritis and Rheumatism 37: 32–40
Chapman CR, Gavrin J 1999 Suffering: the contributions of persistent pain. Lancet 353: 2233–2237
Clark SR 1994 Prescribing exercise for fibromyalgia patients. Arthritis Care Research 7: 221–225
Clark SR, Bennett RM 2000 Supplemental dextromethorphan in the treatment of fibromyalgia: a double-blind, placebo-controlled study of efficacy and side-effects. Arthritis and Rheumatism 43: S333
Clark S, Tindall E, Bennett RM 1985 A double blind crossover trial of prednisone versus placebo in the treatment of fibrositis. Journal of Rheumatology 12: 980–983
Clark SR et al 2001. Exercise for patients with fibromyalgia: risks versus benefits. Current Rheumatology Reports 3: 135–140
Clauw DJ 1995 Fibromyalgia: more than just a musculoskeletal disease. American Family Physician 52: 843–851, 853–854
Coward DM 1994 Tizanidine: neuropharmacology and mechanism of action. Neurology 44: S6–10
Craig AD 1998 A new version of the thalamic disinhibition hypothesis of central pain. Pain Forum 7: 1–14
Crofford LJ et al 1994 Hypothalamic–pituitary–adrenal axis perturbations in patients with fibromyalgia. Arthritis and Rheumatism 37: 1583–1592
Croft P et al 1993 The prevalence of chronic widespread pain in the general population. Journal of Rheumatology 20: 710–713
Drewes AM et al 1991 Zopiclone in the treatment of sleep abnormalities in fibromyalgia. Journal of Rheumatology 20: 288–293
Drewes AM et al 1995 Clustering of sleep electroencephalographic patterns in patients with the fibromyalgia syndrome. British Journal of Rheumatology 34: 1151–1156
Farber L et al 2000 Efficacy and tolerability of tropisetron in primary fibromyalgia—a highly selective and competitive 5-HT3 receptor antagonist. German Fibromyalgia Study Group. 113: 49–54
Fassbender K et al 1997 Tender points, depressive and functional symptoms: comparison between fibromyalgia and major depression. Clinical Rheumatology 16: 76–79
Fishbain D 2000 Evidence-based data on pain relief with antidepressants. Annals of Medicine 32: 305–316
Fogelholm R, Murros K 1992 Tizanidine in chronic tension-type headache: a placebo controlled double-blind cross-over study. Headache 32: 509–513
Forseth KO, Forre O, Gran JT 1999a A 5.5 year prospective study of self-reported musculoskeletal pain and of fibromyalgia in a female population: significance and natural history. Clinical Rheumatology 18: 114–121
Forseth KO et al 1999b Prognostic factors for the development of fibromyalgia in women with self-reported musculoskeletal pain. A prospective study. Journal of Rheumatology 26: 2458–2467
Gibson SJ et al 1994 Altered heat pain thresholds and cerebral event-related potentials following painful CO_2 laser stimulation in subjects with fibromyalgia syndrome. Pain 58: 185–193
Giovengo SL, Russell IJ, Larson AA 1999 Increased concentrations of nerve growth factor in cerebrospinal fluid of patients with fibromyalgia. Journal of Rheumatology 26: 1564–1569
Glass JM, Park DC 2001 Cognitive dysfunction in fibromyalgia. Current Rheumatology Reports 3: 123–127
Goldenberg DL 1987 Fibromyalgia syndrome. An emerging but controversial condition. Journal of the American Medical Association 257: 2782–2787
Goldenberg DL 1989 A review of the role of tricyclic medications in the treatment of fibromyalgia syndrome. Journal of Rheumatology 19 (suppl): 137–139
Goldenberg DL et al 1990 High frequency of fibromyalgia in patients with chronic fatigue seen in a primary care practice. Arthritis and Rheumatism 33: 381–387
Goldenberg DL et al 1994 A controlled study of a stress-reduction, cognitive-behavioral treatment program in fibromyalgia. Journal of Musculoskeletal Pain 2: 53–66
Gowans SE et al 1999 A randomized, controlled trial of exercise and education for individuals with fibromyalgia. British Medical Journal 12: 120–128
Gowers WR 1904 Lumbago: Its lessons and analogues. British Medical Journal 1: 117–121
Granges G, Zilko P, Littlejohn GO 1994 Fibromyalgia syndrome: assessment of the severity of the condition 2 years after diagnosis. Journal of Rheumatology 21: 523–529
Graven-Nielsen T et al 1997 Quantification of local and referred muscle pain in humans after sequential i.m. injections of hypertonic saline. Pain 69: 111–117
Graven-Nielsen T et al 2000 Ketamine reduces muscle pain, temporal summation, and referred pain in fibromyalgia patients. Pain 85: 483–491
Gruber AJ, Hudson JI, Pope HG Jr. 1996 The management of treatment-resistant depression in disorders on the interface of psychiatry and medicine. Fibromyalgia, chronic fatigue syndrome, migraine, irritable bowel syndrome, atypical facial pain, and premenstrual dysphoric disorder. Psychiatric Clinics of North America 19: 351–369
Hauri P, Hawkins DR 1973 Alpha-delta sleep. Electroencephalography and Clinical Neurophysiology 34: 233–237
Haus U et al 2000 Oral treatment of fibromyalgia with tropisetron given over 28 days: influence on functional and vegetative symptoms, psychometric parameters and pain. Scandinavian Journal of Rheumatology 113: 55–58
Henriksson CM 1994 Longterm effects of fibromyalgia on everyday life. A study of 56 patients. Scandinavian Journal of Rheumatology 23: 36–41
Henriksson CM 1995 Living with continuous muscular pain—patient perspectives. Part I: Encounters and consequences. Journal of the Caring Sciences 9: 67–76
Henriksson KG 1994 Chronic muscular pain: aetiology and pathogenesis. Baillière's Clinical Rheumatology 8: 703–719
Hill R 2000 NK1 (substance P) receptor antagonists—why are they not analgesic in humans? Trends in Pharmalogical Sciences 21: 244–246
Jubrias SA, Bennett RM, Klug GA 1994 Increased incidence of a resonance in the phosphodiester region of ^{31}P nuclear magnetic resonance spectra in the skeletal muscle of fibromyalgia patients. Arthritis and Rheumatism 37: 801–807
Kellgren JH 1938. Observations on referred pain arising from muscle. Clinical Science 3: 175–190
Koltzenburg M, Torebjork HE, Wahren LK 1994 Nociceptor modulated central sensitization causes mechanical hyperalgesia in acute chemogenic and chronic neuropathic pain. Brain 117: 579–591
Kosek E, Ekholm J, Hansson P 1996 Sensory dysfunction in fibromyalgia patients with implications for pathogenic mechanisms. Pain 68: 375–383
Kwiatek R et al 2000 Regional cerebral blood flow in fibromyalgia: single-photon-emission computed tomography evidence of reduction in the pontine tegmentum and thalami. Arthritis and Rheumatism 43: 2823–2833
Lapossy E et al 1995 The frequency of transition of chronic low back pain to fibromyalgia. Scandinavian Journal of Rheumatology 24: 29–33
Lautenbacher S, Rollman GB 1997 Possible deficiencies of pain modulation in fibromyalgia. Clinical Journal of Pain 13: 189–196
Lewis KS, Han NH 1997 Tramadol: a new centrally acting

analgesic. American Journal of Health-System Pharmacy 54: 643–652
Liu Z et al 2000 A high-recovery extraction procedure for quantitative analysis of substance P and opioid peptides in human cerebrospinal fluid. Peptides 21: 853–860
Lorenz J, Grasedyck K, Bromm B 1996 Middle and long latency somatosensory evoked potentials after painful laser stimulation in patients with fibromyalgia syndrome. Clinical Neurophysiology 100: 165–168
Lyons TJ, French J 1991 Modafinil: the unique properties of a new stimulant. Aviation Space and Environmental Medicine 62: 432–435
MacFarlane GJ 1999 Generalized pain, fibromyalgia and regional pain: an epidemiological view. Baillieres Best Practice in Clinical Rheumatology 13: 403–414
Magerl W, Wilk SH, Treede RD 1998 Secondary hyperalgesia and perceptual wind-up following intradermal injection of capsaicin in humans. Pain 74: 257–268
Mannerkorpi K et al 2000 Pool exercise combined with an education program for patients with fibromyalgia syndrome. A prospective, randomized study. Journal of Rheumatology 27: 2473–2481
McQuay HJ et al 1994 Dextromethorphan for the treatment of neuropathic pain: a double-blind randomised controlled crossover trial with integral n-of-1 design. Pain 59: 127–133
Mengshoel AM, Vollestad NK, Forre O 1995 Pain and fatigue induced by exercise in fibromyalgia patients and sedentary healthy subjects. Clinical and Experimental Rheumatology 13: 477–482
Mense S 2000 Neurobiological concepts of fibromyalgia—the possible role of descending spinal tracts. Scandinavian Journal of Rheumatology 113: 24–29
Moldofsky H 1989 Sleep and fibrositis syndrome. Rheumatic Diseases Clinics of North America 15: 91–103
Moldofsky H 1994 Chronobiological influences on fibromyalgia syndrome: theoretical and therapeutic implications. Baillière's Clinical Rheumatology 8: 801–810
Moldofsky H,. Scarisbrick P 1976 Induction of neurasthenic musculoskeletal pain syndrome by selective sleep stage deprivation. Psychosomatic Medicine 38: 35–44
Moldofsky H et al 1975 Musculosketal symptoms and non-REM sleep disturbance in patients with 'fibrositis syndrome' and healthy subjects. Psychosomatic Medicine 37: 341–351
Moldofsky H et al 1996 The effect of zolpidem in patients with fibromyalgia: a dose ranging, double blind, placebo controlled, modified crossover study. Journal of Rheumatology 23: 529–533
Montplaisir J et al 1992 The treatment of the restless leg syndrome with or without periodic leg movements in sleep. Sleep 15: 391–395
Morand EF et al 1994 Fibromyalgia syndrome and disease activity in systemic lupus erythematosus. Lupus 3: 187–191
Mountz JM et al 1995 Fibromyalgia in women. Abnormalities of regional cerebral blood flow in the thalamus and the caudate nucleus are associated with low pain threshold levels. Arthritis and Rheumatism 38: 926–938
Nabeshima T et al 1987 Antinociceptive activity induced by tizanidine and alpha-2 adrenoreceptors. Neuropharmacology 26: 1453–1455
O'Malley PG et al 2000 Treatment of fibromyalgia with antidepressants: a meta-analysis. Journal of General Internal Medicine 15: 659–666
Okifuji A, Turk DC, Sherman JJ 2000 Evaluation of the relationship between depression and fibromyalgia syndrome: why aren't all patients depressed? Journal of Rheumatology 27: 212–219
Park DC et al 2001 Cognitive function in fibromyalgia patients. Arthritis and Rheumatology 44: 2125–2133
Park JH, Niermann KJ, Olsen N 2000 Evidence for metabolic abnormalities in the muscles of patients with fibromyalgia. Current Rheumatology Reports 2: 131–140
Pillemer SR et al 1997 The neuroscience and endocrinology of fibromyalgia. Arthritis and Rheumatism 40: 1928–1939
Portenoy RK 1996 Opioid therapy for chronic nonmalignant pain: a review of the critical issues. Journal of Pain and Sympton Management 11: 203–217
Ramos-Remus C et al 2000 How important is patient education? Baillieres Best Practice in Clinical Rheumatology 14: 689–703
Reilly PA, Littlejohn GO 1992 Peripheral arthralgic presentation of fibrositis/fibromyalgia syndrome. Journal of Rheumatology 19: 281–283
Reveille JD 2000 The changing spectrum of rheumatic disease in human immunodeficiency virus infection. Seminars in Arthritis and Rheumatology 30: 147–166
Roth SH 1998 Efficacy and safety of tramadol HCl in breakthrough musculoskeletal pain attributed to osteoarthritis. Journal of Rheumatology 25: 1358–1363
Russell IJ et al 1991 Treatment of primary fibrositis/fibromyalgia syndrome with ibuprofen and alprazolam: a double-blind, placebo-controlled study. Arthritis and Rheumatism 34: 552–560
Russell IJ et al 1994 Elevated cerebrospinal fluid levels of substance P in patients with the fibromyalgia syndrome. Arthritis and Rheumatism 37: 1593–1601
Russell IJ et al 1997 Efficacy of Ultram™ [Tramadol HCL] treatment of fibromyalgia syndrome: Preliminary analysis of a multi-center, randomized, placebo-controlled study. Arthritis and Rheumatism 40: S214
Satrustegui J et al 1988 An in vivo phosphorus nuclear magnetic resonance study of the variations with age in the phosphodiers content of human muscle. Mechanisms of Aging and Development 42: 105–114
Savage SR 1996 Long-term opioid therapy: assessment of consequences and risks. Journal of Pain and Symptom Management 11: 274–286
Schnitzer TJ et al 2000 Efficacy of tramadol in treatment of chronic low back pain. Journal of Rheumatology 27: 772–778
Simms RW 1996 Is there muscle pathology in fibromyalgia syndrome? Rheumatic Disease Clinics of North America 22: 245–266
Smith HS, Barton AE 2000 Tizanidine in the management of spasticity and musculoskeletal complaints in the palliative care population. American Journal of Hospital and Palliative Care 17: 50–58
Sorensen J et al 1995 Pain analysis in patients with fibromyalgia: effects of intravenous morphine, lidocaine and ketamine. Scandinavian Journal of Rheumatology 24: 360–365
Sorensen J et al 1998 Hyperexcitability in fibromyalgia. Journal of Rheumatology 25: 152–155
Spath M, Welzel D, Farber L 2000 Treatment of chronic fatigue syndrome with 5-HT3 receptor antagonists—preliminary results. Scandinavian Journal of Rheumatology 113: 72–77
Sperber AD et al 1999 Fibromyalgia in the irritable bowel syndrome: studies of prevalence and clinical implications. American Journal of Gastroenterology 94: 3541–3546
Sprott H et al 2000 ^{31}P magnetic resonance spectroscopy in fibromyalgic muscle. Rheumatology (Oxford) 39: 1121–1125
Staud R et al 2001 Abnormal sensitization and temporal summation of second pain (wind-up) in patients with fibromyalgia syndrome. Pain 91: 165–175
Stockman R 1904 The causes, pathology and treatment of chronic rheumatism. Edinbugh Medical Journal 15: 107–116
Tecott LH, Maricq AV, Julius D 1993 Nervous system distribution of the serotonin 5-HT3 receptor mRNA. Proceedings of the National Academy of Sciences of the USA 90: 1430–1434
Travell JG, Simons DG 1992 Myofascial pain and dysfunction: the trigger point manual, vol. 2. Williams & Wilkins, Baltimore.

Turk DC et al 1998. Interdisciplinary treatment for fibromyalgia syndrome: clinical and statistical significance. 11: 186–195
Urhausen A, Gabriel HH, Kindermann W 1998 Impaired pituitary hormonal response to exhaustive exercise in overtrained endurance athletes. Medicine and Science in Sports and Exercise 30: 407–414
Urrows S et al 1994 Unique clinical and psychological correlates of fibromyalgia tender points and joint tenderness in rheumatoid arthritis. Arthritis and Rheumatism 37: 1513–1520
Vaeroy H et al 1988 Elevated CSF levels of substance P and high incidence of Raynaud phenomenon in patients with fibromyalgia: new features for diagnosis. Pain 32: 21–26
Wall PD, Cronly-Dillon JR 1960 Pain, itch and vibration. 2: 365–375
Waylonis GW, Ronan PG, Gordon C 1994 A profile of fibromyalgia in occupational environments. American Journal of Physican Medicine and Rahabilitation 73: 112–115
Weissman DE, Haddox JD 1989 Opioid pseudo-addiction: an iatrogenic syndrome. Pain 36: 363–364
White KP et al 1995 Fibromyalgia in rheumatology practice: a survey of Canadian rheumatologists. Journal of Rheumatology 22: 722–726
Willis WD, Westlund KN 1997 Neuroanatomy of the pain system and of the pathways that modulate pain. Journal of Clinical Neurophysiology 14: 2–31
Wolf H 2000 Preclinical and clinical pharmacology of the 5-HT3 receptor antagonists. Scandinavian Journal of Rheumatology 113: 37–45
Wolfe F et al 1990 The American College of Rheumatology 1990 criteria for the classification of fibromyalgia: report of the Multicenter Criteria Committee. Arthritis and Rheumatism 33: 160–172
Wolfe F et al 1995 The prevalence and characteristics of fibromyalgia in the general population. Arthritis and Rheumatism 38: 19–28
Wolfe F et al 1997a Health status and disease severity in fibromyalgia: results of a six-center longitudinal study [see comments]. Arthritis and Rheumatism 40: 1571–1579
Wolfe F et al 1997b Work and disability status of persons with fibromyalgia. Journal of Rheumatology 24: 1171–1178
Younkin DP et al 1987 ^{31}P NMR studies in Duchenne muscular dystrophy: age-related metabolic changes. Neurology 37: 165–169
Yunus MB 1994 Psychological aspects of fibromyalgia syndrome: a component of the dysfunctional spectrum syndrome. Baillière's Clinical Rheumatology 8: 811–837
Yunus M et al 1981 Primary fibromyalgia (fibrositis): clinical study of 50 patients with matched normal controls. Arthritis and Rheumatism 11: 151–171

Chapter 8

Abdominal pain

Laurence M Blendis

Introduction

In the vast majority of patients with the very common symptom of pain in the abdomen, presenting from childhood through to the elderly, no physical cause is apparent and in most cases, the symptoms are short-lived. Thus, although we classify abdominal pain as organic or non-organic, this only refers to the precipitating cause. The fact that a pathological process causes pain may depend on psychological factors, whereas even non-organic pain can often be shown to have a clearcut physical mechanism.

The acute abdomen

Sudden onset of abdominal pain is a very common and important diagnostic problem. Less than 5% of young people presenting with this symptom are admitted to hospital for observation and even fewer undergo surgery (Stevenson 1985). One helpful approach to diagnosis is to divide the abdomen into four quadrants and the central abdomen and to discuss the differential diagnosis for each quadrant.

Right lower quadrant pain

Acute appendicitis

Pain in the right lower quadrant is common, and the main differential diagnosis is that of acute appendicitis, especially in a male child (Michalowski et al 2001). The pain, commonly associated with anorexia, nausea, and frequent vomiting, often starts in the periumbilical area and moves to the right lower quadrant after some hours, often associated with a slight temperature of up to 39°C with or without frequency of bowel action or micturition. The clinical challenge is both to make the correct diagnosis of appendicitis, preventing unnecessary surgery, and to make it early enough to prevent complications, such as perforation, which increase morbidity. It is important to enquire about previous similar attacks since up to 10% may be suffering from recurrent appendicitis (Barber et al 1997). The patient is usually exquisitely tender in the right lower quadrant, with a sensation of a mass, except for patients with retrocaecal appendix, who are especially tender in the right side on rectal examination. Abdominal X-rays are unlikely to show any diagnostic features. Blood tests usually reveal a polymorphonuclear leucocytosis commonly

>20 000/mm (Barber et al 1997, Michalowski et al 2001), and urinalysis shows increased white cells. In one study the >40% incidence of negative surgical explorations was more than halved in uncertain cases by a simple 24-h observation period, during which more than 60% of admissions were found to have an infection not requiring surgery (Wenham 1982).

With the addition of appendiceal ultrasonography, no patients were operated upon unnecessarily for a normal appendix (100% specificity) but the sensitivity was only 75% (Puylaert et al 1987). Since in women the differential diagnosis is longer, laparoscopy has been added. This reduced unnecessary appendicectomy from 37 to 7% (Olsen et al 1993).

Recently, routine appendiceal computed tomography (CT) was performed on 100 consecutive patients and was 98% accurate, changing the proposed management in 59 patients, including unnecessary surgery or admission for 24-h observation (Rao et al 1998). CT involves more irradiation and expense than ultrasound, and although overall savings were $447 per patient, expertise in appendiceal ultrasound should be encouraged, as well as maintenance of clinical skills (McColl 1998).

Mesenteric lymphadenitis

This differential diagnosis is a large one, and the more common disorders are shown in Box 8.1. In children and young adolescents, who are at the commonest age of presentation of acute appendicitis, mesenteric lymphadenitis is a likely alternative. This usually occurs in a setting of an 'epidemic' or contact history of virus infections, usually of the upper respiratory tract. Symptomatically, the patients closely resemble those with acute appendicitis. One helpful differentiating point is that in mesenteric lymphadenitis, the white blood count is usually normal with a relative lymphocytosis, although it may be surprisingly high. Abdominal imaging should reveal a lymphadenopathy and normal appendix, hopefully reducing the number of young people with this condition having a normal appendix removed.

Infective distal ileocaecitis

Infectious ileocaecitis is usually associated with more systemic symptoms than acute appendicitis. Patients with distal ileitis due to Yersinia very often give a history of swimming in a lake or drinking possibly contaminated water. Serial serological studies for Yersinia should be performed (Attwood et al 1987). The differential diagnosis of infective ileocaecitis has been considerably lengthened because of the increase in immuno-suppressed patients (Box 8.2).

BOX 8.1
Some common causes of acute abdomen: differential diagnosis

Right lower quadrant
Acute appendicitis
Mesenteric lymphadenitis
Infective distal ileitis
Crohn's disease
In females, tubo-ovarian disorders
- Ectopic pregnancy
- Rupture of ovarian cyst
- Acute salpingitis

Renal disorders
- Right ureteric calculus
- Acute pyelonephritis
- Acute cholecystitis
- Acute rheumatic fever
- Pyogenic sacroiliitis

Right upper quadrant
Acute cholecystitis
Biliary colic
Acute hepatic distension or inflammation
Perforated duodenal ulcer

Central abdominal pain
Gastroenteritis
Small intestinal colic
Acute pancreatitis

Left upper quadrant
Perisplenitis
Splenic infarct
Disorders of splenic flexure

Left lower quadrant
Acute diverticulitis
Pyogenic sacroiliitis

Crohn's disease

Patients with Crohn's disease usually give a past history of abdominal symptoms such as intermittent discomfort with distension and alteration in bowel habit and weight loss, with or without other systemic manifestations. On examination, the most important differential diagnostic sign is a mass in the right lower quadrant. Barium radiographs are diagnostic in Crohn's disease, but since they are inadvisable in a patient with a differential diagnosis of acute appendicitis, non-invasive imaging is preferable for further diagnostic support.

> **BOX 8.2**
> **Some causes of ileocaecitis**
>
> Infectious
> - Viral—herpes virus, cytomegalovirus
> - Bacterial—salmonella, shigella, yersinia
> - Mycobacterial
> - Protozoal—entamoeba, cryptosporidium
> - Fungal—candida, aspergillus
>
> Ischaemic ileocolitis
> - Vasculitis

Ovarian tubular disorders

In young women in the third and fourth decades, ovariotubal disorders become more important. Thus, it is extremely important to obtain a complete menstrual history. A period of amenorrhoea suggests the possibility of an ectopic pregnancy, whereas a history of promiscuity would suggest the possibility of acute salpingitis. However, this is usually bilateral. These conditions usually give rise to tenderness on vaginal examination.

Renal and ureteric colic

Renal colic starts in either flank and radiates around and down into the groin. It is usually due to a ureteric calculus passing from the renal pelvis into the ureter causing obstruction. The colicky pain, resulting from increasing peristaltic contractions as the calculus is forced distally towards the bladder, characteristically comes in waves that gradually build up in intensity, causing the patient to sweat and to feel nauseated. As the wave of pain recedes, the patient feels considerable relief, despite residual soreness, until the next wave begins. The calculous is usually seen on an abdominal flat plate or ultrasound.

Right upper quadrant pain

Biliary colic and acute cholecystitis

Biliary colic usually starts in the right upper quadrant and radiates around to the back with or without referred pain to the right shoulder tip. Such patients are often tender in the right upper quadrant, particularly on deep inspiration. In contrast, in acute inflammation of the gallbladder or cholecystitis without the passage of a gallstone, the pain is constant and the patient is exquisitely tender in the right upper quadrant. At least two other conditions must be considered in acute right upper quadrant pain: duodenal ulcer perforation and acute hepatic congestion.

Acute duodenal ulcer perforation

Acute perforation of a duodenal ulcer produces pain. Acute ulcers are often precipitated by stress. The sudden onset of severe pain in the region is followed by symptoms and signs of peritonism with 'boardlike' rigidity of the anterior abdominal wall and 'guarding'. A straight abdominal radiograph may show a gas shadow outside the duodenal lumen under the right diaphragm.

Acute hepatic congestion

The major organ in the right upper quadrant, the liver, occasionally causes acute pain that is usually associated with acute enlargement and stretching of the hepatic capsule, due either to inflammation, as in acute viral hepatitis, or to acute congestion secondary to acute heart failure or hepatic vein obstruction, the Budd–Chiari syndrome. All conditions result in a variable degree of jaundice and an acute release into the bloodstream of hepatic enzymes, especially the transaminases with levels rising from less than 50 to greater than 1000 IU/L.

If acute Budd–Chiari syndrome is suspected, a liver–spleen radionuclide scan may show the characteristic pattern of hepatic 'wipe-out' with sparing or hypertrophy of the caudate lobe due to its venous drainage directly into the inferior vena cava. The diagnosis must be confirmed by Doppler ultrasound of the hepatic veins, and hepatic venography to demonstrate the blockage.

Central abdomen

Colic of the small intestine

Intestinal colic is most commonly due to acute inflammation of the bowel, such as acute gastroenteritis, in which the patient suffers from acute nausea, with or without vomiting, and crampy or colicky abdominal pain, repeatedly relieved by defecation of loose or watery stools. The infection is either viral, usually by contact during an epidemic, bacterial or parasitic from contaminated food or water. Microscopic examination of the stool for inflammatory cells, ova, and parasites, and stool culture may be diagnostic. In contrast, intestinal colic may be secondary to intestinal obstruction, the cause of which will depend on the site and on the age of the patient. This is associated with partial or complete constipation and abdominal distension. Vomiting occurs in relation to the site of the obstruction; the more proximal the lesion, the more likely the associated vomiting.

Non-invasive techniques are most useful in the diagnosis of colicky conditions. A flat plate of the abdomen may reveal a calcified stone in the ureter, gallbladder, or bile duct, whereas a non-calcified stone may be seen on ultrasonography. With intestinal obstruction, a supine and erect film will show distension of the bowel proximal to the obstruction whilst the erect film will show multiple air–fluid levels.

Acute pancreatitis

One of the few pains to begin in the centre of the abdomen is pancreatic. Acute pancreatitis is one of the severest of all pains and has a number of causes (Box 8.3). Infrequently none of these causes are present, and a diagnosis of idiopathic acute pancreatitis (IAP) is made. Endoscopic ultrasound may reveal an assortment of unsuspected diagnoses (Box 8.4). The central pain of pancreatitis is constant in nature and commonly bores through to the back so that classically relief may be attained by the patient sitting forward hugging his knees. On examination the patient may be tender on deep palpation. The diagnosis is confirmed by greatly elevated pancreatic enzymes, serum amylase, and especially lipase. This test has a 75% sensitivity and 90% specificity. More recently, a urinary trypsinogen-2 dipstick test was shown to have 95% sensitivity and specificity and 99% negative predictive value (Kemppainen et al 1997).

Abdominal angina

Central abdominal pain associated with large as opposed to small meals may be due to intestinal ischaemia. The diagnosis can only be made by angiographic demonstration of narrowed coeliac or superior mesenteric vessels and confirmed by the demonstration of a pressure difference across the stricture.

BOX 8.3
Some common causes of acute pancreatitis

Alcohol
Gallstones
Drugs, e.g., thiazides, frusemide, the pill
Metabolic: parathyroidism, hyperlipidaemia
Local inflammation: gastric or duodenal ulcer
Postoperative

BOX 8.4
Some causes of idiopathic acute pancreatitis

Microcrystals
Dysfunction of sphincter of Oddi
Pancreatic diversum
CFTR related
Crohn's disease
Celiac disease

Left upper quadrant

Splenic pain

The left upper quadrant is occupied by the spleen, which rarely causes pain except following a splenic infarct or when involved in a serositis, as in familial Mediterranean fever. Much more commonly, the spleen causes discomfort or a dragging sensation when it becomes enlarged due to any cause.

Splenic flexure of colon

The splenic flexure of the colon may cause pain if distended acutely, for example in patients with toxic megacolon secondary to ulcerative colitis, although this usually occurs in the transverse or descending colon. It is a common site of involvement in elderly patients with ischaemic colitis and secondary stricture formation may occur in the area.

Miscellaneous

Pain originating from the stomach due to distension or ulceration, or from the tail of an inflamed pancreas, may radiate to this area.

Left lower quadrant

Acute diverticulitis

The left lower quadrant is the classic site of pain in elderly patients with acute diverticulitis. Characteristically, they suffer from fever, pain, and either bloody stools or constipation. On examination, they may have a painful mass.

Non-specific ulcerative colitis

The commonest site of pain in patients with ulcerative colitis is the left lower quadrant. The patient is often tender over the descending colon. The diagnosis is made by observing the classic characteristics of the colonic and rectal muscosa colonoscopy. However, this condition, by spreading proximally, can involve any amount of the colon and thus cause pain and tenderness over the surface markings of the colon, especially in patients with toxic megacolon.

Peritonitis

Acute peritonitis usually occurs secondarily to perforation of a viscus or from direct involvement with an inflamed organ, such as the pancreas (Boxes 8.3, 8.4). The pain is usually generalized, although it may start in the area of the perforated organ. The patient learns to lie very still, since any movement of the abdomen increases the pain. Thus, on examination, the abdomen is still and the anterior abdominal wall is not involved in respiration. It feels 'boardlike' on palpation as the anterior abdominal wall muscles 'guard' the inflamed mucosa underneath. The secondary effect of peritonitis is a loss of bowel sounds as the bowel becomes paralysed by contact with the inflammation and an ileus develops. Abdominal radiographs and ultrasound show large dilated loops of both large and small bowel, and extraluminal collections.

From the clinical viewpoint, the physician must make the following decisions. Is the cause surgical (e.g., perforation) or medical, infected, or non-infected inflammation? The cause will determine the management.

Diagnosis of difficult cases of acute abdominal pain

All physicians must be aware of the possibility of a generalized medical condition presenting as acute abdominal pain, examples of which are shown in Box 8.5.

When the diagnosis of acute abdominal pain is in doubt and laparotomy is being considered, the diagnostic method of fine catheter aspiration cytology may be used (Stewart et al 1986). Cytological specimens were prepared by the cytosieve technique and the number of neutrophils per 500 cells was counted. Of 27 patients, 25 had a successful test. Prelaparotomy diagnosis was correct in 14 patients before the test, compared to 20 after the test.

BOX 8.5
Some examples of acute abdominal pain in general medical conditions

AIDS
Neutropenic enteropathy (Starnes et al 1986)
Collagen vascular disorders (mesenteric arteritis)
Polyarteritis nodosa and polyangiitis (Jennette and Falk 1997)
Familial Mediterranean fever (Babior and Matzner 1997)
Diabetes mellitus
Tabes dorsalis
Sickle cell anaemia
Acute intermittent porphyria (Kauppinen and Mustajorki 1992)
Opiate withdrawal
Abdominal migraine

Chronic abdominal pain

Chronic abdominal wall pain

Before discussing the causes of chronic visceral pain, it is important to exclude the pain originating from the anterior abdominal wall. This is done first and foremost by considering this diagnosis and then looking for the characteristic findings on examination of this pain, namely, superficial tenderness that persists when the patient tenses the anterior abdominal wall. The pain and tenderness should disappear following injection of local anaesthetic directly into the tender area. The most likely explanation for this pain is entrapment and stretching of the anterior cutaneous branch of the thoracoabdominal nerve, and treatment is by local anaesthetic injection. However, the presence of a small ventral hernia must be excluded.

Organic causes of chronic abdominal pain

Atypical gastro-oesophageal reflux disorders (GERD)

Although the vast majority of patients suffering from GERD present with heartburn and other thoracic symptoms, a minority present with epigastric pain. When suspected, the diagnosis will require some or all of the following tests: barium swallow with video, manometry with 24-h monitoring for acid reflux, radionuclide technetium swallows for reflux, endoscopy with biopsy, especially looking for the presence of *Helicobacter pylori* infection, and serological tests for *H. pylori*. If present, then eradication of the infection with triple therapy, including a proton pump inhibitor, may bring relief (Klinkenberg-Knol et al 2000).

Gastric ulcer

Patients with gastric ulcer complain of periodic upper abdominal pain over a fairly large area, which is frequently related to meals and occurs soon after the patient starts eating. The pain is usually relieved to some extent by antacid medication. Gastric ulcer patients may lose a little weight in association with decreased food intake. It is now clear that the major factor in the aetiology of peptic ulcer disease is infection with *H. pylori*, cagA genotype (Maastricht Consensus Report 1997). This organism infects the mucosal environment and results in inflammation and ulceration. The treatment is one of a number of 1-week courses of triple therapy with two antibiotics and antacid therapy, such as a proton pump inhibitor (Maastricht Consensus Report 1997).

Gastric malignancy

The major differential diagnosis of a gastric ulcer is whether it is benign or malignant. Malignant ulcers are usually associated with atypical, constant pain, unrelated to meals but associated with anorexia and considerable weight loss. Fundic cancer causes dysphagia and regurgitation, whereas prepyloric lesions will cause gastric outlet obstruction with vomiting.

Primary low-grade lymphoma of the mucosa-associated lymphoid tissue (MALT) of the stomach is relatively rare, accounting for up to 10% of gastric malignancies. It is now clear that *H. pylori* infection is involved in the pathogenesis of both gastric cancer and lymphoma, and that eradication of the infection may lead to disappearance of the lymphoma (Sackman et al 1997).

Duodenal ulcer

Patients with duodenal ulcer are often able to localize their epigastric pain with one finger, commonly to the right of the midline or very high up in the midline, with or without radiation through to the back. The pain is also characteristically associated with the fasting state, often waking the patient in the early hours of the morning, and is then relieved by eating or drinking or antacid medication.

Nausea, abdominal distension, and vomiting are these days uncommon symptoms. These patients do not usually lose weight and may actually gain weight due to eating frequently to relieve the pain.

Treatment Once the diagnosis has been made, the aim of therapy is eradication of *H. pylori* infection, with one of the triple-therapy combinations. These generally include two antibiotics such as clarithromycin, amoxicillin, tetracycline, with or without metronidazole, in addition to antacid therapy with a proton pump inhibitor, H2-receptor antagonist, or bismuth compound (Wyeth et al 1996, Maastricht Consensus Report 1997).

Gastroparesis

There is little doubt that gastric distension can cause pain. Some of the best evidence comes from patients with gastroparesis, most of whom are diabetic. At one time this was thought to be only poorly manageable with prokinetic agents. Recently, gastric pacing with cardiac pacing wires implanted on the serosal surface has been used. Pacing entrained the gastric slow wave and converted tachygastria into regular 3-cpm slow waves with an improvement in both gastric emptying and symptoms, including pain (McCallum et al 1998). Furthermore it has recently been shown that symptomatic gastric distension activates structures implicated in somatic pain processing (Ladabaum et al 2001).

Chronic intestinal pseudo-obstruction (Wood et al 1999)

Disorders of the myenteric plexus and smooth muscle result in loss of peristaltic control and the migrating motor complex and intestinal distension. Initially the patient's symptoms may mimic IBS and later chronic intestinal obstruction with abdominal distension and pain, with or without vomiting, and diarrhoea associated with bacterial overgrowth and malabsorption. Or there may be involvement of the oesophagus, stomach, with gastroparesis, or colon, with constipation. There may be a family history or a history of drug ingestion. The numerous causes can be classified in various ways as for example in Box 8.6.

Therefore the diagnosis will involve clinical history, examination, radiology, endoscopy, and finally surgery with full-thickness biopsy of the intestinal wall. Recently antienteric neuron antibodies have been detected in patients with inflammatory degenerative neuropathy. The treatment will depend on the diagnosis.

Chronic pancreatitis and carcinoma of the pancreas

Chronic pancreatitis develops in less than 10% of patients following an attack of acute pancreatitis. The majority of these patients suffer from chronic relapsing pancreatitis with recurrent bouts of pain

BOX 8.6
Some causes of chronic intestinal pseudo-obstruction

1. Disorders of the myenteric plexus
   a. Developmental disorders
   b. Familial visceral disorders
   c. Sporadic visceral disorders
   d. Diffuse small intestinal diverticulosis
   e. Amyloidosis
   f. Toxic damage, e.g., laxatives, anticholinergics
2. Disorders of smooth muscle
   a. Primary (familial) visceral myopathies
   b. Secondary myopathies, e.g., systemic sclerosis

similar to the acute attacks associated with elevation of pancreatic enzymes. In less than 20% the pain is chronically persistent. There are two theories for this pain. The first is that there is involvement of the pancreatic nerves by inflammatory or scar tissue, and therefore the treatment is by medical nerve block. The second is that the pain is due to pancreatic ductular hypertension secondary to stricture formation. The medical treatment for this is to attempt to reduce pancreatic secretion. Patients with alcoholic chronic pancreatitis may benefit from cessation of drinking, so that many can expect cessation of pain by 7 to 10 years (Amman and Muelhaupt 1999).

The pain of carcinoma of the pancreas is usually central abdominal, deep, and radiating through to the back. Unrelated to meals, it is characteristically severe and requires powerful analgesics. Once the diagnosis is suspected, abdominal CT is the test of choice, showing pancreatic enlargement. This can be confirmed by endoscopic retrograde cholangiopancreatography (ERCP) examination. Unfortunately, only a small percentage of such cancers are operable.

Gastrointestinal food hypersensitivity

The evaluation of food allergies has been clarified by the recent publication of the document representing the official recommendation of the AGA (Sampson et al 2001). It is a true entity, most frequently involving cow's milk and soya proteins, eggs, fish, and nuts. There is a clear symptom complex with bloating, abdominal pain, and diarrhoea, especially in atopic infants. Such allergies are rarely confirmed in adults. Whatever the mechanism, recognition of the possibility and withdrawal of the offending food can result in the disappearance of symptoms.

Unusual causes

Finally when unable to make a diagnosis, the physician must always be aware of the long list of unusual causes of chronic abdominal pain such as Leishmaniasis (Magill et al 1993), mesenteric panniculitis (sclerosing mesocolitis, Weber–Christian disease) (Steely and Gooden 1986), and grumbling appendicitis, in which colonoscopy can be diagnostic with the appearance of inflammation localized to the root of the appendix in the caecal region (Johnson and De Cosse 1998).

Carbohydrate maldigestion and malabsorption

Five grams of indigestible carbodydrate can produce 1000 ml carbon dioxide, 400 ml methane (in methane producers), and 200 ml hydrogen via colonic bacterial fermentation (Hightower 1977). However, it has recently been shown that it is important to distinguish excess gas formation, as in hypolactasia, from a sensation of bloating, as in irritable bowel syndrome with normal gas production (Levitt et al 1996).

Hypolactasia

A lack of intestinal lactase is very common in many parts of the world. The result is that on drinking milk or eating certain dairy foods, lactose malabsorption occurs, leading to colonic gaseous fermentation, crampy abdominal pain over the colon and diarrhoea and excessive flatus. The diagnosis can be made from the history and confirmed by the lactose hydrogen breath test (Metz et al 1975). Lactose maldigestion was detected in 24% of 137 children with recurrent abdominal pain, which improved with a lactose free diet (Webster et al 1995). Management consists of treating any underlying pathology such as coeliac syndrome, in this case with a gluten-free diet, and then putting the patient on a lactose-free diet. Alternatively, if the patient needs or likes milk and dairy foods, these can be given together with synthetic lactases.

Hyposucrasia and multiple sugar malabsorptions

Because of their position further down the villi and their greater number and quantity, other disaccharidase deficiencies are either rare or never occur. For example, there are only a few case reports of sucrase deficiency. The patients present in the same way after eating foods containing sucrose, are diagnosed by the sucrose hydrogen breath test (Metz et al 1976a), and are treated by the elimination of sucrose from the diet. However, if symptoms do not improve, other sugars may be involved, such as fructose and sorbitol, with such patients presenting as non-ulcer dyspepsia (Mishkin et al 1997).

Stagnant loop syndrome

Carbohydrate maldigestion may also occur in patients who have bacterial colonization of the small intestine. Normally, the upper small intestine is only significantly colonized after meals and the bacteria are 'swept downstream' with the food. In patients with certain pathologies of the small intestine, luminar contents stagnate and become colonized, resulting in malabsorption. Examples of this are jejunal diverticulosis; systemic sclerosis of the duodenum and jejunum; fistulae producing a blind loop, such as Crohn's disease; and incomplete obstruction, such as radiation enteropathy (Newman et al 1973). These conditions are grouped under the heading of 'stagnant loop syndrome' and if proximal lead to monosaccharide fermentation, causing increased hydrogen production from glucose (Metz et al 1976b). The diagnosis of a stagnant loop can be suspected by evidence of bile acid or vitamin B_{12} malabsorption and confirmed by anatomical demonstration of the lesion by radiology.

Colonic maldigestion

Colonic 'maldigestion' of carbohydrate occurs normally if the diet contains large amounts of indigestible carbohydrate. Excessive amounts of unabsorbed carbohydrate, such as from fruit, vegetable, or sorbitol contained in chewing gum, can cause gaseous abdminal pain.

Constipation

In constipated individuals, increasing amounts of faecal material and gas build up in the colon, causing crampy pain. This may occur in the elderly, in the absence of any colonic pathology, or in association with diverticular disease of the colon. This diagnosis is made by clinical examination, and flat plates of the abdomen and treatment consists of normalizing the bowel action with a combination of diet, laxatives, and if necessary colonic lavage. Constipation is also a particularly common cause of abdominal pain in children, but a long list of causes must be excluded first (Seth and Heyman 1994).

Non-organic or psychogenic pain (Glaser and Engel 1977)

1. The location, distribution, timing, quality, and intensity of the pain do not relate to established pathophysiological patterns.
2. There is often a marked discrepancy between the severity of the pain and the patient's behaviour.
3. The patient usually has or has had multiple pains in many other parts of the body, which may have been fully investigated without any obvious abnormality being discovered. In other words, the patient is 'pain prone'.
4. The onset of pain may bear an obvious temporal relationship to stress. This is particularly the case with bereavement, where the onset may coincide with the death of a close relative or friend in whom abdominal pain may have been a major symptom.

In patients suffering from chronic pain the abdomen is the second commonest site (Merskey 1965). In the majority of older children and adolescents chronic abdominal pain is functional (Daum 1997). Extensive research into brain–gut relationships should lead to further elucidation of this problem and advances in therapy (Aziz and Thompson 1998).

Gaseous distension syndromes

Aerophagy

Aerophagy or excessive air swallowing can be due to organic conditions that cause pain or discomfort of the pharynx and oesophagus and include acute pharyngitis and peptic oesophagitis. The patient experiences relief of discomfort momentarily by swallowing air since, presumably, this results in a 'cushion' of air separating the inflamed surfaces.

The non-organic and far more common causes of aerophagy include anxiety and depression (Song et al 1993). Anxious people tend to swallow more air and tend to eat more quickly and take in excessive amounts of air, whilst swallowing food, which collects in the fundus of the stomach, causing discomfort and eventually pain throughout the gastrointestinal tract by stimulation of stretch receptors in the wall of the viscera. The patient will then gain temporary relief by belching the air out and the process is repeated. In one series there was a high incidence of bereavement of someone close who had died with abdominal pain. In a small group of these patients, the pain responded to antidepressant therapy (Blendis et al 1978).

Non-ulcer dyspepsia

On investigation 30–60% of patients complaining of non-specific upper abdominal discomfort or dyspepsia will be found to be infected with *H. pylori* with or without gastritis. It is still unclear whether this infection is the cause of the symptoms. Although in a percentage of patients the symptoms will disappear with triple therapy, there is no evidence that this is better than placebo (Blum et al 1998, Talley et al 1999). However, this remains a contenious issue, and some authors still advocate triple therapy for *H. pylori* positive functional dyspepsia (McColl et al 1998). If symptoms persist following successful eradication, then alternative therapy such as psychodynamic-interpersonal psychotherapy may be helpful (Hamilton et al 2000). Alternatively another cause may be present. For example, delayed gastric emptying with gastric distension has been detected in up to 35% of dyspeptic patients in a referral centre (Stanghellini et al 1996). This syndrome was associated with the female sex, postprandial fullness, and vomiting and tended to respond to prokinetic agents.

Irritable bowel syndrome (Horwitz and Fisher 2001)

Definition

As indicated at the beginning of the chapter, most people at some time or other suffer from a bout of non-organic abdominal pain associated with stress or after a bout of gastroenteritis. However, in the majority, the symptoms gradually disappear. Therefore, in children, irritable bowel syndrome (IBS) may occur in up to 15%, and has been classified as symptoms lasting for longer than 3 months (Milla 2001). Thus, IBS may be defined as symptoms of abdominal pain and disturbance of bowel action of more than 12 weeks duration without any organic cause. However, separating patients into diagnoses of non-ulcer dyspepsia and IBS may be artificial since 50% of patients may change their symptoms from one category to the other over a 1-year period (Agreus et al 1995).

Incidence

A recent study in the United States indicates that about 20–30% of the population suffer from IBS symptoms. IBS affects females more commonly than males, with ratios in published series varying from 1.5:1. A recent study found that in up to 44% of women presenting with IBS, there is a history of sexual and physical abuse (Drossman et al 1990). The peak age of onset is in the third decade. However, up to 70% of persons with identical IBS symptoms do not seek medical attention (Hahn et al 1997).

Clinical features

Abdominal pain is predominantly periumbilical in children (Milla et al 2001), whereas in adults it tends to occur over the surface markings of the colon with the commonest site in the left lower quadrant, less commonly the right or left upper quadrant over the hepatic or splenic flexures. It varies from a dull ache to attacks of excruciating severity, lasting from minutes to several hours to all day, but it rarely prevents the patient from sleeping through the night. 'Meteorism' is due to 'air trapping' in which segmental accumulation of gas occurs.

Alterations of bowel habit, diarrhoea or constipation occur in up to 90% of the patients. In about half the patients pain is aggravated by eating and relieved by defecation. However, the patient's appetite is rarely affected, and therefore a history of significant weight loss (i.e., more than 3.5 kg) is unusual and should raise suspicions of an alternative diagnosis.

IBS pain is associated with nausea without vomiting, dyspepsia, urinary symptoms, especially dysuria, gynaecological symptoms, especially dysmenorrhoea, and headache; IBS symptoms may begin after an attack of gastroenteritis (Gwee et al 1999). IBS may have been the cause of pelvic pain in 60% women attending gynaecological clinics, having dilatation and curettage for dysmenorrhoea, 40% having elective hysterectomy, compared to 32% of age-matched controls (Crowell et al 1994). They frequently have a past history of appendicectomy for 'chronic appendicitis'. Cancer phobia is another frequent observation in these patients.

Recently at a second conference in Rome on IBS, the Rome II Criteria evolved (Box 8.7). The Rome II Criteria are excellent for standardization of therapeutic trials and the discipline that they brought to the field but their very rigidity brings artificial constraints that will have to be reconsidered in the future (Camilleri 1998). On examination, there is usually a disparity between the severity of the patient's symptoms and his or her physical condition, since they look well. The patient will be tender over an area of the colon, most commonly the descending colon. Some patients are exquisitely tender on rectal examination. Sigmoidoscopic examination is usually normal but it is extremely difficult to proceed beyond the rectosigmoid junction, because of spasm and pain. The patients may also have mucosal hyperalgesia to light touch via the sigmoidoscope. Routine blood tests, including sedimentation rate, should be normal.

Psyche

Historical evidence of an affective disorder is common. Continuous fatigue is almost universal, some patients waking up tired after a full night's

BOX 8.7
The Rome II Criteria for IBS

Abdominal pain or discomfort, for at least 12 weeks out of the previous 12 months, which need not necessarily be consecutive (and cannot be explained by structural or biochemical changes), and has 2 of these 3 features:

a. relieved by defecation
b. onset associated with a change in frequency
c. consistency of stool

sleep, although insomnia may also be a problem. Alternatively, they may feel depressed and frequently close to tears. On formal testing, patients scored higher for anxiety, neuroticism, and introversion than normal controls or than patients with ulcerative colitis, their neurosis score lying midway between normal and frank neurosis, even in those patients with acute gastroenteritis before they have developed IBS (Gwee et al 1999). However, the psychological abnormalities found in IBS may be secondary to their patient status and not primary factors causing IBS (Kumar et al 1990), but they may be the determinants of health care seeking (Smith et al 1990).

Investigations

Any evidence of anaemia, leucocytosis, etc. should be further investigated to exclude other disease such as inflammatory bowel disease. Although it is important psychologically not to overinvestigate these patients, most of them eventually have a barium enema or colonoscopy, which is normal apart from a variable amount of spasm. Up to 25% of patients may have lactose intolerance (Bohmer and Tuynman 1996) or some other form of food intolerance (Nanda et al 1989). Removal of the offending food may lead to a marked improvement in symptoms.

Motility studies

Colonic motility has frequently been shown to be abnormal in IBS patients but motility studies on the small intestine, upper gastrointestinal tract, and even the oesophagus have shown abnormalities associated with hypersensitivity of lumbar splanchnic afferents (Lembo et al 1994, Accarino et al 1995). Distension of the appropriate area of intestine, especially distal colon and rectum, in adults and especially in children, reproduced the pain (van Ginkel et al 2001), with pain thresholds lower than that of normal volunteers, now recognized as the hypersensitivity phenomenon (Mayer and Gebhart 1994).

When patients have been subdivided clinically, the constipated type, with reduced colonic activity, were associated with a cholinergic disorder, and diarrhoeal types, in which colonic motor activity was increased and disordered, with an adrenergic abnormality (Aggarwal et al 1994).

Treatment (Camilleri 2001)

The essence of treatment of IBS is a sympathetic, patient, and even innovative physician who is prepared to spend time discussing the patient's symptoms and the pathogenesis of IBS. A high-fibre diet using soluble, cereal fibre such as natural bran, in an attempt to normalize intestinal transit, has been proposed as the basis of therapy, but is not universally accepted. As abdominal symptoms occur frequently in IBS patients following the ingestion of lactose, fructose, or sorbitol it is worth attempting to exclude these carbohydrates, one at a time, from the diet. In addition, stool-softening agents such as diocyte sodium 100 mg twice daily can be useful in constipated patients. Antispasmodic agents with or without sedatives have been tried with some success for patients with bloating and cramps (Jailwala et al 2000). Tricyclic antidepressants (Jackson et al 2000) and serotonin reuptake antagonists have been advocated for patients with frequent severe pain, since their neuromodulatory and analgesic properties function at lower doses. They have proven to be effective in randomized controlled trials, despite placebo response rates of >50% (Drossman et al 1997). It is still unclear whether the tricyclics have a specific antidepressant action in IBS (Jackson et al 2000). Serotonin plays a major role in the modulation of brain–gut function. The use of 5-HT3 receptor inhibitors, such as ondanstron, in diarrhea-predominant IBS patients improved stool consistency and reduced frequency. Alosetron, acting primarily on extrinsic afferent neurons innervating gut mucosa, decreased diarrhoea, by slowing left colonic transit, and improved pain directly by increasing compliance to distension and indirectly by inhibiting activation of spinal cord neurons by colonic distension. In a randomized controlled trial, alosetron, 1 mg b.i.d. for 12 weeks, caused significant improvement in pain and bowel function, during the entire 3 months, but increased constipation, compared to placebo (Camilleri et al 2000). Unfortunately since FDA approval for this very promising therapy, there have been frequent reports of severe side effects, including complete constipation with fecal impaction and ischaemic colitis (Friedel et al 2001). Tegaserod, a partial 5-HT4 receptor agonist at 2 mg b.i.d., was shown to significantly accelerate proximal colonic filling, a measure of orocaecal transit, at 6 h, compared to placebo (Prather et al 2000), and is superior to placebo in relieving abdominal bloating, discomfort, and constipation (Pandolfino et al 2000). However, in a recent review there was still considerable scepticism about the performance and therefore results of controlled trials in IBS (Klein 1998).

Prognosis

Irritable bowel syndrome is considered a chronic pain condition lasting for many years. However, in a report of the aggressive use of high-fibre diets and bulking agents, nearly 70% of patients were reported to be pain free at 5 years (Harvey et al 1987). Recently advances in the understanding of the gut–brain axis, and in the psychopathology of IBS, have led, and will continue to lead, to major advances in its management.

References

Accarino AM, Azpiroz F, Malagelada J-R 1995 Selective dysfunction of mechanosensitive intestinal afferents in irritable bowel syndrome. Gastroenterology 108: 636–643

Aggarwal A, Cutts TF, Abell TL, Cardoso S, Familoni B et al 1994 Predominant symptoms in irritable bowel syndrome correlate with specific autonomic nervous system abnormalities. Gastroenterology 106: 945–950

Agreus L, Svardsudd K, Nyren O et al 1995 Irritable bowel syndrome and dyspepsia in the general population: overlap and lack of stability. Gastroenterology 109: 671–680

Amman RW, Muelhaupt B 1999 The natural history of pain in alcoholic chronic pancreatitis. Gastroenterology 116: 1132–1140

Attwood SEA, Mealy K, Cafferkey MT et al 1987 *Yersinia* infection and acute abdominal pain. Lancet 1: 529–533

Aziz Q, Thompson DG 1998 Brain–gut axis in health and disease. Gastroenterology 114: 559–578

Babior BM, Matzner Y 1997 The familial Mediterranean fever gene-cloned at last. New England Journal of Medicine 337: 1548–1549

Barber MD, McLaren J, Rainey JB 1997 Recurrent appendicitis. British Journal of Surgery 84: 110–112

Blendis LM, Hill OW, Merskey H 1978 Abdominal pain and the emotions. Pain 5: 179–191

Blum AL, Talley NJ, O'Morain C et al 1998 Lack of effect of treating *Helicobacter pylori* positive functional dyspepsia in patients with nonulcer dyspepsia. New England Journal of Medicine 339: 1875–1881

Bohmer CJM, Tuynman H 1996 The clinical relevance of lactose malabsorption in irritable bowel syndrome. European Journal of Gastroenterology and Hepatology 8: 1013–1016

Camilleri M 1998 What's in a name? Roll on Rome II. Gastroenterology 114: 237

Camilleri M 2001 Management of irritable bowel syndrome. Gastroenterology 120: 652–668

Camilleri M, Northcutt AR, Kong S et al 2000 Efficacy and safety of alosetron in women with irritable bowel syndrome: a randomised, placebo-controlled trial. Lancet 355: 1035–1040

Crowell MD, Dubin NH, Robinson JC et al 1994 Functional bowel disorders in women with dysmenorrhea. American Journal of Gastroenterology 89: 1973–1977

Daum F 1997 Functional abdominal pain in older children and adolescents. Gastrointestinal Diseases Today 6: 7–12

Drossman DA, Leserman J, Nachman G et al 1990 Sexual and physical abuse in women with functional gastrointestinal disorders. Annals of Internal Medicine 113: 808–833

Drossman DA, Whitehead WE, Camilleri M 1997 Irritable bowel syndrome. Gastroenterology 112: 2118–2137

Friedel D, Thomas R, Fisher RS 2001 Ischemic colitis during treatment with alosetron. Gastroenterology 120: 557–560

Glaser JP, Engel GL 1977 Psychodynamics, psychophysiology and gastrointestinal symptomatology. Clinics in Gastroenterology 6: 507–531

Gwee KA, Leong YL, Graham C et al 1999 The role of psychological and biological factors in post-infective gut dysfunction. Gut 44: 400–440

Hahn BA, Saunders WB, Maier WC 1997 Differences between individuals with self-reportable irritable bowel syndrome (IBS) and IBS-like symptoms. Digestive Diseases and Sciences 42: 2585–2590

Hamilton J, Guthrie E, Creed F et al 2000 A randomised controlled trial of psychotherapy in patients with chronic functional dyspepsia. Gastroenterology 119: 661–669

Harvey RF, Mauad EC, Brown AM 1987 Prognosis in the irritable bowel syndrome: a 5-year prospective study. Lancet 1: 963–965

Hightower NC 1977 Intestinal gas and gaseousness. Clinics in Gastroenterology 6: 597–606

Horwitz BJ, Fisher RS 2001 The irritable bowel syndrome. New England Journal of Medicine 344: 1846–1850

Jackson JL, O'Malley PG, Tomkins G et al 2000 Treatment of functional gastrointestinal disorders with antidepressant medications: a meta-analysis. American Journal of Medicine 108: 65–72

Jailwala J, Imperiale TF, Kroenke K 2000 Pharmacological treatment of the irritable bowel syndrome: asystematic review of randomized, controlled trials. Annals of Internal Medicine 133: 136–147

Jennette JC, Falk RJ 1997 Small-vessel vasculitis. New England Journal of Medicine 337: 1512–1523

Johnson TR, De Cosse JJ 1998 Colonoscopic diagnosis of grumbling appendicitis. Lancet 351: 495–496

Kauppinen R, Mustajorki P 1992 Prognosis of acute porphyria. Medicine 71: 1–12

Kemppainen EA, Hedstrom JI, Puolakkainen PA et al 1997 Rapid measurement of urinary trypsinogen-2 as a screening test for acute pancreatitis. New England Journal of Medicine 336: 1788–1793

Klein KB 1998 Controlled treatment trials in the irritable bowel syndrome. A critique. Gastroenterology 95: 232–241

Klinkenberg-Knol EC, Nelis F, Dent J et al 2000 Long-term omeprazole treatment in resistant gastroesophageal reflux disease. Gastroenterology 118: 661–669

Kumar D, Pfeffer J, Wingate DLS 1990 Role of psychological factors in the irritable bowel syndrome. Digestion 45: 80–85

Ladabaum U, Minoshima S, Hasler WL et al 2001 Gastric distension correlates with activation of multiple cortical and subcortical regions. Gastroenterology 120: 369–376

Lembo T, Munakata J, Mertz H et al 1994 Evidence for the hypersensitivity of lumbar splanchnic afferents in irritable bowel syndrome. Gastroenterol 107: 1686–1696

Levitt MD, Furne J, Olsson S 1996 The relation of passage of gas and abdominal bloating to colonic gas production. Annals of Internal Medicine 124: 422–424

Maastricht Consensus Report 1997 The management of *H. pylori* infection. Gut 41: 8–13

Magill AJ, Grogi M, Gasser RA et al 1993 Visceral infection caused by leishmania tropica in veterans of Operation Desert Storm. New England Journal of Medicine 328: 1383–1387

Mayer EA, Gebhart GF 1994 Basic and clinical aspects of visceral hyperalgesia. Gastroenterology 107: 271–293

McCallum RW, Chen J de Z, Lin Z et al 1998 Gastric pacing improves emptying and symptoms in patient with gastroparesis. Gastroenterology 114: 456–461

McColl I 1998 More precision in diagnosing appendicitis. New England Journal of Medicine 338: 190–191

McColl K, Murray L, El-Omar E et al 1998 Symptomatic benefit from eradicating *Helicobacter pylori* infection in patients with nonulcer dyspepsia. New England Journal of Medicine 339: 1869–1874

Merskey H 1965 Psychiatric patients with persistent pain. Journal of Psychosomatic Research 9: 299–309

Metz G, Jenkins DJA, Peters TJ et al 1975 Breath hydrogen as a diagnostic method for hypolactasia. Lancet 1: 1155–1157

Metz G, Jenkins DJA, Peters TJ et al 1976a Breath hydrogen in hyposucrasia. Lancet 1: 119–120

Metz G, Gassull, MA, Draser BS et al 1976b Breath hydrogen test for small intestinal bacterial colonization. Lancet 1: 668–669
Michalowski W, Rubin S, Slowinski R et al 2001 Triage of the child with abdominal pain. Paediatrics and Child Health 6: 23–28
Milla P 2001 Irritable bowel syndrome in childhood. Gastroenterology 120: 287–307
Mishkin D, Sablauskas L, Yalosky M et al 1997 Fructose and sorbitol malabsorption in ambulatory patients with functional dyspepsia. Digestive Diseases and Sciences 42: 2591–2598
Nanda R, James R, Smith H et al 1989 Food intolerance and the irritable bowel syndrome. Gut 30: 1099–1104
Newman A, Katsaris J, Blendis LM et al 1973 Small intestinal injury in women who received pelvis radiotherapy. Lancet 2: 1471–1473
Olsen JB, Myren CI, Haahr PE 1993 Randomised study of the value of laparoscopy before appendectomy. British Journal of Surgery 80: 922–923
Pandolfino JE, Howden CW, Kahrilas PJ 2000 Motility-modifying agents and management of disorders of gastrointestinal motility. Gastroenterology 118: S32–S47
Prather CM, Camilleri M, Zinsmeister AR et al 2000 Tegaserod acclerates orocecal transit in patients with constipation in patients with constipation-predominant irritable bowel syndrome. Gastroenterology 118: 463–468
Puylaert JB, Rutgers PH, Lalisang RI et al 1987 A prospective study of ultrasonography in the diagnosis of appendicitis. New England Journal of Medicine 317: 666–670
Rao PM, Rhea JT, Novelline RA, Mostafavi AA, McCabe CJ 1998 Effect of computerised tomography of the appendix on treatment of patients and use of hospital resources. New England Journal of Medicine 338: 141–146
Sackman M, Morgner A, Rudolph B et al 1997 Regression of gastric MALT lymphoma after eradication of *H. pylori* is predicted by endosonographic staging. Gastroenterology 113: 1087–1090
Sampson HA, Sicherer SH, Birnbaum AH 2001 AGA technical review on the evaluation of food allergy in gastrointestinal disorders. Gastroenterology 120: 1026–1040
Seth R, Heyman MB 1994 Management of constipation and encopresis in infants and children. Gastroenterology Clinics of North America 23: 621–636
Smith RC, Greenbaum DS, Vancouver JB et al 1990 Psychosocial factors are associated with health care seeking rather than diagnosis in irritable bowel syndrome. Gastroenterology 98: 293–301
Song JY, Merskey H, Sullivan S et al 1993 Anxiety and depression in patients with abdominal bloating. Canadian Journal of Psychology 38: 475–479
Stanghellini V, Tosetti C, Paternico A et al 1996 Risk indicators of delayed gastric emptying of solids in patients with functional dyspepsia. Gastroenterology 110: 1036–1042
Starnes HF, Moore FD, Mentzer S et al 1986 Abdominal pain in neutropenic cancer patients. Cancer 57: 616–619
Steely WM, Gooden SM 1986 Sclerosing mesocolitis. Diseases of the Colon and Rectum 29: 266–268
Stevenson RJ 1985 Abdominal pain unrelated to trauma. Surgical Clinics of North America 65: 1181–1215
Stewart RJ, Gupta RK, Purdie GL et al 1986 Fine catheter aspiration cytology of peritoneal cavity in difficult cases of acute abdominal pain. Lancet 2: 1414–1415
Talley NJ, Vakil N, Ballard D et al 1999 Absence of benefit of eradicating *Helicobacter pylori* in patients with nonulcer dyspepsia. New England Journal of Medicine 341: 1106–1111
van Ginkel R, Voskuul WP, Benninga MA et al 2001 Alterations in rectal sensitivity and motility in childhood irritable bowel syndrome. Gastroenterology 120: 31–38
Webster RB, Di Palma JA, Gremse DA 1995 Lactose maldigestion and recurrent abdominal pain in children. Digestive Diseases and Sciences 40: 1506–1510
Wenham PW 1982 Viral and bacterial associations of acute abdominal pain in children. British Journal of Clinical Practice 36: 321–326
Wood JD, Alpers DH, Andrews PLR 1999 Fundamentals of neurogastroenterology. Gut 45: 1–44
Wyeth JW, Pounder RE, Duggan AE et al 1996 The safety and efficiency of ranitidine bismuth citrate in combinaton with antibiotics for the eradication of *Helicobacter pylori*. Alimentary Pharmacology and Therapeutics 10: 623–630

Chapter 9

Heart, vascular, and haemopathic pain

Paolo Procacci, Massimo Zoppi, and Marco Maresca

Introduction

This chapter analyses the clinical aspects of heart pain, vascular pain, and pain in haemopathies. These pains are associated with disease processes that are a major cause of morbidity and mortality.

Heart pain

The main diagnostic problem for a clinician who sees a patient suffering from chest pain is whether he is affected by heart disease. Particular attention is focused on exploring for possible cardiac ischaemia. We must, however, remember that many diseases cause chest pain. Apart from angina pectoris and myocardial infarction, pain can be present in some valvular heart diseases and in pericarditis. Many thoracic diseases may cause chest pain that often resembles pain from the heart, including:

1. some diseases of the aorta, such as dissection and atherosclerotic aneurysms
2. some diseases of the lungs, such as pulmonary embolism, infarction, pneumonia, cancer
3. pleuritis
4. diseases of the oesophagus, such as alterations of motility and inflammation.

Chest wall pain may also accompany or follow herpes zoster, chest injury, or Tietze's syndrome (i.e., discomfort localized in swelling of the costochondral and costosternal joints, which are painful to palpation).

General considerations on pain from ischaemic heart disease

Pain from ischaemic heart disease is a symptom well known to every physician, for it is frequently observed. However, descriptions in textbooks and everyday experience give the impression of a wide variety of symptoms because of different areas of reference, different kinds of pain in the same area, and involvement of areas far away from the heart. This pain, therefore, seems not to follow any rules. We believe that for this reason the attention of the physician is given less to an exact observation of the pain and more to laboratory and instrumental investigations.

The absence of rules for cardiac pain is only apparent if we examine in detail the various types of pain perceived by the patient. Indeed, it is not enough to investigate where pain is felt, but it is also necessary to distinguish between true visceral pain and referred pain and to determine whether pain is referred in deep or superficial parietal structures. Only an adequate and careful investigation of the patient can give us such information. Consequently, the description of cardiac pain should be preceded by a few clinical concepts on the characteristics of visceral pain.

The subsequent discussion on pain from the heart and from other chest organs is mainly based on observations made in the Medical School of Florence over the past 50 years (Teodori and Galletti 1962, Procacci 1969, Procacci et al 1986, Procacci and Maresca 1987a).

Clinical characteristics of visceral pain

The qualities of true visceral pain are clearly different from those of deep pain or cutaneous pain. Visceral pain is dull, aching, or boring, and is not well localized. It is always accompanied by a sense of malaise and of being ill. It is associated with strong autonomic reflexes, such as diffuse sweating, vasomotor responses, changes of arterial pressure and heart rate, and with an intense alarm reaction.

When an algogenic process affecting a viscus recurs frequently or becomes more intense and prolonged, the location is more exact and pain is gradually felt in more superficial structures, even, sometimes, far from the site of origin. This phenomenon is usually called referred pain in English, whereas German authors use the less common but, in our opinion, more appropriate term transferred pain (übertragener Schmerz). Referred pain may be accompanied by autonomic reflexes. Cutaneous hyperalgesia and zones of muscular tenderness are often present.

With unpleasant visceral feelings, the patient often declines to apply the word pain, selecting words such as discomfort, pressure, tightness, or squeezing. Between the lack of sensory symptoms and the true pain we have a continuum of intensity and unpleasantness.

Pain in myocardial infarction

This pain may arise suddenly during stressful activities, after a large meal or during rest or sleep. Occasionally, it is preceded by a feeling of chest discomfort or slight dyspnoea or unpleasant gastric sensations described as fullness of the stomach or indigestion. The patient has often experienced previous paroxysms of angina pectoris. The early pain is deep, central, anterior, and sometimes also posterior; it lasts from a few minutes to a few hours, showing the characteristics of true visceral pain. It is defined by most patients as pressing, constricting, or squeezing or with phrases such as 'a band across the chest'. This kind of pain is central, often behind the lower sternum, less frequently on the epigastrium or in both these sites. Anterior pain may be concomitant with central back pain; in some patients pain is only posterior. Pain is often accompanied by nausea and vomiting and by diffuse sweating. This pain is very intense and often accompanied by a strong alarm reaction, sometimes with a feeling of impending death.

In a following phase, after a period which varies from 10 min to a few hours, the pain reaches the parietal structures, assuming the characteristics of referred pain. It may be the first perceived pain. This pain is often defined as pressing or constricting and tends to radiate. The spatial localization is more exact than for visceral pain; it is often accompanied by sweating and rarely by nausea and vomiting. This pain is often referred beneath the sternum or in the precordial area, sometimes spreading to both sides of the anterior chest or, in a few cases, only to the right. The radiation is accompanied by feelings such as numbness, cramp, or squeezing of the elbow or wrist. Frequently the pain radiates to the whole left arm or to both arms or involves the left forearm and hand; in a few cases it radiates only to the right arm. Another uncommon radiation is to the neck, jaw, and temporomandibular joint on both sides simultaneously. In rare cases a posterior pain is felt in the interscapulovertebral region and may radiate to the ulnar aspect of the left arm. In patients not treated with drugs, the duration of this parietal pain varies from half an hour to 12 or more hours. It always lasts longer than true visceral pain.

Muscular tenderness follows the onset of this pain after a delay that varies from a few hours to half a day. It mainly involves the pectoralis major, the deep muscles of the interscapular region, the muscles of the forearm, and, less frequently, the trapezius and deltoid muscles.

In some patients a superficial referred pain arises, localized within the dermatomes C8–T1, that is, on the ulnar side of the arm and forearm. This pain is rarely the only starting symptom. It lasts from half an hour to 6 h and is intense, stabbing or lancinating. In the areas of reference cutaneous hyperalgesia is often found. There are no clear correlations between the type of infarction (inferior, anterior, transmural, non-transmural) and the pattern of pain.

Pain in angina pectoris

The pain is generally deep, more rarely superficial, with the same qualities and radiations as those described in myocardial infarction, but the intensity and duration are less. Pain is not accompanied by a feeling of impending death and seldom by nausea and vomiting. The alarm reaction with the accompanying symptoms is less intense than in myocardial infarction. In these patients deep muscular tenderness is found in the same areas as in infarction and is constant and independent of pain attacks.

In recent classifications of angina pectoris, the following anginal syndromes are distinguished: stable angina, unstable angina, and variant (Prinzmetal's) angina (Rogers 1996, Gersh et al 1997).

Stable angina

Patients with stable angina usually have angina with effort or exercise or during other conditions in which myocardial oxygen demand is increased. The quality of sensation is sometimes vague and may be described as a mild pressure-like discomfort or an uncomfortable numb sensation. Anginal 'equivalents' (i.e., symptoms of myocardial ischaemia other than angina) such as breathlessness, faintness, fatigue, and belching have also been reported (Gersh et al 1997). A classic feature of stable angina is the disappearance of pain after the use of nitroglycerine or the inhalation of amyl nitrite.

Unstable angina

The term unstable angina, previously also known as preinfarction angina, acute coronary insufficiency, and intermediate coronary syndrome, indicates angina pectoris characterized by one or more of the following features:

1. crescendo angina (more severe, prolonged or frequent) superimposed on a pre-existing pattern of relatively stable, exertion-related angina pectoris
2. angina pectoris at rest as well as with minimal exertion
3. angina pectoris of new onset (usually within 1 month), which is brought on by minimal exertion (Gersh et al 1997).

In unstable angina the chest discomfort is similar in quality to that of chronic stable angina, although it is usually more intense, is usually described as pain, may persist for as long as 30 min, and occasionally awakens the patient from sleep. When it lasts more than 30 min, an infarction should be suspected. One of the characteristics of this pain is that its intensity varies greatly, from very slight to (more frequently) intermediate, sometimes reaching maximal intensity, like that described in infarction.

Several clues should alert the physician to a changing anginal pattern. These include an abrupt reduction in the threshold of physical activity which provokes angina; an increase in the frequency, severity, and duration of angina; radiation of the discomfort to a new site; onset of new features associated with the pain, such as nausea and decreased relief of pain afforded by nitroglycerine.

Variant angina

Variant (Prinzmetal's) angina is an unusual syndrome of cardiac pain that occurs almost exclusively at rest, usually is not precipitated by physical exertion or emotional stress, and is associated with S-T segment elevations on the electrocardiogram (Prinzmetal et al 1959). This syndrome has been demonstrated convincingly to be due to coronary artery spasm. However, in arteriographic studies Maseri et al (1978) observed that in many patients the coronary vasospasm occurring during an anginal attack was associated with S-T segment elevation or depression, blurring the distinction between variant (Prinzmetal's) angina and unstable angina. Selwyn and Braunwald (1998) consider variant angina as a peculiar form of unstable angina.

Syndrome X

Under the broad definition of syndrome X (Kemp 1973), some studies have included a variety of patients with chest pain with a pattern of chronic stable angina and angiographically normal coronary arteries. Some patients, however, may have had a non-cardiac origin of symptoms (Maseri 1995). In some of the subjects ischaemic-appearing S-T segment responses are evident with exercise test, while in some ischaemia is undetectable by currently available techniques (Maseri 1995). It was proposed that patients with cardiac syndrome X have an exaggerated response of small coronary vessels to vasoconstrictor stimuli (Gersh et al 1997).

The absence of definitive evidence of ischaemia in some patients with syndrome X has focused attention upon other causes of chest pain, e.g., upon pain originating from oesophagus. An increased sensitivity to, and decreased tolerance of, forearm tourniquet and electrical skin stimulation were observed in women with typical angina and normal coronary arteries compared with patients with coronary artery obstructions; an exaggerated sensitivity to cardiac, potentially painful stimuli, but also an overlap between increased sensitivity to cardiac and oesophageal pain were also reported (Maseri 1995). Thus, a generalized increase in somatic and visceral pain sensitivity seems to be a common feature in patients with syndrome X. Whether this phenomenon represents an abnormal activation of somatic and visceral receptors or an abnormal processing of afferent neural impulses is unknown.

The problem of painless coronary heart diseases

It is well known that myocardial infarction has been found in electrocardiographic studies or at postmortem examinations in patients in whom there was no history of a well-defined episode of chest pain. The occurrence of painless infarctions has not been correlated with the location, size, or age of the infarction, nor with the age of the patients (Rinzler 1951, Friedberg 1956, Teodori and Galletti 1962, Stern 1998). During long-term follow-up in the Framingham Study, one-quarter of patients had 'unrecognized' myocardial infarction, detected only on routine 2-yearly electrocardiogram, and of these approximately half of the episodes were truly silent (Kannel and Abbott 1984). Other population studies suggest that between 20 and 60% of non-fatal myocardial infarctions are unrecognized by the patient and are discovered only on subsequent routine electrocardiographic or postmortem examination (Antman and Braunwald 1997). These differences are partly due to the use of different methods of investigating and understanding the symptoms. If, indeed, we assemble an accurate history of patients in whom a diagnosis of asymptomatic previous myocardial infarction is suspected in the course of routine examination, we may find a transient episode of chest discomfort or sudden and unusual thoracic paraesthesias (tingling, pricking, numbness) radiating to the left arm or a slight pain that was judged unimportant by the patient or an episode of nausea and vomiting interpreted as due to gastric fullness or indigestion (Procacci et al 1976). The history should be very accurate, since often these episodes are underestimated and have been forgotten by patients. Taking these factors into account, the frequency of asymptomatic myocardial infarction is reduced.

Recently the term and concept of silent myocardial ischaemia have been introduced to indicate all forms of painless myocardial ischaemia. The frequency of silent myocardial ischaemia is higher in patients with diabetes, probably because of neuropathy involving the visceral afferent fibres.

Two forms of silent myocardial ischaemia are recognized (Gersh et al 1997). The first and less common form occurs in patients with obstructive coronary artery disease, sometimes severe, who do not experience angina at any time; some patients do not even experience pain in the course of myocardial infarction. The second and more frequent form occurs in patients with the usual forms of chronic stable angina, unstable angina, and variant angina. When monitored with a dynamic ECG, these patients exhibit some episodes of ischaemia associated with chest discomfort and other episodes that are not, i.e., episodes of silent (asymptomatic) ischaemia.

Painful complications of myocardial infarction

Angina may evolve into myocardial infarction. After myocardial infarction, stable or unstable angina may develop.

Persistent pain after myocardial infarction, especially transmural, may be due to pericarditis. It is important to diagnose the chest pain of pericarditis accurately, since failure to appreciate it may lead to the erroneous diagnosis of recurrent ischaemic pain and/or extension of the infarction and to the inappropriate use of anticoagulants, nitrates, β-adrenergic blocking agents, or narcotics. The pain can often be distinguished from that of an extending infarction by its characteristic pericardial pattern: the pain is relieved by leaning forward and exacerbated by deep breathing.

Pleuropericardial chest pain with fever may begin in a few cases 1–6 weeks after myocardial infarction. This postmyocardial infarction syndrome (or Dressler's syndrome) is thought to be caused by a pericarditis and pleuritis, possibly due to an autoimmune mechanism (Dressler 1956, Lorell 1997). The syndrome usually benefits from treatment with aspirin-like agents or corticosteroids. Since effusions associated with Dressler's syndrome may be haemorrhagic, anticoagulants should be discontinued if they are being administered.

Left scapulohumeral periarthritis, giving a picture of frozen shoulder, with pain, stiffness, and marked limitation of motion of the shoulder joint, may complicate some cases of long-lasting angina and 5% of cases of myocardial infarction. In some cases, 3–6 weeks after myocardial infarction, a progressive reflex dystrophy of the left arm begins. It mainly involves the shoulder, the wrist, and the hand (shoulder–hand syndrome). The evolution may be very severe and includes advanced stages of osteoporosis, muscular and cutaneous atrophy, glossy skin, loss of hair, vasomotor changes, etc. As in other reflex dystrophies, it often improves with blocks of the stellate ganglion.

Functional or psychogenic chest pain

Patients with chest pain and without instrumental signs of ischaemic heart disease are frequently observed. A precordial pain, often radiating with characteristics that resemble those of angina, worries many anxious patients, often with a depressive trait. They frequently undergo medical visits and examinations, the normality of which reassures them for only a short while.

Pain is variously described as stabbing, piercing, burning, dull, squeezing, annoying, slight, intense, variable, and synchronous with the cardiac beats, etc. First of all, the physician must consider other causes of chest pain.

Some characteristics of this pain distinguish it from true angina: the duration varies from a few moments to some days; it is often not related to effort; patients are restless and nervous, while during an attack of angina they remain relatively immobile. The behaviour of patients often differs when they are asked where they feel pain: the patient with angina puts an open hand on the sternum, the anxious patient touches, with his index finger, the left submammary region or often zones of the precordial area.

Despite these differences, great caution should be exercised in diagnosing functional or psychogenic chest pain, because differentiation between a true angina and an anxious depressive syndrome is often difficult.

Other causes of heart pain

Aortic stenosis and insufficiency

Angina pectoris has been noted in about two-thirds of cases of symptomatic aortic stenosis. Angina pectoris occurs more frequently in aortic stenosis than in other valvular lesions. The pain is usually a typical angina of effort. Patients with severe chronic aortic stenosis tend to be free of cardiovascular symptoms until relatively late in the course of the disease. Once patients become symptomatic the average survival is 2–5 years (Braunwald 1997). Obviously the course of this disease changes after cardiac surgery or angioplasty. The pain is generally related to a coronary narrowing or to myocardial hypertrophy with increased oxygen demand.

It is well known that angina pectoris has long been regarded as a symptom of aortic insufficiency. According to Friedberg (1956), angina pectoris is uncommon in uncomplicated aortic insufficiency, but it may occur because of coronary atherosclerosis or because superimposed calcification of the aortic valve leads to stenosis of the coronary arteries.

Mitral stenosis

Braunwald (1997) has pointed out that about 15% of patients suffering from mitral stenosis have a pain with the same characteristics as that of angina pectoris (Braunwald 1997). The observation of pain in mitral stenosis is now rare, following the development of cardiac surgery.

Mitral valve prolapse

In mitral valve prolapse chest pain is sometimes reported. In some cases, in which mitral valve prolapse is associated with coronary heart disease, a typical anginal pain is present.

Inflammatory disease of the heart

Pain can occur in all inflammatory diseases of the heart, i.e., pericarditis, myocarditis, and endocarditis. Pain is, however, much more frequent in pericarditis than in myocarditis or endocarditis; consequently we shall describe only the pain from pericarditis.

Pain in pericarditis is less frequent than in pleurisy, so when pain is present, pleural involvement should be suspected. For these reasons the pericardium is considered to be less sensitive to pain than the pleura (Teodori and Galletti 1962).

In acute pericarditis the onset of pain often coincides with fever or it may follow a shivering chill. Pain is often deep and substernal, usually involving the upper two-thirds of the sternum, less commonly precordial; it is continuous and lasts from a few hours to 3 days. It may appear repeatedly, always for brief periods. It is aggravated by deep inspiration, cough, and lateral movements of the chest. Pain is reduced by sitting up and leaning forward.

In about half the cases, together with this deep pain, there is a superficial referred pain. The pain may radiate to the left shoulder, scapula and arm, the neck, and the epigastrium. It may appear during exertion, resembling angina.

Chronic pericarditis is often painless, but on careful questioning the patient may report a deep, dull, slight pain or sensation of heaviness or fullness in the chest.

Cor pulmonale

In many cases of acute cor pulmonale (pulmonary embolism) a true visceral pain that has the same qualities and radiation as myocardial infarction, including a strong alarm reaction, is observed.

Some patients suffering from chronic cor pulmonale have pain that shows great similarities with that of angina. The pain may be present in all diseases in which pulmonary hypertension is present: chronic cor pulmonale, mitral stenosis, some congenital heart diseases, and idiopathic pulmonary hypertension. Anginal pain in patients with pulmonary hypertension is similar to that of angina pectoris: both types of pain have the same location, radiation, quality, and intensity. A careful analysis, however, will show that during spontaneous or exertional pain in pulmonary hypertension, the severity of cyanosis increases (angor coeruleus), whereas in coronary angina the patient is pale (angor pallidus).

Causes of chest pain (from organs other than the heart)

Diseases of the aorta

Aneurysms

The aneurysms that give rise to chest pain are those of the thoracic aorta, while aneurysms of the abdominal aorta are often asymptomatic but are sometimes accompanied by abdominal and low back pain (Isselbacher et al 1997).

Pain in thoracic aortic aneurysms is probably due to the excitation of aortic end organs and to compression and erosion of adjacent musculoskeletal structures. It is usually steady and boring and occasionally may be pulsating.

Aortic dissection

According to Isselbacher et al (1997), by far the commonest presenting symptom of aortic dissection is severe pain, which is found in 74–90% of cases. The pain of dissection is often unbearable, forcing the patient to writhe in agony or pace restlessly in an attempt to gain some measure of relief. Pain resembles that of myocardial infarction but several features of the pain may arouse suspicion of aortic dissection. The quality of the pain as described by the patient is often remarkably appropriate to the actual event. Adjectives such as 'tearing', 'ripping', and 'stabbing' are frequently used. Another characteristic of the pain of aortic dissection is its tendency to migrate from the point of its origin to other sites, following the path of the dissecting haematoma as it extends through the aorta. Pain felt maximally in the anterior thorax is more frequent with proximal dissection, whereas pain that is most severe in the interscapular area is much more common with the involvement of a distal site. Nausea and vomiting, diffuse sweating, fainting, and hiccup, resistant to drugs and to manoeuvres which would ordinarily stop it, can frequently accompany the pain.

Pleurisy

Chest pain is frequently observed in the course of pleurisy because the pain sensitivity of the pleura is very high.

We shall first consider which kind of stimulus determines the pain in pleuritis. Two components are present: a mechanical component, due both to the friction between the two adjacent pleural surfaces (particularly when they are covered with fibrinous exudate) and to the stretching of the parietal pleura during inspiration; and a chemical component, due to the high algogenic power of the pleural liquid, rich in pain-producing substances (Procacci 1969).

The pain is generally well localized. Its onset is more frequently sudden than progressive, often preceding other symptoms such as fever, dyspnoea, and cough, and lasts a few days.

The location of pain varies according to the location and extent of the inflammation (Teodori and Galletti 1962).

1. In effusive pleurisy, it is felt in a region corresponding to the site of inflammation and frequently referred to the submammary area.
2. In diaphragmatic pleurisy, pain is often felt on the trapezius ridge and on the base of the affected side of the chest.
3. In apical pleurisy, pain is in the interscapulovertebral region.

Almost always, in effusive pleurisies, pain is steady, aggravated by deep inspiration, cough, movements of the chest, and lying on the affected side. Shoulder pain with diaphragmatic pleurisy and interscapulovertebral pain with apical pleurisy are less localized, constrictive, and not aggravated by movement, cough, or deep inspiration. Pain is very intense in effusive pleurisy, especially when it is located in the submammary area, in empyema, in pleurisy that follows a pulmonary or subdiaphragmatic abscess, and in pleurisy that complicates pneumonia or cancer of the lung.

Diseases of the oesophagus

Experimental and spontaneous oesophageal pain shows the typical characteristics of visceral pain: it is poorly localized, accompanied by autonomic reflexes and by emotions and becomes referred.

The fundamental algogenic stimuli for the oesophagus are:

1. strong mechanical stimulation from oesophageal stenosis and motor disorders, such as cancer, achalasia, diffuse oesophageal spasm, nutcracker oesophagus (symptomatic peristalsis), and aspecific motor disorders (Goyal 1998)
2. gastro-oesophageal reflux and inflammation. In patients with gastro-oesophageal reflux, the most common symptom is heartburn. The term 'burning' rather than 'pain' is usually used, although heartburn can increase in intensity until it is perceived as pain. Pain can be long-lasting or present during swallowing (odynophagia).

Oesophageal pain may be induced in routine exams by oesophageal infusion of 0.1 N hydrochloric acid (Bernstein test) or by inflating a balloon.

The areas of reference of oesophageal pain are the higher sternum for diseases of the proximal third of the oesophagus and lower sternum for diseases of the distal third. Diseases of the intermediate third give rise to pain referred to one or other area. The zones to which pain radiates are many and may be the same for diseases of the upper and lower oesophagus. The more frequently observed are the interscapular and central dorsal areas at the level of the sixth and seventh thoracic vertebrae, the neck, the ear, the jaw, the precordium, the shoulders, the upper limbs, and the epigastrium (Teodori and Galletti 1962).

Oesophageal pain can mimic that of myocardial ischaemia. Discomfort is often relieved by nitroglycerine, sometimes by calcium antagonists, and also, unlike angina, by milk or antacids.

Some acute diseases of abdominal organs, such as peptic ulcer, acute cholecystitis and pancreatitis, may simulate heart pain, just as heart pain may simulate those diseases. Sometimes a multifactorial pain is present.

Complex problems

Frequently heart pain is mingled with pain arising from other structures (*angors coronariens intriqués*) (Froment and Gonin 1956). For instance, a myocardial ischaemia may be accompanied by cervicothoracic osteoarthritis (vertebrocoronary syndrome), by chest fibromyalgias, or by many diseases of the gastrointestinal tract, such as diseases of the oesophagus, hiatus hernia, gastroduodenitis, peptic ulcer, and calculous and non-calculous cholecystitis (cholecystocoronary syndrome). It is difficult to ascertain whether these intricate conditions are due to a simple addition of impulses from different sources in the central nervous system or to somatovisceral and viscerosomatic reflexes that may induce a classic 'vicious circle' between different structures (Procacci et al 1986). Pain may vary from typical angina pectoris to chest pain with different patterns.

Mechanisms of cardiac pain

The mechanisms of cardiac pain seem to be partly similar to those of visceral and partly similar to those of skeletal muscles. For instance, a solution of NaCl 5%, a well-known algogenic stimulus for the skeletal muscles, injected in the left ventricular wall of the cat induces a powerful discharge of A-δ afferent fibres from the heart (Brown 1967). The problem of spasm of the coronaries during painful attacks is much debated. The coronary artery spasm is typical of variant angina and can be observed in both stable and unstable angina. Constriction of a small coronary vessel is supposed to be the cause of some cases of syndrome X (Maseri 1995).

According to Aviado and Schmidt (1955), the necessary stimuli in the heart for the onset of pain and of reflex phenomena were the following:

1. reduced coronary arterial pressure distal to an occlusion, acting on coronary arterial pressoreceptors
2. ischaemia, stimulating the myocardial pressoreceptors and chemoreceptors
3. release of pain-producing substances formed by tissue breakdown or platelet disintegration.

The problem of the presence of true cardiac nociceptors is still debated (Cervero 1994, 1995).

Malliani and his school (Malliani and Lombardi 1982, Malliani 1995) observed in animals an increased discharge of cardiac afferent C-fibres after powerful stimuli, such as the intracoronary injection of bradykinin, but never observed that coronary occlusion or bradykinin administration induced a recruitment of silent afferents. Malliani (1995) concluded that the 'intensity mechanism' was the most likely candidate to account for the properties of the neural substrate subserving cardiac nociception.

Together with mechanical factors, the biochemical component of cardiac pain in ischaemic heart disease is relevant. This component is multifactorial; increase of lactic acid, release of potassium ions, and production of kinins and of other pain-producing substances must be considered. In recent years, attention has focused on adenosine as a potential biochemical mediator of anginal pain (Cannon 1995). Malliani (1995) found that adenosine can potentiate the excitation induced by myocardial ischaemia on the impulse activity of ventricular afferent fibres. It is probable that a group of pain-producing substances act in concert.

We believe that another important mechanism is the development of an ischaemic neuropathy of heart nerves. Such a neuropathy is present in atherosclerotic arterial disease of the legs with intermittent claudication (*claudicatio intermittens*) in which, according to Lewis (1942), pain resembles that of effort angina (*claudicatio cordis*).

The various mechanisms for cardiac pain intermingle, one or other being prevalent in different conditions and in different patients (Procacci et al 1986, Maseri 1995). We can endorse the opinion of Malliani (1986) and Cervero (1994) that the link between myocardial ischaemia and cardiac pain is neither strong nor unequivocal, for cardiac pain can occur in the absence of ischaemia and, conversely, episodes of myocardial ischaemia can be painless.

Mnemonic traces

Every level of the central nervous system can hold learned experiences and replay when necessary. It has been demonstrated that the mnemonic process is facilitated if the experience to be retained is repeated many times or is accompanied by pleasant or unpleasant emotions. Like other sensory modalities, pain is, at least in part, a learned experience (Melzack 1973). The processes of retained painful experience were termed memory-like processes by Melzack (1973). Nathan (1962) observed that in some subjects different kinds of stimuli could call to mind forgotten pain experiences.

We performed experiments in patients with previous myocardial infarction but with normal sensibility as judged by accurate examination. Ischaemia of the upper limbs was provoked with two pneumatic cuffs according to the technique of our school (Procacci et al 1986). In most patients ischaemia caused pain with characteristics similar to those of the pain felt during the episode of infarction. Some patients felt common sensations accompanied by alarm reaction with sweating, nausea, tachycardia, and tachypnoea. No ECG changes were observed. The test was promptly interrupted at the onset of these symptoms. We also examined patients with previous painless myocardial infarction. Some of these patients remembered an episode variously defined as fullness of the stomach, nausea, or indigestion, whereas in other patients the history was completely silent. In most of the patients, the ischaemia of the upper limbs provoked the onset of diffuse unpleasant common sensations, often accompanied by autonomic and emotional reactions (Procacci et al 1976).

Ischaemia of the upper limbs was also induced in patients suffering from angina pectoris. Most patients whose anginal pain radiated to the left arm reported pain in the same limb and with the same radiation as their spontaneous pain. Most patients whose anginal pain was felt only in the chest or radiated to both upper limbs reported pain in both limbs (Procacci et al 1986).

These results suggest that ischaemic pain induced in the limbs can evoke mnemonic traces left by heart pain.

Therapy

Pain in angina pectoris is relieved by a group of drugs that are ineffective in other types of pain. The first drugs used were amyl nitrite (Brunton 1867) and, a few years later, nitroglycerine. The relief of pain with nitrates is often dramatic. Other drugs, such as β-blocking agents, long-lasting organic nitrates, and calcium antagonists, are used to prevent ischaemic attacks. The mechanism of these drugs is as controversial as the mechanism of pain.

We should also mention the useful association of antianginal drugs with aspirin, which presumably has a direct action on cardiac pain and contributes to the elimination of the algogenic summation from myalgic spots, often present in patients with angina. This latent afferent input may assume an important role in reflexes that facilitate the attacks of angina. Aspirin is also useful for its antithrombotic effect, due to inhibition of platelet aggregation. Intravenous heparin has been used in the control of myocardial ischaemia in patients with unstable angina (Neri Serneri et al 1995).

The drug of choice in myocardial infarction is morphine, which generally induces relief of pain and good sedation. Morphine in myocardial infarction not only relieves pain but also centrally interrupts reflexes that may worsen the cardiovascular state or induce life-threatening arrhythmias.

In myocardial infarction intracoronary thrombolysis with streptokinase, urokinase, and other drugs is useful in the first hours after the onset of symptoms. When intracoronary thrombolysis cannot be performed, intravenous thrombolysis is used.

As far back as 1955, White and Sweet gave a detailed description of the method of injecting the four upper thoracic sympathetic ganglia with procaine and alcohol for relief of persistent pain in angina pectoris.

Epidural blockade of the upper thoracic sympathetic segments has been shown to offer good pain relief in patients with severe unstable angina or acute myocardial infarction (Blomberg et al 1990, Kirnö et al 1994, Olausson et al 1997). The mechanism of action of this therapy is surely multifactorial, as both visceral afferent fibres and sympathetic efferent fibres are blocked.

In cardiac surgery, it is well known that most patients with angina have good relief of pain after coronary angioplasty or aortocoronary bypass. The disappearance of pain is generally related to an improvement of coronary flow. It should, however, be considered that during the operation of coronary bypass some of the cardiac afferent fibres running in sympathetic nerves are cut. This denervation may be relevant to the relief of heart pain.

Vascular pain

Vascular pain is a complex area. It may be divided into three sections: arterial pain; pain due to lesion or dysfunction of the microvessels (arterioles, capillaries, small venules); and venous pain.

Obviously many traumas, frequent in daily life, can damage the vascular tree with different consequences.

Arterial pain

Pain originating in coronary vessels and in the aorta has been covered in previous sections of this chapter.

Arterial pain may be due to different diseases such as atherosclerosis and/or thrombosis of the arterial bed, arteritis or arteriolitis, and dysfunction of the arterioles.

Atherosclerosis and/or thrombosis of arterial bed

Atherosclerosis and/or thrombosis in the coronary vessels give rise to the pain of angina pectoris and of myocardial infarction. In arterial occlusive diseases of the limbs, it gives rise to intermittent claudication or to rest pain. Intermittent claudication is defined as a pain, ache, cramp, numbness in the muscles; it occurs during exercise and is relieved by rest. As in angina pectoris, in intermittent claudication of lower limbs the onset of pain after a given effort is an important clue for judging the severity of the syndrome. If the free interval before the onset of pain is constant, the condition is stable, as in stable angina pectoris; if the free interval shortens, the condition is similar to unstable angina. This clinical observation is obviously important for medical or surgical therapy.

Leriche's syndrome is due to isolated aortoiliac occlusive arterial disease, which produces a characteristic clinical picture: intermittent claudication of the low back, buttocks, and thigh or calf muscles, impotence, atrophy of the limbs, and pallor of the skin of the feet and legs. In rare cases, when atherosclerotic processes involve abdominal vessels, the patient suffers from angina abdominis. As in angina pectoris, the pain of chronic mesenteric insufficiency occurs under conditions of increased demand for splanchnic blood flow. There is usually intermittent dull or cramping midabdominal pain after eating. The arteriographic studies of angina abdominis demonstrate occlusion or high-grade stenosis of the superior or inferior mesenteric artery or the coeliac axis.

Arteritis or arteriolitis

Some diseases, such as thromboangiitis obliterans, Takayasu's syndrome, and systemic giant cell arteritis, are well known (Rosenwasser 1996, Fauci 1998).

Thromboangiitis obliterans (Bürger's disease) is an obstructive arterial disease caused by segmental inflammatory and proliferative lesions of the medium and small arteries and veins of the limbs (Kontos 1996). The symptoms result mainly from impairment of arterial blood supply to the tissues and to some extent from local venous insufficiency. The symptoms are intermittent claudication, rest pain when severe ischaemia of tissues has developed, pain from ulcerations and gangrene, and pain from ischaemic neuropathy, which must be considered an important component. Raynaud's phenomenon and migratory superficial thrombophlebitis are common.

Takayasu's syndrome (aortic arc syndrome) is due to arteritis and arteriolitis of the vessels of the upper part of the body as far as the arterioles of the eye. It is prevalent in adolescent girls and young women. In a prodromic phase about two-thirds of the patients complain of malaise, fever, limb-girdle stiffness, and arthralgia; this prodromic phase is similar to that seen in giant cell arteritis, rheumatic diseases, and systemic lupus erythematosus. In many instances this is soon followed by local pain over the affected arteries, erythema nodosum, and erythema induratum. In some cases the disease evolves in angina pectoris or myocardial infarction.

Giant cell arteritis (temporal arteritis) is an inflammation of medium and large arteries. It characteristically involves one or more branches of the carotid artery, particularly the temporal artery, hence the name cranial or temporal arteritis. It occurs almost exclusively in individuals older than 55 years and is more common in women than in men. Headaches are often intense and almost unbearable. Headache typically occurs over involved arteries, usually the temporal arteries, but occasionally in the occipital region. A typical tenderness and induration along the vessels is observed. The area around arteries is exquisitely sensitive to pressure. Claudication in the jaw muscles while chewing occurs in up to two-thirds of patients.

Giant cell arteritis is considered a systemic disease and can involve arteries in multiple locations (Fauci 1998). The patient often describes an illness that begins like a 'flu syndrome', with severe malaise, slight fever, and myalgia. The muscle pain progresses and may become severe, involving mainly the neck, shoulder girdle, and pelvic girdle and also the trunk and the distal limbs to a lesser degree; the involvement is bilateral but not necessarily equal in severity. Intermittent claudication, myocardial infarctions, and infarctions of visceral organs have been reported. This syndrome is considered strictly related to polymyalgia rheumatica and consequently it is classified with rheumatic diseases.

The borderline between Takayasu's syndrome and giant cell arteritis is often not clear. Today they are both considered connective tissue diseases. Rosenwasser (1996) classifies cranial or temporal arteritis and Takayasu's arteritis as subgroups of giant cell arteritides.

Dysfunction of arterioles

Raynaud's phenomenon is characterized by episodes of intense pallor of the fingers and toes (ischaemic phase), generally followed by rubor and cyanosis. The phenomenon is due to a sudden arteriolar constriction, followed by a paralytic phase. The patients usually feel an intense burning or throbbing pain during the ischaemic phase and a less intense pain together with paraesthesias during the cyanotic phase. This condition may be classified as primary or idiopathic Raynaud's phenomenon (Raynaud's disease) and as Raynaud's phenomenon secondary to other diseases, trauma, or drugs. In Raynaud's disease, different alterations of the arterioles, characteristic of different kinds of arteriolitis, have been described. Calcium antagonists, adrenergic-blocking drugs, and other sympathicolytic agents are considered the specific therapy for Raynaud's phenomenon (Creager and Dzau 1998).

Erythromelalgia (erythermalgia) is a syndrome characterized by the following symptoms in the extremities: red discoloration and increased temperature of the skin; deep and superficial burning pain, often accompanied by tingling and pricking; and in many cases oedema. The symptoms simultaneously involve the distal part of the lower limbs and, less frequently, of the upper limbs as well. The attacks of erythromelalgia are induced by increased temperature, either in the environment or locally, and are aggravated by a dependent position. The duration of attacks varies from a few minutes to hours. Erythromelalgia may be primary or secondary and is sometimes familial. The most common recognized cause of secondary erythromelalgia is thrombocytosis due to essential thrombocythaemia or to other myeloproliferative disorders (see Pain in Haemopathies, below) (Ball 1996). Other reported associations with erythromelalgia include diabetes mellitus. Arteriolar inflammation and thrombotic occlusions were found on skin punch biopsy samples. Erythromelalgia due to thrombocytosis disappears for 3 or 4 days after a single dose of aspirin, which is the duration of its inhibition of platelet aggregation. It is pertinent to ask whether primary erythromelalgia could be classified with reflex sympathetic dystrophies. As a matter of fact, excellent results, with complete disappearance of the symptoms, were observed with local anaesthetic blocks of the sympathetic chain (Zoppi et al 1985).

Mechanisms of arterial pain

The mechanisms of pain in arterial diseases are many and often intermingle.

1. Ischaemia per se. The most evident examples of diseases due to this mechanism are angina at

rest, pain occurring in arterial embolism, and Raynaud's phenomenon. Ischaemia can give rise to a continuous pain in the limb when:

a. the ischaemia is very severe
b. myalgic spots with the characteristics of trigger points are present in the limbs (Dorigo et al 1979)
c. a reflex sympathetic dystrophy arises, which contributes to pain and dystrophy through different mechanisms: vasomotor changes; fast and slow changes in permeability of microvessels and tissue imbibition; release of active substances; direct control of some enzymatic reactions; and direct modulation of sensory receptors (Procacci 1969, Maresca et al 1984, Geppetti and Holzer 1996, Jänig 1996).

2. Ischaemia occurring during muscular exercise because of a discrepancy between the supply and demand of oxygen carried to muscles. This mechanism, according to Lewis (1942), is typical of effort angina pectoris (stable chronic angina) and intermittent claudication of the limbs. Typical myalgic spots are found in many patients with intermittent claudication and are a component of pain (Procacci 1969, Dorigo et al 1979, Maresca et al 1984).
3. Ischaemia plus inflammation and/or metabolic disorders, typical of thromboangiitis obliterans, inflammatory arteriolitis and diabetic arteriolitis.

The process of vascular thrombosis is generally considered a common arrival point of different pathways. However, in many vascular diseases the two mechanisms, thrombosis and inflammation, are in part overlapping, as is clear from clinical observations, e.g., in thromboangiitis obliterans or in angina or infarction that sometimes occur in giant cell arteritis and in thrombophlebitis.

Pain due to dysfunction of microvessels

Pain originating from microvessels must be distinguished from classic arterial and venous pain for pathophysiological and clinical reasons.

Firstly, both arterial and venous vessels are involved in some classic syndromes, such as Raynaud's phenomenon, pernio (chilblains), and erythromelalgia (erythermalgia) (Kontos 1996, Creager and Dzau 1998). Obviously, in these cases an alteration of capillary filtration is also present, with changes in the microenvironment important for the onset of pain, as stated by Zimmermann (1979) and Jänig (1996). Many substances may be active in inducing pain. Only some of these have been identified: histamine, 5-hydroxytriptamine, kinins, and substance P. The temporal relationships involved in the release of active substances in different cases are unknown. Neurogenic inflammation, i.e., the antidromic release from afferent C-fibres of substance P, calcitonin gene-related peptide (CGRP), neurokin-A, and possibly other substances (Geppetti and Holzer 1996), probably plays a role in many diseases of microvessels; certainly neurogenic phenomena are important in Raynaud's phenomenon and erythromelalgia. It must be noted that Raynaud's phenomenon is often induced by cold, applied not on the hands but on the face; a disorder of the hypothalamic centres of thermoregulation may be considered probable.

Venous pain

A typical venous pain is observed in thrombophlebitis. In superficial thrombophlebitis the vein may be apparent as a red, tender cord. Pain at rest is often observed. In deep vein thrombophlebitis about half of the patients may be asymptomatic. Tenderness to palpation and pain on the voluntary dorsiflexion of the foot can be observed (Kontos 1996, Creager and Dzau 1998). Many factors are active in inducing pain: biochemical factors and mechanical factors, especially venous stasis. Much more than in arterial pain, in venous pain perivascular tissues, muscles and tendons are involved in inflammation and hence are painful. The importance of these additional factors is demonstrated by the fact that, when thrombophlebitis is resolved, a postphlebitis pain often remains in the limbs. We have observed that in many cases pain originates not only from the vein which remains painful, but also from myalgic spots, often accompanied by skin hyperalgesia. In conclusion, a postphlebitic myofascial pain syndrome is observed, which sometimes responds to aspirin-like drugs.

In every vascular disease, as well as in myocardial infarction, a reflex sympathetic dystrophy can arise. In this case skin dystrophy (glossy skin), muscle atrophy, osteoporosis, and clear vasomotor and sudomotor phenomena are observed in the limbs. The classic treatment of reflex sympathetic dystrophies with sympathetic blocks can be opportune (Procacci and Maresca 1987b, Bonica 1990).

Pain in haemopathies

In many haemopathies pain, due to different mechanisms, can be observed. In four haemopathies, pain is a fundamental symptom: sickle cell disease, in which strong pain crises in trunks and limbs are frequent; essential thrombocythaemia, in which an erythromelalgic syndrome is frequently observed; haemophilic disorders; and multiple myeloma, in which bone pain can be observed. We shall describe these four syndromes in detail.

Pain in sickle cell disease

Sickle cell disease is a genetic disorder, inherited with an autosomal recessive pattern that is more frequent in certain African populations, in which the sickle cell gene conferred a selective advantage, i.e., resistance to infection with malaria. The disease is present in black populations of African ancestry in America and in other parts of the world in which the presence of African groups is relevant, i.e., in the United Kingdom.

The main clinical manifestations of sickle cell disease include haemolytic anaemia and different complications related to the rheologic abnormalities: haematuria due to renal papillary necrosis, stroke due to cerebral infarction, and painful crises due to infarctions of different organs (Ballas 1998). Acute pain is often the first symptom of disease and is the most frequent complication after the newborn period. The frequency of pain is highest in the third and fourth decades, and after the second decade frequent pain is associated with increased mortality rates (Embury 1996). Painful crises may be induced by precipitating factors, such as cold, infection, fever, dehydration, menses, alcohol consumption, and exposure to low oxygen tension. However, the majority of painful episodes have no clear precipitant. Apart from these factors, the frequency of painful crises varies greatly from patient to patient.

Pain may be localized in different parts of the body (Ballas 1998). An acute chest syndrome is described, characterized by fever, chest pain, dyspnoea, leucocytosis, and pulmonary infiltrates on radiography (Embury 1996). The syndrome is usually due to vaso-occlusion and infection. The back, extremities, and abdomen are also commonly affected in painful episodes. In the abdominal crises, pain simulates intra-abdominal disorders; consequently it is difficult to distinguish between painful episodes of sickle cell disease and other acute processes as appendicitis, biliary colic, and perforated viscus. The clue to the differential diagnosis is the presence of increased sickling of red cells on peripheral blood smears and evidence of haemolysis. The episodes last from hours to weeks, followed by a return to baseline. Onset and resolution can be sudden or gradual. Some patients may experience chronic, persistent pain. Severe skeletal pain is related to bone infarctions. Periarticular infarctions may provoke arthritic pain, swelling, and effusion. Frequent pain may cause despair, depression, and apathy, with consequent psychosocial problems such as poor family relationships and social isolation. Shapiro et al (1995) observed that the impact of pain on psychosocial function can also affect school attendance of children and adolescents with sickle cell disease.

The treatment of painful episodes of sickle cell disease is mainly based on the administration of steroidal and non-steroidal anti-inflammatory drugs, associated with mild or strong opioids in more severe crises. Antibiotic therapy is also necessary in acute chest syndrome and other cases in which infection is present. Therapy with hydroxycarbamide (hydroxyurea), which induces an improvement of other clinical manifestations of sickle cell disease, may also decrease the incidence of painful episodes.

A comprehensive approach to the problem of pain in sickle cell disease includes the administration of antidepressive drugs and psychosocial support (Ballas 1998).

Pain in essential thrombocythaemia

The predominant disease expression in essential thrombocythaemia is thrombocytosis, a condition also observed in other acute or chronic myeloproliferative disorders such as granulocytic leukaemia and polycythaemia vera (Tefferi and Silverstein 1996). By far the most frequent painful disorder is erythromelalgia but headache, angina, and myocardial infarction can be observed. In the cases we observed, some had a true erythromelalgia while others had attacks of acute pain in the inferior limbs without any cutaneous manifestation. In all cases the symptomatology disappeared with the administration of aspirin.

Pain in haemophilic disorders

Haemophilia is a group of disorders of blood coagulation. Classic haemophilia (haemophilia A) and Christmas disease (haemophilia B) are deficiencies of factor VIII and IX, respectively. Both haemophilia A and B are associated with recurrent spontaneous and traumatic haemarthroses.

Pain may complicate haemophiliac arthropathy in different ways:

1. Haemarthroses characterized by load pain and joint swelling: the most involved joints are the knees, ankles, elbows, and shoulders.

2. Septic arthritis: this complication is not rare and is accompanied by fever and allodynia in the affected joints (Rasner and Bhogal 1991, Gilliland 1998).
3. Subacute or chronic arthritis with intra-articular effusion and synovitis whose typical symptom is morning stiffness and pain on awakening in the morning, lasting up to 2–3 h.
4. Endstage haemophiliac arthritis: pain in this case is continuous and exacerbated by little movements of the joints; the joint appears enlarged and 'knobby' owing to osteophytic bony overgrowth. Pain is due to severe restriction of motion, fibrous ankylosis, subluxation, joint laxity, and malalignment. The joint changes stimulated by repeated intra-articular bleeding resemble those of rheumatoid arthritis (Gilliland 1998).
5. Muscle and soft tissue haemorrhage: bleeding into muscles and soft tissues is common and provokes spontaneous pain, which worsens on moving the affected muscle. The most frequently involved muscles are the iliopsoas and the volar forearm muscles: if the pressure remains elevated for several hours cramp-like pain worsens and the normal function of muscles and nerves is compromised, and over time, muscle infarction and nerve injury lead to Volkman's ischaemic contracture accompanied by a continuous very intense pain on the volar surface of the hand which interferes with sleep (Heck 1997).

The best therapy is infusion of recombinant factor VIII to stop bleeding. Non-steroidal anti-inflammatory drugs are contraindicated as they may worsen bleeding (York 1998).

Pain in multiple myeloma

Multiple myeloma is a malignant proliferation of plasma cells derived from a single clone. The tumour, its products, and the host response to it result in a number of organ dysfunctions and symptoms. Bone pain, due to bone destruction, is the most common symptom, affecting nearly 70% of patients. The pain usually involves the back and ribs and, unlike the pain of metastatic carcinoma which is often worse at night, the pain of myeloma is precipitated by movement. Persistent localized pain in a patient with myeloma usually signifies a pathologic fracture (Longo 1998). Bony damage and collapse may lead to cord compression, radicular pain, and loss of bowel and bladder control. Infiltration of peripheral nerves by amyloid can be a cause of carpal tunnel syndrome and other sensorimotor mono- and polyneuropathies.

References

Antman EM, Braunwald E 1997 Acute myocardial infarction. In: Braunwald E (ed) Heart disease, 5th edn. Saunders, Philadelphia, pp 1184–1288

Aviado DM, Schmidt CF 1955 Reflexes from stretch receptors in blood vessels, heart and lungs. Physiological Reviews 35: 247–300

Ball EV 1996 Erythromelalgia. In: Bennett JC, Plum F (eds) Cecil textbook of medicine, 20th edn. Saunders, Philadelphia, p 1528

Ballas SK 1998 Sickle cell pain. IASP Press, Seattle

Blomberg S, Emanuelsson H, Kvist H et al 1990 Effects of thoracic epidural anesthesia on coronary arteries and arterioles in patients with coronary artery disease. Anesthesiology 75: 840–847

Bonica JJ 1990 Causalgia and other reflex sympathetic dystrophies. In: Bonica JJ (ed) The management of pain, 2nd edn. Lea & Febiger, Philadelphia, pp 220–243

Braunwald E 1997 Valvular heart disease. In: Braunwald E (ed) Heart disease, 5th edn. Saunders, Philadelphia, pp 1007–1076

Brown AM 1967 Excitation of afferent cardiac sympathetic nerve fibers during myocardial ischaemia. Journal of Physiology 190: 35–53

Brunton TL 1867 On the use of nitrite of amyl in angina pectoris. Lancet 2: 97

Cannon RO 1995 Cardiac pain. In: Gebhart GF (ed) Visceral pain. IASP Press, Seattle, pp 373–389

Cervero F 1994 Sensory innervation of the viscera: peripheral basis of visceral pain. Physiological Reviews 74: 95–137

Cervero F 1995 Mechanisms of visceral pain: past and present. In: Gebhart GF (ed) Visceral pain. IASP Press, Seattle, pp 25–40

Creager MA, Dzau VJ 1998 Vascular diseases of the extremities. In: Fauci AS, Braunwald E, Isselbacher KJ et al (eds) Harrison's principles of internal medicine, 14th edn. McGraw–Hill, New York, pp 1398–1406

Dorigo B, Bartoli V, Grisillo D, Beconi D 1979 Fibrositic myofascial pain in intermittent claudication. Effect of anesthetic block of trigger points on exercise tolerance. Pain 6: 183–190

Dressler W 1956 Post-myocardial infarction syndrome; preliminary report of a complication resembling idiopathic, recurrent, benign pericarditis. Journal of the American Medical Association 160: 1379–1383

Embury SH 1996 Sickle cell anemia and associated hemoglobinopathies. In: Bennett JC, Plum F (eds) Cecil textbook of medicine, 20th edn. Saunders, Philadelphia, pp 882–893

Fauci AS 1998 The vasculitis syndromes. In: Fauci AS, Braunwald E, Isselbacher KJ et al (eds) Harrison's principles of internal medicine. McGraw–Hill, New York, pp 1910–1922

Friedberg CK 1956 Disease of the heart, 2nd edn. Saunders, Philadelphia

Froment R, Gonin A 1956 Les angors coronariens intriqués. Expansion Scientifique Française, Paris

Geppetti P, Holzer P (eds) 1996 Neurogenic inflammation. CRC Press, Boca Raton

Gersh BJ, Braunwald E, Rutherford JD 1997 Chronic coronary artery disease. In: Braunwald E (ed) Heart disease, 5th edn. Saunders, Philadelphia, pp 1289–1365

Gilliland BC 1998 Relapsing polychondritis and other arthritides. In: Fauci AS, Braunwald E, Isselbacher KJ et al (eds) Harrison's principles of internal medicine, 14th edn. McGraw–Hill, New York, pp 1951–1963

Goyal RK 1998 Diseases of the esophagus. In: Fauci AS, Braunwald E, Isselbacher KJ et al (eds) Harrison's principles of internal medicine, 14th edn. McGraw–Hill, New York, pp 1588–1596

Heck LV Jr 1997 Arthritis associated with hematologic disorders, storage diseases, disorders of lipid metabolism and dysproteinemias. In: Koopman WJ (ed) Arthritis and allied conditions, 13th edn. Williams & Wilkins, Baltimore, pp 1697–1717
Isselbacher EM, Eagle KA, Desanctis RW 1997 Diseases of the aorta. In: Braunwald E (ed) Heart disease, 5th edn. Saunders, Philadelphia, pp 1546–1581
Jänig W 1996 The puzzle of 'reflex sympathetic dystrophy': mechanisms, hypotheses, open questions. In: Jänig W, Stanton-Hicks M (eds) Reflex sympathetic dystrophy: a reappraisal. IASP Press, Seattle, pp 1–24
Kannel WB, Abbott RD 1984 Incidence and prognosis of unrecognized myocardial infarction. New England Journal of Medicine 311: 1144–1147
Kemp HG 1973 Left ventricular function in patients with the anginal syndrome and normal coronary arteriograms. American Journal of Cardiology 32: 375–376
Kirnö K, Friberg P, Grzegorczyk A et al 1994 Thoracic epidural anesthesia during coronary artery bypass surgery: effects on cardiac sympathetic activity, myocardial blood flow and metabolism, and central hemodynamics. Anesthesia and Analgesia 79: 1075–1081
Kontos HA, 1996 Vascular diseases of the limbs. In: Bennett JC, Plum F (eds) Cecil textbook of medicine, 20th edn. Saunders, Philadelphia, pp 346–357
Lewis T 1942 Pain. Macmillan, New York
Longo DL 1998 Plasma cell disorders. In: Fauci AS, Braunwald E, Isselbacher KJ et al (eds) Harrison's principles of internal medicine, 14th edn. McGraw–Hill, New York, pp 712–718
Lorell BH 1997 Pericardial diseases. In: Braunwald E (ed) Heart disease, 5th edn. Saunders, Philadelphia, pp 1478–1534
Malliani A 1986 The elusive link between transient myocardial ischaemia and pain. Circulation 73: 201–204
Malliani A 1995 The conceptualization of cardiac pain as a nonspecific and unreliable alarm system. In: Gebhart GF (ed) Visceral pain. IASP Press, Seattle, pp 63–74
Malliani A, Lombardi F 1982 Considerations of fundamental mechanisms eliciting cardiac pain. American Heart Journal 103: 575–578
Maresca M, Nuzzaci G, Zoppi M 1984 Muscular pain in chronic occlusive arterial diseases of the limbs. In: Benedetti C, Chapman CR, Moricca G (eds) Recent advances in the management of pain. Raven Press, New York, pp 521–527
Maseri A 1995 Ischemic heart disease. Churchill Livingstone, New York
Maseri A, Severi S, Nes MD et al 1978 'Variant' angina: one aspect of a continuous spectrum of vasospastic myocardial ischemia. Pathogenetic mechanisms, estimated incidence and clinical and arteriographic findings in 138 patients. American Journal of Cardiology 42: 1019–1035
Melzack R 1973 The puzzle of pain. Penguin, Harmondsworth
Nathan PW 1962 Pain traces left in the central nervous system. In: Keele CA, Smith R (eds) The assessment of pain in man and animals. Livingstone, Edinburgh, pp 129–134
Neri Serneri GG, Modesti PA, Gensini GF et al 1995 Randomised comparison of subcutaneous heparin, intravenous heparin, and aspirin in unstable angina. Lancet 345: 1201–1204
Olausson K, Magnusdottir H, Lurje L et al 1997 Anti-ischemic and anti-anginal effects of thoracic epidural anesthesia versus those of conventional medical therapy in the treatment of severe refractory unstable angina pectoris. Circulation 96: 2178–2182
Prinzmetal M, Kennamer R, Merliss R et al 1959 A variant form of angina pectoris. American Journal of Medicine 27: 375–388
Procacci P 1969 A survey of modern concepts of pain. In: Vinken PJ, Bruyn GW (eds) Handbook of clinical neurology, vol 1. North-Holland, Amsterdam, pp 114–146
Procacci P, Maresca M 1987a Clinical aspects of heart pain. In: Tiengo M, Eccles J, Cuello AC, Ottoson D (eds) Advances in pain research and therapy, vol 10: Pain and mobility. Raven Press, New York, pp 127–133
Procacci P, Maresca M 1987b Reflex sympathetic dystrophies and algodystrophies: historical and pathogenic considerations. Pain 31: 137–146
Procacci P, Zoppi M, Padeletti L, Maresca M 1976 Myocardial infarction without pain. A study of the sensory function of the upper limbs. Pain 2: 309–313
Procacci P, Zoppi M, Maresca M 1986 Clinical approach to visceral sensation. In: Cervero F, Morrison JFB (eds) Visceral sensation. Elsevier, Amsterdam, pp 21–28
Rasner SM, Bhogal RS 1991 Infectious arthritis in a hemophiliac. Journal of Rheumatology 8: 519–523
Rinzler SH 1951 Cardiac pain. Thomas, Springfield, IL
Rogers WJ 1996 Angina pectoris. In: Bennett JC, Plum F (eds) Cecil textbook of medicine, 20th edn. Saunders, Philadelphia, pp 296–301
Rosenwasser LJ 1996 The vasculitic syndromes. In: Bennett JC, Plum F (eds) Cecil textbook of medicine, 20th edn. Saunders, Philadelphia, pp 1490–1495
Selwyin AP, Braunwald E 1998 Ischemic heart disease. In: Fauci AS, Braunwald E, Isselbacher KJ et al (eds) Harrison's principles of internal medicine, 14th edn. McGraw–Hill, New York, pp 1365–1375
Shapiro BS, Dinges DF, Orne EC et al 1995 Home management of sickle cell-related pain in children and adolescents: natural history and impact on school attendance. Pain 61: 139–144
Stern S 1998 Silent myocardial ischemia. Martin Dunitz, London
Tefferi A, Silverstein MN 1996 Chronic myeloproliferative diseases. In: Bennett JC, Plum F (eds) Cecil textbook of medicine, 20th edn. Saunders, Philadelphia, pp 922–925
Teodori U, Galletti R 1962 Il dolore nelle affezioni degli organi interni del torace. Pozzi, Roma
White JC, Sweet WH 1955 Pain. Its mechanisms and neurosurgical control. Thomas, Springfield, IL
York JR 1998 Endocrine and hemoglobin-related arthropathies and storage diseases. In: Klippel JH, Dieppe PA (eds) Rheumatology, 2nd edn. Mosby, London, pp 8–24
Zimmermann M 1979 Peripheral and central nervous mechanisms of nociception, pain and pain therapy: facts and hypotheses. In: Bonica JJ, Liebeskind JC, Albe-Fessard D (eds) Proceedings of the Second World Congress on Pain. Raven Press, New York, pp 3–32
Zoppi M, Zamponi A, Pagni E, Buoncristiano U 1985 A way to understand erythromelalgia. Journal of the Autonomic Nervous System 13: 85–89

Chronic pelvic pain

Andrea J Rapkin and Julie A Jolin

Introduction

Chronic pelvic pain (CPP) is defined as pain that persists for more than 6 months. Even after a thorough evaluation, the etiology of the pain may remain obscure, and the relationship between certain types of pathology (such as adhesions, endometriosis, and pelvic congestion) and pain can be inconsistent. This chapter outlines the relevant anatomy and reviews the differential diagnosis and management of chronic pelvic pain.

Biological considerations

The sensory nerves from pelvic visceral organs (such as bowel, bladder, rectum, and uterus) and somatic structures (such as skin, muscles, anus, and urethra) as well as their related sensory spinal roots are listed in Table 10.1 (Kumazawa 1986, Cervero and Tattersall 1986, Wesselmann and Lai 1997). Visceral pain, in contrast to somatic pain, is usually deep and difficult to localize. Moreover, acute visceral pain is associated with various autonomic reflexes such as restlessness, nausea, vomiting, and diaphoresis (Procacci et al 1986). An important aspect of visceral pelvic pain is referred pain, which is superficial and well-localized, and perceived to arise from the dermatome receiving the visceral stimulus. Various acute and chronic gynecologic pain conditions are characterized by referred pain to the dermatomes associated with pelvic organ innervation, i.e., T10–L2 (anterior abdominal wall and anterior thighs) and dorsal rami of L1–L2 (lower back) (Slocumb 1984, Giamberardino et al 1995, Wesselmann and Lai 1997; and see Chaps. 11 and 12).

Peripheral causes of chronic pelvic pain

Table 10.2 lists the differential diagnosis of the peripheral component of pelvic pain.

Adhesions

The role of pelvic adhesions in the genesis of pelvic pain has been debated from various perspectives. Adhesions were found in 16–44% of the patients undergoing laparoscopy for chronic pelvic pain (Kresch et al 1984, Rapkin 1986, Hughes 1990). However, the prevalence of adhesions in the control group depends on the comparison group selected (i.e., sterilization or infertility). Kresch noted adhesions in 51% of CPP patients and 14% of women undergoing sterilization (Kresch et al 1984). In

Table 10.1 Nerves carrying painful impulses from the pelvis

Organ	Spinal Segments	Nerves
Perineum, vulva, lower vagina	S2–S4	Pudendal, inguinal, genitofemoral, posterofemoral cutaneous
Upper vagina, cervix, lower uterine segment, posterior urethra, bladder trigone, uterosacral and cardinal ligaments, rectosigmoid, lower ureters	S2–S4	Pelvic autonomics via pelvic nerve
Uterine fundus, proximal fallopian tubes, broad ligament, upper bladder, caecum, appendix, terminal large bowel	T11–12, L1	Lumbosacral autonomics via hypogastric plexus
Outer two-thirds of fallopian tubes	T9–T10	Thoracolumbar autonomics via renal and aortic plexus and coeliac and mesenteric ganglia
Abdominal wall	T12–L1	Iliohypogastric
	T12–L1	Ilioinguinal
	L1–L2	Genitofemoral

Table 10.2 Peripheral causes of chronic pelvic pain

1. Gynaecologic

Non-cyclic
- Adhesions
- Endometriosis
- Salpingo-oophoritis
- Ovarian remnant syndrome
- Pelvic congestion syndrome (varicosities)
- Ovarian neoplasms
- Pelvic relaxation

Cyclic
- Primary dysmenorrhoea
- Secondary dysmenorrhoea
  - a. Imperforate hymen or transverse vaginal septum
  - b. Cervical stenosis
  - c. Uterine anomalies (congenital malformation, bicornuate uterus, bline uterus horn)
  - d. Intrauterine synechiae (Asherman's syndrome)
  - e. Endometrial polyps
  - f. Uterine leiomyoma
  - g. Adenomyosis
  - h. Pelvic congestion syndrome (varicosities)
  - i. Endometriosis

Atypical cyclic

2. Gastrointestinal

Irritable bowel syndrome
Ulcerative colitis
Granulomatous colitis (Crohn's disease)
Carcinoma
Infectious diarrhoea
Recurrent partial small bowel obstruction
Diverticulitis
Hernia
Abdominal angina
Recurrent appendiceal colic

3. Genitourinary

Recurrent or relapsing cystourethritis
Urethral syndrome
Interstitial cystitis
Ureteral diverticuli or polyps
Carcinoma of the bladder
Ureteral obstruction
Pelvic kidney

4. Neurologic

Nerve entrapment syndrome
Neuroma
Trigger points

5. Musculoskeletal

Low back pain syndrome
- Congenital anomalies
- Scoliosis and kyphosis
- Spondylolysis
- Spondylolisthesis
- Spinal injuries
- Inflammation
- Tumours
- Osteoporosis
- Degenerative changes
- Coccydynia

Myofascial syndrome
Fibromyalgia
Pelvic floor muscle tension/spasm or trigger points

6. Systemic

Acute intermittent porphyria
Abdominal migraine
Systemic lupus erythematosus
Lymphoma
Neurofibromatosis

contrast, Rapkin reported adhesions in 26% of CPP patients and 39% of asymptomatic infertility patients (Rapkin 1986). Furthermore, the location and density of adhesions did not differ between groups (Rapkin 1986). The latter findings were confirmed by Koninckx et al (1991), who laparoscoped 227 patients and noted a similar prevalence and distribution of adhesions between CPP patients and asymptomatic infertility patients.

Although women with CPP have a higher prevalence of adhesions than women undergoing sterilization, one cannot conclude that these findings are causal or even highly associated. If adhesions cause pain, adhesiolysis should relieve pain. There is only one randomized controlled trial of lysis of adhesions in women with CPP (Peters et al 1992). Patients with CPP and laparoscopic diagnosis of stage III to IV adhesions were subjected to adhesiolysis via laparotomy or expectantly managed. Follow-up assessment of pain was performed 16 months postoperatively, showing that no significant benefit of adhesiolysis as compared to expectant management. A prospective non-randomized study of adhesiolysis also showed no improvement in pain at an 8-month follow-up (Steege and Scott 1991). There was, however, significant relief of pain after adhesiolysis in the subgroup of women without 'CPP syndrome'. (CPP syndrome was defined as women manifesting 4 or more of the following: (1) pain duration >6 months; (2) incomplete relief by previous treatments; (3) impaired physical functioning secondary to pain; (4) vegetative signs of depression; and (5) altered family roles.) Steege concluded that lysis of adhesions may be a useful procedure in some women but not those with 'CPP syndrome' (Steege and Scott 1991).

Future studies of laparoscopy under local anesthesia may allow 'pain mapping' to determine which tissues or adhesions would be the most likely to be the cause of the pain. To date, there are no studies of pain symptoms after procedures guided by pain mapping techniques (Howard et al 2000).

Endometriosis

Endometriosis affects about 1–2% of all women and 15–25% of infertile women. Endometriosis is found in approximately 28–74% of the patients undergoing laparoscopy for chronic pelvic pain (Kresch et al 1984, Rapkin 1986, Howard 1993, Reese et al 1996). Endometriosis is defined as the presence of endometrial glands and stroma located outside the uterine cavity, occurring most commonly in the cul-de-sac, ovaries, and pelvic visceral and parietal peritoneum. The favoured theory of aetiology is retrograde menses with implantation of endometrium in susceptible women, and likely involves a local disorder of immune modulation (D'Hooghe and Hill 1996).

The most common symptoms of endometriosis are dysmenorrhoea, dyspareunia, infertility, and abnormal uterine bleeding, usually from a secretory endometrium. Pelvic pain in women with endometriosis may occur at any time in the menstrual cycle, though dysmenorrhoea is the most classic symptom. Dysmenorrhoea may begin 7–10 days before the onset of the menstrual period and persist after the bleeding has ceased. The patient often describes pressure-like or sharp pain in the lower abdomen, back, and rectum with radiation to the vagina, thighs, or perineum. Dyspareunia or dyschezia (pain with bowel movements) is common when the disease involves the cul-de-sac (pouch of Douglas), uterosacral ligaments, or rectovaginal septum. Although the serosa of the intestine is involved in many patients, only rarely is the mucosa affected leading to cyclic haematochezia. Urinary urgency, frequency, bladder pain, and rarely haematuria can also be associated with urinary tract involvement. Rarely, patients may develop bowel or ureteral obstruction. Postmenopausal women on oestrogen replacement can continue to experience symptomatic endometriosis. However, without oestrogen replacement the diagnosis is highly debatable.

Examination of patients with endometriosis often reveals focal tenderness and nodularity on the rectovaginal examination of the uterosacral or broad ligaments and posterior cul-de-sac. Progressive disease will result in obliteration and fibrosis of the cul-de-sac, and fixed retroversion of the uterus. Enlarged ovaries filled with 'chocolate cysts' (endometriomas) with decreased mobility are often noted on examination or ultrasound of the pelvis.

While endometriosis may be suggested by history and pelvic examination, a definitive diagnosis requires laparoscopy. A clinical diagnosis is accurate in 50% of cases (D'Hooghe and Hill 1996). Ultrasound is not diagnostic since small implants are undetectable, and endometriomas can resemble cystic ovarian neoplasms.

Endometriosis is usually progressive if untreated. Medical treatment options include continuous or cyclic oral contraceptive pills, androgenic hormones (Danocrine), high-dose oral or depo progestins, or gonadotropin-releasing hormone analogues (D'Hooghe and Hill 1996, Prentice et al 2000, Olive and Pritts 2001). Laparoscopic electro-dessication or laser vapourization or laparotomy with resection of disease is usually recommended particularly for severe endometriosis or endometriomas. Patients not desiring fertility may undergo total abdominal hysterectomy with bilateral salpingo-oophorectomy and appendectomy, as well as removal of any residual GI, GU, or peritoneal disease. Some women benefit from adjunctive acupuncture or multidisciplinary pain management (Rapkin and Kames 1987).

In many women suffering chronic pelvic pain, endometriosis may not be the cause of the pain or may only represent a contributing factor. At least 30% of patients with recurrent pain after treatment for endometriosis have no residual implants upon repeat laparoscopy. There is no significant correlation between disease amount and pain severity except in higher-stage disease, which tends to be associated with a greater prevalence of and increased intensity of pain. Furthermore, there is no correlation between location of pain and site of endometriotic lesions (Fukaya et al 1993). Pain not responding to adequate medical or surgical management of endometriosis needs careful reevaluation.

Tumours and cysts of the reproductive organs

Most reproductive organ tumours and cysts can cause acute pain from adnexal torsion, torsion of leiomyomata, or degeneration. Chronically, pelvic tumours such as leiomyomata or ovarian neoplasms cause vague lower abdominal discomfort and fullness and require ultrasound to diagnose.

The most common pelvic neoplasms are leiomyomata. Mild pelvic discomfort from myomata usually presents itself when the masses encroach on adjacent bladder or rectum. Surgery, myomectomy or hysterectomy, is warranted for abnormal bleeding or discomfort due to uterine size, usually greater than 14 cm.

Pelvic congestion

For the past 40 years, there has been interest in the role of 'pelvic congestion' or uterine and ovarian vein varicosities in the genesis of chronic pelvic pain. Clinically, the syndrome includes abdominal and low back pain, dysmenorrhoea, dyspareunia, and menorrhagia. The pain is usually bilateral, lower pelvic in distribution, and exacerbated by the luteal phase and the menstrual period. On exam, there is tenderness over the uterus, parametria, and especially the uterosacral ligaments and polycystic ovaries often are noted (Beard et al 1988).

Pelvic congestion, until recently, was only a clinical diagnosis. Transuterine venogram is diagnostic; however, this test is technically not feasible or unreadable in 21% of patients (Beard et al 1988). There are a few small studies examining pelvic ultrasound with Doppler or MRI for diagnosis of pelvic congestion (Stones et al 1990).

Hormonal suppression inducing a hypo-oestrogenic environment has been used to treat pelvic congestion (Farquhar et al 1989, Gangar et al 1993). Medroxyprogesterone acetate (MPA) 30 mg daily for three months was administered in a randomized, placebo-controlled treatment trial, which resulted in a 50% reduction in pain score for those given MPA compared to a 33% reduction for those given placebo (Beard et al 1991). However, after discontinuation of treatment, the pain recurred in the MPA group but did not return in the placebo group. Total abdominal hysterectomy with bilateral salpingo-oophorectomy eliminated pain in 33 of 36 patients followed for one year (Beard et al 1991). Transcatheter embolization of pelvic veins has been performed in a limited number of subjects with promising outcome but the long-term risks and benefits remain unknown (Sichlau et al 1994).

Salphingo-oophoritis

Salpingo-oophoritis can cause chronic pelvic pain, though patients usually present with symptoms and signs of acute or subacute infection before the pain becomes chronic. Patients may report numerous episodes of pain associated with fever, and may have been told they have pelvic inflammatory disease. However, the patient may not have salpingitis at all. Clinical diagnosis leads to error in 50% of the cases (Westrom and Eschenbach 1999). Laparoscopic visualization of pelvic organs and peritoneal fluid cultures are diagnostic. The standard treatment for salpingo-oophoritis is intravenous antibiotics. Only rarely is hysterectomy and salpingo-oophorectomy required, generally for tubo-ovarian abscesses.

Ovarian remnant syndrome

A hysterectomy and bilateral salpingo-oophorectomy performed in the setting of severe anatomic distortion such as with severe endometriosis or pelvic inflammatory disease may result in the ovarian remnant syndrome, in which residual ovarian cortical tissue is left *in situ* (Siddal-Allum et al 1994). While the incidence of ovarian remnants is unknown but suspected to be high, associated pain is rare.

Ovarian remnant syndrome is diagnosed on history, physical examination, and hormonal evaluation (Price et al 1990). Two to five years after surgery, cyclic pain may arise, accompanied by flank pain, and on occasion, urinary tract infection and intermittent, partial bowel obstruction. Pelvic exam may reveal a tender mass in the lateral pelvis. Ultrasound following ovarian stimulation with clomiphene usually confirms a mass with sonographic characteristics of ovarian tissue. In a patient who has had bilateral salpingo-oophorectomy and is not on hormonal replacement, estradiol and follicle stimulating hormone (FSH) levels reveal a characteristic premenopausal picture, though on occasion the remaining ovarian tissue may not be active enough to suppress FSH levels. Laparotomy with removal of residual ovarian tissue is necessary for treatment (Price et al 1990), though commonly complications ensue, including haemorrhage, ureteral, bladder, and bowel injury, and postoperative ileus, and recurrent remnants occur in 15% of cases. Treatment with GnRH agonists and oestrogen and progestin addback therapy may be an appropriate alternative (Carey and Slack 1996).

Cyclic pelvic pain

Cyclic pelvic pain implies pain occurring with a specific relationship to the menstrual cycle. It consists of primary and secondary dysmenorrhoea but also includes atypical cyclic pain, such as pain beginning two weeks prior to menses. Atypical cyclic pain is a variant of secondary dysmenorrhoea. The diagnosis of cyclic pain often depends on the review of a daily pain and menstrual diary.

Dysmenorrhoea or 'painful monthly flow' is a common gynaecologic disorder affecting up to 50% of menstruating women (Rapkin et al 1997). Primary dysmenorrhoea refers to pain with menses when there is no pelvic pathology, whereas secondary dysmenorrhoea is painful menses with underlying pelvic pathology. Primary dysmenorrhoea usually appears one to two years after menarche, with the establishment of ovulatory cycles, but may persist into the 40s. The pain consists of suprapubic cramping radiating down the anterior thighs and to the lumbosacral region often accompanied by nausea, vomiting, and diarrhoea. The pain occurs prior to or just after the onset of menses and lasts for 48–72 h.

Secondary dysmenorrhoea most often starts years after menarche and may occur with anovulatory cycles. The most common causes of secondary dysmenorrhoea are endometriosis and adenomyosis, a condition in which the endometrial glands penetrate the myometrium. Other common causes are listed in Table 10.2 and include vaginal, cervical, uterine, fallopian tube, adnexal, and peritoneal pathology. The distinction between primary and secondary dysmenorrhoea and chronic pelvic pain requires a thorough history as to the timing and duration of the pain, a pain diary, and a careful pelvic examination, with focus on the size, contour, mobility, and tenderness of the uterus, adnexal structures, and nodularity of the uterosacral ligaments and rectovaginal septum. Genital studies for gonorrhoea and chlamydia, complete blood count with ESR, and possibly a transvaginal ultrasound are warranted. If no abnormalities are found and pain is cyclic, a tentative diagnosis of primary dysmenorrhoea can be made.

Prostaglandin synthetase inhibitors are effective for the treatment of primary dysmenorrhoea in up to 80% of the cases and should be initiated premenstrually or at least before the pain begins or becomes severe (Deligeoroglou 2000). For the patient with primary dysmenorrhoea who has no contraindications to oral contraceptive agents, the birth control pill is the second agent of choice. More than 90% of women with primary dysmenorrhoea have relief with oral contraceptive control pills (Chan and Dawood 1980). Narcotic analgesics can be administered for pain control. Prior to the addition of narcotic medication, organic pathology should be ruled out, generally via laparoscopy and, if indicated, hysteroscopy. Other modes of hormonal menstrual suppression include high-dose progestins (oral or depo intramuscular injection), continuous oral contraceptive pill administration, or gonadotropin-releasing hormone agonists with continuous low- (menopausal) dosage hormone addback. Breakthrough bleeding with associated pain are potential problems with these regimens. Acupuncture or transcutaneous electrical nerve stimulation may be successful (Wilson et al 2000). If treatment fails, laparoscopy is warranted to rule out causes of secondary dysmenorrhoea, particularly endometriosis. Surgical approaches to dysmenorrhoea include laparoscopic uterosacral ligament ablation, presacral neurectomy, and in selected cases of secondary dysmenorrhoea, hysterectomy (Malinak 1980).

Gastroenterologic causes of chronic pelvic pain

Many patients referred to gynaecologists with chronic pelvic pain actually have gastroenterologic

(GI) pathology (Reiter 1990, Walker et al 1996). Since the cervix, uterus, adnexa, lower ileum, sigmoid colon, and rectum share the same visceral innervation, with pain signals travelling via the sympathetic nerves to spinal cord segments T10–L1, it is often difficult to determine whether lower abdominal pain is of gynaecologic or enterocolic origin (Mayer and Gebhart 1993). In addition, as is true with other types of visceral pain, pain sensation from the GI tract is often diffuse and poorly localized.

Irritable bowel syndrome (IBS) is one of the more common causes of lower abdominal pain and may account for as many as 7 to 60% of referrals to a gynaecologist for chronic pelvic pain (Reiter 1990). The predominant symptom of irritable bowel syndrome is abdominal pain that is intermittently crampy and predominantly in the left lower quadrant. The Rome II criteria for the diagnosis of IBS are listed in Table 10.3. Symptoms are usually worse after eating, during periods of stress, tension, anxiety, or depression, and with the premenstrual and menstrual phases of the cycle.

History and exclusion of other conditions establishes the diagnosis of IBS. Red flags such as blood in stool, recent antibiotic usage, nocturnal awakening, family history of colon cancer, weight loss, and abnormal pelvic or abdominal exam do not support its diagnosis, but rather warrant colonoscopy or CAT scan with contrast to rule-out pathology. IBS treatment consists of dietary alterations, bulk-forming agents, high-fibre diet, reassurance, education, stress reduction, and medications such as low-dose tricyclic antidepressants (Ringel et al 2001), anxiolytics, anticholinergics, or other antispasmodics.

Another cause of chronic enterocolic pain is diverticular disease of the colon. Five to 40% of individuals over the age of 40 have diverticulosis, although most patients never develop diverticulitis. Though diverticulosis is usually asymptomatic, diverticulitis results in severe, acute left lower quadrant pain associated with fever, a tender mass, and leukocytosis.

Table 10.3 The Rome II Criteria for diagnosing irritable bowel syndrome

Abdominal pain or discomfort, for at least 12 weeks out of the previous 12 months, which need not necessarily be consecutive (and cannot be explained by structural or biochemical changes), and has 2 of these 3 features:

a. relieved by defecation
b. onset associated with a change in frequency
c. consistency of stool

Inflammatory bowel disease (IBD) such as ulcerative colitis or granulomatous disease (Crohn's disease) similarly do not usually present as chronic pelvic pain because their presentation is usually more acute with diarrhoea, fever, vomiting, and anorexia. A colonoscopy or barium study is diagnostic for IBD.

Tumours of the GI tract can cause chronic lower abdominal pain. The most frequent and early symptoms of bowel carcinomas are change in bowel habits (74% of patients) and abdominal pain (65% of patients). Rectal bleeding and weight loss may be signs of advanced disease. Most rectal tumours can be palpated on rectal examination. Endoscopy, barium enema, or CAT scan with contrast are diagnostic.

Hernia

Hernia is included in the differential diagnosis of lower abdominal pain. There is a relatively low incidence of inguinal hernia in females. Anterior and posterior perineal hernias are usually limited to cystocele, rectocele, or enterocele and may cause lower pressure-like abdominal/perineal pain in women. This type of pain will usually respond to a pessary followed by surgical management. Another cause of abdominal pain in women is a Spigelian hernia, which results from weakness in the transversalis fascia (Spangen 1984) and produces lower abdominal pain between the semilunar line and the lateral border of the rectus muscle. Increased pain with valsalva, clinical exam, and ultrasound are helpful for diagnosis. Surgery is necessary for repair.

Urologic causes of chronic pelvic pain

(also see Chap. 12)

Chronic pain of urologic origin may present as pelvic pain due to close development and anatomy of urinary and genital tracts. The urethra and bladder and the vagina and vestibule are all derived from the embryologic urogenital sinus. Recurrent cystoureteritis, urethral syndrome, urethral diverticulae, urgency, frequency syndrome, interstitial cystitis, infiltrating bladder tumours, ectopic pelvic kidney, and various ureteral causes of pelvic pain such as urolithiasis, ureteral obstructions, or endometriosis can present as pelvic pain in approximately 5% of women with chronic pelvic pain (Reiter 1990, Spangen 1984). The medical history should query symptoms such as urgency, frequency, hesitancy, incontinence, nocturia, dyspareunia, and past history of treatment of urinary tract problems.

The patient with infectious cystitis presents with complaints of suprapubic pain, dysuria, frequency, and urgency, and has pyuria and a positive urine culture. The symptoms usually respond to adequate antibiotic therapy. Relapses and reinfection can be diagnosed with the aid of history, urinalysis, and culture. The antibiotic and duration of therapy may have to be adjusted and on occasion, if the patient has recurrent cystoureteritis, antibiotics may have to be administered post-coitally or for a prolonged period of time. Chlamydial infection is responsible for about 25% of cases of pyuria and urethritis in women (Summit 1993).

The urethral syndrome may present as chronic pelvic pain or irritative lower urinary tract symptoms such as dysuria, urinary frequency, and dyspareunia (Bergman et al 1989, Summit 1993). The diagnosis is one of exclusion. A negative urinalysis, negative or a low colony count (e.g., $<10^4$ col/mL) on urine culture, and negative chlamydia study and evaluation for vulvovaginitis will increase the suspicion for the diagnosis of urethral syndrome. The aetiology of the syndrome is unknown: chronic inflammation of the periurethral glands or urethral spasticity with periurethral muscle fatigue has been suggested. Treatment consists of re-education of voiding habits through pelvic floor muscle biofeedback (Bergman et al 1989), chronic suppression with 3–6 month low-dose course of broad spectrum antibiotics, or tetracycline for 2 to 3 weeks if chlamydia is suspected. If without success, urethral dilatation has been utilized. Vaginal oestrogen for peri- and postmenopausal women is important (Karram 1993). Consideration should be given to pelvic floor muscle biofeedback, muscle relaxants, and psychotherapy.

Symptoms of urinary frequency, urgency, nocturia, and suprapubic pain with negative laboratory studies are consistent with both interstitial cystitis (IC) and urgency/frequency syndrome. The consensus criteria for the diagnosis of IC include at least two of the following: pain or bladder filling relieved by emptying; pain in suprapubic, pelvic, urethral, vaginal, or perineal region; glomerulations on endoscopy; or decreased compliance on cystometrogram (Kream and Carr 1999). Symptoms that do not meet IC criteria can be termed urgency/frequency syndrome. Interstitial cystitis is an inflammatory condition of uncertain aetiology although autoimmune disease, defect of the glycosaminoglycan layer of the bladder mucosa, and activated bladder sensory neuropeptides have been proposed (Sant 1998). The evaluation of patients with the above symptoms should include cystoscopy under anaesthesia with hydrodistension and possible biopsy. Therapy consists of bladder diet, intravesical hydrodistension, instillation of dimethylsulfoxide, or analogues of glycosaminoglycan, transcutaneous electrical nerve stimulation (TENS), physical therapy, or biofeedback to the pelvic floor muscles, or repeated anaesthetic blocks (hypogastric plexus). The treatment of the condition remains empiric and less than optimal oral pharmacologic agents such as anticholinergic, antispasmodic, non-steroidal anti-inflammatory agents, tricyclic antidepressants, and narcotics have all been utilized with some success (Sant 1998).

Nerve entrapment or injury

Abdominal cutaneous nerve entrapment or injury should be considered in the differential diagnosis of chronic lower abdominal pain, especially if no visceral aetiology is apparent. The syndrome most commonly occurs months to years after Pfannenstiel skin or other lower abdominal and even laparoscopic incisions (Sippo et al 1987) but can also follow trauma, automobile accidents, or exercise. Commonly involved nerves include ilioinguinal (T12, L1), iliohypogastric (T12, L1), and genitofemoral (L1, L2).

Symptoms of nerve entrapment include pain, typically elicited by exercise and relieved by bedrest. The pain is described as stabbing, colicky, located along the lateral edge of the rectus margin often associated with a burning or aching pain radiating to the hip, or sacroiliac region. Nausea, bloating, menstruation, and a full bladder or bowel exacerbate the pain.

On examination, the pain can be localized with the fingertip (McDonald 1993). The maximal point of tenderness is the neuromuscular foramen at the rectus margin medial and inferior to the anterior iliac spine or, in the case of spontaneous nerve entrapment, at the site of exit from the aponeurosis of the other thoracic/abdominal cutaneous nerves. A manoeuvre that helps to make the diagnosis is to ask the patient to tense the abdominal wall by raising shoulders or raising and extending the lower limbs in a straight leg raising manoeuvre. The outer side of the rectal muscle is then pressed with a single finger. The pain will be exacerbated if abdominal wall pain is present (Thomson and Francis 1977). The tentative diagnosis is confirmed with a diagnostic nerve block consisting of an injection of 2–3 mL of 0.025% Bupivocaine (Slocumb 1990, McDonald 1993). Immediate relief is usually reported and many patients require up to 5 biweekly injections. Only as a last resort should consideration be given to surgical removal of the involved nerves (Hahn 1989). Medications such as tricyclic antidepressants, anticonvulsants, and acupuncture are also useful for pain control. Physical therapy or lifestyle change may be necessary to strengthen other muscles and avoid reinjury.

Musculoskeletal causes of chronic pain

Women complaining of lower back pain without complaints of pelvic pain rarely have gynaecologic pathology as the cause of their pain; however, low back pain may accompany pelvic pathology. Back pain may be caused by gynaecologic, vascular, neurologic, psychogenic, or spondylogenic (related to the axial skeleton and its structures) pathology (Baker 1993). Musculoskeletal abnormalities commonly contribute to the symptoms of chronic pelvic pain. A physical therapist who can evaluate posture, muscle length and strength, and joint range of motion should improve the efficacy of treatment.

Myofascial pain

Reports of the prevalence of myofascial pain as a cause of pelvic pain vary. Reiter and Gambone found myofascial syndrome in 15% of their patients with somatic pathology. (Patients with identifiable somatic pathology represented 47% of all patients referred to their pelvic pain clinic (Reiter 1990).) Slocumb, in comparison, noted 'trigger points' in 89% of women presenting with chronic pelvic pain irrespective of underlying pelvic pathology (Slocumb 1984, 1990).

Myofascial pain is exacerbated by activity within the affected part and by activity in deeper visceral structures that share the same dermatomal innervation (bladder or colon activity or pathology, menses, and cervical motion and intercourse) (Travell 1976; Slocumb 1984, 1990). Any structure or muscle innervated via T12–L4 can refer pain to the lower abdomen (i.e., vertebrae, joint capsule, ligaments, discs, muscles such as the rectus, illiopsoas, quadratus lumborum, piriformis, and obturators). On digital examination of abdominal, back, or vaginal dermatomes, pressure on the trigger point evokes local and referred pain. Pain is exacerbated by the straight leg raising manoeuvre described above. Treatment of myofascial trigger points includes injecting the trigger points with local anaesthetic as well as physical therapy and treatment of associated psychological factors such as depression, anxiety, and learned behaviour patterns that may accompany and exacerbate the condition (Travell 1976; Slocumb 1984, 1990). Medications such as tricyclic antidepressants and anticonvulsants may also be useful.

Psychological factors in chronic pelvic pain

From a psychological perspective, there are various factors that may promote the chronicity of pain. Studies of women with chronic pelvic pain have documented a high level of psychological disturbance (Reiter 1990).

Higher depression scores and family histories of affective disorder were described in women with chronic pelvic pain without pathology compared to women with chronic pelvic pain and pathology as established by laparoscopy (Magni et al 1984). A comparison of women with pelvic pain of unknown aetiology, IBS, and a pain-free control group revealed the pelvic pain group had significantly higher prevalence of major depression, dysthymic disorder, panic disorders, somatization disorder, and sexual abuse. Often, the depression preceded the onset of the pain; however, no prospective studies have been performed (Magni et al 1984, Mayer and Gebhart 1993).

Studies have also examined the role of sexual abuse as a specific risk factor for chronic pelvic pain. A high prevalence (90%) of sexual abuse and physical abuse has been reported in women with chronic pelvic pain (Rapkin et al 1990). A history of childhood sexual abuse and a past history of depression are strongly related to the subsequent persistence of pelvic pain (Harrop-Griffiths et al 1988). Toomey reaffirmed the importance of obtaining sexual and physical abuse histories in chronic pelvic pain patients (Toomey et al 1993).

The diagnosis 'chronic pelvic pain without obvious pathology' has been proposed for patients who lack somatic pathology (Renaer 1980). Often these patients have been considered to have psychogenic pain. The role of neurophysiologic mechanisms within the brain and spinal cord in the maintenance of chronic pain cannot be underestimated (Rapkin 1995). Wall has suggested that it is 'necessary to consider the lability of central transmission pathways as well as seeking peripheral pathology in all painful conditions' (Wall 1988).

Diagnosis and management of chronic pelvic pain

Successful diagnosis and management of patients with chronic pelvic pain as with other chronic pain conditions requires a meticulous yet compassionate, multidisciplinary approach. A thorough history should be obtained. The nature of the pain, location and radiation, aggravating and alleviating factors, timing, effect of menses, exercise, work, stress, intercourse, and orgasm should be queried. Ascertain context in which the pain arose and is maintained including previous episodes of pain, inability to perform family role or occupation, and litigation or worker's compensation. Other somatic symptoms should be noted: genital tract (abnormal vaginal bleeding, discharge, mittelschmerz, dysmenorrhoea, dyspareunia, infertility), enterocolic (constipation, diarrhoea, flatulence, tenesmus, blood, changes in colour or calibre of stool), musculoskeletal (predominant low back distribution, pain radiation, association with injury, fatigue, postural changes), and urologic (dysuria, urgency, frequency, suprapelvic pain). Historical questions specific to all of the peripheral pathologies noted in Table 10.1 should be queried. Past history including medical, surgical, gynaecologic, obstetric, sexual, medication intake, and prior evaluations for the pain should be documented. Operative and pathology reports are important if the patient has had surgery.

Current and past psychological history, including psychosocial factors, history of past (or current) physical, sexual, and/or emotional abuse, history of hospitalization, suicide attempts, and chemical (drug or alcohol) dependency, should be asked. The attitude of the patient and her family towards the pain, resultant behaviour of patient family with respect to the pain, and current upheavals in patient's life should be discussed. The part of the history addressing sensitive issues may have to be reobtained after establishing rapport with the patient.

Symptoms of an acute process such as fever, anorexia, nausea, emesis, significant diarrhoea, recurrent constipation, ascites, uterine bleeding, pregnancy, or recent abortion should alert one as to the possibility of an acute condition requiring immediate medical or surgical intervention, especially if accompanied by orthostasis, peritoneal signs, pelvic or abdominal mass, abnormal CBC, positive genital or urinary tract cultures, or a positive pregnancy test.

One should perform a complete physical examination, with particular attention to the abdominal, back, vaginal, urethrovesicle, bimanual, rectovaginal, and pelvic floor muscle examination. The examination should include evaluation of the abdomen with straight leg raising manoeuvre to discern abdominal wall sources of pain. Abdominal wall pain is augmented and visceral pain is diminished with the above manoeuvres (Slocumb 1990, McDonald 1993). The patient should be examined while standing for hernias, abdominal (inguinal, femoral, and Spigelian) and pelvic (cystocele, enterocele). An attempt should be made to locate by fingertip palpation of the tissues (abdominal, pelvic, external genital, and lower back) that reproduce the patient's pain. The appearance, support, and tenderness of the bladder, urethra, and rectum should be determined. A neurologic exam of the lower extremities and perineum can aide with the assessment of S3–S5 and L2–L4 nerve roots. Vaginal oestrogenization should also be determined when visualizing the vaginal epithelium.

Laboratory studies, if not already performed, include CBC, ESR, urinalysis and culture, cervical and urethral cultures (gonorrhoea and chlamydia), wet mount of vaginal secretions, pap smear, stool guaiac, and, if diarrhoea is present, stool culture. If the pelvic or abdominal examination is inadequate or suggestive of a mass, ultrasound or MRI evaluation is indicated. If symptoms and signs are suggestive of other system involvement, fibreoptic or other appropriate imaging studies of other organ systems should be considered.

A daily pain diary to note the occurrence and intensity of pain and mood should be administered. Medication intake, menses, and aggravating and alleviating factors should be noted in the diary. A simple diary utilizes a visual analogue scale from 1 (no pain) to 10 (most severe pain ever). The diary should be maintained for at least 2 months.

The patient should be evaluated by a psychologist who is familiar with the management of chronic pain. The psychologist should preferably be located within the same clinic suite. Psychological referral accomplishes evaluation, as well as opens the possibility for introducing stress reduction, relaxation, and behavioural therapies. The assessment should be designed to evaluate the pain complaint, its impact on life circumstances, controlling factors, and coping mechanisms.

Pelvic pain is likely to affect sexual functioning, which may have additional repercussions in terms of mood and quality of the relationships and self-esteem. A careful history is needed to establish whether the sexual problems existed before the pain or developed subsequently. Previous or current physical abuse, sexual abuse, or trauma should be evaluated. The impact of the pain on day-to-day functioning should be determined. Standardized psychological testing is helpful to determine whether affective disturbance is present, as well as to establish a baseline against which to measure treatment response and guide treatment approaches.

If specific pathology (Table 10.2) is confirmed, management should proceed. Patients with cyclic or atypical cyclic pain based on evaluation of the pain diary should be evaluated and treated for primary or secondary dysmenorrhoea. Evaluation of pelvic pain, especially cyclic pain, may require a diagnostic laparoscopy. Pelvic ultrasound, MRI, or transuterine venography, if available, may be indicated if pelvic congestion is suspected but treatment can proceed on the basis of clinical suspicion. If trigger points were injected and pain has persisted, injection should be repeated weekly or biweekly up to five injections and consideration should be given to a physical therapy consultation, especially if activity increases the pain or if low back pain is prominent. Pharmacologic management of CPP mirrors that of chronic pain in general. Tricyclic antidepressants and anticonvulsants have been used successfully in pelvic pain patients although controlled studies are lacking. Narcotics administered appropriately and with a narcotic contract are useful in the control of pelvic pain. Depression is treated with selective serotonin reuptake inhibitors. The patient should continue to have scheduled visits with the gynaecologist on a regular basis.

Surgical management of chronic pelvic pain

Only a rare study of the surgical management of CPP is a randomized controlled trial. Postoperative follow-up is often less than 6 months and pain measurement scales are generally not adequate.

Diagnostic laparoscopy

Although exceedingly useful in the diagnosis and management of acute pelvic pain, the role of the laparoscope in the management of chronic pelvic pain has been controversial. Fourteen to 77% of patients have no obvious pathology and two-thirds of patients have findings of adhesions that may or not play a role in their pain (Rapkin 1986, Steege and Scott 1991, Stout et al 1991). Furthermore, non-surgical management of chronic pelvic pain is successful in 65 to 90% of patients regardless of presence of 'pathology' (Rapkin and Kames 1987, Reiter et al 1991, Peters et al 1991). Peters randomized women with chronic pelvic pain to two different management approaches: standard-approach group in which laparoscopy was routinely performed and results guided by findings and an integrated approach group with attention to somatic, psychological, dietary, and physiotherapeutic factors, laparoscopy not routinely performed (Peters et al 1991). Of the 49 patients in the standard group, 65% had no abnormality, 5% had endometriosis, 18% had adhesions, and the remainder had myomata, ovarian cysts, or pelvic varices. The integrated approach was significantly more effective in the reduction of pelvic pain (75% vs 41%; $p < 0.01$) (Peters et al 1991).

Hysterectomy

Nineteen percent of hysterectomies are performed for the sole indication of chronic pelvic pain (Howard 1993). However, 30% of patients presenting to pelvic pain clinics have already undergone hysterectomy without experiencing relief of pain. Patients with cyclic pain or dysfunctional uterine bleeding are excellent candidates for hysterectomy especially if they have relief of pain with hormonal suppression, and hysterectomy remains an option for appropriately selected patients with pain of 'uterine' origin (Hillis et al 1995).

Presacral neurectomy

Presacral neurectomy or sympathectomy (PSN) was first described for the indication of dysmenorrhoea. The presacral nerve, which is actually the superior hypogastric plexus, receives the major afferent supply from the cervix, uterus, and proximal fallopian tubes. Afferents from adnexal structures travel with sympathetic fibres accompanying the spinal cord at T9–T10, and therefore, lateralizing pain of visceral origin will not be relieved by PSN.

PSN has been described for the management of central pelvic pain in the setting of both cyclic (dysmenorrhoea) and non-cyclic pain (Vercellini et al 1991, Candiani et al 1992). PSN can reduce the suprapubic, midline component of menstrual pain (Vercellini et al 1991). The surgery is technically difficult to perform via laparoscopy (Chen and Soong 1997). The laparoscopic transection of the uterosacral ligaments (LUNA), and thus uterine afferents, has been subjected to only one randomized controlled trial (Lichten and Bombard 1987). Eighty-one percent had relief with LUNA but the improvement at the one-year follow-up was only significant in 45% of the 10 subjects. None of the controls improved, however (Lichten and Bombard 1987).

Multidisciplinary pain management

Multidisciplinary pain management is an excellent approach to chronic pelvic pain. The team usually includes a gynaecologist or internist as pain manager, psychologist, and often a physical therapist, anaesthesiologist, and dietitian. Non-steroidal anti-inflammatory medications, narcotics, tricyclic antidepressants, anticonvulsants, and trigger point injections and nerve blocks (i.e., pudendal, ilioinguinal, iliohypogastric, genitofemoral and occasionally hypogastric) are utilized.

One program utilizing cognitive behavioural therapy, acupuncture, and tricyclic antidepressants was successful in reducing pain by at least 50% in 85% of the subjects (Rapkin and Kames 1987, Kames al 1990). Other studies have suggested that similar results may be obtained with a multidisciplinary team (Wood et al 1990, Reiter et al 1991, Peters et al 1991, Milburn et al 1993). In a prospective randomized, controlled study, the multidisciplinary approach combining traditional gynaecologic treatment and psychological, dietary, and physical therapy input was found to be more effective than traditional gynaecologic (medical and surgical) management or cure (Peters et al 1991).

References

Baker PK 1993 Musculoskeletal origins of chronic pelvic pain. In: Ling FW (ed) Obstetrics and gynecology clinics of North America: contemporary management of chronic pain. Saunders, Philadelphia, pp 719–742

Beard RW, Reginald PW, Wadsworth J 1988 Clinical features of women with chronic lower abdominal pain and pelvic congestion. British Journal of Obstetrics and Gynaecology 95: 153–161

Beard RW, Kennedy RG, Gangar KF, Stones RW, Rogers V, Reginald PW, Anderson M 1991 Bilateral oophorectomy and hysterectomy in the treatment of intractable pelvic pain associated with pelvic congestion. British Journal of Obstetrics and Gynaecology 98: 988–992

Bergman A, Karram M, Bhatia NN 1989 Urethral syndrome: a comparison of different treatment modalities. Journal of Reproductive Medicine 34: 157–160

Candiani GB, Fedele L, Vercellini P, Bianchi S, Di Nola G 1992 Presacral neurectomy for the treatment of pelvic pain associated with endometriosis: a controlled study. American Journal of Obstetrics and Gynecology 167: 100–103

Carey MP, Slack MC 1996 GnRH analogue in assessing chronic pelvic pain in women with residual ovaries. British Journal of Obstetrics and Gynaecology 103: 150–153

Cervero F, Tattersall JEH 1986 Somatic and visceral sensory integration in the thoracic spinal cord. In: Cervero F, Morrison J (eds) Visceral sensation. Elsevier, New York, pp 189–205

Chan WY, Dawood MY 1980 Prostaglandin levels in menstrual fluid of non-dysmenorrheic and of dysmenorrheic subjects with and without oral contraceptive or ibuprofen therapy. Advances in Prostaglandin, Thromboxane and Leukotriene Research 8: 1443–1447

Chen F-P, Soong Y-K 1997 The efficacy and complications of laparoscopic presacral neurectomy in pelvic pain. Obstetrics and Gynecology 90: 974–977

D'Hooghe TM, Hill JA 1996 Endometriosis. In: Berek JS, Adashi EY, Hillard PA (eds) Novak's gynecology, 12th edn. Williams & Wilkins, Baltimore pp 887–914

Deligeoroglou E 2000 Dysmenorrhea. Annals of the New York Academy of Science 900: 237–244 (Review)

Farquhar CM, Rogers V, Franks S, Pearce S, Wadsworth J, Bland RW 1989 A randomized controlled trial of medroxyprogesterone acetate and psychotherapy for the treatment of pelvic congestion. British Journal of Obstetrics and Gynaecology 96: 1153–1162

Fukaya T, Hoshiai H, Yajima A 1993 Is pelvic endometriosis always associated with chronic pain? A retrospective study of 618 cases diagnosed by laparoscopy. American Journal of Obstetrics and Gynecology 169: 719–722

Gangar KV, Stones RW, Saunders D, Rogers V, Rae T, Cooper S, Beard RW 1993 An alternative to hysterectomy? GnRH analogue combined with hormone replacement therapy. British Journal of Obstetrics and Gynaecology 100: 360–364

Giamberardino MA, Berkley KJ, Iezzi S, di Bigotina P, Vecchiet L 1995 Changes in skin and muscle sensitivity in dysmenorrheic vs. normal women as a function of body site and monthly cycle. Society of Neuroscience Abstracts 1638

Hahn L 1989 Clinical findings and results of operative treatment in ilioinguinal nerve entrapment syndrome. British Journal of Obstetrics and Gynaecology 96: 1080–1083

Harrop-Griffiths J, Katon W, Walker E, Helm L, Russo J, Hickok C 1988 The association between chronic pelvic pain, psychiatric diagnoses and childhood sexual abuse. Obstetrics and Gynecology 71: 589–594

Hillis SD, Marchbanks PA, Peterson HB 1995 The effectiveness of hysterectomy for chronic pelvic pain. Obstetrics and Gynecology 86: 941–945

Howard FM 1993 The role of laparoscopy in chronic pelvic pain: promise and pitfalls. Obstetrical and Gynecological Survey 48: 357–387

Howard FM, El-Minawi AM, Sanchez RA 2000 Conscious pain mapping by laparoscopy in women with chronic pelvic pain. Obstetrics and Gynecology 96: 934–944

Hughes JM 1990 Psychological aspects of pelvic pain. In: Rocker I (ed) Pelvic pain in women. Diagnosis and management. Springer-Verlag, London, pp 13–20

Kames LD, Rapkin AJ, Naliboff BD, Afifi S, Ferrer-Brechner T 1990 Effectiveness of an interdisciplinary pain management program for the treatment of chronic pelvic pain. Pain 41: 41–46

Karram MM 1993 Frequency, urgency, and painful bladder syndrome. In: Walters MD, Karram MM (eds) Clinical urogynecology. Mosby, St Louis, pp 285–298

Koninckx PR, Meuleman C, Demeyere S, Lesaffre E, Cornillie FJ 1991 Suggestive evidence that pelvic endometriosis is a progressive disease, whereas deeply infiltrating endometriosis is associated with pelvic pain. Fertility and Sterility 55: 759–770

Kream RM, Carr DB 1999 Interstitial cystitis. Pain Forum 8: 139–145

Kresch AJ, Seifer DB, Sachs LB, Barrese I 1984 Laparoscopy in 100 women with chronic pelvic pain. Obstetrics and Gynecology 64: 672–674

Kumazawa T 1986 Sensory innervation of reproductive organs. In: Cervero F, Morrison J (eds) Visceral sensation. Elsevier, New York, pp 115–131

Lichten EM, Bombard J 1987 Surgical treatment of primary dysmenorrhea with laparoscopic uterine nerve ablation. Journal of Reproductive Medicine 32: 37–41

McDonald JS 1993 Management of chronic pain. In: Ling FW (ed) Obstetrics and gynecology clinics of North America: contemporary management of chronic pain. Saunders, Philadelphia, pp 817–839

Magni G, Salmi A, deLeo D, Ceola A 1984 Chronic pelvic pain and depression. Psychopathology 17: 132–136

Malinak LR 1980 Operative management of pelvic pain. Clinical Obstetrics and Gynecology 23: 191–199

Mayer EA, Gebhart GF 1993 Functional bowel disorders and the

visceral hyperalgesia hypothesis. In: Mayer EA, Raybould HE (eds) Pain research and clinical management, vol 9. Elsevier, Amsterdam, pp 3–28
Milburn A, Reiter RC, Rhomberg AT 1993 Multidisciplinary approach to chronic pelvic pain. In: Ling FW (ed) Obstetrics and gynecology clinics of North America: contemporary management of chronic pelvic pain. Saunders, Philadelphia, pp 643–661
Olive DL, Pritts EA 2001 Treatment of endometriosis. New England Journal of Medicine 345: 266–275
Peters AA, Van Dorst E, Jellis B, Van Zuuren E, Hermans J, Trimbos JB 1991 A randomized clinical trial to compare two different approaches in women with chronic pelvic pain. Obstetrics and Gynecology 77: 740–744
Peters AAW, Trimbos-Kemper GCM, Admiraal C, Trimbos JB 1992 A randomized clinical trial on the benefit of adhesiolysis in patients with intraperitoneal adhesions and chronic pelvic pain. British Journal of Obstetrics and Gynaecology 99: 59–62
Prentice A, Deary AJ, Goldbeck-Wood S, Farquhar C, Smith SK 2000 Gonadotrophin-releasing hormone analogues for pain associated with endometriosis (Cochrane Review). The Cochrane Library, issue 4. Update Software, Oxford
Price FV, Edwards R, Buchsbaum HJ 1990 Ovarian remnant syndrome: Difficulties in diagnosis and management. Obstetrical and Gynecological Surgery 45: 151–156
Procacci P, Zoppi M, Maresen M 1986 Clinical approach to visceral sensation. In: Cervero F, Morrison J (eds) Visceral sensation. Elsevier, New York, pp 21–36
Rapkin AJ 1986 Adhesions and pelvic pain: a retrospective study. Obstetrics and Gynecology 68: 13–15
Rapkin AJ 1995 Gynecological pain in the clinic: is there a link with the basic research? In: Gebhart GF (ed) Visceral pain: progress in pain research and management. IASP Press, Seattle, pp 469–488
Rapkin AJ, Kames LD 1987 The pain management approach to chronic pelvic pain. Journal of Reproductive Medicine 32: 323–327
Rapkin AJ, Kames LD, Darke LL 1990 History of physical and sexual abuse in women with chronic pelvic pain. Obstetrics and Gynecology 76: 90–96
Rapkin AJ, Rasgon NL, Berkley KJ 1997 Dysmenorrhea. In: Yaksh TL et al (eds) Anesthesia. Biologic foundations. Lippincott-Raven, Philadelphia, pp 785–793
Reese KA, Reddy S, Rock JA 1996 Endometriosis in an adolescent population: The Emory experience. Journal of Pediatric and Adolescent Gynecology 9: 125–128
Reiter RC 1990 Occult somatic pathology in women with chronic pelvic pain. Clinical Obstetrics and Gynecology 33: 154–160
Reiter RC, Gambone JC, Johnson SR 1991 Availability of a multidisciplinary pelvic pain clinic and frequency of hysterectomy for pelvic pain. Journal of Psychosomatic Obstetrics and Gynaecology 12(suppl): 109
Renaer M 1980 Chronic pelvic pain without obvious pathology in women: Personal observation and a review of the problem. European Journal of Obstetrics and Gynecology 10: 415–463
Ringel Y, Sperber AD, Drossman DA 2001 Irritable bowel syndrome. Annual Review of Medicine 52: 319–338
Sant GR 1998 Interstitial cystitis—a urogynecologic perspective. Contemporary OB/GYN June: 119–130
Sichlau MJ, Yao JST, Vogelzang RL 1994 Transcatheter embolotherapy for the treatment of pelvic congestion syndrome. Obstetrics and Gynecology 83: 892–896
Siddall-Allum J, Rae T, Rogers V, Witherow R, Flanagan A, Beard RW 1994 Chronic pain caused by residual ovaries and ovarian remnants. British Journal of Obstetrics and Gynaecology 101: 979–985
Sippo WC, Burghardt A, Gomez AC 1987 Nerve entrapment after Pfannensteil incision. American Journal of Obstetrics and Gynecology 157: 420–421
Slocumb JC 1984 Neurological factors in chronic pelvic pain: trigger points and the abdominal pelvic pain syndrome. American Journal of Obstetrics and Gynecology 149: 536–543
Slocumb JC 1990 Chronic somatic myofascial and neurogenic abdominal pelvic pain. In: Porreco RP, Reiter RC (eds) Clinical obstetrics and gynecology. Lippincott, Philadelphia, pp 145–153
Spangen L 1984 Spigelian hernia. Surgical Clinics of North America 64: 351–366
Steege JF, Scott AL 1991 Resolution of chronic pelvic pain after laparoscopic lysis of adhesions. American Journal of Obstetrics and Gynecology 165: 278–283
Stones RW, Rae T, Rogers V, Fry R, Beard RW 1990 Pelvic congestion in women: Evaluation with transvaginal ultrasound and observation of venous pharmacology. British Journal of · Radiology 63: 710–711
Stout AL, Steege JF, Dodson WC, Hughes CL 1991 Relationship of laparoscopic findings to self-report of pelvic pain. American Journal of Obstetrics and Gynecology 164: 73–79
Summit RL 1993 Urogynecologic causes of chronic pelvic pain. In: Ling FW (ed) Obstetrics and gynecology clinics of North America: contemporary management of chronic pain. Saunders, Philadelphia, pp 685–698
Thomson H , Francis DMA 1977 Abdominal-wall tenderness: A useful sign in the acute abdomen. Lancet 2: 1053–1055
Toomey TC, Hernandez JT, Gittelman DF, Hulka JF 1993 Relationship of sexual and physical abuse to pain and psychological assessment variables in chronic pelvic pain patients. Pain 53: 105–109
Travell J 1976 Myofascial trigger points: clinical view. Advances in Pain Research and Therapy 1: 919–926
Vercellini P, Fedele L, Bianchi S, Candiani GB 1991 Pelvic denervation for chronic pain associated with endometriosis: fact or fancy? American Journal of Obstetrics and Gynecology 165: 745–749
Walker EA, Gelfand AN, Gelfand MD, Green C, Katon WJ 1996 Chronic pelvic pain and gynecological symptoms in women with irritable bowel syndrome. Journal of Psychosomatic Obstetrics and Gynecology 17: 39–46
Wall PD 1988 The John J. Bonica distinguished lecture. Stability and instability of central pain mechanisms. In: Dubner R (ed) Proceedings of the Fifth World Congress on Pain. Elsevier, Amsterdam, pp 13–24
Wesselmann U, Lai J 1997 Mechanisms of referred visceral pain: uterine inflammation in the adult virgin rat results in neurogenic plasma extravasation in the skin. Pain 73: 209–317
Westrom L, Eschenbach D 1999 Pelvic inflammatory disease. In: Holmes KK et al (eds) Sexually transmitted diseases, third edn. McGraw-Hill, New York, pp 783–809
Wilson M, Farquhar C, Kennedy S, Jin X 2000 Transcutaneous electrical nerve stimulation and acupuncture for primary dysmenorrhoea (Protocol for a Cochrane Review). The Cochrane Library, Issue 4. Update Software, Oxford
Wood DP, Weisner MG, Reiter RC 1990 Psychogenic chronic pelvic pain. Clinical Obstetrics and Gynecology 33: 179–195

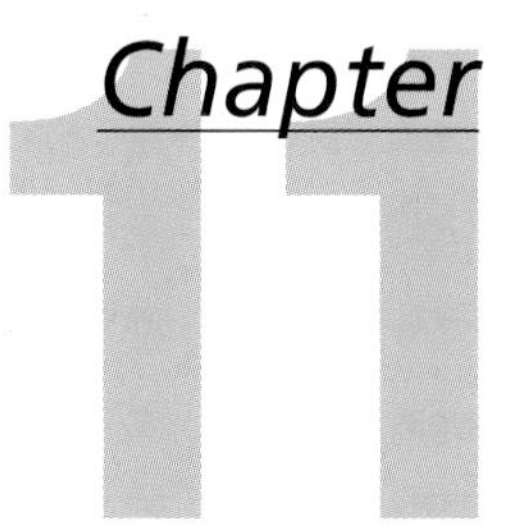

Chapter 11

Obstetric Pain

John S McDonald and Carl R Noback

Introduction

The modern concept of pain management in labour and delivery holds that pain must be relieved effectively because persistent severe pain and its stress generate harmful effects for the mother and, possibly, the fetus. Impressive clinical evidence shows that *properly* administered analgesia reduces maternal and perinatal mortality and morbidity (Shnider and Levinson 1987, Gabbe and Steven 1991, Bonica and McDonald 1995).

Present-day obstetricians have adopted a conservative attitude regarding maternal medication. There is an acute awareness that drugs administered to mothers can have fetal and neonatal depressant effects. Furthermore, mothers are by far more appreciative of a lucid, coherent participation in their childbirth experience (Lamaze and Vellay 1952, Atlee 1956). The obstetric scenario is highly stable and effective, in which patients receive not only antepartum evaluation and consultation, but also careful consideration and management augmented by monitoring during the intrapartum period. A sensitive index of the proficiency of such a system of care is the perinatal mortality rate, which is now at its lowest level in the history of the USA. A systematic study using the McGill Pain Questionnaire found that, prior to administration of analgesic therapy, about 65–68% of primiparas and multiparas rated their labour pain as severe or very severe, and 23% of primiparas and 11% of multiparas rated their pain as 'horrible' (Melzack 1984). Highly developed countries are now cognizant of the benefits of modern analgesia and fully expect effective pain relief throughout labour and delivery.

Mechanisms and pathways of the pain of childbirth

The neural mechanisms of childbirth pain provide foundation to build the logical application of pain relief in labour. The innervation of the reproductive organs can be divided into five general sections: (i) uterus; (ii) lower uterine segment; (iii) cervix; (iv) vagina, and (v) perineum.

The uterus and lower uterine segments are innervated by afferents with cell bodies in the dorsal root ganglia of the T10, T11, T12 and L1 segments. Afferent pathways course alongside the sympathetic nerves that make up the pelvic plexus and cervical plexus. These afferents from the four segments move through the three hypogastric pelvic plexi (inferior, medial, and superior), and finally pass through the posterior roots to make synaptic contact with interneurons in the dorsal horn (Fig. 11.1). Typical of pain arising from the viscera, the pain caused by uterine contractions is referred to the dermatomes supplied by the same spinal cord segments that receive input from the uterus and cervix. The cervix is also innervated by the T10–T12 pathways (Bonica 1969).

Innervation of the perineum, however, is via the sacral nerve roots with input transmitted directly to the spinal dorsal horn via the pudendal nerves.

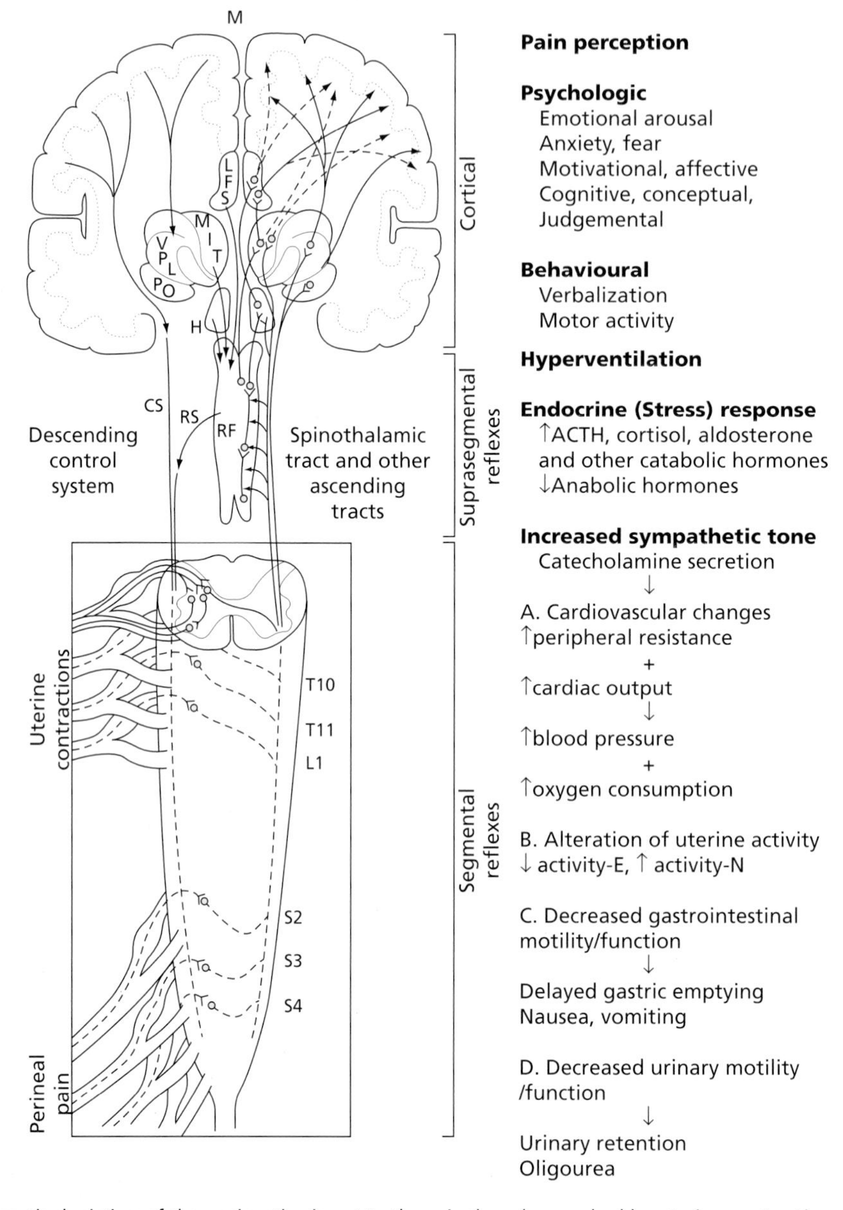

Fig. 11.1 Schematic depiction of the nociceptive input to the spinal cord, provoked by uterine contractions throughout labour and stimulation of the perineum during the second and third stages of labour. The spinothalamic tract and other ascending tracts in the neuraxis are primarily involved in central transmission of nociceptive information to the anterior and anterolateral horn cells of the spinal cord, which provoke segmental reflex responses and impulses that reach the brainstem, provoking the suprasegmental responses listed on the right. The nociceptive impulses that reach the brain provoke the cortical responses that include perception of pain, initiation of psychological mechanisms and behavioural responses. On the left is a simple schematic illustration of descending pathways that convey modulating influence from the brain to the spinal cord. RF = reticular formation; RS = reticulospinal; CS = corticospinal; H = hypothalamus; PO = posterior thalamus; VPL = ventral posterolateral thalamus; MIT = medial and intralaminar thalamic nuclei; LFS = limbic forebrain structures. (Modified from Bonica 1990.)

There are some mixed areas of overlap in the vagina with over 70% of the afferents from the uterine–cervical area linking up with the inferior hypogastric plexus of nerves on each side of the cervix, while the remainder of the afferents from the vagina and lower genital tract link up to the pudendal nerve. Innervation of the uterine horns is also separate, via the sympathetic nerves (Kawatani and de Groat 1991). The fibre types of the reproductive tract are consistent with other visceral organ innervation: small myelinated and unmyelinated fibres.

The vagina and the perineum are therefore innervated by the same neural pathways as the second and third stages of labour, involving the pudendal nerve and other smaller nerves derived from S2, S3, and S4. The peculiar pain caused by pressure on the intrapelvic structures, and which is felt in the thigh and upper legs, usually involves fibres as high as L2 and as low as S3.

Labour pain

The first stage of labour pain is caused by uterine contractions and stretching of the cervix. This continues throughout the first stage until complete dilatation is achieved.

When complete dilatation of the cervix occurs, uterine contractions persist even against impressive forces of resistance. The pain that develops in this second stage emanates from continued distension of the entire vaginal canal as the fetus descends towards the vaginal outlet. During the second stage, there is descent of the fetus until the fetal head begins to negotiate the mid-pelvis at the anatomical level of the ischial spines. The eventual passage of the fetal head through the mid-pelvis results in distension and stretching of the tissues of the mid and lower vagina, distension of the outlet, and eventual dilatation to make way for the passage of the largest portion of the fetus—the head. These anatomical changes are accomplished with maximum stimulation via the nociceptive pathways of the pudendal nerves to the dorsal root ganglia of the at the S2–S4 levels. There is also a significant sensory spillover to other adjacent pathways via the lower sacrum, perianal, and even upper thigh regions. Similar to the pain caused by stimulation of superficial somatic structures, the perineal pain is sharp and well localized. This pain can be eliminated by blockade of the sensory nerves (Klink 1953, Bonica 1967).

As complete dilatation occurs, the pain may be intense and pushing against the strong tension of the perineal muscles may be difficult until analgesia is accomplished with an epidural block that includes the sacral nerves or a caudal injection. In the late part of the first stage of labour and during the second stage, a number of parturients develop aching, burning, or cramping discomfort in the thigh and, less frequently, the legs. This can be the result of the stimulation of pain-sensitive structures in the pelvic cavity including traction on the pelvic peritoneum; stretching of and tension on the bladder, urethra, and rectum; stretching and tension of the ligaments, fascia, and muscles of the pelvic cavity; and abnormal pressure on roots of the lumbosacral plexus. As noted above, the neural pathways for the second and third stages of labour involve the pudendal nerve and other smaller branches, which are derived from S2, S3, and S4.

Physiological and psychological effects of labour pain

Changes in ventilation

The pain experienced at the time of labour and delivery serves as a powerful respiratory stimulus. This results in a marked increase in tidal volume and minute ventilation, and an increase in alveolar ventilation. This physiological change causes a reduction of $PaCO_2$ from the pregnancy level of 32 mmHg to a value of as low as 16–20 mmHg, or occasionally even as low as 10–15 mmHg. This causes an increase in pH to 7.5–7.6 (Bonica 1973, Huch et al 1977, Peabody 1979). This respiratory alkalosis, which occurs at the peak of each uterine contraction, results in decreases in cerebral and uterine blood flow and a shift to the left of the maternal oxygen dissociation curve. With the onset of the relaxation phase, pain no longer stimulates respiration so that the hypocapnia causes a transient period of hypoventilation that decreases the maternal $PaCO_2$ by 10–50% with a mean of 25–30% (Huch et al 1977, Peabody 1979). Mothers who have received an opioid for pain relief have the depressant effect of the respiratory alkalosis then enhanced by the action of the opioids. When the maternal $PaCO_2$ falls below 70 mmHg, it has a significant effect on the fetus, namely a decrease in fetal $PaCO_2$ with late decelerations (Myers 1975).

Neuroendocrine effects

Some of the previously described changes, such as reduced carbon dioxide levels, coupled with the increases in catecholamine levels (20–40%) caused by noxious stimulation, produce a net reduction in uterine blood flow in the animal model (Jouppila 1977, Morishima et al 1978, Shnider and Levinson 1987, Berkley and Wood 1989).

Levels of noradrenaline (NA) are primarily increased, with reductions of uterine blood flow of 35–70%. In human studies, data have shown that severe pain and anxiety during active labour can cause a 300–600% increase in the adrenaline (epinephrine) (A) level, a 200–400% increase in the noradrenaline (norepinephrine) (NA) level, a 200–300% increase in the cortisol level, and significant increases in corticosteroid and ACTH levels. These all reach peak values at or just after delivery (Lederman et al 1977, 1978; Ohno et al 1986). Lederman's work showed adrenaline (epinephrine) level increases of nearly 300%, NA levels of 150%, and the cortisol levels of 200%. Of great interest was the fact that increased A and cortisol levels correlated with anxiety and pain. More recent research in a comprehensive study of catecholamines and cyclic nucleotides during labour and following delivery noted a nearly twofold increase in the dopamine levels, a threefold increase in the A level, and a twofold increase in the NA level, as well as a small increase in the cyclic adenosine monophosphate (cAMP) level. A positive correlation between the A level and heart rate and systolic blood pressure, along with a correlation between NA and cAMP levels, during labour was also noted (Ohno et al 1986).

Cardiovascular changes

In labour, cardiac output increases further above prelabour levels. The percentage increase in cardiac output was higher when the parturient was in the supine position than when she was in the lateral position. With the parturient in the supine position, between contractions, cardiac output during the early first stage was about 15% above that of prelabour, during the late first stage it was increased about 30%, during the second stage the increase was about 45%, and immediately after delivery cardiac output was 65–80% greater than prelabour (Hendricks and Quilligan 1956, Adams and Alexander 1958, Hansen and Ueland 1966). During painful uterine contractions, there was even a further increase of 15–20% in cardiac output.

It is believed that nearly 50% of the increase during contractions is caused by the extrusion of 250–300 ml of blood from the uterus and by increased venous return from the pelvis and lower limbs into the maternal circulation. The remainder is caused by an increase in sympathetic activity provoked by pain, anxiety, apprehension, and the physical effort of labour, which contribute to the progressive rise in cardiac output as labour advances. Uterine contractions in the absence of analgesia also cause increases of 20–30 mmHg in the systolic and diastolic blood pressures. The increase in cardiac output and systolic blood pressure leads to a significant increase in left ventricular work. This is tolerated by healthy parturients, but it can prove deleterious if the parturients have heart disease, pre-eclampsia, essential hypertension, or pulmonary hypertension (Hendricks and Quilligan 1956, Hansen and Ueland 1966, Robson et al 1987).

Metabolic effects

It would be expected during pregnancy that the basal metabolic rate and oxygen consumption progressively increase, and at term, their values rise to an imposing 20% above normal (Bonica 1967, 1969, 1980, Bonica and McDonald 1995). During parturition, the metabolism and oxygen consumption increase further (Bonica and McDonald 1990). It is believed that in labour, free fatty acids and lactate levels increase significantly as a result of pain-induced catecholamine release and the resultant sympathetic-induced lipolytic metabolism (Bonica and McDonald 1990). This is based on the fact that, with complete blockade of nociceptive afferent and efferent pathways with epidural analgesia, only small increases in maternal free fatty acid, lactate levels, and acidosis are observed (Marx and Greene 1964). With poor analgesia during the second stage of labour, maternal acidosis can occur. This is caused by maternal pain and physical exertion inherent in the repetitive active bearing-down efforts. The increased sympathetic nervous system activity caused by labour pain and anxiety also increases metabolic rate and oxygen consumption, as mentioned above. The increased oxygen consumption inherent in the work of labour, along with the loss of bicarbonate from the kidney as compensation for the pain-induced respiratory alkalosis, produces a progressive maternal metabolic acidosis that is transferred to the fetus (Marx and Greene 1964, Buchan 1980, Bonica and McDonald 1990). The maternal pyruvate level increases, alongside a greater increase in the lactate level; soon a progressive accumulation of excess lactate occurs, which is reflected by a progressive offset increase in base excess (Marx and Greene 1964, Buchan 1980, Bonica and McDonald 1990).

Gastrointestinal and urinary function

The pain of labour and the consequent increase in sympathetic activity also affect the function of the gastrointestinal and urinary tracts. Pain during labour stimulates gastrin release and results in increased gastric acid secretion (Marx and Greene 1964). Additionally, pain, anxiety, and emotional stress create segmental and suprasegmental reflex inhibition of gastrointestinal and urinary motility with delays in gastric and urinary bladder function. Such reflex effects of nociception are aggravated by recumbent positions, opioids, and depressant medications (Marx and Greene 1964; Pearson and Davies 1973, 1974; Buchan 1980). The combined effects of pain and depressant drugs can thus cause food and fluids other than water to be retained for as long as 36 h or more. During this period, swallowed air and gastric juices accumulate progressively, with gradual gastric pH decline below the critical value of 2.5. Therefore, delayed gastric emptying of the acidic gastric contents increases the risk of regurgitation and pulmonary aspiration, especially during the induction of general anaesthesia. This hazard has long been, and still today remains, one of the most common causes of maternal mortality and morbidity due to general anaesthesia (Hayes et al 1972).

Effects on uterine activity and labour

The same increased secretion of catecholamines and cortisol caused by pain and emotional stress can either increase or decrease uterine contractility, which, of course, influences the duration of labour. Noradrenaline (norepinephrine) increases uterine activity, whereas it is decreased by adrenaline and cortisol (Nimmo et al 1975). An early animal study revealed nociceptive stimulation increased uterine activity by about 60% that was associated with a decrease in fetal oxygen tension and fetal heart rate characterized by ominous signs of late decelerations (Holdsworth 1978). Lederman and associates (Lederman et al 1977, 1978) noted that in some parturients severe pain and anxiety caused such an increase in adrenaline (epinephrine) and cortisol levels that uterine activity was decreased and labour was prolonged. In a small percentage of parturients, pain and anxiety even produced 'incoordinate uterine contractions' manifested by a decrease in intensity and an increase in frequency and uterine tone with ineffectual labour patterns (Moir and Willocks 1967, Holdsworth 1978, Tomkinson et al 1982).

Psychological effects

There is no question that psychological factors do affect the incidence and intensity of parturition pain and impact the mental attitude and mood of the patient during labour. Fear, apprehension, and anxiety further enhance pain perception and pain behaviour (Moir and Willocks 1967, Bonica and Hunter 1969, Brown et al 1972, Morishima et al 1980, Tomkinson et al 1982). Ignorance or misinformation is the classic generator of fear and anxiety for the parturient. An uninformed patient, especially a primipara, can be disturbed by fear of the unknown, suffering, complications, and even the possibility of death. In addition, she may also be concerned that her fetus may be damaged (Myers 1975, Tomkinson et al 1982, Reading and Cox 1985). Studies have demonstrated patients who have an unplanned or illegitimate pregnancy or have an ambivalent or negative reaction to gestation report more pain during labour and delivery (Reading and Cox 1985).

The relationship between the parturient and her spouse or partner also plays an important role in the degree of pain she experiences. Melzack reported in 1984 that the effective pain scores were higher when the husband was in the labour room than when he was absent. He suggested that this may reflect genuinely higher effective pain scores or may be due to a deliberate choice of descriptors in the attempt to impress the husband or express anger at him, but in any case, the finding was not spurious. Wallach found a similar effect in an independent study in 1982. By contrast, Nettelbladt et al (1976), Norr et al (1977), and Fridh et al (1988) found that positive feelings of the expectant father towards the pregnancy seemed to be an important factor in decreasing the mother's feelings of apprehension during pregnancy. When expectant fathers were very supportive of their mates during pregnancy and labour, the women experienced less pain during parturition.

Other emotional factors, such as intensive motivation and cultural influences, can affect modulation of sensory transmissions and certainly can influence the effective and behavioural dimensions of pain. Cognitive intervention, such as giving the parturient preparatory information about labour, reduces uncertainty, while producing distraction and dissociation from pain reduces pain behaviour. In a study of 134 low-risk parturients at term, Lowe (1989) found that confidence in ability to handle labour was the most significant predictor of all components of pain during active labour. The greater the confidence the parturient had, the less the pain she experienced and vice versa.

Severe labour pain can produce serious long-term emotional disturbances that might impair the parturient's mental health, negatively influence her relationship with her baby during the first few crucial days, and cause a fear of future pregnancies that could affect her sexual relationship with her husband (Marx and Greene 1964). Melzack et al (1981), Gaston-Johansson et al (1988), and Stewart (1982) all reported that a significant number of women who had participated in natural childbirth developed or had aggravation of prelabour depression, or had other deleterious emotional reactions in the postpartum period, consequent to the pain experienced during their childbirth without analgesia. Melzack also noted that some women experienced an added burden of guilt, anger, and failure when they anticipated 'a natural painless childbirth', but had to convert to the use of analgesia when confronted with severe pain. Stewart reported that such patients became miserable, depressed, and even suicidal and lost interest in sex. In some cases, the husbands of women who anticipated 'natural' childbirth had to undergo psychotherapy for serious reactions after seeing their wives experience such severe pain as they themselves developed feelings of guilt and subsequent impotence and phobias.

Current methods to relieve childbirth pain

In centres where anaesthesia coverage is available, regional analgesia is preferred by far to any other technique offered today. In the past there were questions about what was the safest technique for pain relief for the first stage of labour. Regional analgesia by lumbar epidural (LE) method has been heavily scrutinized. The LE method has withstood the test of time and is clearly the favourite of the mother, the nurse, the anaesthetist, and even the obstetrician. Unfortunately, there is not one standard of anaesthesia available in all countries; therefore alternative forms of labour analgesia will be briefly covered. This chapter will emphasize regional anaesthetic techniques. Currently, many drugs and techniques are available to provide for the relief of childbirth pain. All of these can be arbitrarily classified into four categories: psychological analgesia, simple methods of pharmacological analgesia, inhalation analgesia/anaesthesia, and regional analgesia/anaesthesia.

During the past two decades, there have been significant changes in the methods used for the relief of pain of childbirth. This is suggested by four major surveys of the practice of obstetric analgesia/anaesthesia carried out in the USA during the past three decades, and two surveys that included current practice in the UK, Scandinavian countries, and a number of other countries throughout the world (Marx and Green 1964, Bonica and McDonald 1995). These surveys indicate that in major hospitals where obstetric services are well organized and an obstetric anaesthesia service is available, there has been a trend of increasing use of continuous lumbar epidural block with a dilute solution of local anaesthetics and opioids and a decrease in the use of regional analgesia and inhalation analgesia.

In the USA, about 20–30% of parturients select psychological analgesia, but eventually two-thirds of them receive lumbar epidural or other forms of regional analgesia. There has also been a general trend not to use inhalation anaesthesia for labour and vaginal delivery. However, in the UK and in Scandinavian countries, inhalation analgesia is still being used, alone or together with the systemic opioids, in 20–50% of parturients. In the UK, nevertheless, there has been a steady increase in the use of continuous lumbar epidural blocks as opposed to the use of inhalation analgesia for the first stage of labour.

In developing countries there are, as anticipated, still many problems because of the limited availability of regional anaesthesia experts and because of deficient equipment and support systems. Most parturients receive either no analgesia or simple methods of inhalation and local anaesthesia (Marx and Green 1964, Bonica and McDonald 1995). On the basis of these data, psychological analgesia and simple techniques of inhalation and regional anaesthesia are briefly commented upon below, and adequate emphasis is given to the use of continuous lumbar epidural analgesia/anaesthesia (Brownridge 1991).

Psychological analgesia

Natural childbirth

Dick-Read (1953) popularized natural childbirth at a time when little else could be offered for pain relief, and for that contribution he should be appreciated. His original emphasis was centred upon the mother entirely. It was paramount she be in excellent physical condition so that she could endure the challenge of labour. Therefore, conditioning became very important in the early phases of the development of the technique and later on the psychological aspects were added, but this was not a sole emphasis made by Dick-Read himself, who did stress the need for patient control over the process of labour. This method was enhanced greatly by the cooperation of a friendly and helpful nurse who would act as a coach and facilitator for the patient during stressful times.

Psychoprophylactic method

The method was popularized by Lamaze (1956) of France, who successfully introduced it to the USA around the same time that regional anaesthesia was being reintroduced. At this time, various exercises in ventilation were added, and it was understood that control of this aspect of breathing could have a salutary effect on the pain experience. This occurred in the mid 1970s, when there were still not many physicians involved in obstetric anaesthesia. All of these methods demanded the close communication and coordination of the teachers, the nurses, the patient, and the obstetrician. The health care team helped to foster confidence and optimism in the parturient, which was very important in developing a pleasing, fulfilling experience at childbirth.

Hypnotic method

The hypnotic method demands complete cooperation between the obstetric patient and the obstetrician. Often the obstetrician may act as the teacher for the hypnosis sessions. The relationship between the patient and her obstetrician is usually strong and positive, which of course makes learning hypnosis from the physician quite effective. Continued enthusiasm for this method demands time, concentration, dedication to learning a new technique and a belief in the patient's own inner self and strength (see Chap. 37).

Simple techniques of pharmacological analgesia

Systemic analgesics (see Chaps 1, 24, and 25)

Narcotics, or more correct opioids, are the primary agents used for pain relief in labour not managed by regional analgesic methods. These agents are simple to use with intramuscular delivery by a labour nurse who really serves as the primary health care person responsible for decision-making in regard to comfort of the patient. Thus the nurse would establish contact with the patient during regular rounds and contact the patient's physician only when necessary. Often an initial order was given for meperidine (Demerol) after good active labour was established. Additional narcotic drugs, such as morphine, alphaprodine, nalbuphine, and fentanyl, were used. Although these narcotics were initially used via the intramuscular route in earlier years, they are now given in small intravenous doses to decrease the total amount needed for labour pain and thus decrease the amount available for effect upon the fetus.

Morphine was perhaps the oldest and the most long-standing opioid of choice for many obstetricians for many years. When combined with scopolamine to provide twilight sleep, it had a dramatic analgesic effect. This effect was impressive, but so was the depressant effect upon the mother and the neonate. In an attempt to decrease the depressant effect, intravenous boluses of small amounts of morphine were tried. When administered just before uterine contractions, there may have been some fetal protective effect (Gerdin et al 1990).

Nalbuphine or nubain is both an agonist- and antagonist-type opioid. Its respiratory depressant effect is similar to morphine. The advantage of nalbuphine is that its depressant characteristic has a ceiling effect. In other words, a dosage that gives maximum depression can be increased without further evidence of increased depression upon the neonate. This opioid is 80% as potent as morphine. The onset of 2–3 min after intravenous injection was appealing for the management of labour pain.

Fentanyl is a highly lipid soluble synthetic opioid that is 100 times more potent than morphine. It was used primarily for its quick analgesic effect, but its other advantage was that it did produce active metabolites that could act as respiratory depressants. Small doses of 50 μg IV were used with success in the first stage of labour, but there was little if any advantage noted over morphine and the latter had a much longer analgesic effect. Because of its high lipid solubility, it also crossed the placenta and appeared rapidly in the fetal circulation (Rosaeg et al 1992).

Once the first stage of labour is managed, it is time to consider a good second-stage technique that will be reliable and offer full pain relief. With the onset of the moderate pain of the second stage, opioids are required. Narcotics produce adequate relief of moderate pain in 70–80% and relief of severe pain in about 35–60% of parturients (Bonica 1967, 1969). Small doses do not produce significant maternal respiratory depression, but can produce some neonatal depression. For delivery, inhalation analgesia with nitrous oxide can be used with intermittent or continuous administration via a mask connected to an anaesthesia machine. This technique can be useful right at delivery, with the crowning of the fetal head causing maximum dilatation of the perineum (Marx and Katsnelson 1992). An alternative analgesic technique is bilateral pudendal nerve block or infiltration of the perineum for similar pain relief during the delivery of the fetus.

Labour pain is not well appreciated still in many parts of the world and is a major problem today in regard to pain control. There is such a wide variance in care given from modern centres with 90% benefiting from regional analgesic methods to third world countries where no pain relief exists whatsoever. In modern centres, there are even classes to allay the patient's fears and reassure them that they will be cared for with the utmost consideration for their comfort and the baby's safety. Discussions like this emphasize the importance of the nurse who helps both the obstetrician and the anaesthetist by offering support to the patient in a time of need.

Inhalational analgesia/anaesthesia

The next logical step up from systemic analgesia is inhalation analgesia. Today it is still a popular method of relieving labour pain because it rapidly produces moderately effective pain relief at a time when it is sorely needed without causing loss of consciousness or significant maternal/neonatal depression. Commonly agents such as these are 40–50% nitrous oxide in oxygen, or sevoflurane or desflurane in oxygen can be used (Swart et al 1991). Nitrous oxide can be administered intermittently during uterine contractions by the assistant to the anaesthetist or the anaesthetist (Carstoniu et al 1994). Premixed cylinders of 50% nitrous oxide and 50% oxygen are used in some parts of the world just for this purpose, but most of the time it is administered by an anaesthetic machine in the operating room or delivery room setting for safety purposes. Safety and optimal analgesia principles dictate that the inhalation of the drug should be given administered by someone in the specialty of anaesthesia. Inhalation should be given some 10–15 s before the painful period of each contraction. Properly used, inhalational analgesia produces good analgesia in one-third and partial relief in another one-third of parturients (Norman et al 1992).

Inhalational anaesthesia for very brief time periods and for actual delivery is still employed, because it can be rapidly induced and affords maximum control of depth and duration of action and is rapidly eliminated at the end of the procedure. On the other hand, general anaesthesia is very dangerous and carries the risk of maternal mortality caused by difficult endotracheal intubation with consequent asphyxia (Glassenberg 1991). This and regurgitation and pulmonary aspiration are the two leading causes of anaesthesia-related maternal mortality in Britain and the USA. For this reason, general anaesthesia should be avoided but, if necessary, should be given only by a properly trained anaesthetist who has secured the airway by endotracheal intubation prior to the induction of anaesthesia. This is a controversial issue at present as there is not enough experience with the use of the laryngeal mask airway in obstetrics to make claims for the safety of the mother. Furthermore, this is one of the most difficult areas of obstetric anaesthesia. Until more experience is gained with this technique, it should be reserved for those expert in its application and then only under special indications.

Regional analgesia/anaesthesia

The popularity and use of regional analgesia in the form of epidurals for labour and delivery has increased incredibly since the 1970s. Regional analgesia offers excellent pain relief without any central nervous system depression. In other words, the mother can enjoy the beauty of the experience of her lifetime in complete control and with all her faculties intact. With the current methods of delivery and selection of local anaesthetics, there are few if any complications for either the mother or the fetus, and there is little if any deleterious effect upon the pattern or length of labour. By selecting regional techniques, the use of depressant medications during labour that adversely affect the mother and baby, along with the use of general anaesthesia for operative delivery with the complications of aspiration, is avoided.

Maternal hypotension is reduced by infusing fluids before inducing spinal, epidural, or caudal block to compensate for the increased vascular capacitance experienced after sympathetic block; the parturient is also placed in the lateral decubitus position during labour to avoid the aortocaval compression inherent in the supine position. Systemic toxic reactions may be prevented by avoiding excessive doses or accidental intravenous injection of therapeutic doses and by the administration of local anaesthetic doses in small quantities with repeated injections over several small intervals of time. In addition, the use of small quantities of adrenaline (epinephrine) was found to reduce the maternal and fetal exposure to the local anaesthetic agent used for the epidural (McLintic et al 1991). Sometimes this complication can be picked up by use of the test dose and careful monitoring of the maternal heart rate from injection until a 3-min period. The adrenaline in the test dose will cause an acute increase in the heart rate for a transient period of time.

Very high or total spinal anaesthesia may result from accidental subarachnoid injection of a local anaesthetic dose intended for extradural block. Because the dosage of local anaesthetic is huge compared to what would be administered in the subarachnoid space, the effect upon the sympathetic system responsible for the maintenance of tone in the capacitance vessels is profound, and results in a progressive reduction in blood pressure with eventual shock if not diagnosed and treated in a timely fashion.

The latter two complications can be virtually obviated by attempting to aspirate blood or cerebrospinal fluid and injecting a test dose of 2–3 ml of solution containing 5–7.5 mg bupivacaine and 15 mg adrenaline. If the injection is accidentally subarachnoid, the parturient will develop a low (T10–S5) spinal anaesthesia. As mentioned above, if the injection is intravenous the adrenaline (epinephrine) will produce moderate tachycardia and hypertension within 20–30 s of the injection and this will last for 30–60 s (Moore and Batra 1981). Only when neither occurs should large therapeutic doses be injected.

Paracervical and pudendal block

Techniques of paracervical block combined with pudendal block (Fig. 11.2) offer excellent first- and second-stage analgesia if performed by an expert who is skilled in the anatomy of those specific nerve areas. The paracervical block is used in some centres now in dilute local anaesthetic concentrations only. However, in many places, this excellent regional block has been abandoned because of the problems of bradycardia in the fetus after administration of the drug to the mother. Bilateral pudendal block may still be used by obstetricians in those institutions where obstetric anaesthesia services are unavailable.

Epidural analgesia

Over the past several decades epidural analgesia for labour and vaginal delivery and for caesarean section has become increasingly popularized. The technique has undergone a number of modifications since the 1960s. Initially, the method entailed

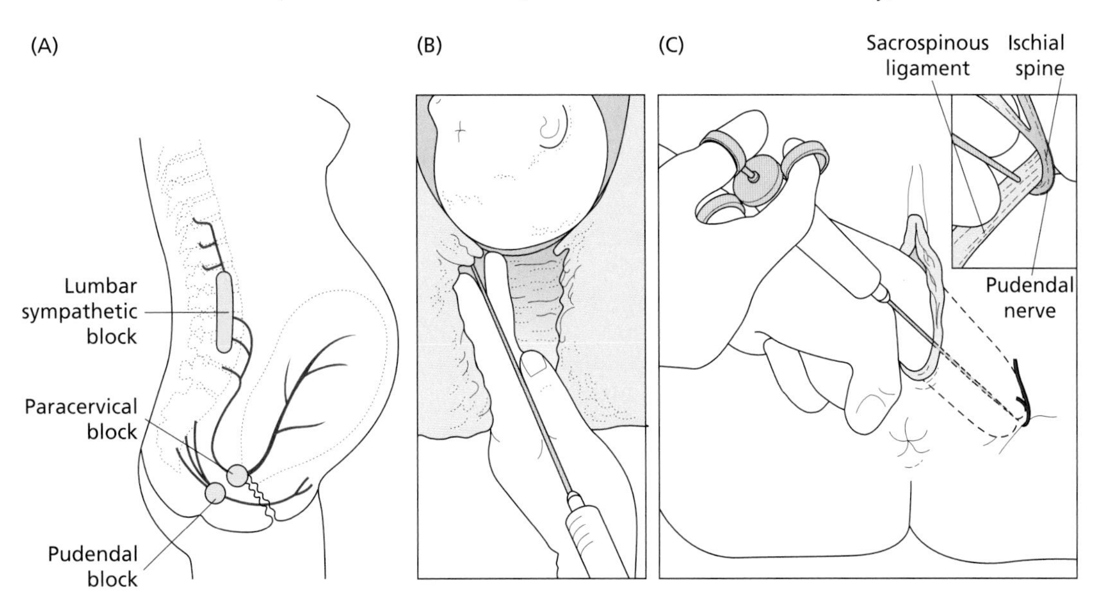

Fig. 11.2 (A) Sites of three regional techniques for obstetric analgesia. Lumbar sympathetic block is rarely used but is highly effective in relieving pain of the first stage and may be preferable to paracervical block, especially in high-risk pregnancies. (B) Schematic coronal section of vagina and lower part of the uterus containing the fetal head, showing the techniques of paracervical block. The 22-gauge needle is within a guide, with its point protruding only 5–7 mm beyond the end of the guide. This prevents insertion of the needle more than 5–7 mm beyond the surface of the mucosa. After negative aspiration, an injection of 8–10 ml of 0.25% bupivacaine at 4 and 8 o'clock of the cervical fornix will produce relief of uterine pain for several hours. (C) Transvaginal technique of blocking the pudendal nerve. The two fingers of the left hand are inserted into the vagina to guide the needle point into the sacrospinous ligament. As long as the bevel of the needle is in the ligament, there is some resistance to the injection of local anaesthetic, but as soon as the bevel passes through the ligament, there is sudden lack of resistance, indicating that the needle point is next to the nerve. (Modified from Bonica 1967.)

the intermittent injection of 12–15 ml of 1–1.5% lidocaine (lignocaine) or equianaesthetic concentrations of another local anaesthetic that usually produced analgesia from T9–T10 to S5 (Fig. 11.3A). While usually effective in providing pain relief throughout labour and delivery, the use of such a relatively high dose of local anaesthetic increased the risk of systemic toxic reactions from accidental intravenous injection or total spinal anaesthesia from accidental subarachnoid injection. In many parturients each injection of local anaesthetic produced a transitory decrease in uterine activity and weakness or even paralysis of the lower limbs and perineal muscles. With loss of control of the lower limbs, this caused discomfort and inconvenience to the patient. Perineal muscle weakness or paralysis diminished resistant forces essential for internal rotation of the presenting part. Sacral anaesthesia also eliminated the afferent limb of the reflex urge to bear down. All of these effects combined to result in prolongation of the second stage and often the need for instrumental delivery (Bonica 1967, 1969, 1980; Bonica and McDonald 1995).

These and other concerns led to a series of modifications (Bonica and McDonald 1995). The first was limiting analgesia to T10–T11 during the first stage and then extended to the sacral segments (Fig. 11.3B). Continuous epidural block provides an excellent form of obstetric analgesia and anaesthesia (Eddleston et al 1992). The advantage of this technique is that less medication is required than with other epidural block techniques mentioned above. It causes no premature numbness or weakness of the lower limbs and no premature weakness of the perineal muscles. Consequently, there is no interference with flexion or internal rotation. Continuous epidural, or its discontinuous counterpart, patient-controlled epidural infusion, is now used routinely for parturients who request epidural analgesia. In the 1980s, at obstetric centres where the anaesthetists have had extensive experience with caudal blocks as well as lumbar epidural blocks, the double catheter technique was also used in some of the parturients who required analgesia (Bonica and McDonald 1995). The norm is now to add opioids (usually fentanyl) to the infusion to enhance the analgesic efficacy of the local anaesthetics and to use infusion pumps that permit more precise administration of the analgesic solution. In many institutions where anaesthetists provide an obstetric anaesthesia service, it has replaced all other regional techniques for labour and vaginal delivery because it has been shown to:

1. Produce more stable levels of analgesia.
2. Lead to a smaller incidence of maternal hypotension.
3. Decrease the risk of systemic toxic reaction or accidental total spinal anaesthesia.
4. Decrease and, in some instances, eliminate the incidence of unintended motor block, thus obviating the problems mentioned above (Bonica and McDonald 1995).

In the early 1970s, the use of modified techniques to try to decrease the amount of drug the fetus would be exposed to came into vogue. Early attempts included the use of smaller volumes of 8–10 ml of local anaesthetic to get only a T10–T12 block for early labour and to increase it slightly to a T10 to L2 block for later labour. This method worked nicely and started the trend in the use of various dosages and agents which has continued. Today the patient gets a very small injection of 8–10 ml of 0.25% bupivacaine followed by a continuous dosage throughout the rest of her labour. The continuous infusion dosage includes a dilute local anaesthetic (0.0625% bupivacaine and adrenaline (epinephrine)), and a dilute concentration of fentanyl or sufentanil (Bonica and McDonald 1995). The combination is delivered via a pump throughout labour until the patient is ready for delivery. More detailed accounts of the lumbar epidural for obstetrics are presented by Bonica (1969), Shnider and Levinson (1987), Gaylard (1990), Candido and Winnie (1992), and Zarzur and Gonzalves (1992).

The caudal epidural block was popularized before lumbar epidural block as a method of pain relief for labour. The caudal block, while being ideal for second-stage analgesia, is not perfectly suited for first-stage pain relief because a generous amount of local anaesthetic must be used to obtain analgesia at the T10 level from where the catheter tip resides at S4 or S2. In some instances as much as a 20- to 25-ml volume has been used to effect first-stage pain relief. Of course, all the intermediary segments are also blocked so that the patient necessarily has a complete sympathetic block with all the attendant complications thereof. Nevertheless, it is mentioned because it is such an effective method of pain relief for labour and was the mainstay for so many years earlier in the history of obstetric anaesthesia. More detailed information on performing caudal analgesia can be found in numerous texts (Bonica 1973, Shnider and Levinson 1987).

Technique of continuous epidural infusion (Fig. 11.4)

A detailed description of the technique of achieving lumbar epidural analgesia is beyond the scope of

(A)
Standard spinal epidural block

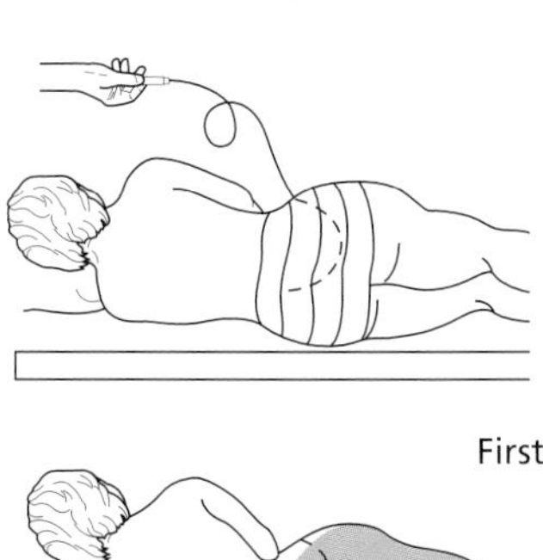
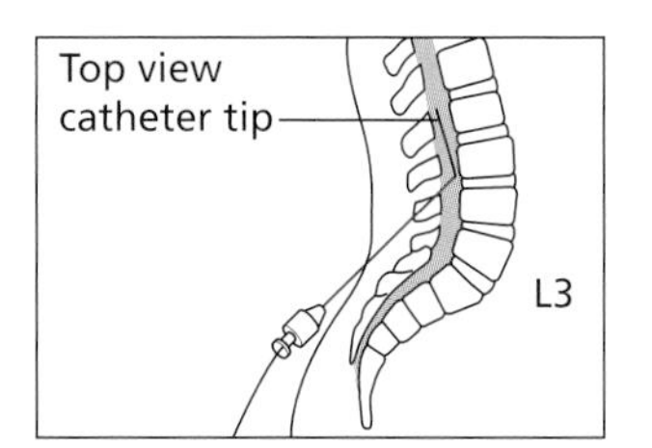

First stage

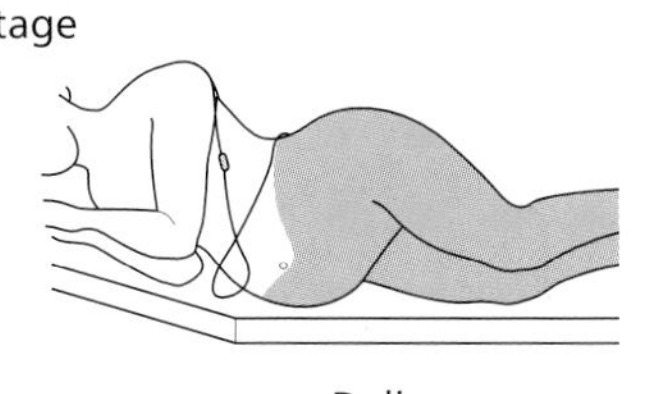

Early second stage

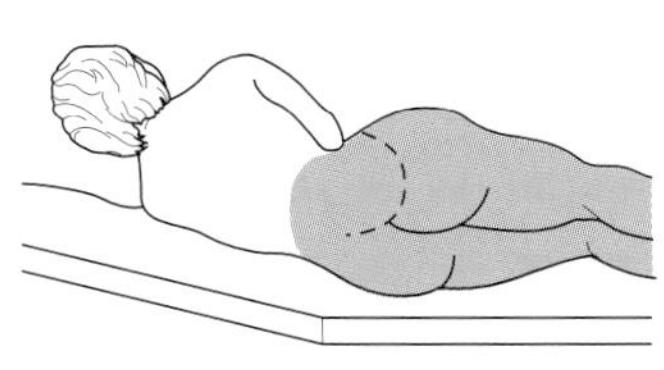

Delivery

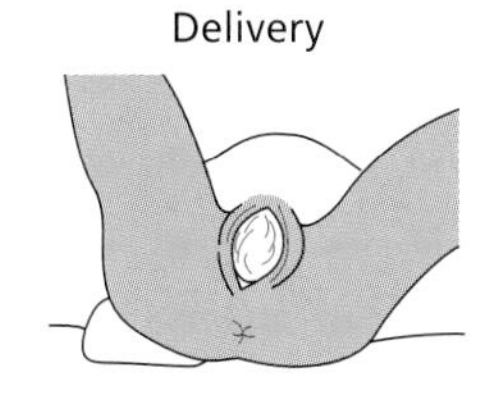

(B)
Segmental spinal epidural block

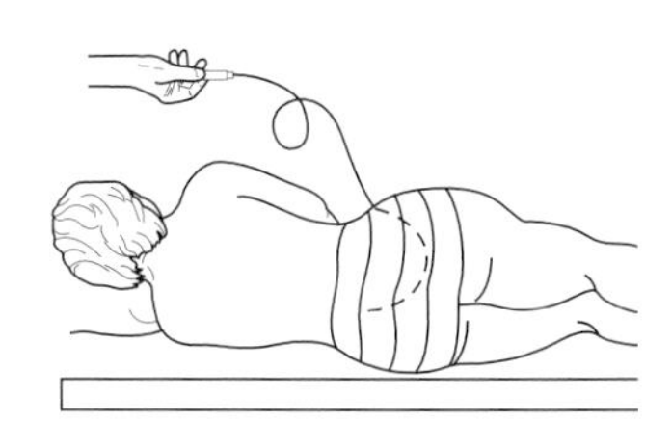
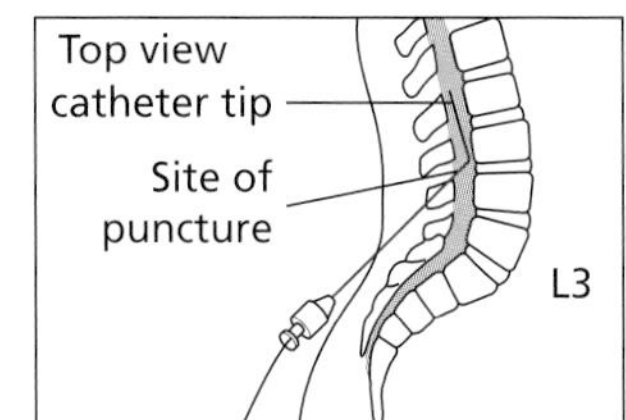

First stage

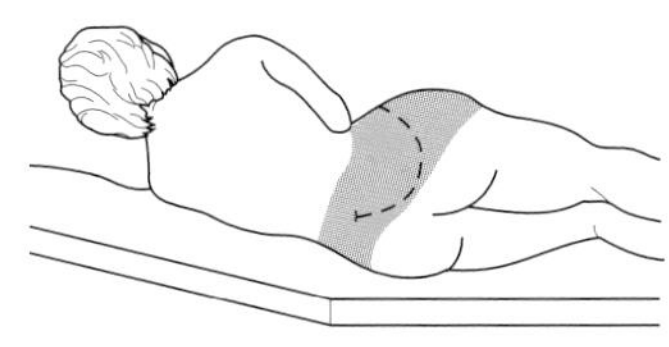
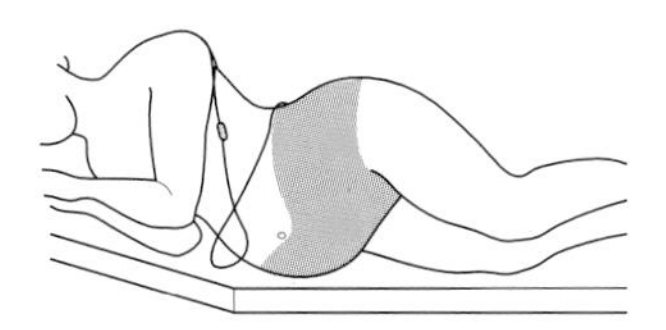

Early second stage

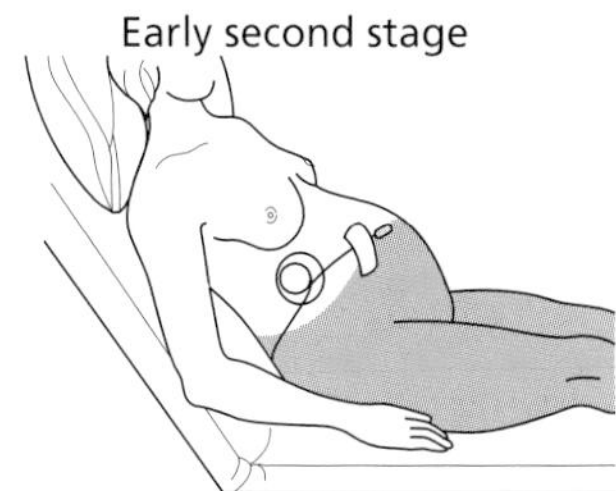

Delivery

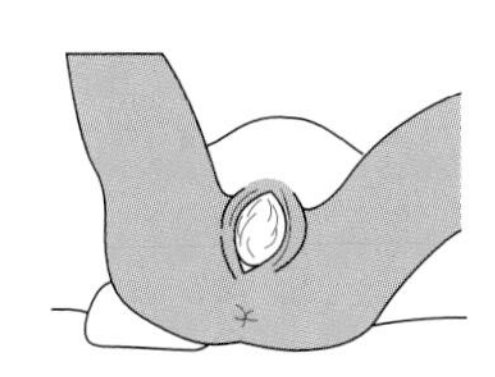

Fig. 11.3 Techniques of lumbar epidural block for labour and vaginal delivery. (A) The standard continuous technique, which is carried out as follows: after starting a preload infusion of fluid, a continuous catheter is inserted through a needle placed in the L4 interspace and advanced until its tip is at the L3 vertebra. With the onset of moderate pain, a test dose is injected and, if negative, 10–12 ml of a local anaesthetic (e.g., 0.25% bupivacaine) is injected to produce analgesia extending from T10–S5. The patient is then made to lie on her side, is given oxygen, and is frequently monitored, and 'top-up' analgesic doses are injected as soon as pain returns, to produce continuous analgesia. After flexion and internal rotation have occurred, a high concentration of local anaesthetic is injected with the patient in the semirecumbent position to produce perineal relaxation and anaesthesia as depicted (black) in the lower right figure. For the delivery, a wedge is placed under the right buttock to displace the uterus towards the left away from the inferior vena cava and aorta. (B) The technique of segmental epidural analgesia differs slightly from the standard technique in that the catheter is placed higher (L2), and for the first stage the dose is limited to 5–6 ml of local analgesic solution. At the onset of perineal pain, analgesia is extended to the lower lumbar and sacral segments by injecting 10–12 ml of local analgesic solution with the patient in Fowler's position.

this chapter. Most clinicians use a single catheter placed with its tip in the upper lumbar epidural space (Gieraerts et al 1992). To introduce the catheter, we prefer the use of a Touhy needle and the paramedian technique (Bonica 1980). Once the catheter is fixed in place and all the monitoring and resuscitation equipment is available for immediate use, anaesthetic consisting of 3 ml 0.25% bupivacaine and 1:200 000 adrenaline (epinephrine) is injected. Alternatively, 10 ml of bupivacaine 0.125% with 12.5 μg of adrenaline (epinephrine) can be used (Williams et al 1990). If no signs of intravenous or subarachnoid injection develop within 5 min, a single bolus of 5 ml of 0.25% bupivacaine is injected as a priming dose. This usually produces analgesia extending from T9–T10 to L1–L2 (Fig. 11.4). As soon

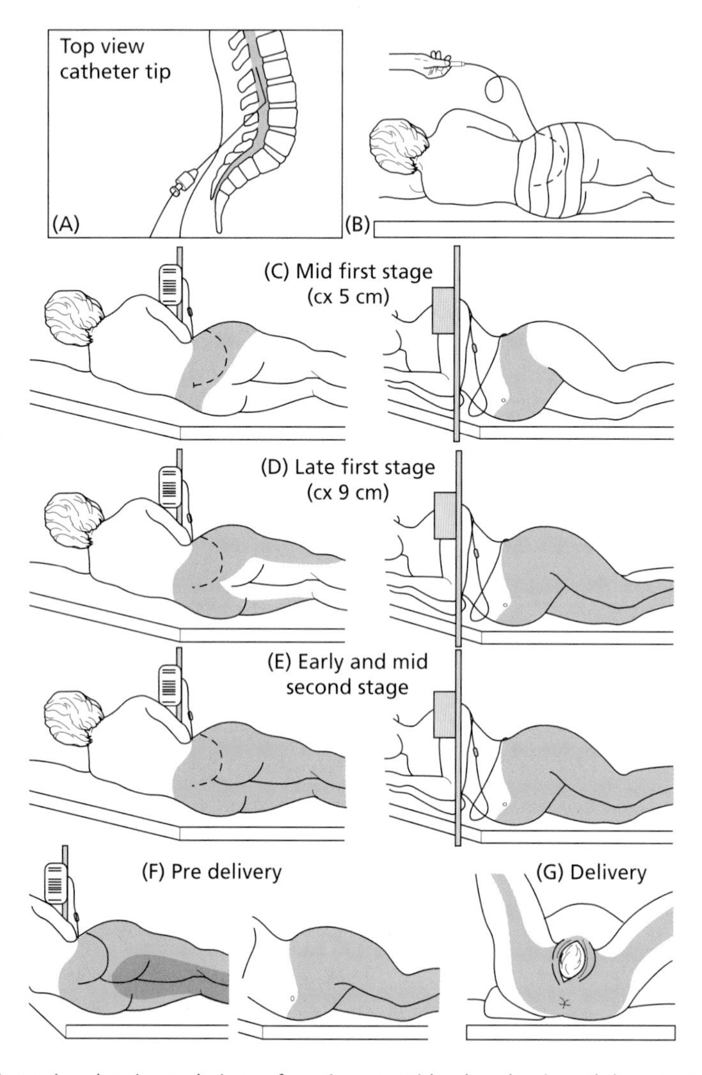

Fig. 11.4 Schematic illustration showing technique of continuous epidural analgesia and the extent and intensity of analgesia during the first and second stages of labour and for delivery. (A) The epidural needle and catheter in place. After removing the needle, the catheter is taped to the patient's back and a test dose of local anaesthetic given. (B) If after 5 min there is no sign of accidental intravenous or subarachnoid injection, a bolus of 5 ml of local anaesthetic is injected while the patient is in the lateral position. (C) After signs of epidural analgesia of T9–T10 to L1–L2 are noted, the catheter is connected to the continuous infusion system and the solution is administered at a rate of 10–12 ml/h with the patient in a 15°–20° head-up position, lying on her side. (D) Extent of analgesia after 1.5–2 h of infusion. (E) Extent of analgesia in the early and mid second stage. (F) After internal rotation has occurred, injection of a bolus of 10 ml of local anaesthetic solution (e.g., 1% lidocaine) produces an increase in the intensity of analgesia indicated by the more heavily shaded area involving the lower sacral segments. (G) The patient is ready for delivery. Note the wedge under the right hip and lower region to help displace the uterus to the left. (See text for details.)

as this is achieved, a continuous infusion of a solution containing 0.0625% bupivacaine and 0.002% fentanyl (2 μg/ml) is initiated at a rate of 10–12 ml/h, and this is subsequently increased or decreased to maintain analgesia with the upper level at T10. Usually a total of 120 ml of solution is prepared. Some clinicians use a mixture of 30 ml of 0.25% bupivacaine, 60 μg of sufentanyl, and 200 μg of adrenaline (epinephrine) in a 120-ml volume (McIntosh and Rayburn 1991). By using a pump, it is easy to deliver precise amounts of drugs. The pumps are small and portable, so ambulation during the early part of labour is feasible. Some obstetricians prefer maternal ambulation in the early first stage because of the belief that it enhances labour. A unique advantage related to portability is that the pump has a self-contained medication cassette with a typical capacity of at least 100 ml of solution, obviating the need to have a separately suspended medication bottle. A wide variety of acceptable pumps is available.

Throughout labour and until delivery, if the patient prefers to lie in bed, she is placed in the left or right lateral position with the upper part of the body raised about 15°–20°. With each subsequent hour, the extent of cephalad level of analgesia remains fairly constant at T10, but the caudal level tends to extend. After about the third or fourth hour, analgesia usually involves all of the lumbar and sacral segments (Fig. 11.4E). In about 50–60% of the parturients, the sacral analgesia is sufficient for perineal analgesia. The patient is examined prior to delivery, and if sacral analgesia is incomplete 10 ml of 1% lidocaine or 2% chloroprocaine are given with the patient in the sitting position. This usually produces sufficient analgesia and perineal relaxation for the actual delivery.

An extension of the continuous epidural infusion is the patient-controlled epidural analgesic delivery system. Studies have compared these two techniques, revealing similar advantages for the patients and no real differences in patient preferences of one over the other (Bonica 1980, Gambling et al 1990, Ferrante et al 1991).

Technique of spinal–epidural

One last technique must be mentioned that has gained momentum recently, the spinal–epidural combination technique where a 27-gauge spinal needle is passed via the standard 18-gauge thin-walled epidural needle for delivery of a small amount of subarachnoid opioid. First the lumbar epidural needle is placed and the usual entry into the epidural space is assured. Next the small-gauge spinal needle is passed through the epidural needle until the dura is contacted. After the spinal needle contacts the dura a puncture is made and a small amount of opioid is injected for the purpose of providing analgesia without significant sympathetic blockade and without significant motor paralysis of the lower extremities. Some refer to this method as the 'walking epidural', because the patient is able to control her legs and has good first-stage pain relief due to the opioid in the subarachnoid space, but has no motor loss of any note (Norris et al 1998). The ability to ambulate is especially important during the second stage because the incidence of lack of rotation of the presenting part is decreased and the mother can voluntarily mobilize her expulsive forces to augment those of labour to achieve spontaneous delivery.

Conclusion

The unnecessary and avoidable pain of childbirth has only been recently effectively tamed. The advantages of maternal analgesia and therefore management of maternal and fetal stress hormone release and effect clearly outweigh the relative risks of analgesic techniques. Such risks are themselves less than the risks of unprepared childbirth. The continuous epidural techniques with local anesthetic and opioid mixtures, or alternatively combined spinal–epidural techniques, are currently the state of the art.

References

Adams JQ, Alexander Jr AM 1958 Alterations in cardiovascular physiology during labour. Obstetrics and Gynecology 12: 542–549

Atlee HB 1956 Natural childbirth. Thomas, Springfield, IL

Berkley KJ, Wood E 1989 Responses to varying intensities of vaginal distension in the awake rat. Society of Neuroscience Abstracts 15: 979

Bonica JJ 1967 Principles and practice of obstetric analgesia and anesthesia, vol 1. Davis, Philadelphia

Bonica JJ 1969 Principles and practice of obstetric analgesia and anesthesia, vols 1, 2. Davis, Philadelphia

Bonica JJ 1973 Maternal respiratory changes during pregnancy and parturition. In: Marx GF (ed) Parturition and perinatology. Davis, Philadelphia

Bonica JJ 1980 Obstetric analgesia and anaesthesia, 2nd edn. World Federation of Societies of Anaesthesiologists, Amsterdam/University of Washington Press, Seattle

Bonica JJ, Hunter Jr CA 1969 Management in dysfunction of the forces of labor. In: Bonica JJ (ed) Principles and practice of obstetric analgesia and anesthesia, vol 2. Davis, Philadelphia

Bonica JJ, McDonald JS 1990 The pain of childbirth. In: Bonica JJ (ed) The management of pain, 2nd edn. Lea & Febiger, Malvern, PA, pp 1313–1343

Bonica JJ, McDonald JS 1995 Principles and practice of obstetric analgesia and anesthesia, 2nd edn. Williams & Wilkins, Baltimore

Brown WA, Manning T, Grodin J 1972 The relationship of antenatal and perinatal variables to the use of drugs in labor. Psychosomatic Medicine 34: 119–127
Brownridge P 1991 Treatment options for the relief of pain during childbirth. Drugs 41: 69–80
Buchan PC 1980 Emotional stress in childbirth and its modification by variations in obstetric management—epidural analgesia and stress in labor. Acta Obstetricia et Gynecologica Scandinavica 59: 319–321
Candido KD, Winnie AP 1992 A dual-chambered syringe that allows identification of the epidural space using the loss of resistance technique with air and with saline. Regional Anesthesia 17: 163–165
Carstoniu J, Levytam S, Norman P et al 1994 Nitrous oxide in labour: safety and efficacy assessed by a double-blind placebo controlled study. Anesthesiology 80: 30–35
Dick-Read G 1953 Childbirth without fear. Harper, New York
Eddleston JM, Maresh M, Horsman EL, Young H 1992 Comparison of maternal and fetal effects associated with intermittent or continuous infusion or extradural analgesia. British Journal of Anaesthesia 69: 154–158
Ferrante FM, Lu L, Jamison SB, Datta S 1991 Patient-controlled epidural analgesia: demand dosing. Anesthesia and Analgesia 73: 547–552
Fridh G, Kopare T, Gaston-Johansson F, Norvell KT 1988 Factors associated with more intense labor pain. Research in Nursing and Health 11: 117–124
Gabbe, Steven G 1991 Obstetrics—normal and problem pregnancies, 2nd edn. Churchill Livingstone, Edinburgh
Gambling DR, McMorland GH, Yu P, Laszlo C 1990 Comparison of patient-controlled epidural analgesia and conventional intermittent 'top-up' injections during labor. Anesthesia and Analgesia 70: 256–261
Gaston-Johansson F, Fridh G, Turner-Norvell K 1988 Progression of labor pain in primiparas and multiparas. Nursing Research 37: 86–90
Gaylard D 1990 Epidural analgesia by continuous infusion. In: Reynolds F (ed) Epidural and spinal blockade in obstetrics. Baillière Tindall, London, pp 49–58
Gerdin A, Salmonson T, Lindberg B, Rane A 1990 Maternal kinetics of morphine during labor. Journal of Perinatal Medicine 18: 479–487
Gieraerts R, Van Zundert A, De Wolf A, Vaes L 1992 Ten ml bupivacaine 0.125% with 12.5μ epinephrine is a reliable epidural test dose to detect inadvertent intravascular injection in obstetric patients. A double-blind study. Acta Anaesthesiologica Scandinavica 36: 656–659
Glassenberg R 1991 General anesthesia and maternal mortality. Seminars in Perinatology 15: 386–396
Hansen JM, Ueland K 1966 The influence of caudal analgesia on cardiovascular dynamics during normal labour and delivery. Acta Anaesthesiologica Scandinavica 23 (suppl 10): 449–452
Hayes JR, Ardill J, Kennedy TL, Shanks RG, Buchanan KD 1972 Stimulation of gastrin release by catecholamines. Lancet i: 819–821
Hendricks CH, Quilligan EJ 1956 Cardiac output during labor. American Journal of Obstetrics and Gynecology 71: 953–972
Holdsworth JD 1978 Relationships between stomach contents and analgesia in labour. British Journal of Anaesthesia 50: 1145–1148
Huch A, Huch R, Schneider H, Rooth G 1977 Continuous transcutaneous monitoring of foetal oxygen tension during labour. British Journal of Obstetrics and Gynaecology 84 (suppl 1): 1–39
Jouppila R 1977 The effect of segmental epidural analgesia on hormonal and metabolic changes during labour. Acta Universitatis Ouluensis, Series D, Medica No 16, Anaesthesiologica No 2
Kawatani M, de Groat WC 1991 A large proportion of afferent neurons innervating the uterine cervix of the cat contain VIP and other neuropeptides. Cell and Tissue Research 266: 191–196
Klink EW 1953 Perineal nerve block: an anatomic and clinical study in the female. Obstetrics and Gynecology 1: 137–146
Lamaze F 1956 Qu'est-ce que l'accouchement sans douleur par la méthode psychoprophylactique? Ses principles, sa réalization, ses résultants. Savoir et Connâitre, Paris
Lamaze F, Vellay P 1952 L'accouchement sans douleur par la methode psycholophysique: premiers resultats portant sur 500 cas. Gazette médicale de France 59: 1445
Lederman RP, McCann DS, Work B, Huber MJ 1977 Endogenous plasma epinephrine and norepinephrine in last-trimester pregnancy and labour. American Journal of Obstetrics and Gynecology 129: 5–8
Lederman RP, Lederman E, Work BA Jr, McCann DS 1978 The relationship of maternal anxiety, plasma catecholamines, and plasma cortisol to progress in labor. American Journal of Obstetrics and Gynecology 132: 495–500
Lowe NK 1989 Explaining the pain of active labor: the importance in maternal confidence. Research in Nursing and Health 12: 237–245
Marx GF, Greene NM 1964 Maternal lactate, pyruvate and excess lactate production during labor and delivery. American Journal of Obstetrics and Gynecology 90: 786–793
Marx GF, Katsnelson T 1992 The introduction of nitrous oxide into obstetrics. Obstetrics and Gynecology 80: 715–718
McIntosh DG, Rayburn WF 1991 Patient-controlled analgesia in obstetrics and gynecology. Obstetrics and Gynecology 70: 202–204
McLintic AJ, Danskin SH, Reid JA, Thorburn J 1991 Effects of adrenaline on extradural anesthesia, plasma lignocaine concentrations and feto-placental unit during elective cesarean section. British Journal of Anaesthesia 67: 683–689
Melzack R 1984 The myth of painless childbirth. The John J. Bonica Lecture. Pain 19: 321
Melzack R, Taenzer P, Feldman P, Kinch RA 1981 Labour is still painful after prepared childbirth training. Canadian Medical Association Journal 125: 357–363
Moir DD, Willocks J 1967 Management of incoordinate uterine action under continuous epidural analgesia. British Medical Journal 3: 396–400
Moore DC, Batra MS 1981 The components of an effective test dose prior to epidural block. Anesthesiology 55: 693–696
Morishima HO, Pedersen H, Finster M 1978 The influence of maternal psychological stress on the fetus. American Journal of Obstetrics and Gynecology 131: 286–290
Morishima HO, Pedersen H, Finster M 1980 Effects of pain on mother, labour and fetus. In: Marx GF, Bassel GM (eds) Obstetric analgesia and anaesthesia. Elsevier/North Holland, Amsterdam, pp 197–210
Myers RE 1975 Maternal psychological stress and fetal asphyxia: a study in the monkey. American Journal of Obstetrics and Gynecology 122: 47–59
Nettelbladt P, Fagerstrom CF, Uddenberg N 1976 The significance of reported childbirth pain. Journal of Psychosomatic Research 20: 215–221
Nimmo WS, Wilson J, Prescott LF 1975 Narcotic analgesics and delayed gastric emptying during labour. Lancet i: 890
Norman PH, Kavanagh B, Daley MD et al 1992 Nitrous oxide analgesia in labour (abstract). Anesthesia and Analgesia 74: S222
Norr KL, Block CR, Charles A, Meyering S, Meyers E 1977 Explaining pain and enjoyment in childbirth. Journal of Health and Social Behavior 18: 260–275
Norris MC, Fogel ST, Holtmann B 1998 Intrathecal sufentantil (5 vs. 10 microg) for labor analgesia: efficacy and side effects. Regional Anesthesia and Pain in Medicine 23: 252–257

Ohno H, Yamashita K, Yahata et al 1986 Maternal plasma concentrations of catecholamines and cyclic nucleotides during labor and following delivery. Research Communications in Chemical Pathology and Pharmacology 51: 183–194
Peabody JL 1979 Transcutaneous oxygen measurement to evaluate drug effect. Clinical Perinatology 6: 109–121
Pearson JF, Davies P 1973 The effect of continuous epidural analgesia on the acid–base status of maternal arterial blood during the first state of labour. Journal of Obstetrics and Gynaecology of the British Commonwealth 80: 218–224
Pearson JF, Davies P 1974 The effect of continuous lumbar epidural analgesia on the acid–base status of maternal arterial blood during the first state of labour. Journal of Obstetrics and Gynaecology of the British Commonwealth 81: 975–979
Reading AE, Cox DN 1985 Psychosocial predictors of labor pain. Pain 22: 309–315
Robson SC, Dunlop W, Boys RJ, Hunter S 1987 Cardiac output during labor. British Medical Journal 295: 1169–1172
Rosaeg OP, Kitts JB, Koren G, Byford LL 1992 Maternal and fetal effects of intravenous patient-controlled fentanyl analgesia during labour in a thrombocytopenic parturient. Canadian Journal of Anesthesia 39: 277–281
Shnider SM, Levinson G 1987 Anesthesia for obstetrics, 3rd edn. Williams & Wilkins, Philadelphia
Stewart DE 1982 Psychiatric symptoms following attempted natural childbirth. Canadian Medical Association Journal 127: 713–716
Swart F, Abboud TK, Zhu J et al 1991 Desflurane analgesia in obstetrics: maternal and neonatal effects (abstract). Anesthesiology 75: A844
Tomkinson J et al 1982 Report on confidential inquiries into maternal death in England and Wales 1976–1978. Report on Health and Social Subjects No 16. HMSO, London
Williams B, Kwan K, Chen B, Wu Y 1990 Comparison of 0.0312% bupivacaine plus sufental and 0.0625% bupivacaine plus sufental for epidural anesthesia during labor and delivery. Anesthesiology 73: A950
Zarzur E, Gonzalves JJ 1992 The resistance of the human dura mater to needle penetration. Regional Anesthesia 17: 216–218

Chapter 12

Genitourinary pain

Ursula Wesselmann and Arthur L Burnett

Introduction

Chronic non-malignant pain syndromes (longer than 6 months' duration) of the genitourinary tract are well described but poorly understood, and are often very frustrating for the patients and their physicians. Pain in these areas of the body is usually very embarrassing for the male and female patient, who may be afraid to discuss his/her symptoms with family members, friends, and health care providers. Except in those cases in which a specific secondary cause can be identified, the aetiology of the chronic genitourinary pain syndromes often remains unknown. The controversy that surrounds these pain syndromes ranges from questioning their existence to dismissing them as purely psychosomatic. This is counterbalanced by an extensive literature attesting to their organicity. Patients with these pain syndromes often suffer for many years, have seen numerous physicians in numerous subspecialties, and are frustrated, embarrassed, and frequently depressed. Despite the challenge inherent in the management of chronic genitourinary pain, many patients can be treated successfully. Effective treatment modalities, although often empirical only, are available to lessen the impact of pain and offer reasonable expectations of an improved functional status. The focus of this chapter is on chronic non-malignant genitourinary pain syndromes. Another very important issue is the management of pain syndromes associated with cancer of the genitourinary tract (see Chap. 45 for a discussion of cancer pain). The present chapter first reviews key points of the neurobiology of the genitourinary tract, which is a prerequisite for trying to understand the chronic pain syndromes in this area. We will then discuss the clinical presentation, aetiology, and differential diagnosis of chronic genitourinary pain and review treatment options.

Neurobiology of the genitourinary tract

The pelvic region including the genitourinary tract is a highly specialized area of the body, responsible for carrying out a host of basic biological functions including micturition, copulation, and reproduction. The display of these diverse functions relies on precise nervous system control, coordinated with endocrine and other local control mechanisms. This paragraph gives a condensed overview of the genitourinary neurobiology, targeted towards health care providers who are evaluating and treating patients with chronic urogenital pain. A detailed review of the neurobiology of the pelvis and genitourinary tract is provided in Burnett and Wesselmann (1999). The innervation of the genitourinary area involves both components of the autonomic nervous system, the sympathetic and parasympathetic divisions, as well as the somatic nervous system (Morrison 1987; de Groat et al 1993, de Groat 1994). In a broad neuroanatomical view, dual projections from the thoracolumbar and sacral segments of the spinal cord carry out this innervation, converging mostly into peripheral neuronal plexuses from which nerve fibres ramify throughout the pelvic floor (Figs. 12.1 and 12.2). Autonomic preganglionic efferents arise for the most part in the intermediolateral cell column, referred to as the sacral parasympathetic nucleus at sacral levels, whereas cell bodies of corresponding afferents are contained within dorsal root ganglia. The sympathetic thoracolumbar outflow to the urogenital tract involves preganglionic projections to the celiac plexus and to the superior hypogastric plexus (Ferguson and Bell 1993, Lincoln and Burnstock 1993). The celiac plexus provides the majority of the autonomic innervation to the adrenal, kidney, renal pelvis, and ureter, as well as some sympathetic input to the testes along the course of the internal spermatic vessels. The majority of the sympathetic input to the pelvic urinary organs and genital tract is through the superior hypogastric plexus. In addition to this route in supplying pelvic structures, thoracolumbar preganglionic nerves also synapse on postganglionic nerves in sympathetic chain ganglia that commingle with autonomic sacral nerve projections as well as with pelvic somatic neuronal pathways (McKenna and Nadelhaft 1986). Parasympathetic sacral outflow (S2–S4) consists of preganglionic nerves that are referred to as the pelvic splanchnic nerves. Parasympathetic afferent cell bodies are located in S2–S4 dorsal root ganglia and also course with the pelvic splanchnic nerve.

The inferior hypogastric plexus is the major neuronal coordinating centre that supplies visceral structures of the pelvis and the pelvic floor (Lincoln and Burnstock 1993). The inferior hypogastric

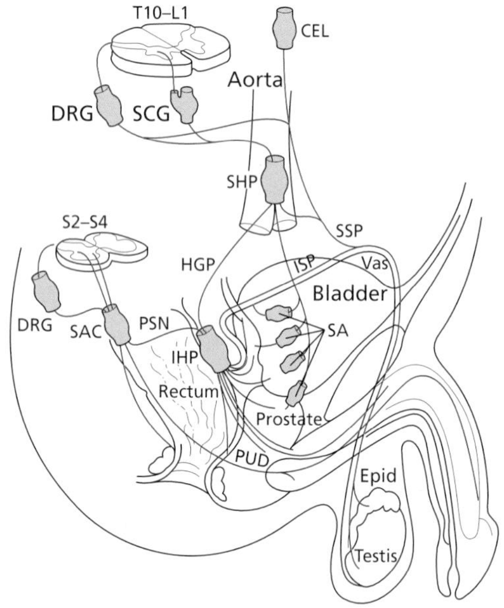

Fig. 12.1 The innervation of the urogenital and rectal area in *males*. Although this diagram attempts to show the innervation in humans, much of the anatomical information is derived from animal data (see text). CEL = coeliac plexus; DRG = dorsal root ganglion; Epid. = epididymis; HGP = hypogastric plexus; IHP = inferior hypogastric plexus; ISP = inferior spermatic plexus; PSN = pelvic splanchnic nerve; PUD = pudendal nerve; SA = short adrenergic projections; SAC = sacral plexus; SCG = sympathetic chain ganglion; SHP = superior hypogastric plexus; SSP = superior spermatic plexus. (Reproduced from Wesselmann et al 1997 with permission.)

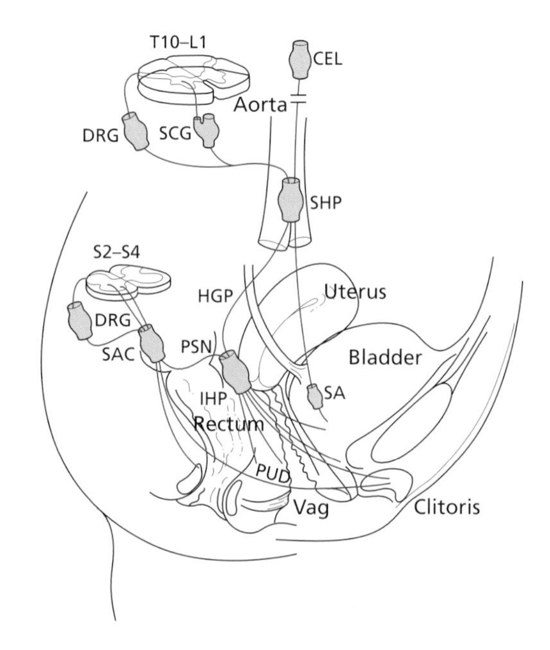

Fig. 12.2 The innervation of the urogenital and rectal area in *females*. Although this diagram attempts to show the innervation in humans, much of the anatomical information is derived from animal data (see text). CEL = coeliac plexus; DRG = dorsal root ganglion; HGP = hypogastric plexus; IHP = inferior hypogastric plexus; PSN = pelvic splanchnic nerve; PUD = pudendal nerve; SA = short adrenergic projections; SAC = sacral plexus; SCG = sympathetic chain ganglion; SHP = superior hypogastric plexus; Vag. = vagina. (Reproduced from Wesselmann et al 1997 with permission.)

plexus receives sympathetic (superior hypogastric plexus and its caudal extension, the hypogastric plexus, the sympathetic chain ganglia) and parasympathetic input (pelvic splanchnic nerve) (de Groat 1994). Both efferent and afferent fibres are carried in these sympathetic and parasympathetic projections (Jänig and Koltzenburg 1993).

Somatic efferent and afferent innervation to the pelvic floor originates from sacral spinal cord levels (S2–S4). Somatic efferents originate within Onuf's nucleus in the ventral horn and afferents have their cell bodies located within dorsal root ganglia at these levels (Lincoln and Burnstock 1993). Overlapping of somatic afferents with pelvic splanchnic nerve afferents on the spinal cord level have been proposed to account for the coordination of somatic and visceral motor activity (McKenna and Nadelhaft 1986). Sacral nerve roots form the sacral plexus. The pudendal nerve arises from the sacral plexus as the primary efferent and afferent somatic distribution with various branches involving pelvic viscera and the pelvic floor musculature (Elbadawi 1996). The pudendal nerve also receives terminations of postganglionic axons arising from the caudal sympathetic chain ganglia (de Groat 1994). Nerve branches originating mainly from sacral level S4 supply the posterior perineal muscles, whereas branches from sacral level S3 primarily supply the anterior perineal musculature. Branches of S4–S5 nerve roots form the coccygeal plexus supplying the perineal, perianal, and scrotal/labial skin.

Sensations from the pelvic floor are mainly conveyed via the sacral afferent parasympathetic system, with a far lesser afferent supply from afferents travelling with the thoracolumbar sympathetics (Jänig and Koltzenburg 1993). However, sensations of the testis and epididymis may predominantly involve thoracolumbar afferents (Jänig and Koltzenburg 1993). Cholinergic nerve release likely governs the somatic mechanisms of the perineal musculature (Vodusek and Light 1983). Neuropeptide release appears to account for perineal sensations (Jänig and Koltzenburg 1993).

Chronic pain syndromes of the genitourinary tract: clinical presentation, aetiology, differential diagnosis, and treatment strategies

Kidney and ureter pain

There are few chronic non-malignant pain syndromes of the upper urinary tract. Most pain syndromes of the kidney and ureter are acute, colicky in character, and caused by acute distension due to an obstructing lesion or by infection. With improved diagnostic techniques cases of idiopathic nephralgia, as they were frequently diagnosed earlier this century (Harris and Harris 1930), have become extremely rare. As in other visceral disease, patients with diseases of the kidney and/or ureter present with true visceral pain and referred visceral pain to somatic structures. The referred pain is typically radiating from the costovertebral angle laterally around to the lower quadrant and into the testicle or labia.

Loin pain/haematuria syndrome is a descriptive diagnosis given to patients with recurrent attacks of unilateral or bilateral loin pain accompanied by microscopic or macroscopic haematuria in whom no cause can be identified (Little et al 1967, Editorial 1992). The syndrome is more frequent in women than men (Little et al 1967, Bultitude et al 1998). No consistent histological changes have been described in renal specimens (Editorial 1992, Weisberg et al 1993). The diagnosis is made by exclusion, and because no aetiological treatment is possible to this date, treatment is symptomatic to relieve pain. Sometimes the syndrome resolves spontaneously. Most patients require large doses of analgesics, usually opioids, for pain control (Bultitude 1995). Transcutaneous electrical nerve stimulation (TENS) has been reported to result in partial pain relief, some women have benefited from stopping birth control pills, and anticoagulation has been beneficial in several patients (Burden et al 1975, Aber and Higgins 1982). Surgical approaches have included renal denervation and even nephrectomy or autotransplantation (with the aim of achieving complete denervation while preserving kidney function). However, after nephrectomy or autotransplantion the pain often returns on the contralateral side (Editorial 1992). Bultitude et al (1998) reported symptomatic pain relief in 65% of patients with loin pain/haematuria syndrome after local irrigation of the renal pelvis and ureter with capsaicin solution, which lasted for several months. This treatment results in degeneration of afferent fibres of the ureter and renal pelvis (Allan et al 1997).

Interstitial cystitis

Interstitial cystitis (IC) is a chronic, painful, and often debilitating disease, whose aetiology and pathophysiology is largely unknown (for review see Hanno et al 2001). It is characterized by pelvic and suprapubic pain, urinary symptoms such as frequency and urgency, and in females often by dyspareunia that may be relieved by voiding. IC subdivides into an ulcerative and non-ulcerative type, as determined by cystoscopic findings of either Hunner's ulcer or glomerulations without ulcer on the bladder wall (Johansson and Fall 1994, Elbadawi 1997, Messing et al 1997, Nigro et al 1997). While prevalence estimates vary widely, it has been suggested that somewhere between 450 000 (Slade et al 1997) and 1 million people (Jones and Nyberg 1997) in the USA suffer from IC or IC-like conditions. The most recent study on the epidemiology of IC used the Nurses' Health Study (NSH) I and II cohort as a study population and reported the prevalence of IC in NSH II as 67/100 000 and in NSH I as 52/100 000 (Curhan et al 1999). A distinguishing feature of IC is the overwhelming burden reported by women. Population prevalence estimates indicate a female to male ratio of 9:1 (Jones and Nyberg 1997).

Aetiologies that have been considered include infection (Ratliff et al 1994, Warren 1994, Duncan and Schaeffer 1997), lymphatic or vascular obstruction (Ratliff et al 1994), immunological deficiencies (Ratliff et al 1994), glycosaminoglycan layer deficiency (Ratliff et al 1994, Mobley and Baum 1996, Parsons 1997), changes in bladder epithelial regeneration (Keay et al 2001), presence of toxic urogenous substance (Ratliff et al 1994), neural factors, and primary mast cell disorders (Elbadawi 1997, Theoharides et al 2001, Wesselmann 2001). It has also been considered that the cause leading to the onset of IC has resolved, leaving in its wake a chronic visceral pain syndrome (Wesselmann 2001). This is consistent with the report of Baskin and Tanagho (1992), where several cases of removal of the bladder in IC patients did not lead to a resolution of pain. Rare cases of the coexistence of vulvodynia and IC have been reported, and it has been proposed that these syndromes represent a generalized disorder of urogenital sinus-derived epithelium (Fitzpatrick et al 1993). In 60% of men with prostate pain without bacteriuria there might be an association with IC or a related condition (Miller et al 1995, Berger et al 1998).

An assortment of oral, intravesical, surgical, local, and behaviourally based treatments have been suggested for the management of IC. Surgical approaches include removal or modification of the bladder (Irwin and Galloway 1994, Peeker et al 1998). Local treatments include laser therapy (Malloy and Shanberg 1994), hydrodistension (Irwin and Galloway 1994, Sant and LaRock 1994, Zimmern 1995) and urethral dilatation (Irwin and Galloway 1994), infusions of various materials into the bladder such as dimethyl sulfoxide (DMSO) (Fowler 1981, Barker et al 1987, Childs 1994, Sant and LaRock 1994, Parkin et al 1997), silver nitrate (Sant and LaRock 1994), heparin (Sant and LaRock 1994), chlorpactin (Sant and LaRock 1994), and hyaluronic acid (Morales et al 1997). Oral medications range from those used for other chronic pain syndromes such as amitriptyline (Hanno 1994, Pontari et al 1997, Pranikoff and Constantino 1998) and calcium channel blockers (Fleischmann 1994), to medications acting against a possible allergic mechanism such as hydroxyzine and other antihistamines (Simmons and Bunce 1958, Theoharides and Sant 1997). Pentosanpolysulphate sodium, a mild anticoagulant with properties of sulphated glycosaminoglycans and an affinity for mucosal membranes, has been used for the treatment of IC based on the hypothesis that a defect in the glycosaminoglycan layer contributes to the pathogenesis (Fritjofsson et al 1987, Hanno 1997, Jepsen et al 1998). Non-medical treatment strategies such as TENS (Fall and Lindstrom 1994), acupuncture (Geirsson et al 1993), behavioural interventions (including the keeping of voiding diaries, pelvic floor muscle training), and acid-lowering diets have been advocated (Chaiken et al 1993, Whitmore 1994). Most reports of treatment of IC so far have suffered from lack of agreement about what constitutes a case and the lack of agreeable, valid outcome data. The National Institutes of Health in the USA have focused several major research initiatives on IC (see Hanno et al 2001 for review). Several multicentre controlled trials comparing different treatment strategies for the management of IC are currently underway, and it is to be hoped that this clinical research will result in improved—logical and systematic—treatment approaches in the near future.

Urethral syndrome

Many women present to the urologist, gynaecologist, or family physician with painful micturition but no evidence of organic disease, and the urine culture is negative by standard techniques. To describe this problem the term 'urethral syndrome' was coined by Gallagher et al (1965). He reported that 41% of women seen in general practice with symptoms of a urinary tract infection had in fact sterile urine. The urethral syndrome is defined as an entity characterized by urinary urgency, frequency, dysuria, and, at times, suprapubic and back pain and urinary hesitancy in the absence of objective urological findings. The urethral syndrome is estimated to account for as many as 5 million office visits a year in the United States (Peters-Gee 1998).

The urethral syndrome typically occurs in women during their reproductive years, but it has also been reported in children (Kaplan et al 1980) and in men (Barbalias 1990).

The aetiology of the urethral syndrome is not clear. Several theories have been proposed, however, with little supporting evidence. One popular theory is that symptoms are caused by urethral obstruction and are thus surgically treatable (Davis 1955, Bergman et al 1989, Sand et al 1989). Although surgical procedures aimed at relieving a urethral obstruction claim excellent results, it must be cautioned that diagnostic criteria were unfortunately poorly documented (Splatt and Weedon 1981). Most importantly, there is rarely evidence to support an anatomically obstructive aetiology (Mabry et al 1981). These procedures involve some risk of incontinence and are of uncertain and usually temporary efficacy (Mabry et al 1981, Schmidt and Tanagho 1981). Many studies have investigated the role of infection in the urethral syndrome, but there is little evidence supporting the concept of an inflammatory or infectious aetiology for the urethral syndrome (reviewed in Messinger 1992). Urinary hesitance, which is often reported by patients with urethral syndrome, might be due to spasms of the external urethral sphincter. Several studies reported a staccato or prolonged flow phase during uroflowmetry and increased external sphincter tone detected on urethral pressure profilometry in patients with urethral syndrome (Raz and Smith 1976, Kaplan et al 1980, Schmidt and Tanagho 1981). However, these urodynamic findings are difficult to interpret in support of a neurogenic aetiology of the urethral syndrome, because they may also be produced voluntarily in a neurologically intact person (Messinger 1992). In contrast to other non-malignant genitourinary pain syndromes, the rates of spontaneous remission are very high in this patient population (85% in Carson et al 1980 and 100% in Zufall 1978).

A thorough diagnostic evaluation is crucial. The urethral syndrome is a diagnosis of exclusion, its symptoms are indistinguishable from those caused by urinary infections, tumours, stones, interstitial cystitis and many other entities, and these conditions must be ruled out. The first diagnostic step is a thorough urological examination including urine analysis, culture, and cytology. In selected patients further radiographic studies, urodynamic studies, and cystoscopy are necessary (Messinger 1992). In females a gynaecological problem needs to be ruled out. The symptoms of the urethral syndrome can be part of the symptoms of systemic diseases affecting the innervation of the urogenital area, including multiple sclerosis, collagen diseases, and diabetes mellitus. A psychological evaluation should be part of the multidisciplinary evaluation to rule out a psychogenic aetiology and to assess for symptoms of depression associated with the chronic pain syndrome.

Various invasive and medical treatment options have been suggested for patients with the urethral syndrome (reviewed in Messinger 1992). Endoscopic and open surgical procedures have been reported with the aim of eliminating a presumed urethral stenosis. Fulguration, scarification, resection, or cryosurgery have been advocated to obliterate cystoscopically apparent urethritis. Bladder instillations with a variety of anti-inflammatory or cauterizing agents and systemic therapy with anticholinergics, α-adrenergic blockers, and muscle relaxants have been considered. Electrical stimulation and biofeedback have been advocated to correct neurogenic causes. High rates of success were found with skeletal muscle relaxants or electrostimulation combined with biofeedback techniques (Kaplan et al 1980, Schmidt and Tanagho 1981). While exercising caution towards invasive and irreversible therapeutic procedures, a conservative approach is recommended because this is usually as effective as surgery, less expensive, and most importantly, less subject to risk.

Vulvodynia (vulvar dysaesthesia)

Interestingly, hyperaesthesia of the vulva was a well-described entity in American (Thomas 1880) and European (Pozzi 1897) gynaecological textbooks of the nineteenth century. Surprisingly, despite early detailed reports, there was little interest in chronic vulvar pain until the early 1980s. In 1982 the International Society for the Study of Vulvar Disease (ISSVD) formed a task force to survey vulvar pain syndromes. This task force coined the term 'vulvodynia' as chronic vulvar discomfort (McKay 1984), characterized by the patient's complaint of burning (and sometimes stinging, irritation, or rawness) in the vulvar area. The term vulvodynia included several disorders, all of which result in chronic vulvar pain: vulvar dermatosis, cyclic vulvovaginitis, vulvar vestibulitis, vulvar papillomatosis, and dysaesthetic vulvodynia (McKay 1988, 1989). At the 1999 World Congress of the ISSVD a new classification system for vulvar dysaethesia was proposed, namely a division into two broad categories: (1) generalized vulvar dysaesthesia and (2) localized vulvar dysaesthesia—vestibulodynia, clitorodynia, and others. This new classification system has not been fully published in the peer-reviewed literature, and most of the studies on vulvar pain so far have used the term vulvodynia. Therefore we will use the term vulvodynia for the purpose of this chapter. However, as the knowledge about the aetiology and treatment of vulvar dysaesthesia is advancing, definitions will probably be modified, based on emerging knowledge of the underlying pathophysiological mechanisms. The recognition of multiple factors in the aetiology of vulvodynia is the key to appropriate evaluation and treatment.

The incidence or prevalence of vulvodynia is not known, but, as was already pointed out by Thomas (1880), this pain syndrome is probably more common than generally thought. A recent survey of sexual dysfunction in the USA, analysing data from the National Health and Social Life Survey, reported that 16% of women between the ages of 18 and 59 years living in households throughout the United States experience pain during sex (Laumann et al 1999). The location and aetiology of pain was not analysed in this study. In a small sample of 303 women aged 20 to 59 years, 18.5% reported a history of lower genital tract discomfort; however the aetiology of the pain was not reported (Harlow et al 2001). The age distribution of vulvodynia ranges from the twenties to late sixties (Lynch 1986, Paavonen 1995a,b).

The aetiology of vulvodynia remains unclear. Despite the fact that many aetiological hypotheses have been proposed, our current understanding of vulvodynia is limited because most of the proposed causal explanations are derived from clinical case reports. Twenty-five to 33% of women with vulvodynia know of a female relative with dyspareunia or tampon intolerance, raising the question of a genetic predisposition (Goetsch 1991, Bergeron et al 1997). The coexistence of vulvodynia and interstitial cystitis has been reported, and it has been proposed that these syndromes represent a generalized disorder of urogenital sinus-derived epithelium (Fitzpatrick et al 1993). Vulvodynia often has an acute onset, but sometimes no associated event can be recalled by the patient. In many cases the onset can be linked to episodes of a vaginal infection, local treatments of the vulvar or vaginal area (application of steroid or antimicrobial cream, cryo- or laser-surgery), or changes in the pattern of sexual activity. However, many of these parameters are quite frequent in women anyway, and controlled prospective studies are necessary in order to assess whether the development of chronic vulvar discomfort is linked to a history of vaginal infection, vaginal irritation, or vaginal trauma. It could be hypothesized that the vaginal tissue is more sensitive to these events in some women than in others.

Histopathological studies of punch biopsies of the vulvar vestibule in patients with vestibulitis in comparison to control cases showed histopathological abnormalities in patients with vulvar vestibulitis as a result of a chronic inflammatory reaction of the mucosa of the vestibule, for which the cause remained unclear. Early reports suggested that human papilloma virus (HPV) plays a major role in the pathogenesis of vulvar vestibulitis, but this could not be confirmed by studies using molecular techniques (De Deus et al 1995). The unique distribution of interleukin 1 receptor antagonist alleles among women with vulvar vestibulitis suggests that polymorphism in this gene might be a factor influencing susceptibility to this pain syndrome (Jeremias et al 2000). Anatomical studies demonstrate that the innervation of the vestibule is different in women with vulvar vestibulitis as compared to controls; there is vestibular neural hyperplasia in patients with vulvar dysaesthesia (Bohm-Starke et al 1998, Weststrom and Willen 1998).

On physical examination patients with vulvodynia usually present with no abnormalities. In patients with vulvar vestibulitis pain can easily be elicited or exacerbated by a simple 'Swabtest' (Goetsch 1991, Paavonen 1995a,b): touching the vulvar vestibule with a cotton swab results in sharp, burning pain. The allodynia and hyperalgesia reported by women suffering from vulvodynia has been quantified with psychophysical assessments, consistent with the hypothesis that there is nocicepetor sensitization (Sonni et al 1995, Bohm-Starke et al 2001). Chronic infections of the vulvar area should be treated, before a diagnosis of vulvodynia is considered. Further, iatrogenic causes must be excluded when evaluating a patient with vulvodynia. Local agents applied to the vulvar region can cause irritant reactions, which resolve after discontinuation of the irritant agent. Thus, vulvodynia is a diagnosis of exclusion.

The first step in the treatment of vulvodynia is to identify and eliminate local irritants and potential allergens. Many patients can be helped with oral medications recommended for neuropathic pain management including antidepressants, anticonvulsants, membrane-stabilizing agents, and opioids. In patients with vulvar vestibulitis, where a small area is painful, topical treatment regimens such as creams with local anaesthetics, aspirin, steroids, or oestrogen might reduce the pain. Glazer et al (1995) reported pain relief in over 80% of patients with vulvar vestibulitis using electromyographic biofeedback of the pelvic floor musculature. Surgical procedures to remove the hyperalgesic skin area in patients with vulvar vestibulitis have been advocated (for review see Wesselmann et al 1997, Bergeron et al 2001). The most commonly used procedure is perineoplasty. A simplified surgical revision, as an alternative to this extensive surgical intervention, where the painful area is excised under local anaesthesia, has been advocated by Goetsch (1996).

Clitoral pain

In contrast to the emerging literature about chronic pain syndromes of the vulva/vagina, very few reports on clitoral pain exist. Occasionally clitoral pain is seen as part of the vulvodynia pain syndrome complex in clinical practice. The patients report a burning stinging sensation that is exacerbated by touch (U Wesselmann, unpublished data). Chronic pain is reported as one of the complications of female circumcision, which involves excision of the clitoris and the labia minora and is still performed on young females in many parts of the world, where it is favoured as an instrument to control female sexuality and maintain cultural pride (Dirie and Lindmark 1992, Hanly and Ojeda 1995, Briggs 1998). With increasing mobility some of these women have moved to western countries. It is estimated that 2000 young women living in the UK undergo this ritual every year (Hanly and Ojeda 1995). However, the incidence of pain in these women is not known, because few of them seek medical attention.

Testicular pain

Chronic testicular pain (orchialgia) can be one of the most vexing pain problems for men and their treating physician. Because pain syndromes in the genital region are often considered taboo in our society, men with testicular pain are usually embarrassed to talk about it, similar to women who suffer from vulvodynia. The incidence and prevalence is not known. Patients from adolescence to old age who suffered from chronic testicular pain have been described (Zvieli et al 1989, Davis et al 1990, Costabile et al 1991): the majority are in their mid to late thirties (Davis et al 1990, Costabile et al 1991). Many patients cannot recall any precipitating event that led to the onset of the chronic pain syndrome (Costabile et al 1991, Wesselmann and Burnett 1996). Chronic testicular pain can be unilateral or bilateral and may be confined to the scrotal contents or can radiate to the groin, penis, perineum, abdomen, legs, and back. Some patients have constant pain; in others the pain is intermittent—either spontaneously or precipitated by certain movements or pressure on the testis. There is usually no sexual dysfunction associated with chronic orchialgia (Davis et al 1990, U Wesselmann and AL Burnett, unpublished observation).

A careful history, physical examination, urological evaluation, and selected imaging studies will uncover most secondary causes of chronic testicular pain. For the physician evaluating a patient with chronic testicular pain it is important to understand the nerve supply of the testis, so that the diagnostic evaluation can be guided by the functional neuroanatomy including the referred pain pattern (see Fig. 12.1). However, in many cases the patients present with a completely normal physical examination of the scrotum, testis, epididymis, and spermatic cord. The pain remains unexplained despite a very thorough diagnostic work-up (Davis et al 1990). Secondary causes of chronic orchialgia include infection, tumour, testicular torsion, varicocele, hydrocele, spermatocele, trauma (such as a bicycle accident), and previous surgical interventions (Davis et al 1990, Costabile et al 1991). Testicular pain can be a sign of referred pain from the ureter or hip (Goldberg and Witchell 1988, Holland et al 1994) or from entrapment neuropathies of the ilioinguinal or genitofemoral nerve (Yeates 1985, Bennini 1992). There have been case reports about referred testicular pain from aneurysms of the common iliac artery or aorta due to pressure on the genitofemoral nerve (Ali 1983, McGee 1993); however, usually this pain is acute rather than chronic. Testicular pain can be due to intervertebral disc protrusion (White and Leslie 1986). Neuropathic testicular pain has been described in men with diabetic neuropathy (Hagen 1993). Vasectomy can result in chronic orchialgia and is probably far more common than realized (Selikowitz and Schned 1985, McCormack 1988, McMahon et al 1992, Hayden 1993). It has been hypothesized that this postvasectomy pain syndrome is due to impairment of the genital branch of the genitofemoral nerve by sperm granuloma (Yeates 1985), but others have questioned this theory (Silber 1981, McCormack 1988). Chronic testicular pain can be one of the symptoms of retroperitoneal fibrosis, usually associated with abdominal pain and low back pain (Mitchinson 1972, Baker et al 1987). There are two case reports in the neurological literature describing episodic testicular pain as a manifestation of epilepsy (York et al 1979, Bhaskar 1987). Schneiderman and Voytovich (1988) reported a patient who was overly concerned about developing testicular cancer and palpated his testis numerous times per day, resulting in 'self-palpation orchitis'.

The diagnostic work-up should include a thorough urological evaluation. If the urological evaluation is unrevealing, further gastroenterological evaluations may be necessary to rule out referred pain from the lower pelvic organs and evaluation for hernia. Ekberg et al (1988) suggested herniography to evaluate for an occult hernia in patients who present with testicular pain. A neurological evaluation is directed towards the lumbosacral roots, the ilioinguinal, genitofemoral, pelvic, and pudendal nerves. Placebo-controlled nerve blocks with local anaesthetic may help to differentiate which nerves are mediating the chronic pain problem. A discogram might be helpful to assess whether a protruding disc is the cause of the pain problem. A psychological evaluation should be included in a multidisciplinary comprehensive work-up to assess for depression or other psychological issues. It is important to be aware that in nearly 25% of patients, despite thorough evaluations, no aetiology of the pain can be found (Davis et al 1990).

The treatment of chronic testicular pain is directed towards the underlying aetiology, if one can be found. We agree with Holland et al (1994) that hydrocele, varicocele, or spermatocele usually are not the cause of chronic testicular pain, but a coincidental finding. We have seen many patients with chronic testicular pain (U Wesselmann and AL Burnett, unpublished observation) who had previously undergone testicular surgery for these conditions without any pain relief. It is important that the physician is not impelled by the lack of findings to institute more invasive procedures in an effort to find a non-existent pathological condition (Costabile et al 1991). Drastic surgical procedures have been recommended for the treatment of chronic orchialgia, including epididymectomy (Davis et al 1990, Chen and Ball 1991) and orchiectomy (Davis et al 1990). Several studies recently suggested microsurgical denervation of the spermatic cord as an alternative to orchiectomy for chronic testicular pain (Choa and Swami 1992, Levine et al 1996). However, before any invasive and irreversible measures are considered for pain relief, medical pain management should be attempted. Traditionally, urologists prescribed only a trial of antibiotics and NSAIDs for men presenting with chronic testicular pain, with the aim of treating a possible occult inflammatory process (Davis et al 1990). Clinical reports indicate that medications used for other chronic pain syndromes (Galer 1995), such as low-dose antidepressants, anticonvulsants, membrane-stabilizing agents, and opiates, often result in excellent pain relief in patients with chronic testicular pain (Costabile et al 1991, Hagen 1993, Hayden 1993, Wesselmann et al 1996). TENS might be helpful (Hayden 1993, Holland et al 1994). The testes receive a rich sympathetic innervation, and sympatholytic procedures such as a lumbar sympathetic block with local anaesthetic or phentolamine infusions have resulted in marked pain relief in a subgroup of men with chronic testicular pain (Wesselmann et al 1995, Wesselmann and Burnett 1996).

Prostatodynia (chronic prostatitis/chronic pelvic pain syndrome)

Prostatodynia is defined as persistent complaints of urinary urgency, dysuria, poor urinary flow, and perineal discomfort, without evidence of bacteria or purulence in the prostatic fluid (Drach et al 1978). Patients report pain in the perineum, lower back, suprapubic area, and groin, as well as pain on ejaculation. They typically range from 20 to 60 years of age (Moul 1993). Often the term 'prostatitis' is used to describe any unexplained symptom or condition that might possibly originate from the prostate gland (Nickel 1998). In the USA approximately 25% of all office visits of male patients for genitourinary tract problems are diagnosed with prostatitis (Lipsky 1989, Meares 1992). The National Institutes of Health (Nickel et al 1999) recently established research guidelines for chronic prostatitis and defined four categories of prostatitis:

1. acute bacterial prostatitis
2. chronic bacterial prostatitis
3. chronic prostatitis/chronic pelvic pain syndrome
   A. inflammatory
   B. non-inflammatory
4. asymptomatic inflammatory prostatitis.

These revised definitions have incorporated and replaced the old term 'prostatodynia' (Drach et al 1978) with the category chronic prostatitis/chronic pelvic pain syndrome. Prostatodynia accounts for approximately 30% of patients presenting with prostatitis (Brunner et al 1983).

On physical examination the prostate is typically normal with no sign of tenderness on palpation (Orland et al 1985). A thorough urological evaluation should include urinalysis, urine culture, urine cytology, and urethral cultures (de la Rosette et al 1992). In selected patients urodynamic evaluation should be performed, because several studies have demonstrated detrusor striated sphincter dyssynergy, abnormalities in urethral closing pressure, and urethral narrowing in patients with prostatodynia (Segura et al 1979, Barbalias et al 1983, Barbalias 1990). Prostatodynia is a diagnosis of exclusion, where it is assumed that the chronic pain syndrome is related to the prostate, but no inflammatory prostatic process can be identified. It is important to consider in the differential diagnosis other diseases that can mimic prostatodynia. A gastroenterological examination is indicated if referred pain from the colon or rectum is suspected. The neurological examination is directed towards the nerve supply of the prostate (Fig. 12.1). Osteitis pubis, a well-recognized disease in active participants in strenuous sports and exercises, can mimic prostatodynia. Pelvic X-ray and bone scan confirm the diagnosis of osteitis pubis (Buck et al 1982). In some patients prostatodynia is one of the presenting symptoms of interstitial cystitis (see above).

Various medical and invasive treatment options have been suggested for patients with prostatodynia, most of which are anecdotal reports. Despite the fact that in patients with prostatodynia no infection can be demonstrated (Brunner et al 1983), the most frequently advocated treatment is antibiotics, probably based on the assumption that there might be an infection that is undiagnosed. De la Rosette et al (1992) reviewed the diagnostic and therapeutic results of 409 patients diagnosed with pain from the prostate: antibiotic treatment resulted in the relief of complaints in 36% of the patients and cure in 24%. Interestingly, however, similar results were found, even if no antibiotic was administered: 32% of the patients reported relief and 30% reported cure. As the urodynamic abnormalities observed in some patients with prostatodynia suggest increased sympathetic activity (Barbalias et al 1983), treatment with oral α-adrenergic blockers to improve the voiding abnormalities as well as the pain has been proposed. Prazosin, terazosin, and doxazosin are the most frequently used agents (Orland et al 1985, Moul 1993, Barbalias et al 1998), but their use is often limited by side effects, most frequently hypotension.

In cases where a functional urinary outlet obstruction can be documented on urodynamic testing, retrograde transurethral balloon dilatation of the prostate has been suggested. This resulted in marked improvement of the voiding symptomatology but no results were given regarding the effect on the pain scores (Lopatin et al 1990). Transurethral microwave hyperthermia has been suggested for non-bacterial prostatitis and prostatodynia (Montorsi et al 1993, Nickel and Sorenson 1994). Pain relief has been reported with pelvic floor relaxation techniques (Segura et al 1979) and muscle-relaxing medications (Moul 1993).

Penile pain

In contrast to other chronic pain syndromes of the genitourinary tract, chronic penile pain seems to be extremely rare. If a patient presents with persistent penile pain, the pain can usually be treated by treating the underlying disease (paraphimosis, priapism, Peyronie's disease, herpes genitalis—see Gee et al 1990). One of the most frequently reported acute penile pain events is the intracavernous injection of drugs for the treatment of erectile dysfunction (Godschalk et al 1996). Acute penile pain has been examined with regards to penile prosthesis (Althof et al 1987, Pedersen et al 1988, Tiefer et al 1988). Patients undergoing penile prostheses surgery report that postoperative pain is one of the most negative sequelae of surgery (Tiefer et al 1988). However, there are no reports indicating that a chronic pain syndrome develops after these acute noxious events. Also, surgical trauma to the penis such as occurs during routine circumcision does not seem to result in a chronic penile pain syndrome. A case report in the British literature described a man with recurrent penile pain attacks (Corder 1989). Physical examination revealed an inguinal hernia, which was surgically repaired. No recurrence of his episodic penile pain attacks was reported, and it was hypothesized that the penile pain in this case was due to irritation of the ilioinguinal nerve in the inguinal canal, which supplies the ventral base of the penis. Pudendal nerve injury in men results in sensory loss over the shaft and bulb of the penis and difficulty with erection, but persistent pain associated with the nerve injury has not been reported (Goodson 1981, Hofmann et al 1982).

Perineal pain

Perineal pain can be part of one of the more specific genitourinary pain syndromes discussed here, such as interstitial cystitis, urethral syndrome, clitoral pain, vulvodynia, testicular pain, or prostatodynia, all of which might present with pain radiating into the perineal region. However, often chronic perineal pain is an entity of its own, although poorly defined. The differential diagnosis of chronic perineal pain is extensive: gastroenterological, proctological, urological, gynaecological, and neurological pathology needs to be excluded. Systemic diseases associated with painful peripheral neuropathies such as diabetes mellitus or AIDS can present with perineal pain. French studies report pudendal nerve entrapment in up to 91% of patients with perineal pain referred to a pain clinic (Bensignor et al 1996). Surgical neurolysis-transposition resulted in pain improvement in 67% of the patients (Robert et al 1993). The best results were seen in patients where the pudendal nerve entrapment was diagnosed early. Local anaesthetic blocks of the pudendal nerve and electromyography and nerve conduction studies of the pelvic floor might be helpful to confirm the diagnosis (Beck et al 1994). Imaging studies of the thoracolumbosacral spine can be considered if there is suspicion of rare cases of meningeal cysts (Van De Kleft and Van Vyve 1993) or meningiomas (Pagni and Canavero 1993) resulting in perineal pain. Surgical resection of sacral meningeal cysts has been reported to result in complete resolution of symptoms in 10/12 patients with perineal pain (Van de Kleft and Van Vyve 1993). Rare cases of perineal pain caused by plexiform neurofibromas involving the nerves of the perineum have been reported (Batta et al 1989). Ford et al (1994, 1996) reported perineal pain as a symptom of movement disorders.

Psychological aspects of chronic genitourinary pain

As with other chronic pain syndromes in the absence of obvious organic pathology, many theories regarding a psychogenic origin of chronic non-malignant genitourinary pain have been entertained (see Wesselmann et al 1997 for review). The location of pain may be a significant predictor for appraisals of pain, affective response, and disclosure of pain complaints. This is likely to play an important role in pain syndromes of the genitourinary region, an area often considered taboo. It is not surprising that subjects asked to imagine pain in their genitals reported that they would be least likely to disclose genital pain and would be more worried, depressed, and embarrassed by pain in the genitals than in all other areas. They appraised themselves more ill than if they were asked to imagine chest, stomach, head, or mouth pain (Klonoff et al 1993). Preliminary psychological research has been published on most of the genitourinary pain syndromes; however most studies have suffered from lack of adequate control groups, retrospective design, lack of standardized measures, small sample size, and samples with significant self-selection factors. Of major concern is that most studies have neglected to assess whether the psychological findings in patients with genitourinary pain were likely to be pre-existing or reactive (see Wesselmann et al 1997 for review). While the traditional psychosocial view of the sexual pain disorders has focused on sexual and marital issues, conflicts and experiences and has tried to dichotomize aetiology between psychological and physiological factors, a pain-centred approach focusing on the major symptom of these problems, the pain, has been suggested in the recent psychological literature (Binik et al 1999). Further, a history of sexual and physical abuse has been associated with a variety of pain syndromes (Kinzl et al 1995), and that association appears to be especially strong with chronic gynaecological pain (Walker and Stenchever 1993). However, these studies may wrongly assume cause and effect between abuse history and the development of chronic pain. Often sexual and physical abuse are symptoms of multiproblem families, characterized by chaos, alcohol and substance abuse, and general neglect, which results in children not being adequately protected. A recent prospective study, aimed at determining whether childhood victimization increases risk for adult pain complaints, indicated that the relationship between childhood victimization and pain symptoms in adulthood is more complex than previously assumed. The odds of reporting unexplained pain symptoms was not associated with childhood victimization; however, it was significantly associated with retrospective self-reports of all specific types of childhood victimization (Raphael et al 2001).

Conclusion

Chronic genitourinary pain syndromes are well described but poorly understood. Patients with chronic genitourinary pain have often suffered for many years and have frequently seen multiple physicians and undergone endless tests without finding a cure or even a diagnosis. A specific secondary cause can only be identified in the minority of patients. For the physician who is consulted by a patient with genitourinary pain, it is important to be familiar with these pain syndromes of body areas that are often considered taboo. The approach to the patient begins with acknowledging that the genitourinary pain syndromes are well described, searching for a secondary cause, and performing a careful physical and psychological evaluation. It is usually very reassuring for the patient to learn that he/she is suffering from a well-described pain syndrome and is not the only case with this syndrome. Some patients present with more than one genitourinary pain syndrome (e.g., interstitial cystitis and vulvodynia). It has been suggested that this might be due to a generalized disorder of urogenital sinus-derived epithelium (Fitzpatrick et al 1993). Realizing the extensive convergence of visceral afferent input on the spinal cord level and in the neuronal plexuses in the pelvis demonstrated in animal studies (Wesselmann 1987, Jänig et al 1991, Cervero 1994, Wesselmann and Lai 1997), it would not be surprising if a chronic pain syndrome in one area of the genitourinary tract could trigger the development of chronic pain and dysfunction in another area of the genitourinary system. Although complete cures are uncommon, some pain relief can be provided to almost all patients using a multidisciplinary approach including pain medications, local treatment regimens, local anaesthetic techniques, physical therapy, and psychological approaches, all the while exercising caution towards invasive and irreversible therapeutic procedures.

The aetiology of most genitourinary pain syndromes is not known and further research is desperately needed. These areas of the body, which are often considered taboo in our society, have been largely neglected in neuroanatomical, neurophysiological, and neuropharmacological research. Current treatment approaches are empirical only. Better knowledge of the underlying pathophysiological mechanisms of chronic genitourinary pain will allow the development of treatment strategies specifically targeted against the pathophysiological mechanisms.

Acknowledgments

Ursula Wesselmann is supported by NIH Grants NS36553 (NINDS, Office of Research for Women's Health), HD39699 (NICHD), and DK57315 (NIDDK). Arthur L Burnett is supported by NIH Grant DK02568 (NIDDK).

References

Aber GM, Higgins PM 1982 The natural history and management of the loin pain/haematuria syndrome. British Journal of Urology 54: 613–615

Ali MS 1983 Testicular pain in a patient with aneurysm of the common iliac artery. British Journal of Urology 55: 447–448

Allan JDD, Bultitude MI, Bultitude MF, Wall PD, McMahon SB 1997 The effect of capsaicin on renal pain signaling systems in humans and Wistar rats. Journal of Physiology 505: 39P

Althof SE, Turner LA, Levine SB et al 1987 Intracavernosal injection in the treatment of impotence: a prospective study of sexual, psychological, and marital functioning. Journal of Sex and Marital Therapy 13: 155–167

Baker LR, Mallinson WJ, Gregory MC et al 1987 Idiopathic retroperitoneal fibrosis. A retrospective analysis of 60 cases. British Journal of Urology 60: 497–503

Barbalias GA 1990 Prostatodynia or painful male urethral syndrome? Urology 36: 146–153

Barbalias GA, Meares EM Jr, Sant GR 1983 Prostatodynia: clinical and urodynamic characteristics. Journal of Urology 130: 514–517

Barbalias GA, Nikiforidis G, Liatsikos EN 1998 Alpha-blockers for the treatment of chronic prostatitis in combination with antibiotics. Journal of Urology 159: 883–887

Barker SB, Matthews PN, Philip PF, Williams G 1987 Prospective study of intravesical dimethyl sulphoxide in the treatment of chronic inflammatory bladder disease. British Journal of Urology 59: 142–144

Baskin LS, Tanagho EA 1992 Pain without pelvic organs. Journal of Urology 147: 683–686

Batta AG, Gundian JC, Myers RP 1989 Neurofibromatosis presenting as perineal pain and urethral burning. Urology 33: 138–140

Beck R, Fowler CJ, Mathias CJ 1994 Genitourinary dysfunction in disorders of the autonomic nervous system. In: Rushton DN (ed) Handbook of neuro-urology. Marcel Dekker, New York, pp 281–301

Bennini A 1992 Die Ilioinguinalis- und Genitofemoralisneuralgie. Schweizerische Rundschau der Medizin 81: 1114–1120

Bensignor MF, Labat JJ, Robert R, Ducrot P 1996 Diagnostic and therapeutic pudendal nerve blocks for patients with perineal non-malignant pain. Abstract, 8th World Congress on Pain, p 56

Berger RE, Miller JE, Rothman I, Krieger JN, Muller CH 1998 Bladder petechiae after cystoscopy and hydrodistension in men diagnosed with prostate pain. Journal of Urology 159: 83–85

Bergeron S, Bouchard C, Fortier M, Binik YM, Khalife S 1997 The surgical treatment of vulvar vestibulitis syndrome: a follow-up study. Journal of Sex and Marital Therapy 23: 317–325

Bergeron S, Binik YM, Khalife S, Pagidas K, Glazer HI, Meana M, Amsel R 2001 A randomized comparison of group-cognitive behavioral therapy, surface electromyographic biofeedback, and vestibulectomy in the treatment of dyspareunia resulting from vulvar vestibulitis. Pain 91: 297–306

Bergman A, Karram M, Bhatia NN 1989 Urethral syndrome: a comparison of different treatment modalities. Journal of Reproductive Medicine 34: 157–160

Bhaskar PA 1987 Scrotal pain with testicular jerking: an unusual manifestation of epilepsy. Journal of Neurology, Neurosurgery and Psychiatry 50: 1233–1234

Binik YM, Meana M, Berkley K, Khalife S 1999 The sexual pain disorders: is the pain sexual or is the sex painful. Annual Reviews of Sex Research 10: 210–235

Bohm-Starke N, Hilliges M, Falconer C, Rylander E 1998 Increased intraepithelial innervation in women with vulvar vestibulitis syndrome. Gynecologic and Obstetric Investigation 46: 256–260

Bohm-Starke N, Hilliges M, Brodda-Jansen G, Rylander E, Torebjörk E 2001 Psychophysical evidence of nociceptor sensitization in vulvar vestibulitis syndrome. Pain 94: 177–183

Briggs LA 1998 Female circumcision in Nigeria—is it not time for government intervention. Health Care Analysis 6: 14–23

Brunner H, Weidner W, Schiefer HC 1983 Studies on the role of *Ureaplasma urealyticum* and *Mycoplasma hominis* in prostatitis. Journal of Infectious Diseases 126: 807–813

Buck AC, Crean M, Jenkins IL 1982 Osteitis pubis as a mimic of prostatic pain. British Journal of Urology 54: 741–744

Bultitude MI 1995 Capsaicin in treatment of loin pain/haematuria syndrome. Lancet 345: 921–922

Bultitude M, Young J, Bultitude M, Allan J 1998 Loin pain haematuria syndrome: distress resolved by pain relief. Pain 76: 209–213

Burden RP, Booth LJ, Ockenden BG, Boyd WN, Higgins P McR, Aber GM 1975 Intrarenal vascular changes in adult patients with recurrent haematuria and loin pain: a clinical, histological and angiographic study. Quarterly Journal of Medicine 175: 433–447

Burnett AL, Wesselmann U 1999 Neurobiology of the pelvis and perineum: Principles for a practical approach. Journal of Pelvic Surgery 5: 224–232

Carson CC, Segura JW, Osborne DM 1980 Evaluation and treatment of the female urethral syndrome. Journal of Urology 124: 609–610

Cervero F 1994 Sensory innervation of the viscera: peripheral basis of visceral pain. Physiological Reviews 74: 95–138

Chaiken DC, Blaivas JG, Blaivas ST 1993 Behavioral therapy for the treatment of refractory interstitial cystitis. Journal of Urology 149: 1445–1448

Chen TF, Ball RY 1991 Epididymectomy for post-vasectomy pain: histological review. British Journal of Urology 68: 407–413

Childs SJ 1994 Dimethyl sulfone in the treatment of interstitial cystitis. Urologic Clinics of North America 21: 85–88

Choa RG, Swami KS 1992 Testicular denervation: a new surgical procedure for intractable testicular pain. British Journal of Urology 70: 417–419

Corder AP 1989 Penile pain and direct inguinal hernia. British Journal of Hospital Medicine 42: 238

Costabile RA, Hahn M, McLeod DG 1991 Chronic orchialgia in the pain prone patient: the clinical perspective. Journal of Urology 146: 1571–1574

Curhan GC, Speizer FE, Hunter DJ, Curhan SG, Stampfer MJ 1999 Epidemiology of interstitial cystitis: a population based study. Journal of Urology 161: 549–552

Davis BE, Noble MJ, Weigel JW, Foret J, Mebust WK 1990 Analysis and management of chronic testicular pain. Journal of Urology 143: 936–939

Davis DM 1955 Vesicle orifice obstruction in women and its treatment by transurethral resection. Journal of Urology 73: 112–117

De Deus JM, Focchi J, Stavale JN, De Lima GR 1995 Histologic and biomolecular aspects of papillomatosis of the vulvar vestibule in relation to human papillomavirus. Obstetrics and Gynecology 86: 758–763

De Groat WC 1994 Neurophysiology of the pelvic organs. In: Rushton DN (ed) Handbook of neuro-urology. Marcel Dekker, New York, pp 55–93

De Groat WC, Booth AM, Yoshimura N 1993 Neurophysiology of micturition and its modification in animal models of human disease. In: Maggi CA (ed) Nervous control of the urogenital system. Harwood Academic, Chur, Switzerland, pp 227–290

De la Rosette JJMCH, Hubregtse MR, Karhaus HFM, Debruyne FMJ 1992 Results of a questionnaire among Dutch urologists and general practitioners concerning diagnostics and treatment of patients with prostatitis syndrome. European Journal of Urology 22: 14–19

Dirie MA, Lindmark G 1992 The risk of medical complications after female circumcision. East African Medical Journal 69: 479–482

Drach GW, Fair WR, Meares EM, Stamey TA 1978 Classification of benign diseases associated with prostatic pain: prostatitis or prostatodynia? Journal of Urology 120: 266

Editorial 1992 Loin pain/haematuria syndrome. Lancet 340: 701–702

Ekberg O, Abrahamsson P-A, Kesek P 1988 Inguinal hernia in urological patients: the value of herniography. Journal of Urology 139: 1253–1255

Elbadawi A 1996 Functional anatomy of the organs of micturition. Urologic Clinics of North America 23: 177–210

Elbadawi A 1997 Interstitial cystitis: a critique of current concepts with a new proposal for pathologic diagnosis and pathogenesis. Urology 49: 14–40

Fall M, Lindstrom S 1994 Transcutaneous electrical nerve stimulation in classic and nonulcer interstitial cystitis. Urologic Clinics of North America 21: 131–139

Ferguson M, Bell C 1993 Autonomic innervation of the kidney and ureter. In: Maggi C A (ed) Nervous control of the urogenital system. Harwood Academic, Chur, Switzerland, pp 1–31

Fitzpatrick CC, Delancey JOL, Elkins TE, McGuire EJ 1993 Vulvar vestibulitis and interstitial cystitis: a disorder of urogenital sinus-derived epithelium? Obstetrics and Gynaecology 81: 860–862

Fleischmann J 1994 Calcium channel antagonists in the treatment of interstitial cystitis. Urologic Clinics of North America 21: 107–112

Ford B, Greene P, Fahn S 1994 Oral and genital tardive pain syndromes. Neurology 44: 2115–2119

Ford B, Louis ED, Greene P, Fahn S 1996 Oral and genital pain syndromes in Parkinson's disease. Movement Disorders 11: 421–426

Fowler JE 1981 Prospective study of intravesical dimethyl sulphoxide in treatment of suspected early interstitial cystitis. Urology 18: 21–26

Fritjofsson A, Fall M, Juhlin R, Persson E, Ruutu M 1987 Treatment of ulcer and nonulcer interstitial cystitis with sodium pentosanpolyphosphate: a multicenter trial. Journal of Urology 138: 508–512

Galer BS 1995 Neuropathic pain of peripheral origin: advances in pharmacologic treatment. Neurology 45: S17–S25

Gallagher DJA, Montgomerie JZ, North JDK 1965 Acute infections of the urinary tract and the urethral syndrome in general practice. British Medical Journal 1: 622–626

Gee WF, Ansell JS, Bonica JJ 1990 Pelvic and perineal pain of urologic origin. In: Bonica JJ (ed) The management of pain, vol 2. Lea & Febiger, Philadelphia, pp 1368–1394

Geirsson G, Wang YG, Lindstrom S, Fall M 1993 Traditional acupuncture and electrical stimulation of the posterior tibial nerve. A trial in chronic interstitial cystitis. Scandinavian Journal of Urology and Nephrology 27: 67–70

Glazer HI, Rodke G, Swencionis C, Hertz R, Young A W 1995 Treatment of vulvar vestibulitis syndrome with electromyographic biofeedback of pelvic floor musculature. Journal of Reproductive Medicine 40: 283–290

Godschalk M, Gheorghiu D, Katz PG, Mulligan T 1996 Alkalization does not alleviate penile pain induced by intracavernous injection of prostaglandin E1. Journal of Urology 156: 999–1000

Goetsch MF 1991 Vulvar vestibulitis: prevalence and historic features in a general gynecologic practice population. American Journal of Obstetrics and Gynecology 164: 1609–1616

Goetsch MF 1996 Simplified surgical revision of the vulvar vestibule for vulvar vestibulitis. American Journal of Obstetrics and Gynecology 174: 1701–1707

Goldberg SD, Witchell SJ 1988 Right testicular pain: unusual presentation of obstruction of the ureteropelvic junction. Canadian Journal of Surgery 31: 246–247

Goodson JD 1981 Pudendal neuritis from biking. New England Journal of Medicine 304: 365

Hagen NA 1993 Sharp, shooting neuropathic pain in the rectum or genitals: pudendal neuralgia. Journal of Pain and Symptom Management 8: 496–501

Hanly MG, Ojeda VJ 1995 Epidermic inclusion cysts of the clitoris as a complication of female circumcision and pharaonic infibulation. Central African Journal of Medicine 41: 22–24

Hanno PM 1994 Diagnosis of interstitial cystitis. Urologic Clinics of North America 21: 63–66

Hanno PM 1997 Analysis of long-term elmiron therapy for interstitial cystitis. Urology 49: 93–99

Hanno PM, Ratner V, Sant G, Wein AJ (eds) 2001 Interstitial cystitis 2001: an evolving clinical syndrome. Urology 57 (suppl 6a)

Harlow BL, Wise LA, Stewart EG 2001 Prevalence and predictors of lower genital tract discomfort. American Journal of Obstetrics and Gynecology 185: 545–550

Harris SH, Harris RGS 1930 Sympathicotonus, renal pain and renal sympathectomy. British Journal of Urology 2: 367–374

Hayden LJ 1993 Chronic testicular pain. Australian Family Physician 22: 1357–1365

Hofmann A, Jones RE, Schoenvogel R 1982 Pudendal nerve neurapraxia as a result of traction on the fracture table. Journal of Bone and Joint Surgery 64: 136–138

Holland JM, Feldman JL, Gilbert HC 1994 Phantom orchalgia. Journal of Urology 152: 2291–2293

Irwin PP, Galloway NTM 1994 Surgical management of interstitial cystitis. Urologic Clinics of North America 21: 145–152

Jänig W, Koltzenburg M 1993 Pain arising from the urogenital tract. In: Maggi CA (ed) Nervous control of the urogenital system. Harwood Academic, Chur, Switzerland, pp 525–578

Jänig W, Schmidt M, Schnitzler A, Wesselmann U 1991 Differentiation of sympathetic neurones projecting in the hypogastric nerve in terms of their discharge patterns in cats. Journal of Physiology (London) 437: 157–179

Jepsen JV, Sall M, Rhodes PR, Schmid D, Messing E, Bruskewitz RC 1998 Long-term experience with pentosanpolysulfate in interstitial cystitis. Urology 51: 381–387

Jeremias J, Ledger WJ, Witkin SS 2000 Interleukin 1 receptor antagonist gene polymorphism in women with vulvar vestibulitis. American Journal of Obstetrics and Gynecology 182: 283–285

Johansson SL, Fall M 1994 Pathology of interstitial cystitis. Urologic Clinics of North America 21: 55–62

Jones CA, Nyberg LM 1997 Epidemiology of interstitial cystitis. Urology 49: 2–9

Kaplan WE, Firlit CF, Schoenberg HW 1980 The female urethral syndrome: external sphincter spasm as etiology. Journal of Urology 124: 48–49

Keay SK, Zhang C-O, Shoenfelt J, Erickson DR, Whitmore K, Warren JW, Marvel R, Chai T 2001 Sensitivity and specificity of antiproliferative factor, heparin-binding epidermal growth factor-like growth factor, and epidermal growth factor as urine markers for interstitial cystitis. Urology 57 (Suppl 6A): 9–14

Kinzl JF, Traweger C, Biebl W 1995 Family background and sexual abuse associated with somatization. Psychotherapy and Psychosomatics 64: 82–87

Klonoff EA, Landrine H, Brown M 1993 Appraisal and response to pain may be a function of its bodily location. Journal of Psychosomatic Research 37: 661–670

Laumann EO, Paik A, Rosen RC 1999 Sexual dysfunction in the United States. Prevalence and Predictors. Journal of American Medical Association 281: 537–544

Levine LA, Matkov TG, Lubenow TR 1996 Microsurgical denervation of the spermatic cord: a surgical alternative in the treatment of chronic orchialgia. Journal of Urology 155: 1005–1007

Lincoln J, Burnstock G 1993 Autonomic innervation of the urinary bladder and urethra. In: Maggi CA (ed) Nervous control of the urogenital system. Harwood Academic, Chur, Switzerland, pp 33–68

Lipsky BA 1989 Urinary tract infections in men. Annals of Internal Medicine 110: 138

Little PJ, Sloper JS, de Wardener HE 1967 A syndrome of loin pain and haematuria associated with disease of peripheral renal arteries. Quarterly Journal of Medicine 36: 253–259

Lopatin WB, Martynik M, Hickey DP, Vivas C, Hakala TR 1990 Retrograde transurethral balloon dilation of prostate: innovative management of abacterial chronic prostatitis and prostadynia. Urology 36: 508–510

Lynch PJ 1986 Vulvodynia: a syndrome of unexplained vulvar pain, psychologic disability and sexual dysfunction. Journal of Reproductive Medicine 31: 773–780

Mabry EW, Carson CC, Older RA 1981 Evaluation of women with chronic voiding discomfort. Urology 18: 244–246

Malloy TR, Shanberg AM 1994 Laser therapy for interstitial cystitis. Urologic Clinics of North America 21: 141–144

McCormack M 1988 Physiologic consequences and complications of vasectomy. Canadian Medical Association Journal 138: 223–225

McGee SR 1993 Referred scrotal pain: case reports and review. Journal of General Internal Medicine 8: 694–701

McKay M 1984 Burning vulva syndrome. Journal of Reproductive Medicine 29: 457

McKay M 1988 Subsets of vulvodynia. Journal of Reproductive Medicine 33: 695–698

McKay M 1989 Vulvodynia. A multifactorial problem. Archives of Dermatology 125: 256–262

McKenna KD, Nadelhaft I 1986 The organization of the pudendal nerve in the male and female cat. Journal of Comparative Neurology 248: 532–549

McMahon AJ, Buckley J, Taylor A, LLoyd SN, Deane RF, Kirk D 1992 Chronic testicular pain following vasectomy. British Journal of Urology 69: 188–191

Meares EMJ 1992 Prostatitis and related disorders. In: Walsh PC, Retik AB, Stanley TA, Vaughan EDJ (eds) Campbell's urology, 6th edn. Saunders, Philadelphia, pp 807–822

Messing E, Pauk D, Schaeffer A et al 1997 Associations among cystoscopic findings and symptoms and physical examination findings in women enrolled in the interstitial cystitis data base study. Urology 49: 81–85

Messinger EM 1992 Urethral syndrome. In: Walsh PC, Retik AB, Stanley TA, Vaughan EDJ (eds) Campbell's urology, 6th edn. Saunders, Philadelphia, pp 997–1005

Miller JL, Rothman I, Bavendam TG, Berger RE 1995 Prostatodynia and interstitial cystitis: one and the same? Urology 45: 587–589

Mitchinson MJ 1972 Some clinical aspects of idiopathic retroperitoneal fibrosis. British Journal of Surgery 59: 58–60

Mobley DF, Baum N 1996 Interstitial cystitis: when urgency and frequency mean more than routine inflammation. Postgraduate Medicine 99: 201–208

Montorsi F, Guazzoni G, Bergamaschi F et al 1993 Is there a role for transrectal microwave hyperthermia of the prostate in the treatment of abacterial prostatitis and prostatodynia. Prostate 22: 139–146

Morales A, Emerson L, Nickel JC 1997 Intravesical hyaluronic acid in the treatment of refractory interstitial cystitis. Urology 49: 111–113

Morrison JFB 1987 Role of higher levels of the central nervous system. In: Torrens M, Morrison JFB (eds) The physiology of the lower urinary tract. Springer-Verlag, London, pp 237–274

Moul JW 1993 Prostatitis: sorting out the different causes. Postgraduate Medicine 94: 191–194

Nickel JC 1998 Prostatitis—myths and realities. Urology 51: 363–366

Nickel JC, Sorenson R 1994 Transurethral microwave thermotherapy of nonbacterial prostatitis and prostatodynia: initial experience. Urology 44: 458–460

Nickel JC, Nyberg LM, Hennenfent M 1999 Research guidelines for chronic prostatitis: consensus report from the first National Institutes of Health International Prostatitis Collaborative Network. Urology 54: 229–233

Nigro DA, Wein AJ, Foy M et al 1997 Associations among cystoscopic and urodynamic findings for women enrolled in the interstitial cystitis data base study. Urology 49: 86–92

Orland SM, Hanno PM, Wein AJ 1985 Prostatitis, prostatosis, and prostatodynia. Urology 25: 439–459

Paavonen J 1995a Diagnosis and treatment of vulvodynia. Annals of Medicine 27: 175–181

Paavonen J 1995b Vulvodynia—a complex syndrome of vulvar pain. Acta Obstetricia et Gynecologica Scandinavica 74: 243–247

Pagni CA, Canavero S 1993 Paroxysmal perineal pain resembling tic douloureux, only symptom of a dorsal meningioma. Italian Journal of Neurological Sciences 14: 323–324

Parkin J, Shea C, Sant GR 1997 Intravesical dimethyl sulfoxide for interstitial cystitis—a practical approach. Urology 49: 105–107

Parsons CL 1997 Epithelial coating techniques in the treatment of interstitial cystitis. Urology 49: 100–104
Pedersen B, Tiefer L, Ruiz M, Melman A 1988 Evaluation of patients and partners 1 to 4 years after penile prosthesis surgery. Journal of Urology 139: 956–958
Peeker R, Aldenborg F, Fall M 1998 The treatment of interstitial cystitis with supratrigonal cystectomy and ileocystoplasty—difference in outcome between classic and nonulcer disease. Journal of Urology 159: 1479–1482
Peters-Gee JM 1998 Bladder and urethral syndromes. In: Steege JF, Metzger DA, Levy BS (eds) Chronic pelvic pain. Saunders, Philadelphia, pp 197–204
Pontari MA, Hanno PM, Wein AJ 1997 Logical and systematic approach to the evaluation and management of patients suspected of having interstitial cystitis. Urology 49: 114
Pozzi SJ 1897 Traite de gynecologie clinique et operatoire. Masson, Paris
Pranikoff K, Constantino G 1998 The use of amitriptyline in patients with urinary frequency and pain. Urology 51 (suppl 5A): 179–181
Raphael KG, Spatz Widom C, Lange G 2001 Childhood victimization and pain in adulthood: a prospective investigation. Pain 92: 283–293
Ratliff TL, Klutke CG, McDougall EM 1994 The etiology of interstitial cystitis. Urologic Clinics of North America 21: 21–30
Raz S, Smith RB 1976 External sphincter spasticity syndrome in female patients. Journal of Urology 115: 443–446
Robert R, Brunet C, Faure A et al 1993 La chirurgie du nerf pudental lors de certaines algies perineales: evolution et resultats. Chirurgie 119: 535–539
Sand PK, Bowen LW, Ostergard DR, Bent A, Panganibaum R 1989 Cryosurgery versus dilation and massage for treatment of recurrent urethral syndrome. Journal of Reproductive Medicine 34: 499–504
Sant GR, LaRock DR 1994 Standard intravesical therapies for interstitial cystitis. Urologic Clinics of North America 21: 73–84
Schmidt RA, Tanagho EA 1981 Urethral syndrome or urinary tract infection? Urology 18: 424–427
Schneiderman H, Voytovich A 1988 Self-palpation orchitis. Journal of General Internal Medicine 3: 97
Segura JW, Opitz JL, Greene LF 1979 Prostatosis, prostatitis or pelvic floor tension myalgia? Journal of Urology 122: 168–169
Selikowitz SM, Schned AR 1985 A late post-vasectomy syndrome. Journal of Urology 134: 494–497
Silber SJ 1981 Reversal of vasectomy and the treatment of male infertility: role of microsurgery, vasoepididymostomy, and pressure-induced changes of vasectomy. Urologic Clinics of North America 8: 53–62
Simmons JL, Bunce PL 1958 On the use of antihistamine in the treatment of interstitial cystitis. American Journal of Surgery 24: 664–667
Slade D, Ratner V, Chalker R 1997 A collaborative approach to managing interstitial cystitis. Urology 49: 10–13
Sonni L, Cattaneo A, De Marco A, De Magnis C, Carli P, Marabini S 1995 Idiopathic vulvodynia clinical evaluation of the pain threshold with acetic acid solutions. Journal of Reproductive Medicine 40: 337–341
Splatt AJ, Weedon D 1981 The urethral syndrome: morphological studies. British Journal of Urology 53: 263–265
Theoharides TC, Sant GR 1997 Hydroxyzine therapy for interstitial cystitis. Urology 49: 108–110
Theoharides TC, Kempuraj D, Sant GR 2001 Mast cell involvement in interstitial cystitis: a review of human and experimental evidence. Urology 57 (Suppl 6A): 47–55
Thomas TG (ed) 1880 Practical treatise on the diseases of woman. Henry C Lea's Son, Philadelphia, pp 145–147
Tiefer L, Pederson B, Melman A 1988 Psychosocial follow-up of penile prosthesis implant patients and partners. Journal of Sex and Marital Therapy 14: 184–201
Van de Kleft E, Van Vyve M 1993 Sacral meningeal cysts and perineal pain. Lancet 341: 500–501
Vodusek DB, Light JK 1983 The motor nerve supply of the external sphincter muscles: an electrophysiological study. Neurourology and Urodynamics 293: 193–200
Walker EA, Stenchever MA 1993 Sexual victimization and chronic pelvic pain. Obstetrics and Gynecology Clinics of North America 20: 795–807
Warren JW 1994 Interstitial cystitis as an infectious disease. Urologic Clinics of North America 21: 31–40
Weisberg LS, Bloom PB, Simmons RL, Viner ED 1993 Loin pain haematuria syndrome. American Journal of Nephrology 13: 229–237
Wesselmann U 1987 Untersuchungen der Impulsübertragung im Ganglion Mesentericum Inferius. Dissertation, Medizinische Fakultät der Christian-Albrechts-Universität zu Kiel, Germany, pp 1–244
Wesselmann U 2001 Interstitial cystitis: a chronic visceral pain syndrome. Urology 57 (suppl 6A): 32–39
Wesselmann U, Burnett AL 1996 Treatment of neuropathic testicular pain. Neurology 46 (suppl): 206
Wesselmann U, Lai J 1997 Mechanisms of referred visceral pain: uterine inflammation in the adult virgin rat results in neurogenic plasma extravasation in the skin. Pain 73: 309–317
Wesselmann U, Burnett AL, Campbell JN 1995 The role of the sympathetic nervous system in chronic visceral pain. Society for Neuroscience (Abstracts) 21: 1157
Wesselmann U, Burnett AL, Heinberg LJ 1996 Chronic testicular pain—a neuropathic pain syndrome: diagnosis and treatment. Abstract, 8th World Congress on Pain, p 256
Wesselmann U, Burnett AL, Heinberg LJ 1997 The urogenital and rectal pain syndromes. Pain 73: 269–294
Westrom LV, Willen R 1998 Vestibular nerve fiber proliferation in vulvar vestibulitis syndrome. Obstetrics and Gynecology 91: 572–576
White SH, Leslie IJ 1986 Pain in scrotum due to intervertebral disc protrusion. Lancet i: 504
Whitmore KE 1994 Self-care regimens for patients with interstitial cystitis. Urologic Clinics of North America 21: 121–130
Yeates WK 1985 Pain in the scrotum. British Journal of Hospital Medicine 33: 101–104
York GK, Gabor AJ, Dreyfus PM 1979 Paroxysmal genital pain: an unusual manifestation of epilepsy. Neurology 29: 516–519
Zimmern PE 1995 Hydrodistension in suspected interstitial cystitis patients: diagnosis and therapeutic benefits. Urology 153: 290A
Zufall R 1978 Ineffectiveness of treatment of urethral syndrome in women. Urology 12: 337–339
Zvieli S, Vinter L, Herman J 1989 Nonacute scrotal pain in adolescents. Journal of Family Practice 28: 226–228

Chapter 13

Orofacial pain

Yair Sharav

Introduction

The most prevalent pain in the orofacial region originates from the teeth and their surrounding structures and is summarized in Table 13.1. Temporomandibular disorders (TMD), subdivided into temporomandibular myofascial pain (TMP) and internal derangement of the temporomandibular joint, is another prevalent entity of orofacial pain. Primary vascular-type craniofacial pain is summarized in Table 13.2 and includes pains such as cluster headache, paroxysmal hemicrania, and a new diagnostic entity, vascular orofacial pain. The ill-defined atypical oral and facial pain is discussed next, including the 'burning mouth' syndrome (BMS), which is considered in detail. Finally, the differential diagnosis of orofacial pain is subclassified into pain associated with defined local injury and pain not related to defined injury and is summarized in Table 13.3.

Oral pain

Oral pain is most frequently associated with the teeth and their supporting structures, i.e., the periodontium. It is subdivided into dental, periodontal, gingival, and mucosal pain, and is summarized in Table 13.1. Usually, dental pain is a sequela of dental caries. Initially, when the carious lesion is confined to the dentine, the tooth is sensitive both to changes in temperature and to sweet substances. As the lesion penetrates deeper into the tooth, the pain produced by these stimuli becomes stronger and lasts longer. Eventually, when the carious lesion invades the tooth pulp, an inflammatory process develops (pulpitis) associated with acute, intermittent *spontaneous* pain. When microorganisms and products of tissue disintegration invade the area around the root apex (periapical periodontitis), the tooth becomes very sensitive to chewing, touch and percussion. At that stage the explosive, intermittent pain, typical of pulpitis, acquires a continuous boring nature and the tooth is no longer sensitive to changes in temperature. In clinical practice the demarcation between these various stages is sometimes indistinct; e.g., the tooth may be sensitive simultaneously to temperature changes and to chewing. Other pains may result from lateral periodontal abscess or acute gingival inflammation. Pain arising from the oral mucosa can be localized to a detectable erosive or ulcerative lesion or be of a diffuse nature all over the oral mucosa. Pain alone is an insufficient diagnostic tool for oral disease and must be validated by other diagnostic procedures for each individual case.

Table 13.1 Differential diagnosis of oral pain

		History		Physical examination			Radiography	
Source of pain	**Ability to locate**	**Character of pain**	**Pain intensified by**	**Pain intensity**	**Associated signs**	**Pain duplicated by**	**Bite-wing**	**Periapical**
Dental								
Dentinal	Poor	Evoked, does not outlast stimulus	Hot, cold, sweet, sour	Mild to moderate	Caries, defective restorations exposed dentine	Hot or cold application, scratching dentine	Interproximal caries, defective restorations	NA
Pulpal	Very poor	Spontaneous, explosive, intermittent	Hot, cold, sometimes chewing	Usually severe	Deep caries, extensive restoration	Hot or cold, caries probing, sometimes percussion	Deep caries and deep restoration with no secondary dentine	Limited use, sometimes periapical change
Periodontal								
Periapical	Good	For hours on same level, deep, boring	Chewing	Moderate to severe	Periapical swelling and redness, tooth mobility	Percussion, palpation of periapical area	Limited use, deep caries and deep restorations	Sometimes periapical changes
Lateral	Good	For hours on same level, boring	Chewing	Moderate to severe	Periodontal swelling, deep pockets with pus exudating, tooth mobility	Percussion, palpation of periodontal area	Sometimes alveolar bone resorpion	Very useful when X-rayed with probe inserted into pocket
Gingival	Good	Pressing, annoying	Food impaction, tooth-brushing	Mild to severe	Acute gingival inflammation	Touch, percussion	NA	NA
Mucosal	Usually good	Burning, sharp	Sour, sharp, and hot food	Mild to moderate	Erosive or ulcerative lesions, redness	Palpation of lesion	N/A	N/A

NA = not applicable.

Dental pain

Dentinal pain

Pain originating in dentine is a sharp, deep sensation, usually evoked by an external stimulus and subsides within a few seconds. Such stimuli are normally produced by food and drinks that are hot, cold, sweet, or sour, and indicate a hyperalgesic state of the tooth. The pain is poorly localized, and the patient may not be able to distinguish whether the pain originates from the lower or the upper jaw. However, patients rarely make localization errors across the midline, and posterior teeth are more difficult to localize than anterior ones (Friend and Glenwright 1968).

Duplication of pain produced by controlled application of cold or hot stimuli to various teeth in the suspected area can aid in identifying the affected, hyperalgesic tooth. Most frequently, this hyperalgesic state is associated with dental caries, which can be found by means of direct observation and probing with a sharp dental explorer. The 'bite-wing' intraoral dental radiograph (Fig. 13.1) is a very useful diagnostic aid in these cases. Defective restorations and any other cavity, e.g., abrasion and erosion of the enamel or roots exposed due to gingival recession, are other causes for pain. In these instances, scratching the exposed dentine with a sharp probe can evoke pain and aid in locating its source.

In addition to these symptoms, the patient may also complain of a sharp pain, elicited by biting, that ceases immediately when pressure is removed from the teeth. Localization of the source of pain is not precise, although the affected area can often be limited to two or three adjacent teeth. The patient complains of pain and discomfort associated with cold and hot stimuli in the area. These complaints indicate that there may be a crack in the dentine, the so-called 'cracked tooth syndrome' (Cameron 1976, Goose 1981). Although the diagnosis is frequently difficult because the affected tooth is not readily localized and radiographs are unhelpful, diagnosis and localization of the affected tooth can be achieved by the following:

1. percussing the cusps of the suspected teeth at different angles
2. asking the patient to bite on individual cusps using a fine wooden stick
3. probing firmly around margins of fillings and in suspected fissures.

Additional possible diagnoses include occlusal abrasion with exposed dentine or a cracked filling. These can be detected visually and with the aid of a sharp explorer.

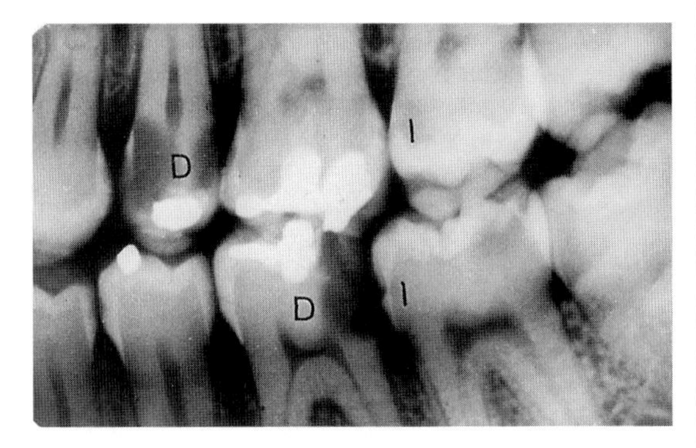

Fig. 13.1 Bite-wing radiograph demonstrating the coronal parts of the posterior teeth on the left. I=initial caries associated with dentinal pain; D= deep caries associated with pulpal pain.

Treatment Dentinal pain due to caries is best treated by removal of the carious lesion and restoring the tooth by a filling. Sensitivity usually disappears within a day. Treatment of the 'cracked tooth' is achieved by 'crowning' the tooth. Treatment of exposed, hypersensitive dentine is somewhat less satisfactory. Some fluoride-containing preparations are available, and recently acrylic-based sealing materials have been suggested. Treatment can be enhanced by good oral hygiene and avoiding acidic foods and beverages.

Pulpal pain

Pain associated with pulp disease is spontaneous, strong, and often throbbing and is exacerbated by temperature change, sweet foods, and pressure on the carious lesion. When pain is evoked it outlasts the stimulus (unlike stimulus-induced dentinal pain) and can be excruciating for many minutes. Similarly to dentinal pain, localization is poor and seems to be even poorer when pain becomes more intense. Pain tends to radiate or refer to the ear, temple and cheek but does not cross the midline. Pain may be described by patients in different ways and a continuous dull ache can be periodically exacerbated (by stimulation or spontaneously) for short (minutes) or long (hours) periods (Cohen 1996). Pain may increase and throb when the patient lies down and in many instances wakes the patient from sleep (Sharav et al 1984). The pain of pulpitis is frequently not continuous and abates spontaneously; the precise explanation for such abatement is not clear.

This interrupted, sharp, paroxysmal, non localized pain may lead to the misdiagnosis of other conditions that may mimic pain of pulpal origin (e.g., trigeminal neuralgia). The initial aim of the diagnostic process is to identify the affected tooth and then to assess the state of the tooth pulp in order to determine treatment. Localization of the affected tooth is achieved through hot and cold application, which should be done carefully because it may cause excruciating pain. Percussion also aids in localizing the affected tooth. The state of the pulp cannot be judged from one single symptom and should be based on the combination of several signs and symptoms (Cohen 1996).

Treatment Depending on the prognosis of the pulp, treatment may aim at conserving the pulp, extirpating it, or extracting the tooth. Pulpal pain usually disappears immediately after treatment.

Differential diagnosis of odontalgia

Diagnosis of toothache is challenging because teeth often refer pain to other teeth as well as to other craniofacial locations (Sharav et al 1984) and other craniofacial pain disorders (Benoliel et al 1997), or pain from more remote structures (Tzukert et al 1981) may refer to teeth. The latter may mimic the symptoms of a toothache. In this respect vascular orofacial pain, to be discussed later, is of great diagnostic importance.

Periodontal pain

Periodontal pain usually results from an acute inflammatory process of the gingiva, the periodontal ligament, and alveolar bone due to bacterial infection. Pain is readily localized, and the affected teeth are very tender to pressure. Aetiologically, two modes of affection are most common:

1. a sequela of pulp infection and pulp necrosis that results in periapical inflammation
2. periodontal infection with pocket formation that result in a lateral periodontal abcsess.

Although pain characteristics, ability to localize, and pain-producing situations are similar in both cases (Table 13.1), treatment differs for aetiological reasons, and these categories are therefore discussed separately.

Acute periapical periodontitis

Pain is spontaneous and moderate to severe in intensity for extended periods of time (hours). Pain is exacerbated by biting on the tooth and, in more advanced cases, even by closing the mouth and bringing the affected tooth into contact with the opposing teeth. In these cases, the tooth feels extruded and is sensitive to touch. Frequently the patient reports that pulpal pain preceded the pain originating from the periapical area. The latter, although of a more continuous nature, is usually better tolerated than the paroxysmal and excruciating pulpal pain. Localization of pain originating from the periapical area is usually precise and the patient is able to indicate the affected tooth. In this respect periodontal pain differs from the poorly localized dentinal and pulpal pain. However, although localization of the affected tooth is usually precise, in approximately half the cases the pain is diffuse and spreads into the jaw on the affected side of the face (Sharav et al 1984).

During examination the affected tooth is readily located by means of tooth percussion. The periapical vestibular area may be tender to palpation. The pulp of the affected tooth is non-vital; i.e., it does not respond to thermal changes or to electrical pulp stimulation. However, as mentioned above, in clinical practice pulpitis may not be sharply distinguished from acute periapical periodontitis, and pulpal as well as periapical involvement could occur at the same time. In these cases, although the periapical area has been invaded by endogenous pain-producing substances due to pulp tissue damage (e.g., 5HT, histamine, bradykinin) and exogenous pain-producing substances (e.g., bacterial toxins) the pulp has not yet completely degenerated and can still react to stimuli such as temperature changes. These instances are fairly common (Okeson 1995). In more severe, purulent cases, swelling of the face associated with cellulitis is present and can be associated with fever and malaise. The affected tooth may be extruded and mobile. Usually, when swelling of the face occurs, pain diminishes in intensity due to rupture of the periostium of the bone around the affected tooth and the decrease in pus pressure.

The radiographic picture is of limited use in the diagnosis of acute periapical periodontitis as no periapical radiographic changes are detected in the early stages. If a radiographic periapical rarefying osteitis is noticed in a tooth that is sensitive to touch and percussion, the condition is then classified as reacutization of chronic periapical periodontitis. Often, however, such a rarefying osteitis lesion is present in an otherwise symptomless situation.

Treatment The source of insult and infection usually lies within the pulp chamber and the root canal, although the pain originates from the periodontal periapical tissues. Treatment, therefore, is aimed at the source of irritation in the pulp chamber and the root canal that are opened and cleansed. Grinding the tooth to prevent contact with the opposing teeth helps to relieve pain. If cellulitis, fever, and malaise are present, systemic administration of antibiotics is recommended. Incision and drainage are very effective when a fluctuating abscess is present. Pain usually subsides within 24–48 h.

Lateral periodontal abscess

Pain characteristics are very similar to those of acute periapical periodontitis. Pain is continuous, well localized, moderate to severe in intensity, and exacerbated by biting on the affected tooth. During examination swelling and redness of the gingiva may be noticed, usually located more gingivally than in the case of the acute periapical lesion. The affected tooth is sensitive to percussion and is often mobile and slightly extruded. In more severe cases, cellulitis, fever, and malaise may occur. A deep periodontal pocket (over 6 mm) is usually located around the tooth; once probed there is pus exudation and usually, subsequent relief from pain. The tooth pulp is usually vital; i.e., it reacts to temperature changes and electrical stimulation. The pulp may occasionally be slightly hyperalgesic in these cases, and sometimes pulpitis and pulpal pain may develop due to retrograde infection (Fig. 13.2). Abscess formation usually results from a blockage of drainage from a periodontal pocket and is frequently associated with a deep infrabony pocket and teeth with root furcation involvement (Fig. 13.2).

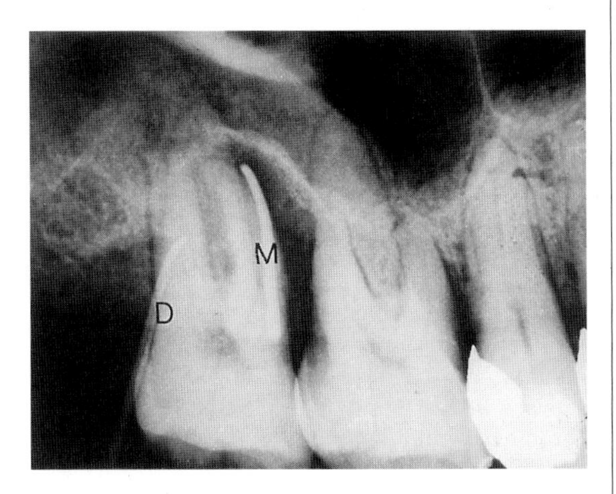

Fig. 13.2 Periapical radiograph of the molar area in the right maxillary region. Radiopaque probes were inserted into mesial (M) and distal (D) periodontal pockets of the second molar to demonstrate the depth of these pockets. Lateral periodontal and pulpal pain were both present. Pulpal pain in this case was not associated with caries but with 'retrograde' infection of the pulp through the deep mesial pocket.

Treatment Gentle irrigation and curettage of the pocket should be performed. The tooth is ground in order to avoid contact with the opposing teeth. When cellulitis, fever, and malaise are present, systemic antibiotic administration is recommended. Direct incision and drainage are recommended when the abscess cannot be approached through the pocket, and is ripe for incision. Pain usually subsides within 24 h of treatment.

Gingival pain

Gingival pain may occur as a result of mechanical irritation, acute inflammation associated with a gingival pocket, or gingival acute bacterial or viral infection.

Food impaction

The patient complains of localized pain between two adjacent teeth especially after meals, particularly when food is fibrous (e.g., meat, celery). The pain is associated with a very annoying feeling of pressure and discomfort. The patient reports that the pain may gradually disappear until evoked again at the next meal. Pain may be relieved by removing the food impacted between the teeth. Upon examination, a faulty contact between two adjacent teeth is noticed. Food is usually trapped between these teeth; the gingival papilla is inflammed, tender to touch and bleeds easily. The two adjacent teeth are usually sensitive to percussion. The cause of the faulty contact between the teeth is often a carious lesion and restoring the tooth will eliminate pain.

Pericoronitis

Pain is severe, and is usually located at the distal end of the arch of teeth in the lower jaw. Pain is spontaneous and may be exacerbated by closing the mouth. In more severe cases, pain is aggravated by swallowing and be associated by trismus. Acute pericoronal infections are common in teeth that are incompletely erupted, and are partially covered by flaps of gingival tissue.

Upon examination, the flap of gingiva is acutely inflamed, red and oedematous. Frequently, an indentation of the opposing tooth can be seen imprinted on the oedematous gingival flap. Occasionally, fever and malaise are associated with this infection.

Treatment includes irrigation of debris between the flap and the affected tooth and eliminating trauma by the opposing tooth (by grinding or extraction). Systemic antibiotic administration is commonly recommended, especially when trismus occurs.

Acute necrotizing ulcerative gingivitis

Soreness and pain are felt at the margin of the gums. Pain is intensified by eating and brushing the teeth and is accompanied by gingival bleeding. Metallic taste is sometimes experienced and usually there is a foetid smell from the mouth. Pain is fairly well localized to the affected areas, but in cases when lesions are spread all over the gums pain is experienced all over the mouth. Fever and malaise are sometimes present. Necrosis and ulceration are noticed upon examination on the marginal gingiva with different degrees of gingival papillary destruction. An adherent greyish slough represents the so-called pseudomembrane present in the acute stage of the disease. Swabbing this slough is associated with pain and bleeding. Although basically a bacterial disease that responds to antibiotics, it is not clear whether the bacteria actually initiate the disease or are merely secondary to some underlying factors. Local as well as systemic factors are suggested as possible underlying factors. These include, locally, gross neglect of oral hygiene, heavy smoking, and mouth breathing. Systemically, any underlying debilitating factors are suggested, but there is no doubt that these are secondary to the more important local factors.

Treatment includes swabbing and gentle irrigation of the ulcerative lesions, preferably with an oxidizing agent (hydrogen peroxide), and scaling and cleaning the teeth. Systemic antibiotics are recommended when fever and malaise are present.

Intensity and location of acute oral pain

Acute dental and periodontal pain is frequently rated as moderate to severe in intensity or from 60–100 on a 100-mm visual analogue scale (Sharav et al 1984). Pain is conceived of as deep and unpleasant. In about 60% of cases pain is not localized only at the affected site but spreads into remote areas in the head and face. There is a considerable overlap in pain reference locations for maxillary and mandibular sources. Pain spread is correlated positively with pain intensity and unpleasantness. Two factors that may be important for this pain spread are the large receptive fields of wide dynamic-range neurons with extensive gradient sensitivity and the somatotopic organization (Sharav et al 1984).

Mucosal pain

Pain originating from the oral mucosa can be either localized or of a more generalized diffuse nature. The localized pain is usually associated with a detectable erosive or ulcerative lesion; the diffuse pain may be associated with a widespread infection, a systemic underlying deficiency disease or other unknown factors.

Only the most common lesion, recurrent aphthous stomatitis, will be described briefly.

Recurrent aphthous stomatitis is characterized by a prodromal burning sensation from 2 to 48 h before an ulcer appears. Although small in diameter (0.3–1.0 cm) this lesion may be quite painful. In the mild form, healing occurs within 10 days and pain is usually mild to moderate in severity. In the more severe forms (major aphthous ulcers), deep ulcers that may be confluent, are extremely painful, and interfere with speech and eating occur. Such lesions may last for months, heal slowly, and leave scars. Treatment is mostly symptomatic, including the application of a topical protective emollient for the mild form and the use of topical corticosteroids and tetracycline to decrease healing time for the severe form. In the 'major' type systemic corticosteroids are often needed.

The diffuse pain in the oral mucosa has usually a burning nature and may be accompanied by a change in taste, predominantly of a bitter metallic quality. This pain may result from a direct insult to the tissues due to bacterial, viral, or fungal infection, which can be identified by the characteristic appearance of the oral mucosa. Diagnosis is aided by microbiological laboratory examinations. In cases of chronic fungal infection (candidiasis), possible underlying aetiological factors such as prolonged broad-spectrum antibiotic therapy, immunodeficiencies, and other debilitating factors should be investigated. Radiation therapy to the head and neck region may result in acute mucositis with severe generalized mucosal pain (Kolbinson et al 1988). Decreased salivary flow is a later sequela that may result in chronic pain and discomfort of the oral mucosa.

Burning sensation of the oral mucosa, particularly the tongue, may result from systemic deficiency disease, such as chronic iron deficiency anaemia. This is usually associated with observable atrophic changes, in particular that of the filiform and fungiform papillae of the tongue. However, there is a large proportion of patients, mostly women between the ages of 50 and 70 years, who complain of a burning sensation in the mouth and the tongue, with no observable changes in the oral mucosa and with no detectable underlying systemic changes. This condition is discussed below under 'burning mouth syndrome'.

Temporomandibular disorders

This prevalent entity of orofacial pain and mandibular dysfunction (Helkimo 1979, Dworkin et al 1990a) has acquired more than a dozen names (De Boever 1979, McNeill 1997) since it was first described by Costen in 1934. In addition to a variety of names, a variety of different criteria have been used for defining this disorder (Rugh and Solberg 1979). Indeed, the criteria for the syndrome were such that they encompassed disorders that under today's concepts would be diagnosed differently (Eversole and Machado 1985, McNeill 1997, Okeson 1997). By the 1950s it was becoming obvious that many of these patients suffered from a masticatory muscle disorder apparently unrelated to the temporomandibular joint (TMJ). However, it was only during the 1980s that, with the aid of modern TMJ imaging techniques (Dolwick et al 1983), we began to understand that there was also a temporomandibular disorder of the joint proper that justified separate classification. The definition of internal derangements of the TMJ finally dissociated the temporomandibular joint from this 'syndrome', and the justification for a separate entity of temporomandibular myofascial pain (unrelated to TMJ pathology), as opposed to the 'general' myofascial pain dysfunction (MPD) syndrome, was further questioned. The justification for segregation of temporomandibular myofascial pain and dysfunction from other myofascial pain disorders of a more generalized type, such as primary fibromyalgia, has more recently been questioned (Widmer 1991). The question of whether temporomandibular pain is a localized symptom of a more generalized condition or a discrete entity will be addressed in more detail later.

Recently, the American Academy of Orofacial Pain recommended that orofacial pain and mandibular dysfunction be termed temporomandibular disorders (TMD) (Okeson 1996). TMD are defined as a collective term embracing a number of clinical problems that involve the masticatory musculature, the temporomandibular joint and associated structures, or both. These are characterized by pain usually aggravated by manipulation or function, limited range of motion, asymmetric mandibular movement, and/or locking and joint sounds. It is felt, however, that such 'an all-embracing collective term' is too wide to be usefully discussed. I have chosen therefore to approach TMD as two distinct entities: one associated primarily with pain and dysfunction of myofascial origin, which will be referred to as temporomandibular myofascial pain (TMP), the other associated primarily with intra-articular disorders and referred to as internal derangement (ID) of the TMJ.

Temporomandibular myofascial pain

Patients usually describe a poorly localized, dull, continuous ache, typically around the ear, the angle of the mandible, and the temporal area. However, pain has also been described in the jaws, teeth, and diffusely throughout one side of the face (Okeson 1995). Pain may also occur bilaterally; there is some evidence that bilateral pain is more commonly associated with underlying psychogenic factors (Gerschman et al 1990). Pain may be aggravated during function with transient spikes of pain occurring spontaneously or induced by jaw movements (Okeson 1995). Pain rarely wakes the patient from sleep.

Associated signs are deviation of the mandible on opening, fullness of the ear, dizziness, and soreness of the neck (Sharav et al 1978, Blasberg and Chalmers 1989).

Examination may reveal limited mouth opening (less than 40 mm, interincisal). Masticatory and neck muscles are tender to palpation (Sharav et al 1978) and pain often refers (Okeson 1995). Trigger points in the muscles may also be detected (Travell and Simons 1983). Clinical signs are difficult to measure with consistency (Kopp and Wenneberg 1983, Carlsson et al 1980), and inter-rater reliability for some signs of TMD is not good (Dworkin et al 1990b).

Epidemiology

Temporomandibular pain and dysfunction disorders are recognized as the most common *chronic* orofacial pain condition (Dworkin et al 1990a). In the available epidemiological studies of the general population, TMD signs and symptoms appear to be equally distributed between the sexes (Helkimo 1979, Christensen 1981) or the differences are minor (Locker and Slade 1988). In Agerberg and Carlsson's classic cross-sectional study (1972), about half of the 15- to 44-year-old population had at least one symptom of dysfunction and one-third had two or more symptoms. Reporting symptoms in a population over 18 years old, Locker and Slade (1988) describe a prevalence of 48.8% while the percentage of those needing treatment was estimated at

3.5–9.7%. Of much interest in this respect is the study of Wanman and Agerberg (1986a), who reported a prevalence of 20% in a study group of 17-year-olds. They followed up this group for 2 years and found that although the incidence was 8%, there was no general increase in the severity or number of symptoms in this study period; the explanation offered was that new symptoms appear as often as old ones disappear (Wanman and Agerberg 1986b). Thus, spontaneous remission seems to be quite prevalent in this disorder.

While signs and symptoms of TMD are equally distributed between the sexes in the general population, the majority of patients who seek treatment (up to 80%) are females (Sharav et al 1978, Helkimo 1979, Rugh and Solberg 1985). Signs and symptoms of mandibular dysfunction have been found in all age groups (Helkimo 1979, Nielsen et al 1990), with a tendency to increase with age (Rugh and Solberg 1985, Torvonen and Knuuttila 1988). Dworkin et al (1990a,b) report that TMJ pain, however, is less common among the elderly. Signs of mandibular dysfunction have been described in children and adolescents with a higher prevalence than was previously suspected (Perry 1973, Nielsen et al 1990). The syndrome occurs also in edentulous patients (Carlsson 1976, Agerberg 1988).

Aetiological factors

Bruxism and occlusal derangement The association between TMP, the teeth, and dental occlusion stems back to Costen (1934), who believed that overclosure of the mandible due to loss of teeth was responsible for TMJ pain. More recent theories consider occlusal disturbances a prerequisite for the development of dysfunction and pain. Whilst the extent of the occlusal 'interference' may be minute, the important fact is that such interference can upset proprioceptive feedback and thus cause bruxism and spasm of masticatory muscles (Krogh-Poulsen and Olsson 1968). These assumptions were later refuted by Rugh et al (1984), who demonstrated that occlusal discrepancies, produced experimentally, tend to reduce bruxism rather than enhance it. Furthermore, data by Thomson (1971), Solberg et al (1972), and Clarke (1982) indicate that there are no significant differences between the occlusal relationship in patients and in asymptomatic controls. Finally, in a recent paper, Clark et al (1997) state that the relationship made between occlusion and TMD is not convincing, powerful, or practical enough to make any recommendations about a causal association.

Bruxism is no longer perceived as related to occlusal 'disharmonies' but rather as a physiological behaviour that may sometimes be associated with TMP (Rugh and Harlan 1988). Clark et al (1980) suggest that bruxism is stress related. They demonstrated a positive relationship between increased urinary epinephrine and high levels of nocturnal masseter muscle activity. The forces exerted during nocturnal tooth grinding are quite high and were found to exceed maximal conscious clenches (Clarke et al 1984). However, the association between bruxism and TMP is not entirely clear. Bruxism is viewed as an arousal phenomenon (Satoh and Harada 1973) or as a sleep parasomnia (American Sleep Disorder Association 1990). Some preliminary results suggest that a majority of patients with bruxism have pain levels and sleep quality comparable with TMP patients (Lavigne et al 1991). Patients having bruxism without muscle pain did not show differences in any of the sleep variables compared to matched controls (Velly-Miguel et al 1991).

Psychosocial correlates On the basis of an extensive literature review, Rugh and Solberg (1979) concluded that there was little evidence suggesting that TMP is related to any specific personality trait. Thus, Marbach et al (1978) found no significant difference in either state anxiety or trait anxiety between patients with intractable facial pain and groups of general dental and general medical patients. In a later study Marbach and Lund (1981) found no difference in depression and anhedonia between TMP patients and a normal, non-patient group. Salter et al (1983) challenge the idea that TMP patients represent a population whose pain results from their emotional state. They found that the comparison of TMP patients and patients with facial pain and lesions or pathophysiological disorders showed little evidence of neuroticism in either group. Furthermore, examining the premorbid characteristics of TMP patients did not reveal abnormal parental bonding attitudes in this group (Salter et al 1983) nor did they show any other measures of previous premorbid personality traits (Merskey et al 1987). Sharav et al (1987) found that only 2 out of 32 patients with chronic facial pain were cortisol non-suppressors on the dexamethasone suppression test (DST). In a recent study Schnurr et al (1990) classified their TMD patients according to the diagnostic criteria of Eversole and Machado (1985), enabling a separate comparison of myogenic (TMP) and of TMJ facial pain to non-facial injury 'pain controls' and healthy controls. The results of Schnurr et al (1990) suggested that TMP and TMJ pain patients do not appear to be significantly different from other pain patients or healthy controls in personality type, response to illness, attitudes towards health care, or ways of coping with stress.

While psychological factors seem to play a minor role in the aetiology of TMP, research supports the appropriateness of a dual diagnostic approach for TMD based on physical and psychological axes that allows for treatment to be customized to address the physical as well as the psychological characteristics of the patient (Turk 1997).

Vascular mechanisms and headache Muscle tenderness is a frequent finding in headache patients (Raskin and Appenzeller 1980) and the distribution may be distinctly similar to that in TMP patients (Sharav et al 1978, Tafelt-Hansen et al 1981, Clark et al 1987). Patients with signs of TMP report a significantly higher incidence of tension headache than controls (Magnusson and Carlsson 1978, Watts et al 1986); indeed, epidemiological data suggest great similarity and possible overlap between patients suffering from headache and TMP (Magnusson and Carlsson 1978). The sex ratio is similar—about 75% females in both groups; age distribution and contributing psychophysiological mechanisms are also shared (Rugh and Solberg 1979, Raskin and Appenzeller 1980). It seems, therefore, that two of the fundamental symptoms of TMP, i.e., pain of daily occurrence and tenderness of muscles to palpation, fail to properly differentiate between tension-type headache and TMP patients. As previously mentioned, the 1986 IASP classification combines these two under 'craniofacial pain of musculoskeletal origin'. However, most TMP patients have pain and muscle tenderness on palpation unilaterally (Sharav et al 1978) while tension-type headache causes pain bilaterally.

The association between migraine and temporomandibular dysfunction was studied by Watts et al (1986). The authors stated that the rate of migraine in the TMP group did not differ from that in the general population and concluded that TMP and migraine patients are two segregated groups. That TMP and vascular headache are two distinct entities can also be inferred from studies of sleep physiology. Bruxism, associated with TMP (Lavigne et al 1991), occurred mostly in non-rapid eye movement (N-REM) stages of sleep (Satoh and Harada 1973, Wieselmann et al 1986, Rugh and Harlan 1988), while vascular headache is REM 'locked' (Dexter and Weizman 1970). Recently, however, a severe tooth-destructive form of bruxism has been found in REM sleep (Ware and Rugh 1988), which may suggest that in some cases vascular mechanisms could be associated with TMP.

Fibromyalgia Much controversy exists in the medical literature concerning muscle tenderness and its diagnosis in specific cases. In the light of the possibility that on the one hand fibromyalgia (FM) may begin as a localized pain disorder and later become widespread, and on the other hand that persistent myofascial pain dysfunction (MPD) may involve multiple sites and cause systemic symptoms (Bennet 1986, Wolfe 1988), some authors believe that all local 'syndromes' of myofascial pain should be conflated to form one entity. Thus, it is claimed by Widmer (1991) that when the symptoms of FM patients are compared with those of patients with temporomandibular disorders without joint pathology, no symptoms are specific to TMP. TMP seems to be a localized condition but the evidence needs to be examined carefully. Blasberg and Chalmers (1989) conclude that there are great similarities between TMP patients and primary fibromyalgia (PFM) patients. Eriksson et al (1988) also support the hypothesis that a connection may exist between TMP and PFM entities.

These conclusions should be viewed very carefully; PFM, by definition, is characterized by a widespread pain on both sides of the body and in both the upper and the lower parts of the body in 97.6% of PFM patients (Henriksson and Bengtsson 1991), whereas TMP is mostly a local, unilateral, pain syndrome (Sharav et al 1978, Okeson 1995).

TMJ damage Theoretically, trauma or noxious stimulation of TMJ tissues can produce a sustained excitation of masticatory muscles that may serve to protect the masticatory system from potentially damaging movements and stimuli (Sessle and Hu 1991). However, injection into the TMJ of algesic chemicals resulted in sustained reflex increase in EMG activity of jaw-opening muscles; excitatory effects were also seen in jaw-closing muscles but were generally weaker (Broton and Sessle 1988). While such effects might be related to clinically based concepts of myofascial dysfunction (e.g., splinting, myospastic activity, and trigger points), the weak effects in muscles invoked clinically to show such dysfunction (jaw closing) and the stronger effects in antagonist muscles (jaw opening) suggest associations more in keeping with protective, withdrawal-type reflexes (Sessle and Hu 1991). Based upon the available data, it seems that pain originating in the TMJ contributes minimally to the development of TMP.

Implications Bruxism and TMJ derangements do not seem to be primary aetiological factors of TMP. The role that vascular mechanisms, related to other craniofacial pains (e.g., migraine, cluster headache, paroxysmal hemicrania), play in TMP is not entirely clear. Whilst the importance of vascular mechanisms may not yet be fully appreciated, one should not dismiss their contribution to TMP. Some data (Ware and Rugh 1988) point to a REM-locked destructive form of bruxism that may link certain forms of TMP with vascular mechanisms. Recent findings strongly suggest that neurogenic inflammation may play the major role in vascular headache (Moskowitz et al 1989). In view of the cardinal role of the trigeminal system in conveying vascular headache (Dostrovsky et al 1991), the possibility of interrelated central mechanisms of headache and facial pain cannot be discounted. Research in the area of TMP should concentrate more on central generators of pain mechanisms rather than peripheral inputs such as occlusal interferences and 'muscle hyperactivity'. One attractive way to understand TMP better is to study the role of trigeminal neurogenic inflammation and the contribution of the sympathetic nervous system (Basbaum and Levine 1991) regarding the pain mechanisms of TMP.

Differential diagnosis

TMP should be differentiated from pain due to TMJ derangement and other specific TMJ diseases (e.g., psoriasis, rheumatoid arthritis). Of particular importance are instances where TMP can mask underlying malignancies such as nasopharyngeal carcinoma (Sharav and Feinsod 1977, Roistacher and Tanenbaum 1986).

Treatment

Like other chronic pain syndromes, TMP is a complex entity associated with behavioural changes, secondary psychological gains, changes in mood and attitudes to life, and drug abuse. While alleviation of pain and dysfunction remain the primary goals of therapy, restoring the patient's attitudes by modelling behavioural changes and controlling drug abuse should also be achieved. Often reassurance of the patient, combined with simple muscle exercises for masticatory and neck muscles, will result in pain alleviation and restored mandibular function (Selby 1985). Muscle tenderness may be treated with vapocoolant sprays and injections of local anaesthetics into identified trigger points (Travell and Simons 1983). Diazepam is significantly more effective than placebo in the relief of pain, while ibuprofen has had minimal therapeutic benefit in TMP patients (Singer et al 1987). Sharav et al (1987) demonstrated the beneficial effect of low doses of amitriptyline (less than 30 mg/day) in patients with chronic facial pain of myofascial origin. The efficacy of amitriptyline in relieving chronic facial pain, such as TMP, is through a direct analgesic effect not associated with the antidepressive effect of the drug (Sharav et al 1987). Occlusal splint therapy is a widely used mode of treatment (Clarke et al 1984), and may be associated with the reduction of nocturnal bruxism (Clark et al 1979). Some investigators found occlusal splint therapy to be superior to relaxation procedures (Okeson et al 1983).

It is widely believed that chronic pain patients lack psychological insight and therefore do not respond to psychodynamic interpretation (Sternbach 1978). Consequently other psychological interventions such as relaxation training, biofeedback, and cognitive behaviour approaches (Carlsson and Gale 1976, Stem et al 1979) would be more appropriate for these patients.

Prognosis in the majority of patients is good and remission of pain and dysfunction is readily achieved for long periods.

Internal derangement of the temporomandibular joint

Internal derangement (ID) of the TMJ is defined as an abnormal relationship of the articular disc to the mandibular condyle, fossa, and articular eminence. Usually the disc is displaced in an anteromedial direction (Dolwick and Riggs 1983). In addition to pain, limited mouth opening, or deviation of mouth opening, patients complain of clicking in the TMJ. Clicking refers to a distinct cracking, snapping sound associated with opening and closing of the mouth. Farrar (1971) introduced the term 'reciprocal clicking' to describe patients with opening and closing clicks. Reciprocal click is considered pathognomonic to internal derangement. Patients may report an increase in the intensity of the pain prior to the click with relief after the click occurs. Pain is usually limited to the TMJ area. Crepitus and multiple scraping sounds are best detected with the aid of a stethoscope placed over the TMJ while the patient opens and closes the mouth. Crepitus frequently indicates a disruption of the disc or its posterior attachment and heralds more advanced disease.

The final, definitive diagnosis of ID is made by arthrography of the TMJ using radiopaque contrast material injected into the joint space, usually the lower one (Katzberg et al 1979). While the diagnostic 'gold standard' has been arthrography, MRI is now the imaging technique of choice for the TMJ IDs (Rao 1995) and CT for hard tissue imaging

(Larheim 1995). However, these seem justified only in appropriately selected cases (doubtful or suspicion of tumour) or in candidates for surgery. In combination with SPECT, MRIs demonstrate a sensitivity of 0.96 for IDs. The invasive nature of arthrography and the high cost involved in MRIs that would otherwise need to be performed routinely support a conservative approach.

On the basis of clinical signs and arthrographic findings, ID of the TMJ has been further classified (Dolwick and Riggs 1983, Eversole and Machado 1985, Roberts et al 1985). This classification includes:

1. disc displacement with reduction
2. disc displacement with intermittent locking
3. disc displacement without reduction
4. disc displacement with perforation.

Clinical signs and arthrographic findings are usually in good agreement (Roberts et al 1985).

Recent findings may challenge the relationship between TMJ pain dysfunction and the concept of disc displacement (Westesson et al 1989, Nitzan et al 1991). Westesson et al (1989) demonstrated that 15% of healthy asymptomatic volunteers were radiographically abnormal with displacement of the disc; Nitzan and Dolwick (1991) showed that more than 50% of patients in a most advanced stage of ID (closed-locked) had normally shaped discs. Although in both studies there may be a sample selection bias, they still indicate that factors other than disc position may be considered, at least in some patients, for the genesis of pain and dysfunction associated with the TMJ. These may include decreased volume of synovial fluid with high viscosity or a 'vacuum effect' (Nitzan et al 1991, 1992).

Treatment

Conservative treatment modalities recommended for TMP are utilized for ID of the TMJ. Unfortunately, as has long been known, the elimination of joint sounds is the single most resistant feature in most studies dealing with these patients (Eversole and Machado 1985). If joint sounds with no pain or dysfunction are present, no treatment is indicated. Interocclusal anterior repositioning splints are of value in eliminating clicks, but are of short-term benefit with no known long-term effect (Lundh et al 1985). In more advanced cases that do not respond to non-surgical treatment, surgery is recommended (Dolwick and Riggs 1983). However, long-term evaluation of non-surgical treatment of advanced cases demonstrated favourable results (Yoshimura et al 1982), and it seems that most individuals with internal derangement do not deteriorate and, indeed, demonstrate remarkable adaptive potential (Okeson 1995). In selected cases, arthrographic surgery or rinsing and lavage seems to be the treatment of choice (Nitzan et al 1991). On the basis of current data, one is unable to conclusively recommend any specific treatment modality.

Primary vascular-type craniofacial pain

The differential diagnosis of primary vascular-type craniofacial pain includes migraine-type headaches, cluster headaches, paroxysmal hemicranias, SUNCT, cold stimulus ('ice cream') headache, and a recently proposed (Sharav et al 1996) vascular orofacial pain (Table 13.2). Each diagnostic entity has specific criteria for diagnosis (Headache Classification Committee 1988, Mersky and Bogduk 1994) but in general craniofacial vascular pains have some common signs and symptoms:

Pain is:	Accompanied by:
a. Periodic	a. Ocular: tearing, redness
b. Severe	b. Nasal: rhinorrhoea, congestion
c. Unilateral	c. Local swelling and redness
d. Pulsatile	d. Nausea, vomiting
e. Wakes from sleep	e. Photo/phonophobia

Migraine

Migraine with or without aura is a periodic, unilateral headache mostly in the forehead and temple areas. Pain may persist from a couple of hours to 2 days. Pain intensity is moderate to severe, usually throbs and may be accompanied by photo- and phonophobia and is associated with nausea and occasional vomiting (Table 13.2).

As migraine headache is discussed in detail in Chapter 15, it will not be further discussed here.

Cluster headache

Cluster headache (CH) was first recognized in the 1950s. Episodic CH refers to a temporal pattern consisting of a series of pain attacks, or 'active' episodes, occurring in succession over a period of 4–12 weeks with 'inactive' periods that last from 6 to 18 months. In the active period pain occurs daily or almost daily. Patients with continuous cluster headache, or constantly 'active', were also recognized and are termed 'chronic CH' (Nappi and Russell 1993).

Table 13.2 Differential diagnosis of primary vascular-type craniofacial pain

	Migraine headache	Cluster headache	Paroxysmal hemicrania	Vascular orofacial pain
Onset (age)	20–40	30–40	30–40	40–50
M:F	1:2	5:1	1:2	1:2.5
Location (mostly unilateral)	Forehead, temple	Orbital and periorbital	Temporal and periauricular	Intraoral/lower face
Duration	Hours to days	15–120 min	Minutes	Minutes to hours
Time course	Periodic	Periodic/chronic	Chronic	Periodic/chronic
Character of pain	Throbbing, deep, continuous	Paroxysmal, boring in clusters	Paroxysmal, lancinating	Throbbing, may be paroxysmal
Pain intensity	Moderate to severe	Severe	Severe	Moderate to severe
Precipitating factors	Stress, hunger, menstrual period, etc.	Alcohol	Movement of head	Sometimes cold foods
Associated signs	Nausea, photophobia, visual aura	Lacrimation, rhinorrhoea, ptosis, miosis	Lacrimation, rhinorrhoea, eye redness	Cheek swelling and redness, tearing
Treatment: *abortive*	NSAID, ergot, sumatriptan	Oxygen, ergot, sumatriptan	Indometacin	NSAID
Treatment: *prophylactic*	Amitriptyline, β-blockers, valproates	Ergot, methysergide, lithium carbonate	Indometacin	Amitriptyline, β-blockers

Pain pattern

Pain is unilateral, occurs in the ocular, frontal, and temporal areas, is excruciatingly severe and paroxysmal and may last from 15 to 120 min. Nocturnal attacks are typical.

Accompanying phenomena

Pain attacks are accompanied by ipsilateral conjunctival injection, lacrimation, stuffiness of the nose, and/or rhinorrhoea. Ipsilateral ptosis and miosis may be associated with some attacks; occasionally they persist after attacks and may remain permanently (Mersky and Bogduk 1994). Onset is at 30–40 years, with predominantly a male population. Alcohol precipitates attacks in the active period (Table 13.2).

Treatment

Treatment consists of abortive and prophylactic approaches. Most effective abortive treatment is the administration of 100% oxygen at a rate of 7–8 l/min for 15 min during an attack (Nappi and Russell 1993). Ergot preparations and sumatriptan (s.c.) have a beneficial effect. Prophylactic treatment is administered during the active period. Ergot preparations should not exceed 10 mg per week. Methysergide can be administered for short (weeks) periods. Lithium carbonate is utilized for the chronic-type cluster headache.

Paroxysmal hemicrania

Paroxysmal hemicrania (PH) was first described by Sjaastad and Dale in 1974 and was thought initially to be a rare variant of cluster headache. As new cases appear and the clinical features of this syndrome (Table 13.2) are further defined, it is doubtful that subclassifying PH under CH will be justified (Benoliel and Sharav 1998b). The International Association for the Study of Pain (IASP), in their most recent classification (Mersky and Bogduk 1994), thus defined a separate category for PH. This seems justified, based on a number of features that distinguish PH from CH (Table 13.2).

Temporal pattern

The attacks in PH are short (10–25 min), sharp and excruciating; hence the term 'paroxysmal' (Antonaci and Sjaastad 1989). Frequency is higher than that usually seen in cluster headaches; about eight attacks per 24 h in PH, but with as many as 30 (Haggag and Russell 1993). The first reported cases of PH were of a continuous nature and were categorized as chronic paroxysmal hemicrania (CPH). In contrast to CH, only a scant number of PHs behaved episodically (EPH) and many of these eventually developed into a chronic form (CPH:EPH = 4:1) (Antonaci and Sjaastad 1989). A high number of patients report nocturnal attacks of PH that wake the patient from sleep (Antonaci and Sjaastad 1989). However, the same nocturnal tendency as in CH is not apparent. Like most vascular-type craniofacial pain, PH is considered to be REM sleep related (Sahota and Dexter 1990).

Location

Pain occurs typically in the temporal, periauricular, and periorbital areas, hence the term hemicrania. Referral to the shoulder, neck, and arm has been reported. Unlike CH that may change sides, the vast majority of PH cases do not. Most cases in PH are unilateral and do not become bilateral but strong pain may cross the midline.

Accompanying phenomena

As in other primary vascular-type headaches, PH is accompanied by a number of usually ipsilateral autonomic phenomena. These may occur bilaterally but the symptomatic side is more pronounced. The most commonly seen are lacrimation (62%), nasal congestion (42%), conjunctival injection, and rhinorrhoea (36% each) (Benoliel and Sharav 1998b).

Treatment

The response to indometacin in PH is usually absolute and clearly distinguishes it from CH, which is non-responsive. Recently, however, the inclusion of an absolute indometacin response as part of PH's criteria has been questioned.

SUNCT

*S*hort-lasting, *u*nilateral, *n*euralgiform, headache attacks with *c*onjunctival injection and *t*earing (SUNCT) syndrome was introduced by Sjaastad (Sjaastad et al 1989). It is a unilateral headache/ facial pain characterized by brief, triggered, paroxysmal pain accompanied by ipsilateral local autonomic signs, usually conjunctival injection and lacrimation (Benoliel and Sharav 1998a). Multiple attacks occur usually during daytime, with less than 2% occurring at night. Each attack lasts from 15 to 120 s (Pareja et al 1996).

Triggering

SUNCT may be triggered by light mechanical stimuli in the areas innervated by the trigeminal nerve, in a way similar to trigeminal neuralgia. Neck movements have also been shown to trigger attacks (Mersky and Bogduk 1994).

Pain typically appears in the ocular and periocular regions, corresponding to the area innervated by the first branch (ophthalmic) of the trigeminal nerve. However, pain may be felt in the temporal and auricular regions.

Accompanying phenomena

By definition, SUNCT is accompanied by marked ipsilateral conjunctival injection and lacrimation, but these can also be seen in trigeminal neuralgia (Benoliel and Sharav 1998c). Nasal stuffiness, rhinorrhoea, and sweating may also accompany attacks, but are rarer and may be subclinical.

Treatment

A further distinct factor in SUNCT is its absolute resistance to both antineuralgic and antivascular drug therapy.

Cold stimulus ('ice cream') headache

Application of ice to the palate or to the posterior pharyngeal mucosa produces facial pain in the midfrontal region or around the ears, referred probably by the trigeminal and glossopharyngeal nerves respectively (Lance 1993). Pain follows the passage of cold material over the palate and posterior pharyngeal wall and does not originate in the teeth. It is postulated that incoming impulses due to cold cause disinhibition of central pain pathways. Cold stimulus headache or 'ice cream' headache occurs particularly in individuals with a history of migraine and is not associated with dental pathology.

Treatment

No treatment is needed other than sensible caution in ingestion of cold substances.

Vascular orofacial pain

Vascular orofacial pain (VOP), possibly a new diagnostic entity (Sharav et al. 1996, Benoliel et al. 1997), shares many of the signs and symptoms common to other vascular-type craniofacial pain. However, the rational for introducing VOP is based on its specific features that segregate it from other primary vascular-type craniofacial pain and justify a unique diagnosis. Furthermore, orofacial pain of vascular origin is of great diagnostic and therapeutic importance. The similarities between dental pulpitis and VOP, especially when it affects only the oral structures, has obviously caused diagnostic difficulties (Rees and Harris 1979, Benoliel et al 1997, Cherninsky et al 1999).

Vascular orofacial pain is characterized by strong, episodic, unilateral, intraoral pain. In about half of cases the pain throbs, and wakes the patient from sleep. Pain may last from minutes to hours (70% of cases) or can go on for days (30% of cases). Pain can be accompanied by various local autonomic signs, such as tearing or nasal congestion, or by other phenomenon, such as photo- or phonophobia and nausea (Benoliel et al 1997) The onset of VOP is around 40–50 years of age, and it affects females at a rate of 2.5 times more than males.

Differential diagnosis of VOP

Dental pain The extensive involvement of the teeth and oral structures accompanied with common dental symptomatology (e.g., thermal hypersensitivity) in VOP often leads to confusion with pulpitis.

Primary vascular-type headaches Although exhibiting some similarities to other primary vascular headaches there may be enough differentiating factors to define VOP separately. If VOP was simply a migraine-variant one would expect to see the majority of patients with long pain attacks (hours–days) and no local autonomic signs. Cluster headache is often misdiagnosed as pain of dental origin, but is usually located primarily periocularly (Nappi and Russell 1993). The similarities to the cluster headache group are limited by the fact that systemic symptoms (such as nausea and photo/phonophobia) are often present in VOP, with an overwhelming female preponderance and treatment response is not similar.

Neuropathic-type pains Trigeminal neuralgia is a short-lasting pain with a particular triggering pattern not usually accompanied by frank autonomic signs, making it clinically distinct from VOP.

Treatment

Successful abortive treatment in VOP has been attained with non-steroidal anti-inflammatory drugs. No particularly preferential response to indometacin (cf. paroxysmal hemicrania) has been noted and sodium naproxen (275–550 mg stat) has proved very effective abortive therapy. Prophylactic treatment using amitriptyline at doses up to 50 mg and the use of β-adrenergic blocking agents (in antihypertensive dosage) are effective (Cherninsky et al 1999).

Atypical oral and facial pain

This ill-defined category includes a variety of pain descriptions such as phantom tooth pain (Marbach 1978), atypical odontalgia (Rees and Harris 1979, Brooke 1980), and atypical facial neuralgia (Marbach et al 1982). Chronic pain, usually at a constant intensity, is a common feature of all the above. The pain has a burning quality that occasionally intensifies to produce a throbbing sensation. The pain is not triggered by remote stimuli, but may be intensified by stimulation of the painful area itself. Autonomic phenomena are usually not seen. The pain does not usually wake the patient from sleep. The location is ill defined. Although the pain usually starts in one quadrant of the mouth, it often spreads across the midline to the opposite side. Frequently, the pain changes location, which may result in extensive dental work, alcohol nerve blocks, and surgery; this does not usually alleviate the pain. Unfortunately, it has been the author's experience and that of others (Marbach et al 1982) to see patients who have had more than 70(!) operations performed in their mouth (e.g., pulp extirpation, apicoectomy, tooth extraction) for the relief of this type of pain.

Typically in most of these patients there is a lack of objective signs and all other tests are negative. The age range is wide (20–82 years), but the mean age of patients with atypical odontalgia is around 45–50 years (Marbach 1978, Rees and Harris 1979, Brooke 1980, Vickers et al 1998), and of patients with sore mouth and other oral complaints (e.g., burning sensation) around 55 years (Grushka et al 1987a). All reports indicate an overwhelming majority of females (82–100%) in the series of atypical oral and facial pain studied.

There is no identified uniform aetiology of atypical oral and facial pain (Loeser 1985). Several underlying mechanisms have been proposed. A number of reports have suggested that atypical facial pain is a psychiatric disorder (Engel 1951, Lascelles 1966, Feinmann et al 1984, Remick and Blasberg 1985). Depression is considered the most likely diagnosis and is explained on the basis of the catecholamine hypothesis of affective disorders (Rees and Harris 1979). However, Sharav et al (1987) showed that only 2 of their 28 patients were cortisol non-suppressors on the dexamethasone suppression test and that half the patients were not depressed at all. Grushka et al (1987a) conclude that the personality characteristics of patients with burning mouth syndrome are similar to those seen in other chronic pain patients and that these personality disturbances tend to increase with increased pain. Marbach (1978) postulates that phantom tooth pain associated with previous trauma such as tooth extraction and tooth pulp extirpation interferes with central nervous system pain modulatory mechanisms. This idea is supported by the observation that experimental tooth extraction produces lesions in the trigeminal nucleus caudalis (Westrum et al 1976, Gobel and Binck 1977). It was also found that more extensive tooth pulp injury is associated with greater excitatory changes of central trigeminal neurons (Hu et al 1990). Although far from proven, a deafferentation associated with peripheral nerve injury may be responsible for some types of atypical facial pain.

Vascular changes are other possible underlying mechanisms for atypical facial pain (Reik 1985). Rees and Harris (1979) and Brooke (1980) found a history of migraine in about a third of their patients (and see previous section on vascular orofacial pain).

Atypical facial pain should be differentiated from pains associated with a causative lesion. Chronic atypical facial pain can be a presenting symptom of a slow-growing cerebellopontine angle tumour (Nguyen et al 1986).

While various treatment modalities are used for atypical oral and facial pain, the predominant trends are clear. All authors firmly recommend against any surgical or dental interventions for the relief of pain (Loeser 1985). Since such interventions usually exacerbate the condition, reassurance, psychological counselling, and the use of antidepressants, particularly from the tricyclic group, have been found to be a very promising mode of therapy. Two double-blind controlled studies demonstrated that tricyclic antidepressive drugs were superior to placebo in reducing chronic facial pain (Feinmann et al 1984, Sharav et al 1987). Furthermore, Sharav et al (1987) showed that amitriptyline was effective in a daily dose of 30 mg or less and that the relief of pain was independent of the antidepressive activity. Vickers et al (1998) suggest a possible neuropathic pain mechanism, but point out that it cannot explain all cases, and suggest that some may fit the diagnosis of complex regional pain syndrome.

The burning mouth syndrome

The burning mouth syndrome (BMS) is an intraoral pain disorder unaccompanied by clinical signs. Its vague definition and unknown aetiology warrant its inclusion under atypical oral and facial pain. Inclusion criteria of patients with BMS may differ in different studies; e.g., the presence of systemic disorders may or may not be an exclusion criterion (Grushka 1987, Van der Ploeg et al 1987).

The prevalence of BMS is in the range of 1.5–2.5% of the general population but may be as high as 15% in women over 40 years of age (Grushka and Sessle 1991).

Clinical features

Burning pain often occurs at more than one oral site, with the anterior two-thirds of the tongue, the anterior hard palate, and the mucosal aspect of the lower lip most frequently affected (Main and Basker 1983, Grushka et al 1987a). The pain is intense and quantitatively similar to toothache pain but differs from toothache in quality. While toothache was mostly described as annoying and sharp, BMS pain was most commonly described as burning (Grushka et al 1987a). Burning pain is constant throughout the day or begins by mid-morning and reaches maximum intensity by early evening, but is not usually present at night and does not disturb sleep (Gorsky et al 1987, Grushka 1987). Many studies indicate, however, that BMS patients have difficulty falling asleep (Grushka 1987, Lamey and Lamb 1988, Zilli et al 1989). Grushka (1987) reported no significant difference between BMS and controls in any clinical oral features including number of teeth, oral mucosal conditions, presence of Candida, and parafunctional habits.

Psychophysical assessment

There is evidence for taste dysfunction in BMS, especially in those individuals with self-reported dysgeusia (Grushka et al 1987c). Sweet thresholds were significantly higher for BMS than control subjects. No differences were found between BMS and control subjects in somatosensory modalities such as two-point discrimination, temperature perception, and stereognostic ability at any of eight intraoral and facial sites tested (Grushka et al 1987b). Grushka et al (1987b) did, however, find that heat pain tolerance was significantly reduced at the tongue tip of BMS subjects, and suggested that hyperalgesia in these patients may depend on prolonged temporal or spatial central summation.

Recently, Jaaskelainen et al (1997) studied the blink reflex (BR) in 11 patients with BMS. As a group, the BMS patients demonstrated higher stimulus thresholds for the R1 component of the BR, indicating altered tactile sensation. These findings were explained as correlates of allodynia; stimulus intensities were not noxious (Jaaskelainen et al 1997). BMS patients thus demonstrated changes on the BR similar to other atypical facial pain subjects (Jaaskelainen et al 1999).

Aetiology

Many possible aetiologies have been suggested and include local, intraoral factors as well as general, systemic ones.

Local factors These include galvanic currents, denture allergy and mechanical irritation, and decreased salivary secretion or change in saliva composition. No difference was found in electric currents, potential, or energy capacity in the dental metallic restorations between BMS patients and controls (Hampf et al 1987). Most studies have not supported an allergic or mechanical irritation cause for BMS (Grushka and Sessle 1991). Most salivary flow rate studies have not demonstrated a significant decrease in salivary output, stimulated or unstimulated (Glick et al 1976, Syrjanen et al 1984, Lamey and Lamb 1988). On the other hand, some studies found significant alterations in salivary components such as proteins, immunoglobulins, and phosphates as well as differences in saliva pH buffering capacity (Glick et al 1976, Syrjanen et al 1984, Hampf et al 1987, Grushka and Sessle 1991). Whether these alterations in salivary composition are a causal or a coincidental event in BMS is unknown (Grushka and Sessle 1991).

Systemic factors Among these are menopause and hormonal imbalance, nutritional deficiencies, and psychogenic factors. A wide range of prevalence rates (18–80%) was given to BMS during menopause or after oophorectomy (Storer 1965, Ferguson et al 1981, Wardrop et al 1989), pointing to different definition criteria and possibly to various sampling methods. In a recent study Wardrop et al (1989) found significantly more oral discomfort in menopausal women. The oral discomfort was not associated with any of the vasomotor symptoms of menopause nor did it show any relationship to mucosal health. The presence of oral discomfort bore no relationship to follicle-stimulating hormone (FSH) or oestradiol levels measured in menopausal women, but hormone replacement therapy was accompanied with a significant reduction in oral discomfort (Wardrop et al 1989). However, as no control group was utilized it was difficult to assess how much of this reduction was due to a placebo effect. Despite the conflicting data on the effect of menopause and oestrogen replacement therapy on oral discomfort, the high frequency of oral complaints in menopausal women clearly indicates a significant, although poorly understood, association between menopause and BMS (Grushka and Sessle 1991).

A double-blind placebo-controlled study (Hugoson and Thorstensson 1991) could not demonstrate any effect of B_1, B_2, and B_6 vitamin replacement therapy in vitamin-deficient BMS patients. Recently serum zinc levels were found to be significantly lower in BMS patients than in matched controls (Maragou and Ivanyi 1991). However, only 9 out of 30 BMS patients demonstrated zinc levels less than the minimum normal levels. There is certainly a need for more controlled studies in order to determine the role of these nutrient elements in BMS.

Numerous studies have used psychological questionnaires and psychiatric interviews to demonstrate psychological disturbances such as depression, anxiety, and irritability in patients with BMS (Grushka et al 1987a, Van der Ploeg et al 1987, Hammaren and Hugoson 1989, Zilli et al 1989). BMS patients showed elevation in certain personality characteristics which were similar to those seen in other chronic pain patients (Grushka et al 1987a). Zilli et al (1989) indicate that psychiatric illness, especially depression, may play an important role in BMS. However, most investigators cannot say whether depression and other personality characteristics are causative or the result of the pain (Grushka et al 1987a, Van der Ploeg et al 1987, Zilli et al 1989, Grushka and Sessle 1991).

In conclusion, no clear aetiology is available today, and it is possible that a further subclassification of this 'syndrome' is needed. A more rigorous definition of inclusion and exclusion criteria may help in future studies of aetiology and possible therapy.

Treatment

Before treatment is instigated, local and systemic underlying factors should be ruled out and treated. Thus, faulty irritating prosthetic devices should be corrected and underlying diseases, such as diabetes or anaemia, should be treated. Unfortunately, as noted above, in many instances these corrections may not improve the burning sensation and oral discomfort. Symptomatic treatment with psychotropic drugs, such as amitriptyline or clonazepam, may be of some benefit, but no good controlled studies are available to demonstrate a real effect of these drugs. The local application of various medications was recently examined. Interestingly, burning sensation increased after local application of topical anaesthesia, while dysgeusia symptoms were more likely to decrease (Ship et al 1995). Ship et al (1995) suggested a centrally based neuropathic condition for the burning sensation and that the topical anaesthesia may be releasing peripheral inhibition of central sensory pathways. However, the application of capsaicin to oral mucosa in patients with intraoral neuropathic pain was beneficial in about 50% of patients (Epstein and Marcoe 1994). The potential importance of a placebo effect cannot be ruled out in this open study (Epstein and Marcoe 1994), and double-blind controlled studies are warranted before this treatment can be recommended for BMS.

Differential diagnosis of orofacial pain

Pain and defined local injury

Diagnosis of pain in the orofacial region is complicated by the density of anatomical structures, rich innervation, high vascularity of the area, and the important psychological meaning attributed to the face and the oral cavity. Most prevalent is pain in the area that results from local injury to fairly well-defined anatomical structures. Injury can result from trauma, infection, and neoplasia. Pain in these cases can be defined and described in terms of anatomical structures and thus originates from the oral cavity, the jaws, salivary glands, paranasal sinuses, or the TMJ. Oral pain has been extensively reviewed above and can be divided into dental, periodontal, and mucosal pain. These have been summarized in Table 13.1.

Pain from the jaws can be associated with acute infection, malignancies, and direct trauma. Unless infected, cysts, retained roots, or impacted teeth are usually not responsible for pain in the jaws. Radiation therapy to this area may result in severe pain due to infection and osteomyelitis associated with osteoradionecrosis. Odontogenic and other benign tumours of the bone do not normally produce pain in the jaws except for the osteoid osteoma, which is known to be associated with severe pain. However, this tumour is extremely rare in the jaws (Shafer et al 1974). Malignant tumours, both primary and those metastasized to the jaws, usually produce deep, boring pain associated with paraesthesia (Massey et al 1981).

Pain from salivary glands is localized to the affected gland, may be quite severe, and, when associated with a blocked salivary duct, is intensified by increased saliva production, such as that occurring before meals. The salivary gland is swollen and extremely sensitive to palpation. Salivary flow from the affected gland is usually reduced and sometimes abolished completely. Pain may be associated with fever and malaise. In children, the most common causes are acute recurrent parotitis and mumps. In adults, pain from salivary glands usually results from blockage of a salivary duct by calculus or mucin plug formation. Pain results from salivary retention, resulting in pressure and sometimes ascending infection. In acute parotitis, mouth opening exerts pressure on the gland by the posterior border of the mandible, resulting in severe pain (see Table 13.3).

Pain from the maxillary sinus is deep and boring and may become quite severe. Usually the maxillary posterior teeth on the affected side are tender to pressure and percussion. Pain is commonly felt all over the maxillary sinus. In some cases, the infraorbital nerve on the affected side is very sensitive to pressure, and there is hyperaesthesia in the area supplied by this nerve. Pain is intensified either by moving the head rapidly or by lowering the head. Pain may be associated with fever and malaise (Table 13.3).

Pain from the TMJ is usually intensified by movement of the mandible; the joint is tender when palpated via the external auditory meatus. Pain may result from acute infection, trauma, rheumatoid arthritis, psoriasis, and primary or secondary malignant tumours. When acutely inflamed the joint may be swollen and warm to touch. A splinting protective mechanism by the masticatory muscles may result in muscle spasm, producing secondary pain.

Pain not related to defined injury

Pain in the orofacial area can result from mechanisms other than local injury described above. These are usually associated with chronic orofacial pain and can be generated by musculoskeletal, vascular, neuropathic, referred, and psychogenic mechanisms (Okeson 1995). Trauma to the head and neck, especially high-velocity trauma, may be associated with a combination of mechanisms (Benoliel et al 1994).

Musculoskeletal pain is related to TMP and was discussed extensively above.

Vascular pain was discussed under the section on primary vascular-type craniofacial pain. In addition, pain in the facial area may also be associated with occlusive vascular disease, such as temporal arteritis (Paine 1977). External carotid occlusive disease has been described as a cause of facial pain (Herishanu et al 1974), and carotid system arteritis is an important entity in the differential diagnosis of facial pain (Troiano and Gaston 1975).

Table 13.3 Differential diagnosis of orofacial (excluding primary vascular-type) pain

	Dental	TMP	TMJ (ID)	Sinusitis (maxillary)	Salivary glands	Trigeminal neuralgia	Atypical deafferent
Location	Mouth, ear, jaws, cheek	Angle of mandible, temple, jaws	TMJ, ear	Cheek, zygomatic area	Area of gland	Nerve distribution	Diffuse, may cross midline
Localization	Poor, radiating, does not cross midline	Diffuse but usually unilateral	Localized, usually good	Usually localized, may radiate	Usually good	Good, in the trigeminal distribution	Poor, may change location
Duration	Minutes to hours	Weeks to years	Weeks to years	Days to weeks	Hours to days	Seconds	Weeks to years
Character of pain	Intermittent, sharp, paroxysmal	Dull, continuous, annoying	Deep, boring	Dull, boring, pressing	Drawing, pulling	Lancinating, paroxysmal	Dull, boring, continuous
Pain intensity	Mild to severe	Mild to moderate	Mild to moderate	Mild to severe	Moderate to severe	Severe	Mild to severe
Precipitating factors	Hot and cold foods	Yawning, chewing	Yawning, chewing	Bending, head movement	Eating, especially sour food	Touch, vibration, cold wind	Stress, fatigue
Associated signs	Caries	Limited mouth opening	Click in TMJ, deviation of mouth opening	Cheek oedema, infraorbital nerve hypoaesthesia	Blockage of salivary flow, salivary gland swelling	Facial tic	Sometimes scarring
Pain duplication	Cold/hot application	Masticatory muscle palpation	TMJ palpation	Pressure on sinus wall, head bending	Pressure to gland, citric acid to tongue	Touch of trigger point	Rubbing of scar if present
Sleep association	May disturb	Does not disturb	May disturb	May disturb	May disturb	Does not disturb	Does not disturb
Treatment	Endodontic, tooth restoration	Physiotherapy behavioural TCA	Bitegaurd, NSAID, TCA	Antibiotic decongestants	Antibiotics, blockage removal	Carbamazepine baclofen, nerve block, neurosurgery	TCA, clonazepam behavioural

TMP = temporomandibular pain; ID = internal derangement; TMJ = temporomandibular joint; NSAID = non-steroidal anti-inflammatory drugs; TCA = tricyclic antidepressant drugs.

Neuropathic pain is primarily expressed in the facial area as idiopathic trigeminal neuralgia, also known as tic douloureux. Classic features are paroxysmal pain that lasts only seconds, pain produced by non-noxious stimuli applied to a trigger zone, and pain confined to the trigeminal nerve and unilateral in any one paroxysm; the patient is pain free between attacks and there is no accompanying sensory loss (Dubner et al 1987). A rare form of facial neuralgic pain, associated with sweet food intake, was recently described (Sharav et al 1991, Helcer et al 1998). Neuralgic pain of a completely different type may be associated with herpes zoster, which is a boring, burning pain of long duration and high intensity. Postherpetic neuralgia may develop in some of these cases.

Referred pain is a frequent feature in the facial area: pain may refer from teeth to remote areas in the head and face (Sharav et al 1984), and muscle pain from both neck and masticatory muscle is referred to the oral and facial areas (Travell 1960). Pain in the teeth may also be referred from the ear (Silverglade 1980). Of special interest is pain due to cardiac ischaemia that is referred to the orofacial area (Tzukert et al 1981). Facial pain can also be an expression of a central nervous system lesion (Bullitt et al 1986).

Psychogenic pain in the orofacial area is associated with many emotional disorders; however, depression is apparently the most frequent (Lascelles 1966, Remick and Blasberg 1985). Psychogenic pain overlaps many of the features of atypical oral and facial pain that have been described previously. It is possible that apparent atypical oral and facial pain is often psychogenic in nature.

References

Agerberg G 1988 Mandibular function and dysfunction in complete denture wearers – a literature review. Journal of Oral Rehabilitation 15: 237–249

Agerberg G, Carlsson GE 1972 Functional disorders of the masticatory system. Distribution of symptoms accordings to age and sex as judged from investigation by questionnaire. Acta Odontologica Scandinavica 30: 597–613

American Sleep Disorder Association 1990 International classification of sleep disorders: diagnosis and coding manual. American Sleep Disorder Association, Rochester, MN, pp 181–185

Antonaci F, Sjaastad O 1989 Chronic paroxysmal hemicrania (CPH): a review of the clinical manifestations. Headache 29: 648–656

Basbaum AI, Levine JD 1991 The contribution of the nervous system to inflammation and inflammatory disease. Canadian Journal of Physiology and Pharmacology 69: 647–651

Bennet RM 1986 Current issues concerning management of the fibrositis/fibromyalgia syndrome. American Journal of Medicine (suppl 3A): 1–115

Benoliel B, Sharav Y 1998a SUNCT syndrome: case report and literature review. Oral Surgery, Oral Medicine, Oral Pathology, Oral Radiology and Endodontics 85: 158–161

Benoliel R, Sharav Y 1998b Paroxysmal hemicrania: case studies and review of the literature. Oral Surgery, Oral Medicine, Oral Pathology, Oral Radiology and Endodontics 85: 285–292

Benoliel R, Sharav Y 1998c Trigeminal neuralgia with lacrimation or SUNCT syndrome? Cephalalgia 18: 85–90

Benoliel R, Eliav E, Elishoov H, Sharav Y 1994 The diagnosis and treatment of persistent pain following trauma to the head and neck. Journal of Oral and Maxillofacial Surgery 52: 1138–1147

Benoliel R, Elishoov H, Sharav Y 1997 Orofacial pain with vascular-type features. Oral Surgery, Oral Medicine, Oral Pathology, Oral Radiology and Endodontics 84: 506–512

Blasberg B, Chalmers A 1989 Temporomandibular pain and dysfunction syndrome associated with generalized musculoskeletal pain: a retrospective study. Journal of Rheumatology (suppl 19): 87–90

Brooke RI 1980 Atypical odontalgia. Oral Surgery 49: 196

Broton JG, Sessle BJ 1988 Reflex excitation of masticatory muscles induced by algesic chemicals applied to the temporomandibular joint of the cat. Archives of Oral Biology 33: 741–747

Bullitt E, Tew J, Boyd J 1986 Intracranial tumors in patients with facial pain. Journal of Neurosurgery 64: 865–871

Cameron CE 1976 The cracked tooth syndrome: additional findings. Journal of the American Dental Association 93: 971

Carlsson GE 1976 Symptoms of mandibular dysfunction in complete denture wearer. Journal of Dentistry 4: 265

Carlsson GE, Gale EN 1976 Biofeedback treatment for muscle pain associated with the temporomandibular joint. Journal of Behavioural, Therapeutic and Experimental Psychiatry 7: 383

Carlsson GE, Egermark-Eriksson I, Magnusson T 1980 Intra- and inter-observer variation in functional examination of the masticatory system. Swedish Dental Journal 4: 187–194

Cherninsky R, Benoliel R, Sharav Y 1999 Odontalgia in vascular orofacial pain. Journal of Orofacial Pain 13: 196–200

Christensen LV 1981 Facial pains and the jaw muscles: a review. Journal of Oral Rehabilitation 8: 193

Clark GT, Beemsterboer PL, Solberg WK, Rugh JD 1979 Nocturnal electromyographic evaluation of myofascial pain dysfunction in patients undergoing occlusal splint therapy. Journal of the American Dental Association 99: 607–611

Clark GT, Rugh JD, Handelman SL 1980 Nocturnal masseter muscle activity and urinary acid catecholamine levels in bruxers. Journal of Dental Research 59: 1571–1576

Clark GT, Green EM, Dornan MR, Flack VF 1987 Craniocervical dysfunction levels in a patient sample from a temporomandibular joint clinic. Journal of the American Dental Association 115: 251–256

Clark GT, Tsukiyama Y, Baba K, Simmons M 1997 The validity and utility of disease detection methods and of occlusal therapy for temporomandibular disorders. Oral Surgery, Oral Medicine, Oral Pathology, Oral Radiology and Endodontics 83: 101–116

Clarke NG 1982 Occlusion and myofascial pain dysfunction: is there a relationship? Journal of the American Dental Association 85: 892

Clarke NG, Townsend GC, Carey SE 1984 Bruxing patterns in man during sleep. Journal of Oral Rehabilitation 11: 123–127

Cohen S 1996 Endodontic diagnosis. In: Cohen S, Burns RC (eds) Pathways of the pulp, 7th edn. Mosby, St Louis

Costen JB 1934 Syndrome of ear and sinus symptoms dependent upon disturbed function of the temporomandibular joint. Annals of Otorhinolaryngology 43: 1

De Boever JA 1979 Functional disturbances of the temporomandibular joint. In: Zarb GA, Carlsson GE (eds) Temporomandibular joint. Munksgaard, Copenhagen, p 193

Dexter JD, Weizman ED 1970 The relationship of nocturnal headaches to sleep stage patterns. Neurology 20: 513–518

Dolwick MD, Riggs RR 1983 Diagnosis and treatment of internal derangements of the temporomandibular joint. Dental Clinics of North America 27: 561
Dolwick MF, Katzberg RW, Helms CA 1983 Internal derangements of the temporomandibular joint: fact or fiction? Journal of Prosthetic Dentistry 49: 415
Dostrovsky JO, Davis KD, Kawakita K 1991 Central mechanisms of vascular headaches. Canadian Journal of Physiology and Pharmacology 69: 652–658
Dubner R, Sharav Y, Gracely RH, Price DD 1987 Idiopathic trigeminal neuralgia: sensory features and pain mechanisms. Pain 31: 23–33
Dworkin SF, Huggins KH, LeResche L et al 1990a Epidemiology of signs and symptoms in temporomandibular disorders: clinical signs in cases and controls. Journal of the American Dental Association 120: 273–281
Dworkin SF, LeResche L, DeRouen T, Von-Kroff M 1990b Assessing clinical signs of temporomandibular disorders: reliability of clinical examiners. Journal of Prosthetic Dentistry 63: 574–579
Engel GL 1951 Primary atypical facial neuralgia. An hysterical conversion symptom. Psychosomatic Medicine 13: 375
Epstein JB, Marcoe JH 1994 Topical application of capsaicin for treatment of oral neuropathic pain and trigeminal neuralgia. Oral Surgery, Oral Medicine and Oral Pathology 77: 135–140
Eriksson PO, Lindmen R, Stal P, Bengtsson A 1988 Symptoms and signs of mandibular dysfunction in primary fibromyalgia syndrome (PSF) patients. Swedish Dental Journal 12: 141
Eversole LR, Machado L 1985 Temporomandibular joint internal derangements and associated neuromuscular disorders. Journal of the American Dental Association 110: 69
Farrar W 1971 Diagnosis and treatment of anterior dislocation of the articular disc. New York Journal of Dentistry 41: 348
Feinmann C, Harris M, Cawley R 1984 Psychogenic facial pain: presentation and treatment. British Medical Journal 288: 436
Ferguson MM, Carter J, Boyle P et al 1981 Oral complaints related to climacteric symptoms in oophorectomized women. Journal of the Royal Society of Medicine 74: 492
Friend LA, Glenwright HD 1968 An experimental investigation into the localisation of pain from the dental pulp. Oral Surgery 25: 765
Gerschman JA, Reade PC, Hall W, Wright J, Holwill B 1990 Lateralization of facial pain, emotionality and affective disturbance. Pain 5 (suppl): S42
Glick D, Ben Aryeh H, Gutman D et al 1976 Relation between idiopathic glossodynia and salivary flow rate and content. International Journal of Oral Surgery 5: 161
Gobel S, Binck JM 1977 Degenerative changes in primary trigeminal axons and in neurons in nucleus caudalis following tooth pulp extirpations in the cat. Brain Research 132: 347
Goose DH 1981 Cracked tooth syndrome. British Dental Journal 2: 224
Gorsky M, Silverman S Jr, Chinn H 1987 Burning mouth syndrome: a review of 98 cases. Journal of Oral Medicine 42: 7
Grushka M 1987 Clinical features of burning mouth syndrome. Oral Surgery 63: 30
Grushka M, Sessle BJ 1991 Burning mouth syndrome. Dental Clinics of North America 35: 171
Grushka M, Sessle BJ, Miller R 1987a Pain and personality profiles in burning mouth syndrome. Pain 28: 155
Grushka M, Sessle BJ, Howley TP 1987b Psychophysical assessment of tactile pain and thermal sensory functions in burning mouth syndrome. Pain 28: 169
Grushka M, Sessle BJ, Howley TP 1987c Taste dysfunction in burning mouth syndrome (BMS). Annals of the New York Academy of Sciences 510: 321
Haggag KJ, Russell D 1993 Chronic paroxysmal hemicrania. In: Olesen J, Tafelt-Hansen P, Welch KMA (eds) The headaches. Raven Press, New York, pp 601–608
Hammaren M, Hugoson A 1989 Clinical psychiatric assessment of patients with burning mouth syndrome resisting oral treatment. Swedish Dental Journal 13: 77–88
Hampf G, Ekholm A, Salo T et al 1987 Pain in oral galvanism. Pain 29: 301
Headache Classification Committee of the International Headache Society 1988 Classification and diagnostic criteria for headache disorders, cranial neuralgias and facial pain. Cephalalgia 8(suppl 7): 19–41
Helcer M, Schnarch A, Benoliel R, Sharav Y 1998 Trigeminal neuralgic-type pain and vascular-type headache due to gustatory stimulus. Headache 38: 129–131
Helkimo M 1979 Epidemiological surveys of dysfunction of the masticatory system. In: Zarb GA, Carlsson GE (eds) Temporomandibular joint. Munksgaard, Copenhagen, p 175
Henriksson KG, Bengtsson A 1991 Fibromyalgia—a clinical entity? Canadian Journal of Physiology and Pharmacology 69: 672–677
Herishanu Y, Bendheim P, Dolberg M 1974 External carotid occlusive disease as a cause of facial pain. Journal of Neurology, Neurosurgery and Psychiatry 8: 963
Hu JW, Sharav Y, Sessle BJ 1990 Effect of one- or two-stage deafferentation of mandibular and maxillary tooth pulps on the functional properties of trigeminal brainstem neurons. Brain Research 516: 271–279
Hugoson A, Thorstensson B 1991 Vitamin B status and response to replacement therapy in patients with burning mouth syndrome. Acta Odontologica Scandinavica 49: 367–375
Jaaskelainen SK, Forsssell H, Tenovuo O 1997 Abnormalities of the blink reflex in burning mouth syndrome. Pain 73: 455–460
Jaaskelainen SK, Forsssell H, Tenovuo O 1999 Electrophysiological testing of the trigeminofacial system: aid in the diagnosis of atypical facial pain. Pain 80: 191–200
Katzberg RW, Dolwick MF, Bles DJ, Helms CA 1979 Arthrography of the temporomandibular joint: new technique and preliminary observations. American Journal of Roentgenology 132: 949
Kolbinson DA, Schubert MM, Flournoy N, Truelove EL 1988 Early oral changes following bone marrow transplantation. Oral Surgery, Oral Medicine and Oral Pathology 66: 130–138
Kopp S, Wenneberg B 1983 Intra- and interobserver variability in the assessment of signs of disorder in the stomatognathic system. Swedish Dental Journal 7: 239–246
Krogh-Polsen WG, Olsson A 1968 Management of the occlusion of the teeth, Part 1: Background, definitions, rationale. In: Schwartz L, Chayes CM (eds) Facial pain and mandibular dysfunction. Saunders, Philadelphia, pp 239–249
Lamey PJ, Lamb AB 1988 Prospective study of aetiological factors in burning mouth syndrome. British Medical Journal 296: 1243
Lance JW 1993 Miscellaneous headaches unassociated with a structural lesion. In: Olesen J, Tafelt-Hansen P, Welch KMA (eds) The headaches. Raven Press, New York, pp 609–617
Larheim TA 1995 Current trends in temporomandibular joint imaging. Oral Surgery, Oral Medicine, Oral Pathology, Oral Radiology and Endodontics 80: 555–576
Lascelles RG 1966 Atypical facial pain and psychiatry. British Journal of Psychiatry 112: 654
Lavigne GJ, Velly-Miguel AM, Montplaisir J 1991 Muscle pain, dyskinesia, and sleep. Canadian Journal of Physiology and Pharmacology 69: 678–682
Locker D, Slade G 1988 Prevalence of symptoms associated with temporomandibular disorders in a Canadian population. Community Dental and Oral Epidemiology 16: 310–313
Loeser JD 1985 Tic douloureux and atypical facial pain. Journal of the Canadian Dental Association 12: 917

Lundh H, Westesson P-L, Kopp S, Tillström B 1985 Anterior repositioning splint in the treatment of temporomandibular joints with reciprocal clicking: comparison with a flat occlusal splint and untreated control group. Oral Surgery 60: 131
Magnusson T, Carlsson GE 1978 Comparison between two groups of patients in respect of headache and mandibular dysfunction. Swedish Dental Journal 2: 85–92
Main DMG, Basker RM 1983 Patients complaining of a burning mouth. British Dental Journal 154: 206
Maragou P, Ivanyi L 1991 Serum zinc levels in patients with burning mouth syndrome. Oral Surgery, Oral Medicine and Oral Pathology 71: 447–450
Marbach JJ 1978 Phantom tooth pain. Journal of Endodontics 4: 362
Marbach JJ, Lund P 1981 Depression, anhedonia and anxiety in temporomandibular joint and other facial pain syndromes. Pain 11: 73–84
Marbach JJ, Lipton J, Lund P et al 1978 Facial pains and anxiety levels: considerations for treatment. Journal of Prosthetic Dentistry 40: 434–437
Marbach JJ, Hulbrock J, Hohn C, Segal AG 1982 Incidence of phantom tooth pain: a typical facial neuralgia. Oral Surgery 53: 190
Massey EW, Moore J, Schold SC 1981 Dental neuropathy from systemic cancer. Neurology 13: 1227
McNeill C 1997 History and evolution of TMD concepts. Oral Surgery, Oral Medicine, Oral Pathology, Oral Radiology and Endodontics 83: 51–60
Merskey H, Bogduk N (eds) 1994 Classification of chronic pain: descriptions of chronic pain syndromes and definition of pain terms, 2nd edn. IASP Press, Seattle, pp 68–71
Merskey H, Lau CL, Russel ES et al 1987 Screening for psychiatric morbidity. The pattern of psychological illness and premorbid characteristics in four chronic pain populations. Pain 30: 141–157
Moskowitz MA, Buzzi MG, Sakas DE, Linik MD 1989 Pain mechanisms underlying vascular headaches. Revue Neurologique (Paris) 145: 181–193
Nappi G, Russell D 1993 Cluster headache clinical features. In: Olesen J, Tafelt-Hansen P, Welch KMA (eds) The headaches. Raven Press, New York, pp 577–584
Nguyen M, Maciewicz R, Bouckoms A, Poletti C, Ojemann R 1986 Facial pain symptoms in patients with cerebellopontine angle tumors: a report of 44 cases of cerebellopontine angle meningioma and review of the literature. Clinical Journal of Pain 2: 3
Nielsen LL, McNeil C, Danzig W, Goldman S, Levy J, Miller AJ 1990 Adaption of craniofacial muscles in subjects with craniomandibular disorders. American Journal of Orthodontics and Dentofacial Orthopedics 97: 20–34
Nitzan DW, Dolwick MF 1991 An alternative explanation for the genesis of closed-lock symptoms in the internal derangement process. Journal of Oral and Maxillofacial Surgery 49: 810–815
Nitzan DW, Dolwick MF, Martinez GA 1991 Temporomandibular joint arthrocentesis: a simplified treatment for severe, limited mouth opening. Journal of Oral and Maxillofacial Surgery 49: 1163–1167
Nitzan DW, Mahler Y, Simkin A 1992 Intra-articular pressure measurements in patients with suddenly developing severely limited mouth opening. Journal of Maxillofacial Surgery 50: 1038
Okeson JP 1995 Bell's orofacial pains, 5th edn. Quintessence, Chicago, pp 135–184
Okeson JP (ed) 1996 Orofacial pain: guidelines for assessment, diagnosis and management. Quintessence, Chicago
Okeson JP 1997 Current terminology and diagnostic classification schemes. Oral Surgery, Oral Medicine, Oral Pathology, Oral Radiology and Endodontics 83: 61–64
Okeson JP, Moody PM, Kemper JT, Haley JV 1983 Evaluation of occlusal splint therapy and relaxation procedures in patients with temporomandibular disorders. Journal of the American Dental Association 107: 420
Paine R 1977 Vascular facial pain. In: Alling CC III, Mahan PE (eds) Facial pain, 2nd edn. Lea & Febiger, Philadelphia, p 57
Pareja JA, Shen JM, Kruszewski P, Caballero V, Pamo M, Sjaastad O 1996 SUNCT syndrome: duration, frequency, and temporal distribution of attacks. Headache 36: 161–165
Perry HT 1973 Adolescent temporomandibular dysfunction. American Journal of Orthodontics 63: 517
Rao VM 1995 Imaging of the temporomandibular joint. Seminars in Ultrasound, CT and MRI 16: 513–526
Raskin NH, Appenzeller O (1980) Headache. WB Saunders, Philadelphia, pp 132–136
Rees RT, Harris M 1979 Atypical odontalgia. British Journal of Oral Surgery 16: 212–218
Reik L 1985 Atypical facial pain: a reappraisal. Headache 25: 30
Remick RA, Blasberg B 1985 Psychiatric aspects of atypical facial pain. Journal of the Canadian Dental Association 12: 913
Roberts CA, Tallents RH, Espeland MA, Handelman SL, Katzberg RW 1985 Mandibular range of motion versus arthrographic diagnosis of the temporomandibular joint. Oral Surgery 60: 244
Roistacher SL, Tanenbaum D 1986 Myofascial pain associated with oropharyngeal cancer. Oral Surgery 61: 459
Rugh JD, Harlan J 1988 Nocturnal bruxism and temporomandibular disorders. Advances in Neurology 49: 329–341
Rugh JD, Solberg WK 1979 Psychological implications in temporomandibular pain and dysfunction. In: Zarb GA, Carlosson GE (eds) Temporomandibular joint. Munksgaard, Copenhagen, p 239
Rugh JD, Solberg WK 1985 Oral health status in the United States: temporomandibular disorders. Journal of Dental Education 49: 398–405
Rugh JD, Barghi N, Drago CJ 1984 Experimental occlusal discrepancies and nocturnal bruxism. Journal of Prosthetic Dentistry 51: 548
Sahota PK, Dexter JD 1990 Sleep and headache syndromes: a clinical review. Headache 30: 80–84
Salter M, Brooke RL, Merskey H et al 1983 Is the temporomandibular pain and dysfunction syndrome a disorder of the mind? Pain 17: 151–166
Satoh T, Harada Y 1973 Electrophysiological study on tooth grinding during sleep. Electroencephalography and Clinical Neurophysiology 35: 267–275
Schnurr RF, Brooke RI, Rollman GB 1990 Psychosocial correlates of temporomandibular joint pain and dysfunction. Pain 42: 153–165
Selby A 1985 Physiotherapy in the management of temporomandibular disorders. Australian Dental Journal 30: 273–280
Sessle BJ, Hu JW 1991 Mechanisms of pain arising from articular tissues. Canadian Journal of Physiology and Pharmacology 69: 617–626
Shafer WG, Hine MK, Levy BM 1974 A textbook of oral pathology, 3rd edn. Saunders, Philadelphia, p 152
Sharav Y, Feinsod M 1977 Nasopharyngeal tumor manifested as myofascial pain dysfunction syndrome. Oral Surgery 44: 54
Sharav Y, Tzukert A, Refaeli B 1978 Muscle pain index in relation to pain dysfunction and dizziness associated with myofascial pain-dysfunction syndrome. Oral Surgery 46: 742
Sharav Y, Leviner E, Tzukert A, McGrath PA 1984 The spatial distribution, intensity and unpleasantness of acute dental pain. Pain 20: 363
Sharav Y, Singer E, Schmidt E, Dionne RA, Dubner R 1987 The analgesic effect of amitriptyline on chronic facial pain. Pain 31: 199
Sharav Y, Benoliel R, Schnarch A, Greenberg L 1991 Idiopathic

trigeminal pain associated with gustatory stimuli. Pain 44: 171–174
Sharav Y, Benoliel R, Elishoov H 1996 Vascular orofacial pain: diagnostic features. 8th World Congress on Pain, Vancouver. IASP Press, Seattle, p 155
Ship J, Grushka M, Lipton J, Mott AE, Sessle BJ, Dionne RA 1995 Burning mouth syndrome: an update. Journal of the American Dental Association 126: 842–853
Silverglade D 1980 Dental pain without dental etiology: a manifestation of referred pain from otitis media. Journal of Dentistry for Children 47: 358
Singer EJ, Sharav Y, Dubner R, Dionne RA 1987 The efficacy of diazepam and ibuprofen in the treatment of the chronic myofascial orofacial pain. Pain 4 (suppl): 583
Sjaastad O, Dale I 1974 Evidence for a new (?) treatable headache entity. Headache 14: 105–108
Sjaastad O, Saunte C, Salvesen R, Fredrikson TA, Seim A, Roe OD et al 1989 Short-lasting unilateral neuralgiform headache attacks with conjunctival injection, tearing, sweating and rhinorrhea. Cephalalgia 9: 1947–1956
Solberg WK, Flint RT, Brantner JP 1972 Temporomandibular joint pain and dysfunction: a clinical study of emotional and occlusal components. Journal of Prosthetic Dentistry 28: 412
Stem PG, Mothersill KJ, Brooke RI 1979 Biofeedback and a cognitive behavioral approach to treatment of myofascial pain dysfunction syndrome. Behavioural Therapy 10: 29
Sternbach RA 1978 Clinical aspects of pain. In: Sternbach RS (ed) The psychology of pain. Raven Press, New York, p 241
Storer R 1965 The effects of the climacteric and of aging on prosthetic diagnosis and treatment planning. British Dental Journal 119: 340–354
Syrjanen S, Piironen P, Yli-Urpo A 1984 Salivary content of patients with subjective symptoms resembling galvanic pain. Oral Surgery 58: 387
Tafelt-Hansen P, Lous I, Olesen J 1981 Prevalence and significance of muscle tenderness during common migraine attacks. Headache 21: 49–54
Torvonen T, Knuuttila M 1988 Prevalance of signs and symptoms of mandibular dysfunction among adults aged 25, 35, 50 and 60 years in Osthrobotnia, Finland. Journal of Oral Rehabilitation 15: 455–463
Thomson H 1971 Mandibular dysfunction syndrome. British Dental Journal 130: 187
Travell J 1960 Temporomandibular joint pain referred from muscles of head and neck. Journal of Prosthetic Dentistry 10: 475
Travell J, Simons D 1983 Myofascial pain and dysfunction: the trigger point manual. Williams & Wilkins, Baltimore, pp 165–182
Troiano MF, Gaston GW 1975 Carotid system arteritis: an overlooked and misdiagnosed syndrome. Journal of the American Dental Association 91: 589
Turk DC 1997 Psychosocial and behavioral assessment of patients with temporomandibular disorders: diagnostic and treatment implications. Oral Surgery, Oral Medicine, Oral Pathology, Oral Radiology and Endodontics 83: 65–71
Tzukert A, Hasin Y, Sharav Y 1981 Orofacial pain of cardiac origin. Oral Surgery 51: 484
Van der Ploeg HM, Van der Wal N, Ejkman MAJ et al 1987 Psychological aspects of patients with burning mouth syndrome. Oral Surgery 63: 664
Velly-Miguel A, Montplaisir J, Lavigne G 1991 Nocturnal bruxism, jaw movements and sleep parameters: a controlled pilot study. Journal of Dental Research 70 (abstract): 1970
Vickers ER, Cousins MJ, Walker S, Chisholm K 1998 Analysis of 50 patients with atypical odontalgia. Oral Surgery, Oral Medicine, Oral Pathology, Oral Radiology and Endodontics 85: 24–32
Wanman A, Agerberg G 1986a Mandibular dysfunction in adolescents. I. Prevalence of symptoms. Acta Odontologica Scandinavica 44: 47–54
Wanman A, Agerberg G 1986b Two year longitudinal study of symptoms of mandibular dysfunction in adolescents. Acta Odontologica Scandinavica 44: 321–331
Wardrop RW, Hailes J, Burger H et al 1989 Oral discomfort at menopause. Oral Surgery 67: 535
Ware JC, Rugh JD 1988 Destructive bruxism: sleep state relationship. Sleep 11: 172–181
Watts PG, Peet KM, Juniper RP 1986 Migraine and the temporomandibular joint: the final answer? British Dental Journal 161: 170–173
Westesson PL, Eriksson L, Kurita K 1989 Reliability of negative clinical temporomandibular joint examination: prevalence of disc displacement in asymptomatic temporomandibular joints. Oral Surgery, Oral Medicine and Oral Pathology 68: 551–554
Westrum LE, Canfield RC, Black RG 1976 Transganglionic degeneration in the spinal trigeminal nucleus following removal of tooth pulps in adult cats. Brain Research 101: 137
Widmer CG 1991 Introduction III. Chronic muscle pain syndromes: an overview. Canadian Journal of Physiology and Pharmacology 69: 659–661
Wieselmann G, Permann R, Korner E 1986 Distribution of muscle activity during sleep in bruxism. European Neurology 25 (suppl 2): 111–116
Wolfe F 1988 Fibrositis, fibromyalgia, and musculoskeletal disease: the current status of the fibrositis syndrome. Archives of Physical Medicine and Rehabilitation 69: 527–531
Yoshimura Y, Yoshida Y, Oka M, Miyoshi M, Uemura S 1982 Long-term evaluation of non-surgical treatment of osteoarthrosis of temporomandibular joint. International Journal of Oral Surgery 11: 7
Zilli C, Brooke RI, Lau CL et al 1989 Screening for psychiatric illness in patients with oral dysaesthesia by means of the General Health Questionnaire—twenty-eight item version (GHQ-28) and the Irritability, Depression and Anxiety Scale (IDA). Oral Surgery 67: 384

Chapter 14

Trigeminal, eye, and ear pain

Joanna M Zakrzewska

Introduction

This chapter covers pain that can occur in the area of the face bounded by the distribution of the trigeminal nerve. It includes pain in and around the eyes and ears but excludes pain in the oral cavity or associated with the temporomandibular joint and deals primarily with chronic pain.

An evidence-based approach to the management of facial pain is presented. Readers are encouraged to regularly use updated resources when deciding on the optimal treatment. These resources include *Best Evidence*, *The Cochrane Library*, *Clinical Evidence*, evidence-based journals that summarize data, online databases, and nationally produced guidelines. The data found must then be critically appraised (Sackett et al 2000). The diagnostic criteria proposed by the International Association for the Study of Pain (IASP) (Anonymous 1994) or the International Headache Society (IHS) (Anonymous 1988) are listed in Table 14.1, and will be used throughout this chapter. The epidemiology of facial pain has been reviewed in *Epidemiology of Pain* (Zakrzewska and Hamlyn 1999).

Trigeminal neuralgia

Background information

The IASP definition of trigeminal neuralgia is 'sudden, usually unilateral, severe, brief, stabbing, recurrent pains in the distribution of one or more branches of the fifth cranial nerve'. Secondary or symptomatic trigeminal neuralgia is caused by a demonstrable, structural lesion such as a tumour, aneurysm, or multiple sclerosis. It is a rare disease (Zakrzewska and Hamlyn 1999) most commonly linked with multiple sclerosis. Its aetiology and pathophysiology remain controversial, and it is postulated that a blood vessel compresses the trigeminal nerve in the root entry zone in the posterior fossa (Burchiel and Slavin 2000).

Clinical features

The validity and reliability of the various diagnostic criteria have not been ascertained using evidence-based methodology. Drangshott and Truelove (2001) have shown that the key diagnostic

Table 14.1 Differential diagnosis of facial pain by location or type

	Condition	Prevelance incidence
Eye	Corneal abrasions	Relatively common
	Iritis, ant. uveitis	Relatively rare
	Optic neuritis	Relatively rare
	Acute angle closure glaucoma	Relatively common
	Tolosa–Hunt	Rare
	Raeder's syndrome	Rare
Otolaryngological	Sinusitis	Very common
	Otitis externa	Relatively common
	Otitis media	Relatively common
Orodental	Salivary gland	Rare
	TMJ	Common
	Dental disease	Very common
Neuralgias	Trigeminal	Relatively rare
	Glossopharyngeal	Very rare
	Postherpetic trigeminal	Relatively rare
	Pretrigeminal	Rare
	SUNCT	Rare
	Cluster headaches	Relatively rare
	Geniculate neuralgia (Ramsay Hunt)	Relatively rare
Psychogenic/ somatizers	Atypical facial pain	Infrequent
Vascular	Migraine	Common
	Giant cell arteritis	Relatively rare
	Aneurysym	Rare
Neoplasia	Sinus, posterior fossa, ear	Rare
Referred	From other organs	Rare

Table 14.2 Trigeminal neuralgia: diagnostic clinical criteria

1. [a]Character	Shooting, electric shock, sharp, superficial
2. [a]Severity	Moderate to most severe
3. Duration	Each episode of pain lasts less than a few seconds, numerous episodes during the day
4. [a]Periodicity	Periods of weeks, months when no pain; also, pain-free periods between attacks
5. [a]Site	Distribution of the trigeminal nerve area, mostly unilateral
6. Radiation	Within trigeminal nerve area, rarely beyond
7. [a]Provoking features	Light touch such as eating, talking, washing
8. Relieving features	Often sleep, anticonvulsant drugs
9. Associated features	Trigger areas, weight loss, poor quality of life, depression

[a]The IHS classification suggests that at least four of these must be present to make the diagnosis.

features have a high sensitivity and these are summarized in Table 14.2. At present the diagnosis of trigeminal neuralgia is made principally on the history, which must be taken with utmost care and non-verbal behaviour should be noted. Patients should be encouraged to 'tell their own story' as the words used to describe the character of the pain, such as shock-like, lightning, shooting, and an electric current, its severity, and periodicity are often pathognomonic of the condition. This can then be supplemented by the McGill Pain Questionnaire, which discriminates well between trigeminal neuralgia and atypical facial pain (Melzack et al 1986). Not only does the McGill Pain Questionnaire provide details of the characteristics of the pain but it also gives an indication of its severity. The most frequently used words are sharp, shooting, unbearable, stabbing, exhausting, tender, vicious, terrifying, and torturing. The McGill Pain Questionnaire has also shown that some patients additionally have a dull, aching, continuous component to their pain (Zakrzewska et al 1999).

The severity of trigeminal neuralgia varies from moderate to most severe. It is generally accepted that pain severity increases with time but there have been no formal studies to validate this. During an attack of severe pain the face may be distorted or 'freeze' and hands may be put in front of the face as if to protect it without touching it. Patients may also cry out with pain. These non-verbal behaviours are useful clues as to the severity of the pain.

Another important characteristic is the siting of the pain, unilaterally distributed along the trigeminal nerve. Around 4% of patients will have bilateral pain but it rarely occurs simultaneously. There is a slight right-sided predominance, around 60%, but there seems to be no relationship to handedness (Rothman and Wepsic 1974). All three divisions may be affected, and the most commonly affected divisions are the second and third, together. The rarest division is that of the ophthalmic branch.

The timing of the pain attacks is highly significant. Each single burst of severe pain usually lasts for seconds but several of these may follow in quick succession before the nerve becomes refractory so making it feel like minutes. After such attacks patients often report residual, dull ache or burning sensations. These attacks of pain diminish at night, and patients can be free of pain for years (6%), months (36%), weeks (16%), or only days (16%). Diurnal constant pain can be present in 4% of patients and 23% had no recordable pain-free intervals (Rasmussen 1990, 1991). Katusic et al (1990), in their epidemiological survey of 75 patients, found that the median length of an episode of pain was 49 days and the mean was 116 days with a range of 1–462 days. Up to 58% of patients have long, spontaneous remission periods and these tend to occur early in the disease process (Kurland 1958).

Pain is characteristically triggered by light touch with the major precipitating factors being chewing and talking (76%), touching (65%), and cold (48%) (Rasmussen 1991). A trigger zone can be identified in 50% of these patients. Apart from avoiding touching and moving their faces, patients can do little to gain relief without recourse to drug therapy.

It is important to enquire how patients cope with the pain and what strategies they adopt to deal with it. Many patients will avoid precipitating factors and so will lose weight, avoid cleaning their teeth on the affected side, and reduce their socializing, especially if it involves eating and talking. Patients with trigeminal neuralgia, especially when going through a bout of severe pain, will suffer from anhedonia and even depression (Zakrzewska and Thomas 1993, Zakrzewska et al 1999).

Using a variety of measures, including the Spielberger State-Trait Anxiety Inventory, Marbach and Lund (1981) failed to differentiate between different facial pain syndromes. On the Illness Behaviour Questionnaire patients with trigeminal neuralgia scored higher on denial and low on affective inhibition when compared to other facial pain patients. They had normal scores on hypochondriasis and irritability but were convinced that there was a physical cause for their disease (Gordon and Hitchcock 1983). Patients with trigeminal neuralgia also score lower on neuroticism when tested on the Eysenck Personality Inventory (Gordon and Hitchcock 1983).

Examination

Gross neurological examination rarely shows up any abnormalities in idiopathic trigeminal neuralgia. However, instrumental examination shows that over 50% of patients may have at least one abnormal measure of sensation, not only in the trigger zone division but also in the adjacent division (Nurmikko 1991). There is currently no evidence to suggest that these subtle findings reflect severity of disease or predict the presence of compression. Patients with neurological abnormalities or developing or progressive intractable pain often have secondary trigeminal neuralgia. Nurmikko and Eldridge (2001) suggest that there are several types of trigeminal neuralgia and call these typical and atypical trigeminal neuralgia and trigeminal neuropathy. This latter group has pain that is more continuous, and on examination large allodynic areas as well as sensory loss are found.

Investigations

There is, as yet, no highly specific or sensitive test to confirm the diagnosis of trigeminal neuralgia. Computer tomography (CT) and magnetic resonance imaging (MRI) are used to identify patients with multiple sclerosis or tumours and should be done in those patients with neurological changes that are progressive or develop as new features. Magnetic resonance angiography with weighted spin echo sequences is used prior to surgery to assess compression of the trigeminal nerve in the posterior fossa. These techniques have not been evaluated according to evidence-based medicine methodology (Sackett et al 2000) but an evaluation of the current status can be found in a review article of diagnosis and differential diagnosis of trigeminal neuralgia (Zakrzewska 2002). Baseline haematological and biochemical tests (urea and electrolytes, liver function) are essential prior to use of drugs.

Management

The wide range of treatments currently in use for trigeminal neuralgia and lack of randomized controlled multinational trials are ample evidence that there is no simple answer to how trigeminal neuralgia should be managed. Trials in patients with trigeminal neuralgia are difficult to conduct for a number of reasons: its relative rarity, its unknown aetiology, its natural history of spontaneous remissions, its varying severity, and lack of an objective diagnostic test. Currently, there are no agreed guidelines on the conduct of trials such as have been prepared in other disciplines, e.g., cluster headaches (Lipton et al 1995). There is no consensus on what outcome parameters should be used and how they should be measured. No surveys have been done to ascertain what outcomes the patients themselves would expect given that a complete cure is rarely achieved and most treatments have side effects.

Medical management

A systematic review of the use of anticonvulsants in the management of acute and chronic neuropathic pain, which includes trigeminal neuralgia, has been completed (McQuay et al 1995) and is kept updated on the Cochrane database. There is also a regularly updated review in *Clinical Evidence* (Zakrzewska 2002). The results are listed in Table 14.3.

Carbamazepine is likely to be beneficial and remains the gold standard. The incidence of side effects is often higher in the elderly and those in whom the drug and dose escalations are introduced rapidly. Haematological adverse reactions include a lowering of the white cell count and megaloblastic anaemia associated with folic acid deficiency. Carbamazepine hypersensitivity in the form of an allergic rash may occur in up to 10% of patients. At high concentrations, fluid retention can occur in patients with cardiac problems and the risk of hyponatraemia increases with age, higher carbamazepine serum concentrations, and the use of diuretics. As carbamazepine is a potent hepatic enzyme inducer, it results in numerous drug interactions that can result in variable side effects.

The effectiveness of the following drugs is based on the review in *Clinical Evidence* (Zakrzewska 2002). Tizanidine's, lamotrigine's, and baclofen's effectiveness have not been proven due to lack of large trials. Pimozide produced better results than carbamazepine but 40 out of 48 patients reported adverse reactions, which limits its use (Lechin et al 1989). Tocainide is harmful and proparacaine is unlikely to be beneficial. Numerous other drugs that have never been evaluated in any form of trial are being used and some of these are listed in Table 14.4, with proposed maximum dosages.

Anticonvulsant drugs, especially initially, are the treatment of choice but the timing of surgery is controversial. Most physicians and patients opt for surgery when medical management either fails to give pain relief or results in unacceptable side effects. However, some surgeons argue that surgery reduces damage to the trigeminal nerve and results in fewer recurrences if done early and that fewer postoperative complications occur, as patients are younger and medically fitter (Burchiel and Slavin 2000, Zakrzewska 2002).

Surgical management

Hundreds of reports on the surgical management of trigeminal neuralgia have been published but

Table 14.3 Drugs used in the management of trigeminal neuralgia which have been evaluated in randomized controlled trials or controlled trials

Report	Type of study	Drug daily dose/control	No. of patients	Efficacy NNT	NNH
Campbell et al 1998	RCT	Carbamazepine 400–800 mg/placebo	77	2.8	4.3
Killian and Fromm 1968	RCT	Carbamazepine 400 mg–1 g/placebo	30	1.4	1.6
Nicol 1969	RCT	Carbamazepine 100 mg–2.4 g/placebo	54	-9.3	3.7
Vilming et al 1986	RCT	Tizanidine 18 mg/carbamazepine 900 mg	12	Worse tizanidine	NS
Fromm et al 1993	CT	Tizanidine 12 mg/carbamazepine	11	2**	NS
Lindstrom and Lindblom 1987	RCT	Tocainide 20 mg/kg/carbamazepine	12	Equal result	3
Lechin et al 1989	RCT	Pimozide 4–12 mg/carbamazepine 300 mg–1.2 g	68	1	2.9
Zakrzewska et al 1997	RCT	*Lamotrigine 400 mg/placebo	13	2.1	NS
Fromm et al 1984	CT	Baclofen 40–80 mg/placebo	10	1.4	NS
Fromm and Terrence 1987	CT	Racemic baclofen 60 mg/L-baclofen 6–12 mg	15	2	2
Kondziolka et al 1994	RCT	Proparcaine eyedrops 0.5%/placebo	25	NS	—

RCT, randomized controlled trial; CT, controlled trial, not randomized double blind; *, add on therapy; **, short term; NNT, number needed to treat; NNH, number needed to harm; NS, not significant.

Table 14.4 Reported daily dosages of drugs used in trigeminal neuralgia. Many of these have not been evaluated in trials and dosages are based on case series (Nurmikko et al 2001, Zakrzewska 2002)

Drug	Daily dose
Baclofen[a]	50–80 mg[b]
Carbamazepine[a]	300–1000 mg
Clonazepam	4–8 mg
Gabapentin	1800–3600 mg
Lamotrigine[a]	200–400 mg[b]
Oxcarbazepine	300–1200 mg
Phenytoin	200–300 mg
Topiramate	25–250 mg
Tizanidine[a]	6–18 mg
Valproic acid	600–1200 mg

[a]Evaluated in randomized controlled trials.
[b]Slow dose escalation is recommended.

there are only two randomized controlled trials, each on peripherally injected streptomycin. There are no well-designed cohort studies performed prospectively with concurrent or even historical controls. Most of the cohort studies are retrospective and have no controls. There is only one prospective, longitudinal study and a few prospective ones. Most of the available data are in the form of descriptive studies and few have used independent observers to assess outcome. The expertise of the surgeon is known to affect outcome. Very few studies give full details of diagnostic criteria, including inclusion and exclusion criteria. Rarely are the criteria for classification of recurrences given and few authors provide definitions of the terminology used, e.g., anaesthesia dolorosa, dysaesthesia, hyperaesthesia. An outcome measure is rarely defined, and in the vast majority pain is measured solely on a verbal rating scale using an ordinal scale of 1–3. Only a handful of papers give measurements of preoperative pain. Length of follow-up is extremely variable, some series do not even provide details, and others exclude patients lost to follow-up. Timings of the assessments are extremely variable as most studies are conducted at a particular time point and so the patients are at different stages of follow-up. Data analysis is very variable, and it is only possible to compare those series that have used analysis such as the Kaplan–Meier probability methodology. No studies have assessed outcome in terms of quality of life or ability to carry out daily activities. No economic evaluations are available for a single surgical procedure (Zakrzewska 2002).

The ideal procedure should fulfil the following criteria: be easy to perform, require no sophisticated equipment, be repeatable if necessary, give immediate pain relief, have no or low recurrence rates, be free of risks and side effects, provide excellent quality of life, and be low cost. The following account of surgical management at three different levels, peripheral, Gasserian ganglion, and posterior fossa, is, unfortunately, biased due to lack of evidence. The major procedures will be described next, and they are compared in Table 14.5 using data only from larger, more complete studies.

Peripheral surgery

Two randomized controlled trials have been done to assess the value of injections of streptomycin with lidocaine (lignocaine) as compared to lidocaine (lignocaine) on its own (Stajcic et al 1990, Bittar and Graff-Radford 1993). Both studies showed that lidocaine (lignocaine) on its own was as effective as streptomycin. Table 14.6 lists, in general, the advantages and disadvantages of peripheral treatments, which vary depending on whether the nerve is visualized, as in cryotherapy or neurectomy, or whether the procedures are done using a blind technique, e.g., alcohol, streptomycin injections, peripheral radiofrequency thermocoagulation.

Most of these procedures can be done under local anaesthesia with sedation although in some it is technically easier to use a general anaesthetic. The various techniques used for each of the individual procedures are described in greater detail in the chapter on *Trigeminal Neuralgia* (Zakrzewska 2002) but personally I think there are currently very few indications for these techniques.

Surgery at the level of the Gasserian ganglion

Surgery at this level relies on the principle that a needle is guided through the foramen ovale into the Gasserian ganglion or the surrounding trigeminal cistern. This is done utilizing fluoroscopic techniques, and then other instruments or substances can be passed through this wide-bore needle. These techniques are mostly done under sedation or a brief general anaesthetic, which rarely requires endotracheal intubation. Patients, therefore, can have these procedures done as day cases or, at the most, a 1- to 2-day inpatient stay. The reader is referred to more surgical details in

Table 14.5 Comparison of different surgical techniques used for the management of trigeminal neuralgia at the level of the Gasserian ganglion (procedures 1–3) or posterior fossa (procedures 4, 5) (Burchiel 1996, Nurmikko and Eldridge 2001, Zakrzewska 2002)

	1. Radiofrequency thermocoagulation	**2. Glycerol decompression**	**3. Microcompression**	**4. Stereotactic surgery**	**5. Microvascular**
Age of patient years	Any age	Any age	Any age	Any age	Preferably under 65
Medical fitness of patient	Care needed if bleeding problems	Care needed if bleeding problems	Care needed with cardiac patients	Any patient	Medically fit only
Ease of technique	Need to wake patient during procedure	No need to wake patient	Need a larger bore needle so may be more difficult to cannulate	Multidisciplinary team	Needs considerable skill
Specialized equipment	Lesioning machine	None needed	None needed	Very specialized equipment	Operating microscope
Type of anaesthesia	Short-acting GA, sedation	Light GA, sedation, no need to wake patient	Light GA, sedation, no need to wake patient	Local anaesthesia with sedation	Full general anaesthesia
Perioperative complications	Haemorrhage	Bradycardia, hypotension	Bradycardia, hypertension	None reported	All the usual reported with neurosurgical procedures
Repeatability	Easy	Easy	Easy	Probably can be repeated	Rarely repeated
Length of stay in hospital	Day stay	Day stay	Day stay	24 hours	One week
Specificity of area lesioned	Difficult to be specific	Can vary area of treatment	Difficult to be specific	Specific with MRI	Highly specific
Immediacy of pain relief	Immediate	Can be delayed for days	Immediate	Median time 4 weeks up to 6 months	May be delayed
Recurrence rates	Mean 3–5 years	Mean 2–3 years	Mean 4–5 years	48–32% recurrence at 36 months	Low, 10 years 70% pain free
Morbidity	Low outside trigeminal nerve	Low outside trigeminal nerve	Low outside trigeminal nerve	Low outside trigeminal nerve, little long-term data	Transient cranial nerve, may be up to 10%
Mortality	Very low	One reported	None reported	None reported	Up to 0.5%
Sensory loss	Always present, related to temperature used	Little	V3 often affected	12% partial loss	None
Anaesthesia dolorosa	0.3–4%	None reported	None reported	One reported	None reported
Eye complications	Keratitis, 0.5–3%	None reported	Very rare	None reported	Diplopia rare
Hearing complications	1% transient	None reported	None reported	None reported	4% may have hearing loss
Masticatory complications	10%	None reported	Common, 100% for 3 months, permanent 3%	One reported	Rare
Number of treatments reported	Very large series	Reasonably large	Small	Small	Large

Table 14.6 Advantages and disadvantages of peripheral treatments

Advantages	Disadvantages
Most do not require general anaesthesia	Short-term relief—months
Can be done at any age	Often need adjuvant therapy
Patients do not need to be medically fit	Repeat procedures common
Relatively easy to perform	Sensory loss can occur
Most reversible	Only possible if there is a discrete trigger point
Can be repeated	
Minor side effects	
No mortality	
Immediate treatment in the case of injections	

textbooks on trigeminal neuralgia (Rovit et al 1990) or to neurosurgical articles (Burchiel 1996). Mortalities with these techniques are very rare and morbidity is mainly in relation to damage to the trigeminal nerve, the major complication being sensory loss. These are neurodestructive procedures. Recurrence rates are between 3 and 5 years.

Radiofrequency thermocoagulation

A precisely controlled heat source differentially destroys pain fibres, A-δ and C, while preserving light-touch A-fibres. Once the needle is in place and its position confirmed on fluoroscopy, the stilette is removed and a radiofrequency electrode thermistor, of varying length and curvature depending on the number of divisions to be treated, is inserted. The patient is woken while small pulses are passed so that details can be obtained as to the stimulation of the trigger zone and the potential area of anaesthesia to be achieved. The patient is then anaesthetized more fully and the lesions are made at temperatures varying from 69 to 90°C for periods varying from 30 to 300 s.

Percutaneous retro-Gasserian glycerol injection

Glycerol is a chemoneurotoxic substance that has a slow, non selective neurolytic effect as it diffuses slowly out of the cistern around the surface of the nerve. Once the needle is introduced into the cistern, this is visualized by the injection of radiocontrast medium. The radiocontrast medium is then drained out and glycerol slowly injected by the same amount as previously estimated on cisternography. By the use of careful positioning and injection, the ophthalmic branch may be spared.

Microcompression of the Gasserian ganglion

The trigeminal nerve is compressed with a small balloon and the ischaemia damages the rootlets and ganglion cells.

Once entry has been gained into the Gasserian ganglion, a Fogarty embolectomy catheter is inserted through the needle and inflated with nonionic water-soluble radiocontrast until it assumes a pear shape. The length of time for inflation varies from 0.5 to 1 min.

Posterior fossa surgery

Apart from the use of the gamma knife, surgery at the level of the posterior fossa is major surgery that, inevitably, carries with it a risk of mortality, which may be up to 0.5% in some less experienced centres, and a morbidity of around 26%.

Microvascular decompression

Microvascular decompression entails entry into the posterior fossa and visualization of the trigeminal nerve at its junction with the pons. Using microscopic techniques, blood vessels and lesions are identified and removed from direct contact with the trigeminal nerve. A pre-operative MRI helps to identify these vessels. This is a non destructive procedure.

If no compression of the nerve is identified, some neurosurgeons will proceed to partial sensory rhizotomy. This involves the division of the sensory root of the trigeminal nerve. It will, inevitably, result in sensory loss.

Stereotactic radiosurgery—gamma knife

The procedure is carried out under local anaesthesia with light sedation and patients can be discharged within 24 h. MRI sequencing is performed in order to identify the trigeminal nerve in its course from the pons into the Gasserian ganglion. Radiosurgical doses of between 70 and 90 Gy are normally used. The radiosurgery planning and dose selection are performed by a combination of neurosurgeons, radiation oncologists, and medical physicists. The morbidity from gamma knife irradiation is much smaller given that this is a noninvasive procedure but its long-term effects have not been evaluated (Nurmikko and Eldridge 2001).

Additional management

It is inevitable that severe and intractable chronic pain leads to psychological and behavioural disturbances. Little attention has been paid to this aspect of management when describing medical or surgical procedures (Zakrzewska et al 1999). Referral to a psychiatrist or clinical psychologist may, in some patients, be of more importance than other forms of treatment, especially in those patients who do not present with classic features or have a recurrence of pain.

Allaying fear and anxiety and reducing depression, if present, can have considerable effect on reducing pain. Patients should be taught how to develop coping strategies and pain diaries are extremely useful in monitoring response to drugs. Patients in control of their management are likely to do better. Support or self-help groups fulfil an important role as they allow consumers to have a greater say in the direction of research. In the USA and UK there are national Trigeminal Neuralgia Associations, which provide access to information and patient contacts and both have internet sites (http://www.tna-support.org/ and http://www.tna-uk.org.uk). All patients should be given adequate information, both verbally and in writing, e.g., leaflet on facial pain available from the Brain and Spine Foundation, 7 Winchester House, Kennington Park, Cranmer Road, London SW9 6EJ. Physicians and surgeons must avoid bias and be prepared to explain all forms of treatment even if they do not do the full range, as only then will patients be able to give fully informed consent.

Guidelines for management

1. Detailed history and examination.
2. MRI on patients with rapidly progressing, severe trigeminal neuralgia, sensory loss, or other symptoms in relation to possible lesion or multiple sclerosis. Very young patients.
3. Medical management initially with carbamazepine up to 1 g daily. Then trial of other drugs.
4. Surgical management is proposed if drug therapy becomes ineffective or quality of life is adversely affected by side effects. In deciding which surgery to choose, the age of the patient, medical history, recurrence rate, and sensory loss, with its effect on quality of life, need to be taken into account. Surgery at the posterior fossa level is advocated for the medically fit patient. Patients need to be aware of the risks and balance these against a high chance of long-term but not permanent relief of pain.
5. Psychological support, treatment of anxiety, and depression is important. Contact with a support group can be extremely helpful.

Trigeminal neuralgia remains an enigma and its management is controversial, not least because of the lack of multicentre, randomized controlled trials.

Glossopharyngeal neuralgia

Background information

Sudden, severe, brief, stabbing, recurrent pains in the distribution of the glossopharyngeal nerve is the definition provided by the IASP. This is a rare condition and there are no data on its prevalence. Its incidence is 0.7 per 100,000 (Katusic et al 1991). The mechanism may be similar to that of trigeminal neuralgia with compression of nerve roots.

Clinical features

The pain is usually unilateral predominantly left sided, distributed within the posterior part of the tongue, tonsillar fossa, and pharynx or beneath the angle of the jaw or even the ear and may radiate to the mandibular area, eye, nose, and maxilla.

The pain is:

- sharp, shooting in quality but a dull, aching, burning pain is often present
- extremely severe but less severe than trigeminal neuralgia
- episodic but has fewer recurrences than in patients with trigeminal neuralgia
- provoked by factors such as swallowing, contact with fluids, especially cold ones, yawning, talking, and moving the head
- immediately relieved by the application of a 10% solution of cocaine to the trigger zone
- may be associated with syncope and cardiac arrhythmias.

Examination shows no gross neurological deficits (Rushton et al 1981, Katusic et al 1991, Ceylan et al 1997).

Investigation

MRI of the posterior fossa or vertebral angiograms have been used but there have been no studies specifically to investigate glossopharyngeal neuralgia and assess their specificity and sensitivity.

Guidelines for management

Not a single randomized controlled trial has been carried out in this group of patients. Treatment, therefore, is based on case series and relies on comparison with trigeminal neuralgia. Drugs used are the same as for trigeminal neuralgia while surgery has included radiofrequency thermocoagulation and microvascular decompression, not without complications (Resnick et al 1995).

Acute herpes zoster trigeminal

Background information

Pain in the distribution of the trigeminal nerve is associated with acute herpes zoster. Its annual incidence in the UK is 3.4/1000, and it changes with age (Hope-Simpson 1975). From these up to 20% of patients may have trigeminal herpes zoster and out of this group, 50% will have involvement of the eye itself. Acute and long-term complications are common, especially in the elderly.

Clinical features

The mouth is involved in maxillary and mandibular cases, whereas the nasolabial area is often involved in ophthalmic division pain. The continuous pain in any division (mainly unilateral) is extremely severe and described as burning and tingling with sharp, shooting exacerbation. Pain may occur at any time, either before the eruption of the vesicles, during the eruption, or after, and last from one to several weeks. It can gradually merge into postherpetic neuralgia pain. There are no provoking factors and only drug therapy provides relief of symptoms. Associated with the pain are a generalized fever, headaches, and malaise.

The eye may initially be red prior to the eruption of the vesicles. Vasculitis occurs within the ophthalmic division. Any structure within or surrounding the orbit may be involved, leading to any of the following: eyelid scarring, keratitis and scleritis, iritis, glaucoma, and retinal necrosis. Ulceration and chronic scarring of the cornea can result in future blindness. Involvement of extraocular muscles occurs if optic neuritis develops.

On the skin the small cluster of vesicles in the distribution of the affected nerve slowly enlarge, become pustular and later haemorrhagic. The lesions take 1–2 weeks to crust over. The lymph nodes draining the area may become tender and enlarged. Immunocompromised patients are at risk of more systemic complications such as pneumonia, encephalitis, polyneuritis, and motor neuropathies.

Investigation

In most patients laboratory confirmation is not necessary although immunocompromised patients and those who have an unusual form or progression may need further investigations, which would include polymerase chain reactions on vesicle scrapings, CSF, or vitreous aspirates.

Guidelines for acute management

The aim of treatment is to reduce the duration and spread of the rash. It is also important to attempt to reduce the frequency and severity of complications, including those of postherpetic neuralgia. Lancaster et al (1995) carried out a systematic review of primary care management of acute herpes zoster from randomized controlled trials up until 1993, which has been reviewed for the *Cochrane Library*. Since then, the British Society for the Study of Infection has also produced guidelines for the management of shingles (Anonymous 1995). The following are suggested:

1. Oral antiviral agent, e.g., aciclovir 800 mg tds or valaciclovir 100 mg tds or famciclovir 500 mg tds within 72 h of onset, continued for 7 days may be of value.
2. Ophthalmic involvement requires an opinion within 72 h and all need treatment.
3. Topical eye steroids—only under the guidance of an ophthalmologist.

Postherpetic neuralgia

Background information

The IHS and IASP have varying definitions for this pain subsequent to acute herpes zoster. The risk of postherpetic neuralgia (PHN) may be as high as 20% in those over 60 years with it rising to 34% in those over 80 years (Hope-Simpson 1975).

Clinical features

Patients may present with three different types of pain, all in the distribution of the affected cranial nerve or division. The pain does not radiate extensively, may be described as aching, burning, or lancinating, and is usually of moderate severity although it can become intolerable. The pain can last from months to years. The allodynia is often triggered by light touch such as clothing or washing the face. It can be cold induced. Associated with the pain is a sensory deficit in all modalities including perception of warmth, cold, heat, pain, touch, pinprick, vibration, and two-point discrimination. Patients will often be anxious and depressed. Cutaneous scarring and pigmentary changes may be seen. Abnormal responses are noted on sensory testing.

Guidelines on management

A review of interventions to prevent PHN and the effects of treatments in established PHN have been published and are kept updated in *Clinical Evidence* (Lancaster et al 2002). The Cochrane database of reviews of effectiveness as well as the CRD databases have reviews with appraisals. These are summarized in Table 14.7.

Sinusitis

Background

Sinusitis is defined as inflammation of any sinus, leading to a constant burning pain over the site of the sinus with a nasal discharge. Sinusitis, especially maxillary sinusitis, is extremely common and is not gender or age specific. The infection in most cases is due to bacterial causes, and the common organisms are *Haemophilus influenzae* and *Streptococcus pneumoniae*. Acute sinusitis is reviewed in *Best Evidence* under diagnostic strategies for Common Medical Problems (Chodosh 1999).

Clinical features

Williams et al (1992) have shown that a diagnosis of sinusitis is likely to be correct in 92% of patients if all the following are present: no improvement on use of decongestants, report of coloured nasal discharge, maxillary toothache, presence of coloured discharge, and transillumination.

Investigations

Chodosh (1999) in his review in *Best Evidence* suggests that radiological investigations should be reserved for complicated cases and those failing to respond to treatment as underlying systemic disease or carcinoma may be present.

Management

Del Mar et al (2002) have published a review of treatments of upper respiratory tract infection

Table 14.7 Management of postherpetic neuralgia: drugs and daily dosage

Beneficial	Likely to be beneficial or beneficial	Unknown effectiveness	Unlikely to be effective	Likely to be ineffective or harmful
Preventing postherpetic neuralgia	Oral antivirals: aciclovir 4 g daily for 7 days; famciclovir 500 mg–1 g; valaciclovir 3 g; SE: headache, nausea; AR: nil reported			Corticosteroids may disseminate herpes zoster
	Amitriptyline 25 mg for 90 days; SE: dry mouth, sedation, urinary difficulties; AR: nil	Levadopa, amantadine, adenosine, monophosphate, isoprinosine	Topical idoxuridine	
Relieving established postherpetic neuralgia	Amitriptyline; desipramine; SE: dry mouth, sedation, urinary difficulties; AR: heart block and syncope in desipramine patient			Epidural morphine—poorly tolerated; dextro-methorphan—no relief
	Gabapentin; SE: drowsiness, ataxia, peripheral oedema; AR: nil	Topical lidocaine (lignocaine), topical capsaicin, oxycodone —		

Based on review in *Clinical Evidence*, Issue 6 (Lancaster et al 2002)

Table 14.8 Rare conditions that cause pain in the trigeminal, ear, and eye regions (most recent references cited)

	Tolosa–Hunt syndrome	**SUNCT[a]**	**Geniculate neuralgia (Ramsay Hunt)**	**Raeder's syndrome (paratrigeminal)**	**Pretrigeminal neuralgia**
Definition	Episodic unilateral orbital pain associated with ophthalmoplegia	Repetitive paroxysms of short-lasting pain associated with eye and nasal symptoms	Severe pain in external auditory meatus following herpes zoster	Painful type of Horner's syndrome	Prodromal pain prior to trigeminal neuralgia
Epidemiology	Rare, mean age of onset 40 yrs, M=F	Very rare, middle age M:F, 4:0.25	Rare, incidence 5/100 000 per year	Rare, mainly males, middle age	Rare, 52 cases reported, age late 50s
Aetiology	Fibrous tissue formation in the cavernous sinus and surrounding area, venous vasculitis	Unknown, may be abnormal cerebral circulation	Related to herpes zoster infection	Tumour, trauma for type 1, unknown for type 2	As for trigeminal neuralgia
Site:	Eye, unilateral	Ocular, periocular, unilateral	Deep in external auditory meatus	Unilateral	Unilateral, trigeminal distribution
Radiation	Periorbital, behind the eye	Frontotemporal, upper jaw, palate	Postauricular	Upper part of face, forehead	Other divisions, teeth
Character	Ache	Burning, electrical, stabbing	Sharp, lancinating	Aching, non-pulsatile	Dull, aching, toothache-like
Severity	Moderate to severe	Moderate to severe	Severe	Mild to severe, fluctuates	Moderate
Duration	Average 8 weeks	5–250 s, mean 61 s	Several days to weeks	Long-lasting pain that gradually builds up and then diminishes	Up to several hours
Periodicity	Average 1 year, not all recur	Several attacks a day, mean 28, periods of weeks to months and then remissions	Continuous, a week or so after eruption	Weeks to months, rarely recurs	3 months to 10 yrs before trigeminal neuralgia develops
Provoking factors	May be stress	Mechanical, neck movements		Strenuous exercise, cardiovascular factors but not always	Movement, temperature
Relieving factors	Drugs	Drugs slightly	Drugs	Analgesia	Carbamazepine
Associated factors	Back pain, cold feet, arthralgia, gut problems, may get other facial pain in between without ophthalmoplegia, nasal, hearing deficit may also occur	Conjunctival injection, lacrimation, nasal stuffiness, rhinorrhoea	These may also be present: hearing loss, tinnitus, hyperacusis, vertigo, Bell's palsy, dysgeusia, epiphora	Ptosis, miosis, hypohidrosis in type 1, also involvement of any of the following cranial nerves II, III, IV, V, VI	Often thought to have dental problems
Clinical signs	Paralysis of one or more nerves 3rd, 4th, 6th occurs either at time of pain or later	Conjunctival injection, forehead sweating unilateral	Nil	Cranial nerve abnormalities, most commonly discrete involvement of V	Nil

Table 14.8 Rare conditions that cause pain in the trigeminal, ear, and eye regions (most recent references cited) (*cont'd*)

	Tolosa–Hunt syndrome	SUNCT[a]	Geniculate neuralgia (Ramsay Hunt)	Raeder's syndrome (paratrigeminal)	Pretrigeminal neuralgia
Investigations	Orbital phlebography shows venous, collateral venous flow and obstruction of cavernous sinus, ESR, serum inflammatory changes may be raised, MRI may need to be repeated	Orbital phlebography shows venous vasculitis, MRI	MRI shows enhancement of geniculate ganglion and facial nerve, auditory tests to assess hearing loss	Type 1 numerous to find underlying pathology, MRI	Nil
Medical treatment	Steroids during an episode, rapid response, resistant cases azothioprine, follow-up with MRI	Poor response, to all drugs including indometacin	Aciclovir-prednisolone (not RCT)	Analgesia for type 2	Carbamazepine, baclofen
References	Anon (1994), Forderreuther and Staube (1999)	Anon (1994), Goadsby and Lipton (1997)	Anon (1994), Sweeney and Gilden (2001)	Anon (1994), Grimson and Thompson (1980)	Fromm et al (1990)

[a]SUNCT = short-lasting, unilateral neuralgiform pain with conjunctival infection and tearing. Other conditions that need to be considered in the differential diagnosis, such as cluster headaches, paroxysmal hemicrania, cluster tic syndrome, and cranial arteritis are discussed in Chap. 15. Atypical facial pain and TMJ pain are covered in Chap. 13.

including sinusitis, which is regularly updated, and the *Cochrane Library* carries systematic reviews. The reviews suggest that antibiotics are likely to be beneficial, although they must be balanced against the potential for adverse effects. Decongestants are useful for short-term relief.

Guidelines for management

1. Careful assessment of symptoms and signs.
2. Sinus radiography, either plain or CT only in refractory cases.
3. Nasal decongestants.
4. Antibiotics in those patients with bacterial maxillary sinusitis: penicillin V and amoxicillin are most commonly used for 7–10 days (Williams et al 2001).

Rare pains of the face

Table 14.8 lists the principal features of some rare pains of the face that need to be considered if other common causes are excluded. The data for all these conditions are based on case series and there is very little evidence at present on how these conditions should be managed (Chong 2002). Both IASP and IHS provide lists of their diagnostic criteria.

Eye pain

Eye pain may be from eye disease itself or from other extraocular structures or may be referred to the region of the eye. The majority of ocular diseases are not painful and referred pain may be from structures as distant as the neck, jaws, sinuses, or teeth (see Table 14.9). Most eye pain needs to be evaluated by an ophthalmologist because of the specialized nature of the disease and the equipment required to evaluate the problem.

Eye pain can originate from the surface or from the deeper structures of the globe. Superficial pain originating from structures like the cornea typically result in acute, sharp pain that is easily relieved by local anaesthetic solutions. Diseases within the globe cause a dull, aching, deep type of pain that results in tenderness of the globe on palpation. Iritis and keratitis can cause reflex spasm of the ciliary muscles and the iris sphincter, and this can lead to pain over the brow area and painful light sensitivity. These deeper pains are more difficult to treat.

Refractory errors due to hypermetropia, astigmatism, or presbyopia or the wearing of incorrect glasses can result in pain either in the eyes or referred to the frontal region, which develops throughout the day as more prolonged visual tasks

Table 14.9 Causes, presentation, and management of eye pain (most recent references cited)

Location	Cause	Signs and symptoms	Principles of management	References RCTs
Corneal abrasion	Foreign body, metallic fragments, scratch, contact lens	Sharp stabbing, severe pain, worse on blinking, often acute, blepharospasm, photophobia, red eye, lacrimation	Local anaesthesia may aid removal of foreign body, topical antibiotic, mydriatic, may patch the eye if no overt infection	Kaiser (1995), Jayamanne et al (1997)
Corneal infection, keratitis, peripheral corneal ulcers	Viral, e.g., herpes simplex, bacterial, chronic use of eye medication	Dull, throbbing, persistent severe pain, worse on moving eyelid, photophobia, tearing, ulceration	Antibiotics, antivirals, topical steroids	Barker (2002)R
Episcleritis, scleritis	Often associated with rheumatoid arthritis, herpes zoster	Ocular discomfort, dull, throbbing photophobia, lacrimation, vision normal or reduced, cornea clear, pupil normal or miosed	Nil to topical steroids of varying strength and frequency, non-steroidal anti-inflammatories, cycloplegic agents	Watson et al (1973)
Iritis, anterior uveitis, granulomatous or non-granulomatous	Granulomatous caused by infective agents, non-granulomatous due to hypersensitivity reaction	Pain most marked in non-granulomatous, red eye, photophobia, blurred vision, often reduced vision, pupil miosed, fixed	Topical steroid eye drops may be beneficial	Curi et al (2002)R
Acute angle closure glaucoma	Elevated intraocular pressure due to impaired access of aqueous to the drainage system	Sudden onset, pain: throbbing, dull, very severe at times; vomiting, dehydrated, blurring, halos, red eye, raised intraocular pressure, oedematous cornea, mid dilated oval fixed pupil, with pupillary block, reduced vision, cornea cloudy, tender to touch, swollen	Emergency, carbonic anhydrase inhibitors, hyperosmotics, topical β-blockers, miotic drops, topical steroids, may need surgery. Review showed no treatments to be effective	Rossetti et al (1993), O'Brien and Diamond (2001)R
Optic neuritis	Associated with multiple sclerosis	Pain with eye movements, tenderness of the globe	High-dose steroids	Beck et al (1992, 2001), Rodriguez et al (1995)

R = recent reviews

are undertaken. Typically, the patient has no pain on wakening. Uncorrected squints can also lead to mild-to-moderate headaches in the frontal region and can also be associated with intermittent blurred vision or diplopia and difficulty in adjusting focus from near to distant objects. Closing an eye often relieves the symptoms. These conditions can easily be rectified by an ophthalmologist.

Conditions that most often cause eye pain are summarized in Table 14.9. The general principles of management are given but the reader is referred to data from randomized controlled trials for more evidence-based treatments.

Optic neuritis

Background

This is a broad term denoting inflammation or demyelination of the optic nerve. One form of optic neuritis is retro-bulbar neuritis, which is often diagnosed late, as the optic disc is involved deeply and so signs are not seen on ophthalmological examination. The median age of onset is 31 years and the age- and sex-adjusted prevalence rate is 115.3 per 100 000 (95% CI, 95.2–135.4/100 000) (Rodriguez et al 1995). Optic neuritis is most closely linked with multiple sclerosis and progression increases with length of follow-up. It is regarded as an immune-mediated inflammatory disorder.

Clinical features

Pain is a prominent feature, often beginning 2 weeks before loss of visual function and resolving before visual improvement. The pain is deep-seated, of a dull, throbbing character, and is made worse with specific eye movements. Other symptoms include loss of vision, which can vary and last

Table 14.10 Causes, presentation and management of primary otalgia

Location	Condition	Clinical features	General principles of management	References to RCTs on management or reviews (R)
Pinna	Haematoma	Blow to ear results in haematoma, ballooned blue pinna	Aspiration of clot and compression	
Pinna	Perichondritis	Pain on moving pinna or tragus	Antibiotic, incision	
Pinna	Acute dermatitis	Oedematous, red auricle, serous fluid, painful when pinna moved	Debridement, topical steroids	
	Frostbite or burn to pinna	Itchiness		
External auditory meatus	Foreign body	History of insertion often by children	Removal of foreign body by otologist	Browning (2002)R
	Wax impaction	Deafness, itchiness	Soften wax, remove	
	Otitis externa	Bacterial or fungal, pain moderate to severe, increased by jaw movement, irritation, scanty discharge, deafness, tender on compression of tragus, red desquamated meatal skin	Swab for culture and sensitivity, aural toilet, appropriate topical therapy	
	Furunculosis	Infection of hair follicle in meatus, severe pain worse with jaw movement and movement of pinna, deafness, tenderness on compression of tragus, boils seen in meatus on examination	Analgesics, aural dressing, only in severe cases systemic antibiotic	
	Malignant disease	Pain becomes intractable and very severe, bloodstained discharge from the ear, presents as ulcer or friable mass	Radiotherapy and/or surgery	
	Acute otitis media	Earache is severe, throbbing, not exacerbated by movement of pinna or tragus, child will cry and scream, deafness, pyrexia, tenderness, depending on stage of disease tympanic membrane may be bulging or perforated	Analgesics. If bacterial antibiotics, myringotomy, aural toilet if discharge, follow-up, xylitol chewing gum	Glasziou et al (1998), Williamson (2002)R
	Chronic otitis media		Topical antibiotics, in children adenoidectomy	
	Acute mastoiditis	Persistent throbbing pain with tenderness over the mastoid antrum, creamy discharge, increasing deafness, pyrexial, malaise, swelling over mastoid	Antibiotics, cortical mastoidectomy if indicated	
	Petrositis (Gradenigo's syndrome)	Pain in trigeminal area, diplopia, headache, signs of middle ear infection	Antibiotics and mastoidectomy	
	Secretory otitis media (glue ear)	Deafness, stuffy feeling in the ear, transient pain, fluid in the middle ear, common in children	Systemic steroids combined with antibiotics, myringotomy, grommets, adenoidectomy	Rosenfeld and Post (1992), Acuin et al (2001)

RTC = randomized controlled trials, R = recent reviews.

for 2–6 weeks, central scotomas, or any unilateral field change. The pupillary light reflex is sluggish and there may also be impairment of colour vision. The optic disc is initially normal in 65% of patients. Hyperaemia of the optic disc with distension of large veins is common (Beck et al 1992, 1993).

The main differential diagnosis is that of papilloedema. Although multiple sclerosis is the most likely disease, lupus erythematosus or optic neuropathy due to other demyelinating diseases such as diabetes or B_{12} deficiency may also occur. Optic neuritis may also be drug induced or related to syphilis, sarcoidosis, and vascular disorders.

Investigations

Abnormal visual evoked potentials are noted.

Management

Treatment of acute optic neuritis with intravenous methylprednisolone (1 g/day) improves short-term (6 months) visual outcome but this tends not to influence the final disability or rate of further relapse (Beck et al 1992). Oral steroid therapy, however, results in a high incidence of recurrent optic neuritis when compared with either intravenous steroids or placebo (Beck et al 1993).

Phantom eye pain

Background

Phantom eye pain occurs following ocular bulb amputation, most commonly for orbital cancer.

Clinical features

In the series of Nicolodi et al (1997), 62% of patients complained of non-painful phantom sensations, 43% had photopsia (appearance of sparks or flashes within the eye), and 28% complained of phantom pain. They also found that these patients were more likely to suffer from headaches than those who were non-headache sufferers prior to surgery.

Treatment

None has been described but it would be expected that these patients would respond to neuropathic-type drugs.

Ear pain

Otalgia can be due to primary causes or may be referred pain (see Table 14.10). The primary causes of otalgia are summarized in Table 14.10. Most patients will need to be seen by an ear, nose, and throat specialist for specific management.

Conclusion

Pain in the trigeminal, ear, and eye regions is extremely complex and may be due to a wide variety of causes. Diagnosis may be difficult but in most cases is based on a careful history. Treatments involve a wide range of specialists and currently, in some conditions, there are very few randomized controlled trials to help a clinician in managing the condition.

References

Anonymous 1988 Classification and diagnostic criteria for headache disorders, cranial neuralgias and facial pain. Headache Classification Committee of the International Headache Society. Cephalalgia 8 (suppl 7): 1–96

Anonymous 1994 In: Merskey H, Bogduk N (eds) Classification of chronic pain: descriptors of chronic pain syndromes and definitions of pain terms. IASP Press, Seattle

Anonymous 1995 Guidelines for the management of shingles. Report of a working group of the British Society for the Study of Infection (BSSI). Journal of Infection 30(3): 193–200

Acuin J, Smith A, Mackenzie I 2001 Interventions for chronic suppurative otitis media. Cochrane Library, Issue 3 (CD-ROM)

Barker N 2002 Ocular herpes simplex. Clinical Evidence 7: 597–604

Beck RW, Henshaw K 2001 Corticosteroids for optic neuritis protocol for Cochrane Review. Cochrane Library, Issue 3 (CD-ROM)

Beck RW, Cleary PA, Anderson MM Jr et al 1992 A randomized, controlled trial of corticosteroids in the treatment of acute optic neuritis. The Optic Neuritis Study Group. New England Journal of Medicine 326(9): 581–588

Beck RW, Cleary PA, Trobe JD et al 1993 The effect of corticosteroids for acute optis neuritis on the subsequent development of multiple sclerosis. The Optic Neuritis Study Group. New England Journal of Medicine 329(24): 1764–1769

Bittar GT, Graff-Radford SB 1993 The effects of streptomycin/lidocaine block on trigeminal neuralgia: a double blind crossover placebo controlled study. Headache 33(3): 155–160

Browning G 2002 Wax in ear. Clinical Evidence 7: 490–497

Burchiel KJ 1996 Pain in neurology and neurosurgery: tic douloureux (trigeminal neuralgia). In: Campbell JN (ed) Pain 1996—an updated review. IASP Press, Seattle, pp 41–60

Burchiel KJ, Slavin KV 2000 On natural history of trigeminal neuralgia. Neurosurgery 46(1): 152–154

Campbell FG, Graham JG, Zilkha KJ 1998 Clinical trial of carbamazepine (Tegretol) in trigeminal neuralgia. Journal of Neurology, Neurosurgery and Psychiatry 29: 265–267

Ceylan S, Karakus A, Duru S, Baykal S, Koca O 1997 Glossopharyngeal neuralgia: a study of 6 cases. Neurosurgical Review 20(3): 196–200

Chodosh J 1999 Acute sinusitis—diagnostic strategies for common medical problems. Best Evidence: 293–302

Chong MS 2002 Chapters 12 and 17. In Zakrzewska JM, Harrison SD Assessment and Management of Orofacial Pain. Elsevier Sciences, Amsterdam

Curi A, Matos K, Pavesio C 2002 Acute anterior uveitis. Clinical Evidence 7: 555–559

Del Mar CB, Glasziou PP 2002 Upper respiratory tract infections. Clinical Evidence 7: 1391–1399

Drangshott M, Truelove EL 2001 Trigeminal neuralgia mistaken as a temperomandibular disorder. Journal of Evidence Based Dental Practice 1: 40–50

Forderreither S, Straube A 1999 The criteria of the International

Headache Society for Tolosa–Hunt syndrome need to be revised. Journal of Neurology 246: 371–377
Fromm GH, Terrence CF 1987 Comparison of L-baclofen and racemic baclofen in trigeminal neuralgia. Neurology 37(11): 1725–1728
Fromm GH, Terrence CF, Chattha AS 1984 Baclofen in the treatment of trigeminal neuralgia: double-blind study and long-term follow-up. Annals of Neurology 15(3): 240–244
Fromm GH, Graff-Radford SB, Terrence CF, Sweet WH 1990 Pre-trigeminal neuralgia. Neurology 40(10): 1493–1495
Fromm GH, Aumentado D, Terrence CF 1993 A clinical and experimental investigation of the effects of tizanidine in trigeminal neuralgia. Pain 53(3): 265–271
Glasziou PP, Del Mar CB, Sanders SL 2001 Antibiotic for acute otitis media in children. Cochrane Library, Issue 3 (CD-ROM)
Goadsby PJ, Lipton RB 1997 A review of paroxysmal hemicranias, SUNCT syndrome and other short-lasting headaches with autonomic features, including new cases. Brain 120(Pt 1): 193–209
Gordon A, Hitchcock ER 1983 Illness behaviour and personality in intractable facial pain syndromes. Pain 17(3): 267–276
Grimson BS, Thompson HS 1980 Raeder's syndrome. A clinical review. Survey of Ophthalmology 24(4): 199–210
Hope-Simpson RE 1975 Postherpetic neuralgia. Journal of the Royal College General Practitioner 25: 571–575
Jayamanne DG, Fitt AW, Dayan M, Andrews RM, Mitchell KW, Griffiths PG 1997 The effectiveness of topical diclofenac in relieving discomfort following traumatic corneal abrasions. Eye 11(Pt 1): 79–83
Kaiser PK 1995 A comparison of pressure patching versus no patching for corneal abrasions due to trauma or foreign body removal. Corneal Abrasion Patching Study Group. Ophthalmology 102(12): 1936–1942
Katusic S, Beard CM, Bergstralh E, Kurland LT 1990 Incidence and clinical features of trigeminal neuralgia, Rochester, Minnesota, 1945–1984. Annals of Neurology 27(1): 89–95
Katusic S, Williams DB, Beard CM, Bergstralh EJ, Kurland LT 1991 Incidence and clinical features of glossopharyngeal neuralgia, Rochester, Minnesota, 1945–1984. Neuroepidemiology 10(5–6): 266–275
Killian JM, Fromm GH 1968 Carbamazepine in the treatment of neuralgia. Use of side effects. Archives of Neurology 19(2): 129–136
Kondziolka D, Lemley T, Kestle JR, Lunsford LD, Fromm GH, Jannetta PJ 1994 The effect of single-application topical ophthalmic anesthesia in patients with trigeminal neuralgia. A randomized double-blind placebo-controlled trial. Journal of Neurosurgery 80(6): 993–997
Kurland LT 1958 Descriptive epidemiology of selected neurological and myopathic disorders with particular reference to a survey in Rochester, Minnesota. Journal of Chronic Diseases 8: 378–418
Lancaster T, Silagy C, Gray S 1995 Primary care management of acute herpes zoster: systematic review of evidence from randomized controlled trials. British Journal of General Practice 45(390): 39–45
Lancaster T, Yaphe J, Wareham D 2002 Postherpetic neuralgia. Clinical Evidence 7: 733–746
Lechin F, Van der Dijs B, Lechin ME et al 1989 Pimozide therapy for trigeminal neuralgia. Archives of Neurology 46: 960–963
Lindstrom P, Lindblom V 1987 The analgesic effect of tocainide in trigeminal neuralgia. Pain 28: 45–50
Lipton RB, Micieli G, Russell D, Solomon S, Tafelt-Hansen P, Waldenlind E 1995 Guidelines for controlled trials of drugs in cluster headache. Cephalalgia 15(6): 452–462
Marbach JJ, Lund P 1981 Depression, anhedonia and anxiety in temporomandibular joint and other facial pain syndromes. Pain (11): 73–84
McQuay H, Carroll D, Jadad AR, Wiffen P, Moore A 1995 Anticonvulsant drugs for management of pain: a systematic review. British Medical Journal 311(7012): 1047–1052
Melzack R, Terrence C, Fromm G, Amsel R 1986 Trigeminal neuralgia and atypical facial pain: use of the McGill Pain Questionnaire for discrimination and diagnosis. Pain 27(3): 297–302
Nicol CF 1969 A four year double-blind study of tegretol in facial pain. Headache 9(1): 54–57
Nicolodi M, Frezzotti R, Diadori A, Nuti A, Sicuteri F 1997 Phantom eye: features and prevalence. The predisposing role of headache. Cephalalgia 17(4): 501–504
Nurmikko TJ 1991 Altered cutaneous sensation in trigeminal neuralgia. Archives of Neurology 48(5): 523–527
Nurmikko TJ, Eldridge PR 2001 Trigeminal neuralgia—pathophysiology diagnosis and current treatment. British Journal of Anaesthesia 87: 117–132
O'Brien C, Diamond J 2001 Glaucoma. Clinical Evidence 5: 442–448
Rasmussen P 1990 Facial pain. II. A prospective survey of 1052 patients with a view of: character of the attacks, onset, course, and character of pain. Acta Neurochirurgica (Wien) 107(3–4): 121–128
Rasmussen P 1991 Facial pain. IV. A prospective study of 1052 patients with a view of: precipitating factors, associated symptoms, objective psychiatric and neurological symptoms. Acta Neurochirurgica (Wien) 108(3–4): 100–109
Resnick DK, Jannetta PJ, Bissonnette D, Jho HD, Lanzino G 1995 Microvascular decompression for glossopharyngeal neuralgia. Neurosurgery 36(1): 64–68; discussion 68–69
Rodriguez M, Siva A, Cross SA, O'Brien PC, Kurland LT 1995 Optic neuritis: a population-based study in Olmsted County, Minnesota. Neurology 45(2): 244–250
Rosenfeld RM, Post JC 1992 Meta-analysis of antibiotics for the treatment of otitis media with effusion. Otolaryngology–Head and Neck Surgery 106(4): 378–386
Rossetti L, Marchetti I, Orzalesi N, Scorpiglione N, Torri V, Liberati A 1993 Randomized clinical trials on medical treatment of glaucoma. Are they appropriate to guide clinical practice? Archives of Ophthalmology 111(1): 96–103
Rothman KJ, Wepsic JG 1974 Site of facial pain in trigeminal neuralgia. Journal of Neurosurgery 40(4): 514–523
Rovit RL, Murali R, Jannetta PJ (eds) 1990 Trigeminal neuralgia. Williams and Wilkins, Baltimore
Rushton JG, Stevens JC, Miller RH 1981 Glossopharyngeal (vagoglossopharyngeal) neuralgia: a study of 217 cases. Archives of Neurology 38(4): 201–205
Sackett DL, Straus SE, Richardson WS, Rosenberg W, Haynes RB 2000 Evidence based medicine. How to practice and teach EBM. Churchill Livingstone, Edinburgh
Stajcic Z, Juniper RP, Todorovic L 1990 Peripheral streptomycin/lidocaine injections versus lidocaine alone in the treatment of idiopathic trigeminal neuralgia. A double blind controlled trial. Journal of Craniomaxillofacial Surgery 18(6): 243–246
Sweeney CJ, Gilden DH 2001 Ramsay Hunt Syndrome. Journal of Neurology, Neurosurgery and Psychiatry 71: 149–154
Vilming ST, Lyberg T, Latase X 1986 Tizanidine in the management of trigeminal neuralgia. Cephalalgia 6: 181–182
Watson PG, McKay DA, Clemett RS, Wilkinson P 1973 Treatment of episcleritis. A double-blind trial comparing betamethasone 0.1 per cent, oxyphenbutazone 10 per cent, and placebo eye ointments. British Journal of Ophthalmology 57(11): 866–870
Williams JW Jr, Simel DL, Roberts L, Samsa GP 1992 Clinical evaluation for sinusitis: making the diagnosis by history and physical examination. Annals of Internal Medicine 117: 705–710
Williams JW Jr, Aguilar C, Makela H, Cornell J, Hollman DR, Chiquette E, Simel DL 2001 Antibiotics for acute maxillary sinusitis. Cochrane Library, Issue 3 (CD-ROM)

Williamson I 2002 Otitis media with effusion. Clinical Evidence 7: 469–476
Zakrzewska JM 1995 Trigeminal neuralgia. Saunders, London
Zakrzewska JM 2002 Trigeminal neuralgia. Clinical Evidence 7: 1221–1231
Zakrzewska JM 2002 Diagnosis and differential diagnosis of trigeminal neuralgia. Clinical Journal of Pain 18: 14–21
Zakrzewska JM 2002 Trigeminal neuralgia. In Zakrzewska & Harrison (eds) Assessment & management of orofacial pain. Elsevier Sciences, Amsterdam
Zakrzewska JM, Hamlyn P 1999 Facial pain. In: Crombie IK, Croft PR, Linton SJ, LeResche L, Von Korff M (eds) Epidemiology of pain. IASP, Seattle
Zakrzewska JM, Thomas DG 1993 Patient's assessment of outcome after three surgical procedures for the management of trigeminal neuralgia. Acta Neurochirurgica (Wien) 122(3–4): 225–230
Zakrzewska JM, Chaudhry Z, Nurmikko TJ, Patton DW, Mullens EL 1997 Lamotrigine (lamicatal) in refractory trigeminal neuralgia: results from a double blind placebo controlled crossover trial. Pain 73: 223–230
Zakrzewska JM, Sawsan J, Bulman JS 1999 A prospective, longitudinal study on patients with trigeminal neuralgia who underwent radiofrequency thermocoagulation of the Gasserian ganglion. Pain 79: 51–58

Chapter 15

Headache

Jean Schoenen and Peter S Sándor

Introduction

Headache is the most common pain syndrome in middle-aged adults. It is also the most frequent symptom in neurology where it may indicate an underlying local or systemic disease (secondary or symptomatic headache) or be a disorder in itself (primary or idiopathic headache). In this chapter, we follow the headache classification of the International Headache Society (IHS 1988) although it is about to be revised, but the new version will probably not contain fundamental changes. For each of the most common types of headache this chapter will briefly summarize clinical features, diagnosis, epidemiology, and pathogenesis and give a more detailed overview of the current knowledge of therapeutic options.

The IHS Headache Classification is hierarchically constructed and based on operational diagnostic criteria for all headache disorders and makes it possible to make diagnoses at different levels of sophistication (overview Table 15.1). The second edition of the IHS classification is about to be published in 2003. It will contain some modifications. Codes 1–4 comprise most of the primary headaches. Because of space limitations, we will cover only the primary and the most frequent secondary headaches, leaving aside some very common but generally obvious causes of pain in head or face, such as systemic infections (Code 9), metabolic disorders (Code 10), eye disorders (Code 11.3), or nose and sinus diseases (Code 11.5).

1. Migraine

Diagnosis and clinical features

Migraine is a multifaceted disorder, of which the head pain is only one component. It is a paroxysmal disorder characterized by attacks, which are separated by symptom-free intervals. The clinical diagnosis of migraine is based on the repetition and characteristics of the attack. The *heterogeneity* of the clinical phenotype, however, is underestimated.

The diagnostic criteria for *migraine without aura* (Code 1.1) (formerly common migraine) are illustrated in Table 15.2. In *migraine with aura* (Code 1.2) the headache phase is immediately preceded by focal neurological symptoms (Table 15.3). Visual disturbances are the most *common aura* symptoms, occurring in 90% of patients. Aura symptoms of sensory, motor, or speech disturbances seldom occur without preexisting visual symptoms (Rasmussen and Olesen 1992).

Migrainous aura symptoms can be distinguished from those produced by a seizure or by a transient

Table 15.1 Classification and diagnostic criteria for headache disorders, cranial neuralgias and facial pain (Cephalalgia 1988) (*& ICD-10 codes*)

1. Migraine (*G43*)

1.1 Migraine without aura (*G43.0*)

1.2 Migraine with aura (*G43.1*)
- 1.2.1 Migraine with typical aura (*G43.10*)
- 1.2.2 Migraine with prolonged aura (*G43.11*)
- 1.2.3 Familial hemiplegic migraine (*G43.1×5*)
- 1.2.4 Basilar migraine (*G43.1×3*)
- 1.2.5 Migraine aura without headache (*G43.1×4*)
- 1.2.6 Migraine with acute onset aura (*G43.12*)

1.3 Ophthalmoplegic migraine (*G43.80*)

1.4 Retinal migraine (*G43.81*)

1.5 Childhood periodic syndromes that may be precursors to or associated with migraine (*G43.82*)
- 1.5.1 Benign paroxysmal vertigo of childhood (*G43.821*)
- 1.5.2 Alternating hemiplegia of childhood (*G43.822*)

1.6 Complications of migraine
- 1.6.1 Status migrainosus (*G43.2*)
- 1.6.2 Migrainous infarction (*G43.3*)

1.7 Migrainous disorder not fulfilling above criteria (*G43.83*)

2. Tension-type headache (*G44.2*)

2.1 Episodic tension-type headache
- 2.1.1 Episodic tension-type headache associated with disorder of pericranial muscles (*G44.20*)
- 2.1.2 Episodic tension-type headache unassociated with disorder of pericranial muscles (*G44.21*)

2.2 Chronic tension-type headache
- 2.2.1 Chronic tension-type headache associated with disorder of pericranial muscles (*G44.22*)
- 2.2.2 Chronic tension-type headache unassociated with disorder of pericranial muscles (*G44.23*)

2.3 Headache of the tension-type not fulfilling above criteria (*G44.28*)

3. Cluster headache and chronic paroxysmal hemicrania

3.1 Cluster headache (*G44.0*)
- 3.1.1 Cluster headache periodicity undetermined (*G44.00*)
- 3.1.2 Episodic cluster headache (*G44.01*)
- 3.1.3 Chronic cluster headache (*G44.02*)
  - 3.1.3.1 Unremitting from onset (*G44.020*)
  - 3.1.3.2 Evolved from episodic (*G44.021*)

3.2 Chronic paroxysmal hemicrania (*G44.03*)

3.3 Cluster headache-like disorder not fulfilling above criteria (*G44.08*)

4. Miscellaneous headaches unassociated with structural lesion (*G44.8*)

4.1 Idiopathic stabbing headache (*G44.800*)

4.2 External compression headache (*G44.801*)

4.3 Cold stimulus headache (*G44.802*)
- 4.3.1 External application of a cold stimulus (*G44.8020*)
- 4.3.2 Ingestion of a cold stimulus (*G44.8021*)

4.4 Benign cough headache (*G44.803*)

4.5 Benign exertional headache (*G44.804*)

4.6 Headache associated with sexual activity (*G44.805*)
- 4.6.1 Dull type (*G44.8050*)
- 4.6.2 Explosive type (*G44.8051*)
- 4.6.3 Postural type (*G44.8052*)

5. Headache associated with head trauma

5.1 Acute post-traumatic headache (*G44.880*)
- 5.1.1 With significant head trauma and/or confirmatory signs (*S06*)
- 5.1.2 With minor head trauma and no confirmatory signs (*S09.9*)

5.2 Chronic post-traumatic headache (*G44.3*)
- 5.2.1 With significant head trauma and/or confirmatory signs (*G44.30*)
- 5.2.2 With minor head trauma and no confirmatory signs (*G44.31*)

6. Headache associated with vascular disorders (*G44.81*)

6.1 Acute ischaemic cerebrovascular disease
- 6.1.1 Transient ischaemic attack (TIA)
- 6.1.2 Thromboembolic stroke

6.2 Intracranial haematoma
- 6.2.1 Intracerebral haematoma
- 6.2.2 Subdural haematoma
- 6.2.3 Epidural haematoma

6.3 Subarachnoid haemorrhage

6.4 Unruptured vascular malformation
- 6.4.1 Arteriovenous malformation
- 6.4.2 Saccular aneurysm

6.5 Arteritis
- 6.5.1 Giant cell arteritis
- 6.5.2 Other systemic arteritides
- 6.5.3 Primary intracranial arteritis

6.6 Carotid or vertebral artery pain
- 6.6.1 Carotid or vertebral dissection
- 6.6.2 Carotidynia (idiopathic)
- 6.6.3 Postendarterectomy headache

6.7 Venous thrombosis

6.8 Arterial hypertension
- 6.8.1 Acute pressor response to exogenous agent
- 6.8.2 Phaeochromocytoma
- 6.8.3 Malignant (accelerated) hypertension
- 6.8.4 Pre-eclampsia and eclampsia

6.9 Headache associated with other vascular disorder

Table 15.1 Classification and diagnostic criteria for headache disorders, cranial neuralgias and facial pain (Cephalalgia 1988) (*& ICD-10 codes*) (*cont'd.*)

7. Headache associated with non-vascular intracranial disorder (*G44.82*)

- 7.1 High cerebrospinal fluid pressure
  - 7.1.1 Benign intracranial hypertension
  - 7.1.2 High pressure hydrocephalus
- 7.2 Low cerebrospinal fluid pressure
  - 7.2.1 Postlumbar puncture headache
  - 7.2.2 Cerebrospinal fluid fistula headache
- 7.3 Intracranial infection
- 7.4 Intracranial sarcoidosis and other non-infectious inflammatory diseases
- 7.5 Headache related to intrathecal injections
  - 7.5.1 Direct effect
  - 7.5.2 Due to chemical meningitis
- 7.6 Intracranial neoplasm
- 7.7 Headache associated with other intracranial disorder

8. Headache associated with substances or their withdrawal (*G44.4*)

- 8.1 Headache induced by acute substance use or exposure (*G44.40*)
  - 8.1.1 Nitrate/nitrite-induced headache
  - 8.1.2 Monosodium glutamate-induced headache
  - 8.1.3 Carbon monoxide-induced headache
  - 8.1.4 Alcohol-induced headache
  - 8.1.5 Other substances
- 8.2 Headache induced by chronic substance use or exposure (*G44.41*)
  - 8.2.1 Ergotamine-induced headache
  - 8.2.2 Analgesics abuse headache
  - 8.2.3 Other substances
- 8.3 Headache from substance withdrawal (acute use)
  - 8.3.1 Alcohol withdrawal headache (hangover)
  - 8.3.2 Other substances
- 8.4 Headache from substance withdrawal (chronic use)
  - 8.4.1 Ergotamine withdrawal headache
  - 8.4.2 Caffeine withdrawal headache
  - 8.4.3 Narcotics abstinence headache
  - 8.4.4 Other substances
- 8.5 Headache associated with substances but with uncertain mechanism
  - 8.5.1 Birth control pills or oestrogens
  - 8.5.2 Other substances

9. Headache associated with non-cephalic infection (*G44.881*)

- 9.1 Viral infection
  - 9.1.1 Focal non-cephalic
  - 9.1.2 Systemic
- 9.2 Bacterial infection
  - 9.2.1 Focal non-cephalic
  - 9.2.2 Systemic (septicaemia)
- 9.3 Headache related to other infection

10. Headache associated with metabolic disorder (*G44.882*)

- 10.1 Hypoxia
  - 10.1.1 High-altitude headache
  - 10.1.2 Hypoxic headache
  - 10.1.3 Sleep apnoea headache
- 10.2 Hypercapnia
- 10.3 Mixed hypoxia and hypercapnia
- 10.4 Hypoglycaemia
- 10.5 Dialysis
- 10.6 Headache related to other metabolic abnormality

11. Headache or facial pain associated with disorder of cranium, neck, eyes, ears, nose, sinuses, teeth, mouth or other facial or cranial structures (*G44.84*)

- 11.1 Cranial bone (*G44.840*)
- 11.2 Neck
  - 11.2.1 Cervical spine (*G44.841*)
  - 11.2.2 Retropharyngeal tendinitis (*G44.842*)
- 11.3 Eyes (*G44.843*)
  - 11.3.1 Acute glaucoma
  - 11.3.2 Refractive errors
  - 11.3.3 Heterophoria or heterotropia
- 11.4 Ears (*G44.844*)
- 11.5 Nose and sinuses (*G44.845*)
  - 11.5.1 Acute sinus headache
  - 11.5.2 Other diseases of nose or sinuses
- 11.6 Teeth, jaws and related structures (*G44.846*)
- 11.7 Temporomandibular joint disease

12. Cranial neuralgias, nerve trunk pain and deafferentation pain

- 12.1 Persistent (in contrast to tic-like) pain of cranial nerve origin (*G44.848*)
  - 12.1.1 Compression or distortion of cranial nerves and second or third cervical roots
  - 12.1.2 Demyelinization of cranial nerves
    - 12.1.2.1 Optic neuritis (retrobulbar neuritis)
  - 12.1.3 Infarction of cranial nerves
    - 12.1.3.1 Diabetic neuritis
  - 12.1.4 Inflammation of cranial nerves
    - 12.1.4.1 Herpes zoster
    - 12.1.4.2 Chronic postherpetic neuralgia (*G53.00*)
  - 12.1.5 Tolosa–Hunt syndrome (*G44.850*)
  - 12.1.6 Neck–tongue syndrome
  - 12.1.7 Other causes of persistent pain of cranial nerve origin
- 12.2 Trigeminal neuralgia (*G50.0*)
  - 12.2.1 Idiopathic trigeminal neuralgia (*G50.00*)
  - 12.2.2 Symptomatic trigeminal neuralgia (*G50.09*)

Table 15.1 Classification and diagnostic criteria for headache disorders, cranial neuralgias and facial pain (Cephalalgia 1988) (*& ICD-10 codes*) (*cont'd.*)

Code	Description
12.	**Cranial neuralgias, nerve trunk pain and deafferentation pain (*Contd*)**
12.2.1	Idiopathic trigeminal neuralgia (*G50.00*)
12.2.2	Symptomatic trigeminal neuralgia (*G50.09*)
12.2.2.1	Compression of trigeminal root or ganglion
12.2.2.2	Central lesions
12.3	Glossopharyngeal neuralgia (*G52.1*)
12.3.1	Idiopathic glossopharyngeal neuralgia
12.3.2	Symptomatic glossopharyngeal neuralgia
12.4	Nervus intermedius neuralgia (*G51.80*)
12.5	Superior laryngeal neuralgia (*G52.20*)
12.6	Occipital neuralgia (*G52.80*)
12.7	Central causes of head and facial pain other than tic douloureux
12.7.1	Anaesthesia dolorosa (*G97.8*)
12.7.2	Thalamic pain (*G46.21*)
12.8	Facial pain not fulfilling criteria in groups 11 or 12
13.	**Headache non-classifiable**

ischaemic attack (TIA) by their progressive onset, march over time, and quality (Table 15.4).

In about 10% of patients unspecific *premonitory symptoms* (or prodromes) like sudden mood changes, repetitive yawning, or craving for special foods may precede the migraine attack by hours or by a day or two (Blau 1980). The migraine attack can be followed by so-called 'postsyndromes', such as fatigue.

There are several rare, but distinct clinical subtypes of migraine. In *migraine with prolonged aura* (Code 1.2.2) at least one aura symptom lasts more than 60 min and less than a week. Migraine *aura* can present *without headache* (Code 1.2.5). In *basilar migraine* (Code 1.2.4) aura symptoms suggest disturbed brainstem function. The differential diagnosis between *migraine with acute onset aura* (Code 1.2.6) and thromboembolic transient ischaemic attacks may be difficult.

Familial hemiplegic migraine (FHM) is a rare autosomal dominant subtype of migraine characterized by hemiparesis/-plegia during the aura. It is caused in most families by mutations in the CACNA1A gene on chromosome 19 (Ophoff et al 1996).

There are two major complications of migraine. In *status migrainosus* (Code 1.6.1) the headache lasts more than 72 h without interruption, despite treatment, or headache-free intervals do not exceed 4 h. In *migrainous infarction* (Code 1.6.2), a neurological deficit has to occur during a migraine attack that is typical of those previously experienced by a patient, to last more than 7 days, and/or to be associated with ischaemic infarction in the relevant area on neuroimaging techniques. Other causes of infarction must be ruled out (Welch and Levine 1990). In the IHS-II classification, 'chronic migraine' will be included as a complication of migraine to classify patients who have ≥15 days of migraine headaches per month.

In *children* below the age of 12 years, migraine often presents differently from adult migraine with shorter attacks, predominant GI symptoms or, in contrast, unremarkable associated symptoms. In the latter case the differential diagnosis with tension-type headache may be difficult.

Epidemiology

Epidemiological data from various countries are similar with a *prevalence* of migraine around 15% (Rasmussen et al 1991) to 23.3% (Stewart et al 1992).

Migraine without aura is more than twice as frequent as migraine with aura, but both types of attacks may coexist in the same patients. *Female preponderance* is a characteristic feature of migraine. While in children there is no gender difference (Bille 1962, Chu and Shinnar 1991), from age 16 on migraine is 2–3 times more frequent in females than in males. Onset is nearly always below age 50 (Stewart et al 1994b).

About 50% of migraineurs have less than two attacks per month, the median *attack frequency* being 1.5 per month. At least 10% of patients have weekly attacks (Stewart et al 1994a). Five percent of the general population has at least 18 migraine days per year and 1% at least one day per week (Ferrari 1998). The annual cost of migraine-related productivity loss is therefore enormous (Lipton et al 1994).

Trigger (or precipitating) or aggravating factors are manifold and may vary between patients and during the disease course. The most common ones are stress or hassles, the perimenstrual period (Stewart et al 2000), and alcohol (Amery and Vandenbergh 1987). Changes of weather condition

Table 15.2 Migraine without aura (MO) (Code 1.1): diagnostic criteria

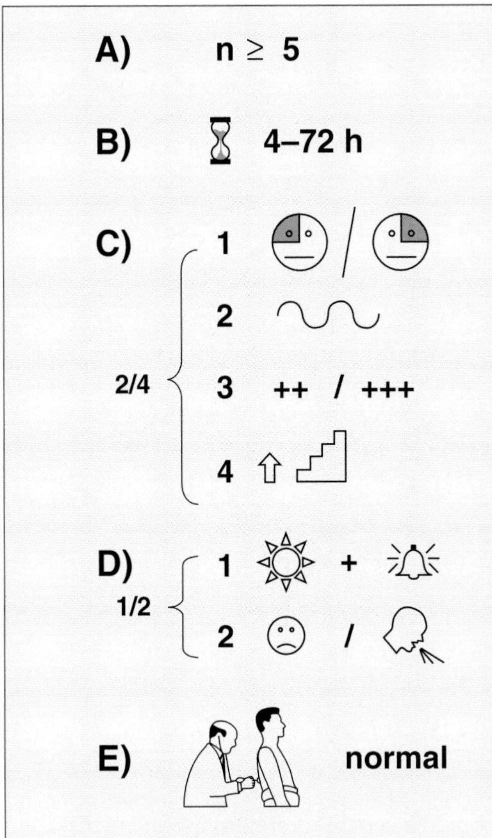

A. – At least 5 attacks fulfilling B–D

B. – Headache attacks lasting 4–72 h (untreated or unsuccessfully treated)

C. – Headache has at least 2 of the 4 following characteristics:
1. Unilateral location
2. Pulsating quality
3. Moderate or severe intensity (inhibits or prohibits daily activities)
4. Aggravated by walking stairs or similar routine physical activity

D. – During headache at least 1 of the 2 following symptoms occur:
1. Phonophobia and photophobia
2. Nausea and/or vomiting

E. – At least 1 of the following 3 characteristics is present:
1. History and physical and neurological examinations do not suggest 1 of the disorders listed in groups 5–11 (please see Table 33.1)
2. History and/or physical and/or neurological examinations do suggest such a disorder, but it is ruled out by appropriate investigations
3. Such a disorder is present, but migraine attacks do not occur for the first time in close temporal relation to the disorder

Table 15.3 Migraine with aura (MA) (Code 1.2): diagnostic criteria

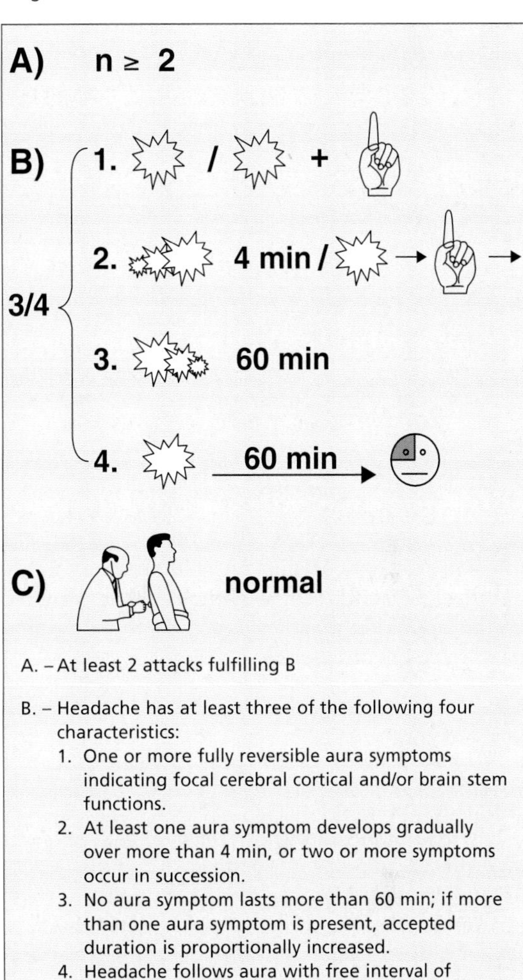

A. – At least 2 attacks fulfilling B

B. – Headache has at least three of the following four characteristics:
1. One or more fully reversible aura symptoms indicating focal cerebral cortical and/or brain stem functions.
2. At least one aura symptom develops gradually over more than 4 min, or two or more symptoms occur in succession.
3. No aura symptom lasts more than 60 min; if more than one aura symptom is present, accepted duration is proportionally increased.
4. Headache follows aura with free interval of <60 min (it may also simultaneously begin with the aura.)

C. – At least one of the following three characteristics is present:
1. History, physical and neurological examinations do not suggest one of the disorders listed in groups 5–11 (please see IHS classification and diagnostic criteria)
2. History and/or physical and/or neurological examinations do suggest such a disorder, but it is ruled out by appropriate investigations.
3. Such a disorder is present, but migraine attacks do not occur for the first time in close temporal relation to the disorder.

like Chinook winds (Cooke et al 2000) and circannual influences (Salvesen and Bekkelund 2000) have been shown to play a role. Overuse of acute antimigraine drugs, in particular of combination analgesics and ergotamine is another—highly underestimated—aggravating factor. There is a

Table 15.4 Differential diagnosis of focal paroxysmal neurological symptoms

	TIA	Epilepsy	Migraine
Onset	Sudden	Sudden	Progressive
Progression rate	None	Fast	Slow
Different symptoms	Simultaneous	In succession	In succession
Type of symptoms if visual	Negative	Positive coloured	Negative/ positive b&w, grey
Territory	Vascular	Cortical	Cortical
Duration	Short (10–15 min)	Short (min)	Longer ($\frac{1}{2}$–1 h)

complex *interrelation between migraine and depression*. As confirmed by recent epidemiological studies (Breslau et al 2000, Joish et al 2000), they are highly *comorbid*. Episodic *vertigo* without other signs of basilar migraine might belong to the migraine phenotype (Neuhauser et al 2001).

Genotype

A number of genes have been implicated in migraine pathogenesis.

Up to now, the only known *monogenic* subtype of migraine is familial hemiplegic migraine (FHM) (Ophoff et al 1996). The more common migraine phenotypes appear to be *complex genetic disorders*, where additive genetic effects (susceptibility genes) and environmental factors are interrelated (Gervil et al 1999a, b). For a full discussion of this topic see Schoenen and Sándor (1999).

Pathophysiology

Migraine is considered to be a *neurovascular headache*, which implies that both neuronal and vascular components are relevant and most probably interrelated (Lance et al 1983, Welch 1987, Olesen 1991, Ferrari 1998).

The migraine aura

There is indirect but growing evidence that the migraine aura is the clinical manifestation of a cortical phenomenon similar to spreading depression and not of ischaemia (Laritzen 1992, Dahlem et al 2000). This hypothesis is supported by the similarity of f-MRI patterns observed during the aura phase in migraineurs (Cao et al 1999, Chabriat et al 2000) and during experimental spreading depression in animals (James et al 1999), but also by the therapeutic effect on the aura of ketamine (Kaube et al 2000) or furosemide (Rozen 2000). As mentioned above, the pathogenesis of the aura and that of the headache may not be necessarily linked.

Role of the brainstem

During attacks of migraine without aura, an area of increased blood flow has been identified in the dorsolateral part of the brainstem opposite to the hemicrania in one study using positron emission tomography (PET) (Weiller et al 1995). Since this increase persisted after headache relief with sumatriptan, it was hypothesized that a 'migraine generator' could exist in the brainstem, but more research is needed (Schoenen and Sándor 1999).

Role of the cortex

During the headache-free interval, an abnormal functioning of the migrainous brain can be demonstrated by neurophysiological and metabolic studies. Neurophysiological methods show that cortical information processing in migraineurs is characterized by a *deficient habituation (or dishabituation)* during repetition of visual or auditory stimulation (Schoenen 1998b, Lahat et al 1999, Siniatchkin et al 2000a). The cortical abnormality is likely to be genetically determined (Sándor et al 1999). Although not specific for migraine and not found under certain conditions in all patients (Sand and Vanagaite Vingen 2000), it may represent an endophenotypic vulnerability marker. It could be due to low activity in raphe-cortical serotonergic pathways which would reduce preactivation levels of sensory cortices, allowing a wider range for suprathreshold cortical activation and thus enhancing intensity dependence and reducing habituation (Hegerl and Juckel 1993).

In the headache-free interval migraineurs present subtle cognitive dysfunctions that may contribute to the burden of the disorder. For instance, memory defects have been found and are thought to be related to strategically and organizationally defective aspects of learning (Le Pira et al 2000). Whether the latter could be a consequence of the electrophysiologically demonstrated abnormalities in cortical information processing seems plausible, but remains to be proven.

Role of the trigeminovascular system

The trigeminovascular system is the major pain-signalling pathway of the visceral organ brain (Moskowitz 1984), but there is still no definite proof that an activation of its peripheral components is necessary to produce a migraine attack. It is not known what activates the trigeminovascular nociceptive pathway in migraine. Contrary to previous reports, no evidence for a direct activation of trigeminal nociceptors by repeated episodes of cortical spreading depression was found in a recent study in rats (Ebersberger et al 2001). This was felt to support the hypothesis that aura and headache may be independent expressions of the migraine diathesis (Goadsby 2001).

Role of nitric oxide

Nitric oxide (NO) donors like glyceryl trinitrate (GTN) are able to induce attacks in patients suffering from migraine with or without aura (Olesen et al 1993, Christiansen et al 1999) but the underlying mechanisms are not well established.

For further analysis of *pathophysiology* see Schoenen and Sándor (1999).

Treatment

Any therapeutic regimen in migraine must be *tailored to the individual patient*, taking into account his demands, disability, previous medical history, and psychosocial profile. The flowchart in Fig. 15.1 is an example of treatment decisions made on basis of attack severity and disability, the so-called stratified approach. One must keep in mind that attack severity may vary in the same patient; in this case the option for a step-wise approach within the attack can be given.

Migraine therapy can be divided into acute treatment of the attack and prophylactic treatment. A US Headache Consortium has recently proposed evidence-based treatment guidelines with a hierarchical classification of acute and prophylactic medications into groups 1 (the best) to 4 (the worst) (Silberstein 2000). Though being a useful reference

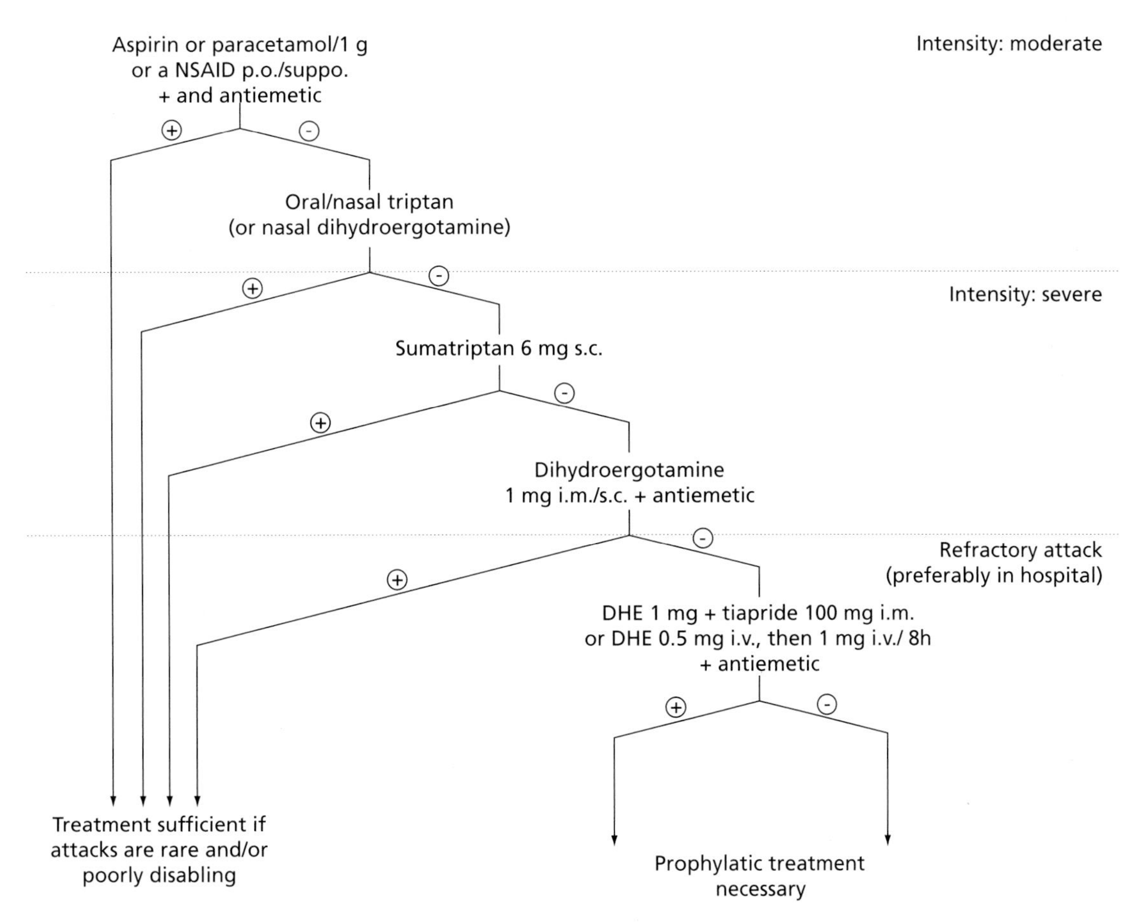

Fig. 15.1 Schematic flowchart of management for migraine. Assessing the disability produced by the disorder makes it possible to apply a stratified care approach or a stepwise approach within attacks.

for migraine management, these guidelines are not a panacea because some methodologically flawed trials have been taken into account and they must be adapted to the individual patient's needs and history.

Whenever possible, individual *precipitating factors* should be avoided or treated. Strategies for coping with stress or dietary measures can be advised. Attacks occurring during the perimenstrual period can sometimes be prevented by treatment with transdermal oestradiol and/or a non-steroidal anti-inflammatory drug (NSAID), or, as shown more recently, with naratriptan (Newman et al 2001).

Acute treatment

All the acute treatments of migraine are more effective if combined with a short resting period or a nap.

Mild migraine attacks can be effectively treated with high doses of *aspirin, paracetamol (at least 1000 mg), or NSAIDs*. There is no evidence of superiority for one NSAID over another as long as a sufficient dose (e.g., *1200 mg ibuprofen*) is used. The new COX2 inhibitors, like rofecoxib, seem also effective. Because of the gastroparesis that accompanies the attack, all these drugs are more effective when administered by the rectal or parenteral route and usually need to be associated with an antiemetic/prokinetic such as metoclopramide or domperidone (Tfelt-Hansen et al 1995).

During the past decade the advent of highly effective 5-$HT_{1B/1D}$ agonists, the *triptans*, has been a major breakthrough in the attack treatment. Triptans are able to act as vasoconstrictors via vascular 5-HT_{1B} receptors and to inhibit neurotransmitter release on the peripheral as well as central ending of trigeminal nociceptors via 5-HT_{1D} receptors. The site of action relevant for their efficacy in migraine is still a matter of controversy; it cannot be excluded that their high efficacy rate is due to their capacity of acting at all three sites in contrast to other antimigraine drugs. *Sumatriptan*, the first triptan, was followed by several *second generation triptans* (zolmi-, nara-, riza-, ele-, almo-, frovatriptan), which were thought to be able to correct some of the shortcomings of sumatriptan (Schoenen 1997).

The therapeutic gain is clearly higher for the triptans than for simple analgesics or NSAIDs, such as acetaminophen 1000 mg po (Lipton et al 2000b), effervescent aspirin 1000 mg (Lange et al 2000), or ibuprofen 600 mg (Kellstein et al 2000). Triptans are also much more efficient and much better tolerated than the classical ergotamine–caffeine combination, leaving little space for the latter in the antimigraine armamentarium (Tfelt-Hansen et al 2000).

A number of comparative trials between neotriptans and sumatriptan and several meta-analyses have been published. Taken together, they confirm that the subcutaneous auto-injectable form of sumatriptan (6 mg) has the best efficacy whatever outcome measure is considered, but also the highest adverse event incidence (Sheftell and Fox 2000, Gawel et al 2001). In severely disabled migraineurs the efficacy rate of injectable sumatriptan for pain-free at 2 h is twice that of high oral doses of ergotamine or NSAIDs (Schoenen et al 1994) and of IV acetylsalicylic acid lysinate (Diener 1999).

Except for naratriptan which acts more slowly, the therapeutic score of oral triptans is quite similar as long as headache relief at 2 h is concerned. When pain-free rates at 2 h or earlier time points and sustained pain-free responses over 24 h are compared, rizatriptan 10 mg and eletriptan 80 mg appear slightly more efficacious (Ferrari et al 2001, Gawel et al 2001). Oral, rectal, or nasal formulations of triptans have over injectable sumatriptan the advantages of better patient acceptability and lower adverse event rates. The choice of a triptan must be adapted to the patients' individual needs and personal experience.

Preliminary post hoc analyses of protocol violators in sumatriptan trials suggest that efficacy, in particular pain-free rates, are much greater if the drug is taken at a stage where the headache is mild (Cady et al 2000). Triptans are also effective for mild headache episodes resembling tension-type headache that occur in migraineurs between typical attacks (Lipton et al 2000a). This suggests that mild migraine may present as tension-type headache, although inferring diagnosis from triptan efficacy is risky, as subcutaneous sumatriptan may also reduce certain symptomatic headaches (Manfredi et al 2000).

At present the major reason for not considering the triptans as first choice treatments for migraine attacks is their high cost. However, stratifying care by prescribing a triptan to the most disabled patients has been proven cost-effective (Lipton et al 2000b). Combining analgesics or NSAIDs with caffeine or codeine increases their efficacy, which explains in part why non-specific antimigraine drugs are still listed together with triptans in the first group of acute therapies for migraine in the US Headache Consortium guidelines. Unfortunately, overuse of combination analgesics or ergotamine are the most frequent cause of the insiduous transformation of migraine into chronic daily headache. Among the ergot derivatives, only dihydroergotamine administered via parenteral injections or nasal spray still has utility in managing some patients.

As expected, the triptans have not solved the

patients' problems. For instance 2 h after intake of one of the most effective oral triptans, rizatriptan 10 mg, 60% of patients still have at the least a mild headache and 68% nausea and/or sensoriphobia (Adelman et al 2001); 55% still have not returned to normal activity; and 45% have adverse effects of some kind. There is thus room for more efficient oral acute anti-migraine treatments, among which those that activate the 5-HT_{1F} receptor (Goldstein et al 2001) or antagonize CGRP, glutamate, or NO are the most promising.

Prophylactic treatment

Prophylactic antimigraine treatment should be considered when attacks are frequent and/or disabling. A useful rule of thumb is to discuss prophylaxis when attacks occur on average twice per month.

Long-term efficacy of prophylactic treatments does not exceed 50–60%. *Classical* drugs effective for preventing migraine attacks include *beta-blockers* devoid of intrinsic sympathomimetic activity (Massiou and Bousser 1992), *sodium valproate* (Jensen et al 1994), *calcium channel blockers*, such as flunarizine or verapamil, and *serotonin antagonists* such as pizotifen or methysergide (Ollat 1992). In some patients *tricyclics* may be useful. A major drawback of all these prophylactics are side effects, many of which, like weight gain, fatigue, or hypotension, are not well tolerated by migraineurs.

In recent years some *new prophylactics* with less side effects have been studied. High-dose *magnesium* (24 mmol/day) was found to be effective (Peikert et al 1996), while a trial with 10 mmol (Pfaffenrath et al 1996) was discontinued because of a lack of effect. *Cyclandelate*, which is well tolerated at a dosage of 1200 mg/d, was found comparable to propranolol in one study (Diener et al 1996). In another trial using 1600 mg/d, it was preferred by patients and physicians, but failed to demonstrate superiority over placebo in classical endpoints (Diener et al 2001).

A novel preventive treatment for migraine is high dose (400 mg/d), *riboflavin*, which has an excellent efficacy/side effect ratio (Schoenen et al 1998). Riboflavin may improve the reduced mitochondrial phosphorylation potential while the other anti-migraine prophylactics are chiefly acting on neuro-transmission. Along the same rationale promising results were obtained with coenzyme Q10 in a preliminary study.

Lisinopril (10 mg b.i.d.), an inhibitor of angiotensin converting enzyme well known for the treatment of hypertension, was found to reduce migraine days by 21% in a placebo-controlled crossover trial of 47 patients (Schrader et al 2001). Recent preliminary but promising results with novel antiepileptic compounds like gabapentin and topiramate (Jimenez et al 1999, Shuaib et al 1999) or with pericranial botulinum toxin type-A injections (Binder et al 2000) need to be confirmed in randomized controlled trials.

Among the *non-pharmacological treatments* of migraine, behavioural therapies, such as relaxation and biofeedback, have proved some efficacy in many studies (Holroyd et al 1984). Acupuncture is considered effective in a Cochrane review (Melchart et al 2001) in which both migraine and tension-type headache were considered. Petasites hybridus was also found effective (Grossmann and Schmidramsl 2000), as was feverfew, while the situation seems to be less clear for homeopathy (Whitmarsh et al 1997).

2. Tension-type headache

Diagnosis and clinical features

The headaches formerly described as 'muscle contraction', 'psychogenic', 'stress', or 'essential' are classified in this heterogeneous group. The term 'tension type' has been chosen to underline the uncertainties about the precise pathogenesis, but to indicate nevertheless that some kind of mental or muscular tension may play a causative role.

The diagnostic criteria of *episodic tension-type headache* (Code 2.1) (ETH) are illustrated as visual symbols in Table 15.5.

In *chronic tension-type headache* (Code 2.2) (CTH) the average headache frequency is at least 15 days per month or 180 days per year. In CTH, nausea can be accepted as an isolated associated symptom.

Tension headache can be associated (Codes 2.1.1 and 2.2.1) or unassociated (2.1.2 and 2.2.2) with disorder of the pericranial muscles (tenderness by manual palpation or pressure algometer, increased electromyographic levels). Clinical presentation, pathogenesis of pain, or response to therapy (Schoenen et al 1991b) are similar between the two groups.

The single episode of tension-type headache is the least distinct of all headache types since clinical diagnosis is chiefly based on negative features (cf. Table 15.6). As a substantial proportion of patients may present with atypical symptoms (Rasmussen and Olesen 1992), episodic tension-type headache can be difficult to distinguish from migraine without aura (IHS Code 1.1) or from organic brain disease. The diagnosis of chronic tension-type headache on the other hand seems straightforward in most cases with a long enough clinical course,

Table 15.5 Tension-type headache (TH) (Code 2.1): diagnostic criteria

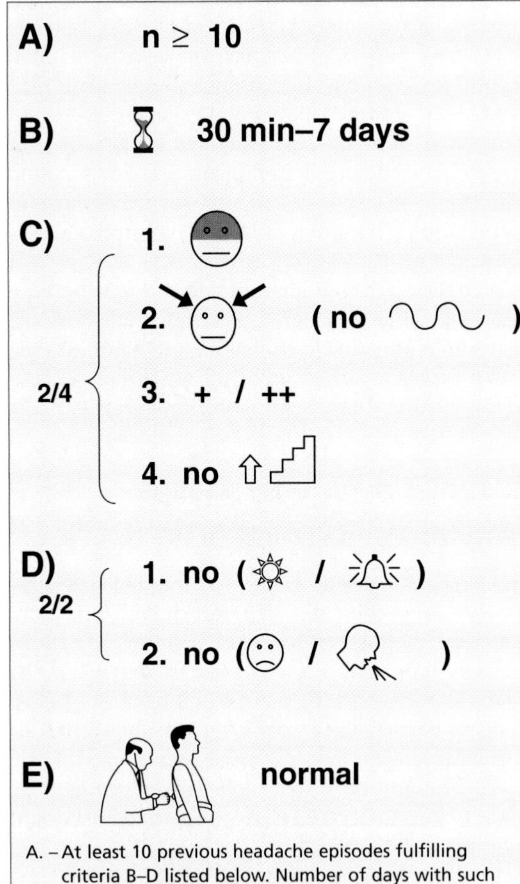

A. – At least 10 previous headache episodes fulfilling criteria B–D listed below. Number of days with such headache, 180/year (<15/month).

B. – Headache lasting from 30 min to 7 days

C. – At least 2 of the following pain characteristics:
1. Pressing/tightening (non-pulsating) quality
2. Mild or moderate intensity (may inhibit, but does not prohibit activities)
3. Bilateral location
4. No aggravation by walking up/downstairs or similar routine physical activity

D. – Both of the following:
1. No nausea or vomiting (anorexia may occur)
2. Photophobia and phonophobia are absent, or one but not both is present

E. – At least one of the following:
1. History, physical- and neurological examinations do not suggest one of the disorders listed in groups 5–11 (please see Table 15.1)
2. History and/or physical- and/or neurological examinations do suggest such disorder, but it is ruled out by appropriate investigations
3. Such disorder is present, but tension-type headache does not occur for the first time in close temporal relation to the disorder

although some patients may have migrainous features (see above).

So-called 'chronic daily headache' may affect up to 4% of the general population (Solomon et al 1992). It comprises patients with chronic migraine or tension-type headache due to medication overuse, those with chronic tension-type headache, and a puzzling minority of patients with new daily persistent headache.

Epidemiology

In a population-based study (Rasmussen and Olesen 1992) the lifetime prevalence of tension-type headache was 79% with 3% suffering from CTH, i.e., headache on more than 15 days per month. Prevalence of tension headache seems to be higher in women than in men, declining with age.

Pathophysiology

From the clinical heterogeneity of TH one may infer that pathophysiological mechanisms are multiple, involving, e.g., muscular, neuronal, and psychological factors. The controversy between peripheral and central pathogenesis may indeed not be decided as both aspects could be at work, interacting and varying in importance between patients, between TH subtypes, or even during the course of the disorder (Schoenen and Wang 1997).

Peripheral aspects

There is evidence both for and against a *myofascial origin* of pain. While EMG levels in pericranial muscles may be on average increased in TH, there is no correlation between EMG activity and headache severity. Palpation tenderness is increased in patients, more so during an actual headache. Lower pressure pain thresholds (PPTs) are found at pericranial sites in CTH patients (Schoenen et al 1991a, Jensen et al 1993a, Schoenen and Wang 1997)—the characteristics of the stimulus–response function suggesting a sensitization of nociceptors (Bendtsen et al 1996b). In ETH, however, cephalic PPTs are usually normal (Drummond 1987, Bovim 1992, Göbel et al 1992, Schoenen and Wang 1997). Taken together, the studies of extracephalic pain thresholds (Jensen and Olesen 1996, Proietti Cecchini et al 1997) suggest that in addition to sensitization of peripheral nociceptors, central factors may play a role in the increased pericranial tenderness of TH patients.

Central nervous system aspects

EEG and *evoked potentials* are normal in TH (Schoenen 1992). Many *psychological abnormalities* have been associated with TH, although it could not be determined whether as cause or consequence (Andrasik and Passchier 1993). Though not confirmed in all studies (Lipchick et al 1996), abnormalities of *exteroceptive suppression* (or silent period) in jaw-closing muscles, an inhibitory brain stem reflex, suggest that the descending control systems, and not the inhibitory interneurons themselves, are dysfunctioning in TH (Wang and Schoenen 1994).

A model for TH pathogenesis

Considering the heterogeneity of pathophysiological abnormalities found in TH, the following model was proposed as a working hypothesis (Olesen and Schoenen 1999). TH may be the result of an interaction between changes of the descending control of second-order trigeminal brainstem nociceptors and interrelated peripheral changes, such as myofascial pain sensitivity and strain in pericranial muscles. An acute episode of ETH may occur in many individuals otherwise perfectly normal. It can be brought on by physical stress usually combined to psychological stress or by non-physiological working positions. In such cases, increased nociception from strained muscles may be the primary cause of the headache, possibly favoured by a central temporary change in pain control due to stress. Emotional mechanisms increase muscle tension via the limbic system and at the same time reduce tone in the endogenous antinociceptive system. With more frequent episodes of headache central changes become increasingly more important. Long-term potentiation/sensitization of nociceptive neurons and decreased activity in the antinociceptive system gradually leads to CTH. These central changes probably predominate in frequent ETH and in CTH.

The relative importance of peripheral and central factors may, however, vary between patients and over time in the same patient. The complex interrelation between various pathophysiological aspects in TH may explain why this disorder is so difficult to treat. Management of TH should primarily try to prevent chronification.

Treatment

Therapies for TH can be schematically subdivided into short-term, abortive (mainly pharmacologic) treatments of the individual attack and long-term, prophylactic (pharmacologic or nonpharmacologic) treatments that may prevent headache.

Acute pharmacotherapy

NSAIDs are the drugs of first choice (Fig. 15.2) (see Mathew and Schoenen 1993 for a review). Ibuprofen, 400 or 800 mg, is significantly more effective than placebo or aspirin (Schachtel et al 1996). Other NSAIDs such as naproxen, ketoprofen (Dahlöf and Jacobs 1996), ketoralac, or indomethacin are also effective, but less well studied. Because of the overall lower prevalence of gastrointestinal side-effects (Ryan 1977), ibuprofen (800 mg) is probably the first choice, followed by naproxen sodium (825 mg). The new NSAIDs with selective COX2 inhibition are probably also effective in TH, but no studies are available yet.

In some patients, combination of analgesics with caffeine, sedatives, or tranquillizers may be more effective than simple analgesics or NSAIDs. Before turning to a combination drug, the analgesic or NSAID must be given in a high enough dosage, as there is a clear dose–effect relationship (see Fig. 15.2). Whenever possible, combination analgesics for TH should be avoided because of the risk of dependency, abuse, and chronification of the headache. There is at present no scientific basis for the use of muscle relaxants, such as the mephenesin-like compounds, baclofen, diazepam, tizanidine, cyclobenzaprine, or dantrolene sodium, in the treatment of TH.

Prophylactic pharmacotherapy

The *tricyclic antidepressants* are the most widely used first-line therapeutic agents for CTH. Surprisingly, few controlled studies have been performed and not all of them have found an efficacy superior to placebo.

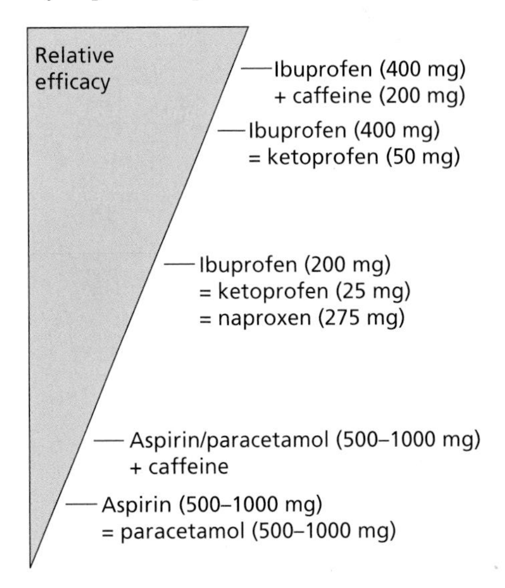

Fig. 15.2 Hierarchy of NSAIDs according to their relative efficiency in aborting tension-type headache episodes. Summary of 8 comparative, randomized controlled trials performed between 1995 and 1997.

One major problem that arises with trials showing statistical superiority of tricyclics over placebo is to evaluate whether the observed effect is clinically relevant. Nonetheless, in clinical practice the tricyclic antidepressants remain useful prophylactic drugs for CTH or frequent ETH. Amitriptyline is the most commonly used, with an average dose in CTH of 75–100 mg per day (Mathew and Bendtsen 1999), but many patients will be satisfied with a lower dose. Clomipramine may be slightly superior, but has more side effects. Other antidepressants, such as doxepin, maprotiline, or mianserin, can be used as a second choice. In clinical practice, the final choice of these drugs also depends on their side-effect profile. If the headache is improved by at least 80% after 4 months, it is reasonable to attempt discontinuation of the medication. Decreasing the daily dose by 20–25% every 2–3 days may avoid rebound headache. Selective 5-HT reuptake inhibitors have little usefulness (Bendtsen et al 1996a).

The mechanism of action of antidepressants in CTH remains to be determined. Their effect on the headache may be partly independent from their antidepressant effect. Tricyclics have a variety of pharmacological activities. Serotonin increase by inhibition of its reuptake and subsequent down-regulation of 5-HT receptors, endorphin release, or inhibition of NMDA receptors that play a role in pain transmission may all be relevant for the pathophysiology of TH.

Non-pharmacological treatments

Psychological and behavioral techniques There is solid scientific support for the usefulness of *relaxation* and *EMG biofeedback* therapies in the management of TH (Blanchard et al 1987, Bogaards and ter Kuile 1994) with significant improvement in headache in near 50% of patients. Each treatment modality seems to lead to similar improvements, but patients may subjectively prefer one or the other (Holroyd and Penzien 1986). Cognitive behavioural interventions, such as stress management programmes, can effectively reduce TH activity, but they seem to be most useful when added to biofeedback or relaxation therapies in patients with higher levels of daily hassles. A recent randomized controlled trial demonstrated that combining stress management therapy (relaxation plus cognitive coping) and amitriptyline (up to 100 mg/d) or nortriptyline (up to 75 mg/d) produced greater benefit than either treatment alone: reduction in headache index scores of at least 50% in 64% of patients with the combination, as opposed to 38% of patients for the tricyclics, 35% for stress management, and 29% for placebo (Holroyd et al 2001).

Limited contact treatment based on the patient's guidance at home by audiotapes and written materials with only 3 or 4 monthly clinical sessions may be a cost-effective alternative to fully therapist-administered treatment in many patients (Haddock et al 1997). Despite this alternative, behavioural therapies are time-consuming for patients and therapists. Although there is no infallible means of *predicting treatment outcome*, a number of factors that may have some predictive value have been identified. Excessive analgesic or ergotamine use limits the therapeutic benefits. Short duration of headache complaints and young age improve treatment outcome (Holroyd and Penzien 1986, Bogaards and ter Kuile 1994). Patients with continuous headache are less responsive to relaxation or biofeedback therapies, and patients with elevated scores on psychological tests that assess depression or psychiatric disturbance have done poorly with behavioural treatment in some studies (Holroyd 1993).

Other non-pharmacologic treatments *Physical therapy* techniques include positioning, ergonomic instruction, massage, transcutaneous electrical nerve stimulation, heat or cold application, and manipulations. None of these techniques has been proven to be effective in the long term. Physical treatment such as massage may be useful for acute episodes of TH. In the long term, it reduced headache intensity on average only by 23% in one study, which was nonetheless superior to acupuncture given as a comparator treatment (Carlsson et al 1990, Bove and Nielsson 1998).

Oromandibular treatment may be helpful in selected TH patients. Unfortunately, most studies claiming efficacy of treatments such as occlusal splints, therapeutic exercises for masticatory muscles, or occlusal adjustment are uncontrolled. Two controlled trials (Forsell et al 1985, Schokker et al 1990) have shown effective reduction of headache after occlusal equilibration. Considering the large number of headache-free subjects who display signs and symptoms of oromandibular dysfunction (Jensen et al 1993b), caution should be taken not to advocate irreversible dental treatments in TH.

3. Cluster headache

Diagnosis and clinical features

The diagnostic criteria of cluster headache are listed in Table 15.6.

Table 15.6 Cluster headache (Code 3.1): diagnostic criteria

A. At least five attacks fulfilling B–D

B. Severe unilateral orbital, supraorbital and/or temporal pain lasting 15–180 minutes untreated

C. Headache is associated with at least one of the following signs which have to be present on the pain side.
1. Conjunctival injection
2. Lacrimation
3. Nasal congestion
4. Rhinorrhoea
5. Forehead and facial sweating
6. Miosis
7. Ptosis
8. Eyelid oedema

D. Frequency of attacks: from one every other day to eight per day

The most typical feature of cluster headache is the temporal clustering of attacks during several weeks separated by remissions of at least 14 days, but usually of several months (*episodic cluster headache*, Code 3.1.2.). In *chronic cluster headache* (Code 3.1.3) remissions of at least 14 days are absent for more than 1 year.

Cluster headache is a primary neurovascular headache that is unilateral and shows features different from migraine. Characteristics distinguishing the cluster headache attack from migraine are short duration (average: 30–45 min), presence of autonomic symptoms around the eye, absence of gastrointestinal disturbances, and the extreme intensity of the pain, which is the most unbearable among the primary non-symptomatic headaches. Patients tend to be agitated and to pace the floor, which is clearly different from migraineurs who lie down and seek rest during the attack. Cluster headache attacks tend to occur in the evening or during sleep. Cluster headache also must be distinguished from trigeminal neuralgia, which is characterized by short-lasting, explosive pains, trigger points, and absent autonomic signs. It shares some characteristics with other disorders grouped under the heading 'trigeminal autonomic cephalalgias' (see below).

Epidemiology

The overall prevalence is around 0.04–0.09% (Sjaastad 1986). The relative incidence of the chronic form (Code 3.1.3) is on average 10% (Ekbom 1986). There is a clear preponderance of the male sex (male-to-female ratio 5:1). Most often the first attack occurs between 20 and 40 years. Cluster headache is associated with cigarette smoking, head trauma (about 16%; Turkewitz et al 1992), and a positive family history for headache (ICECH 1995).

Genetic influences seem to be less pronounced than those in migraine with an autosomal dominant inheritance pattern in some families.

Pathophysiology

There is at present no pathogenetic theory of cluster headache that accounts for all aspects of this disorder, i.e., the pain location and characteristics, autonomic features, temporal profile of attacks and clusters, and the male preponderance. Several pathophysiological abnormalities have been demonstrated both during and between attacks. A central *hypothalamic dysfunction* regarding the circadian and circannual pattern of attacks, the disruption of neuroendocrine tests, and neurophysiological data has been suggested. With positron emission tomography an area of increased blood flow was recently found in the ventro-medial hypothalamus ipsilateral to nitroglycerin-provoked attacks (May et al 1998, Schoenen 1998a). The activated area may comprise the suprachiasmatic nucleus where biological rhythms are generated and is ictally activated. Furthermore, in a subsequent study using voxel-based morphometry in MRI, a structural change consisting of increased tissue amounts was found in the same hypothalamic area. On the other hand the cavernous sinus has been pinpointed as a potential crossroad where nociceptive peptidergic afferents of the ophthalmic nerve, preganglionic parasympathetic fibres running through the greater superficial petrosal nerve, and postganglionic sympathetic fibres of the pericarotid plexus can be impaired and give rise both to the pain and the autonomic symptoms of the cluster headache attack (Ollat 1992). Interestingly, cluster-like headaches can be due to organic lesions among which the most frequent are pituitary adenomas (Goldstein et al 2001). Hypothalamic-driven vascular changes in the cavernous sinus loggia may reconcile the peripheral and central theories of cluster headache pathophysiology (Schoenen 1998a).

Treatment

Acute treatment To abate the single attack inhalation of 100% *oxygen* (7–10 L/min) using a face mask is effective within 10–15 min in 60–70% of cases.

At present, subcutaneous injection of *sumatriptan* is the most efficient treatment of cluster headache attacks. At a dose of 6 mg, it alleviates the attack within 15 min in more than 90% of patients without tachyphylaxis in the long term (Wilkinson et al 1995). Sumatriptan is not able to prevent attacks when given on a daily prophylactic basis (Monstad et al 1995).

Intranasal application of dihydroergotamine is effective in less than 50% of patients. Recently, oral and intranasal triptans were found to have some utility in cluster attacks, but, because of their limited speed of action compared to injectable sumatriptan, only in those who have a long duration (Hardebo and Dahlöf 1998, Bahra et al 2000).

Prophylactic treatment There is no general agreement on a standard prophylactic therapy for cluster headache (Ekbom 1995).

Verapamil is probably the most effective preventative treatment (Lewis and Solomon 1996). The average dose is 240 mg b.i.d., but daily doses up to 960 mg, or more if tolerated, may be necessary in some patients. The most common adverse effects are constipation, fatigue, and hypotension.

Lithium carbonate is effective at doses inducing plasma levels between 0.7 and 1 mmol/L. The effectiveness of lithium may decrease during successive clusters. Lithium may be more effective in the chronic form.

Methysergide has been used with success in cluster headache for many years. Daily dosage should be as low as possible, preferably 3–4 mg. Methysergide must be interrupted every 5–6 months for 1 month to avoid retroperitoneal fibrosis.

Ergotamine tartrate given orally at bedtime may be useful to prevent nocturnal attacks.

Corticosteroids at high doses are able to interrupt a cluster in most patients. However, their use should be restricted to incapacitated and resistant patients with the episodic form. Tapering or interruption of cortisone treatment is indeed frequently followed by recurrence of attacks. *Suboccipital* injection of a mixture of short- and long-acting corticosteroids, associated or not with a local anaesthetic, is used as an adjuvant therapy in some centers. It offers the advantage of a 'one-shot' corticotherapy and may by itself interrupt a cluster in a number of patients.

In more resistant patients, it can be helpful to combine two of the above-mentioned substances. Other drugs like pizotifen, indometacin, or sodium valproate may have some effect.

Various invasive treatments have been proposed in cluster headache: alcoholization, corticosteroid infiltrations, radiofrequency lesions (Sanders and Zuurmond 1997), cryosurgery or resection of the pterygopalatine ganglion, radiofrequency lesions or glycerol injections of the Gasserian ganglion, and gamma knife radiosurgery of the trigeminal nerve root entry zone (Ford et al 1998). None of these procedures gives consistent long-lasting relief and some of them are not yet sufficiently validated. They should therefore be considered only in the minority (±1%) of patients who resist a full trial of medical therapy. Recently stimulation of the postero-inferior hypothalamus with deep electrodes was found effective.

Pain syndromes related to cluster headache

Paroxysmal hemicrania is a rare disorder first described by Sjaastad and Dale (1974), affecting preferentially adult females. It has an absolute responsiveness to indometacin and belongs therefore to the 'indometacin-responsive headaches', which comprise also benign coital headache, exertional headache, and hemicrania continua and idiopathic stabbing headache. Attacks resemble those of cluster headache, but with a shorter duration (mean 15 min), with a much higher frequency (more than 5 a day for more than half of the time; mean of about 12 per day), and without nocturnal preponderance. The chronic form (CPH), which characterizes most reported cases, may be preceded by an episodic, 'pre-CPH', stage.

The exact pathogenesis of CPH is not known. Various abnormalities (e.g., corneal indentation or temperature changes, intraocular pressure changes) are similar to those reported in cluster headache (Sjaastad 1986). Several symptomatic cases occurring with sellar or parasellar neoplasms have been reported.

The absolute responsiveness of CPH to indometacin is part of the diagnostic criteria. The effective oral dosage varies between patients and may be as high as 200 mg. An IV injection of indometacin, the so-called 'indo-test' may be rapidly effective. On discontinuation of the drug attacks frequently reappear, but long-lasting remissions have been observed. Recently other NSAIDs, such as ketoprofen, have been found effective in a few patients.

*S*hort-lasting, *u*nilateral, *n*euralgiform orbital pain with *c*onjunctival injection, *t*earing, sweating, and rhinorrhoea, the so-called SUNCT syndrome, is a rare entity, mostly affecting males, which has similarities both with CPH and trigeminal neuralgia (Sjaastad et al 1989). SUNCT is characterized by a multiplicity of short (usually less than 120 s) paroxysms of moderate to severe pain with massive autonomic symptoms in the eye.

4. Miscellaneous headaches unassociated with structural lesion

This section comprises rather characteristic headaches that are benign in nature. They are triggered by stimulation of the trigeminal nerve territory or changes in intracranial pressure. Some of them have been more frequently reported in migraineurs.

Idiopathic stabbing headache (Code 4.1) (ice-pick pains or 'jabs and jolts') is characterized by short-lasting pains at irregular intervals, in the distribution of the first division of the trigeminal nerve. It was found in 2% of the general population (Rasmussen et al 1991) and is more prevalent in migraineurs. If treatment is necessary, indometacin or other NSAIDs are usually effective.

External compression headache (Code 4.2) ('swim-goggle headache') is a dull constant pain felt in an area of the scalp subjected to prolonged pressure. It affects up to 4% of the population (Rasmussen et al 1991), preferentially individuals suffering also from migraine.

Cold stimulus headache (Code 4.3) develops during external exposure to cold (e.g., cold water) or during ingestion of a cold food or drink ('ice-cream headache'). It seems to be frequent in the general population, affecting 15% of individuals; it is also more frequent in migraineurs.

Benign cough headache (Code 4.4) and benign exertional headache (code 4.5) are rare (1% of the population) and not associated with migraine or tension-type headache (Rasmussen et al 1991). Note that cough headache is benign in only about 50% of cases, with a male preponderance and an onset after 45 years of age. For the other 50%, cough headache is most often due to Chiari Type-I malformation, equally distributed in both sexes and begins under age 50 (Pascual et al 1996). Benign exertional headache has an earlier onset than benign cough headache and is frequently related to benign sexual headache. It can be prevented by taking indometacin before exercise. Ergotamine tartrate, methysergide, and propranolol have also been used.

Headache associated with sexual activity (Code 4.6) is rare (<1%) (Rasmussen et al 1991, Pascual et al 1996) and may present under three different forms: a dull pain in the head and neck that intensifies as sexual excitement increases (Code 4.6.1) or a postural headache resembling that of low cerebrospinal fluid pressure developing after coitus (Code 4.6.3). The third form, a sudden severe, explosive, headache, occurs at orgasm (Code 4.6.2). Indometacin may prevent these benign sexual headaches, especially the last type. Spontaneous remissions are also frequent.

When a sudden severe headache occurs for the first time during sexual activity or exertion, an intracranial aneurysm must be excluded (see the section on Code 6.4).

5. Headache associated with head trauma

Diagnosis and clinical features

The diagnostic criteria for *acute posttraumatic headache* (Code 5.1) are listed in Table 15.7. In the *chronic form* (Code 5.2) the headache continues for more than 8 weeks after regaining consciousness or after trauma. Acute posttraumatic headache is often moderate to severe, throbbing, with accompanying nausea, vomiting, photo- and phonophobia, memory impairment, irritability or drowsiness, or vertigo. It is usually exacerbated by physical exercise, described as incapacitating by the patient, and bears many similarities to migraine, except the attack pattern.

Chronic posttraumatic headache is usually a generalized headache, almost permanent like chronic tension-type headache, but aggravated by physical effort and mental strain. The pain may be focused on the area that the patient believes to have been damaged. Migrainous features, such as a pulsating quality or nausea, may occur.

Table 15.7 Acute post-traumatic headache (Code 5.1): diagnostic criteria

5.1.1 *With significant head trauma and/or confirmatory signs*

A. Significance of head trauma documented by at least one of the following:
   1. Loss of consciousness
   2. Post-traumatic amnesia lasting more than 10 minutes
   3. At least two of the following exhibit relevant abnormality: clinical neurological examination, X-ray of skull, neuroimaging, evoked potentials, spinal fluid examination, vestibular function test, neuropsychological testing

B. Headache occurs less than 14 days after regaining consciousness (or after trauma, if there has been no loss of consciousness)

C. Headache disappears within 8 weeks after regaining consciousness (or after trauma, if there has been no loss of consciousness)

5.1.2 *With minor head trauma and no confirmatory signs*

A. Head trauma that does not satisfy 5.1.1.

B. Headache occurs less than 14 days after injury

C. Headache disappears within 8 weeks after injury

Many patients with chronic posttraumatic headache fulfil DSM-III-R criteria for posttraumatic stress disorder. Depressive features are common (Hickling et al 1992).

Migraine or cluster headache may appear de novo after a head trauma. The incidence of posttraumatic migraine was as high as 3% in one study (Solomon and Newman 1998).

Epidemiology and pathophysiology

Headache is a major factor in the symptomatology of head trauma. Interestingly, there is some evidence that the incidence of posttraumatic headache is inversely related to the severity of head injury (Kay et al 1971). In one study severe posttraumatic headache was found in 72% of mildly injured and 33% of severely injured patients (Yamaguchi 1992).

Acute posttraumatic headache is very common and reported by more women than men. The incidence of chronic posttraumatic headache varies from 15 to 40% (Jensen and Nielsen 1990). Patients suffering from headache before the trauma are not at greater risk of having posttraumatic headache.

The correlation between persistence of posttraumatic symptoms and litigation remains controversial (Russell 1932, Cook 1972, Kelly 1986, Schrader et al 1996, Warner and Fenichel 1996).

Treatment

Treatment of acute posttraumatic headache is part of the general management of the cerebral concussion syndrome: physical and mental rest in a supine position and simple analgesics or anti-inflammatory drugs. After the immediate acute stage, the practitioner frequently must deal with the other symptoms of the postconcussion syndrome such as memory impairment, mood and personality changes, and social dysfunctioning.

Treatment of chronic posttraumatic headache is difficult because of the complex interrelation between organic and psychosocial factors. *Daily consumption of analgesics are a well-established, but often neglected, chronifying factor* (Warner and Fenichel 1996; see the section on Code 8.2). It can be prevented by using NSAIDs as symptomatic treatment for the headache. Moreover, there is often an outstanding claim for compensation from the employer (when trauma occurred at work) or from insurance companies (for traffic accidents), and until this claim is settled, a complete failure of any proposed treatment may be observed. The first, and possibly major, step is to recognize that the condition does exist and is not always a 'figment of the patient's cupidity' (Kelly 1986). Once this is accepted, therapeutic strategy must be planned for each patient individually. In patients who have migrainous features, prophylactic antimigraine drugs can be useful (see above). Behavioural treatments, such as biofeedback, have provided persistent relief in some patients. In many of them antidepressants, tricyclics, or MAO inhibitors are necessary. In all cases of resistant posttraumatic headache, psychosocial guidance is the cornerstone of management with the objective of helping the patient to recover progressively his social and professional status.

Unfavourable prognostic factors in chronic forms are age higher than 40, low intellectual, educational, and socio-economic level, previous head trauma, and a history of alcohol abuse. Initial severe headache, extensive mobility decrease of the cervical spine, depressive mood, and vegetative symptoms are additional factors that tend to prolong headache after whiplash injury (Keidel and Diener 1997).

6. Headache associated with vascular disorder

All headaches coded to this group fulfill the following criteria: symptoms and/or signs of vascular disorder, including appropriate investigations; and headache as a new symptom or of a new type occurring in close temporal relation to onset of vascular disorder.

Acute ischaemic cerebrovascular disease (Code 6.1)

The importance of headache as a symptom of occlusive cerebrovascular disease is still neglected by many physicians. The major conclusions of two comprehensive reviews (Edmeads 1986, Mitsias and Ramadan 1992) can be summarized as follows:

1. The incidence of headache accompanying transient ischaemia attacks (TIAs) or strokes varies from 15 to 65% (average: 30%); it is less frequent in lacunar infarcts. Headache is more likely to occur in patients with posterior circulation ischaemia.
2. The headache can precede the ischaemic event in about 10% of cases ('sentinel headache').
3. The headache is usually on the side of the affected artery when the carotid circulation or the posterior cerebral artery are involved and mostly frontal. In basilar artery or vertebral involvement it is most often occipital and nonlateralized.

4. The quality of headache in ischaemic cerebrovascular disease may be continuous or throbbing. It is usually of moderate intensity.
5. Headache at the onset of the ischaemic stroke does not help to distinguish embolic from atherothrombotic stroke.

Recent surveys suggest that migraine is an independent risk factor for ischaemic stroke only in females younger than 45 years of age (Tzourio et al 1995, 2000). This risk is greatly enhanced by adding the contraceptive pill and/or smoking.

Intracranial haematoma (Code 6.2)

The overall incidence of headache as a major symptom of *intracerebral haemorrhages* (Code 6.2.1) ranges from 36 to 66% (Edmeads 1986). There is a proportion of non-comatose, non-aphasic patients, ranging from 10% in putaminothalamic to 30% in lobar haemorrhages, who do not have headaches. The occurrence, acuity, and severity of headache will depend largely on characteristics of the haemorrhage.

Headache is a useful indicator of the late development of an acute *epidural* (Code 6.2.3) or *subdural* (Code 6.2.2) haematoma in patients who have recovered consciousness and subsequently appear to deteriorate. It may be similar to that due to raised intracranial pressure (see the section on Code 7.1). Subdural haematomata can sometimes produce a paroxysmal headache that returns on and off irregularly throughout the day, lasts only minutes, and is accompanied by generalized sweating and an increase in pulse rate (Kelly 1986). The headache is usually frontal, but when the subdural haematoma is in the posterior fossa, it is likely to be occipital. Occipital headache associated with neck stiffness may indicate the onset of cerebellar pressure coning.

Subarachnoid haemorrhage (Code 6.3)

The headache of subarachnoid haemorrhage is typically abrupt in onset and incapacitating in severity. Time from onset to maximal pain intensity is less than 60 min in the case of ruptured aneurysm and less than 12 h if it is an arteriovenous malformation. The headache is diffuse, often posterior, and radiating into the neck. It can be accompanied by blunting of consciousness, vomiting, stiff neck, and sometimes subhyaloid haemorrhages. The diagnosis is confirmed by CT scan, which may be normal in 10% of cases, and CSF examination.

Unruptured vascular malformation (Code 6.4)

About one-quarter of patients with an intracranial aneurysm present prerupture manifestations. The most frequent of these is the so-called 'sentinel headache' (or 'premonitory headache', 'minibleeds', or 'warning leaks'), suggesting that an aneurysm might leak intermittently into the subarachnoid space. Fortunately, not every severe global headache of abrupt onset, the so-called 'thunderclap' headache, is the first symptom of an *intracranial aneurysm* (Code 6.4.1). At least two studies have shown that patients struck by thunderclap headache, who have normal CT scan and lumbar puncture results, do not subsequently develop subarachnoid haemorrhage (Wijdicks et al 1988, Markus 1991). Some of these patients may subsequently develop typical migraine attacks. Others may have at the time of the event radiological signs of diffuse, multifocal, reversible vasospasm of cerebral arteries (Dodick et al 1999). Consequently, the following guidelines may be helpful in patients with an abrupt 'worst headache of my life' thunderclap and a normal neurological examination: perform CT scan; if normal, perform lumbar puncture; if normal, the patient can be reassured and the headache considered to be benign (but it may recur in some patients). If the patient consults at a later stage, angio-magnetic resonance imaging is necessary to search for an aneurysm.

Arteriovenous malformations (AVM) (Code 6.4.1) often cause focal seizures or neurological deficits. There are several case reports of AVMs mimicking attacks of migraine with aura.

Arteritis (Code 6.5)

Giant cell arteritis (Code 6.5.1)

Diagnosis and clinical features In the IHS classification, the diagnostic criteria for giant cell arteritis (temporal arteritis or Horton's disease) are the presence of typical histopathological features on temporal artery biopsy, and one or more of the following: swollen and tender scalp artery, elevated erythrocyte sedimentation rate, and disappearance of headache within 48 h of steroid therapy.

Other clinical characteristics may be helpful for the diagnosis at an earlier stage. Giant cell arteritis is a disease of the elderly. Its prevalence increases after the age of 50 years and was found to be 78.1 per 100 000 in the ninth decade (Ross Russell 1986). The mean age was reported to be over 65 years and women predominated by 2:1 (Berlit 1992, Chmelewski et al 1992). The headache is usually temporal, of variable severity, of a constant boring quality, and temporarily relieved by analgesics such as aspirin. Pulsation in branches of the superficial temporal artery or the facial artery may be absent. Symmetrical arthralgia–myalgia in shoulder or pelvic girdle areas ('polymyalgia rheumatica') frequently accompanies this systemic disease as well as general malaise, anorexia, or mild fever, but early morning large joint stiffness may be the only manifestation. Typical complications are claudication of jaw muscles, tongue paraesthesias, and visual loss due to ischaemia of the optic nerve and retina, which is reported with a frequency varying between 7 and 60% (Ross Russell 1986). Visual disturbances require immediate and energetic treatment, because the prognosis for recovery of vision lost for more than a few hours is poor. Stroke due to involvement of cerebral arteries may occur.

Pathology Temporal artery biopsy confirms the diagnosis of a granulomatous arteritis but treatment should nevertheless be undertaken if the clinical picture of the disease is suggestive (Berlit 1992).

Treatment The first choice treatment of giant cell arteritis is corticosteroids. Initial steroid dosage ranges from 40 to 90 mg/d prednisone. The clinical response to treatment is rapid and severe headache disappears within 48 h. Whenever necessary, corticosteroid treatment can be initiated before temporal artery biopsy is performed. This does not immediately suppress histopathologic abnormalities.

Once symptoms are controlled, doses of steroids should gradually be reduced over a period of weeks to months. The erythrocyte sedimentation rate is helpful for determining the lowest effective dose. With doses of steroids below 20 mg of prednisone, 30% of patients have a relapse. The prednisone dosage should be brought down to 10–15 mg/d by the third month (side effects!), while monitoring the erythrocyte sedimentation rate value as an early indication of potential relapse. If side effects of corticosteroids are severe, immunosuppressive drugs such as azathioprine can be used.

Carotid or vertebral artery pain (Code 6.6)

Ipsilateral headache and/or cervical pain may be the only manifestation of *carotid or vertebral dissection* (Code 6.6.1) or accompany the neurological symptoms (Biousse et al 1992). *Carotidynia* (Code 6.6.2) is a controversial entity. A number of diseases of the carotid artery or of the neck are able to produce symptoms suggestive of carotidynia, such as tenderness, swelling, and increased pulsation of the carotid artery.

Postendarterectomy headache (Code 6.6.3) is defined as an ipsilateral headache beginning within 2 days of carotid endarterectomy, in the absence of carotid occlusion or dissection. In a prospective study of 50 patients, 62% reported headache, which occurred in the first 5 days after surgery in 87% of cases. The headache was mostly bilateral (74%), mild or moderate (78%), and requiring no treatment (77%) (Tehindrazanarivelo et al 1992).

Venous thrombosis (Code 6.7)

Headache is the most frequent symptom in cerebral venous thrombosis and most often the first one. It is more frequently diffuse than localized and more often subacute than acute. Its intensity is highly variable. Associated neurological signs (focal deficit or seizures), and/or raised intracranial pressure-causing papilloedema, are present in the majority of cases. Headache can, however, occasionally be the only symptom of cerebral venous thrombosis. This is thus another reason why recent, persisting headache should prompt appropriate investigations including cerebral imaging and, if necessary, angiography. The condition is treated with intravenous anticoagulation, later switched to the oral form for at least 6 months in most centres.

Arterial hypertension (Code 6.8)

There is convincing evidence that chronic hypertension of mild or moderate degree does not cause headache. Arterial hypertension is considered to be the cause of headache in four conditions that are usually not difficult to diagnose: acute pressor response to exogenous agent (Code 6.8.1), phaeochromocytoma (Code 6.8.2), malignant hypertension with hypertensive encephalopathy (Code 6.8.3), and preeclampsia and eclampsia (Code 6.8.4).

7. Headache associated with nonvascular intracranial disorder

In the IHS classification this category comprises mainly headaches associated with changes in intracranial pressure. The diagnosis of disorders, such as intracranial infections, is usually straightforward. Others will be considered in the following section, because they are frequent and/or because their diagnosis can be difficult. This is the case for benign intracranial hypertension, postlumbar puncture headache, and headache associated with brain tumour.

High cerebrospinal fluid pressure (Code 7.1)

Benign intracranial hypertension (Code 7.1.1)

Diagnosis and clinical features The diagnostic criteria for benign or idiopathic intracranial hypertension (pseudotumour cerebri) are listed in Table 15.8.

The headache accompanying this condition may mimic migraine. It is usually increased on suddenly jolting or rotating the head. In the study by Wall (1990) the following features were found to be characteristic for the diagnosis: predominant occurrence in young obese women (93%), the most severe headache ever experienced by the patient (93%), pulsatile character (83%), nausea (57%), vomiting (30%), tinnitus (55%), orbital pain (43%), transient visual obscuration (71%), diplopia (38%), and visual loss (31%). Papilloedema, without neuroradiological abnormalities (except for a possible 'empty sella'), is pathognomonic for this condition (Marcelis and Silberstein 1991), but cases without papilloedema have been reported. The resting CSF pressure in the lying position varies from 220 to 600 mm H_2O. CSF cytology is normal, but protein content may be low. Computerized axial tomography may show narrow, 'slit-like' ventricles.

Pathogenesis Pathogenetic factors that may be associated with benign intracranial hypertension include, in addition to intracranial venous occlusion, menstrual dysfunction, deficiency of the adrenals, corticosteroid therapy, hypoparathyroidism, vitamin A intoxication, insecticides, and administration of tetracycline in infants. In many cases no precise cause is found.

Table 15.8 High cerebrospinal fluid pressure (Code 7.1): diagnostic criteria

A. Patient suffers from benign intracranial hypertension fulfilling the following criteria:
1. Increased intracranial pressure (>200 mm H_2O) measured by epidural or intraventricular pressure monitoring or by lumbar puncture
2. Normal neurological examination except for papilloedema and possible VI nerve palsy
3. No mass lesion and no ventricular enlargement on neuroimaging
4. Normal or low protein concentration and normal white cell count in CSF
5. No clinical or neuroimaging suspicion of venous sinus thrombosis

B. Headache intensity and frequency related to variations of intracranial pressure with a time lag of less than 24 hours

Treatment The treatment of elevated intracranial pressure syndromes depends on the underlying cause. Benign intracranial hypertension has been reported to respond to, e.g., β-adrenergic blockers, calcium channel antagonists, antidepressants, MAO inhibitors, anticonvulsants, analgesics, and ergotamine preparations. If such therapy is unsuccessful, then a 4- to 6-week trial of furosemide or a potent carbonic anhydrase inhibitor (acetazolamide) should be tried. The use of high-dose corticosteroid may be effective. Lumbar puncture typically relieves headache, but the long-term usefulness of repeated lumbar puncture is uncertain.

Careful ophthalmological follow-up is necessary. Surgical treatment has been directed toward preventing visual loss secondary to papilloedema. Optic nerve sheath fenestration can produce improvement of headache as a felicitous side effect. Ventriculoperitoneal shunts can be performed successfully.

High-pressure hydrocephalus (Code 7.1.2)

High-pressure hydrocephalus may not cause headache when it develops progressively. The acute increase in intracranial pressure that occurs, for example, with ventricular obstruction or shunt malfunction in a treated hydrocephalic usually causes severe headache followed by visual disturbance.

Low cerebrospinal fluid pressure (Code 7.2)

Diagnosis and clinical features

The clinical hallmark of low CSF pressure headache is that the pain is aggravated by upright position and relieved when lying down ('orthostatic headache'). The headache may be frontal, occipital, or diffuse. The pain is severe, dull, or throbbing in nature and not usually relieved with analgesics. Other symptoms include anorexia, nausea, vomiting, vertigo, and tinnitus. The pain is aggravated by head shaking and jugular compression. Physical examination may show mild neck stiffness and a slow pulse rate, but is most often normal. Spinal fluid pressure usually ranges from 0 to 30 mm H_2O in the lateral supine position.

Etiology

The most frequent cause of low CSF pressure is lumbar puncture. Most likely, the pathogenesis of *post lumbar puncture headache* (Code 7.2.1) is related to a loss of CSF secondary to leakage through the dural hole. However, other factors may favour the syndrome: post lumbar puncture headache, with a prevalence of up to 40–50%, is more frequent in young, healthy, female patients with low body mass and in subjects who have a history of previous headaches (Kuntz et al 1992).

There are many other causes of low-pressure headache syndrome like posttraumatic, postoperative, or idiopathic *cerebrospinal fluid leak* (Code 7.2.2) or systemic illnesses such as dehydration, diabetic coma, hyperpnoea, or uraemia. *Spontaneous intracranial hypotension* is also well established, but remains underdiagnosed (Silberstein and Marcelis 1992). Pachymeningeal enhancement on magnetic resonance imaging is a hallmark of intracranial hypotension. CSF leaks at the spinal level can be detected by isotopic cisternography on which early bladder visualization is also a characteristic finding.

Treatment

The incidence of post lumbar puncture headache may be lower when small-diameter (20 or 22 G) or 'atraumatic' needles are used, but this lacks definitive proof (Kuntz et al 1992, Lenaerts et al 1993). Contrary to previous belief, recommendation of a resting period in the supine position after the procedure makes no difference to the incidence (Vilming et al 1988).

Treatment of postlumbar puncture headache and spontaneous intracranial hypotension is similar. It begins with non-invasive therapeutic modalities of bed rest and, if necessary NSAIDs. Intravenous or oral caffeine may produce significant relief. If not, a short course of corticosteroids or ACTH can be used, but if the patient remains disabled, one should not hesitate in applying an epidural autologous blood patch. If the headache of intracranial hypotension recurs, the epidural blood patch can be repeated, or a continuous intrathecal saline infusion may be attempted (Silberstein and Marcelis 1992).

Intracranial neoplasm (Code 7.6)

Headache occurs at presentation in 36–50% of adult patients with brain tumours and develops in the course of the disease in 60% (Silberstein and Marcelis 1992). The headache is usually generalized, of the dull, deep aching type. It may be intermittent and relieved by simple analgesics. If there is any variation in intensity during the 24-h cycle, it is worse in the early morning and ameliorated by breakfast. Elevation of intracranial pressure is not necessary for its occurrence. It is not always more prominent with rapidly growing tumours than with those of slower growth. Headache is a rare initial symptom in patients with pituitary tumours, craniopharyngiomas, or cerebellopontine angle tumours.

Some general rules concerning headache as an aid to localization in patients with brain tumour have been proposed by Dalessio (1989):

1. The headache of brain tumour approximately overlies the tumour in about one-third of patients.
2. If the tumour is above the tentorium, the pain is frequently at the vertex or in the frontal region.
3. If the tumour is below the tentorium, the pain is often occipital and cervical muscle spasms may be present.
4. Headache is always present with posterior fossa tumour.
5. If the tumour is midline, it may be increased with cough or strain or sudden head movement.
6. If the tumour is hemispheric, the pain is usually felt on the same side of the head.
7. If the tumour is chiasmal, at the sella, the pain may be referred to the vertex.

Headache is a more common symptom of brain tumour in children (>90%). The following characteristics were found to occur frequently in children with brain tumour headache: headache awakening from sleep or present on arising, high severity or frequency of headache, and vomiting. The majority of children presenting with headache because of a brain tumour have abnormal signs on neurological examination.

In specialized headache or pain clinics, brain tumours account for less than 1% of cases. There is significant overlap between the headache of brain tumour and migraine and tension-type headache. The following clues indicate that a thorough neuroradiological examination is recommended: any headache of recent onset; a headache that has changed in character; a focalized headache not resembling one of the primary headaches; and morning or nocturnal headache, associated with vomiting, in a nonmigraineur.

8. Headache associated with substances or their withdrawal

A new headache including migraine, tension-type headache, or cluster headache, in close temporal relation to substance use or substance withdrawal is coded to this group. Effective doses and temporal relationships have not yet been determined for most substances. The most significant and intriguing headaches in clinical practice are those induced by misuse of antiheadache medications, i.e., ergotamine, analgesic compounds, and triptans.

Headache induced by acute substance use or exposure (Code 8.1)

A vast number of chemicals can cause headaches (Askmark et al 1989), e.g., nitrates/nitrites ('hot dog headache') (Code 8.1.1), monosodium glutamate ('Chinese restaurant syndrome') (Code 8.1.2), carbon monoxide (Code 8.1.3), or alcohol (Code 8.1.4).

Headache induced by chronic substance use or exposure (Code 8.2)

Diagnosis and clinical features (Table 15.9)

Around 10% of patients attending a specialized headache clinic, of whom most originally had migraine, suffer from this condition (Kudrow 1982, Schoenen et al 1989, Henry 1992). Drug-induced headache is a chronic, usually daily, headache involving the whole skull ('pressing helmet'). Pain is exacerbated by physical exercise and intellectual effort and is often accompanied by asthenia, irritability, sleep, and memory disturbances. The characteristics of chronic drug-induced headache resemble those of tension-type headache, except that nausea and photo- and phonophobia are much more frequent. These patients have a long-lasting history of abortive drug intake, with escalation over months or years of the doses needed to provide some relief. Some use analgesics even before the headache appears. Depression or anxiety are common, as is the tendency towards tranquillizer abuse. Ergotamine, usually associated with caffeine, and combination analgesics containing codeine and/or caffeine are most often involved, but recently abuse of the selective antimigraine drugs, the triptans, was also reported (Limmroth et al 1999).

Pathophysiology

So far, headache induced by chronic use of ergotamine and analgesics has only been described when the drugs were taken for headaches and not when they were taken for other disorders such as chronic low back pain. It remains to be determined whether pain syndromes such as the latter might also be rendered chronic by analgesic abuse. Although some side effects of ergotamine and analgesics are well known, many physicians still ignore the fact that use of these drugs in large amounts can induce chronic headaches. Moreover, analgesic abuse seems to nullify the effects of prophylactic drugs given for the original headache condition.

In the criteria of the IHS classification (Table 15.9), the cumulative doses of ergotamine or analgesics capable of inducing chronic headaches are obviously overestimated. The mechanisms of drug-abuse headache are still poorly understood. A familial predisposition is possible. A similar clinical pattern is encountered in patients using such different drugs as analgesics, ergotamine, triptans, barbiturates, or opiates. These drugs might modify central neurotransmitter systems (e.g., noradrenaline (norepinephrine), serotonin, and endorphins) playing a role in the control of nociception and mood by changing receptor sensitivity.

Treatment

The only effective treatment of drug misuse headache is withdrawal of the substance(s) involved (Kudrow 1982, Dichgans et al 1984, Saper 1987, Schoenen et al 1989, Mathew et al 1990, Henry 1992, Steiner et al 1992, Limmroth et al 1999). For a better management of withdrawal a hospital setting can be chosen, but it does not provide better outcome than an ambulatory setting. Withdrawal reactions include increased headaches, nervousness, restlessness, nausea, vomiting, insomnia, diarrhoea, tremor, autonomic dysfunction, and even seizures in the

Table 15.9 Headache induced by chronic substance use or exposure (Code 8.2): diagnostic criteria

A. Occurs after daily doses of a substance for >3 months
B. A certain minimum dose should be indicated
C. Headache is chronic (15 days or more a month)
D. Headache disappears within 1 month after withdrawal of the substance

8.2.1 *Ergotamine-induced headache*
A. Is preceded by daily ergotamine intake (oral >2 mg, rectal >1 mg)
B. Is diffuse, pulsating and distinguished from migraine by absent attack pattern and/or absent associated symptoms

8.2.2 *Analgesic abuse headache*
One or more of the following:
1. >50 g of aspirin a month or equivalent of other analgesics
2. >100 tablets a month of analgesics combined with barbiturates or other non-narcotic compounds
3. One or more narcotic analgesics

case of barbiturate or benzodiazepine abuse. Their duration is shorter for triptans than for ergotamine or analgesic preparations (Katsavara et al 2001). They can be alleviated by temporary prescription of neuroleptics or tranquillizers, e.g., tiapride (75–100 mg/d) or acamprosate (333 mg t.i.d. or q.i.d.). NSAIDs may be allowed as symptomatic headache treatment and triptans for 'breakthrough' migraine attacks, but no more than twice per week. Intravenous dihydroergotamine is also an effective strategy for withdrawal in inpatients. Prophylactic antimigraine drugs like valproate or beta blockers should be prescribed concomittantly if the patient suffers from migraine, and tricyclics and behavioural therapy if he has chronic tension-type headache (see above). In a study of 121 drug-misusers with chronic daily headache where we used tiapride and clomipramine IV for inpatients, orally for outpatients, in combination with prophylactic therapy, results of withdrawal were excellent in the short term (73% at 10 days, 65% at 90 days), but there was a recurrence in about 20% of patients at 6 months (Schoenen et al 1989). Long-term (<3 years) relapse rates up to 50% were reported in other series. One important aspect of long-term prognosis is appropriate psychological support.

Education of patients and their physicians is obviously important in the prevention of this syndrome. Important steps include limiting the prescription of acute antimigraine drugs (useful rule of thumb: intake on no more than 2 days per week); avoiding treatment with combined analgesics containing codeine, caffeine, and/or ergotamine; using preferentially simple NSAIDs, aspirin or paracetamol compounds, and triptans for acute headache treatment; and considering prophylactic therapy whenever headache is frequent and/or disabling despite acute drug use (Schoenen et al 1989).

9. Headache or facial pain associated with disorder of cranium, neck, eyes, ears, nose, sinuses, teeth, mouth, or other facial or cranial structures

Cervical spine (Code 11.2.1)

Diagnosis and clinical features

The diagnostic criteria of so-called 'cervicogenic headache' remain controversial (Edmeads 1988, Sjaastad et al 1990). In the first IHS Classification functional and/or structural abnormalities on X-rays of the cervical spine are a mandatory diagnostic criterion, which may be disputable. On the other hand, among the unilateral headaches a cervicogenic origin may be overdiagnosed, if strict diagnostic criteria are missing.

Pathophysiology

Pain (also in the supraorbital area) can be transiently relieved by anaesthetic blockade of the greater occipital nerve (GON) (Bovim and Sand 1992), suggesting that the GON and projections from upper cervical root (C2–C3) to second-order nociceptors in the spinal trigeminal complex (Kerr 1961) might play a role, producing referred pain in the area of the ophthalmic division of the trigeminal nerve. However, other structures like bones, muscles, and arteries in the neck area can induce pain. Like tension-type headache, cervicogenic headache (although triggered initially by peripheral mechanisms) might be caused in its chronic form by dysfunction of central rather than peripheral nociceptive structures.

Treatment

Pharmacological treatment of cervicogenic headache is often disappointing. NSAIDs and analgesics can be effectively used for short periods. Tricyclic antidepressants can also produce some benefit. As with tension-type headaches, physical therapy, relaxation, and biofeedback can be useful (Jaeger 1989). Besides blockade of the GON, neurolysis of this nerve or of C2 roots has been performed, but results were short-lasting (Bovim et al 1992). Radiofrequency electrocoagulation of joint facets has also been proposed (Blume et al 1982, van Suijlekom et al 1998), but is not an evidence-based alternative yet.

Temporomandibular joint disease (Code 11.7)

Diagnosis and clinical features

Temporomandibular joint disease produces pain in the jaw, located to the temporomandibular joint and/or radiating from there, usually of mild to moderate intensity. It is precipitated by movement and/or clenching the teeth. Range of movement of the joint is reduced, with palpation tenderness of the capsule and noise ('click') during joint movements. CT scan or MRI of the temporomandibular joint can be abnormal.

Pathophysiology and treatment

Pain from temporomandibular joints is rarely due to definable organic disease. Patients with rheumatoid arthritis or generalized osteoarthrosis often show X-ray involvement of the temporomandibular joints but do not experience significantly more pain in that area than the normal population (Chalmers and Blair 1974). The so-called 'Costen's syndrome' (Costen 1934), including head pain and additional features, was attributed to retroposition of the head of the mandibular condyle, causing irritation of the adjacent nerves. However, sixty years later pathological proof is still missing.

In most cases temporomandibular pain is associated with oromandibular dysfunction and can be consecutive to myofascial involvement, which relates it to tension-type headache (Schokker 1989) (see Code 2). Occlusional splints may help these patients, but additional drug or non-drug treatment for tension-type headache is usually necessary on the long term. Moreover, there is strong evidence that many patients with temporomandibular pain syndrome suffer from concomitant anxiety or depression and should be treated accordingly (Feinmann et al 1984).

10. Cranial neuralgia, nerve trunk pain and deafferentation pain

Herpes zoster (Code 12.1.4.1), chronic postherpetic neuralgia (Code 12.1.4.2)

Herpes zoster affects the trigeminal ganglion in 10–15% of patients, with particular affinity for the ophthalmic division (80%). Third, fourth, or sixth cranial nerve palsies are rare. Herpes zoster may also involve the geniculate ganglion, with an eruption in the external auditory meatus ('Ramsay-Hunt's zone') often associated with facial nerve palsy or acoustic symptoms.

Postherpetic neuralgia (Code 12.1.4.2) is a chronic pain developing during the acute phase of infection, but persisting more than 6 months. It is a frequent sequel of herpes zoster infection (up to 50%), particularly in older patients (Watson and Evans 1988). Its incidence is reduced by acyclovir treatment at the acute phase. Pain is felt in the area formerly involved by the infection. It is constant, moderate to severe, and often described as burning. Paraesthesia or hypoaesthesia is frequent.

Treatment rests on tricyclic antidepressants (e.g., amitryptiline; Watson and Evans 1988) or other classes of antidepressants (Watson et al 1992) improving symptoms in about half of the patients (Watson et al 1991). Better outcome seems to be related to early treatment. Topical administration of capsaicin or analgesics can be tried in refractory cases, and recently new generation antiepileptics like lamotrigine or gabapentin were found effective (Delaux and Schoenen 2001).

Trigeminal neuralgia (tic douloureux) (Code 12.2)

Idiopathic trigeminal neuralgia (Code 12.2.1)

Diagnosis and clinical features Trigeminal neuralgia or 'tic douloureux' is described in detail in Chap. 14. In summary, it is characterized by very short-lasting (up to a few seconds) attacks of intense, electric shock-like pain limited to the distribution of one or more divisions of the trigeminal nerve (usually the second or third divisions), female preponderance (ratio 3:2 over males), onset after 50 years of age, and presence in the affected territory of trigger points where trivial stimuli such as washing, shaving, chewing, brushing the teeth, or speaking can elicit the pain. The pain often induces reflex spasms of facial muscles on the affected side, hence the name 'tic douloureux'. Paroxysms may recur dozens of times in a single day but interfere little with sleep. Remissions of variable duration are described (see Table 15.9).

Pathophysiology It is currently believed that in many cases so-called idiopathic trigeminal neuralgia might result from local demyelination of the trigeminal root entry zone due to compressions in the posterior fossa, usually by small tortuous arteries or veins (Jannetta 1970).

Treatment More than two-thirds of patients with idiopathic trigeminal neuralgia respond favourably to treatment with carbamazepine (200–400 mg t.i.d.) or in refractory cases, carbamazepine plus baclofen (25 mg t.i.d.) or plus clonazepam (2 mg t.i.d.). Phenytoin (200–300 mg/d), lamotrigine, or gabapentin (Delaux and Schoenen 2001) are alternatives. For refractory cases, radiofrequency thermocoagulation or gamma-knife surgery of the Gasserian ganglion or microsurgical decompression (Jannetta 1981, Taarnhoj 1995) of the trigeminal root in the posterior fossa can be proposed. Each of these methods has proven efficacy, but each may be followed by relapses. Each method also may be associated with complications or failures. As a consequence, the choice of an invasive treatment for resistant trigeminal neuralgia must take into account previous experience and expertise in a given centre.

Symptomatic trigeminal neuralgia (Code 12.2.2)

Several diseases can produce trigeminal neuralgia, such as acoustic neurinomas, brainstem infarcts, and, chiefly, multiple sclerosis. The main differences from the idiopathic form are a younger age at onset, persistence of aching between paroxysms, and signs of sensory impairment in the distribution of the corresponding trigeminal division.

Glossopharyngeal (Code 12.3) and nervus intermedius (Code 12.4) neuralgias

These forms of neuralgia are uncommon. Pain characteristics, pathophysiology, and treatment are similar to those of trigeminal neuralgia. In glossopharyngeal neuralgia the pain is localized in the ear, base of tongue, or tonsillar fossa or beneath the angle of the jaw. It is provoked by swallowing, talking, and coughing. Neuralgia of the nervus intermedius is felt deeply in the ear, lasting for seconds or minutes, with a trigger zone in the posterior wall of the auditory canal.

Facial pain not fulfilling criteria in groups 11 and 12 (Code 12.8)

Many patients, usually middle-aged women, complain of facial pain that cannot be put into one of the previous categories ('atypical facial pain'). Pain is described as burning or aching, is present daily, and persists for most of the day. It is poorly localized and does not fit with the sensory distribution of a trigeminal branch. Clinical examination and paraclinical investigations are normal. Pain may be triggered by operations or injuries to the face or dental problems, but becomes chronic without any demonstrable lesion. Such patients often exhibit depressive traits (Lascelles 1966). Tricyclic antidepressants may provide some relief.

Exceptionally, unilateral facial pain mimicking atypical facial pain is due to lung cancer compressing the vagus nerve (Schoenen et al 1992). This referred pain is typically located in the ear and upper teeth.

Conclusions

The operational diagnostic criteria of the IHS Headache Classification allow a more uniform grouping of headache types for research purposes. Their usefulness in routine clinical practice is limited. When confronted with a headache patient, the practitioner first must decide whether the headache is symptomatic of an underlying disease or whether it is a 'primary' headache.

With few exceptions, any headache of recent onset should, as a rule, be considered to be symptomatic. Recognizing the cause needs, above all, clinical skill and an adequate choice of paraclinical investigations.

Most chronic headaches correspond to one of the primary headache types. Many, if not all, are probably biobehavioural disorders, resulting from a complex, variable interplay between neurobiological (in part genetically determined) mechanisms and behavioural processes influenced by environmental factors. Treatment of these patients, besides alleviating the symptom 'head pain', must be directed towards both body and mind.

In primary headaches, the most important recent advances were achieved for the pathogenesis and treatment of *migraine*. The genetic 'Pandora's box' has been opened and detectable interictal nervous system dysfunctions contribute to understanding the neurobiological consequences of the migraine genotypes and to better geno-phenotype correlations. New triptans are on the market for more efficient acute therapy, and some novel prophylactic drugs with few side effects, like riboflavine, lisinopril, and new antiepileptics, were found to be effective. In *tension-type headache*, unfortunately, there has been little pathophysiologic or therapeutic progress. Nonetheless, the advantage of combining behavioural (stress management) and drug (tricyclics) treatment for chronic tension-type headache has been proven. It remains to be proven, however, whether certain tension-type headaches fulfilling IHS criteria are in fact migrainous in origin, as suggested by some recent studies. *Drug-misuse headache*, caused by the overuse of acute headache medications, mainly that of combination analgesics and ergotamine preparations, is still underrecognized by the medical community and largely unknown to patients.

References

Adelman JU, Lipton RB, Ferrari MD, Diener H-C, McCarroll KA, Vandormael K, Lines CR 2001 Comparison of rizatriptan and other triptans on stringent measures of efficacy. Neurology 57: 1377–1383

Amery WK, Vandenbergh V 1987 What can precipitating factors teach us about the pathogenesis of migraine? Headache 27: 146–150

Andrasik F, Passchier J 1993 Tension-type headache, cluster headache, and miscellaneous headaches: psychological aspects. In: Olesen J, Tfelt-Hansen P, Welch KMA (eds) The headaches. Raven Press, New York, pp 489–492

Askmark H, Lundberg O, Olsson S 1989 Drug related headache. Headache 29: 441–444

Bahra A, Gawel MJ, Hardebo JE, Millson D, Breen SA, Goadsby PJ 2000 Oral zolmitriptan in the acute treatment of cluster headache. Neurology 54: 1832–1839

Bendtsen L, Jensen R, Olesen J 1996a A non-selective (amitriptyline), but not a selective (citalopram), serotonin reuptake inhibitor is effective in the prophylactic treatment of chronic tension-type headache. Journal of Neurology,

Neurosurgery and Psychiatry 61: 285–290
Bendtsen L, Jensen R, Olesen J 1996b Qualitatively altered nociception in chronic myofascial pain. Pain 65: 259–264
Berlit P 1992 Clinical and laboratory findings with giant cell arteritis. Journal of the Neurological Sciences 111: 1–12
Bille B 1962 Migraine in school children. Acta Paediatrica 51 (suppl 136): 3–151
Binder WJ, Brin MF, Blitzer A, Schoenrock LD, Pogoda JM 2000 Botulinum toxin type A (BOTOX) for treatment of migraine headaches: an open-label study. Otolaryngol Head Neck Surg 123: 669–676
Biousse V, Woimant F, Amarenco P et al 1992 Pain as the only manifestation of internal carotid artery dissection. Cephalalgia 12: 314–317
Blanchard EB, Appelbaum KA, Guarnieri P et al 1987 Five year follow-up on the treatment of chronic headache with biofeedback and/or relaxation. Headache 27: 580–583
Blau JN 1980 Migraine prodromes separated from the aura: complete migraine. British Medical Journal 281: 658–660
Blume H, Kakolewski R, Richardson R 1982 Radiofrequency denaturation in occipital pain: results in 450 cases. Applied Neurophysiology 45: 54–548
Bogaards MC, ter Kuile MM 1994 Treatment of recurrent tension headache: a meta-analytic review. Clinical Journal of Pain 10: 174–190
Bove G, Nielsson N 1998 Spinal manipulation in the treatment of episodic tension-type headache. A randomized controlled trial. Journal of American Medical Association 280: 1576–1579
Bovim G 1992 Cervicogenic headache, migraine and tension-type headache. Pressure pain thresholds measurements. Pain 1: 169–173
Bovim G, Sand T 1992 Cervicogenic headache, migraine without aura and tension-type headache. Diagnostic blockade of greater occipital and supraorbital nerves. Pain 51: 43–48
Bovim G, Fredriksen TA, Stolt-Nielsen A, Sjaastad O 1992 Neurolysis of the greater occipital nerve in cervicogenic headache. A follow-up study. Headache 32: 175–179
Breslau N, Schultz LR, Stewart WF, Lipton RB, Lucia VC, Welch KM 2000 Headache and major depression: is the association specific to migraine? Neurology 54: 308–313
Cady RK, Sheftell F, Lipton RB, O'Quinn S, Pharmd, Jones M, Putnam DG, Crip A, Metz A, McNeal S 2000 Effect of early intervention with sumatriptan on migraine pain: retrospective analyses of data from three clinical trials. Clin Ther 22: 1035–1048
Cao Y, Welch KM, Aurora S, Vikingstad EM 1999 Functional MRI-BOLD of visually triggered headache in patients with migraine. Archives of Neurology 56: 548–554
Carlsson J, Fahlcrantz A, Augustinsson L-E 1990 Muscle tenderness in tension headache treated with acupuncture or physiotherapy. Cephalalgia 10: 131–141
Chabriat H, Vahedi K, Clark CA, Poupon C, Ducros A, Denier C, Le Bihan D, Bousser MG 2000 Decreased hemispheric water mobility in hemiplegic migraine related to mutation of CACNA1A gene. Neurology 54: 510–512
Chalmers IM, Blair GS 1974 Is the temporomandibular joint involved in primary osteoarthrosis? Oral Surgery, Oral Medicine, Oral Pathology 38: 74–79
Chmelewski WL, McKnight AM, Agudelo CA, Wise CM 1992 Presenting features and outcomes in patients undergoing temporal artery biopsy: a review of 98 patients. Archives of Internal Medicine 152: 1690–1695
Christiansen I, Thomsen LL, Dauggard D, Ulrich V, Olesen J 1999 Glyceryl trinitrate induces attacks of migraine without aura in sufferers of migraine with aura. Cephalalgia 19: 660–667
Chu ML, Shinnar S 1991 Headaches in children younger than 7 years of age. Archives of Neurology 49: 79–82
Cook JB 1972 The postconcussional syndrome and factors influencing after minor head injury admitted to hospital. Scandinavian Journal of Rehabilitation Medicine 4: 27–30
Cooke LJ, Rose MS, Becker WJ 2000 Chinook winds and migraine headache. Neurology 54: 302–307
Costen JB 1934 A syndrome of ear and sinus symptoms dependent upon disturbed function of the temporomandibular joint. Annals of Otology, Rhinology and Laryngology 43: 1–15
Dahlem MA, Engelmann R, Lowel S, Muller SC 2000 Does the migraine aura reflect cortical organization? European Journal of Neuroscience 12: 767–770
Dahlöf CGH, Jacobs LD 1996 Ketoprofen paracetamol and placebo in the treatment of episodic tension-type headache. Cephalalgia 16: 117–123
Dalessio DJ 1989 Headache. In: Wall PD, Melzack R (eds) Textbook of pain, 2nd edn. Churchill Livingstone, Edinburgh, pp 386-401
Delaux V, Schoenen J 2001 New generation anti-epileptics for facial pain and headache. Acta Neurologica Belgica 101: 41–46
Dichgans J, Diener HC, Gerber WD et al 1984 Analgetikainduzierter Dauerkopfsschmerz. Deutsche Medizinische Wochenschrift 109: 369–373
Diener HC for the ASASUMAMIG Study Group 1999 Efficacy and safety of intravenous acetylsalicylic acid lysinate compared to subcutaneous sumatriptan and parenteral placebo in the acute treatment of migraine. A double-blind, double-dummy, randomized, multicenter, parallel group study. Cephalalgia 19: 581–588
Diener HC, Föh M, Iaccarino C et al on behalf of the Study Group 1996 Cyclandelate in the prophylaxis of migraine: a randomized, parallel, double-blind study in comparison with placebo and propranolol. Cephalalgia 16: 441–447
Diener HC, Krupp P, Schmitt T et al 2001 Cyclandelate in the prophylaxis of migraine: a placebo-controlled study. Cephalalgia 21: 66–70
Dodick DW, Brown RD, Britton JW, Huston J 1999 Nonaneurysmal thunderclap headache with diffuse, multifocal, segmental, and reversible vasospasm. Cephalalgia 19: 118–123
Drummond PD 1987 Scalp tenderness and sensitivity to pain in migraine and tension-type headache. Headache 27: 45
Ebersberger A, Schaible HG, Averbeck B, Richter F 2001 Is there a correlation between spreading deperssion, neurogenic inflammation, and nociception that might cause migraine headache? Annals of Neurology 49: 7–13
Edmeads J 1986 Headache in cerebrovascular disease. In: Viken PJ, Bruyn GW, Klawans HL (eds) Handbook of clinical neurology, vol 4(48). Elsevier, Amsterdam, pp 273–290
Edmeads J 1988 The cervical spine and headache. Neurology 38: 1874–1878
Ekbom K 1986 Chronic migrainous neuralgia. In: Vinken PJ, Bruyn GW, Klawans HL (eds) Handbook of clinical neurology, vol 4(48). Elsevier, Amsterdam, pp 247–255
Ekbom K 1995 Treatment of cluster headache: clinical trials, design and results. Cephalalgia 15: 33–36
Feinmann C, Harris M, Cawley R 1984 Psychogenic facial pain: presentation and treatment. British Medical Journal 88: 436–438
Ferrari MD 1998 Migraine. Lancet 351: 1043–1051
Ferrari MD, Roon KI, Lipton RB, Goadsby PJ 2001 Oral triptans (serotonin 5-HT1B/1D agonists) in acute migraine treatment: a meta-analysis of 53 trials. Lancet 358: 1668–1675
Ford ERG, Ford KT, Swaid S et al 1998 Gamma knife treatment of refractory cluster headache. Headache 38: 3–9
Forsell H, Kirveskari P, Kangasniemi P 1985 Changes in headache after treatment of mandibular dysfunction. Cephalalgia 5: 229–236
Gawel MJ, Worthington I, Maggisano A 2001 Progress in clinical neurosciences: a systematic review of the use of triptans in acute migraine. Canadian Journal of Neurological Sciences 28: 30–41

Gervil M, Ulrich V, Kaprio J, Olesen J, Russell MG 1999a The relative role of genetic and environmental factors in migraine without aura. Neurology 53: 995–999

Gervil M, Ulrich V, Kyvik KO, Olesen J, Russell MG 1999b Migraine without aura: a population-based twin study. Annals of Neurology 46: 606–611

Goadsby PJ 2001 Migraine, aura, and cortical spreading depression: why are we still talking about it? Annals of Neurology 49: 4–6

Göbel H, Weigle L, Kropp P et al 1992 Pain sensitivity and pain reactivity of pericranial muscles in migraine and tension-type headache. Cephalalgia 12: 142–151

Goldstein DJ, Roon KI, Offen WW et al 2001 Selective serotonin 1F (5-HT1f) receptor agonist LY334370 for acute migraine: a randomised controlled trial. Lancet 358: 1230–1234

Grossmann M, Schmidramsl H 2000 An extract of *Petasites hybridus* is effective in the prophylaxis of migraine. Int J Clin Pharmacol Ther 38: 430–435

Haddock CK, Rowan AB, Andrasik F et al 1997 Home-based behavioral treatments for chronic benign headache: a meta-analysis of controlled trials. Cephalalgia 17: 113–118

Hardebo JE, Dahlöf C 1998 Sumatriptan nasl spray (20 mg:dose) in the acute treatment of cluster headache. Cepahalalgia 18: 487–489

Hegerl U, Juckel G 1993 Intensity dependence of auditory evoked potentials as an indicator of central serotonergic neurotransmission: a new hypothesis. Biological Psychiatry 33: 173–187

Henry P 1992 Drug abuse in headache. Functional Neurology 6 (suppl 7): 5–6

Hickling EJ, Blanchard EB, Silverman DJ et al 1992 Motor vehicle accidents, headaches and post-traumatic stress disorder: assessment findings in a consecutive series. Headache 32: 147–151

Holroyd KA 1993 Tension-type headache, cluster headache, and miscellaneous headaches: Psychological and behavioral techniques. In: Olesen J, Tfelt-Hansen P, Welch KMA (eds) The headaches. Raven Press, New York, pp 515–520

Holroyd KA, Penzien DB 1986 Client variables and behavioral treatment of recurrent tension headaches: a meta-analytic review. Journal of Behavioural Medicine 9: 515–536

Holroyd KA, Penzien DB, Holm JE et al 1984 Behavioural treatment of tension and migraine headache: what does the literature say? Headache 24: 167–168

Holroyd KA, O'Donnell FJ, Stensland M, Lipchik GL, Cordingley GE, Carlson BW 2001 Management of chronic tension-type headache with tricyclic antidepressant medication, stress management therapy, and their combination: a randomized controlled trial. Journal of American Medical Association 285: 2208–2215

International Headache Society (IHS) 1988 Classification and diagnostic criteria for headache disorders, cranial neuralgias and facial pain. Cephalalgia 8 (suppl 7): 1–96

Italian Cooperative Study Group on the Epidemiology of Cluster Headache (ICECH) 1995 Case–control study on the epidemiology of cluster headache. I: Etiological factors and associated conditions. Neuroepidemiology 14: 123–127

Jaeger B 1989 Are 'cervicogenic' headaches due to myofascial pain and cervical spine dysfunction? Cephalalgia 9: 157–164

James MF, Smith MI, Bockhorst KH et al 1999 Cortical spreading depression in the gyrencephalic feline brain studied by magnetic resonance imaging. Physiology 519: 415–425

Jannetta PJ 1970 Observations on the etiology of trigeminal neuralgia, hemifacial spasm, acoustic nerve dysfunction and glossopharyngeal neuralgia: definitive microsurgical treatment and results in 117 cases. Neurochirurgia 20: 145–154

Jannetta PJ 1981 Vascular decompression in trigeminal neuralgia. In: Samii M, Jannetta PJ (eds) The cranial nerves. Springer, Berlin, pp 331–340

Jensen OK, Nielsen FF 1990 The influence of sex and pre-traumatic headache on the incidence and severity of headache after head injury. Cephalalgia 1: 285–294

Jensen R, Olesen J 1996 Initiating mechanisms of experimentally induced tension-type headache. Cephalalgia 16: 175

Jensen R, Rasmussen BK, Pedersen B et al 1993a Cephalic muscle tenderness and pressure pain threshold in headache. Pain 52: 193–199

Jensen R, Rasmussen BK, Pedersen B et al 1993b Oromandibular disorders in a general population. Journal of Craniomandibular Disorders, Facial and Oral Pain 7: 175–182

Jensen R, Brinck T, Olesen J 1994 Sodium valproate has a prophylactic effect in migraine without aura: a triple-blind, placebo-controlled crossover study. Neurology 44: 647–651

Jimenez MD, Friera G, Manjon T.and the Study Group of Gabapentin-Migraine 1999 Efficacy and safety of gabapentin in prophylaxis migraine headache. A pilot study. Cephalalgia 19: 376 (abstract)

Joish V, Cady P, Bennett D, Harris R 2000 An epidemiological case–control study of migraine and its associated comorbid conditions. Annals of Epidemiology 10: 460

Katsavara Z, Fritsche G, Muessig M, Diener HC, Limmroth V 2001 Clinical features of withdrawal headache following overuse of triptans and other headache drugs. Neurology 57: 1694–1698

Kaube H, Herzog J, Kaufer T, Dichgans M, Diener HC 2000 Aura in some patients with familial hemiplegic migraine can be stopped by intranasal ketamine. Neurology 55: 139–141

Kay DWK, Kerr TA, Lassman LP 1971 Brain trauma and the postconcussional syndrome. Lancet 2: 1052–1055

Keidel M, Diener HC 1997 Post-traumatic headache. Nervenarzt 68: 769–777

Kellstein DE, Lipton RB, Geetha R et al 2000 Evaluation of a novel solubilized formulation of ibuprofen in the treatment of migraine headache: a randomized, double-blind, placebo-controlled, dose-ranging study. Cephalalgia 20: 233–243

Kelly RE 1986 Post-traumatic headache. In: Vinken PJ, Bruyn GW, Klawans HL (eds) Handbook of clinical neurology, vol 4(48). Elsevier, Amsterdam, pp 383–390

Kerr FWL 1961 Structural relation of the trigeminal spinal tract to upper cervical roots and the solitary nucleus in cat. Experimental Neurology 4: 134–148

Kudrow L 1982 Paradoxical effects of frequent analgesic use. Advances in Neurology 3: 335–341

Kuntz KM, Kohmen E, Stevens JC et al 1992 Post-lumbar puncture headaches: experience in 501 consecutive procedures. Neurology 42: 1884–1887

Lahat E, Barr J, Barzilai A, Cohen H, Berkovitch M 1999 Visual evoked potentials in the diagnosis of headache before 5 years of age. European Journal of Pediatrics 158: 892–895

Lance JW, Lambert GA, Goadsby PJ et al 1983 Brain-stem influences on the cephalic circulation: experimental data from cat and monkey of relevance to mechanisms of migraine. Headache 23: 258–265

Lange R, Schwarz JA, Hohn M 2000 Acetylsalicylic acid effervescent 1000 mg (Aspirin®) in acute migraine attacks; a multicentre, randomised, double-blind, single-dose, placebo-controlled parallel group study. Cephalalgia 20: 663–667

Lascelles RG 1966 Atypical facial pain and depression. British Journal of Psychiatry 112: 651–659

Lauritzen M 1992 Spreading depression and migraine. Pathology et Biologie 40: 332–337

Lenaerts M, Pepin J-L, Tombu S, Schoenen J 1993 No significant effect of an 'atraumatic' needle on incidence of post-lumbar puncture headache or traumatic tap. Cephalalgia 13: 296–297

Le Pira F, Zappala G, Giuffrida S, Lo Bartolo ML, Reggio E, Morana R, Lanaia F 2000 Memory disturbances in migraine with and without aura: a strategy problem? Cephalalgia 20: 475–478

Lewis TA, Solomon GD 1996 Advances in cluster headache management Cleveland Clinic Journal of Medicine 63: 237–244
Limmroth V et al 1999 Headache after frequent use of serotonin agonists zolmitriptan and naratriptan. Lancet 353: 378
Lipchick GL, Holroyd KA, France CR et al 1996 Central and peripheral mechanisms in chronic tension-type headache. Pain 64: 467–475
Lipton RB, Stewart WF, Von Korff M 1994 The burden of migraine: a review of cost to society. Pharmacoeconomics 6: 215–221
Lipton RB, Stewart WF, Cady R, Hall C, O'Quinn S, Kuhn T, Gutterman D 2000a Sumatriptan for the range of headaches in migraine sufferers: results of the spectrum study. Headache 40: 783–791
Lipton RB, Stewart WF, Stone AM, Lainez MJ, Sawyer JP 2000b Stratified care vs step care strategies for migraine: the disability in strategies of care (DISC) study: a randomized trial. Journal of American Medical Association 284: 2599–2605
Manfredi PL, Shenoy S, Payne R 2000 Sumatriptan for headache caused by head and neck cancer. Headache 40: 758–760
Marcelis J, Silberstein SD 1991 Idiopathic intracranial hypertension without papilloedoma. Archives of Neurology 48: 392–399
Markus HS 1991 A prospective follow-up of thunderclap headache mimicking subarachnoid haemorrhage. Journal of Neurology, Neurosurgery and Psychiatry 54: 1117–1118
Massiou H, Bousser MJ 1992 Bêta-bloquants et migraine. Pathologie et Biologie 40: 373–380
Mathew NT, Bendtsen L 1999 Pharmacotherapy of tension-type headache. In Olesen J, Tfelt-Hansen P, Welch KMA (eds): The headaches, 2nd edn. Lippincott-Williams & Wilkins, Philadelphia, pp 667–674
Mathew NT, Schoenen J 1999 Acute pharmacotherapy of tension-type headache. In Olesen J, Tfelt-Hansen P, Welch KMA (eds): The headaches, 2nd edn. Lippincott-Williams & Wilkins, Philadelphia, pp 661–666
Mathew N, Kurman R, Perez F 1990 Drug induced refractory headache. Headache 30: 634–638
May A, Bahra A, Büchel C et al 1998 First direct evidence for hypothalamic activation in cluster headache attacks. Lancet 352: 275–278
Melchart D, Linde K, Fischer P, Berman B, White A, Vickers A, Allais G 2001 Acupuncture for idiopathic headache (Cochrane Review). The Cochrane Library, issue 1
Mitsias P, Ramadan NM 1992 Headache in cerebrovascular disease. Part I: clinical features. Cephalalgia 12: 269–274
Monstad I, Krabbe A, Micieli G et al 1995 Preemptive oral treatment with sumatriptan during a cluster period. Headache 35: 607–613
Moskowitz MA 1984 Neurobiology of vascular head pain. Annals of Neurology 6: 157–168
Neuhauser H, Leopold M, von Brevern M, Arnold G, Lempert T 2001 The interrelations of migraine, vertigo, and migrainous vertigo. Neurology 56: 436–441
Newman L, Mannix LK, Landy S et al 2001 Naratriptan as a short-term prophylaxis of menstrually associated migraine: a randomized, double-blind, placebo-controlled study. Headache 41: 248–256
Olesen J 1991 Clinical and pathophysiological observations in migraine and tension-type headache explained by integration of vascular, supraspinal and myofascial inputs. Pain 46: 125–132
Olesen J, Schoenen J 1999 Tension-type headache, cluster headache, and miscellaneous headaches. Synthesis of tension-type headache mechanisms. In: Olesen J, Tfelt-Hansen P, Welch KMA (eds) The headaches, 2nd edn. Lippincott-Williams & Wilkins, Philadelphia, pp 615–618
Olesen J, Iversen HK, Thomsen LL 1993 Nitric oxide supersensitivity. A possible molecular mechnism of migraine pain. Neuroreport 4: 1027–1030
Ollat H 1992 Agonistes et antagonistes de la sérotonine et migraine. Pathologie et Biologie 40: 389–396
Ophoff RA, Terwindt GM, Vergouwe MN et al 1996 Familial hemiplegic migraine and episodic ataxia type-2 are caused by mutations in the Ca^{2+} channel gene CACNL1A4. Cell 87: 543–552
Pascual J, Iglesias F, Oterino A et al 1996 Cough, exertional, and sexual headaches: an analysis of 72 benign and symptomatic cases. Neurology 46: 1520–1524
Peikert A, Wilimzig C, Köhne-Volland R 1996 Prophylaxis of migraine with oral magnesium: results from a prospective, multi-center, placebo-controlled and double-blind randomized study. Cephalalgia 16: 257–263
Pfaffenrath V, Wessely P, Meyer C, Isler HR, Evers S, Grotemeyer KH, Taneri Z, Soyka D, Gobel H, Fischer M 1996 Magnesium in the prophylaxis of migraine—a double-blind placebo-controlled study. Cephalalgia 16: 436–440
Proietti Cecchini A, Áfra J, Maertens de Noordhout A et al 1997 Modulation of pressure pain thresholds during isometric contraction in patients with chronic tension-type headache and/or generalized myofascial pain compared to healthy volunteers. Neurology 48: 118 (abstract)
Rasmussen BK, Olesen J 1992 Migraine with aura and migraine without aura: an epidemiological study. Cephalalgia 12: 221–228
Rasmussen BK, Jensen R, Schroll M et al 1991 Epidemiology of headache in a general population—a prevalence study. Journal of Clinical Epidemiology 44: 1147–1157
Ross Russell RW 1986 Giant cell (cranial) arteritis. In: Vinken PJ, Bruyn GW, Klawans HL (eds) Handbook of clinical neurology, vol. 4(48). Elsevier, Amsterdam, pp 309–328
Rozen TD 2000 Treatment of a prolonged migrainous aura with intravenous furosemide. Neurology 55: 732–733
Russell WR 1932 Cerebral involvement in head injury; a study based on the examination of 200 cases. Brain 55: 549–570
Ryan RE 1977 Motrin—a new agent for symptomatic treatment of muscle contraction headache. Headache 16: 280–283
Salvesen R, Bekkelund SI 2000 Migraine, as compared to other headaches, is worse during midnight-sun summer than during polar night. A questionnaire study in an Arctic population. Headache 40: 824–829
Sand T, Vanagaite Vingen J 2000 Visual, long-latency auditory and brainstem auditory evoked potentials in migraine: relation to pattern size, stimulus intensity, sound and light discomfort thresholds and pre-attack state. Cephalalgia 20: 804–820
Sanders M, Zuurmond WW 1997 Efficacy of sphenopalatine ganglion blockade in 66 patients suffering from cluster headache: a 12- to 70-month follow-up evaluation. Journal of Neurosurgery 87: 876–880
Sándor PS, Áfra J, Proietti-Cecchini A, Albert A, Schoenen J 1999 Familial influences on cortical evoked potentials in migraine. NeuroReport 10: 1235–1238
Saper JR 1987 Ergotamine dependency. A review. Headache 27: 435–438
Schachtel BP, Furey SA, Thoden WR 1996 Nonprescription ibuprofen and acetaminophen in the treatment of tension-type headache. Journal of Clinical Pharmacology 36: 1120–1125
Schoenen J 1992 Clinical neurophysiology studies in headache: a review of data and pathophysiological hints. Functional Neurology 7: 191–204
Schoenen J 1997 Acute migraine therapy: the newer drugs. Current Opinion in Neurology 10: 237–243
Schoenen J 1998a Cluster headaches—central or peripheral in origin? Lancet 352: 253–255
Schoenen J 1998b Cortical electrophysiology in migraine and possible pathogenetic implications. Clinical Neuroscience 5: 10–17
Schoenen J, Sándor PS 1999 Headache. In: Wall PD, Melzack R (eds)

Textbook of pain, 4th edn. Churchill Livingstone, Edinburgh, pp 761–798
Schoenen J, Wang W 1997 Tension-type headache. In: Goadsby PJ, Silberstein SJ (eds) Headache. Butterworth-Heinemann, Boston, pp 177–200
Schoenen J, Lenarduzzi P, Sianard-Gainko J 1989 Chronic headaches associated with analgesics and/or ergotamine abuse: a clinical survey of 434 consecutive out patients. In: Clifford Rose F (ed) New advances in headache research. Smith Gordon, London, pp 255–259
Schoenen J, Bottin D, Hardy F, Gérard P 1991a Cephalic and extracephalic pressure pain thresholds in chronic tension-type headache. Pain 47: 145–149
Schoenen J, Gérard P, De Pasqua V, Sianard-Gainko J 1991b Multiple clinical and paraclinical analyses of chronic tension-type headache associated or unassociated with disorder of pericranial muscles. Cephalalgia 11: 135–139
Schoenen J, Broux R, Moonen G 1992 Unilateral facial pain as the first symptom of lung cancer: are there diagnostic clues? Cephalalgia 12: 178–179
Schoenen J, Bulcke J, Caekebeke J et al 1994 Self-treatment of acute migraine with subcutaneous sumatriptan using an auto-injector device: comparison with customary treatment in an open, longitudinal study. Cephalalgia 14: 55–63
Schoenen J, Jacquy J, Lenaerts M 1998 Effectiveness of high-dose riboflavin in migraine prophylaxis: a randomized controlled trial. Neurology 50: 466–470
Schokker P 1989 Craniomandibular disorders in headache patients. Thesis. University of Amsterdam
Schokker RP, Hansson TL, Ansink BJ 1990 The results of treatment of the masticatory system of chronic headache patients. Journal of Craniomandibular Disorders, Facial and Oral Pain 4: 126–130
Schrader H, Obelieniene D, Bovim G et al 1996 Natural evolution of late whiplash syndrome outside the medicolegal context. Lancet 347 (9010): 1207–1211
Schrader H, Stovner LJ, Helde G, Sand T, Bovim G 2001 Prophylactic treatment of migraine with angiotensin converting enzyme angiotensin converting enzyme inhibitor (lisinopril): randomised, placebo controlled, crossover study. British Medical Journal 322: 19–22
Sheftell FD, Fox AW 2000 Acute migraine treatment outcome measures: a clinician's view. Cephalalgia 20 (suppl 2): 14–24
Shuaib A, Ahmed F, Muratoglu M, Kochanski P 1999 Topiramate in migraine prophylaxis: a pilot study. Cephalagia 19: 379 (I-G2-20)
Silberstein SD 2000 Practice parameter: evidence-based guidelines for migraine headache (an evidence-based review): report of the quality standards subcommittee of the American Academy of Neurology. Neurology 55: 754–562
Silberstein SD, Marcelis J 1992 Headache associated with changes in intracranial pressure. Headache 32: 84–94
Siniatchkin M, Kropp P, Neumann M, Gerber W, Stephani U 2000 Intensity dependence of auditory evoked cortical potentials in migraine families. Pain 85: 247–254
Sjaastad O 1986 Cluster headache. In: Vinken PJ, Bruyn GW, Klawans HL (eds) Handbook of clinical neurology, vol 4(48). Elsevier, Amsterdam, pp 217–246
Sjaastad O, Dale I 1974 Evidence for a new (?) treatable headache entity. Headache 14: 105–108
Sjaastad O, Saunte C, Salvesen R et al 1989 Shortlasting, unilateral, neuralgiform headache attacks with conjunctival injection, tearing, sweating, and rhinorrhea. Cephalalgia 9: 147–156
Sjaastad O, Fredriksen TA, Pfaffenrath V 1990 Cervicogenic headache diagnostic criteria. Headache 30: 25–26
Solomon S, Newman LC 1998 Classification of post-traumatic migraine. Neurology 48: PO4.128
Solomon S, Lipton RB, Newman LO 1992 Evaluation of chronic daily headache—comparison to criteria for chronic tension-type headache. Cephalalgia 12: 365–368
Steiner TJ, Couturier EGM, Catarci T, Hering R 1992 Social aspects of drug abuse in headache. Functional Neurology 6 (suppl): 11–14
Stewart WF, Lipton RB, Celentano DD et al 1992 Prevalence of migraine headache in the United States. Journal of the American Medical Association 267: 64–69
Stewart WF, Schechter A, Lipton RB 1994a Migraine heterogeneity: disability, pain intensity, and attack frequency and duration. Neurology 44 (suppl 4): S24–S39
Stewart WF, Schechter A, Rasmussen BK 1994b Migraine prevalence: a review of population-based studies. Neurology 44 (suppl 4): S17–S23
Stewart WF, Lipton RB, Chee E, Sawyer J, Silberstein SD 2000 Menstrual cycle and headache in a population sample of migraineurs. Neurology 55: 1517–1522
Taarnhoj P 1995 Decompression of the posterior trigeminal root in trigeminal neuralgia: a 30 year follow-up review. Journal of Neurosurgery 57: 14–17
Tehindrazanarivelo AD, Lutz G, Petitjean C, Bousser M-G 1991 Headache following carotid endarterectomy: a prospective study. Cephalalgia 12: 380–382
Tfelt-Hansen P, Henry P, Mulder LJ et al 1995 The effectiveness of combined oral lysine acetylsalicylate and metoclopramide compared with oral sumatriptan for migraine. Lancet 346: 923–926
Tfelt-Hansen P, Dahlof C, Pascual J et al 2000 Ergotamine: current place in the treatment of acute migraine attacks—European Consensus. Brain 123: 9–18
Turkewitz JL, Wirth O, Dawson GA, Casaly JS 1992 Cluster headache following head injury: a case report and review of the literature. Headache 32: 504–506
Tzourio C, Tehindrazanarivelo A, Iglésias S et al 1995 Case–control study of migraine and risk of ischaemic stroke in young women. British Medical Journal 310: 830–833
Tzourio C, Kittner SJ, Bousser MG, Alperovitch A 2000 Migraine and stroke in young women. Cephalalgia 20: 190–199
van Suijlekom HA, van Kleef M, Barendse GA, Sluijter ME, Sjaastad O, Weber WE 1998 Radiofrequency cervical zygapophyseal joint neurotomy for cervicogenic headache: a prospective study of 15 patients. Functional Neurology 13: 297–303
Vilming ST, Schrader H, Monstad I 1988 Post-lumbar puncture headache: the significance of body posture. A controlled study of 300 patients. Cephalalgia 8: 75–78
Wall M 1990 The headache profile of idiopathic intracranial hypertension. Cephalalgia 10: 331–335
Wang W, Schoenen J 1994 Reduction of temporalis ES2 by peripheral electrical stimulation in migraine and tension-type headaches. Pain 59: 327–334
Warner JP, Fenichel GB 1996 Chronic posttraumatic headache often a myth? Neurology 46: 915–916
Watson CPN, Evans RJ 1988 Post-herpetic neuralgia: 208 cases. Pain 35: 289–297
Watson CPN, Watt VR, Chipman M, Birkett N, Evans RJ 1991 The prognosis with post-herpetic neuralgia. Pain 46: 195–199
Watson CPN, Chipman M, Reed K et al 1992 Amitriptyline versus maprotiline in post-herpetic neuralgia: a randomized, double blind, cross-over trial. Pain 8: 29–36
Weiller C, May A, Limmroth V et al 1995 Brain stem activation in spontaneous human migraine attacks. Nature Medicine 1: 658–660
Welch KMA 1987 Migraine, a biobehavioural disorder. Archives of Neurology 44: 323–327
Welch KMA, Levine SR 1990 Migraine-related stroke in the context of the International Headache Society Classification of head pain. Archives of Neurology 47: 458–462

Whitmarsh TE, Coleston-Shields DM, Steiner TJ 1997 Double-blind randomized placebo-controlled study of homoeopathic prophylaxis of migraine. Cephalalgia 17: 600–604

Wijdicks EF, Kerkhoff H, van Gijn J 1988 Long-term follow-up of 71 patients with thunderclap headache mimicking subarachnoid haemorrhage. Lancet 2: 68–70

Wilkinson M, Pfaffenrath V, Schoenen J et al 1995 Migraine and cluster headache their management with sumatriptan: a critical review of the current clinical experience. Cephalalgia 15: 337–357

Yamaguchi M:1992 Incidence of headache and severity of head injury. Headache 32: 427–431

Chapter 16

Postamputation pain

Lone Nikolajsen and Troels Staehelin Jensen

Introduction

The first medical description of postamputation phenomena was reported by Ambroise Paré (sixteenth century) who noticed that amputees may complain of severe pain in the missing limb a long time after amputation (Keil 1990). Subsequent studies provided detailed descriptions of the phenomenon and, in 1871, Mitchell coined the term 'phantom limb'. In the twentieth century, World War II, Vietnam, Israeli, and other wars provided many cases of amputations, and today, landmine explosions all over the world are still responsible for many traumatic amputations. In Western countries the main reasons for amputation are peripheral vascular disease and, less often, tumours. The mechanisms underlying pain in amputees are still not fully understood and although a large number of treatments have been suggested treatment results are often poor.

The present chapter describes the clinical characteristics of postamputation phenomena, followed by a short review of possible mechanisms underlying pain in amputees. Finally, treatment possibilities and the controversial issue—whether phantom pain can be prevented—will be discussed.

It is useful to distinguish between the following three elements of the phantom complex:

- *phantom pain*: painful sensations referred to the missing limb
- *stump pain*: pain referred to the stump
- *phantom sensation*: any sensation of the missing limb except pain.

Clinical characteristics

Phantom pain

Incidence

Recent studies agree that the incidence of phantom pain is in the range of 60–80% (Parkes 1973, Carlen et al 1978, Jensen et al 1983, Sherman and Sherman 1983, Houghton et al 1994, Nikolajsen et al 1997a, Wartan et al 1997, Kooijmann et al 2000).

The incidence of phantom pain seems to be independent of age in adults, gender, side, or level of amputation and cause of amputation (civilian versus traumatic) (Jensen et al 1983, Sherman and Sherman 1985, Houghton et al 1994, Montoya et al 1997). Phantom pain is less frequent in young children and in congenital amputees (Wilkins et al 1998).

Onset and duration

Onset of phantom pain is usually within the first week after amputation (Parkes 1973, Carlen et al 1978, Jensen et al 1983, Krane and Heller 1995,

Nikolajsen et al 1997a). In a prospective study by Nikolajsen et al (1997a), 56 lower limb amputees were interviewed about phantom pain 1 week and 3 and 6 months after the amputation. Sixty-seven percent of patients reported phantom pain after one week and only two patients developed phantom pain later in the course. However, case reports suggest that the onset of phantom pain may be delayed for several years after amputation (Rajbhandari et al 1999).

Although phantom pain may diminish with time and eventually fade away, prospective studies indicate that even 2 years after amputation the incidence is almost the same as at onset (Jensen et al 1985, Nikolajsen et al 1997a). In a survey of 526 veterans with longstanding amputations, phantom pain had disappeared in 16%, decreased markedly in 37%, remained similar in 44%, and increased in 3% of respondents reporting phantom pain (Wartan et al 1997).

Character and localization

Phantom pain is usually intermittent; only few patients are in constant pain. Episodes of pain are reported to occur daily or at daily or weekly intervals with only a few reporting monthly, yearly, or rarer episodes. Duration of individual pain attacks is seconds, minutes, and hours, but rarely days or longer. The pain is described as shooting, stabbing, pricking, boring, squeezing, throbbing, and burning. Some patients have more vivid and colourful descriptions as for example 'my foot is pinched by a tight shoe' or '50 devils are stabbing needles into my foot'. Phantom pain is primarily localized in distal parts of the missing limb (Parkes 1973; Carlen et al 1978; Jensen et al 1983, 1985; Sherman and Sherman 1983, 1985; Katz and Melzack 1990; Krane and Heller 1995; Wartan et al 1997; Montoya et al 1997; Kooijman 2000).

Preamputation pain and phantom pain

Several retrospective studies (Riddoch 1941, Appenzeller and Bicknell 1969, Parkes 1973, Houghton 1994, Krane and Heller 1995)—but not all (Henderson and Smyth 1948, Wall et al 1985, Kooijmann et al 2000)—have pointed to preamputation pain as a risk factor for postoperative phantom pain. Houghton et al (1994) studied 176 amputees: in vascular amputees there was a significant relation between preamputation pain and phantom pain immediately after the amputation and after 6 months and 1 and 2 years. In traumatic amputees phantom pain was only related to preamputation pain immediately after the amputation. Similar findings have been described in prospective studies (Jensen et al 1983, 1985; Nikolajsen et al 1997a). Nikolajsen et al (1997a) found that phantom pain was more frequent after 1 week and 3 months, but not after 6 months, in patients who had moderate or severe preamputation pain compared to patients with less preamputation pain.

The literature contains numerous case reports that show that phantom pain may mimick preamputation pain both in character and location (Bailey and Moersch 1941, Nathan 1962, Katz and Melzack 1990, Hill et al 1996). For example, Hill et al (1996) described a woman who had recurrent infections of a leg wound. The most distressing preamputation pain consisted of cleaning and packing the wound twice daily. After the amputation the patient reported severe phantom pain similar to the pain she experienced before the amputation and localized to the open drainage site of the wound which was no longer there. Other descriptions include the reactivation of pains perceived prior to the amputation. Nathan (1962) described an amputee who, following a noxious stimulus to the stump, re-experienced pain from a skating injury that he had sustained 5 years earlier.

The frequency with which preamputation pain persists as phantom pain varies from 12.5 to nearly 80% (Appenzeller and Bicknell 1969, Parkes 1973, Jensen et al 1985, Wall et al 1985, Katz and Melzack 1990). In a retrospective study by Katz and Melzack (1990), 68 amputees were questioned about preamputation pain and phantom pain from 20 days to 46 years after the amputation. Fifty-seven of those who experienced phantom pain claimed that their phantom pain resembled the pain they had before the amputation. The incidence was much lower in two prospective studies (Jensen et al 1985, Nikolajsen et al 1997a). Nikolajsen et al (1997a) recorded location and character of pain before the amputation and after 1 week and 3 and 6 months. Although 42% of patients claimed that their phantom pain resembled the pain they had experienced before the amputation, there was no relation between the patient's own opinion about similarity and the actual similarity found when comparing pre- and postoperative recordings of pain. It is possible that some patients with phantom pain would try to explain their pain by comparing it to pain experienced previously, thus giving a false high estimate of the number of patients with identical preamputation pain and phantom pain.

Modulating factors

Phantom pain may be modulated by several internal and external factors. Attention, anxiety, and autonomic reflexes such as coughing and urination may increase pain, whereas rest and distraction ameliorate may pain. Phantom pain may be provoked by changes in the weather and cooling and pressure at the stump (Jensen et al 1984, Krebs et al 1985). In a group of upper limb amputees, Weiss et al (1999) reported that phantom pain was decreased by the use of a prosthesis that allowed extensive use of the affected limb, whereas a cosmetic prosthesis had no effect. Coping strategies and rehabilitation also play a role for the pain experience (Hill et al 1995, Pezzin et al 2000) but there is no evidence that phantom pain represents a psychological disturbance (Sherman et al 1987, Katz and Melzack 1990).

Case reports have suggested that spinal anaesthesia in amputees may cause appearance of phantom pain in otherwise pain-free subjects (Mackenzie 1983). However, in a prospective study of 23 spinal anaesthetics in 17 amputees, only one developed transient phantom pain (Tessler and Kleiman 1994).

An existing phantom limb experience, whether painful or not, may be altered by spinal cord or brain lesions (Brihaye 1958, Appenzeller and Bicknell 1969). A focal brain infarct in the posterior internal capsule made a former phantom limb disappear (Yarnitsky et al 1988).

Evidence is growing that the individual´s genetic predisposition to develop phantom pain may be important (Devor and Raber 1990, Mogil et al 1999). However, Schott (1986) described a family in which five members sustained traumatic amputations of their limbs. The development of phantom phenomena, including pain, was unpredictable, despite their being first-degree relatives.

Stump pain

Incidence, time course, and character

Virtually all amputees experience stump pain immediately after the amputation. This is expected and is a normal result of major surgery. If the pain does not decrease substantially within the first few days or if it subsides and then worsens, there is usually a problem with the amputation. In some patients, however, stump pain persists despite proper healing of the stump. Persistent stump pain is reported to occur in 5–21% of patients (Finch et al 1980; Abramson and Feibel 1981; Jensen et al 1983, 1985; Pohjolainen 1991). Nikolajsen et al (1997a) prospectively recorded incidence and intensity of postamputation stump pain in 56 amputees. All patients had some stump pain during the first week after amputation, but in most patients pain subsided. However, in two patients stump pain worsened. Kooijman et al (2000) studied 99 upper-limb amputees and found that 49% experienced some pain in the stump. In most patients the pain was intermittent.

Stump pain is often described as either pressing, throbbing, burning, or squeezing (Jensen et al 1985). Other descriptions include a stabbing sensation or an electric current (Browder and Gallagher 1948). A variant of this type is what Sunderland (1978) termed 'nerve storms', with painful attacks of up to 2 days' duration. Several amputees complain of spontaneous movements of the stump, which range from painful, hardly visible, myoclonic jerks to severe clonic contractions (Sliosberg 1948).

Stump and phantom pain are interrelated phenomena

Parkes (1973) studied 46 amputees and found that stump pain within the first 3 weeks after amputation was significantly associated to phantom pain 1 year later. In a survey of 648 amputees, Sherman and Sherman (1983) found that stump pain was present in 61% of amputees with phantom pain but only in 39% of those without phantom pain. Carlen et al (1978) noted that phantom pain was decreased by the resolution of stump-end pathology. Jensen et al (1985) found that 2 years after amputation phantom pain was significantly more frequent in patients with stump pain than in patients without stump pain. Nikolajsen et al (1997a) found that stump and phantom pain were significantly related 1 week after amputation. Other clinical studies have shown that temperature and muscle activity at the stump are related to phantom pain (Sherman and Glenda 1987, Sherman et al 1992, Katz 1992). Nikolajsen et al (2000a) studied 35 amputees and found that low mechanical thresholds (pressure algometry) at the stump were associated with stump and phantom pain one week after amputation.

The association between stump and phantom pain is consistent with experimental studies in amputees. Nystrøm and Hagbarth (1981) observed abnormal activity in peroneal and median nerve fibres of two amputees with ongoing pain in their phantom foot and hand, respectively. Percussion of neuromas in these two patients produced increased nerve fibre discharges and an augmentation of their phantom pain.

Stump pathology associated with pain

Examinations of stumps often disclose definite pathological findings that may account for the pain in the stump and/or the phantom such as skin pathology, circulatory disturbances, infection of the skin or underlying tissue, bone spurs, or neuromas. Although stump and phantom pain is significantly more frequent in patients with obvious stump pathology than in those without pathological findings, pain may occur in perfectly healed stumps. Careful examination of stump sensibility has revealed areas of altered sensitivity (e.g. hypoalgesia, hyperalgesia, hyperpathia, or allodynia) in almost all amputees (Jensen et al, unpublished data; Nikolajsen et al 1998).

Phantom limb

Phantom limb sensation

Non-painful phantom sensations are rarely a clinical problem. Phantom pain and phantom sensation often coexist but phantom sensations are more frequent than phantom pain. Most reports indicate that 80–100% of all amputees will experience phantom sensations following amputation (Carlen et al 1978, Jensen et al 1983, Krane and Heller 1995, Montoya et al 1997, Wilkins et al 1998, Kooijman et al 2000). The onset is usually within the first days after amputation (Henderson and Smyth 1948, Carlen et al 1978, Jensen et al 1983, 1984). The amputee often wakes up from the anaesthesia with a feeling that the amputated limb is still there. In some cases phantom sensations may be very vivid and include feelings of movement and posture (Riddoch 1941, Henderson and Smyth 1948, Cronholm 1951); in other cases only weak sensations of the phantom are felt. In a prospective study of 58 amputees, the incidence of phantom limb sensation was 84, 90, and 71% 8 days, 6 months, and 2 years after amputation, respectively. While the incidence of phantom sensation did not decrease during follow-up, both duration and frequency of phantom phenomena declined significantly. Approximately three-quarters of patients had kinaesthetic sensations in the limb during the first 6 months after amputation (i.e. feeling of length, volume, or other spatial sensation) but less than half of patients had this later in the course (Jensen et al 1984).

Telescoping (shrinkage of the phantom) is reported to occur in about half of patients (Fig. 16.1). It has been postulated that phantom pain prevents or retards shrinkage of the phantom but Montoya et al (1997) failed to find such a relation: 12 of 16 patients with phantom pain and 5 of 10 patients without pain reported telescoping.

Aetiology and pathophysiological mechanisms

The mechanisms underlying pain in amputees are not known exactly, but both peripheral and central neuronal mechanisms are likely to occur. Although nerve section is associated with clear changes in the periphery, which represents an obvious origin for pain, it is clear that the phantom limb with its complex perceptual qualities is ultimately integrated in the brain. An extensive experimental and clinical literature documents that nerve injury induces a number of morphological, physiological, and chemical changes in both the peripheral and central nervous systems. These changes will be described briefly in the following.

Peripheral mechanisms

Several clinical observations suggest that mechanisms in the periphery (i.e. in the stump or in central parts of sectioned primary afferents) may play a role in the phantom limb percept:

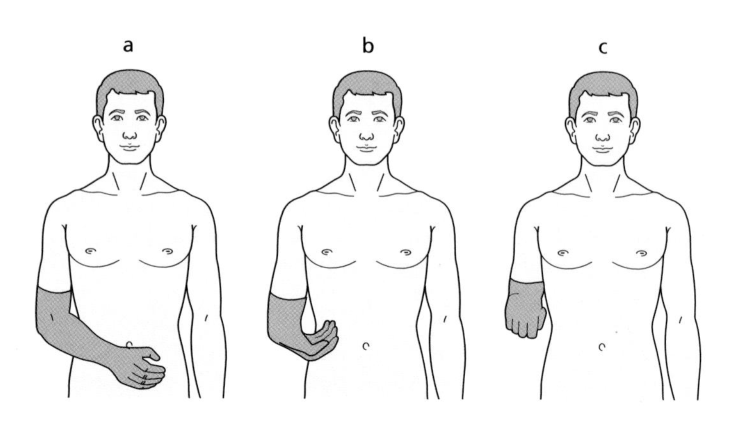

Fig. 16.1 (a–c) Telescoping.

- Phantom limb sensations can be modulated by various stump manipulations.
- Phantom limb sensations are temporarily abolished after local stump anaesthesia.
- Stump revisions and removal of tender neuromas often reduce pain transiently.
- Phantom pain is significantly more frequent in those amputees with long-term stump pain than in those without persistent pain.
- Although obvious stump pathology is rare, altered cutaneous sensibility in the stump is a common if not universal feature.
- Finally, changes in stump blood flow alter the phantom limb perception.

These clinical observations are supported by experimental studies. Following a nerve cut, nerve-end neuromas, which show spontaneous and abnormal evoked activity following mechanical or neurochemical, e.g. noradrenaline (norepinephrine), stimulation, are created (Wall and Gutnick 1974, for review see Devor and Seltzer 1999). This increased activity is assumed to be the result of a novel expression or upregulation of sodium channels (Devor et al 1993, Novakovic et al 1998). The increased sensitivity of neuromas to noradrenaline (norepinephrine) may in part explain the exacerbation of phantom pain by stress and other emotional states associated with increased catecholamine release from sympathetic efferent terminals which are in close proximity to afferent sensory nerves and sprouts.

In addition to abnormal activity from nerve-end neuromas, cell bodies in the dorsal root ganglion show similar abnormal spontaneous activity and increased sensitivity to mechanical and neurochemical stimulation (Kajander et al 1992). Thus, abnormal activity from at least two sources—neuromas and dorsal root ganglion cell bodies—may contribute to the phantom limb percept, including pain.

Spinal cord mechanisms

The increased barrage from neuromas and from dorsal root ganglia cells is thought to induce long-term changes in central projecting neurons in the dorsal horn, including spontaneous neuronal activity, induction of immediate early genes, increases in spinal cord metabolic activity (Price et al 1997), and expansion of receptive fields (Cook et al 1987).

The pharmacology of spinal sensitization involves an increased activity in *N*-methyl-D-aspartate (NMDA) receptor-operated systems (for review see Doubell et al 1999), and many aspects of the central sensitization can be reduced by NMDA receptor antagonists. In human amputees one aspect of such central sensitization, the evoked stump or phantom pain produced by repetitive stimulation of the stump by non-noxious pinprick, can be reduced by the NMDA receptor antagonist ketamine (Nikolajsen et al 1996).

Beside the functional changes in the dorsal horn an anatomical reorganization has been described recently (Woolf et al 1992). Peripheral nerve transection results in a substantial degeneration of afferent C-fibre terminals in lamina II, thus reducing the number of synaptic contacts with second-order neurons in lamina II which normally respond best to noxious stimulation. As a consequence central terminals of Aβ mechanoreceptive afferents, which normally terminate in deeper laminae, sprout into lamina II and may form synaptic contacts with vacant nociceptive second-order neurons. The result of this reorganization could be the evocation of pain by Aβ-fibre input, e.g. touch.

Supraspinal mechanisms

In view of the plasticity in nociceptive and anti-nociceptive systems, it is reasonable to assume that amputation not only produces a cascade of events in the periphery and in the spinal cord, but that these changes eventually sweep more centrally and alter neuronal activity in cortical and subcortical structures.

Davis et al (1998) have shown in a small series of amputees that thalamic stimulation results in phantom sensation and pain. Normally such stimulation does not evoke pain. This suggests that plastic changes in the thalamus are involved in the generation of chronic pain. Other studies in humans have documented a cortical reorganization after amputation using different cerebral imaging techniques. In a series of studies Flor and colleagues (1995, 1998) have shown a correlation between phantom pain and the amount of reorganization in the somatosensory cortex. They therefore suggested that phantom limb pain may be a result of plastic changes in the somatosensory cortex. Birbaumer et al (1997) studied the effect of regional anaesthesia on cortical reorganization in upper limb amputees and found that a brachial plexus blockade abolished pain and reorganization in three out of six amputees. Huse et al (2001) recently showed in a small group of amputees that cortical reorganization and pain was reduced during treatment with morphine.

Therapy

General

Treatment of chronic pain following amputation is difficult and has generally not been successful. In a survey of 764 amputees, Sherman and Sherman (1983) found that 44% of those who discussed their phantom pain with the physician were told that they were mentally disturbed. Only 17% were offered treatment.

Various treatments have been and are currently in use for chronic pain after amputation. In another survey, Sherman et al (1980) identified 68 different treatment methods. Only a few were described as being effective, and today the majority of these treatments have been abandoned.

Most studies dealing with pain treatment in amputees suffer from severe methodological errors:

- samples are small, heterogeneous, and non-randomized
- studies are open
- controls are often lacking
- follow-up periods are short.

With a pathophysiology that is still unclear, it is not possible to give precise directions for pain treatment in amputees. Some cases of phantom pain may be resistent to any treatment. Until more direct data become avaible, guidelines in analogy with treatment regimens for other neuropathic pain states are probably the best approximation (Baron et al 1998, for review). Medical treatment is most effective and can be combined with other non-invasive techniques. Invasive treatment methods should probably be avoided or restricted to patients with an expected short survival time. Surgery on the peripheral or the central nervous system in cases of deafferentation pain always implicates further deafferentation and thereby a risk of increased pain.

Suggestions for treatment of postamputation pain (not evidence based) are presented in Table 16.1.

Non-invasive techniques

Medical

A large number of randomized, controlled clinical trials have shown a beneficial effect of TCA and

Table 16.1 Suggestions for treatment of postamputation pain (not evidence based)

Early postoperative pain	
Stump pain	Conventional analgesics (paracetamol, NSAIDs, opioids), perhaps combined with epidural pain treatment.
Stump and phantom pain	If there are clear signs of neuropathic pain, paroxyms, or abnormal stump sensitivity, TCA or anticonvulsants in a small dose can be tried.
Chronic pain	
Stump pain	Local stump surgery: If obvious stump pathology is present, stump revision should be considered. Surgery should be avoided in cases of sympathetically maintained pain. Local medical treatment: Topical lidocaine (lignocaine)/capsaicin can be tried in cases with stump pain without clear stump pathology
Stump and phantom pain (medical treatment, listed in order of preference):	(1) Gabapentin 1200–900 mg/day. Start dose 300 mg, daily increments of 300 mg/day until effect, max dose 3600 mg/day. (2) Tricyclic antidepressants (imipramine, amitriptyline, nortriptyline) 100–125 mg/day. Start dose 25 mg/day, weekly increments of 25 mg. Check ECG before start. Monitor plasma levels with dose > 100 mg/day. If sedation is wanted amitriptyline should be preferred. (3) In cases of mainly radiating, lancinating, or paroxysmal pain: Oxcarbazepine 600–900 mg/day. Start dose 300 mg, daily increments of 300 mg. Carbamazepine 450 mg/day. Start dose 150 mg, daily increments of 150 mg. Monitor plasma levels after 10 days on max dose. Lamitrigine 100–200 mg/day. Start dose 50 mg/day, slow titration with increments of 50 mg/10–14 days. (4) Opioids (long-acting or sustained release preparations) or tramadol. (5) If no effect from the above, consider referral to pain clinic. (6) In pain clinic: Perform IV lidocaine (lignocaine) test or ketamine test. Positive lidocaine (lignocaine) test: reconsider anticonvulsants. Positive ketamine test: Consider memantine or amandatine.

Practical issue: It is important to distinguish between: (1) early postoperative pain and chronic pain (pain persisting more than 3–4 weeks), and (2) stump and phantom pain.

sodium channel blockers under different neuropathic pain conditions (Sindrup and Jensen 1999). No controlled trials in phantom pain have been performed but the drugs are generally considered to be effective—at least in some patients (Elliott et al 1976, Patterson 1988). Others have reported a beneficial effect of benzodiazepines (Iacono et al 1987, Bartusch et al 1996). However, the general impression is that benzodiazepines do not produce substantial pain relief. Permanent phantom pain should not be accepted until opioids have been tried. It is our experience, as well as that of others (Urban et al 1986, Baron et al 1998, Dellemijn 1999) that opioids can be used safely for years with a limited risk of drug dependence. Huse et al (2001) in a placebo-controlled trial found that morphine reduced pain significantly. Calcitonin has been reported to be effective in phantom pain (Jaeger and Maier 1992). The effect of NMDA receptor antagonists have been examined in different studies (Stannard and Porter 1993, Nikolajsen et al 1996, 1997b, 2000b). In a double-blind placebo-controlled study, IV ketamine reduced pain, hyperalgesia, and 'wind-up' like pain in 11 amputees with stump and phantom pain (Nikolajsen et al 1996). In another controlled trial 19 patients received memantine, a NMDA receptor antagonist avaible for oral use, in a blinded, placebo-controlled cross-over fashion. Memantine failed to have any effect on spontaneous pain, allodynia, and hyperalgesia (Nikolajsen et al 2000b). A large number of other treatments, for example β-blockers (Ahmed 1979, Marsland et al 1982), mexiletine (the oral congener of lidocaine (lignocaine)) (Davis 1993), topical application of capsaicin (Rayner et al 1989), intrathecal opioids (Jacobsen et al 1990, Omote et al 1995), and various anaesthetic blocks (Wassef 1997, Lierz et al 1998) have been claimed to be effective in phantom pain but none of them have proven to be effective in well-controlled trials with a sufficient number of patients.

Non-medical

Transcutaneous electrical nerve stimulation (TENS) has been used with some success in the treatment of phantom pain (Lundeberg 1985, Katz and Melzack 1991). The advantage of peripheral nerve stimulation is the absence of side effects and complications and the fact that the treatment can be easily repeated. Physical therapy involving massage, manipulation, and passive movements may prevent trophic changes and vascular congestion in the stump. Induction of sensory input from the stump area by physical therapy could play a role in the ameliorating effect of such types of treatment. Others have found an effect of acupuncture, relaxation training, ultrasound, and hypnosis. Rasmussen and Rummans (2000) recently described two patients with severe phantom pain refractory to conventional therapy. Both patients experienced substantial pain relief following electric convulsive therapy.

Invasive techniques

The results of invasive techniques such as, for example, stump revision, dorsal root entry zone lesions (DREZ), sympathectomy, and cordotomy have generally been unfavourable and most of them have been abandoned today. Surgery may produce short-term pain relief but pain often reappears. Spinal cord stimulation may also have limited effect.

Prevention

Some previous studies found that patients who had severe pain before the amputation had a higher risk of developing phantom pain than patients who had less or no pain before the amputation (Riddoch 1941, Appenzeller and Bicknell 1969, Parkes 1973, Jensen et al 1983, 1985). Also, early case reports suggested that pain experienced before the amputation (i.e. a painful ulcer) might continue to be present in the phantom (Bailey and Moersch 1941, Nathan 1962).

These observations prompted Bach et al (1988) to carry out a controlled study in which patients scheduled for amputation of the lower limb were randomized to receive either epidural pain treatment for 3 days before the amputation or conventional pain treatment. They found that the incidence of phantom pain was significantly lower after 6 months among 11 patients who received epidural pain treatment than among 14 patients who received conventional pain treatment. Subsequent clinical trials have confirmed their findings (Jahangiri et al 1994, Schug et al 1995, Katsuly-Liapis et al 1996). Jahangiri et al (1994) examined the effect of perioperative epidural infusion of diamorphine, bupivacaine, and clonidine on post-amputation stump and phantom pain. Thirteen patients received the epidural treatment 24–48 h preoperatively and for at least 3 days postoperatively. A control group of 11 patients received opioid analgesia on demand. All patients had general anaesthesia for the amputation. The incidence of severe phantom pain was lower in the epidural group 7 days, 6 months, and 1 year after amputation. No effect was seen on stump pain. In another prospective study by Schug et al (1995), 23 patients had either epidural analgesia before, during, and after the amputation (n=8), intra- and postoperative epidural analgesia (n=7), or general anaesthesia plus systemic analgesia (n=8). After 1 year the incidence of phantom pain was significantly lower among the patients who received pre-, intra-, and postoperative epidural analgesia relative to patients who received general anaesthesia plus systemic analgesia. Katsuly-Liapis et al (1996) presented in abstract form a study in which 45 patients were allocated to one of three groups: group A (n=15) received epidural bupivacaine and morphine for 3 days prior to amputation and the infusion was maintained for 72 h postoperatively; group B (n=12) received conventional analgesics before the amputation and epidural pain treatment after the amputation; group C (n=18) had conventional analgesics both before and after the amputation. After 6 months the incidence of phantom pain was significantly lower in group A than that in groups B and C.

Others have examined the effect of peri- or intraneural blockade on phantom pain. Fischer and Meller (1991) introduced a catheter into the transsected nerve sheath at the time of amputation and infused bupivacaine for 72 h in 11 patients. None developed phantom pain during a 12-month follow-up. In a retrospective study Elizaga et al (1994) found no effect of such a treatment. Pinzur et al (1996) prospectively randomized 21 patients to continuous postoperative infusion of either bupivacaine or saline, but failed to find any difference between the two groups with regard to the incidence of phantom pain after 3 and 6 months.

However, a number of methodological problems, such as small sample sizes, no or insufficient randomization, and non-blinded assessment of pain, limit the validity of all these studies. Nevertheless, the impact of the Bach et al (1988) study is immense and in many anaesthesiological departments procedures have been changed so that patients undergoing amputation are offered an epidural catheter before amputation in order to prevent phantom pain. Starting an epidural treatment before rather than at the time of the amputation is associated with extra hospital costs so simply from a cost–benefit point of view, it is important to know whether patients should be taken into the anaesthesiological department for epidural pain treatment before the amputation.

We therefore carried out a randomized, double-blind, and placebo-controlled study to clarify whether postoperative stump and phantom pain is reduced by preoperative pain treatment with epidural bupivacaine and morphine (Nikolajsen et al 1997c). Sixty patients scheduled for lower limb amputation were randomly assigned into one of two groups:

1. a blockade group that received epidural bupivacaine and morphine before the amputation and during the operation (29 patients)
2. a control group that received epidural saline and oral/intramuscular morphine (31 patients).

Both groups had general anaesthesia for the amputation and all patients received epidural analgesics for postoperative pain management. Patients were interviewed about preamputation pain on the day before the amputation and about stump and phantom pain after 1 week and 3, 6, and 12 months. Median duration of preoperative epidural blockade (blockade group) was 18 h. After 1 week the percentage of patients with phantom pain was 51.9 in the blockade group and 55.6 in the control group. Subsequently the figures were (blockade/control) at 3 months, 82.4/50; at 6 months, 81.3/55; and at 12 months, 75/68.8. Intensity of stump and phantom pain and consumption of opioids were also similar in the two groups at all four postoperative interviews. Thus, we were not able to confirm the findings by others that perioperative epidural blockade prevents phantom pain.

In a recent study, Lambert et al (2001) randomized 30 patients scheduled for amputation of the lower limb to receive either epidural bupivacaine and diamorphine started 24 h before the amputation and continued three days postoperatively or an intraoperative perineural catheter for intra- and postoperative administration of bupivacaine. All patients had general anaesthesia for the amputation. The pre-, peri-, and postoperative epidural pain treatment was not superior to the intra- and postoperative perineural pain treatment in preventing phantom pain as the incidence of phantom pain was similar in the two groups after 3 days and 6 and 12 months.

The above-mentioned studies provide conflicting results. Of the nine studies, five produced positive results and four failed to show that perioperative epidural blockade prevents phantom pain.

Conclusion

Phantom pain is a common consequence of limb amputation. Approximately two-thirds of patients complain of phantom pain following limb removal, but in less than 10% of amputees does pain represent a severe incapacitating condition. The incidence of severe phantom pain is therefore similar to other chronic neuropathic pain states. Experimental studies within the past two decades have shown that a nerve cut gives rise to a series of morphological, physiological, and biochemical changes that result in a hyperexcitability in the nervous system. Spontaneous pain and abnormally evoked pain from the stump of amputees reflect this hyperexcitability, which is amenable for modulation and treatment by the same remedies used for neuropathic pain in general. Although it was thought that phantom pain could be prevented by pre-emptive types of treatments, e.g. epidurally administered local anaesthetics and opioids before amputation, recent data suggest that a short-lasting blockade of afferent input before amputation is not sufficient to prevent the development of central sensitization, hyperalgesia, and pain. Further studies are needed to determine the role of peripheral and central mechanisms in phantom limb phenomena, including phantom pain, in order to find better types of treatments.

References

Abramson AS, Feibel A 1981 The phantom phenomenon; its use and disuse. Bulletin of the New York Academy of Medicine 57: 99–122

Ahmed S 1979 Phantom limb pain and propranolol. British Medical Journal 1: 415

Appenzeller O, Bicknell JM 1969 Effects of nervous system lesions on phantom experience in amputees. Neurology 19: 141–146

Bach S, Noreng MF, Tjéllden NU 1988 Phantom limb pain in amputees during the first 12 months following limb amputation after preoperative lumbar epidural blockade. Pain 33: 297–301

Bailey AA, Moersch FP 1941 Phantom limb. Canadian Medical Association Journal 45: 37–42

Baron R, Wasner G, Lindner V 1998 Optimal treatment of phantom limb pain in the elderly. Drugs and Aging 12: 361–376

Bartusch SL, Sanders J, Dálessio JG, Jernigan JR 1996 Clonazepam for the treatment of lancinating phantom limb pain. Clinical Journal of Pain 12: 59–62

Birbaumer N, Lutzenberger W, Montoya P, Larbig W, Unertl K, Topfner S, Grodd W, Taub E, Flor H 1997 Effects of regional anesthesia on phantom limb are mirrored in changes in cortical reorganization in upper limb amputees. Journal of Neuroscience 17: 5503–5508

Brihaye J 1958 Extinction of phantom limb in leg amputated during medullary compression by cervical discal hernia: revival of phantom after surgical removal of hernia. Acta Neurologica et Psychiatrica Belgica 58: 536

Browder J, Gallagher JP 1948 Dorsal cordotomy for pain phantom limbs. Annals of Surgery 128: 456–469

Carlen PL, Wall PD, Nadvorna H, Steinbach T 1978 Phantom limbs and related phenomena in recent traumatic amputations. Neurology 28: 211–217

Cook AJ, Woolf CJ, Wall PD, McMahon SB 1987 Dynamic receptive field plasticity in rat spinal cord dorsal horn following C-primary afferent input. Nature 325: 151–153

Cronholm B 1951 Phantom limb in amputees. Acta Psychiatrica et Neurologica Scandinavica 72 (suppl): 1–310

Davis KD, Kiss ZH, Luo L 1998 Phantom sensations generated by thalamic microstimulation. Nature 391 (6665): 385–387

Davis RW 1993 Successful treatment for phantom pain. Orthopedics 16: 691–695

Dellemijn P 1999 Are opioids effective in relieving neuropathic pain? Pain 80: 453–462

Devor M, Raber P 1990 Heritability of symptoms in an experimental model of neuropathic pain. Pain 42: 51–67

Devor M, Seltzer Z 1999 Pathophysiology of damaged nerves in relation to chronic pain. In: Wall PD, Melzack R (eds) Textbook of pain, 4th edn. Churchill Livingstone, Edinburgh, pp 129–164

Devor M, Govrin-Lippman R, Angelides K 1993 Na^+ channels immunolocalization in peripheral mammalian axons and changes following nerve injury and neuroma formation. Journal of Neuroscience 135: 1976–1992

Doubell TP, Mannion RJ, Woolf CJ 1999 The dorsal horn: state-dependent sensory processing, plasticity and the generation of pain. In: Wall PD, Melzack R (eds) Textbook of pain, 4th edn. Churchill Livingstone, Edinburgh, pp 165–181

Elizaga AM, Smith DG, Sharar SR, Edwards T, Hansen ST 1994 Continuous regional analgesia by intraneural block: effect on postoperative opioid requirements and phantom limb pain following amputation. Journal of Rehabilitation Research and Development 31: 179–187

Elliott F, Little A, Milbrandt W 1976 Carbamazepine for phantom limb phenomena. New England Journal of Medicine 295: 678

Finch DRA, MacDougal M, Tibbs DJ, Morris PJ 1980 Amputation for vascular disease: the experience of a peripheral vascular unit. British Journal of Surgery 67: 233–237

Fischer A, Meller Y 1991 Continuous postoperative regional analgesia by nerve sheath block for amputation surgery—a pilot study. Anesthesia and Analgesia 72: 300–303

Flor H, Elbert T, Knecht S 1995 Phantom limb pain as a perceptual correlate of cortical reorganization following arm amputation. Nature 375: 482–484

Flor H, Elbert T, Mühlnickel W 1998 Cortical reorganization and phantom phenomena in congenital and traumatic upper-extremity amputees. Experimental Brain Research 119: 205–212

Henderson WR, Smyth GE 1948 Phantom limbs. Journal of Neurology, Neurosurgery and Psychiatry 11: 88–112

Hill A, Niven CA, Knussen C 1995 The role of coping in adjustment to phantom limb pain. Pain 62: 79–86

Hill A, Niven CA, Knussen C 1996 Pain memories in phantom limbs: a case story. Pain 66: 381–384

Huse E, Larbig W, Flor H, Birbaumer N 2001 The effect of opioids on phantom limb pain and cortical reorganization. Pain: 90: 47–55

Houghton AD, Nicholls G, Houghton AL, Saadah E, McColl L 1994 Phantom pain: natural history and association with rehabilitation. Annals of the Royal College of Surgeons of England 76: 22–25

Iacono RP, Sandyk R, Baumford CR, Awerbuch G, Malone JM 1987 Post-amputation phantom pain and autonomous stump movements responsive to doxepin. Functional Neurology 2: 343–348

Jacobsen L, Chabal C, Brody MC 1990. A comparison of the effects of intrathecal fentanyl and lidocaine on established postamputation stump pain. Pain 40: 137–141

Jaeger H, Maier C 1992 Calcitonin in phantom limb pain: a double-blind study. Pain 48: 21–27

Jahangiri M, Jayatunga AP, Bradley JWP, Dark CH 1994 Prevention of phantom pain after major lower limb amputation by

epidural infusion of diamorphine, clonidine and bupivacaine. Annals of the Royal College of Surgeons of England 76: 324–326
Jensen TS, Krebs B, Nielsen J, Rasmussen P 1983 Phantom limb, phantom pain and stump pain in amputees during the first 6 months following limb amputation. Pain 17: 243–256
Jensen TS, Krebs B, Nielsen J, Rasmussen P 1984 Non-painful phantom limb phenomena in amputees: incidence, clinical characteristics and temporal course. Acta Neurologica Scandinavica 70: 407–414
Jensen TS, Krebs B, Nielsen J, Ramussen P 1985 Immediate and long-term phantom limb pain in amputees: incidence, clinical characteristics and relationship to preamputation limb pain. Pain 21: 267–278
Kajander KC, Wakisaka S, Bennett GJ 1992 Spontaneous discharge originates in the dorsal root ganglion at the onset of a painful peripheral neuropathy in the rat. Neuroscience Letters 138: 225–228
Katsuly Liapis I, Georgakis P, Tierry C 1996 Preemptive extradural analgesia reduces the incidence of phantom pain in lower limb amputees. British Journal of Anaesthesia 76: 125
Katz J 1992 Psychophysical correlates of phantom limb experience. Journal of Neurology, Neurosurgery and Psychiatry 50: 811–821
Katz J, Melzack R 1990 Pain 'memories' in phantom limbs: review and clinical observations. Pain 43: 319–336
Katz J, Melzack R 1991 Auricular transcutaneous electrical nerve stimulation (TENS) reduces phantom limb pain. Journal of Pain and Symptom Management 6 (2): 73–83
Keil G 1990 Sogenannte erstbeschreibung des phantomschmerzes von Ambroise Paré. Fortschritte der Medicine 108: 58–66
Kooijman CM, Dijkstra PU, Geertzen JHB, Elzinga A, Schans CP 2000 Phantom pain and phantom sensations in upper limb amputees: an epidemiological study. Pain 87: 33–41
Krane EJ, Heller LB 1995 The prevalence of phantom sensation and pain in pediatric amputees. Journal of Pain and Symptom Management 10: 21–29
Krebs B, Jensen TS, Krøner K, Nielsen J, Jørgensen HS 1985 Phantom limb phenomena in amputees 7 years after limb amputation. In: Fields HL, Dubner R, Cervero F (eds) Advances in pain research and therapy 9. Raven Press, New York, pp 425–429
Lambert AW, Dashfield AK, Cosgrove C, Wilkins DC, Walker AJ, Ashley S 2001 Randomised prospective study comparing preoperative epidural and intraoperative perineural analgesia for the prevention of post stump and phantomoperative limb pain following major amputation. Regional Anesthesia and Pain Medicine 26: 316–321
Lierz P, Schroegendorfer K, Choi S, Felleiter P, Kress HG 1998 Continous blockade of both brachial plexus with ropivacaine in phantom pain: a case report. Pain 78: 135–137
Lundeberg T 1985 Relief of pain from nine phantom limbs by peripheral stimulation. Journal of Neurology 232: 79–82
Mackenzie N 1983 Phantom limb pain during spinal anaesthesia. Anaesthesia 38: 886–887
Marsland AR, Weekes JWN, Atkinson RL, Leong MG 1982 Phantom limb pain: a case for beta blockers? Pain 12: 295–297
Mitchell SW 1872 Injuries of nerves and their consequences. Lippincott, Philadelphia
Mogil JS, Wilson SG, Bon K, Eun Lee S, Chung K, Raber P, Pieper JO, Hain HS, Belknap JK, Hubert L, Elmer GI, Chung JM, Devor M 1999 Heritability of nociception I: responses of 11 inbred mouse strains on 12 measures of nociception. Pain 80: 67–82
Montoya P, Larbig W, Grulke N 1997 Relationship of phantom limb pain to other phantom limb phenomena in upper extremity amputees. Pain 72: 87–93
Nathan PW 1962 Pain traces left in the central nervous system. In: Keele CA, Smith R (eds) The assessment of pain in man and animals. E & S Livingstone, Edinburgh, pp 129–134
Nikolajsen L, Hansen CL, Nielsen J, Keller J, Arendt-Nielsen L, Jensen TS 1996 The effect of ketamine on phantom pain: a central neuropathic disorder maintained by peripheral input. Pain 67: 69–77
Nikolajsen L, Ilkjær S, Krøner K, Christensen JH, Jensen TS 1997a The influence of preamputation pain on postamputation stump and phantom pain. Pain 72: 393–405
Nikolajsen L, Hansen PO, Jensen TS 1997b Oral ketamine therapy in the treatment of postamputation stump pain. Acta Anaesthesiologica Scandinavica 41: 427–429
Nikolajsen L, Ilkjær S, Krøner K, Christensen JH, Jensen TS 1997c Randomised trial of epidural bupivacaine and morphine in prevention of stump and phantom pain in lower-limb amputation. Lancet 350: 1353–1357
Nikolajsen L, Ilkjær S, Jensen TS 1998 Effect of preoperative epidural bupivacaine and morphine on stump sensations in lower limb amputees. British Journal of Anaesthesics 81: 348–354
Nikolajsen L, Ilkjær S, Jensen TS 2000a Relationship between mechanical sensitivity and postamputation pain: A prospective study. European Journal of Pain 4: 327–334
Nikolajsen L, Gottrup H, Kristensen AGD, Jensen TS 2000b Memantine (a N-methyl D-aspartate receptor antagonist) in the treatment of neuropathic pain following amputation or surgery: a randomised, double-blind, cross-over study. Anesthesia and Analgesia 91: 960–966
Novakovic SD, Tzoumaka E, McGivern JG, Haraguchi M, Sangameswaran L, Gogas KR, Eglen RM, Hunter JC 1998 Distribution of the tetrodotoxin-resistant sodium channel PN3 in rat sensory neurons in normal and neuropathic pain conditions. Journal of Neuroscience 18: 2174–2187
Nyström B, Hagbarth KE 1981 Microelectrode recordings from transected nerves in amputees with phantom limb pain. Neuroscience Letters 27: 211–216
Omote K, Ohmori H, Kawamata M, Matsumoto M, Namiki A 1995 Intrathecal buprenorphine in the treatment of phantom limb pain. Anesthesia and Analgesia 80: 1030–1032
Parkes CM 1973 Factors determining the persistence of phantom pain in the amputee. Journal of Psychosomatic Research 17: 97–108
Patterson JF 1988 Carbamazepine in the treatment of phantom limb pain. Southern Medical Journal 81: 1100–1102
Pezzin LE, Dillingham TR, Mackenzie EJ 2000 Rehabilitation and the long-term outcomes of persons with trauma-related amputations. Archives of Physical Medicine and Rehabilitation 81: 292–300
Pinzur MS, Garla PGN, Pluth T, Vrbos L 1996 Continuous postoperative infusion of a regional anaesthetic after an amputation of the lower extremity. Journal of Bone and Joint Surgery 78: 1501–1505
Pohjolainen T 1991 A clinical evaluation of stumps in lower limb amputees. Prosthetics and Orthotics International 15: 178–184
Price DD, Mao J, Mayer DJ 1997 Central consequences of persistent pain states. In: Jensen TS, Turner JM, Wiesenfeld-Hallin Z (eds) Proceedings of the 8th World Congress on Pain, Progress in Pain Research and Management, vol. 8. IASP Press, Seattle, pp 155–184
Rajbhandari SM, Jarett JA, Griffiths PD, Ward JD 1999 Diabetic neuropathic pain in a leg amputated 44 years previously. Pain 83: 627–629
Rasmussen KG, Rummans 2000 Electroconvulsive therapy for phantom limb pain. Pain 85: 297–299
Rayner HC, Atkins RC, Westerman RA 1989 Relief of local stump pain by capsaicin cream. Lancet 2: 1276–1277
Riddoch G 1941 Phantom limbs and body shape. Brain 64: 197–222
Schott GD 1986 Pain and its absence in an unfortunate family of amputees. Pain 25: 229–231

Schug SA, Burell R, Payne J, Tester P 1995 Preemptive epidural anaesthesia may prevent phantom limb pain. Regional Anesthesia 20: 256

Sherman RA, Glenda GM 1987 Concurrent variation of burning phantom limb and stump pain with near surface blood flow in the stump. Orthopedics 10: 1395–1402

Sherman R, Sherman C 1983 Prevalence and characteristics of chronic phantom limb pain among American veterans: results of a trial survey. American Journal of Physical Medicine 62: 227–238

Sherman RA, Sherman CJ 1985 A comparison of phantom sensations among amputees whose amputations were of civilian and military origins. Pain 21: 91–97

Sherman RA, Sherman CJ, Gall NG 1980 A survey of current phantom limb pain treatment in the United States. Pain 8: 85–99

Sherman RA, Sherman CJ, Bruno GM 1987 Psychological factors influencing chronic phantom limb pain: an analysis of the literature. Pain 28: 285–295

Sherman RA, Vernice GD, Evans CB 1992. Temporal relationship between changes in phantom limb pain intensity and changes in surface electromyogram of the residual limb. International Journal of Psychophysiology 13: 71–77

Sindrup SH, Jensen 1999 Efficacy of pharmacological treatments of neuropathic pain: an update and effect related to mechanism of drug action. Pain 83: 389–400

Sliosberg A 1948 Les algies des amputés. Masson, Paris

Stannard CF, Porter GE 1993 Ketamine hydrochloride in the treatment of phantom limb pain. Pain 54: 227–230

Sunderland S 1978 Nerves and nerve injuries. Williams & Wilkins, Baltimore

Tessler MJ, Kleiman SJ 1994 Spinal anaesthesia for patients with previous lower limb amputations. Anaesthesia 49: 439–441

Urban BJ, France RD, Steinberger EK, Scoot DL, Maltbie AA 1986 Long-term use of narcotic/antidepressant medication in the management of phantom limb. Pain 24: 191–196

Wall PD, Gutnick M 1974 Ongoing activity in peripheral nerves: the physiology and pharmacology of impulses originating from a neuroma. Experimental Neurology 43: 580–593

Wall R, Novotny-Joseph P, Macnamara TE 1985 Does preamputation pain influence phantom limb pain in cancer patients? Southern Medical Journal 78: 34–36

Wartan SW, Hamann W, Wedley JR, McColl I 1997 Phantom pain and sensation among British veteran amputees. British Journal of Anaesthesia 78: 652–659

Wassef MR 1997 Phantom pain with probable reflex sympathetic dystrophy. Efficacy of fentanyl infiltration of the stellate ganglion. Regional Anesthesia 22: 287–290

Weiss T, Miltner WH, Adler T, Bruckner L, Taub E 1999 Decrease in phantom limb pain associated with prosthesis-induced increased use of an amputation stump in humans. Neuroscience Letters 272: 131–134

Wilkins KL, McGrath PJ, Finley GA, Katz J 1998 Phantom limb sensations and phantom limb pain in child and adolescent amputees. Pain 78: 7–12

Woolf CJ, Shortland P, Coggeshaal RE 1992 Peripheral nerve injury triggers central sprouting of myelinated afferents. Nature 355: 75–78

Yarnitsky D, Barron SA, Bental E 1988 Disappearance of phantom pain after focal brain infarction. Pain: 32: 285–287

Chapter 17

Peripheral neuropathies

J W Scadding

Introduction

Many terms may be used by patients with neuropathies to describe their painful sensations. The symptoms may be divided into those that are unprovoked (spontaneous) and those that are provoked by manoeuvres such as skin stimulation, pressure over affected nerves, changes in temperature, or emotional factors. The most commonly described spontaneous symptoms are a deep aching in the extremities and a superficial burning, stinging, or prickling pain. Some patients also report paroxysmal, shock-like lancinating pains, sometimes radiating through a whole limb (Dyck et al 1976, Thomas and Ochoa 1993).

Allodynia may be particularly incapacitating in some neuropathies and accompanying hyperpathia is not uncommon (Lindblom 1979, Noordenbos 1979). In the following descriptions of the different neuropathies, the major painful complaints typical of each condition are given, but it should be emphasized that, within a single aetiological or pathological diagnostic category, considerable symptom variation occurs in different individuals. The clinical features of neuropathic pain are summarized in Table 17.1, and the neuropathies commonly associated with pain are listed in Table 17.2.

Investigation of peripheral neuropathies

The cause of some neuropathies may become apparent after a few simple tests and there is no need for specialized investigation. Nevertheless, as pointed out by Thomas and Ochoa (1993), even after extensive investigation the cause of a substantial minority of neuropathies remains uncertain. Detailed discussion of basic clinical diagnostic aspects of peripheral neuropathies and of specialized investigative techniques is beyond the scope of this chapter, and full accounts of these topics are to be found in reviews by Kimuna (1993), Lambert and Dyck (1993), and Dyck et al (1993). A careful and detailed neurological examination is always the starting point, followed by nerve conduction studies, and in some patients, quantitative sensory testing. In a small minority, nerve biopsy is needed for diagnosis. Systemic investigation is essential in all patients with multifocal neuropathies and polyneuropathies.

Mechanisms of pain in neuropathy

It is beyond the scope of this chapter to discuss the evidence from basic neuroscience, which has

Table 17.1 Clinical features of neuropathic pain due to peripheral neuropathy

Clinical features
Abnormal quality: raw, burning, gnawing
Paroxysmal pains
Sensory impairment
Associated allodynia, hyperalgesia, hyperpathia
Evidence of abnormal sympathetic function
Sometimes associated with changes of complex regional pain syndrome (causalgia)
Immediate or delayed onset of pain following injury in mononeuropathy
Intensity of pain markedly altered by emotion and fatigue

provided important insights into the mechanisms of neuropathic pain (NP); for a full account see Devor and Seltzer (1999) and Doubell et al (1999).

Mononeuropathies and multiple mononeuropathies

Postherpetic neuralgia

Definition and description

Postherpetic neuralgia (PHN) is one of the commonest intractable conditions seen in pain clinics. There is no generally agreed definition of PHN. Pain persisting past the stage of healing of the rash, at 1 month after the onset, was the time chosen in some previous investigations (e.g. Hope-Simpson 1965). However, as PHN tends to diminish in severity with time and may cease to be troublesome many months or even years later (see below), most now accept the longer interval of 3 months minimum after the onset of the acute eruption (Watson et al 1988).

It is unusual for shingles to be entirely painless in middle-aged or older people. Pre-eruptive pain for up to 3 weeks is well described (Juel-Jensen and MacCallum 1972), though pain for more than 2 days before the rash is uncommon. Acute herpetic

Table 17.2 Neuropathies commonly associated wth pain

Traumatic mononeuropathies		
Entrapment neuropathies	Painful scars	
Transection (partial or complete)	Post-thoracotomy	
Causalgia	Stump pain	
Other mononeuropathies and multiple mononeuropathies		
Diabetic mononeuropathy	Neuralgic amyotrophy	
Diabetic amyotrophy	Malignant nerve/plexus invasion	
Postherpetic neuralgia	Radiation plexopathy	
Trigeminal neuralgia	Connective tissue disease	
Glossopharyngeal neuralgia		
Polyneuropathies		
Metabolic/nutritional:	Diabetic	Strachan's (Jamaican neuropathy)
	Alcoholic	Cuban neuropathy
	Pellagra	Tanzanian neuropathy
	Amyloid	Burning feet syndrome
	Beriberi	
Drugs:	Isoniazid	Nitrofurantoin
	Cisplatin	Disulfiram
	Vincristine	
Toxic:	Thallium	
	Arsenic	
	Clioquinol	
Infective:	HIV	
Hereditary:	Fabry's disease	
	Dominantly inherited sensory neuropathy	
Malignant:	Myeloma	
	Carcinomatous	
Others:	Acute idiopathic polyneuropathy (Guillain–Barré)	
	Idiopathic	

neuralgia is often severe. There are no features of the pain unique to the acute neuralgia and it merges into PHN. The pain is most often of two types: an ongoing pain described as burning, raw, severe aching or tearing, and superimposed paroxysmal pains, stabbing or electric shock-like. Both the ongoing and paroxysmal pains may be present throughout the whole of the affected dermatome, but commonly become concentrated in one part of the dermatome, particularly after a period of more than 6 months.

The pain is frequently accompanied by a very unpleasant sensitivity of the skin, which again is often most severe in part of the dermatome. The scars themselves tend to be hypoaesthetic, but elsewhere there is hyperaesthesia, allodynia, and sometimes hyperpathia (Watson et al 1988). Allodynia may take the form of an exacerbation of the underlying ongoing pain or the evoked dysaesthesiae may be different, often a severe itching sensation. These evoked sensations constitute the most unbearable part of PHN for many patients, usually produced by clothes contact and skin stretching with movement. The patient's emotional state (there is often associated depression), environmental temperature, and fatigue may profoundly affect the severity of the ongoing and evoked pains.

Incidence of PHN

PHN, defined as pain persisting at 1 month, has an incidence of between 9% (Ragozzino et al 1982) and 14.3% (Hope-Simpson 1975). Of these patients, the number with pain at 3 months is between 35 and 55% and at 1 year is between 22 and 33% (Raggozzino et al 1982). Watson et al (1988) draw attention to an incidence at 1 year of only 3%, and in a further study of 91 patients with PHN defined as pain persisting at more than 3 months Watson et al found that at a median of 3 years follow-up (range 3 months to 12 years), 52 patients (56%) had either no pain or pain that had decreased to a level of no longer being troublesome. More than half of these 52 patients had had PHN for longer than 1 year at the time of first being seen.

This study underlines the tendency of PHN to gradually improve in many patients even after long periods, an important fact that has often been overlooked in studies of treatment for PHN. It is also of interest that Watson et al (1988) found that a good or bad outcome did not depend on age, sex, or affected dermatome. In a further study of prognosis of PHN, Watson et al (1991a) in general confirmed these findings, but found that those patients with longer duration PHN at the time of presentation tended to do worse and some patients whose pain appeared to gradually worsen, despite all attempts at pain relief, were identified.

The commonest sites for PHN are the mid-thoracic dermatomes and the ophthalmic division of the trigeminal nerve, but may occur in any dermatome. Women are more often affected than men, in a ratio of approximately 3:2 (Hope-Simpson 1975, Watson et al 1988).

Pathology and pathogenesis of pain

There have been few pathological studies in PHN. Head and Campbell (1900) were the first to document the changes in the DRG and sensory roots but of 21 patients only one was reported to have PHN. Lhermitte and Nicholas (1924) studied a patient with acute zoster myelitis, who had acute haemorrhagic inflammatory in DRG, posterior roots and peripheral nerve, with demyelination and axonal degeneration. Denny-Brown et al (1944) observed similar changes in three patients, with marked lymphocytic infiltration at the sites of inflammation. Noordenbos (1959) found a reduction in the large myelinated fibre population in intercostal nerves. In peripheral nerves of patients biopsied early and late after the acute eruption, Zachs et al (1964) found Wallerian degeneration, followed by marked fibrotic change, leading to severe myelinated fibre depletion with preservation of small myelinated fibres only in some patients.

In an autopsy study of a 67-year-old man with PHN for 5 years before death in a right T7–T8 dermatome, Watson et al (1988) found atrophy of the dorsal horn on the right from T4 to T8 with loss of myelin and axons. Only the T8 DRG and dorsal root were affected by fibrosis and cell loss. Markers of unmyelinated fibres (substance P levels), substantia gelatinosa neurons (opiate receptors), glial cells (glial fibrillary acidic protein), and monoaminergic descending spinal projections (dopamine β-hydroxylase and serotinin levels) were all normal.

In a further autopsy study, Watson et al (1991b) examined spinal cords, DRG, dorsal roots, and peripheral nerves from five patients, three of whom had had severe persistent PHN and two of whom had had no pain. Dorsal horn atrophy was only found in those patients with PHN. Axonal and myelin loss and fibrosis were found in one DRG from all the patients without pain. In all patients the peripheral nerve showed severe loss of myelin and axons. In these nerves, there was a relative loss of larger myelinated fibres. The dorsal roots in all patients with PHN and in one patient without pain showed loss of myelin and axons, but in the other pain-free patient the dorsal root was normal.

Substance P and CGRP levels were measured in two patients with PHN. Staining was absent in the affected DRG but apparently normal in the dorsal horn. Quantitative study of the unmyelinated fibres was not performed in either study, so the degree to which unmyelinated afferents were affected in patients with PHN remains uncertain. An additional finding of interest in one patient who had had PHN for 22 months prior to death was marked inflammatory change with lymphocytic infiltration bilaterally in the DRG of four adjacent segments and in the respective peripheral nerves, suggesting that an ongoing inflammatory process may result following acute zoster in some patients.

Clearly, further studies of this type are needed in a larger number of patients, before the interpretation of the findings of Watson et al (1988, 1991a, b) in relation to pain pathogenesis. As yet, the pathological studies have not revealed a specific change present in patients with PHN and absent in patients without pain, which might offer a clue as to the mechanism of pain. Preferential loss of larger myelinated fibres appears to be a feature common to patients both with and without PHN. Watson et al (1991a) speculate whether the persistent inflammation found in one patient at a longer interval after acute zoster might indicate continuing low-grade infection and might be a feature of those patients whose pain gradually worsens.

Prevention

Treatment options for PHN are discussed in Chap. 44. The important issue of prevention of PHN has received considerable attention. There are obvious difficulties in conducting an adequate trial of any treatment to answer this question, given the low and decreasing incidence of PHN at intervals between 3 and 12 months after the acute eruption. In a trial of 40% idoxuridine in DMSO in a fairly small group of patients, Juel-Jensen et al (1970) showed a reduction in incidence of PHN. However, subsequent widespread use of this treatment has been disappointing. Systemic corticosteroids may be effective, as suggested in two controlled trials (Keczkes and Basheer 1980). There is a danger of dissemination (Merselis et al 1964), although this may be confined to those patients with underlying malignancy or other serious disease leading to immune suppression. Acyclovir has been advocated as an effective preventive drug but controlled studies have not confirmed earlier hopes that it would substantially reduce the incidence of PHN, although some studies have shown shorter periods of acute zoster neuralgia and faster healing of the rash (Balfour et al 1983).

Diabetic mononeuropathy and amyotrophy

Mononeuropathies occur more frequently in diabetes than in the normal population, affecting particularly the motor nerves to the extraocular muscles but also single peripheral nerves including median, ulnar, peroneal, femoral, and lateral cutaneous nerve of the thigh. It is particularly interesting that approximately half the patients with acute lesions of the third, fourth, and sixth cranial nerves have pain, which may precede the ocular palsy by a few days (Zorilla and Kozak 1967). Third nerve palsy is the most common and is usually pupil sparing. Pain is felt around or behind the eye and may be severe. Since there are no somatosensory fibres in these nerves, where is the pain arising? Two suggestions have been put forward: the first is that the lesions involve the nervi nervorum, producing pain (Thomas 1974), and the second is that there may be concurrent lesions of the branches of the trigeminal nerve in the cavernous sinus, in support of which Zorilla and Kozak (1967) reported discrete facial sensory impairment in some of their patients. With regard to the acute peripheral nerve lesions, pain is a common symptom, though usually transient. Thomas (1979) reported a diabetic patient with an acute radial nerve palsy that was heralded by severe pain in the upper arm, but there was no pain distally. A fascicular biopsy of the nerve in the upper arm showed only small-diameter regenerating myelinated fibres and the endoneurial vessels showed the changes of diabetic microangiopathy. This case is again suggestive of pain arising as a result of activity in nervi nervorum, also termed nerve trunk pain (Asbury and Fields 1984).

Postmortem studies of the pathology of diabetic mononeuropathy include a patient reported by Dreyfus et al (1957), who died 5 weeks after developing a unilateral third cranial nerve palsy. The nerve was swollen retro-orbitally, with degenerative changes in the central parts of the nerve and Wallerian degeneration distally. This lesion was considered to have a vascular cause, on the basis of arteriolar changes observed, although no vessel occlusion was seen. Raff et al (1968) reported the presence of punctate lesions in the nerve of a diabetic patient who had developed mononeuritis multiplex in the legs 6 weeks before death, which also suggested a vascular pathology. A particularly interesting patient who died a month after the onset of a third nerve palsy and who had had a contralateral transient third nerve palsy 3 years earlier was studied by Asbury et al (1970). As in the patient of Dreyfus et al (1957), the changes in the acutely affected nerve were maximal in the central parts of the nerve, although they were less severe, consisting mainly of demyelination. The contralateral previously affected nerve was structurally normal.

Diabetic amyotrophy, also now known as painful proximal diabetic neuropathy (PDN), is an asymmetrical predominantly motor neuropathy, sometimes related to poor diabetic control, found in middle-aged and elderly diabetics (Thomas and Tomlinson 1993). In a clinical and pathological study of PDN, Said et al (1997) examined nerve biopsies of the intermediate cutaneous nerve of the thigh. Inflammatory changes and ischaemic lesions associated with vasculitis of epineurial and perineurial vessels were found. There was an associated mixed axonal and demyelinating neuropathy, with degeneration of unmyelinated axons, together with evidence of regeneration. Endoneurial and perineurial inflammatory infiltrates were common. The findings were considered by Said et al (1997) to be in keeping with an ischaemic mechanism secondary to occlusion of blood vessels. In view of the marked inflammatory component of PDN, it is likely that the pain may in part be another example of pain mediated by nervi nervorum, nerve trunk pain (Thomas 1979).

Entrapment neuropathies

Entrapment neuropathies or sensory or mixed nerves, such as carpal tunnel syndrome, are usually characterized in the early stages by paraesthesiae and pain. Morphologically, entrapment lesions cause damage to myelinated fibres in the first instance (Ochoa and Noordenbos 1979), with a near absence of myelinated fibres only in severe lesion, in which there is preservation only of C fibres. Local pain and tenderness at the site of nerve entrapment in many patients is likely to be nerve trunk pain, mediated by nervi nervorum, as discussed in relation to diabetic mononeuropathy. Paraesthesiae of non-painful type with entrapment neuropathies presumably reflect activity in damaged myelinated fibres, as demonstrated microneurographically in experimental nerve ischaemia in man by Ochoa and Torebjork (1980).

The explanation of pain in entrapment neuropathies (other than nerve trunk pain) is more difficult. Severe pain, sometimes with a burning quality, is frequently a symptom, albeit often in short-lived episodes in electrophysiologically mild carpal tunnel syndrome, in which myelinated fibre conduction is relatively mildly affected and thus it is difficult to imagine that C fibres are damaged. Whether pain is due to activity in myelinated afferents alone in this situation remains uncertain.

Morton's neuralgia is an example of a frequently histologically severe entrapment neuropathy in which a plantar digital nerve becomes compressed in the region of the metatarsal heads in the foot. In badly affected nerves, many myelinated fibres may be disrupted within the region of compression, producing a nerve that is populated almost exclusively by C fibres. However, explanations of pain pathogenesis based on these findings must take account of the fact that similar changes are often found in control nerves from subjects who never suffered this type of neuralgia (Scadding and Klenerman 1987).

Ischaemic neuropathy

Polyarteritis nodosa, rheumatoid arthritis, and systemic lupus erythematosus may all be associated with painful peripheral mononeuropathies, which probably have a microangiopathic basis (Chalk et al 1993). In a study of nerves involved in rheumatoid arthritis, Dyck et al (1972) found degenerative changes in the central parts of fascicles in nerves from the upper arm and thigh and postulated that these represented watershed areas in these nerves. The probable ischaemic basis for these changes is supported by the experimental ischaemic peripheral nerve lesions produced by injection of arachidonic acid in rats (Parry and Brown 1982), which produced similar central fascicular degenerative changes, in which small myelinated fibres and unmyelinated fibres were affected to a greater extent than large myelinated fibres. Lacomis et al (1997) reported two patients with small-fibre neuropathies, found on biopsy to be due to vasculitis. One patient had systemic lupus erythematosus. It was proposed that the mechanism of the pain might be preferential affection of small fibres by ischaemia.

The effects of whole-limb ischaemia on peripheral nerves were shown by Eames and Lange (1967), who found clinical signs of sensory neuropathy in 87.5% of patients undergoing amputation for major vessel atheromatous disease and observed loss of myelinated fibres with segmental demyelination, remyelination, and Wallerian degeneration in nerves from these patients. Ischaemia to the nerves of a limb may, of course, be associated with ischaemia to non-neural structures, which may be the source of pain rather than the neuropathic changes.

There is good evidence that ischaemia may precipitate or potentiate painful symptoms in nerves already damaged by other factors. Gilliatt and Wilson (1954) demonstrated an abnormally rapid onset of paraesthesiae with cuff ischaemia in patients with carpal tunnel syndrome, and Harding and Le Fanu (1977) reported precipitation of symptoms of carpal tunnel syndrome in patients during haemodialysis with antebrachial arterio-venous fistulae.

Neuralgic amyotrophy

Neuralgic amyotrophy, or cryptogenic brachial plexus neuropathy, is a condition characterized by acute onset of severe pain around the shoulder girdle or in the arms, often in a root distribution, which is followed within 2 weeks by weakness in the limb. This is most frequently distributed around the shoulder girdle and upper limb but may involve distal muscle groups. A minority of patients report a minor, possibly viral, preceding illness (Wilbourn 1993). The ensuing paralysis is extremely variable in severity and duration, but good recovery is usual within 2 years. Little is known about the pathology of the condition or even whether the site of the initial lesion is in the roots or more distally in the brachial plexus, although the patchy distribution favours involvement of the plexus and its branches rather than the roots in the majority of patients. The time course of milder lesions suggests demyelination without axonal disruption, whereas that of severe lesions indicates that axonal degeneration probably occurs. There are similarities between neuralgic amyotrophy and the brachial neuritis that occurs in serum sickness. In the latter condition, severe lancinating pain around the shoulder girdle and in the arms is a leading symptom, tending to be more common on the side of handedness, though it may be bilateral. Pathological studies are few, but marked swelling of roots has been observed (Roger et al 1934), and it has been suggested that in some patients the swollen roots may become entrapped in the cervical exit foraminae and that this is the cause of the radicular pain. Neuralgic amyotrophy is reviewed by Wilbourn (1993).

Carcinomatous neuropathies

Neuropathies of various types are well documented as non-metastatic complications of malignant disease, the commonest being a progressive sensory neuropathy that is only occasionally painful (Croft and Wilkinson 1969). However, it was subsequently reported that causalgia may occur as a result of direct invasion of peripheral nerves by carcinoma, responding to sympathectomy (Hupert 1978).

Polyneuropathies

As demonstrated in Table 17.3, there is no clear correlation between type of fibre loss and painfulness in human polyneuropathy. This section discusses the commonly painful neuropathies, preceded by consideration of two remarkable painless neuropathies.

Polyneuropathies with loss of pain sensation

These comprise a rare, poorly defined group of inherited disorders in which, from an early age, an insensitivity to pain is evident. It is important to distinguish those disorders in which the peripheral and central nervous systems are intact, where the problem appears to be a lack of recognition of pain, an indifference or asymbolia, from insensitivity (Schilder et al 1931), which can be explained on the basis of observed structural abnormalities. In the former group, patients are able to identify noxious stimuli and sensory thresholds are normal but they do not react behaviourally or physiologically in the expected way (Ogden et al 1959, Winkelmann et al 1962). Peripheral nerves, spinal cord, and thalamus

Table 17.3 Painful and painless polyneuropathies

Painful and painless polyneuropathies
Polyneuropathies with selective loss of pain sensation
Congenital analgesia with anhidrosis
Congenital analgesia with other sensory impairment
Tangier disease (familial α-lipoprotein deficiency)
Painful polyneuropathies with selective large-fibre loss
Isoniazid neuropathy
Pellagra neuropathy
Painless polyneuropathies with selective large-fibre loss
Friedreich's ataxia
Chronic renal failure
Painful polyneuropathies with selective small-fibre loss
Diabetic neuropathy
Amyloid neuropathy
Fabry's disease
Dominantly inherited sensory neuropathy
Painful polyneuropathies with non-selective fibre loss
Alcoholic neuropathy
Myeloma neuropathy
Miscellaneous painful polyneuropathies
Acute inflammatory polyneuropathy
Nutritional neuropathies
Beriberi
Strachan's syndrome
Burning feet syndrome
Arsenic neuropathy
Subacute myelo-optic neuropathy

are all normal in these patients (Feindel 1953, Baxter and Olszewski 1960). Asymbolia for pain may also be acquired, recent evidence suggesting a crucial role for the insular cortex, damage to which may lead to disconnection between sensory cortex and the limbic system (Berthier et al 1988).

Leaving such cases aside, two major subgroups may be recognized. In congenital analgesia with anhidrosis (Swanson 1963), impairment of pain sensation predisposes to tissue-damaging injury, leading on occasion to loss of fingers (Mazar et al 1976) or severe mutilation of the tongue (Pinsky and DiGeorge 1966). Sweet (1981) reviewed reports of 15 such patients. Typically, pain and, to a lesser extent, thermal sensation are severely defective, while other sensory modalities remain intact. The associated anhidrosis may lead to episodes of hyperpyrexia. Of the 15 patients, only four were of normal intelligence and these children mutilated themselves less severely. Pathologically, a case coming to autopsy showed evidence of a severe sensory neuropathy with a total absence of small dorsal root ganglion cells, of small fibres in dorsal roots, and of Lissauer's tract, together with a reduction in size of the spinal tract of the trigeminal nerve (Swanson et al 1965).

In the second group, an insensitivity to pain is evident in childhood, accompanied by symptoms and signs of a sensory polyneuropathy, but the impairments of pain sensation is out of proportion to impairment of other modalities; 21 such cases were reviewed by Sweet (1981), in which the degree of selectivity of pain sensation impairment was variable. The case reports of a brother and sister aged 6 and 2½ years by Haddow et al (1970) exemplify the most extreme form. Both siblings had extensive mutilating lesions of the fingers and in the 6-year-old a pin was not painful anywhere, while there was a much milder distal loss to other modalities. The pathological peripheral nerve changes in this group range from a complete absence of myelinated fibres to a marked non-selective reduction, with normal unmyelinated fibres (Sweet 1981). It seems likely that some of these cases were examples of dominantly inherited sensory neuropathy, considered below.

Tangier disease

Tangier disease, familial α-lipoprotein deficiency, is an extremely rare lipid disorder in which a neuropathy occurs in at least half those affected (Yao and Herbert 1993). Patients with a remarkable dissociated sensory loss of pain, and temperature sensation over most of the body have been reported. Nerve biopsy findings included decrease in small myelinated fibres and virtual absence of unmyelinated fibres (see Yao and Herbert 1993).

Painful polyneuropathies

Isoniazid neuropathy

Isoniazid neuropathy was first recognized by Pegum (1952), and clinical features were described by Gammon et al (1953). Initial symptoms of distal numbness and tingling paraesthesiae are later accompanied by pain, which may be felt as a deep ache or burning. The calf muscles are often painful and tender and the exacerbation of symptoms produced by walking may prevent the patient from walking. Spontaneous pain and paraesthesiae may be particularly troublesome at night. Examination shows signs of a sensorimotor neuropathy, often confined to the legs. Cutaneous hyperaesthesia is a frequent finding. Ochoa (1970) examined sural nerve biopsies from nine patients, reporting a primary axonal degeneration in myelinated fibres with evidence of degeneration in unmyelinated fibres and regeneration in both types, together with degeneration of regenerated myelinated fibres. Using several ultrastructural criteria, Ochoa (1970) was able to distinguish as yet unmyelinated sprouts of myelinated fibres from unmyelinated fibres and was also able to make an accurate assessment of differential myelinated fibre damage, finding that large fibres were preferentially lost. The relative resistance of unmyelinated fibres to isoniazid was shown by Hopkins and Lambert (1972), who reported preservation of the C-fibre compound action potential in severe experimental isoniazid neuropathy. Prevention and treatment with pyridoxine was described by Biehl and Wilter (1954); the biochemical pathogenesis is discussed by Windebank (1993).

Hypothyroid neuropathy

Pollard et al (1982) reported the pathological changes in sural nerve biopsies from two patients with untreated hypothyroidism. One presented with a long history of pain in the feet and progressive difficulty in walking, the other with pain and paraesthesiae in the hands. In both there were signs of a sensorimotor neuropathy. The biopsies showed a mainly axonal degeneration with occasional segmental demyelination. In both patients, myelinated fibre densities were decreased with a relative loss of large fibres, but there were regenerating myelinated fibres, which may have contributed to the small-fibre bias, although probably not to a significant extent. Unmyelinated fibre densities were increased, due to small-diameter regenerating axons.

Dyck and Lambert (1970) also found reduced myelinated fibre densities in two hypothyroid patients, associated with reduced A α and δ potentials in vitro, with normal C-fibre potentials. Teased fibres showed more marked segmental demyelination and remyelination with less axonal degeneration than in the patients of Pollard et al (1982).

Diabetic neuropathies

Diabetes is associated with several types of polyneuropathy of which the commonest is a symmetrical sensory polyneuropathy (Thomas 1973). Numbness and paraesthesiae are common presenting complaints, the paraesthesiae sometimes having a burning quality. In addition, some patients complain of a spontaneous deep, aching pain and lightning pain may be reported. The prevalence of these severe dysaesthetic symptoms is not known but in the experience of Thomas and Tomlinson (1993), pain is frequently troublesome, even when sensory and motor deficits are mild. Severe sensory neuropathy in diabetes may lead to painless perforating foot ulcers, and in such patients the upper limbs may also be involved and there may be an associated autonomic neuropathy. The pathology and biochemical factors in the sensory neuropathy due to diabetes are complex controversial topics (Thomas and Tomlinson 1993). As with other neuropathies, uncertainty as to whether the pathology is primarily an axonal degeneration of Schwann cell dysfunction leading to demyelination has been the major issue. Segmental demyelination and remyelination, sometimes leading to onion bulb formation, has been reported, but axonal loss has also been observed. In addition, dorsal root ganglion cell degeneration occurs (Olsson et al 1968), and loss of anterior horn cells has been reported. Overall, the evidence indicates that demyelination is the predominant pathology in the majority of patients and axonal degeneration in a minority. Earlier suggestions that the neuropathy might result from a diabetic microangiopathy have not been supported by more recent observations (Thomas and Tomlinson 1993), although a vascular pathology in diabetic mononeuropathy is likely.

Brown et al (1976) reported clinical and pathological findings in three patients with severe pain due to diabetic polyneuropathy. Two of the patients had shooting pains in the legs. In all three there was a distal sensory impairment, but tendon reflexes were preserved. Nerve biopsies suggested a predominant axonal degeneration affecting mainly small myelinated and unmyelinated fibres. There were also myelinated fibre sprouts, and their presence in appreciable numbers led Brown et al (1976) to suggest that the pain in these patients might have been due to abnormal impulse generation, as in sprouts forming experimental neuromas (Wall and Gutnick 1974).

They also reviewed patients with diabetic polyneuropathy with attention to painfulness in relation to physical signs. Patients without pain tended to have areflexia with distal sensory loss particularly involving joint position sense, while patients with severe burning pain and hyperaesthesia tended to have sensory loss with a relative preservation of position sense and intact reflexes and more often had evidence of an accompanying autonomic neuropathy.

Said et al (1983) reported three patients similar to those of Brown et al (1976), with a striking selective loss of pain and temperature sensation, producing a pseudosyringomyelic picture. However, some of the patients with chronic sensorimotor neuropathy reported by Behse et al (1977) had pain. Nerve biopsies showed a non-selective fibre loss. A similar non-selective fibre loss, but accompanied by evidence of regeneration, characterized the nerve biopsies of the patients with the acute painful neuropathy reported by Archer et al (1983).

Britland et al (1992) reported a morphometric study of sural nerve biopsies from six diabetics, four with active acute painful neuropathy and two with recent remission from this type of neuropathy. Myelinated and unmyelinated fibre degeneration and regeneration were present in all of the nerves, the only discernible differences between the nerves from patients with and those without pain being that those with remission from the pain had a less abnormal axon: Schwann cell calibre ratio, more successful myelinated fibre regeneration, and less active myelinated fibre regeneration. However, these were all differences in the severity, and the authors emphasize the similarity of the pathological changes in the two groups.

In a cross-sectional study, Guy et al (1985) found that loss of thermal sensation occurred in isolation or in combination with loss of vibration sensation but the reverse pattern, selective loss of vibration sensation, did not occur. These observations indicate that small fibres are affected early and large fibres later in diabetic polyneuropathy. However, no longitudinal studies have been reported.

Over and above the structural and physiological alterations common to many types of peripheral nerve damage that may lead to pain, two other factors may be of importance in diabetic neuropathy. Hyperglycaemia in diabetics may itself lower pain threshold and tolerance, compared with non-diabetic controls (Morley et al 1984). Further, it has been found in animal experiments that hyperglycaemia reduces the antinociceptive effect of morphine (Simon and Dewey 1981), indicating a possible effect of glucose on opiate receptors. This raises the further possibility that hyperglycaemia might modulate the abnormal properties, such as ectopic impulse generation, that develop in damaged nerve.

The other factor is blood flow. Autonomic involvement in diabetic neuropathy increases peripheral blood flow. Archer et al (1984) compared peripheral blood flow and its response to sympathetic stimulation in diabetics with severe non-painful sensory polyneuropathy and diabetics with acute severe painful neuropathies of the type described by Archer et al (1983). High flow was present in both groups, but was reduced by sympathetic stimulation in the group with painful neuropathy and this reduction was accompanied by an improvement in pain. The explanation of this effect is uncertain; a decrease in temperature may be important. The observations seem to conflict with the experimental observation of an increase in ectopic impulse generation in neuromas produced by sympathetic stimulation (Devor and Janig 1981).

The primary prevention and treatment of diabetic neuropathy is good control of the diabetes, although neuropathies have occasionally developed soon after initiation of treatment with either insulin or oral hypoglycaemic drugs (Thomas and Tomlinson 1993).

Amyloid neuropathy

A second example of a painful small-fibre neuropathy is that caused by amyloid, both the inherited and sporadic varieties (Dyck and Lambert 1969, Dyck et al 1971, Thomas and King 1974). Patients typically present with a distal sensory loss that initially affects pain and thermal sensations, often with autonomic involvement. As the neuropathy progresses, all modalities are affected, reflexes are lost, and there is motor involvement. The physiological and morphological findings of Dyck and Lambert (1969) and Dyck et al (1971), referred to earlier, showed that small myelinated and unmyelinated fibres are selectively lost and this was confirmed by Thomas and King (1974). It is thus a surprising but common experience that this type of polyneuropathy is often very painful, the pain usually having a deep aching quality, sometimes with superimposed shooting pains.

Fabry's disease

Fabry's disease, angiokeratoma corpus diffusum, is a rare lipid storage disorder in which a painful peripheral neuropathy is the usual presenting feature. The dermatological manifestation is telangiectasia with proliferation of keratin and epidermal cells (Wise et al 1962) and most tissues, including heart, kidneys, and lungs, may be involved (Brady 1993). There is a deficiency of ceramide trihexosidase in this sex-linked recessive disease, leading to accumulation of ceramide trihexoside in the tissues (Brady et al 1967). Typically, boys or young men present with tenderness of the feet and spontaneous burning pain in the legs, which may be extremely severe (Wise et al 1962), occasionally leading to suicide (Thomas 1974). The accompanying sensorimotor deficit is often mild. A rash is usually present early on and this should always suggest the diagnosis of Fabry's disease in a young man. Heterozygous carrier females occasionally develop symptoms later in life (Brady 1993). The central nervous system is relatively spared, although patients with mental retardation have been reported. Dorsal root ganglion cells are variably affected, but in peripheral nerves there is a selective loss of small myelinated fibres and a decrease in unmyelinated axons, particularly those of larger diameter (Kocen and Thomas 1970). On electron microscopy the accumulated lipid appears as lamellated, often concentric inclusions known as zebra bodies.

Hereditary sensory neuropathy

The last example of a painful small-fibre neuropathy is dominantly inherited sensory neuropathy, in which symptoms develop slowly from the second decade onwards, mainly in the feet. Distal sensory impairment, particularly affecting pain and temperature sensation in the early stages, with little motor involvement and distal autonomic involvement are the major clinical features. The selective loss of pain sensation may lead to painless penetrating foot ulcers and eventually loss of large parts of the feet (Dyck 1993). Severe lancinating pains are well recognized in this condition and are not related to the severity or the rate of progression of the disease. In their combined electrophysiological and morphological study, Dyck et al (1971) found a preferential reduction in Aδ and C-fibre potentials associated with a selective loss of unmyelinated and small myelinated fibres, although there was also a considerable reduction of larger myelinated fibres. It is interesting to compare this neuropathy with recessively inherited sensory neuropathy, in which touch-pressure sensation is initially preferentially impaired, although in which a painless mutilating acropathy may eventually occur. Pain is not a feature. Recordings in vitro showed absent myelinated fibre potentials with reduced C-fibre potentials, associated with a histological absence of myelinated fibres and reduced numbers of unmyelinated axons (Ohta et al 1973).

Alcoholic neuropathy

The incidence of neuropathy in chronic alcoholism is in the region of 9% (Victor and Adams 1953), including asymptomatic patients. Of the symptomatic patients, approximately one-quarter complain of pain or paraesthesiae as the first symptom (Windebank 1993). Burning pain and tenderness of the feet and legs are the characteristic complaints, the upper limbs being only rarely involved. Examination reveals a sensorimotor neuropathy, and the occurrence of painful symptoms is not related to the severity of the deficit. In a pathological study, Walsh and McLeod (1970) examined sural nerve biopsies from 11 patients who were divided into those with acute and those with chronic neuropathies and, in addition, their diet was assessed. Myelinated fibre densities were decreased in all the biopsies. Fibre-size histograms in five biopsies showed reduction of all fibre sizes in three, but in two there was a relative excess of small-diameter fibres. Teased-fibre preparations showed that these were regenerating sprouts. Patients presenting with an acute neuropathy and a poor diet had active axonal degeneration, whereas those with chronic neuropathies and a better diet had less degeneration and regeneration was present. However, Walsh and McLeod (1970) did not relate this to painfulness in their patients.

In the early stages of alcoholic neuropathy in some patients, clinical evidence of large sensory fibre involvement is slight or even absent, and abnormal thermal thresholds indicate a preferential affectation of unmyelinated afferent fibres. This is thus another example of a painful neuropathy with selective small-fibre involvement.

Treatment of alcoholic neuropathy consists of stopping drinking and ensuring an adequate diet. Poor diet is a major contributory factor to the development of the neuropathy, and there are obvious clinical similarities to the neuropathies caused by specific vitamin deficiencies; pellagra along with some further examples are considered below. The therapeutic effect of thiamine in alcoholic peripheral neuropathy was demonstrated by Victor and Adams (1961). Victor (1975) drew attention to the causalgic nature of the pain in alcoholic neuropathy and reported good temporary pain relief with sympathetic blockade.

Myeloma

Both multiple and solitary myeloma may be associated with a peripheral sensorimotor neuropathy (Walsh 1971, Kyle and Dyck 1993). The neuropathy is extremely variable in severity and rate of progression, ranging from mild, predominantly sensory neuropathy to a complete tetraplegia. Bone pain is of course a common symptom but, in addition, pain attribution to the associated neuropathy occurs. In reviewing reported patients, Davis and Drachman (1972) calculated an incidence of painful symptoms of 59% in patients with neuropathy. In five sural nerve biopsies from patients with neuropathies but without painful symptoms, Walsh (1971) found a loss of myelinated fibres of all sizes, and in teased fibres the appearances suggested a primary axonal degeneration. Unmyelinated axon counts in two patients showed a substantial decrease in numbers, without regeneration. Amyloid has only occasionally been found in nerves of patients with myeloma neuropathy and is not the cause of the neuropathy (Davies-Jones and Esiri 1971). The neuropathy responds well to myeloma chemotherapy or radiotherapy for solitary myeloma and this includes resolution of the painful symptoms.

HIV neuropathy

Peripheral neuropathy is commonly associated with human immunodeficiency virus (HIV) infection. By far the commonest is AIDS-associated sensory neuropathy, in which neuropathic pain is a major symptom in at least 30% of patients. The polyradiculopathy due to cytomegalovirus infection is characteristically painful, and painful neuropathies resulting from antiretroviral therapy are well described. Nutritional neuropathies with HIV infection are occasionally painful, and herpes zoster infection and resultant post-herpetic neuralgia is a common complication of AIDS. The clinical, electrophysiological, and pathological features of the neuropathies associated with HIV infection are reviewed by Griffin et al (1998).

Acute inflammatory polyneuropathy (AIP)

In AIP of the Guillain–Barré type, pain is a common early symptom, often preceding sensory impairment or weakness. It may present in a distal distraction, as generalized muscular pain or as root pain, which sometimes leads to diagnostic difficulties. It has been suggested by Thomas (1979) that such pain may be due to local inflammation in roots, mediated by the nervi nervorum, rather than neuropathic pain due to the pathological processes involving the root fibres themselves. Pain in AIP may be severe but is usually transient. Persisting pain is more often in a distal distribution. In patients with chronic relapsing and chronic progressive inflammatory polyneuropathy, pain is not usually a prominent symptom. The pathology of AIP is demyelination, usually predominantly affecting the roots, and in the great majority of patients full recovery occurs.

Nutritional neuropathies

In addition to nutritional factors in the pathogenesis of alcoholic neuropathy already discussed, several other painful neuropathies attributed to specific nutritional deficiencies have been described (reviewed by Windebank 1993). Many accounts in the literature provide descriptions of clinical features but lack biochemical or neuropathological investigation. Other problems of aetiological differentiation are that nutritional deficiency of a single vitamin seldom occurs and that in some cases, for example alcoholic neuropathy, a known neurotoxin is also involved. Four painful polyneuropathies of probable or possible nutritional origin are relevant here: pellagra, beriberi, Strachan's syndrome (Jamaican neuropathy) and the burning feet syndrome.

Pellagra neuropathy Peripheral neuropathy is one of the many neurological manifestations of pellagra, due to niacin deficiency. A predominant feature of the sensorimotor neuropathy is spontaneous pain in the feet and lower legs, with tenderness of the calf muscles and cutaneous hyperaesthesia of the feet (Lewy et al 1940). There are no recent pathological studies of this neuropathy and no ultrastructural study. Wilson (1913–1914) reported changes suggesting a predominant axonal degeneration and, in a later investigation, Aring et al (1941) observed a decreased density of myelinated fibres, with a preferential loss of larger fibres. In spinal cord, extensive degeneration was found in the dorsal and lateral tracts by Anderson and Spiller (1940) in two patients at autopsy, while others, for example Greenfield and Holmes (1939), observed degeneration mainly in the posterior columns, with less marked changes in the pyramidal tracts. Pellagra neuropathy would thus appear to be a further example of a painful neuropathy in which large fibres are selectively lost. The possibility that regenerated myelinated fibres biased the fibre population studies of Aring et al (1941) is made less likely, but is not excluded, by the overall decrease in fibre density. The spinal cord changes suggest that this is an example of a central–peripheral distal axonopathy (see such section below).

Beriberi neuropathy In beriberi, a painful sensorimotor polyneuropathy is very common. There is spontaneous pain in the feet and sometimes the hands, often with a burning character. The calf muscles may be particularly painful, and although sensory thresholds are raised, skin stimulation may produce extremely unpleasant paraesthesiae. It is likely, though not completely proven, that thiamine deficiency is the cause of this neuropathy, and the associated cardiac disorder and improvement with thiamine is well recorded (Victor 1975). In experimental studies, Swank (1940) showed peripheral nerve degeneration in thiamine-deficient pigeons and North and Sinclair (1956) and Prineas (1970) in rats. In Swank's (1940) investigation, the large myelinated fibres degenerated before the smaller fibres and the longest fibres were preferentially affected. In man, the reported pathological studies are all in the older literature. In an extensive postmortem study, Peklharing and Winkler (1889; quoted by Victor 1975) described degenerative changes that were most marked in the distal part of peripheral nerves and in the posterior columns and their nuclei. Wright (1901) observed degeneration of dorsal root ganglion cells and anterior horn cells. The animal and human pathology suggest that beriberi neuropathy is primary axonal degeneration of the central peripheral distal type. Reversal of the experimental neuropathy with thiamine was shown by Swank and Prados (1942).

Strachan's syndrome (Jamaican neuropathy) In 1897, Strachan described 510 cases of a neuropathy observed in Jamaica. Patients presented with pain, paraesthesiae, and sensory impairment in the feet and hands, together with pains proximally around the shoulder and hip girdles, visual impairment, deafness, and orogenital dermatitis, in some cases resembling the lesions of pellagra. Many of the patients were ataxic, though whether this was peripheral or central in origin is not clear. More recent studies have shown that the neuropathy of Jamaican neuropathy is accompanied by features of spinal cord disease (Montgomery et al 1964) and that a pure peripheral disorder of the type described by Strachan (1897) is not now seen.

There is no evidence that the patients described by Strachan (1897) had a specific nutritional deficiency, although nutritional or toxic factors may have been important in some patients included in this clinically heterogeneous group. Those patients with spinal cord disturbances almost certainly included what is now recognized as tropical spastic paraparesis, due to HTLV1 infection (Gessain and Gout 1992).

Burning feet syndrome This syndrome was seen in many prisoners of war during the Second

World War (Cruickshank 1946, Simpson 1946). The symptoms were severe aching or causalgic-like burning pains with unpleasant paraesthesiae, starting on the soles of the feet and sometimes spreading up the legs. The symptoms were often worse at night and were relieved by cold. Objective signs of neuropathy were not always present in these patients, some of whom also had amblyopia and orogenital dermatitis (Simpson 1946). Hyperhidrosis of the feet was sometimes a prominent feature. A single nutritional deficiency was not identified in this condition, and most patients responded to an improvement in general diet and vitamin B-rich foods.

Cuban neuropathy A very large epidemic of painful sensory neuropathy and bilateral optic atrophy occurred in western Cuba between 1991 and 1993, with more than 45 000 people reported to have been affected. Clinical features in 25 patients are reported by Thomas et al (1995) and include bilateral optic neuropathy with centrocaecal scotomas or a predominantly sensory polyneuropathy, sometimes associated with deafness, or a combination of optic and peripheral neuropathies. There are clearly similarities between the Cuban disease and Strachan's syndrome. In a further study the Cuban Neuropathy Field Investigation Team (1995) examined 123 patients and assessed dietary factors and exposure to potential toxins. It was found that smoking, particularly cigars, was associated with an increased risk of optic neuropathy, and the risk was lower amongst patients with higher dietary intakes of methionine, vitamin B_{12}, riboflavin, and niacin and higher serum concentrations of antioxidant carotenoids. In support of a nutritional basis for Cuban neuropathy is the fact that the numbers of new cases began to decrease after vitamin supplementation was initiated in the population.

Tanzanian neuropathy A syndrome similar to Strachan's syndrome and Cuban neuropathy has also been observed in coastal Tanzania since 1988. The clinical features in 38 affected patients have been described by Plant et al (1997). An optic neuropathy, with primary retinal involvement in some patients, was associated with a dysaesthetic peripheral neuropathy. It was suspected, but not proven, that the condition had a nutritional basis.

Arsenic neuropathy

The polyneuropathy caused by arsenic may be painful, although it is as often painless. It is the commonest of the heavy metal neuropathies and presents as a pure sensory or mixed sensorimotor neuropathy (Goldstein et al 1975). Patients may complain of intense pain or painful paraesthesiae of the extremities (the feet more than the hands) with tenderness. Nerve biopsies show axonal degeneration involving fibres of all classes (Goldstein et al 1975).

Central-peripheral distal axonopathies

An advance in the understanding of diseases affecting the primary sensory neuron was the recognition that some pathological processes may have differential effects on the peripheral and central axons. Several references have already been made to the process of dying back or distal axonopathy, and it seems likely that this is a common pattern in peripheral neuropathies in which axonal degeneration is the primary pathology. The process of distal axonopathy is now well established in a number of experimental neuropathies, for example those caused by triortho-cresyl phosphate (Cavanagh 1954) and acrylamide (Fullerton and Barnes 1966), and the underlying cellular processes involved have been the subject of several investigations (Spencer and Schaumburg 1976). In man, anatomical information concerning the central processes of primary sensory neurons is rather more difficult to obtain than that concerning the peripheral processes, but there is now physiological evidence that central processes may be selectively involved in some diseases, for example in subacute myelo-optic neuropathy (SMON) due to clioquinol poisoning in Japan and in pure hereditary spastic paraplegia (Thomas 1982). A more common pattern in distal axonopathies is probably affectation of both central and distal axons but, as pointed out by Thomas (1982), differential recovery of function in peripheral and central axons may occur, as is probably the case in SMON, where there is poor resolution of the painful symptoms after removal of the toxin, and in a patient with vitamin E deficiency, in whom differential electrophysiological recovery was documented by Harding et al (1982). The implications of differential vulnerability and recovery in relation to pain in neuropathies other than SMON are at present not clear.

Summary of human evidence

The emphasis of most investigations of human neuropathy has been on morphological correlation of fibre size distribution with nerve conduction and painfulness, but review of the data shows that there are too many exceptions to a general hypothesis of fibre size imbalance as a cause of pain for it to be tenable. This has been recognized for some time (Thomas 1974, 1979). Dyck et al (1976) reviewed the nerve biopsies of 72 patients, looking at the type and rate of myelinated fibre degeneration and correlating this with painfulness. There was inevitably bias in the diseases represented in this study, but it was concluded that pain was a feature of those neuropathies in which there was acute axonal degeneration, and this bore no relationship to fibre size distribution. It is interesting to note in this context that a morphological study of an animal model of hyperalgesia due to nerve injury produced by loose ligatures (Bennett and Xie 1988) revealed very acute degenerative changes in both myelinated and unmyelinated fibres (Basbaum et al 1991).

Overall, the human evidence concerning the pathophysiology of pain in the many different types of neuropathy may be summarized as follows:

1. Pain is not related to fibre size distribution alone, if at all.
2. Those neuropathies in which there is rapid degenerative change are more likely to be painful.
3. Neuropathies involving small fibres, with or without large-fibre involvement, are often painful.
4. The coexistence of degenerative and regenerative changes appears to be an important factor (e.g. in some diabetic neuropathies).
5. Some pain may be sympathetic dependent. This evidence derives from studies in traumatic mononeuropathies in man, particularly causalgia (see Chap. 18). The extent to which this is important in polyneuropathies remains uncertain.
6. Ischaemia in nerves may exacerbate paraesthesiae and pain due to peripheral damage and, in certain circumstances, severe ischaemia is the cause of neuropathies that may be very painful.
7. Nerve trunk pain is a feature of mononeuropathies, and this mechanism may also be important in certain polyneuropathies.

References

Anderson PV, Spiller WG 1940 Pellagra, with a report of two cases with necropsy. American Journal of the Medical Sciences 141: 307–312

Archer AG, Watkins PJ, Thomas PK, Sharma AK, Payan J 1983 The natural history of acute painful neuropathy in diabetes mellitus. Journal of Neurology, Neurosurgery and Psychiatry 46: 491–499

Archer AG, Roberts VC, Watkins PJ 1984 Blood flow patterns in painful diabetic neuropathy. Diabetologia 27: 563–567

Aring CD, Bean WB, Roseman E, Rosenbaum M, Spies TD 1941 Peripheral nerves in cases of nutritional deficiency. Archives of Neurology and Psychiatry 45: 772–787

Asbury AK 1993 Neuropathies with renal failure, hepatic disorders, chronic respiratory insufficiency, and critical illness. In: Dyck PJ, Thomas PK, Griffin JW, Low PA, Poduslo JF (eds) Peripheral neuropathy, 3rd edn. Saunders, Philadelphia, pp 1251–1265

Asbury AK, Fields HL 1984 Pain due to peripheral nerve damage: an hypothesis. Neurology 34: 1587–1590

Asbury AK, Aldredge H, Hershberg R, Fisher CM 1970 Oculomotor palsy in diabetes mellitus: a clinico-pathology study. Brain 93: 555–556

Balfour H, Bean B, Laskin OL et al 1983 Acyclovir halts progression of herpes zoster in immunocompromised patients. New England Journal of Medicine 308: 1453

Basbaum AI, Gautrum M, Jazat F, Mayes M, Guilbaud G 1991 The spectrum of fibre loss in a model of neuropathic pain in the rat: an electron microscopic study. Pain 47: 357–367

Baxter DW, Olszewski J 1960 Congenital universal insensitivity to pain. Brain 83: 381–393

Behse F, Buchthal F, Carlsen F 1977 Nerve biopsy and conduction studies in diabetic neuropathy. Journal of Neurology and Psychiatry 40: 1072–1082

Bennett GJ, Xie Y-K 1988 A peripheral mononeuropathy in rat that produces disorders of pain like those seen in man. Pain 33: 87–108

Berthier M, Starkstein S, Leignarda R 1988 Asymbolia for pain: a sensory-limbic disconnection syndrome. Annals of Neurology 24: 41–49

Biehl JP, Wilter RW 1954 The effect of isoniazid on vitamin B6 metabolism, and its possible significance in producing isoniazid neuritis. Proceedings of the Society for Experimental Biology and Medicine 85: 389–392

Brady RO 1993 Fabry disease. In: Dyck PJ, Thomas PK, Griffin JW, Low PA, Poduslo JF (eds) Peripheral neuropathy, 3rd edn. Saunders, Philadelphia, pp 1169–1178

Brady RO, Gal AE, Bradley RM, Martensson E, Warshaw AL, Laster L 1967 Enzymatic defect in Fabry's disease: ceramidetrihexosidase deficiency. New England Journal of Medicine 276: 1163–1167

Britland ST, Young RJ, Sharma AK, Clarke BF 1992 Acute and remitting painful diabetic polyneuropathy: a comparison of peripheral nerve fibre pathology. Pain 48: 361–370

Brown MJ, Martin JR, Asbury AK 1976 Painful diabetic neuropathy. A morphometric study. Archives of Neurology 33: 164–171

Cavanagh JB 1954 The toxic effects of tri-ortho-cresyl phosphate on the nervous system. Journal of Neurology, Neurosurgery and Psychiatry 17: 163–172

Chalk CH, Dyck PJ, Conn DL 1993 Vasculitic neuropathy. In: Dyck PJ, Thomas PK, Griffin JW, Low PA, Poduslo JF (eds) Peripheral neuropathy, 3rd edn. Saunders, Philadelphia, pp 1424–1436

Croft PB, Wilkinson M 1969 The course and prognosis in some types of carcinomatous neuromyopathy. Brain 92: 1–8

Cruickshank EK 1946 Painful feet in prisoners of war in the Far East. Lancet ii: 369–381

Cuban Neuropathy Field Investigation Team 1995 Epidemic optic neuropathy in Cuba—clinical characterization and risk factors. New England Journal of Medicine 333: 1176–1182

Davies-Jones GAB, Esiri MM 1971 Neuropathy due to amyloid in myelomatosis. British Medical Journal 2: 444

Davis LE, Drachman DB 1972 Myeloma neuropathy: successful treatment of two patients and a review of cases. Archives of Neurology 27: 507–511

Denny-Brown D, Adams RD, Fitzgerald PJ 1944 Pathologic features of herpes zoster: a note on 'geniculate herpes'. Archives of Neurology and Psychiatry 77: 337–349
Devor M, Janig W 1981 Activation of myelinated afferents ending in a neuroma by stimulation of the sympathetic supply in the rat. Neuroscience Letters 24: 43–47
Devor M, Seltzer Z 1999 Pathophysiology of damaged nerves in relation to chronic pain. In: Wall PD, Melzack R (eds) Textbook of pain, 4th edn. Churchill Livingstone, Edinburgh, pp 129–164
Doubell TP, Mannion RJ, Woolf CJ 1999 The dorsal horn: state-dependent sensory processing, plasticity and the generation of pain. In: Wall PD, Melzack R (eds) Textbook of pain, 4th edn. Churchill Livingstone, Edinburgh, pp 165–182
Dreyfus PM, Hakim S, Adams RD 1957 Diabetic ophthalmoplegia. Archives of Neurology and Psychiatry 77: 337–347
Dyck PJ 1982 Current concepts in neurology: the causes, classification and treatment of peripheral neuropathy. New England Journal of Medicine 307: 283–285
Dyck PJ 1993 Neuronal atrophy and degeneration predominantly affecting peripheral sensory and autonomic neurons. In: Dyck PJ, Thomas PK, Griffin JW, Low PA, Poduslo JF (eds) Peripheral neuropathy, 3rd edn. Saunders, Philadelphia, pp 1065–1093
Dyck PJ, Lais AC 1973 Evidence for segmental demyelination secondary to axonal degeneration in Friedreich's ataxia. In: Kakulas BA (ed) Clinical studies of myology. Excerpta Medica, Amsterdam, pp 253–263
Dyck PJ, Lambert EH 1969 Dissociated sensation in amyloidosis. Archives of Neurology 20: 490–507
Dyck PJ, Lambert EH 1970 Polyneuropathy associated with hypothyroidism. Journal of Neuropathology and Experimental Neurology 29: 631–658
Dyck PJ, Lambert EH, Nichols PC 1971 Quantitative measurement of sensation related to compound action potentials and number of sizes of myelinated and unmyelinated fibres of sural nerve in health, Friedreich's ataxia, hereditary sensory neuropathy and tabes dorsalis. In: Remond A (ed) Handbook of electroencephalography and clinical neurophysiology, vol. 9. Elsevier, Amsterdam, pp 83–118
Dyck PJ, Conn DL, Okazaki H 1972 Necrotizing angiopathic neuropathy: three-dimensional morphology of fibre degeneration related to sites of occluded vessels. Mayo Clinic Proceedings 47: 461
Dyck PJ, Lambert EH, O'Brien PC 1976 Pain in peripheral neuropathy related to rate and kind of fibre degeneration. Neurology 28: 466–471
Dyck PJ, Giannini C, Lais A 1993 Pathologic alteration of nerves. In: Dyck PJ, Thomas PK, Griffin JW, Low PA, Poduslo JF (eds) Peripheral neuropathy, 3rd edn. Saunders, Philadelphia, pp 515–595
Dyck PJ, Thomas PK, Griffin JW, Low PA, Poduslo JF (eds) 1999 Peripheral neuropathy, 3rd edn. Saunders, Philadelphia
Eames RA, Lange LS 1967 Clinical and pathological study of ischaemic neuropathy. Journal of Neurology, Neurosurgery and Psychiatry 30: 215–226
Feindel W 1953 Note on nerve endings in a subject with arthropathy and congenital absence of pain. Journal of Bone and Joint Surgery 35B: 402–407
Fullerton PM, Barnes JM 1966 Peripheral neuropathy in rats produced by acrylamide. British Journal of Industrial Medicine 25: 210–221
Gammon GD, Burge FW, King G 1953 Neural toxicity in tuberculous patients treated with isoniazid (isonicotinic acid hydrazide). Archives of Neurology and Psychiatry 70: 64–69
Gessain A, Gout O 1992 Chronic myelopathy associated with human T-lymphotropic virus type I (HTLV-1). Annals of Internal Medicine 117: 933–946
Gilliatt RW, Wilson TG 1954 Ischaemic sensory loss in patients with peripheral nerve lesions. Journal of Neurology, Neurosurgery and Psychiatry 17: 104–123
Goldstein NP, McCall JT, Dyck PJ 1975 Metal neuropathy. In: Dyck PJ, Thomas PK, Lambert EH (eds) Peripheral neuropathy, 2nd edn. Saunders, Philadelphia, pp 1227–1262
Greenfield JG, Holmes JM 1939 A case of pellagra: the pathological changes in the spinal cord. British Medical Journal 815–819
Griffin JW, Crawford TO, McArthur JC 1998 Peripheral neuropathies associated with HIV infection. In: Gendelman HE, Lipton SA, Epstein L, Swindells S (eds) The Neurology of AIDS. Chapman and Hall, New York, pp 275–291
Guy RJC, Clark CA, Malcolm PN, Watkins PJ 1985 Evaluation of thermal and vibration sensation in diabetic neuropathy. Diabetologia 28: 131–137
Haddow JE, Shapiro SR, Gall DG 1970 Congenital sensory neuropathy in siblings. Paediatrics 45: 651–655
Harding AE, Le Fanu J 1977 Carpal tunnel syndrome related to antebrachial Cimmino-Brescia fistula. Journal of Neurology, Neurosurgery and Psychiatry 40: 511–513
Harding AE, Muller DPR, Thomas PK, Willison HJ 1982 Spinocerebellar degeneration secondary to chronic intestinal malabsorption: a vitamin E deficiency syndrome. Annals of Neurology 12: 419–424
Head H, Campbell AW 1900 The pathology of herpes zoster and its bearing on sensory localisation. Brain 23: 353–523
Hope-Simpson RE 1965 The nature of herpes zoster: a long term study and a new hypothesis. Proceedings of the Royal Society of Medicine 58: 9–20
Hope-Simpson RE 1975 Post-herpetic neuralgia. Journal of the Royal College of General Practitioners 25: 571–575
Hopkins AP, Lambert EH 1972 Conduction in unmyelinated fibres in experimental neuropathy. Journal of Neurology, Neurosurgery and Psychiatry 35: 63–69
Hupert C 1978 Recognition and treatment of causalgic pain occurring in cancer patients. Pain Abstracts 1: 47
Juel-Jensen BE, MacCallum FO 1972 Herpes simplex varicella and zoster. Lippincott, Philadelphia
Juel-Jensen BE, MacCallum FO, MacKenzie AMR, Pike MC 1970 Treatment of zoster with idoxuridine in dimethyl sulphoxide. Results of two double blind controlled trials. British Medical Journal 4: 776–780
Keczkes K, Basheer AM 1980 Do corticosteroids prevent post-herpetic neuralgia? British Journal of Dermatology 102: 551–555
Kimuna J 1993 Nerve conduction studies and electromyography. In: Dyck PJ, Thomas PK, Griffin JW, Low PA, Poduslo JF (eds) Peripheral neuropathy, 3rd edn. Saunders, Philadelphia, pp 598–644
Kocen RS, Thomas PK 1970 Peripheral nerve involvement in Fabry's disease. Archives of Neurology 22: 81–87
Kocen RS, King RHM, Thomas PK, Haas LF 1973 Nerve biopsy findings in two cases of Tangier disease. Acta Neuropathologica 26: 317–327
Kyle RA, Dyck PJ 1993 Neuropathy associated with the monoclonal gammopathies. In: Dyck PJ, Thomas PK, Griffin JW, Low PA, Poduslo JF (eds) Peripheral neuropathy, 3rd edn. Saunders, Philadelphia, pp 1275–1287
Lacomis D, Giuliani MJ, Steen V, Powell HC 1997 Small fibre neuropathy and fasculitis. Arthritis and Rheumatism 40: 1173–1177
Lambert EH, Dyck PJ 1993 Compound action potentials of sural nerve in vitro in peripheral neuropathy. In: Dyck PJ, Thomas PK, Griffin JW, Low PA, Poduslo JF (eds) Peripheral neuropathy, 3rd edn. Saunders, Philadelphia, pp 672–684
Lewy FH, Spies TD, Aring CD 1940 Incidence of neuropathy in pellagra; effect of carboxylase upon its neurologic signs. American Journal of the Neurological Sciences 199: 840–849

Lhermitte J, Nicholas M 1924 Les lesions spinales du zona. La myelite zosterienne. Revue Neurologique 1: 361–364
Lindblom U 1979 Sensory abnormalities in neuralgia. In: Bonica JJ, Liebeskind JC, Albe-Fessard DG (eds) Advances in pain research and therapy, vol 3. Raven Press, New York, pp 111–120
Mazar A, Herold HZ, Vardy PA 1976 Congenital sensory neuropathy with anhidrosis. Orthopaedic complications and management. Clinical Orthopaedics 118: 184–187
Melzack R, Wall PD 1965 Pain mechanisms: a new theory. Science 150: 971–979
Merselis JG, Kaye D, Hook EW 1964 Disseminated herpes zoster. Archives of Internal Medicine 113: 679–686
Montgomery RD, Cruickshank EK, Robertson WB, McMenemey WH 1964 Clinical and pathological observations on Jamaican neuropathy—a report on 206 cases. Brain 87: 425–462
Morley GK, Mooradian AD, Levine AL, Morley LE 1984 Mechanisms of pain in diabetic peripheral neuropathy: effect of glucose on pain perception in humans. American Journal of Medicine 77: 79
Noordenbos W 1959 Pain. Elsevier, Amsterdam
Noordenbos W 1979 Sensory findings in painful traumatic nerve lesions. In: Bonica JJ, Liebeskind JC, Albe-Fessard DG (eds) Advances in pain research and therapy, vol 3. Raven Press, New York, pp 91–102
North JDK, Sinclair HM 1956 Nutritional neuropathy: chronic thiamine deficiency in the rat. Archives of Pathology 62: 341–353
Ochoa J 1970 Isoniazid neuropathy in man. Brain 93: 831–850
Ochoa J, Noordenbos W 1979 Pathology and disordered sensation in local nerve lesions: an attempt at correlation. In: Bonica JJ, Liebeskind JC, Albe-Fessard DG (eds) Advances in pain research and therapy, vol 3. Raven Press, New York
Ochoa J, Torebjork HE 1980 Paraesthesiae from ectopic impulse generation in human sensory nerves. Brain 103: 835
Ogden TE, Robert F, Carmichael EA 1959 Some sensory syndromes in children: indifference to pain and sensory neuropathy. Journal of Neurology, Neurosurgery and Psychiatry 22: 267–276
Ohta M, Ellefson RD, Lambert EH, Dyck PJ 1973 Hereditary sensory neuropathy type II: clinical, electrophysiologic, histologic and biochemical studies in a Quebec kinship. Archives of Neurology 29: 23–37
Olsson Y, Save-Soderbergh J, Sourander P, Angervaall L 1968 A pathoanatomical study of the central and peripheral nervous system in diabetes of early and long duration. Pathologia Europaea 3: 62–79
Parry GJ, Brown MJ 1982 Selective fibre vulnerability in acute ischaemic neuropathy. Annals of Neurology 11: 147–154
Pegum JS 1952 Nicotinic acid and burning feet. Lancet ii: 536
Pinsky L, Di George AM 1966 Congenital familial sensory neuropathy with anhidrosis. Journal of Paediatrics 68: 1–13
Plant GT, Mtanda AT, Arden GB, Johnson GJ 1997 An epidemic of optic neuropathy in Tanzania: characterisation of the visual disorder and associated peripheral neuropathy. Journal of Neurological Sciences 145: 127–140
Pollard JD, McLeod JG, Honnibal TGA, Verheijden MA 1982 Hypothyroid polyneuropathy. Clinical, electrophysiological and nerve biopsy findings in two cases. Journal of Neurological Sciences 53: 461–471
Prineas J 1970 Peripheral nerve changes in thiamine-deficient rats. Archives of Neurology 23: 541–548
Raff MC, Sangaland V, Asbury AK 1968 Ischaemic mononeuropathy multiplex associated with diabetes mellitus. Archives of Neurology 18: 487
Ragozzino MW, Melton LJ, Kurland LT et al 1982 Population based study of herpes zoster and its sequelae. Medicine 21: 310–316
Roger H, Poursines Y, Recordier M 1934 Polynevrite apres serotherapie antitetanique curative, avec participation due nevraxe et des meninges (observation automoclinique). Revue Neurologique 1: 1078–1088
Said G, Slama G, Selva J 1983 Progressive centripetal degeneration of axons in small fibre diabetic polyneuropathy. A clinical and pathological study. Brain 106: 791–807
Said G, Elgrably F, Lacroix C 1997 Painful proximal diabetic neuropathy: inflammatory nerve lesions and spontaneous favourable outcome. Annals of Neurology 41: 762–770
Scadding JW 1999 Peripheral neuropathies. In: Wall PD, Melzack R (eds) Textbook of pain, 4th edn. Churchill Livingstone, Edinburgh, pp 815–834
Scadding JW, Klenerman LE 1987 Light and electron microscopic observations in Morton's neuralgia. Pain 5 (suppl 4): 246
Schilder P, Schmidt BJ, Leon L 1931 Asymbolia for pain. Archives of Neurology and Psychiatry 25: 598–600
Simon GS, Dewey WL 1981 Narcotics and diabetes. The effect of streptozoticin-induced diabetes on the antinociceptive potency of morphine. Journal of Pharmacology and Experimental Therapeutics 218: 318–323
Simpson J 1946 'Burning feet' in British prisoners of war in the Far East. Lancet i: 959–961
Spencer PS, Schaumburg HH 1976 Central peripheral distal axonopathy—the pathology of dying back polyneuropathies. Progress in Neuropathology 3: 253–295
Strachan H 1897 On a form of multiple neuritis prevalent in the West Indies. Practitioner 59: 477–484
Swank RL 1940 Avian thiamine deficiency. Journal of Experimental Medicine 71: 683–702
Swank RL, Prados M 1942 Avian thiamine deficiency. II. Pathologic changes in the brain and cranial nerves (especially vestibular) and their relation to the clinical behaviour. Archives of Neurology and Psychiatry 47: 97–131
Swanson AG 1963 Congenital insensitivity to pain with anhidrosis. Archives of Neurology 8: 299–306
Swanson AG, Buchan GC, Alvord EC 1965 Anatomic changes in congenital insensitivity to pain. Archives of Neurology 12: 12–18
Sweet WH 1981 Animal models of chronic pain: their possible validation from human experience with posterior rhizotomy and congenital analgesia. Pain 10: 275–295
Thomas PK 1971 Morphological basis for alterations in nerve conduction in peripheral neuropathy. Proceedings of the Royal Society of Medicine 64: 295–298
Thomas PK 1973 Metabolic neuropathy. Journal of the Royal College of Physicians of London 7: 154–160
Thomas PK 1974 The anatomical substratum of pain. Canadian Journal of Neurological Science 1: 92
Thomas PK 1979 Painful neuropathies. In: Bonica JJ, Liebeskind JC, Albe-Fessard DG (eds) Advances in pain research and therapy, vol 3. Raven Press, New York, pp 103–110
Thomas PK 1982 The selective vulnerability of the centrifugal and centripetal axons of primary sensory neurons. Muscle and Nerve 5: S117–121
Thomas PK, King RHM 1974 Peripheral nerve changes in amyloid neuropathy. Brain 97: 395–406
Thomas PK, Ochoa J 1993 Clinical features and differential diagnosis. In: Dyck PJ, Thomas PK, Griffin JW, Low PA, Poduslo JF (eds) Peripheral neuropathy, 3rd edn. Saunders, Philadelphia, pp 749–774
Thomas PK, Tomlinson DR 1993 Diabetic and hypoglycaemic neuropathy. In: Dyck PJ, Thomas PK, Griffin JW, Low PA, Poduslo JF (eds) Peripheral neuropathy, 3rd edn. Saunders, Philadelphia, pp 1219–1250
Thomas PK, Plant GT, Baxter P, Bates C, Santiago Luis R 1995 An epidemic of optic atrophy and painful sensory neuropathy in Cuba: clinical aspects. Journal of Neurology 242: 629–638
Victor M 1975 Polyneuropathy due to nutritional deficiency and

alcoholism In: Dyck PJ, Thomas PK, Lambert EH (eds) Peripheral neuropathy, 2nd edn. Saunders, Philadelphia, pp 1030–1066

Victor M, Adams RD 1953 The effect of alcohol on the nervous system. Research Publications—Association for Research in Nervous and Mental Disease 32: 526–573

Victor M, Adams RD 1961 On the aetiology of the alcoholic neurologic diseases. With special reference to the role of nutrition. American Journal of Clinical Nutrition 9: 379–397

Wall PD, Gutnick M 1974 Ongoing activity in peripheral nerves: the physiology and pharmacology or impulses originating from a neuroma. Experimental Neurology 43: 580–593

Walsh JC 1971 The neuropathy of multiple myeloma. Archives of Neurology 25: 404–414

Walsh JC, McLeod JG 1970 Alcoholic neuropathy. An electrophysiological and histological study. Journal of the Neurological Sciences 10: 457–469

Watson CPN, Morshead C, Van der Koog D, Deck JH, Evans RJ 1988 Post-herpetic neuralgia: post mortem analysis of a case. Pain 34: 129–138

Watson CPN, Watt VR, Chipman M, Birkett N, Evans R 1991a The prognosis with post-herpetic neuralgia. Pain 46: 195–199

Watson CPN, Deck JH, Morshead C, Van der Koog D, Evans RJ 1991b Post-herpetic neuralgia: further post mortem studies of cases with and without pain. Pain 44: 105–117

Wilbourn AJ 1993 Brachial plexus disorders. In: Dyck PJ, Thomas PK, Griffin JW, Low PA, Poduslo JF (eds) Peripheral neuropathy, 3rd edn. Saunders, Philadelphia, pp 911–950

Wilson SAK 1913–1914 The pathology pellagra. Proceedings of the Royal Society of Medicine 7: 31–41

Windebank AJ 1993 Polyneuropathy due to nutritional deficiency and alcoholism. In: Dyck PJ, Thomas PK, Griffin JW, Low PA, Poduslo JF (eds) Peripheral neuropathy, 3rd edn. Saunders, Philadelphia, pp 1310–1321

Winkelmann RK, Lambert EH, Hayes AB 1962 Congenital absence of pain. Archives of Dermatology 85: 325–339

Wise D, Wallace HJ, Jellinek EH 1962 Angiokeratoma corporis diffusum. Quarterly Journal of Medicine 31: 177–206

Wright H 1901 Changes in the neuronal centres in beri-beri neuritis. British Medical Journal i: 1610–1616

Yao JK, Herbert PN 1993 Lipoprotein deficiency and neuromuscular manifestations. In: Dyck PJ, Thomas PK, Griffin JW, Low PA, Poduslo JF (eds) Peripheral neuropathy, 3rd edn. Saunders, Philadelphia, pp 1179–1193

Zachs SI, Langfit TW, Elliot FA 1964 Herpetic neuritis: a light and electron microscopic study. Neurology 14: 644–750

Zorilla E, Kozak GP 1967 Ophthalmoplegia in diabetes mellitus. Annals of Internal Medicine 67: 968–976

Chapter 18

Complex regional pain syndrome

J W Scadding

Introduction

Complex regional pain syndrome (CRPS) is the name now given to a group of conditions previously described as reflex sympathetic dystrophy (RSD), causalgia, algodystrophy, Sudeck's atrophy, and a variety of other diagnoses (Box 18.1; see Rizzi et al 1984). These conditions share a number of clinical features including pain with associated allodynia and hyperalgesia, autonomic changes, trophic changes, oedema, and loss of function. The term causalgia was retrospectively applied by Mitchell to describe a syndrome of burning pain, hyperaesthesia, glossy skin, and colour changes in the limbs of soldiers sustaining major nerve injuries from gunshot wounds, seen during the American Civil War (Mitchell et al 1864, Richards 1967a, b). It was later recognized that a very similar clinical picture could be produced by a variety of other illnesses and injuries that did not include major limb nerve injury, and the term RSD has, for many years, been used to embrace these conditions (Evans 1946, Bonica 1979).

BOX 18.1
Conditions comprising complex regional pain syndrome

Reflex sympathetic dystrophy
Post-traumatic sympathetic dystrophy
Algodystrophy
Algoneurodystrophy
Causalgia (major, minor)
Sudeck's atrophy
Post-traumatic painful osteoporosis
Transient osteoporosis
Acute bone atrophy
Migratory osteolysis
Post-traumatic vasomotor syndrome
Shoulder–hand syndrome

Involvement of the sympathetic nervous system in causalgia and reflex sympathetic dystrophy: historical aspects

It is worthwhile re-examining the early observations that led to a widespread acceptance that the sympathetic nervous system is crucially involved in the pathogenesis and maintenance of these syndromes. This has influenced subsequent thinking to the extent that some have even proposed response of the conditions to sympathetic blockade or sympathectomy as diagnostic criteria. However, this illogical and scientifically unjustified approach to conditions of uncertain, and quite possibly heterogeneous, pathogenesis has now been abandoned.

Leriche (1916) described the relief of causalgia in a patient with a brachial plexus injury and thrombosis of the brachial artery by surgical sympathectomy, resecting the adventitia of a length of the brachial artery. In this and subsequent patients, pain relief combined with an improvement in discolouration and sweating changes led Leriche to conclude that the sympathetic nervous system was involved in the pathogenesis of causalgia (Leriche 1939). As described by Schott (1995), periarterial sympathectomy was replaced by preganglionic sympathectomy and became standard treatment for painful nerve injuries sustained during the two World Wars, although without further critical evaluation of effectiveness.

For the conditions without major nerve or blood vessel injury, later described by the term RSD, in which very similar clinical features to causalgia are present, attempts to relieve pain and restore function by sympathectomy or repeated sympathetic blockade have, for many years, been standard treatment. Evidence of efficacy is examined later but it is recognized by those regularly treating these patients that while temporary pain relief may occur, long-term results are poor. It is probable that sympathetic block has only survived as standard treatment because of the lack of more effective therapy.

Causes of complex regional pain syndrome

According to the previous IASP definitions of causalgia and RSD, causalgia referred to the syndrome associated with nerve injury, while RSD included patients whose pain and associated features followed a variety of insults, most commonly relatively minor, and normally fully recoverable injuries. These are listed in Box 18.2 (Richards 1967a, Schwartzman and McLellan 1987).

BOX 18.2
Causes of complex regional pain syndrome

Peripheral tissues
- Fractures and dislocations
- Soft-tissue injury
- Fasciitis, tendonitis, bursitis, ligamentous strain
- Arthritis
- Mastectomy
- Deep vein thrombosis
- Immobilization

Peripheral nerve and dorsal root
- Peripheral nerve trauma
- Brachial plexus lesions
- Post-herpetic neuralgia
- Root lesions

Central nervous system
- Spinal cord lesions, particularly trauma
- Head injury
- Cerebral infarction
- Cerebral tumour

Viscera
- Abdominal disease
- Myocardial infarction

Idiopathic

Definition and taxonomy of complex regional pain syndrome

The need for a new classification and terminology stems from a poor understanding of the clinical limits of the conditions concerned, the underlying pathophysiology and how variable this may be, and the unsatisfactory existing terminology and particularly RSD with its clear pathogenic implication. The term 'sympathetically maintained pain' (SMP) is discussed later in this chapter.

The new definition results from an IASP consensus conference (Stanton-Hicks et al 1995) and is summarized in Box 18.3, reproduced from Boas (1996). The first criterion for CRPS is that there is an initiating noxious event. However, there are a few patients otherwise fulfilling the diagnostic criteria for CRPS in whom there is no history of any such initiating event (Veldman et al 1993).

Clinical features of complex regional pain syndrome

It can be seen from Box 18.3 that CRPS II is in all respects similar to CRPS I, except that included in the definition is the additional condition that it follows a nerve injury and thus corresponds to the condition previously known as causalgia.

The symptoms and signs of CRPS are found in a regional distribution, often widely in a limb, and in both types of CRPS the symptoms and signs often spread well beyond the limits of the causative injured territory.

Pain

Spontaneous and evoked pain (allodynia and hyperalgesia) coexist in the great majority of

BOX 18.3
Diagnostic criteria for complex regional pain syndrome (Reproduced from Boas 1996)

CRPS describes a variety of painful conditions that usually follow injury, occur regionally, have a distal predominance of abnormal findings, exceed in both magnitude and duration the expected clinical course of the inciting event, often result in significant impairment of motor function, and show variable progression over time.

CRPS Type I (RSD)
1. Follows an initiating noxious event.
2. Spontaneous pain and/or allodynia and hyperalgesia occur beyond the territory of a single peripheral nerve(s), and is disproportionate to the inciting event.
3. There is or has been evidence of oedema, skin blood flow abnormality, or abnormal sudomotor activity in the region of the pain since the inciting event.
4. The diagnosis is excluded by the existence of conditions that would otherwise account for the degree of pain and dysfunction.

CRPS II (Causalgia)
This syndrome follows nerve injury. It is similar in all other respects to CRPS type I.
1. It is a more regionally confined presentation about a joint or area, associated with a noxious event.
2. Spontaneous pain and/or allodynia and hyperalgesia are usually limited to the area involved, but may spread variably distal or proximal to the area, not in the territory of a dermatomal or peripheral nerve distribution.
3. Intermittent and variable oedema, skin blood flow change, temperature change, abnormal sudomotor activity, and motor dysfunction, disproportionate to the inciting event, are present about the area involved.

patients with CRPS. Pain is disproportionate to the initiating cause in distribution, severity, and duration, and may have various qualities. Patients commonly describe burning, aching, or throbbing pain, and in the case of CRPS II, superimposed paroxysmal pains are common. Allodynia, hyperalgesia, and hyperpathia are often so severe that any contact with the affected part and active or passive movement may be extremely painful, leading to protection of the limb and loss of function. This in turn may lead to secondary effects of prolonged immobilization, including muscle wasting and joint stiffness with contracture, which are frequent compounding factors in CRPS.

Autonomic signs

The definition of CRPS is careful to state that autonomic signs are, or have at some time, been present, but are not necessarily constant features in a particular patient. Abnormalities of temperature, colour, and sweating are common. Oedema is often present as an early sign (Blumberg and Janig 1994), which later resolves in about half of patients. These autonomic changes could, in part, be secondary to immobilization.

Motor signs

Objective motor signs are variable, but loss of function of the affected part is almost universal. Wasting and weakness are common; tremor and dystonia are observed in a small proportion of patients.

Dystrophic changes

Some dystrophic changes may simply result from prolonged disuse. Skin changes include thinning, with a shiny appearance, or flaky, thickened skin. Hair may be lost or abnormally coarse and the nails may be thickened. Osteoporosis, explicable on the basis of disuse, is a frequent finding in many patients, but a more profound loss of bone mineral content also occurs (Sudeck's atrophy).

Predisposition to CRPS

It has been postulated that certain individuals might be predisposed to the development of CRPS but there is no conclusive evidence in favour of this (Covington 1996).

Psychological factors

The absence of a clear pathogenesis and pathophysiological basis for CRPS and the disproportionate pain and loss of function have led to examination of potential psychological aetiology. Patients with conversion disorder and factitious illnesses may present with symptoms that can closely resemble CRPS and indeed, because diagnosis of CRPS is based on assessment of symptoms and signs, it is not surprising that some patients with primary psychiatric morbidity are erroneously diagnosed as having CRPS. A diagnosis of CRPS as distinct from conversion disorder may only emerge after a series of diagnostic assessments.

The severe pain of CRPS with loss of function and lack of a clear diagnosis produces anxiety, fear, and depression in many patients. Whether such secondary psychological features developing early following an injury might then predispose to the development of CRPS remains controversial (Covington 1996).

Some of the patients reported by Ochoa and Verdugo (1995) with so-called pseudoneuropathy mimicking CRPS type I undoubtedly had primarily psychiatric illnesses, emphasizing the need for careful and often repeated clinical assessment over a period of time.

Relative frequency of clinical features in CRPS

Case ascertainment is clearly a difficulty in CRPS and all the large series reported in the literature suffer from referral bias. Prospective studies examining patients after a particular known cause, for example Colles fracture (Bickerstaff and Kanis 1994), avoid such bias but only provide a single cause perspective of the condition. A report from a centre known to have an interest in CRPS, and thus attracting referrals from many other hospitals in The Netherlands, inevitably suffered from referral bias to some extent, but analysis of 829 patients with CRPS from all causes provides a fairly reliable insight into the relative frequency of the various symptoms and signs composing CRPS (Veldman et al 1993). These were categorized by Veldman et al (1993) as inflammatory, neurological, dystrophic, and sympathetic and were evaluated with respect to duration of CRPS. Table 18.1 presents data from Veldman et al (1993).

Staging of clinical features in CRPS

Earlier studies of RSD suggested that three stages could be recognized: an acute warm phase in which pain and oedema predominated, a dystrophic phase categorized by muscle wasting and vasomotor instability with pale cyanotic skin, and a later cold, atrophic stage categorized particularly by bone and skin changes (Blumberg and Janig 1994). The value of staging has been questioned as patients do not all follow the same course, the duration of the recognizable phases is variable, and not all patients progress to the third stage (Walker and Cousins 1997). Veldman et al (1993) found that in 95% of their patients the acute phase was categorized by

Table 18.1 Symptoms and signs of complex regional pain syndrome[a]

Symptom/sign	Duration of CRPS 2–6 months (%)	>12 months (%)
Inflammatory		
Pain	88	97
Colour difference	96	84
Temperature difference	91	91
Limited movement	90	83
Exacerbation with exercise	95	97
Oedema	80	55
Neurological		
Hyperaesthesia	75	85
Hyperpathia	79	81
Incoordination	47	61
Tremor	44	50
Involuntary spasms	24	47
Muscle spasm	13	42
Paresis	93	97
Pseudoparalysis	7	26
Dystrophy		
Skin	37	44
Nails	23	36
Muscle	50	67
Bone	41	52
Sympathetic		
Hyperhidrosis	56	40
Changed hair growth	71	35
Changed nail growth	60	52

[a]Data adapted from Veldman et al (1993).

pain, oedema, vasomotor changes, changes in temperature, and loss of function, all of which were intensified by exercise of the affected limb, signs that they interpreted as characteristic of inflammation. With regard to temperature, patients with longer duration symptoms were more likely to have a cold limb. Of those patients seen from the onset of the illness, 13% had primarily cold limbs without any initial warm phase. More than half their patients did not develop signs of tissue dystrophy or atrophy in the later stages.

Less common clinical features of CRPS

Very infrequently, CRPS may be migratory or relapsing or occur in two or more extremities (Johnson 1943, Bentley and Hameroff 1980, Veldman et al 1993). In 53% of the patients with relapsing or multiple RSD described by Velman et al (1993), no initiating injury or illness could be identified, raising the possibility that very rarely a predisposition to develop CRPS may exist in certain subjects. Other less common features of CRPS include intractable or relapsing skin infections (associated with chronic oedema), spontaneous haematomas, increased skin pigmentation, nodular fasciitis of palmar or plantar skin, and clubbing of the nails (Veldman et al 1993).

CRPS in children

It is only relatively recently that the occurrence of CRPS in children has been recognized (Wilder 1996). The lower limb is much more frequently affected than the upper limb (ratio about 5:1), whereas the opposite is true in adults. Most studies of CRPS in adults show a female preponderance, but this is more marked in children (ratio about 4:1). Sufferers are typically pubertal adolescent girls. Approximately half the children affected will get better with complete resolution of symptoms and signs, and only a small proportion continue to experience severe pain. Recovery may be helped by physiotherapy, transcutaneous electrical stimulation, and cognitive and behavioural pain management techniques. Many children with CRPS participate in competitive sports, putting them at greater risk of musculoskeletal injury.

Interest has focused on the role of psychological factors with the suggestion that injury and persistent pain provide a means of escape from stressful competition and the parental expectations associated with this (Sherry and Weisman 1988). Sympatholytic treatment is as unpredictable in its efficacy as it is in adults and long-term results are disappointing, although comparisons are not easy due to the higher rate of spontaneous resolution or cure in children than in adults.

Diagnostic tests: sympathetically maintained pain and sympathetically independent pain

There are no diagnostic tests for CRPS. Three-phase isotope bone scans are frequently abnormal (Goldsmith et al 1989), but a normal bone scan does not exclude the diagnosis. Although the existence of a sympathetic influence on pain in CRPS and other pain states has been questioned (Ochoa et al 1994, Schott 1995), there is substantial experimental and clinical evidence of such an influence (see later discussion; Loh and Nathan 1978, Loh et al 1980, Torebjork et al 1995). Sympathetically maintained pain (SMP) is the component of pain maintained by efferent noradrenergic sympathetic activity and circulating catecholamines; sympathetically independent pain (SIP) is the component that is not (Roberts 1986). Neurogenic pains, central as well as peripheral, may be partly responsive to sympathetic blockade (Loh et al 1980, Bonica 1990, Arner 1991, Raja et al 1991, Wahren et al 1991). A conceptual framework for the relationship between SMP and some painful conditions is shown in Fig. 18.1 (Boas 1996). SMP as assessed clinically by the effect of sympathetic blockade is a variable component of pain in CRPS I and II. SMP is correctly not included

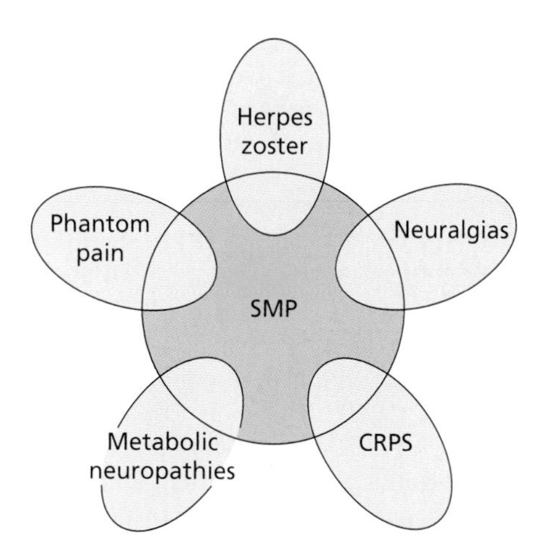

Fig. 18.1 Diagrammatic representation of the relationship of sympathetically maintained pain (SMP) and some painful conditions, demonstrating the existence of SMP in these conditions. (Reproduced from Boas 1996 with permission.)

in the diagnostic criteria for either type of CRPS. A useful algorithm for the diagnosis of CRPS is shown in Box 18.4.

Indicence and natural history of complex regional pain syndrome

One of the problems with the current defining diagnostic criteria for CRPS of both types is establishing the limits of the diagnosis. When is pain judged to be disproportionate in severity, distribution, and duration to the initiating event? Furthermore, some degree of oedema or vasomotor or sudomotor change following many injuries is extremely common. At what stage can these changes be said to be excessive and indicative of the development of CRPS? These uncertainties, together with the fact that there are very few prospective studies, limit conclusions about incidence and natural history.

In a prospective study of 274 patients with Colles fractures of varying severity, Bickerstaff and Kanis (1994) measured tenderness of the fingers, hand swelling, and grip strength, together with symptomatic assessment of pain, vasomotor symptoms, and finger stiffness at intervals up to 1 year following the fracture. At 2 weeks following removal of the plaster cast, 54% had one of the measured features, swelling being the most common (45%). However, only 28% had all four features (bone tenderness, vasomotor symptoms, swelling, and stiffness). These patients were more likely to complain of pain in the hand or shoulder and had a more markedly impaired grip strength. At 1 year 18, 14, and 12% still had finger tenderness, pain, and swelling respectively, and these features were usually found in the same patients. Some 50% of patients still had finger stiffness. These authors' conclusion that each of these symptoms indicated the presence of algodystrophy is at variance with the new diagnostic criteria for CRPS (Stanton-Hicks et al 1995), and it would not be accepted that about 20% of their patients had developed CRPS at 1 year. However, the study of Bickerstaff and Kanis (1994) does indicate that careful prospective study, following a common fracture usually considered to be associated with excellent recovery, presents a truer picture and draws attention to the underestimation of continuing painful symptoms. Prospective study has yielded similar results in other conditions potentially giving rise to chronic painful symptoms, for example amputation (Carlen et al 1978).

Other estimates for the incidence of CRPS, not from prospective studies, include 1–2% after fractures

BOX 18.4
Algorithm for the diagnosis of complex regional pain syndrome (Reproduced from Wilson et al 1996)

Pain
The diagnosis of CRPS cannot be made in the absence of pain; it is a pain syndrome. However, the characteristics of the pain may vary with the initiating event and other factors. The pain is often described as burning, and might be spontaneous or evoked in the context of hyperalgesia or allodynia. Both spontaneous and evoked pain may occur together.

History
- Develops after an initiating noxious event or immobilization
- Unilateral extremity onset (rarely may spread to another extremity)
- Symptom onset usually within a month

Exclusion criteria:
- Identifiable major nerve lesion (CRPS II)
- Existence of anatomical, physiological, or psychological conditions that would otherwise account for the degree of pain and dysfunction

Symptoms (patient report)
A. Pain (spontaneous or evoked)
   Burning
   Aching, throbbing
B. Hyperalgesia or allodynia (at some time in the disease course) to mechanical stimuli (light touch or deep pressure), to thermal stimulation, or to joint motion
C. Associated symptoms (minor)
   Swelling
   Temperature or colour: asymmetry and instability
   Sweating: asymmetry and instability
   Trophic changes: hair, nails, skin

Signs (observed)
Hyperalgesia or allodynia (light touch, deep pressure, joint movement, cold)
Oedema (if unilateral and other causes excluded)
Vasomotor changes: colour, temperature instability, asymmetry
Sudomotor changes
Trophic changes in skin, joint, nail, hair
Impaired motor function (may include components of dystonia and tremor)
Criteria required for diagnosis of CRPS I

History of pain:
- Plus allodynia, hyperalgesia, or hyperaesthesia
- Plus two other signs from the above list

Characteristics of spontaneous pain:
Sympathetically maintained pain (SMP)
Sympathetically independent pain (SIP)
Combined SMP + SIP

(Bohm 1985), 1–5% after peripheral nerve injury (Veldman et al 1993), and the shoulder–hand syndrome in 5% of patients with myocardial infarction (Rosen and Graham 1957).

Pathophysiology of complex regional pain syndrome

Animal and human investigations into the underlying mechanisms of CRPS have focused on three areas: firstly, evidence of abnormal coupling between the efferent sympathetic nervous system and sensory afferents; secondly, the nature and importance of inflammatory processes in peripheral tissues, both with and without nerve injury; and, thirdly, the development of secondary central changes, explaining the wide radiation of the clinical features of CRPS and the maintenance of the syndrome long after the initiating cause has healed or been removed. While it is not yet possible to build a complete picture of pathophysiology and still less possible to translate this into effective treatment, several lines of investigations have provided important insights.

The sympathetic nervous system and pain: nerve damage

Three sites of sympathetic sensory interaction after nerve injury have been identified: the region of the nerve damage itself, undamaged fibres distal to the nerve lesion, and the dorsal root ganglion.

Following severe injury, for example nerve section with neuroma formation, somatosensory fibres develop an abnormal sensitivity to catecholamines, an effect mediated by α receptors. Both circulating catecholamines and endogenously released transmitter following sympathetic trunk stimulation can be shown to stimulate damaged sprouting sensory fibres. This also occurs when continuity of the nerve is restored by resuture following nerve section and other, milder forms of nerve injury (Shyu et al 1990, Sato and Perl 1991). The noradrenergic sensitivity can be reduced by sympathectomy, phentolamine, or guanethidine (Kim et al 1993). All classes of afferent fibre, from both skin and deep tissue, including C fibres, are affected (Janig 1996, Devor and Seltzer 1999).

The normal spontaneous discharge of dorsal root ganglion neurons is enhanced by peripheral nerve injury (Kirk 1974, Wall and Devor 1983), and this may be further increased by sympathetic stimulation (Devor et al 1994). However, subsequent studies have indicated that this sympathetic sensory coupling occurs mainly in non-nociceptive afferents and is present only transiently following nerve injury. Furthermore, at later intervals, sympathetic stimulation may exert an inhibitory effect on dorsal root ganglion neuron activity (Michaelis et al 1996).

There are limited but important human investigations that indicate a sympathetic influence on pain following peripheral nerve injury. Walker and Nulsen (1948) showed that intraoperative sympathetic chain stimulation exacerbated pain in patients with causalgia. In patients with successfully treated causalgia, Wallin et al (1976) found that the patient's original pain could be rekindled by cutaneous application of noradrenaline (norepinephrine). Injection of noradrenaline (norepinephrine) around amputation stump neuromas may cause severe pain (Chabal et al 1992).

In the investigation of Torebjork et al (1995) some of the patients examined in the earlier study of Wallin et al (1976), and who at that time had SMP, were found at the later examination to have pain that did not respond to sympathetic blockade. In addition, only 28% of patients with nerve injury and pain previously responsive to sympathetic blockade (SMP) experienced an increase in their pain when noradrenaline (norepinephrine) was injected into their sensitive skin. This indicates changing pathophysiology in CRPS over long periods of time, presenting further difficulties in targeting treatments.

In a clinical condition that may be likened to experimental situations in which partly damaged regenerated or undamaged afferents in partial nerve injury become sensitive to catecholamines, Choi and Rowbotham (1997) showed that intracutaneous injections of noradrenaline (norepinephrine) or adrenaline (epinephrine) in an area affected by postherpetic neuralgia increased both spontaneous pain and allodynia.

The sympathetic nervous system and pain: without nerve damage

Investigation of possible sympathetic influences on painful sensation without nerve injury, in other words, in conditions more representative of the clinical situations in which CRPS type I may develop, has been more recent than the studies of nerve injury. The complex mechanisms underlying the development of spontaneous pain, hyperalgesia, and allodynia to various types of stimulation following experimental heat and chemically induced cutaneous inflammation using irritants such as mustard oil and capsaicin are summarized by

Koltzenburg (1996). Both peripheral and central factors are involved. Some components of experimental cutaneous inflammation have been shown to be influenced by noradrenergic α-receptor agonists or antagonists. Drummond (1995) reported an increase in heat-induced hyperalgesia in skin inflamed by topical capsaicin after iontophoresis of noradrenaline (norepinephrine). In inflammation produced by intradermal capsaicin, Kinman et al (1997) showed that spontaneous pain could be reduced by locally injected phentolamine, although evoked pain in capsaicin-induced inflammation was not reduced by intravenous phentolamine in the experiments of Liu et al (1996).

It might be argued that the demonstrated sympathetic influence occurred as a secondary effect of altered local blood supply in the area of inflammation. However, in a microneurographic study, Elam et al (1996) found that the discharge from axons sensitized by cutaneous application of mustard oil was not influenced by physiological reflex alterations of sympathetic vasoconstrictor neurons. In addition, Baron et al (1998) have reported that cutaneous sympathetic vasoconstrictor activity does not alter the intensity of ongoing pain induced by capsaicin inflammation.

The sensitization of somatosensory afferents may be caused by direct stimulation by noradrenaline (norepinephrine) or indirectly through release of inflammatory substances, particularly prostaglandins. Levine and others have shown that in certain experimental situations, noradrenaline (norepinephrine) released from sympathetic postganglionic neurons causes release of prostaglandins (Levine et al 1986, Gold et al 1994). In an experimental sciatic neuropathy in rats, Tracey et al (1995) found hyperalgesia was enhanced by local injection of noradrenaline (norepinephrine) and decreased by injection of indometacin, strongly suggesting mediation of the hyperalgesia by prostaglandins and possibly other inflammatory substances.

Pain in CRPS related to inflammation and independent of the sympathetic nervous system

The experimental animal and human evidence outlined above would appear to indicate an important adrenergic sympathetic postganglionic influence in the processes that may lead to pain, both with and without nerve injury. The singular lack of long-term effectiveness of sympathetic blockade and sympathectomy in clinical practice in CRPS, both type I and type II in the majority of patients, has led some to question the existence of any significant sympathetic involvement in CRPS or indeed any type of pain syndrome. Arguments are based on the poor quality of clinical investigations, including lack of proper controls and the questionable relevance of animal models to the human situation, together with possible underestimation of psychological factors (Ochoa and Verdugo 1995; Schott 1995, 1997). Schott (1995, 1997) proposes a mechanism for the analgesic effect of sympathetic blockade that does not depend on a reduction of peripheral noradrenergic activity. He suggests that pain relief after sympathectomy may be explained by a reduction of activity of visceral afferent fibres that travel in sympathetic nerves (Cervero 1994, Schott 1994), rather than any peripheral effect on efferent noradrenergic function.

Schott (1995) proposes inflammatory mechanisms that are independent of noradrenergic efferent function as the cause of pain in CRPS (Dray 1996). In a subsequent paper Schott (1997) draws attention to the evidence indicating an inflammatory basis for the bone atrophy that occurs in CRPS, leading in its extreme form to Sudeck's atrophy. This evidence is reviewed by Kozin (1992) and Oyen et al (1993). Treatments, including calcitonin to reverse the marked osteopenia that may occur in CRPS, have been advocated in the past but without adequate controlled trials. Interest recently has focused on the bisphosphonates, which prevent bone resorption by inhibiting osteoclast activity and dissolution of calcium apatite crystals. However, this property of biphosphonates is unlikely to explain the very rapid relief of bone pain that has been observed in bone pain due to cancer, and it is possible that additional effects of bisphosphonates on prostaglandin E2 and other inflammatory mediators may be responsible for analgesia (Strang 1996). Further investigation may clarify the mechanisms of bone atrophy in CRPS and possibly atrophic changes in other tissues, which are frequent features of CRPS.

Histopathological studies in limbs amputated in patients with CRPS have shown microangiopathic changes, leading to the suggestion that free radical damage may be an important component of the pathogenesis of the condition (van der Laan et al 1998).

Relevant to the issue of visceral and somatic afferents in sympathetic nerves, Kramis et al (1996) review a curious but well-recognized consequence of sympathetic chain interruption, the development of a new pain that occurs days to weeks after sympathectomy, and propose mechanisms for such pain. This so-called sympathalgia, or postsympathectomy pain, tends to be distributed in the proximal parts of the sympathectomized limb and extends onto the trunk. Distally in the limb there is usually evidence of sympathetic denervation, but proximally there may be excessive sweating and other features include deep muscular tenderness and proximal cutaneous allodynia and hyperalgesia (Raskin et al 1974). The incidence of postsympathectomy pain following sympathetic trunk lesioning, but not after local anaesthetic block or more distal sympathetic nerve blockade with either local anaesthetic or guanethidine, is estimated to occur in 30–50% of patients, although it is not usually severe. Kramis et al (1996) propose that postsympathectomy pain develops as a result of transection of paraspinal somatic and visceral afferents travelling within the sympathetic trunk, and that this in turn leads to cell death of many of the axotomized neurons, causing central deafferentation. Pain related to the deafferentation may be worse as a result of prior sensitization of dorsal horn cells produced by the painful state for which the sympathectomy was performed.

Central nervous system changes

Central nervous system physiological changes secondary to nerve injury are reviewed in Chap. 17. There is evidence indicating that prolonged nociceptive inputs, not resulting from nerve injury, are capable of inducing similar secondary central changes (Doubell et al 1999).

Such changes may clearly be important in relation to the pain of CRPS.

Summary of mechanisms in CRPS

The pathophysiology of pain and other clinical features in CRPS remains poorly understood, and although experimental studies outlined here represent a considerable advance in knowledge, we are still some way from a clear understanding of these conditions. The diagrammatic representation in Fig. 18.2 sets out some components of CRPS currently thought to be of importance in pathogenesis. The basic concept of a vicious circle, first proposed by Livingston (1943), remains evident. The importance of the sympathetic nervous system

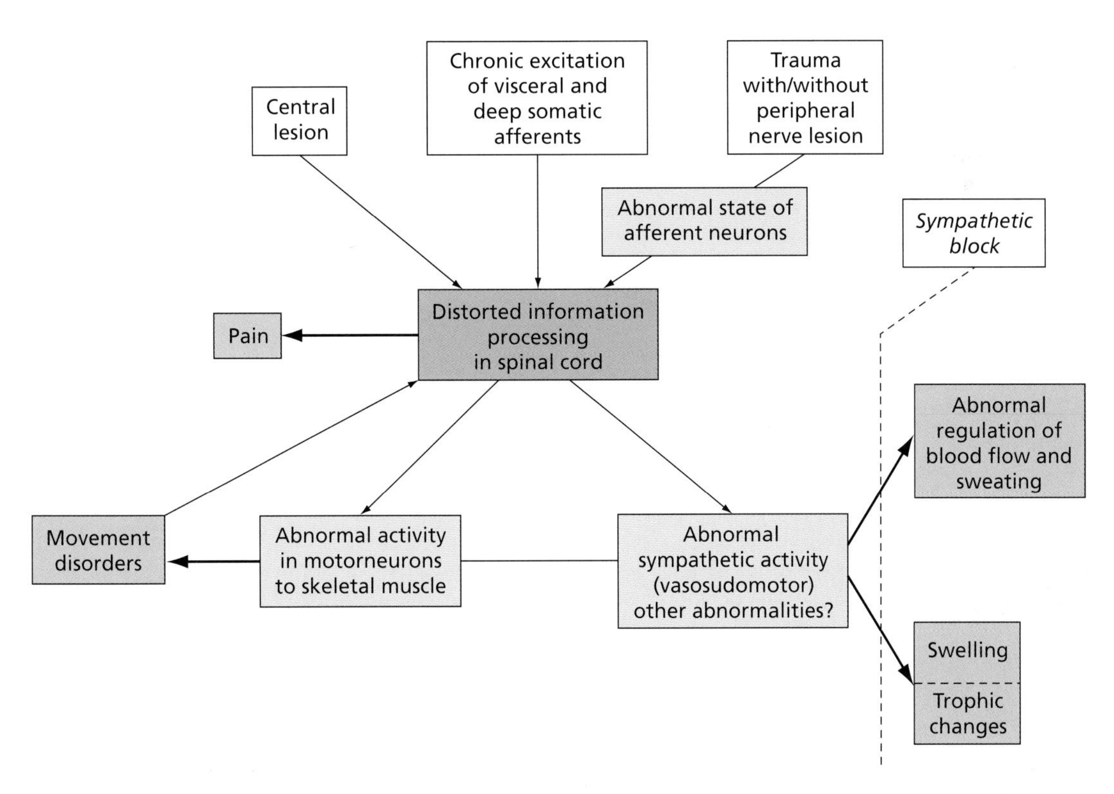

Fig. 18.2 Relationship of various peripheral and central factors important in the mechanisms of pain and other clinical features of CRPS types I and II. See text for further explanation. (Reproduced from Janig 1996 with permission.)

may be overrated, and that of chronic inflammatory changes in deeper tissues underestimated, in the scheme presented. The potential for some central changes to become permanent, and thus possibly limit the effectiveness of any treatment directed towards the initiating peripheral event, is not shown in Fig. 18.2. These factors, together with further knowledge of the somatic and visceral sensory sympathetic coupling in peripheral tissues, require elucidation through further research.

Treatment of complex regional pain syndrome

Few conditions can match CRPS types I and II for the variety of treatment modalities and drugs suggested—a sure indication that no single treatment is superior to others and that nothing is consistently successful. Controlled trials have been few and comparisons of treatments in different reports are made difficult by patient populations heterogeneous in causation, clinical features, and severity. This is not surprising in a condition that has proved so difficult to define and whose limits, even with the now generally accepted definition provided by the IASP consensus conference, are uncertain. The older term, RSD, has focused undue attention upon sympatholytic procedures to the exclusion of consideration of other treatments, although this is now changing. The research on mechanisms of CRPS types I and II is recent, particularly for type I, and many treatments suggested have previously been based on ideas and speculation rather than fact. This state of affairs is now set to change. Controlled trials of treatment in CRPS are reviewed by Kingery (1997) and Perez et al (2001).

Does early treatment improve outcome

It has long been accepted that early recognition and institution of active treatment improves the outcome in CRPS. While this seems intuitively correct, it has never been subjected to systematic study. Clearly, the management of injuries and diseases known to have the potential of leading to the development of CRPS should be optimally managed in the acute stages, but again there is no evidence that it is only badly managed patients who are prone to develop CRPS. However, immobilization and disuse are undoubtedly factors that contribute to the development of CRPS, and it makes sense to minimize these factors by instituting physiotherapy at an early stage after injury.

This raises an important point about the aims of treatment in established cases of CRPS. It is always gratifying, both to patient and clinician, to obtain analgesia by whatever means, but pain relief alone is insufficient. A hallmark of CRPS is loss of function of the affected part, and every period of even partial analgesia should be utilized to begin mobilization and rehabilitation. This emphasizes the importance of a multidisciplinary approach to treatment.

Sympatholytic procedures

Intravenous regional guanethidine blocks

Guanethidine reduces noradrenaline (norepinephrine) concentrations in adrenergic neurons and blocks reuptake. The technique of intravenous regional guanethidine block (IVRGB) described by Hannington-Kiff (1974) quickly became established as a simple and reliable method of peripheral sympathetic blockade and is now widely used. The treatment has, however, only been subject to controlled study in recent years. In open studies it has been common experience that some patients respond, usually transiently, for hours or days, but many patients do not and some patients report a transient increase in pain following IVRGB. Multiple blocks over a period of time have been advocated in the hope of producing a cumulative effect (Girgis and Wynn Parry 1989).

Two recent studies of IVRGB have been helpful in evaluating the treatment in patients with CRPS. Many other studies have used patients with a number of painful conditions and the results are difficult to assess. Jadad et al (1995) reviewed seven randomized controlled trials from the literature. In most of these guanethidine was used, but reserpine, bretylium, droperidol, and ketanserin were used in some as alternatives. In the four guanethidine studies, none demonstrated a difference in analgesia between guanethidine and control, and none of the studies was designed to determine a dose–response effect. Jadad et al (1995) criticized the methodology of these investigations, with problems identified including poor defined diagnostic criteria, inadequate wash-out periods, an incomplete cross-over, open administration of some treatments, and a high proportion of withdrawals. In a subsequent controlled trial, Jadad et al (1995) recruited patients with CRPS who had reported analgesia following an open trial of IVRGB. Nine patients completed the trial and no significant difference was shown between guanethidine and saline control (lidocaine (lignocaine) was not used in this study).

Ramamurthy and Hoffman (1995) randomized 60 patients to receive up to four IVRGBs with lidocaine (lignocaine), control injections being lidocaine (lignocaine) and saline. Although there was no difference between guanethidine- and control-treated patients, patients in all treatment groups showed a decrease in oedema and pseudomotor, trophic, and vasomotor changes. All patients had at least one IVRGB and those receiving up to four blocks gained no greater degree of pain relief. Campbell et al (1988) investigated the effects of a tourniquet inflated to suprasystolic pressure as used in IVRGB. Hyperalgesia was relieved but temperature sensation was not affected. It was suggested that hyperalgesia was mediated via Aβ-mechanoreceptor fibres, these being most susceptible to pressure block.

Sympathetic ganglion block

Local anaesthetic stellate ganglion or lumbar chain blocks have been much used in the treatment of CRPS but no adequately controlled study has been done, and indeed would be difficult to do. Aggressive early treatment has often been suggested (Wang et al 1985, Bonica 1990) but without clear supporting evidence. Kozin (1992) analysed reports in seven studies of sympathetic blocks in more than 500 patients and concluded that 46% of patients had significant prolonged analgesia. Again, these were uncontrolled observations. Wang et al (1985) compared 71 patients with CRPS treated over a 3-year period. Twenty-seven patients did not receive sympathetic blocks and 43 patients did. At 3 years 41 and 65%, respectively, had improved, suggesting some effect from the treatment.

In patients with early CRPS associated with severe limb swelling, sympathetic blocks may dramatically reduce swelling and produce pain relief. It is suggested that this is due to interruption of vasoconstrictor activity with opening of venules (Blumberg and Janig 1994).

The intravenous phentolamine test has been advocated as a test to assess the likely efficacy of subsequent sympathetic blocks (Arner 1991). Patients who may obtain pain relief with IVRGB or sympathetic ganglion block may not respond to phentolamine due to the less complete α-noradrenergic receptor blockade achievable with systemic rather than local administration. The phentolamine test is widely used in many centres to identify those likely to respond to more prolonged local sympathetic blockade.

Sympathectomy

Surgical, chemical, or radiofrequency sympathectomy may produce good short-term results but long-term pain relief is poor (Tasker 1990, Rocco 1995), leading most to abandon these procedures. The problems of sympathalgia following sympathectomy have already been discussed.

Other drugs used in regional blocks

Ketanserin, a selective serotonin type II receptor blocker, and bretylium, which reduces release of noradrenaline (norepinephrine), have both been given by the Biers block technique and in controlled trials have been found to be analgesic in CRPS (Ford et al 1988, Hanna and Peat 1989). Clonidine was not effective by the same root (Glynn and Jones 1990). The non-steroidal anti-inflammatory drug ketorolac, which reduces prostaglandin release, has been reported to be effective in a small group of patients with CRPS, of interest in relation to pathophysiology (Vanos et al 1992).

Calcitonin and corticosteroids

Evidence for an analgesic effect of calcitonin and corticosteroids in CRPS is conflicting, but in controlled trials, a therapeutic effect for calcitonin (Gobelet et al 1992) and for corticosteroid (Christensen et al 1982) has been reported.

Epidural and intrathecal drugs

The role of long-term administration of drugs by the epidural or intrathecal root is uncertain. When CRPS involves the lower limb opiates, with or without local anaesthetic, will produce partial analgesia, although often at the cost of impaired bladder and bowel sphincter function and some degree of weakness. In patients with severe allodynia and hyperalgesia, short-term percutaneous infusions for 1–2 weeks may help by allowing weight bearing on a previously useless leg and the start of rehabilitation. Long-term intrathecal morphine has been reported to produce useful analgesia in CRPS (Becker et al 1995).

Clonidine, an alpha-2 receptor agonist given epidurally, has been reported to relieve pain in CRPS affecting both upper and lower limbs over long periods (Rauck et al 1993, Walker and Cousins 1997). Given orally, clonidine is limited by adverse effects and does not produce analgesia in CRPS (Walker and Cousins 1997).

Oral drugs

Numerous drugs have been tried in CRPS by the oral route. Many patients report analgesic effects from simple analgesics, codeine, and non-steroidal anti-inflammatory drugs, and continue to take these drugs in the absence of more effective treatment. No controlled trials substantiate the effectiveness of these drugs in CRPS. Of the anticonvulsant drugs, recent interest has focused on gabapentin, which is reported to help in CRPS, but again controlled trials are awaited (Mellick and Mellick 1997). Other reports of benefit in uncontrolled studies include phenoxybenzamine (Ghostine et al 1984, Muizelaar et al 1997), tricyclic antidepressants (Wilder et al 1992), phenytoin (Chaturvedi 1989), and nifedipine (Prough et al 1985, Muizelaar et al 1997). Biphosphonates via the intravenous route have been reported to relieve pain in CRPS in open label studies (Adami et al 1997, Cortet et al 1997). Trials with oral bisphosphonates are awaited.

Transcutaneous and dorsal column stimulation

Transcutaneous electrical nerve stimulation has been reported to be beneficial in children with CRPS (Wilder et al 1992) but not in adults. Dorsal column stimulation may be helpful (Law 1993).

Psychological measures and rehabilitation

As in all chronic pain syndromes, psychological interventions may have a vital part to play in treatment. Fear, anxiety, depression, loss of function, job, and income, and domestic and marital stresses may all take their toll in CRPS. Many patients find psychological management extremely helpful, particularly when, as is often the case, physical treatments fail. Efforts to rehabilitate the patient as far as is possible should be initiated at an early stage and pursued with vigour. The role of straightforward support for these unfortunate patients cannot be overemphasized. Patients with established CRPS should always be referred to a centre where a multidisciplinary programme of pain management is available.

References

Adami S, Fossaluzza V, Gatti D, Fracassi E, Braga V 1997 Biphosphonate therapy of reflex sympathetic dystrophy syndrome. Annals of the Rheumatic Disease 56: 201–204

Arner S 1991 Intravenous phentolamine test: diagnostic and prognostic use in reflex sympathetic dystrophy. Pain 46: 17–22

Baron R, Wasner GL, Borgstedt R 1998 Interaction of sympathetic nerve activity and capsaicin evoked spontaneous pain and vasodilatation in humans. Neurology 50: 45

Becker WJ, Ablett DP, Harris CJ, Dold ON 1995 Long term treatment of intractable reflex sympathetic dystrophy with intrathecal morphine. Canadian Journal of Neurological Sciences 22: 153–159

Bentley JB, Hameroff SR 1980 Diffuse reflex sympathetic dystrophy. Anaesthesiology 53: 256–257

Bickerstaff DR, Kanis JA 1994 Algodystrophy: an under-recognised complication of minor trauma. British Journal of Rheumatology 33: 240–248

Blumberg H, Janig W 1994 Clinical manifestation of reflex sympathetic dystrophy and sympathetically maintained pain. In: Wall PD, Melzack R (eds) Textbook of pain, 3rd edn. Churchill Livingstone, Edinburgh, pp 685–698

Boas RA 1996 Complex regional pain syndromes: symptoms, signs, and differential diagnosis. In: Janig W, Stanton-Hicks M (eds) Reflex sympathetic dystrophy: a reappraisal. Progress in pain research and management, vol 6. IASP, Seattle, pp 79–92

Bohm E 1985 Das Sudecksche Syndrom. Hefte zur Unfallheilkunde 174: 241–250

Bonica JJ 1979 Causalgia and other reflex sympathetic dystrophies. In: Bonica JJ, Liebeskind JC, Albe-Fessard DG (eds) Proceedings of the Second World Congress on Pain. Advances in pain research and therapy, vol 3. Raven, New York, pp 141–166

Bonica JJ 1990 Causalgia and other reflex sympathetic dystrophies. In: Bonica JJ (ed) The management of pain, 2nd edn. Lea and Febriger, Philadelphia, pp 230–243

Campbell JN, Raja SN, Meyer RA, Mackinnon SE 1988 Myelinated afferents signal the hyperalgesia associated with nerve injury. Pain 32: 89–94

Carlen PL, Wall PD, Nadvorna H, Steinbach T 1978 Phantom limbs and related phenomena in recent traumatic amputations. Neurology 28: 211–217

Cervero F 1994 Sensory innervation of the viscera: peripheral basis of visceral pain. Physiological Reviews 74: 95–138

Chabal C, Jacobson L, Russell LC, Burchiel KJ 1992 Pain response to perineuronal injection of normal saline, epinephrine, and lidocaine in humans. Pain 49: 9–12

Chaturvedi SK 1989 Phenytoin in reflex sympathetic dystrophy. Pain 36: 379–380

Choi B, Rowbotham MC 1997 Effects of adrenergic receptor activation on post-herpetic neuralgia pain and sensory disturbances. Pain 69: 55–63

Christensen K, Jensen EM, Noer I 1982 The reflex sympathetic dystrophy syndrome response to treatment with systemic corticosteroids. Acta Chirurgica Scandinavica 148: 653–655

Cortet B, Flipo R-M, Coquerelle P, Duquesnoy B, Delcambre B 1997 Treatment of severe, recalcitrant reflex sympathetic dystrophy: assessment of efficacy and safety of the second generation biphosphonate pamidronate. Clinical Rheumatology 16: 51–56

Covington EC 1996 Psychological issues in reflex sympathetic dystrophy. In: Janig W, Stanton-Hicks M (eds) Reflex sympathetic dystrophy: a reappraisal. Progress in pain research and management, vol 6. IASP, Seattle, pp 191–216

Devor M, Seltzer Z 1999 Pathophysiology of damaged nerves in relation to chronic pain. In: Wall PD, Melzack R (eds) Textbook of pain, 4th edn. Churchill Livingstone, Edinburgh, pp 129–164

Devor M, Janig W, Michaelis M 1994 Modulation of activity in dorsal root ganglion neurons by sympathetic activation in nerve-injured rats. Journal of Neurophysiology 71: 38–47

Doubell TP, Mannion RJ, Woolf CJ 1999 The dorsal horn: state-dependent sensory processing, plasticity and the generation of pain. In: Wall PD, Melzack R (eds) Textbook of pain, 4th edn. Churchill Livingstone, Edinburgh, pp 165–182

Dray A 1996 Neurogenic mechanisms and neuropeptides in chronic pain. Progress in Brain Research 110: 85–94

Drummond PD 1995 Noradrenaline increases hyperalgesia to heat in skin sensitised by capsaicin. Pain 60: 311–315

Elam M, Skarphedinsson JO, Olhausson B, Wallin BG 1996 No apparent modulation of single C-fiber afferent transmission in

human volunteers. In: Abstract of the 8th World Congress on Pain. IASP, Seattle, p 398
Evans JA 1946 Reflex sympathetic dystrophy. Surgery, Gynecology and Obstetrics 82: 36–43
Ford SR, Forrest WH, Eltherington L 1988 The treatment of reflex sympathetic dystrophy with intravenous regional bretylium. Anesthesiology 68: 137–140
Ghostine SY, Comair YG, Turner DM, Kassell NF, Azar CG 1984 Phenoxybenzamine in the treatment of causalgia. Journal of Neurosurgery 60: 1263–1268
Girgis FL, Wynn Parry CB 1989 Management of causalgia after peripheral nerve injury. International Disability Studies 11: 15–20
Glynn CJ, Jones PC 1990 An investigation of the role of clonidine in the treatment of reflex sympathetic dystrophy. In: Stanton-Hicks, M, Janig W, Boas RA (eds) Reflex sympathetic dystrophy. Kluwer Academic, Norwell, MA, pp 187–196
Gobelet C, Waldburger M, Meir JL 1992 The effect of adding calcitonin to physical treatment of reflex sympathetic dystrophy. Pain 48: 171–175
Gold MS, White DM, Ahlgeru SC, Guo M, Levine JD 1994 Catecholamine-induced mechanical sensitisation of cutaneous nociceptors in the rat. Neuroscience Letters 175: 166–170
Goldsmith DP, Vivino FB, Eichenfield AH, Athreya BH, Heyman S 1989 Nuclear imaging and clinical features of childhood reflex neurovascular dystrophy: comparison with adults. Arthritis and Rheumatism 32: 480–485
Hanna MH, Peat SJ 1989 Ketanserin in reflex sympathetic dystrophy. A double blind placebo controlled cross-over trial. Pain 38: 145–150
Hannington-Kiff JG 1974 Intravenous regional sympathetic block with guanethidine. Lancet i: 1019–1020
Jadad AR, Carroll D, Glynn CJ, McQuay HJ 1995 Intravenous regional sympathetic blockade for pain relief in reflex sympathetic dystrophy: a systematic review and a randomised, double-blind crossover study. Journal of Pain and Symptom Management 10: 13–20
Janig W 1996 The puzzle of 'reflex sympathetic dystrophy' mechanisms, hypotheses, open questions. In: Janig W, Stanton-Hicks M (eds) Reflex sympathetic dystrophy: a reappraisal. Progress in Pain Research and Management, vol 6. IASP, Seattle, pp 1–24
Johnson AC 1943 Disabling changes in the hands resembling sclerodactylia following myocardial infarctions. Annals of Internal Medicine 19: 433–456
Kim SH, Na HS, Sheen K, Chung JM 1993 Effects of sympathectomy on a rat model of peripheral neuropathy. Pain 55: 85–92
Kingery WS 1997 A critical review of controlled clinical trials for peripheral neuropathic pain and complex regional pain syndromes. Pain 73: 123–139
Kinman E, Nygards EB, Hausson P 1997 Peripheral alpha-adrenoreceptors are involved in the development of capsaicin induced ongoing and stimulus evoked pain in humans. Pain 69: 79–85
Kirk EJ 1974 Impulses in dorsal spinal nerve rootlets in cats and rabbits arising from dorsal root ganglia isolated from the periphery. Journal of Comparative Neurology 155: 165–176
Koltzenburg M 1996 Afferent mechanisms mediating pain and hyperalgesias in neuralgia. In: Janig W, Stanton-Hicks M (eds) Reflex sympathetic dystrophy: a reappraisal. Progress in pain research and management, vol 6. IASP, Seattle, pp 123–150
Kozin F 1992 Reflex sympathetic dystrophy: a review. Clinical and Experimental Rheumatology 10: 401–409
Kramis RC, Roberts WJ, Gillette RG 1996 Post-sympathectomy neuralgia: hypotheses on peripheral and central neuronal mechanisms. Pain 64: 1–9
Law JD 1993 Spinal cord stimulation for intractable pain due to reflex sympathetic dystrophy. CNI Review 17–22
Leriche R 1916 De la causalgie envisagee comme au nevrite de sympathique et de son traitement par la denudation et l'excision des plexus nerveax peri-arteriels. Presse Medicin 24: 177–180
Leriche R 1939 The surgery of pain (transl Young A). Baillière, Tindall and Cox, London
Levine JD, Taiwo YO, Collins SD, Tam JK 1986 Noradrenaline hyperalgesia is mediated through interaction with sympathetic postganglionic neurone terminals rather than activation of primary afferent nociceptors. Nature 323: 158–160
Liu M, Max MB, Parada S, Rowan JS, Bennett GJ 1996 The sympathetic nervous system contributes to capsaicin-evoked mechanical allodynia but not pinprick hyperalgesia in humans. Journal of Neuroscience 16: 7331–7335
Livingston WK 1943 Pain mechanisms: a physiological interpretation of causalgia and its related symptoms. Macmillan, London
Loh L, Nathan PW 1978 Painful peripheral states and sympathetic blocks. Journal of Neurology, Neurosurgery and Psychiatry 41: 664–671
Loh L, Nathan PW, Schott GD, Wilson PG 1980 Effects of regional guanethidine infusion in certain pain states. Journal of Neurology, Neurosurgery and Psychiatry 43: 446–451
Mellick GA, Mellick LB 1997 Reflex sympathetic dystrophy treated with gabapentin. Archives of Physical Medicine and Rehabilitation 78: 98–105
Michaelis M, Devor M, Janig W 1996 Sympathetic modulation of activity in dorsal root ganglion neurons changes over time following peripheral nerve injury. Journal of Neurophysiology 76: 753–763
Mitchell SW, Morehouse GR, Keen WW 1864 Gunshot wounds and other injuries of nerves. Lippincott, Philadelphia.
Muizelaar JP, Kleyer M, Hertogs IAM, De Lange DC 1997 Complex regional pain syndrome (reflex sympathetic dystrophy and causalgia): management with the calcium channel blocker nifedipine and/or the alpha-sympathetic blocker phenoxybenzamine in 59 patients. Clinical Neurology and Neurosurgery 99: 26–30
Ochoa JL, Verdugo RJ 1995 Reflex sympathetic dystrophy. A common clinical avenue for somatoform expression. Neurologic Clinics 13: 351–363
Oyen WJM, Arntz IE, Claessens RAMJ, Van der Meer JWM, Corstens FHM, Goris RJA 1993 Reflex sympathetic dystrophy of the hand: an excessive inflammatory response? Pain 55: 151–157
Perez RSGM, Kwakkel G, Zuurmond WWA, de Lange JJ 2001. Treatment of reflex sympathetic dystrophy (CRPS type 1): A research synthesis of 21 randomized clinical trials. Journal of Pain and Symptom Management 21: 511–526
Prough DS, McLeskey CH, Poehling GG et al 1985. Efficacy of oral nifedipine in the treatment of reflex sympathetic dystrophy. Anesthesiology 62: 796–799
Raja SN, Treede RD, Davis KD, Campbell JN 1991 Systemic alpha-adrenergic blockade with phentolamine: a diagnostic test for sympathetically maintained pain. Anesthesiology 74: 691–698
Ramamurthy S, Hoffman J 1995 Intravenous regional guanethidine in the treatment of reflex sympathetic dystrophy/causalgia: a randomised, double-blind study. Anaesthesia and Analgesia 81: 718–723
Raskin NH, Levinson SA, Hoffman PM, Pickett JBE, Fields HL 1974 Post-sympathectomy neuralgia. American Journal of Surgery 128: 75–78
Rauck RL, Eisenach JC, Jackson K, Young LD, Southern J 1993 Epidural clonidine treatment for refractory reflex sympathetic dystrophy. Anesthesiology 79: 1163–1169

Richards RL 1967a Causalgia: a centennial review. Archives of Neurology 16: 339–350
Richards RL 1967b The term 'causalgia'. Medical History 11: 97–99
Rizzi R, Visentin M, Mazzetti G 1984 Reflex sympathetic dystrophy. In: Benedetti C, Chapman CR, Moricca G (eds) Recent advances in the management of pain. Advances in pain research and therapy, vol 7. Raven, New York, pp 451–465
Roberts WJ 1986 A hypothesis on the physiological basis for causalgia and related pains. Pain 24: 297–311
Rocco AG 1995 Radiofrequency lumbar sympatholysis. The evolution of a technique for managing sympathetically maintained pain. Regional Anaesthesia 20: 3–12
Rosen PS, Graham W 1957 The shoulder–hand syndrome: historical review with observations on 73 patients. Canadian Medical Association Journal 77: 86–91
Sato J, Perl ER 1991 Adrenergic excitation of cutaneous pain receptors induced by peripheral nerve injury. Science 251: 1608–1610
Schott GD 1994 Visceral afferents: their contribution to 'sympathetic dependent pain'. Brain 117: 397–413
Schott GD 1995 An unsympathetic view of pain. Lancet 345: 634–636
Schott GD 1997 Biphosphonates for pain relief in reflex sympathetic dystrophy. Lancet 350: 1117
Schwartzman RJ, McLellan TL 1987 Reflex sympathetic dystrophy: a review. Archives of Neurology 44: 555–561
Sherry DD, Weisman R 1988 Psychologic aspects of childhood reflex neurovascular dystrophy. Pediatrics 81: 572–578
Shir Y, Seltzer Z 1991 Effects of sympathectomy in a model of causalgiform pain produced by partial sciatic nerve injury in rats. Pain 45: 309–320
Shyu BC, Danielsen N, Andersson SA, Dahlin LB 1990 Effects of sympathetic stimulation on C-fibre response after peripheral nerve compression: an experimental study in the rabbit common peroneal nerve. Acta Physiologica Scandinavica 140: 237–243
Stanton-Hicks M, Janig W, Hassenbusch S, Haddox JD, Boas R, Wilson P 1995 Reflex sympathetic dystrophy: changing concepts and taxonomy. Pain 63: 127–133
Strang P 1996 Analgesic effect of biphosphonates on bone pain in breast cancer patients. Acta Oncologica 35 (Suppl): 50–54
Tasker RR 1990 Reflex sympathetic dystrophy – neurosurgical approaches. In: Stanton-Hicks M, Janig W, Boas RA (eds) Reflex sympathetic dystrophy. Kluwer Academic, Norwell, MA, pp 125–134
Torebjork HE, Wahren LK, Wallin BG, Hallin RG, Koltzenburg M 1995 Noradrenaline-evoked pain in neuralgia. Pain 63: 11–20
Tracey DJ, Cunningham JE, Romm MA 1995 Peripheral hyperalgesia in experimental neuropathy: mediation by alpha-2 adreno-receptors on post-ganglionic sympathetic terminals. Pain 60: 317–327
van der Laan L, ter Laak HJ, Gabreels-Festen A, Gabreels F, Goris RJA 1998 Complex regional pain syndrome type 1 (RSD). Pathology of skeletal muscle and peripheral nerve. Neurology 51: 20–25
Vanos DN, Ramamurthy S, Hoffman J 1992 Intravenous regional block using ketorolac: preliminary results in the treatment of reflex sympathetic dystrophy. Anesthesia and Analgesia 74: 139–141
Veldman PJHM, Reynen HM, Arntz IE, Goris JA 1993 Signs and symptoms of reflex sympathetic dystrophy: prospective study of 829 patients. Lancet 342: 1012–1016
Wahren LK, Torebjork HE, Nystrom B 1991 Quantitative sensory testing before and after regional guanethidine block in patients with neuralgia in the hand. Pain 46: 23–30
Walker AE, Nulsen F 1948 Electrical stimulation of the upper thoracic portion of the sympathetic chain in man. Archives of Neurology and Psychiatry 59: 559–560
Walker SM, Cousins MJ 1997 Complex regional pain syndromes: including 'reflex sympathetic dystrophy' and 'causalgia'. Anaesthesia and Intensive Care 25: 113–125
Wall PD 1995 Noradrenaline-evoked pain in neuralgia. Pain 63: 1–2
Wall PD, Devor M 1983 Sensory afferent impulses from dorsal root ganglia. Pain 17: 321–339
Wallin BG, Torebjork HE, Hallin RG 1976 Preliminary observations on the pathophysiology of hyperalgesia in the causalgic pain symdrome. In: Zolterman Y (ed) Sensory functions of the skin in primates. Pergamon, Oxford, pp 489–499
Wang JK, Johnson KA, Ilstrap DM 1985 Sympathetic blocks for reflex sympathetic dystrophy. Pain 23: 13–17
Wilder RT 1996 Reflex sympathetic dystrophy in children and adolescents: differences from adults. In: Janig W, Stanton-Hicks M (eds) Reflex sympathetic dystrophy: A reappraisal. Progress in pain research and management, vol 6. IASP, Seattle, pp 67–77
Wilder RT, Berde CB, Wolohan M, Vieyra MA, Masele BJ, Michell LJ 1992 Reflex sympathetic dystrophy in children. Clinical characteristics and follow-up of seventy patients. Journal of Bone and Joint Surgery 74(A): 910–919
Wilson PR, Low PA, Bedder MD, Covington EC, Rauck RL 1996 Diagnostic algorithm for complex regional pain syndromes. In: Janig W, Stanton-Hicks M (eds) Reflex sympathetic dystrophy: a reappraisal. Progress in pain research and management, vol 6. IASP, Seattle, pp 93–106

Chapter 19

Nerve root disorders and arachnoiditis

David Dubuisson

This chapter reviews painful conditions of the spinal and lower cranial nerve roots (Table 19.1). Some of these conditions may be self-limited, responsive to medications and physical treatment modalities, or curable by surgical decompression. Others, such as chronic postoperative nerve root damage with epidural fibrosis and arachnoiditis, rank among the most refractory causes of severe chronic pain. Few generalities apply to pain of root damage. Lesions of single roots are usually of recent onset in young individuals, while multiradicular syndromes are apt to be of chronic duration in an older age group. Pain of individual root origin is often due to benign mechanical lesions which compress or distort. Pain of multiradicular origin suggests a diffuse degenerative, neoplastic, or inflammatory cause, frequently intradural. In general, pain due to mechanical distortion of a single root is more amenable to surgery than is pain of multiple-root damage.

Pain is not the only issue of clinical importance in nerve root disorders. Root compression and injury can lead to muscle weakness, loss of sensation, gait disorder, restriction of motion, or occasionally loss of bowel and bladder control. In individual patients, the extent of these deficits does not necessarily parallel the severity of pain and disability. The neurological examination should be carefully documented and followed, because progression of neurological damage may sometimes require surgery even at a time when pain is resolving.

The essential quality of pain associated with nerve root damage is referral along the peripheral distribution of fibres in the root. In many cases but not in all, this follows one of the dermatomes (skin sensory territories of nerve roots) down the arm or leg or around the trunk. Dermatomes are certainly not constant from individual to individual. Moreover, no two dermatomal charts agree in all details. Lack of agreement of dermatomal charts is due to the wide variety of clinical and experimental observations that have been used to compile these charts. Unfortunately, commercially available dermatome charts that are so common in clinics tend to be oversimplified and sometimes frankly misleading. Studies by Sherrington (1898) in monkeys and by Foerster (1933) in humans made it clear that extensive overlap and individual variation of dermatomes was present. Physiological studies have shown that the size and shape of individual dermatomes is under dynamic control within the central nervous system. The implications for sensory examination of human patients are not fully understood. Foerster's diagrams (see Figs. 19.1 and 19.2) still provide some of our best information about the location, extent, and variability of the dermatomes in man.

Table 19.1 Some common aetiologies of radicular pain

Lower cranial roots
Glossopharyngeal neuralgia
Idiopathic
Associated with vascular anomaly
Cerebellopontine angle tumour
Skull base tumour
Geniculate neuralgia
Upper cervical roots
Occipital neuralgia
Idiopathic
Associated with C1–C2 arthrosis
Associated with rheumatoid arthritis
Post-traumatic
Postherpetic neuralgia
Metastatic spine tumour
Chiari malformation
Lower cervical roots
Cervical disc protrusion
Cervical spondylosis
Metastatic spine tumour
Brachial plexus avulsion injury
Cervical spine fracture or dislocation
Intradural tumour
Thoracic roots
Postherpetic neuralgia
Intercostal neuralgia
Idiopathic
Following thoracotomy
Associated with systemic malignancy
Thoracic disc protrusion
Metastatic spine tumour
Intradural tumour
Meningeal carcinomatosis, lymphoma, leukaemia
Spinal epidural abscess
Diabetic neuropathy
Thoracic spine fracture or dislocation
Tabes dorsalis
Lumbar and first sacral roots
Lumbar disc protrusion
Lumbar spondylosis
Spinal stenosis
Superior facet syndrome
Postsurgical epidural scarring
Arachnoiditis
Spondylolisthesis
Occult postoperative facet fracture
Metastatic spine tumour
Intradural tumour
Meningeal carcinomatosis, lymphoma, leukaemia
Spinal epidural abscess
Lumbar spine fracture or dislocation
Perineurial or leptomeningeal cyst
Tabes dorsalis
Sacrococcygeal roots
Coccygodynia
Metastatic sacral tumour
Meningeal carcinomatosis, lymphoma, leukaemia
Perineurial cyst

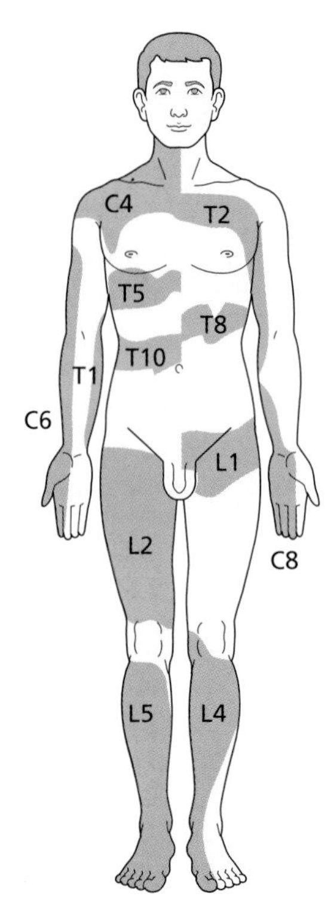

Fig. 19.1 Examples of dermatomes isolated by multiple-root section: anterior aspect (after Foerster 1933).

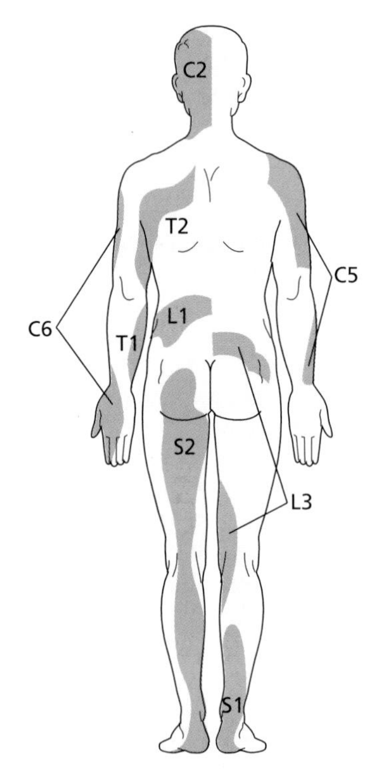

Fig. 19.2 Further examples of dermatomes isolated by multiple-root section: posterior aspect (after Foerster 1933).

The pattern of innervation in muscles and other deep structures often does not conform to the overlying dermatomes. For example, at the cervicothoracic and lumbosacral junctions, the radicular sensory innervation of muscles and fascial structures is largely within the trunk and proximal limb while the corresponding cutaneous territories of the same nerve roots extend distally to the hand or foot. A clinical situation that illustrates this principle is pain referred to the anterior chest or scapular region in compression of lower cervical roots. Another example would be the referral of pain down the leg from pathology of the lumbar spinal facet joints. Although charts of sensory innervations of muscles and fascia are available, it is not usually practical in a clinical setting to test for preservation of sensation in deep structures. Instead, nerve root injury is typically diagnosed by a segmental, radicular pattern of motor deficits, such as weakness, atrophy, fasciculation, or electromyographic changes. A detailed compilation of individual muscles, including their radicular motor innervations, is given by Kendall et al (1971) in their excellent monograph on muscle function and testing.

Syndromes of individual roots

Geniculate neuralgia

Recurrent stabbing or shooting pain of a paroxysmal nature felt deep in the ear and sometimes in the ipsilateral face, neck, or occiput suggests the possibility of geniculate neuralgia. The nervus intermedius may be involved. This neural structure, consisting of fine filaments between the roots of the seventh and eight cranial nerves, contains sensory afferents whose cell bodies are located in the geniculate ganglion. Their axons supply part of the external auditory canal and tympanic membrane, the skin in the angle between ear and mastoid process, the tonsillar region, and some other deep structures of the head and neck.

Patients with geniculate neuralgia are typically young or middle-aged adults. In many cases, a vesicular rash in the external ear and mastoid, typical of herpes zoster, precedes the onset of pain by several days. This has been called the Ramsay Hunt syndrome when it is accompanied by ipsilateral facial paralysis. Attacks of pain lasting seconds, minutes, or sometimes hours may be entirely spontaneous. Less commonly, they can be triggered by touching the external ear canal. Dull background pain may persist between attacks. Other possible symptoms include tenderness in or near the external ear, salivation, nasal discharge, tinnitus, vertigo, or a bitter taste during attacks (White and Sweet 1969).

Geniculate neuralgia is seldom encountered in most clinics, so there is no consensus on management. Detailed CT or MR imaging can help to exclude a tumour or other structural lesion of the posterior fossa and temporal bone. Consultation with an otolaryngologist is appropriate to evaluate for pathology or dysfunction of the facial, auditory, and vestibular nerves. Because of the paroxysmal nature of attacks, it is reasonable to initiate treatment with carbamazepine or other agents of the type used to manage trigeminal neuralgia. Refractory cases sometimes require intracranial sectioning of the nervus intermedius or excision of the geniculate ganglion. In addition, because multiple cranial nerves supply sensation to the ear, some neurosurgeons recommend exploration of the 5th, 9th, and 10th cranial nerves in the posterior fossa for possible microvascular decompression in cases of primary ear pain.

Glossopharyngeal neuralgia

Pain in the afferent distribution of the glossopharyngeal and vagus nerves may be felt in the larynx, base of the tongue, tonsillar region, ear, and occasionally ipsilateral face, neck, or scalp. Paroxysms of pain in this distribution may be due to glossopharyngeal neuralgia (vagoglossopharyngeal neuralgia). The attacks are usually described as stabbing, sharp, 'like a knife', 'like an electric shock', and sometimes hot or burning. They are usually less intense than typical bouts of trigeminal neuralgia, which is 70–100 times as common (Rushton et al 1981). Patients with glossopharyngeal neuralgia are almost always above the age of 20. Men and women are about equally affected. There is a slight predominance of left-sided cases in most large series. Attacks are bilateral in less than 2% of cases. Individual attacks commonly last seconds or minutes and rarely occur at night (Deparis 1968). Constant dull aching, burning, or pressure may persist between attacks. It is characteristic of glossopharyngeal neuralgia that the pain is triggered by such innocuous stimuli as swallowing, yawning, coughing, and chewing. Other reported triggers are laughing, touching the throat, ear, or neck, turning the head, or moving the arm. In unusual cases, particular tastes may trigger attacks (White and Sweet 1969). Spontaneous remissions lasting as long as 20 years were described in 161 of 217 cases of glossopharyngeal neuralgia (Rushton et al 1981).

A variety of cardiovascular and other symptoms may accompany the attacks. They include cardiac arrhythmias or cardiac arrest, hiccups, spells of intractable coughing, inspiratory stridor, excessive salivation, and seizures. These accompanying symptoms can be especially troublesome during and after surgical manipulation of the 10th nerve in the posterior fossa (White and Sweet 1969, Nagashima et al 1976).

Glossopharyngeal neuralgia is most easily distinguished from third division trigeminal neuralgia by the location of pain trigger zones. While trigeminal neuralgia is sometimes triggered from the oral mucosa and teeth, vagoglossopharyngeal neuralgia is more typically triggered from the tonsillar region. Attacks may sometimes be aborted by spraying the tonsil with a topical anaesthetic (Rushton et al 1981). Pain due to vagal involvement tends to be deeper in the throat and may be inactivated by superior laryngeal nerve block. Non-paroxysmal pain in the throat and deep in the ear is not typical of glossopharyngeal neuralgia and should raise concern about possible tumour involvement. The initial investigation of tonsillar or throat pain should include an otolaryngological consultation and detailed, contrast-enhanced CT or MR imaging of the skull base, posterior cranial fossa, and neck to exclude the possibility of tumour, abscess, vascular malformation, or elongated and calcified styloid processes. As with trigeminal neuralgia, appropriate medical management of glossopharyngeal neuralgia might include anticonvulsant drugs such as carbamazepine, phenytoin, or gabapentin. Opiates often fail to prevent the paroxysms of pain. Intractable cases should be considered for referral to a neurosurgeon with special expertise in microsurgery of cranial nerves. Distortion of the 9th and 10th nerve rootlets in the posterior fossa is thought to be a frequent causative factor since microvascular decompression can provide long-term pain relief in 89–95% of cases (Resnick et al 1995, Kondo 1998). The vessels most likely to compress the 9th and 10th cranial nerves are the posterior inferior cerebellar artery, the vertebral artery, and, less often, the anterior inferior cerebellar artery.

Occipital neuralgia

Pain in the territory of the C1–C4 roots may involve the posterior scalp; the periorbital, temporal, and mandibular regions; the external ear and mastoid region; and the neck and shoulder. Posterior roots are frequently absent at the C1 level. The C2 dermatome mainly involves the territory of the greater occipital nerve, which is a direct extension of the C2 root. This territory includes the occipital region from foramen magnum to skull vertex, and from the midline to the mastoid. The C3 dermatome involves mainly the territory of the lesser occipital nerve, which includes the ear, mastoid, and angle of the jaw, and side of the head. C4 radicular pain involves mainly the neck and upper shoulder.

Pain at the craniocervical junction is frequently associated with trauma or structural abnormalities of the upper cervical spine and is not infrequently bilateral. Occipital neuralgia is a syndrome of recurrent attacks of pain in the C2 and C3 territory. Patients sometimes report frontal or periorbital radiation of pain. Attacks of occipital neuralgia may be paroxysmal and lancinating in some cases or prolonged for hours in others. Discrete trigger zones are seldom found, but pain can often be reproduced by pressure over the greater occipital nerve. In some cases, pain may be triggered by pressure over the site of an old craniectomy or depressed skull fracture. Pain may sometimes be produced by neck movements, pressure on the C2 spinous process, or downward pressure on the head. Tingling paraesthesias may be felt in the scalp or ear. Blunting of sharp point sensation is commonly found in the scalp if the patient is examined carefully.

Diagnostic studies in cases of occipital or upper cervical radicular pain should include radiological imaging of the skull vault, skull base, and upper cervical spine, keeping in mind that aetiological factors may include metastatic tumours, old skull fractures and surgical sites, posterior fossa tumours and vascular malformations, Chiari malformation, demyelinating disease, cervical spondylosis or arthropathy, and vertebral instability. Even though many cases are idiopathic, investigation may logically include CT or MR imaging of the skull and upper cervical region, and cervical spine films to look for foraminal constriction or upper cervical joint instability on flexion and extension. In most instances, neuralgias of the upper cervical roots can be managed conservatively with oral analgesic and anti-inflammatory medications and injections of local anaesthetics and steroids at intervals. Frank instability of the upper cervical vertebrae may require referral to a spine surgeon for stabilization.

In typical cases of occipital neuralgia, evidence of radicular involvement may be obtained by observing relief of pain following local anaesthetic block of the greater occipital nerve or fluoroscopically guided block of the C2 ganglion on the involved side. When pain is in the side of the head or neck, local anaesthetic block of the C3 or C4 root at the foramen can be informative. In severe cases refractory to medical management, these temporary blocks may point the way to more definitive treatment by surgical decompression or sectioning of the appropriate roots. Successful blocks do not infallibly predict good results from surgery, but rhizotomy or ganglionectomy for occipital neuralgia offers at least 70% long-term success with low morbidity (White and Sweet 1969, Dubuisson 1995, Lozano et al 1998). Electrical spinal cord stimulation and peripheral nerve stimulation have also been used to treat chronic occipital pain. The long-term effectiveness of this approach remains to be determined.

Lower cervical, thoracic, and lumbar radiculopathy

In nerve root lesions associated with herniated cervical discs, certain patterns of pain are fairly constant. These patterns, and some typical neurological signs that may accompany them, are summarized in Table 19.2. Numbness and tingling paraesthesias ('pins and needles') are often described in a wider zone than the painful one. These innocuous but annoying sensations frequently radiate into the fingers while the pain does not. As noted above, chest pain may sometimes result from lower cervical roots, and when severe, it may imitate the pain of angina or myocardial infarction. Pain associated with cervical disc protrusions is usually constant with daily exacerbations related to activity, especially movements of the neck. Coughing, sneezing, pushing, and any type of straining may severely aggravate the pain and reproduce the paraesthesias. When the intervertebral foramina are narrowed by protruding discs and by spondylotic changes of the vertebral bodies and articular facets ('osteophytes'), the contained roots may be subject to marked compression during extension of the neck, turning in either direction, or tilting of the head.

Root lesions from T2 to L1 mainly involve the trunk. Radicular pain at truncal levels often appears as a discrete band around the chest or abdomen. Disc herniation and spinal tumour metastases are two common causes of radiculopathy in this territory. When truncal radicular pain is due to a spinal tumour, it may be constant, becoming worse at night when the patient is recumbent for hours. Radicular pain of thoracic spinal tumours or disc protrusions is typically aggravated by coughing, sneezing, and straining. Root pain accompanied by fever, spinal ache with local warmth, and tenderness or paraparesis is a warning of spinal epidural abscess, which is most common in the thoracic region (Baker et al 1975). When due to postherpetic neuralgia, truncal pain is apt to be described as sharp, tender, tugging, or pulling (Dubuisson and Melzack 1976). The skin may be exquisitely sensitive in the involved dermatome. Characteristic vesicles usually appear as viral particles and are distributed along peripheral branches of the spinal nerve. In cases of herpes zoster, segmental pain may precede the appearance of cutaneous vesicles by 3–4 days. Healing of the skin lesions takes place over 2–3 weeks. Pain lasts an additional week or two in young patients and usually disappears, leaving hypo- or hyperaesthesia. Pain persists for over 2 months in 70% of patients over 60 years of age, even though the skin lesions heal normally (Ray 1980). Intractable postherpetic neuralgia occurs mainly in elderly patients. When it has been present

Table 19.2 Typical findings in cervical root compression[a]

C5 root compression (C4–C5 disc)
Pain—neck, shoulder, medial scapula, anterior chest, lateral aspect of upper arm
Numbness—sometimes lateral upper arm or area over deltoid
Weakness—deltoid, supraspinatus, infraspinatus, biceps, brachioradialis
Hyporeflexia—biceps, brachioradialis reflexes
C6 root compression (C5–C6 disc)
Pain—neck, shoulder, medial scapula, anterior chest, lateral aspect of upper arm, dorsal aspect of forearm
Numbness—thumb and index finger (sometimes absent)
Weakness—biceps (mild to moderate), extensor carpi radialis
Hyporeflexia—biceps reflex
C7 root compression (C6–C7 disc)
Pain—same as in C6 root compression
Numbness—index and middle fingers (sometimes absent)
Weakness—triceps
Hyporeflexia—triceps reflex
C8 root compression (C7–T1 disc)
Pain—neck, medial scapula, anterior chest, medial aspect of arm and forearm
Numbness—fourth and fifth fingers, occasionally middle finger
Weakness—triceps, all extensors of wrist and fingers except extensor carpi radialis; all flexors of wrist and fingers except flexor carpi radialis and palmaris longus; all intrinsic hand muscles
Hyporeflexia—triceps reflex
T1 root compression (T1–T2 disc)
Pain—same as in C8 root compression
Numbness—ulnar aspect of forearm (usually subjective)
Weakness—only intrinsic muscles of hand
Hyporeflexia—none
Miscellaneous—Horner's syndrome

[a]After Murphey et al (1973)

for 6 months or more, the prognosis for recovery is very poor (Lipton 1979). Postherpetic neuralgia, meaning persistent radicular pain 3 or more months after an acute attack of herpes zoster, can be prevented in about 50% of cases by pre-emptive use of amitriptyline or nortriptyline at time of diagnosis of shingles, according to Bowsher (1997). Treatment with oral acyclovir within 72 h of the appearance of a zoster rash reduces the incidence of residual neuralgic pain at 6 months by 46% (Jackson et al 1997). In a randomized, double-blind, placebo-controlled trial (Tyring et al 1995), famciclovir prescribed for acute herpes zoster led to approximately two times faster resolution of postherpetic neuralgia and decreased the median duration of pain by about 2 months. In established postherpetic neuralgia, chronic radicular pain may still sometimes respond to amitriptyline or topical lidocaine (lignocaine) gel (Rowbotham et al 1995). High doses of the putative NMDA receptor blocker dextromethorphan are not more effective than placebo (Nelson et al 1997). Some cases benefit from transcutaneous electrical nerve stimulation (Nathan and Wall 1974) or epidural steroid injections (Forrest 1980). In 3960 patients with postherpetic neuralgia, dermatomal subcutaneous infiltrations with a combination of local anaesthetics and dexamethasone were said to give relief in 28%; another 57% had relief after two injections and 11% after three injections, while 4% had no response (Bhargava et al 1998). Ablative surgical procedures have not been conspicuously successful in treating postherpetic neuralgia. Dorsal rhizotomy carries about a 29% long-term success rate, similar to the long-term outcome after DREZ lesions (Iskandar and Nashold 1998). Somewhat better results have been reported for electrical spinal cord stimulation. In a review of literature on treatment of postherpetic neuralgia with cord stimulation through 1991, it was noted that 19 out of 21 reported cases responded well to this modality beyond the first 3 months (Spiegelmann and Friedman 1991).

As with cervical root lesions, patterns of pain, numbness, weakness, and loss of reflexes are fairly consistent in the lumbosacral region. These features are summarized in Table 19.3. Radicular pain associated with lumbosacral disc protrusions is described as sharp, tender, and shooting by a majority of patients given a verbal questionnaire (Dubuisson and Melzack 1976). Other descriptive terms commonly chosen are cramping, throbbing, aching, heavy, and stabbing. A majority of patients report feelings of numbness, tingling, 'pins and needles', or a wooden sensation in the involved territory. Due to the overlap of dermatomes, zones of objective sensory loss defined by touch and pinprick are usually small or absent but occasional patients show hypoaesthesia over a large part of a dermatome (Keegan and Garrett 1948). Paraesthesias and loss of sensation help to define the root involved, because they frequently extend distally in the dermatome when the pain does not. In typical sciatica caused by disc herniation, pain radiates from the lumbar region to the buttock, hip, or thigh, and sometimes beyond the knee but usually not into the foot itself. Tingling and feelings of numbness are often perceived more distally than is the pain itself. Bending at the waist is usually restricted in painful lumbosacral radiculopathies of any cause. Passive straight-leg raising in the supine position is almost always painful in the presence of mechanical L4, L5, or S1 root lesions. This manoeuvre, which stretches the sciatic nerve and its tributaries, causes pain to radiate into the appropriate dermatome or muscles. In the apprehensive patient and in the malingerer, the same postural manipulation can often be produced without the patient's knowledge by passively extending his knee while he is seated. Passive reverse-leg raising with the knee flexed stretches the femoral nerve and is often painful when the L2, L3, or L4 root is involved (Dyck 1976).

At lower cervical, thoracic, and lumbar levels, spinal nerve roots may be compressed and distorted in a variety of ways (Figs. 19.3, 19.4). An enlarged facet joint and thickened ligamentum flavum may compress the root posteriorly and laterally. Free fragments of herniated disc material may be trapped within the spinal canal or in an intervertebral foramen. In the lumbar spine, spondylotic changes of the facet joints may entrap roots passing caudally in the lateral recess of the spinal canal, producing lateral recess stenosis, also known as 'superior facet syndrome' (Epstein et al 1972), with symptoms indistinguishable from those of disc herniation. Compression of roots within the foramina may be produced, or aggravated, by spinal instability, due to disc and joint degeneration (degenerative spondylolisthesis) or to a congenital lytic defect of the pars interarticularis of a vertebra (congenital spondylolisthesis with spondylolysis). The portion of the defective arch still attached to the upper vertebra may be dragged forward against the root in the foramen (Fig. 19.3, lower right). Further root entrapment can result from chronic fibrosis around the root near the site of the bony defect. A less frequently diagnosed cause of radicular pain following surgery is an occult fracture of the inferior articular process of a vertebra. This typically follows overly aggressive bone removal around the medial aspect of the facet joint (medial facetectomy)

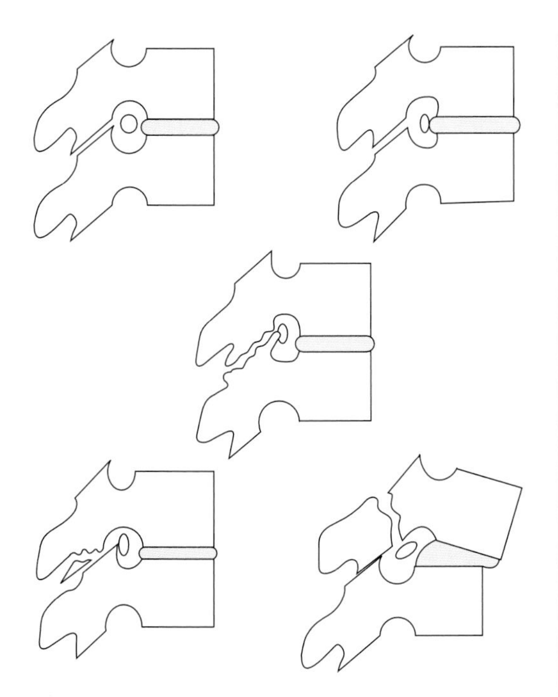

Fig. 19.3 Mechanical root lesions (lateral view). Upper left, normal relationship of nerve root to disc and vertebrae; upper right, disc protrusion and osteophytes; centre facet, joint degeneration; lower left, fracture of inferior articular process; lower right, spondylolysis with spondylolisthesis.

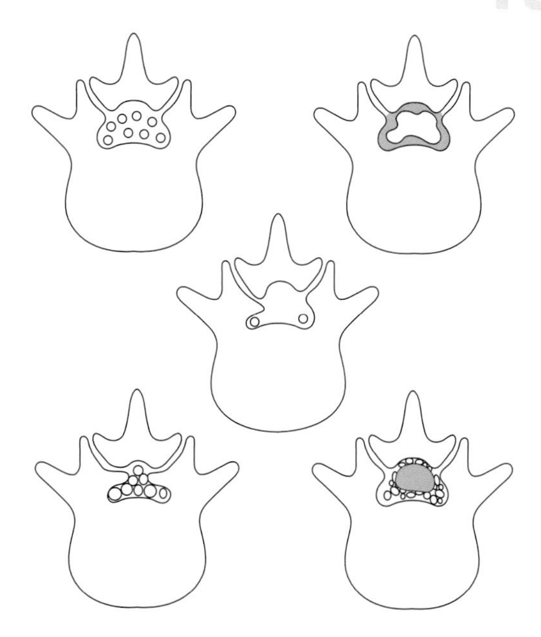

Fig. 19.4 Lumbosacral root lesions (horizontal view). Upper left, normal configuration of the spinal canal and cauda equina; upper right, chronic adhesive arachnoiditis and atrophic roots; centre, entrapment of a root descending in narrow lateral recess ('superior facet syndrome'); lower left, lumbar spinal stenosis due to spondylosis; lower right, intradural tumour compressing the cauda equina.

at the time of disc removal or laminectomies for spinal stenosis and may not develop until the patient resumes activities in an upright posture. The unopposed superior articular process of the vertebra below may encroach into the foramen to pinch an exiting root (Fig. 19.3, lower left). Occult facet fractures were found on routine postoperative CT scans in 6% of patients undergoing lumbar spine surgery (Rothman et al 1985). This type of occult facet fracture is not easily identified on axial images and is probably best seen on sagittally reformatted CT.

The sacrococcygeal dermatomes are known mainly from stimulation of the roots at the time of rhizotomy for painful sacral and pelvic disorders. Stimulation of S2 produces pain in the buttock, groin, posterior thigh, and genitalia. Foerster (1933) mapped portions of an isolated S2 dermatome on the sole of the foot (see Fig. 19.2). During stimulation of S3, pain is felt in the perianal region, rectum, and genitalia. Stimulation of S4 may evoke pain in the vagina. Pain in the anus and around the coccyx is felt with stimulation of S4, S5, and coccygeal roots (Bohm and Franksson 1959, White and Sweet 1969).

Severe burning pain around the coccyx in the absence of tumour or other disease is termed coccygodynia. The pain can be unilateral or bilateral and usually occurs in middle-aged or elderly women. The S4, S5, and coccygeal roots are involved in some cases (White and Sweet 1969). In others, the pain may be referred from lower lumbar spine pathology (Long 1982). Sensory deficits are not typical, nor are signs of bowel and bladder involvement, despite the known innervation of the bladder and anal sphincter by the S2–S4 roots. Objective loss of sensation or diminished anal or bladder sphincter tone suggests destruction of the roots.

A particularly intractable type of pain can occur in the sacral dermatomes in association with the finding of sacral cysts. These cysts are in fact abnormal dilatations of the meninges around the sacral nerve roots, filled with cerebrospinal fluid, expanding the sacral neural canal and foramina. On surgical exploration, which the author rarely advises, the sacral roots are found to be embedded in the meningeal wall of the cyst, stretched and thinned from growth of the fluid-filled compartment. There may or may not be a visible spinal fluid communication with the rest of the subarachnoid space. Terminology used to describe this condition includes 'sacral arachnoid cyst', 'sacral meningocele', and 'sacral root sleeve diverticula'. The anatomy of the meningeal cystic anomaly varies from case to case, but the symptomatology seems to have in common some unusual and relentless, painful sensations and dysaesthesias around the saddle region, rectum, or vagina. The symptoms may be positional, with bizarre-sounding descriptions of pulsation or formication in the region.

Investigation of patients with persistent radicular pain at cervical, thoracic, or lumbosacral levels should include imaging of the relevant portion of the spine by MR or CT myelographic technique. Plain CT imaging can be helpful for demonstrating bony pathology. Intravenous contrast usually brightens the appearance of scar tissue in cases with prior surgery or trauma, whereas herniated disc fragments typically fail to enhance with contrast. Radiological surveys have shown that nerve root compression due to disc protrusions is frequently asymptomatic (Hitselberger and Witten 1968, Wiesel et al 1984). Therefore, evidence of minimal nerve root contact by a protruding disc or osteophyte is usually considered to be insufficient to establish a compressive aetiology of the pain, although it is sometimes difficult to know whether an observed small disc protrusion was previously larger, leaving behind an injured root. It is likely that many instances of root compression by protruding discs are transient and that healing of the torn annulus takes place (Davis 1982). In a study of 47 patients followed prospectively for symptomatic disc herniations, without significant joint disease or stenosis, 42 patients tolerated conservative management without surgery until signs of radiculopathy subsided (Maigne et al 1992). Serial CT scans documented shrinkage of the disc herniations over periods of 1–40 months, with the largest herniations tending to decrease the most. Conservative management of radicular pain due to disc herniation or other benign spine changes typically includes a period of rest and reduced physical activities, and narcotic analgesic medication gradually tapering to non-narcotic over 3–6 weeks. When reactive muscle spasm is problematic, muscle relaxants such as methocarbamol, cyclobenzaprine, or carisoprodol can be useful. Short, tapering courses of oral corticosteroids can be quite helpful, although there is a tendency for the pain to recur. Substitution of nonsteroidal anti-inflammatory agents at the conclusion of the steroid taper may help to avoid this rebound effect.

Epidural steroid injection is sometimes advocated for pain associated with nerve root compression due to disc protrusions and spondylosis. Unfortunately, most of the available literature suffers from poor methodological design, usually with inadequate radiological documentation of the sites of root compression. The presence of inflammatory mediators associated with herniated disc material (Saal et al 1990) suggests a role for early use of anti-inflammatory drugs including corticosteroids in these cases. However, it appears that when frank root damage is already present, the chances of benefit from epidural steroids are greatly diminished. Following mild disc protrusions prior to surgery, reported success rates range from 0 to 70% using rather lenient criteria for success (Dilke et al 1973, Brevik et al 1976, Snoek et al 1977, Cuckler et al 1985). In patients with cervical radicular pain persisting more than 12 months but who are not considered candidates for disc surgery, a randomized comparison of epidural lidocaine (lignocaine) and triamcinolone versus the same combination plus epidural morphine showed no significant difference in outcome (Castagnera et al 1994). Patients with chronic sciatica do not fare too well with epidural steroids and those with previous surgery, entrapment of nerve roots by bone or scar tissue, or demonstrable behavioural disturbances are even less likely to respond (White et al 1980). In successful cases, as many as three injections may be needed and the beneficial effects are often delayed for 2–6 days (Green et al 1980). Steroids given in this way are absorbed systemically and can suppress adrenal function for 3 weeks (Gorski et al 1982).

Most subacute radiculopathies benefit from physical therapy or from treatment with steroids, but it is unwise to withhold decompressive surgery for months if an obvious source of nerve root compression is identified and the patient is failing to improve. Among spine surgeons, it is widely agreed that the likelihood of success from discectomy drops off markedly after herniated disc material becomes fibrosed within the epidural space, as is often the case after the first two months. The usual indication to proceed with discectomy or foramenotomy in a case of single-level radiculopathy is a combination of persistent root pain inadequately controlled by medications and confirmatory signs of root injury by neurological examination. In cases of disc herniation, there is a good correlation between the degree of pain relief and the size of the disc herniation. It is well established that, with current microsurgical techniques, discectomy and foramenotomy carry high success rates. However, even with meticulous surgical technique, persistent root injury is not uncommon With failed disc surgery, one of four chronological patterns may emerge (Bertrand 1975, Auld 1978). The sequence radicular 'pain→operation→relief for weeks or months→ return of pain in the same or in a different distribution' does not usually indicate permanent root damage but rather suggests the presence of recurrent root compression at the same level or at a different level. The sequence 'radicular pain→operation→no change' suggests that the cause of pain was not identified at surgery. Even if surgery was carried out at the correct location, a disc fragment may have migrated out of reach or the root may have been trapped in a hidden zone. The sequence 'radicular pain→operation→relief of pain but severe numbness' suggests surgical trauma to the root or its vascular supply. The pattern 'radicular pain→operation→increased radicular pain and severe bilateral leg cramps→temporary improvement→chronic bilateral pain' suggests the development of arachnoiditis. In this syndrome, severe cramps and spasms in both legs, sometimes accompanied by fever and chills, begin on the first, second, or third postoperative day and last for 4–20 days. There is usually some improvement but signs of chronic arachnoiditis develop over the following months or years with new neurological deficits and relentless bilateral back and leg pain.

Multisegmental root syndromes

Cervical spondylosis

Cervical spondylosis is a condition of the cervical spine characterized by multiple disc protrusions with marginal osteophyte formation, facet joint degeneration, and thickening of ligaments within the spinal canal. Narrowing of the spinal canal and intervertebral foramina are typical. Cervical spondylosis sometimes declares its presence by pain in the distribution of one root, but more often the picture is multisegmental, diffuse, and bilateral. A clinical hallmark of cervical spondylosis is restriction of neck motion with discomfort on attempting a complete range of movement. Multiple root constriction in the intervertebral foramina leads to symptoms of numbness in the hands and forearms, in a pattern not conforming to that of any peripheral nerve territory. Weakness and diminished reflexes point to loss of innervation of muscles. Weakness of the wrist extensors, triceps, and shoulder girdle is typical. Long-tract signs such as upgoing plantar reflexes, difficulty maintaining balance on attempting to walk a straight line in heel-to-toe fashion, and clumsy fine movements of the toes and fingers may indicate myelopathy due to cord compression in the stenotic spinal canal. In cases with coexisting cervical and lumbar spondylosis, there may be loss of tendon reflexes in the lower limbs, instead of the expected hyperreflexia due to cervical cord compression. Occasionally, paraesthesias such as tingling or electrical sensations can occur in the trunk and legs with cervical spondylosis, particularly during neck extension. Frank pain in the legs is rarely if ever due to cervical spondylosis; at least, this author has never seen a believable example of it. Occipital pain due to bony encroachment on the upper cervical roots may add to the confusing picture of a patient with widespread pain and paraesthesias.The character of pain in cervical spondylosis resembles that of chronic compression of individual roots and the same aggravating factors may be present (Wilkinson 1971). In general, patients with single lateral cervical disc protrusions of soft nucleus pulposus tend to form a younger group than patients with multiple degenerated cervical discs and extensive bony spurs and ridges.

Lumbar spondylosis

Pain distributed in several dermatomes of the lower extremities, often bilateral and otherwise resembling the pain of a solitary lumbar disc protrusion, may be due to widespread spondylotic changes of the lumbar spine. Regardless of whether disc protrusions are present, back pain and leg pain are prominent complaints. Weinstein et al (1977) found that 66% of patients with narrowed lumbar canals due to spondylosis suffered from back pain; 36% had unilateral leg pain, and 36% had bilateral leg pain. Painful muscle spasms and cramps in the back and legs were frequent but the localization of pain was not consistent or helpful in diagnosis. Of 227 cases, pain was felt in the buttock or hip in 25, in the thigh in 23, and in the groin or genitalia in 9. In many cases, the pain was aggravated by extension of the lumbar spine. Twenty cases were classified as 'neurogenic claudication', which is discussed below. Objective sensory abnormalities were present in only half of the cases and often did not follow a discrete dermatomal pattern. In a few cases, perianal or 'saddle' hypoaesthesia was noted. Muscle weakness was observed in 64% and was often most marked in the extensor hallucis longus and tibialis anterior, suggesting predominant L5 root involvement. Tendon stretch reflexes in the ankles or knees were decreased or absent in 70% of cases. In about 10% there was additional evidence of cauda equina involvement consisting of bowel or bladder incontinence, urinary retention, or impotence. A positive response to straight-leg raising was found in only 30% of the 227 cases, a useful point in distinguishing the pain of lumbar spondylosis and canal stenosis from that of simple disc protrusion.

A common problem associated with lumbar spondylosis and spinal stenosis is the inability to continue walking or to maintain upright posture for more than a short time. This is known as neurogenic claudication. Typically, pain, aching, numbness, heaviness, or other unpleasant sensations in the legs appear after standing erect for some time, or after walking a certain distance. The symptoms may begin in the feet and spread proximally or vice versa, and are relieved by sitting or by lying in a flexed posture. Patients may learn to assume a flexed posture while walking, or to lean over a shopping cart in stores. These points help to distinguish the syndrome from peripheral vascular claudication, in which cramps affect the leg muscles after exercise regardless of posture. Also, in cases of vascular insufficiency, the peripheral pulses are diminished. While a variety of radicular signs may be present, some patients with disabling neurogenic claudication may have little or no objective deficit of strength, reflexes, or sensation when examined sitting in the office. Neurogenic claudication is usually relieved by decompressive laminectomy, partial removal of hypertrophic facet joints, and excision of thickened ligamentum flavum at the levels of stenosis, as indicated on preoperative MRI or CT myelography studies.

Arachnoiditis and epidural fibrosis

Arachnoiditis is a chronic condition of inflammation and sometimes atrophy of neural structures within the subarachnoid space. Multiple predisposing factors have been identified (Table 19.4). Arachnoiditis is usually an aseptic process seen in patients who have undergone multiple spine surgeries and myelographies. Although cases of focal arachnoiditis affecting only one or two nerve roots are not uncommon, more often there is diffuse involvement of nerve roots. Most reported cases are lumbosacral, but any part of the spine may be affected. Pain is almost always the first symptom. The pain of arachnoiditis may obey a radicular pattern but more often it involves portions of two or more root distributions. The pain territory is typically lumbar with bilateral leg radiation, but may be complex with widely separated zones, irregular distribution, and shifting boundaries. It tends to be aggravated by physical activity, movement of the extremities, and neck flexion. Numbness and paraesthesias are common. They are often widespread, poorly localized, and inconstant from day to day. Occasional patients complain of an inexorable feeling of fullness in the rectum. Objective sensory examination by touch and pinprick may be vague or entirely normal despite bizarre subjective complaints. Arachnoiditis affects men more often than women in a ratio of almost 2:1. The typical age of onset is between 25 and 65 (French 1946).

Table 19.4 Some factors predisposing to arachnoiditis

Chronic lumbosacral root compression
Disc protrusion
Spinal stenosis
Spine surgery
Infection
Bacterial meningitis, including tuberculous
Fungal meningitis
Cryptococcal meningitis
Viral meningitis
Syphilis
Haemorrhage
From spinal vascular malformation
Following trauma
Following lumbar puncture
Following surgery
Implanted epidural catheters
Irritant chemicals
Myelographic contrast agents
Iophendylate
Meglumine iocarmate
Methiodal
? Metrizamide
Anaesthetic agents
Amphotericin B
Methotrexate
? Steroids
Polyethylene glycol
2-Chloroprocaine

In chronic arachnoiditis, some or all of the lumbosacral roots may be encased by dense leptomeningeal adhesions within the dura. The final stage of this process is a lumbar canal in which the roots are bound circumferentially to the dura. Burton (1978) suggested the following sequence of events:

1. The pia of individual roots is inflamed, with root swelling and hyperaemia (radiculitis).
2. The roots adhere to each other and to the surrounding arachnoid trabeculae, and fibroblasts proliferate.
3. There is atrophy of the roots, which are displaced circumferentially and encased in collagen deposits.

The changes characteristic of arachnoiditis can often be demonstrated by MRI or CT. The lumbar nerve roots can sometimes be shown to cluster together and to adhere to the surrounding meninges, leaving the centre of the spinal canal void. With long-standing cases of arachnoiditis, evidence of trapped radiographic contrast material may be found. Magnetic resonance imaging does accurately diagnose arachnoiditis, comparing favourably with CT myelography and plain film myelography for that purpose (Delamarter et al 1990). However, use of gadolinium during MR imaging does not reveal significant additional information about the condition (Johnson and Sze 1990).

Although symptoms may improve or resolve in milder cases, the long-range prognosis of arachnoiditis is poor in that the neurological deficits tend to persist permanently. Late onset of urinary frequency, urgency, or frank incontinence was noted in 23% of a group of arachnoiditis patients followed over 10–21 years (Guyer et al 1989). Of the patients in that study, 90% had undergone Pantopaque myelography and disc surgery prior to developing arachnoiditis. Progression of neurological disability did not appear to be the typical natural course of the disease. When increased neurological deficits were seen, they were most often due to surgical intervention. A majority of the patients depended on daily narcotic analgesics; alcohol abuse, and depression, and two deaths by suicide were also noted.

Epidural fibrosis is scarring on the outside of the meninges. While it is not infrequently coexistent with arachnoiditis, it is a distinct entity. It is quite possible to have severe intradural pathology from arachnoiditis with little or no epidural fibrosis, and vice versa. Postoperative epidural fibrosis is a common finding after laminectomies and disc surgery. Reasons for scar formation probably include reaction to foreign matter such as fibres from cotton pledgets, and root inflammation induced by chemical mediators released by exposed disc fragments or joint synovium. Epidural fibrosis in the lumbosacral region, and probably at other levels of the spine, binds the nerve root sheaths and dural tube to surrounding structures such as the disc annulus and posterior longitudinal ligament and prevents normal elastic stretch and sliding motion of the root sleeves during spine motion and leg elevation. Extensive epidural fibrosis can also cause compression and constriction of nerve roots. All of these processes lead to recurrent radicular pain and physical impairment. Six months after surgery, the extent of epidural fibrosis as shown by contrast-enhanced MRI correlates with the severity of persistent radicular pain (Ross et al 1996). Epidural fibrosis has also been reported as a complication of implanted epidural catheters, appearing 21–320 days after implantation and manifested by pain or resistance to flow on injection of the catheter (Aldrete 1995). This appears to be a type of foreign body reaction due to the presence of the catheter in the epidural space and may limit the permanency of the catheter.

Repeated exploration and decompression of traumatized roots is usually futile and may further increase the patient's pain. In a study of 34 patients with failed back surgery syndrome, some with MRI-documented epidural fibrosis, trials of epidurography and attempted lysis of adhesions by fluid injection produced some improvement of contrast spread without any lasting improvement of pain (Devulder et al 1995). Rhizotomy at the time of re-exploration is not apt to be beneficial (Bertrand 1975) and may lead to a very unpleasant deafferentation syndrome. Approximately 2–3% of patients with chronic low back pain and sciatica due to failed back surgery syndrome may be relieved temporarily by local anaesthetic block of one or two lumbosacral roots (Taub et al 1995). Dorsal root ganglionectomy in these cases was said to relieve sciatica, but not back pain, in 59% of cases. However, there was a high incidence of dysaesthesias often requiring additional treatment measures afterwards. Other authors have found ganglionectomy to be ineffective for chronic sciatica in failed back surgery syndrome (Gybels and Sweet 1989, North et al 1991).

Currently the most promising treatment for chronic radicular pain associated with epidural fibrosis or arachnoiditis is electrical spinal cord stimulation (SCS). Technological advances in stimulation equipment have made this procedure increasingly attractive for large numbers of patients. In particular, bilateral electrode arrays and multichannel stimulator systems make it feasible to treat bilateral sciatica and even low back pain in cases of failed back surgery syndrome. Implantation of a spinal cord stimulator is a reversible procedure very unlikely to leave permanent dysaesthesias or other neurological complications. Electrode placements for lumbar radiculopathy are typically between T8 and T12. Therefore, patients wary of further spinal surgery are usually relieved to learn that a trial of cord stimulation will not require surgical reopening of the laminectomy site. SCS is somewhat more effective for unilateral than for bilateral sciatica (Meilman et al 1989, Kumar et al 1991). When arachnoiditis is present, the outcome of SCS appears to be primarily related to the number of roots involved (Meilman et al 1989). As might be expected, patients with injury to a single root respond more favourably than do patients with multiple-root damage.

Meningeal carcinomatosis

Multiple nerve roots may be involved at different levels by leptomeningeal metastases from solid tumours. The subject of nerve and root pain in cancer is reviewed elsewhere in this volume and will be mentioned only briefly here. The typical clinical syndrome of meningeal carcinomatosis consists of neurological dysfunction at several levels of the neuraxis without radiological evidence of brain metastasis or of epidural spinal metastasis. About two-thirds of the patients in one reported series were women (Wasserstrom et al 1982). Patients ranged in age from 30 to 74 years in this series. Breast cancer was the commonest primary source, followed by lung cancer and malignant melanoma. Spinal root infiltrates are also a common problem in leukaemic patients, who are frequently children (Neiri et al 1968).

Root symptoms, including radicular pain, may be the first sign of meningeal carcinomatosis. Olson et al (1974) found that 25% of patients whose leptomeninges were infiltrated by metastatic cancer had only root symptoms initially. Another 15% had spinal root symptoms plus symptoms of other sites of neurological damage. In a series of 90 patients with known carcinomatous invasion of the meninges, Wasserstrom et al (1982) reported that 74 had spinal symptoms and signs. Pain in a radicular pattern was a prominent feature in 19, while back pain or neck pain was present in 23. Other frequent complaints were of weakness, usually of the legs, paraesthesias in the extremities, and bowel or bladder dysfunction. Seven patients had nuchal rigidity and 11 had back pain on straight-leg raising; 30 patients had signs of cauda equina involvement. The tendency for lumbosacral root involvement has also been noted in leukaemic patients (Neiri et al 1968). It is thought to be due to the gravitation of malignant cells in the cerebrospinal fluid as well as the relatively long course of the lumbosacral roots within the subarachnoid space (Little et al 1974). Headaches are a frequent accompanying complaint. Some patients experience pain when the neck is manipulated; others show tenderness to percussion over the spine. Absence of one or more of the tendon stretch reflexes is typical, as is muscle wasting and fasciculation. Additional signs and symptoms due to systemic cancer may complicate the picture.

Cervical and lumbar plexus nerve root avulsion

A unique type of pain is seen in cases of traumatic avulsion of cervical or lumbosacral nerve roots from the spinal cord in cases of brachial plexus or lumbosacral plexus injury (Wynn Parry 1980, Moossy et al 1987). Avulsion of spinal nerve roots tends to produce a severe deafferentation pain syndrome, whereas traumatic plexus injuries distal to the dorsal root ganglia tend not to produce intractable pain. Patients with plexus root avulsion pain are typically young men between the ages of 18 and 30 involved in motorcycle accidents or industrial injuries. Segmental motor deficits in the involved limb are strikingly obvious. With brachial plexus nerve root avulsion injury, pain is almost invariably felt in the hand and forearm after C6, C7, C8, or T1 root avulsions, conforming fairly well to the dermatomes of the avulsed roots. Some patients with an avulsed C5 root feel pain in the shoulder. Almost all the patents use the term 'hot' or 'burning' to describe the pain; many report a feeling as if the hand were on fire or boiling water were being poured over it. Some describe severe pressure, pounding, or 'electric shock'. There tends to be a constant background of severe pain in which additional sudden paroxysms occur. Paraesthesias are also common, including tingling, 'pins and needles', feelings of electricity, or a phantom limb. The pain of root avulsion is often aggravated by worry and emotional stress and relieved by relaxation and by distraction. Some patients report less pain when gripping, striking, or massaging the painful limb. Others have moderate relief when moving the neck or the paralysed arm. Investigation should include CT myelography of the involved portion of the spine to detect abnormal outpouching of nerve root sleeves at sites of root avulsion. Pain and dysaesthesias associated with avulsion injuries of the brachial or lumbosacral plexus are usually unresponsive to medications. This syndrome is usually best managed by a programme of behavioural pain management and vocational rehabilitation (Wynn Parry 1980). For severe and intractable cases, dorsal root entry zone (DREZ) lesions of the relevant segments of the spinal cord have now been shown to be effective in many surgical series, with long-term pain relief reported in 37–100% of cases (Iskandar and Nashold 1998). A majority of authors report success rates above 65%.

Pseudoradicular syndromes

Multiple sclerosis

Limb pain and paroxysmal pain are not uncommon in patients with multiple sclerosis (Clifford and Trotter 1984, Moulin et al 1988). In some cases, this takes the form of a radicular syndrome mimicking the pain of nerve root compression and prompting a diagnostic search for disc protrusion or other spine disease. Ramirez-Lassepas et al (1992) described 11 patients presenting with acute radicular pain, in whom root compression was ruled out by careful imaging studies. Multiple sclerosis was eventually determined to be the cause of the pseudoradicular pain, which was lumbosacral in six cases, cervical in three, and thoracic in two. In about half the cases, acute radicular symptoms appeared in association with trauma. These patients represented only 4% of newly diagnosed cases of MS in the authors' practices over a 15-year interval. Uldry and Regli (1992) reported four additional cases of pseudoradicular pain associated with demyelinating plaques in the cervical spinal cord diagnosed with MRI. It is important not to ignore the fact that disc protrusions and spondylosis are still the most common causes of radicular pain in the MS population, and the diagnosis of demyelinating disease does not necessarily preclude surgical decompression of these roots. The diagnosis of pseudoradicular pain due to MS is best established by MRI, which is quite sensitive to the presence of demyelinating plaques in the spinal cord (Gebarski et al 1985, Paty et al 1988). The author has seen one instance in which a tiny demyelinating plaque in the high cervical cord of a patient with MS was associated with pain otherwise indistinguishable from occipital neuralgia.

Neurosyphilis and diabetes

In tabetic neurosyphilis (tabes dorsalis), degeneration of dorsal roots and dorsal columns is associated with a clinical syndrome of lancinating pains and visceral crises. Patients are typically 40–60 years of age because the symptoms rarely appear less than 10–20 years after the disease begins (Storm-Mathisen 1978). The most frequent complaint is of 'lightning pains': sudden intense, fleeting pains in the legs, less often in the back and arms. They are described as cramping, crushing, burning, lancinating, or 'like an electric shock'. They tend to occur in clusters and may shift unpredictably in location. Occipital neuralgia has been reported as an unusual presenting feature of neurosyphilis (Smith et al 1987). Numbness or tingling and aching paraesthesias are common in the trunk and soles of the feet. Hyperaesthesia to touch may occur. Objective sensory loss is said to appear in characteristic patterns: the middle of the face, ulnar forearm, nipple area, and perianal region (Storm-Mathisen 1978). Additional signs of neurosyphilis may include Charcot joints, absent joint position sense in the legs, ataxia, and Argyll Robertson pupil.

Diabetic pseudotabes is a pseudoradicular pain syndrome seen in diabetes mellitus. Brief, shooting pains may be restricted to a single dermatome. Paraesthesias and other signs of dorsal column dysfunction may be found. The presence of an irregular pupil that accommodates but reacts poorly to light may sometimes further confuse the clinical picture (Gilroy and Meyer 1975).

Pelvic lesions

Pelvic tumours and inflammatory diseases affecting the lumbosacral plexus may closely mimic lumbosacral radicular syndromes. When adequate CT or MRI studies of the lumbosacral spine fail to show a cause for sciatica, it is probably wise to proceed to imaging of the pelvic region. In patients with advanced vascular disease, atherosclerotic aneurysms of the hypogastric or common iliac arteries may produce sciatica, sometimes with abrupt onset (Chapman et al 1964).

Referred pain from spinal joints

Because the spinal facet joints are innervated by medial branches of the posterior primary rami of nerve roots, there is an anatomical substrate for referred pain to the limb from abnormalities of these joints. Injections into the facet joints may produce apparent radicular pain, as may injections into a variety of ligamentous, fascial, and other soft tissue structures in and around the spine (North et al 1994). Diagnosis of chronic referred pain is somewhat complicated and depends upon a process of elimination. Imaging of the discs and intervertebral foramina should fail to demonstrate direct root compression, and objective radicular neurological deficits should not be found. It may be possible to elicit tenderness to palpation over the involved facet joints. Pain may be provoked by injection into the joint and should be consistently relieved by repeated, selective local anaesthetic blocks directed at the nerve branches innervating the joints (Bogduk and Long 1979, Barnsley et al 1993).

Peripheral nerve entrapment

Peripheral nerve entrapment syndromes may produce symptomatology closely resembling limb pain of nerve root compression. Saal et al (1988) identified 45 patients with peripheral nerve entrapments as the primary cause of pseudoradicular leg pain, out of a population of approximately 4000 patients evaluated for sciatica. Sites of nerve entrapment included the femoral nerve proximal to the inguinal ligament in 9 cases, the saphenous nerve around the knee in 7, the common peroneal nerve at or above the popliteal space in 20, and the tibial nerve within the popliteal space in 9. Diagnosis was established by electromyography and nerve conduction studies and by selective spinal and peripheral nerve blocks. Back pain was noted in 49% of these patients, and 44% showed a positive straight-leg raising sign.

Piriformis syndrome is a form of entrapment of the sciatic nerve at the greater sciatic notch due to an abnormality of the piriformis muscle that can sometimes be identified by MRI. Pain is usually located in the buttock and upper thigh but may radiate distally to resemble radicular pain. Pain is said to be aggravated by prolonged hip flexion, adduction, and internal rotation, and there is typically tenderness around the buttock and sciatic notch (Barton 1991).

References

Aldrete JA 1995 Epidural fibrosis after permanent catheter insertion and infusion. Journal of Pain Symptom Management 10: 624–631

Auld AW 1978 Chronic spinal arachnoiditis. A postoperative syndrome that may signal its onset. Spine 3: 88–91

Baker AS, Ojemann RG, Swartz MN, Richardson EP 1975 Spinal epidural abscess. New England Journal of Medicine 293: 463–468

Barnsley L, Lord SM, Bogduk N 1993 Comparative local anaesthetic blocks in the diagnosis of cervical zygapophyseal joint pain. Pain 55: 99–106

Barron KD, Rowland LP, Zimmerman HM 1960 Neuropathy with malignant tumour metastases. Journal of Nervous and Mental Diseases 131: 10–31

Barton PM 1991 Piriformis syndrome: a rational approach to management. Pain 47: 345–352

Bertrand G 1975 The 'battered' root problem. Orthopedic Clinics of North America 6: 305–309

Bhargava R, Bhargava S, Haldia KN, Bhargava P 1998 Jaipur block in postherpetic neuralgia. International Journal of Dermatology 37: 465–468

Bogduk N, Long DM 1979 The anatomy of the so-called 'articular nerves' and their relationship to facet denervation in the treatment of low back pain. Journal of Neurosurgery 51: 172–177

Bohm E, Franksson C 1959 Coccygodynia and sacral rhizotomy. Acta Chirurgica Scandinavica 116: 268–274

Bowsher D 1997 The management of postherpetic neuralgia. Postgraduate Medical Journal 73: 623–629

Brevik H, Hesla PE, Molnar I, Lind B 1976 Treatment of chronic low back pain and sciatica: comparison of caudal epidural steroid injections of bupivacaine and methylprednisolone with bupivacaine followed by saline. In: Bonica J J, Albe-Fessard D (eds) Advances in pain research and therapy, vol 1. Raven Press, New York, pp 927–932

Burton CV 1978 Lumbosacral arachnoiditis. Spine 3: 24–30

Castagnera L, Maurett P, Pointilart V, Vital JM, Erny P, Senegas J 1994 Long-term results of cervical epidural steroid injection with and without morphine in chronic cervical radicular pain. Pain 58: 239–243

Chapman EM, Shaw RS, Kubik CS 1964 Sciatic pain from arteriosclerotic aneurysm of pelvic arteries. New England Journal of Medicine 271: 1410–1411

Clifford DB, Trotter JL 1984 Pain in multiple sclerosis. Archives of Neurology 41: 1270–1272

Cuckler JM, Bernini PA, Wiesel SW, Booth RE, Rothman RH, Pickens GT 1985 The use of epidural steroids in the treatment of lumbar radicular pain: a prospective, randomized, double-blind study. Journal of Bone and Joint Surgery 67A: 63–66

Davis CH 1982 Extradural spinal cord and nerve root compression from benign lesions of the lumbar area. In: Youmans J R (ed) Neurological surgery. Saunders, Philadelphia, pp 2535–2561

Delamarter RB, Ross JS, Masaryk TJ, Modic MT, Bohlman HH 1990 Diagnosis of lumbar arachnoiditis by magnetic resonance imaging. Spine 15: 304–310

Deparis M 1968 Glossopharyngeal neuralgia. In: Vinken P J, Bruyn G W (eds) Handbook of clinical neurology, vol 5. Headaches and cranial neuralgias. North-Holland, Amsterdam, pp 350–361

Devulder J, Bogaert L, Castille F, Moerman A, Rolly G 1995 Relevance of epidurography and epidural adhesiolysis in chronic failed back surgery patients. Clinical Journal of Pain 11: 147–150

Dilke TFW, Burry HC, Grahame R 1973 Extradural corticosteroid injection in management of lumbar nerve root compression. British Medical Journal 2: 635–637

Dubuisson D 1995 Treatment of occipital neuralgia by partial posterior rhizotomy at C1–3. Journal of Neurosurgery 82: 581–586

Dubuisson D, Melzack 1976 Classification of clinical pain descriptions by multiple group discriminant analysis. Experimental Neurology 51: 480–487

Dyck P 1976 The femoral nerve traction test with lumbar disc protrusions. Surgical Neurology 6: 163–166

Epstein JA, Epstein BS, Rosenthal AD, Carras R, Lavine LS 1972 Sciatica caused by nerve root entrapment in the lateral recess: the superior facet syndrome. Journal of Neurosurgery 36: 584–589

Foerster O 1933 The dermatomes in man. Brain 56: 1–39

Forrest JR 1980 The response to epidural steroid injections in chronic dorsal root pain. Canadian Anesthetists Society Journal 27: 40–46

French JD 1946 Clinical manifestations of lumbar spinal arachnoiditis. Surgery 20: 718–729

Gebarski SS, Gabrielsen TO, Gilman S, Knake JE, Latack JT, Aisen AM 1985 The initial diagnosis of multiple sclerosis: clinical impact of magnetic resonance imaging. Annals of Neurology 17: 469–474

Gilroy J, Meyer JS 1975 Medical neurology, Macmillan, New York

Gorski DW, Rao TLK, Glisson SN, Chintagada M, El-Etr A 1982 Epidural triamcinolone and adrenal response to hypoglycemic stress in dogs. Anesthesiology 57: 364–366

Green PWB, Burke AJ, Weiss CA, Langan P 1980 The role of epidural cortisone injection in the treatment of discogenic low back pain. Clinical Orthopedics 153: 121–125

Guyer DW, Wiltse LL, Eskay ML, Guyer BH 1989 The long-range prognosis of arachnoiditis. Spine 14: 1332–1341

Gybels JM, Sweet WH 1989 Neurosurgical treatment of persistent pain. Physiological and pathological mechanisms of human pain. Karger, New York

Hitselberger WE, Witten RM 1968 Abnormal myelograms in asymptomatic patients. Journal of Neurosurgery 28: 204–206

Iskandar BJ, Nashold BS 1998 Spinal and trigeminal DREZ lesions. In: Gildenberg PL, Tasker RR (eds) Textbook of stereotactic and

functional neurosurgery. McGraw–Hill, New York, pp 1573–1583
Jackson JL, Gibbons R, Meyer G, Inouye L 1997 The effect of treating herpes zoster with oral acyclovir in preventing postherpetic neuralgia. Archives of Internal Medicine 157: 909–912
Johnson CE, Sze G 1990 Benign lumbar arachnoiditis: MR imaging with gadopentetate dimeglumine. American Journal of Neuroradiology 11: 763–770
Keegan JJ, Garrett FD 1948 The segmental distribution of the cutaneous nerves in the limbs of man. Anatomical Record 102: 409–437
Kendall HO, Kendall FP, Wadsworth GE 1971 Muscles: testing and function. Williams & Wilkins, Baltimore
Kondo A 1998 Follow-up results of using microvascular decompression for treatment of glossopharyngeal neuralgia. Journal of Neurosurgery 88: 221–225
Kumar K, Nath R, Wyant GM 1991 Treatment of chronic pain by epidural spinal cord stimulation: a 10 year experience. Journal of Neurosurgery 75: 402–407
Lipton S 1979 Relief of pain in clinical practice. Blackwell, Oxford, pp 231–248
Little JR, Dale AJD, Okazaki H 1974 Meningeal carcinomatosis: clinical manifestations. Archives of Neurology 30: 138–143
Long DM 1982 Pain of spinal origin. In: Youmans JR (ed) Neurological surgery. Saunders, Philadelphia, pp 3613–3626
Lozano AM, Vanderlinden G, Bachoo R, Rothbart P 1998 Microsurgical C2 ganglionectomy for chronic intractable occipital pain. Journal of Neurosurgery 89: 359–365
Maigne J-Y, Rime B, Deligne B 1992 Computed tomographic follow-up study of forty-eight cases of nonoperatively treated lumbar intervertebral disc herniation. Spine 17: 1071–1074
Meilman PW, Leibrock LG, Leong FT 1989 Outcome of implanted spinal cord stimulation in the treatment of chronic pain: arachnoiditis versus single nerve root injury and mononeuropathy. Clinical Journal of Pain 5: 189–193
Moossy JJ, Nashold BS, Osborne D, Friedman AH 1987 Conus medullaris nerve root avulsions. Journal of Neurosurgery 66: 835–841
Moulin DE, Foley KM, Ebers GC 1988 Pain syndromes in multiple sclerosis. Neurology 38: 1830–1834
Murphey F, Simmons JCH, Brunson B 1973 Ruptured cervical discs, 1939 to 1972. Clinical Neurosurgery 20: 9–17
Nagashima C, Sakaguchi A, Kamisasa A, Kawanuma S 1976 Cardiovascular complications on upper vagal rootlet section for glossopharyngeal neuralgia. Journal of Neurosurgery 44: 248–253
Nathan P, Wall PD 1974 Treatment of postherpetic neuralgia by prolonged electric stimulation. British Medical Journal 14: 645–647
Neiri RL, Burgert EO, Groover RV 1968 Central nervous system leukemia: a review. Mayo Clinic Proceedings 43: 70–79
Nelson DA, Vates TS, Thomas RB 1973 Complications from intrathecal steroid therapy in patients with multiple sclerosis. Acta Neurologica Scandinavica 49: 176–188
Nelson KA, Park KM, Robinovitz E, Tsigos C, Max MB 1997 High-dose oral dextromethorphan versus placebo in painful diabetic neuropathy and pstherpetic neuralgia. Neurology 48: 1212–1218
North RB, Kidd DH, Campbell JN, Long DM 1991 Dorsal root ganglionectomy for failed back surgery syndrome: a 5-year follow-up study. Journal of Neurosurgery 74: 236–242
North RB, Han M, Zahurak M, Kidd DH 1994 Radiofrequency lumbar facet denervation: analysis of prognostic factors. Pain 57: 77–83
Olson ME, Chernik NL, Posner JB 1974 Infiltration of the leptomeninges by systemic cancer. A clinical and pathologic study. Archives of Neurology 30: 122–137
Paty DW, Oger JJF, Kastrukoff LF et al 1988 MRI in the diagnosis of MS: a prospective study with comparison of clinical evaluation, evoked potentials, oligoclonal banding, and CT. Neurology 38: 180–185
Ramirez-Lassepas M, Tulloch JW, Quinones MR, Snyder BD 1992 Acute radicular pain as a presenting symptom in multiple sclerosis. Archives of Neurology 49: 255–258
Ray CG 1980 Chickenpox (varicella) and herpes zoster. In: Isselbacher K J et al (eds) Harrison's principles of internal medicine. McGraw-Hill, New York, pp 801–804
Resnick DK, Jannetta PJ, Bisonette D, Jho H-D, Lanzino G 1995 Microvascular decompression for glossopharyngeal neuralgia. Neurosurgery 36: 64–69
Ross JS, Robertson JT, Frederickson RCA et al 1996 Association between peridural scar and recurrent radicular pain after lumbar discectomy: magnetic resonance evaluation. Neurosurgery 38: 855–863
Rothman SLG, Glenn WV, Kerber CW 1985 Postoperative fractures of lumbar articular facets: occult cause of radiculopathy. American Journal of Neuroradiology 145: 779–784
Rowbotham MC, Davies PS, Fields HL 1995 Topical lidocaine gel relieves postherpetic neuralgia. Annals of Neurology 37: 246–253
Rushton JG, Stevens JC, Miller RH 1981 Glossopharyngeal (vagoglossopharyngeal) neuralgia. Archives of Neurology 38: 201–205
Saal JA, Dillingham MF, Gamburd RS, Fanton GS 1988 The pseudoradicular syndrome. Lower extremity peripheral nerve entrapment masquerading as lumbar radiculopathy. Spine 13: 926–930
Saal JS, Franson RC, Dobrow R, Saal JA, White AH, Goldthwaite N 1990 High levels of inflammatory phospholipase A2 activity in lumbar disc herniations. Spine 15: 674–678
Sherrington CS 1898 Experiments in the examination of the peripheral distribution of the fibres of the posterior roots of some spinal nerves. Part II. Philosophical Transactions B 190: 45–186
Smith DL, Lucas LM, Kumar KL 1987 Greater occipital neuralgia: an unusual presenting feature of neurosyphilis. Headache 27: 552–554
Snoek W, Weber H, Jorgensen B 1977 Double blind evaluation of extradural methylprednisolone for herniated lumbar disc. Acta Orthopaedica Scandinavica 48: 635–641
Spiegelmann R, Friedman WA 1991 Spinal cord stimulation: a contemporary series. Neurosurgery 28: 65–71
Storm-Mathisen A 1978 Syphilis. In: Vinken PJ, Bruyn G W (eds) Handbook of clinical neurology. North-Holland, Amsterdam, pp 337–394
Taub A, Robinson F, Taub E 1995 Dorsal root ganglionectomy for intractable monoradicular sciatica. In: Schmidek HH, Sweet WH (eds) Operative neurosurgical techniques, 3rd edn. Saunders, Philadelphia, pp 1585–1593
Tyring S, Barbarash RA, Nahlik JE et al 1995 Famciclovir for the treatment of acute herpes zoster: effects on acute disease and postherpetic neuralgia. A randomized, double-blind, placebo-controlled trial. Collaborative Famciclovir Herpes Zoster Study Group. Annals of Internal Medicine 123: 89–96
Uldry PA, Regli F 1992 Pseudoradicular syndrome in multiple sclerosis. Four cases diagnosed by magnetic resonance imaging. Revue Neurologique 148: 692–695
Wasserstrom WR, Glass JP, Posner JB 1982 Diagnosis and treatment of leptomeningeal metastases from solid tumours. Cancer 49: 759–772
Weinstein PR, Ehni G, Wilsou CB 1977 Lumbar spondylosis. Year Book, Chicago
White AA, Derby R, Wynne G 1980 Epidural injections for the diagnosis and treatment of low back pain. Spine 5: 78–86

White JC, Sweet WH 1969 Pain and the neurosurgeon. Thomas, Springfield, IL
Wiesel SW, Tsoumas N, Feffer HL, Citrin CM, Patronas N 1984 A study of computer-assisted tomography. The incidence of positive CAT scans in an asymptomatic group of patients. Spine 9: 549–551
Wilkinson M 1971 Cervical spondylosis. Heinemann, London
Wynn Parry CB 1980 Pain in avulsion lesions of the brachial plexus. Pain 9: 41–53

Chapter 20

Central pain

Jörgen Boivie

Introduction

The International Assocation for the Study of Pain (IASP) has defined central pain as pain caused by a lesion or dysfunction in the central nervous system (CNS) (Merskey and Bogduk 1994). Note that the cause is a primary process in the CNS. Thus peripherally induced pain with central mechanisms is not central pain, even if the central mechanisms are prominent. As with all definitions, there are conditions that may or may not be included. In the present context pain due to brachial plexus avulsion and phantom pain are such examples. They will not be discussed in this chapter. Painful epileptic seizures are evoked by primary processes in the CNS and may thus be considered central pain.

The term 'thalamic pain' is often used in a general sense for all central pain and the expression 'pseudothalamic pain' is sometimes used for central pain caused by extrathalamic lesions. The term 'dysaesthetic pain' is also sometimes used for central pain in general, probably due to the belief that all or almost all central pain has a predominantly dysaesthetic character, which is incorrect. Dysaesthetic pain can have either central or peripheral causes. It is recommended that the general term central pain be used in most instances, and that only central pain caused by lesions in the thalamus should be labelled thalamic pain.

The term 'anaesthesia dolorosa' has chiefly been used for head and face pain, and in particular for the neuropathic pain that sometimes develops after neurosurgical lesions of the trigeminal nerve or ganglion, or after destructive nerve blocks carried out to treat trigeminal neuralgia. It has also been used for central pain in an anaesthetic region caused by neurosurgical brain lesions created in the treatment of severe pain.

The term 'deafferentation pain' is used for similar conditions, but it is more commonly used in patients with lesions of spinal nerves.

Central pain is commonly thought of as being excruciating pain with bizarre character, and covering large areas of the body. This is only part of the truth, however, because central pain can appear in many guises. It can have a trivial character and be restricted to a relatively small area, such as distal pain in one arm, or in the face. It is true, though, that central pain is mostly severe in the sense that it causes the patient much suffering, even though its intensity may be relatively low. This is because central pain is usually very irritating and constant.

Aetiology and epidemiology

Lesions causing central pain

Structure and location of the lesion

It appears that all kinds of lesion in the brain and spinal cord can cause central pain (Box 20.1). These lesions and dysfunctions are caused by many different disease processes. The macrostructure of the lesion is probably less important than its location as regards the probability that it will induce central pain. This does not mean that the structure of the lesion has no significance, because it is conceivable that the microstructure of the lesion in some instances is critical, but there is to date no information from research on this matter.

Pain in Parkinson's disease has previously not been considered central pain. Recent surveys show that pain is common in this disease, but it is at present not clear to what extent this pain is caused directly by the brain pathology. It is possible though that some of the pain is of central origin and thus is central pain.

The lesions that lead to central pain include rapidly and slowly developing lesions. There appears to be no difference in the tendency to cause central pain between rapidly developing haemorrhages, infarcts (Leijon et al 1989, Bowsher et al 1998), and traumatic spinal cord lesions and slowly developing demyelination or arteriovenous malformations. As the prevalence of central pain is very low in patients with intracranial tumours and spinal tumours, it is difficult to know whether they differ in this respect, and whether there is any difference between intra- and extraparenchymal tumours. Besides the common kind of constant central pain, tumours may also cause painful epileptic seizures.

BOX 20.1
Causes of central pain

- Vascular lesions in the brain and spinal cord
  - Infarct
  - Haemorrhage
  - Vascular malformation
- Multiple sclerosis
- Traumatic spinal cord injury
  - Cordotomy
- Traumatic brain injury
- Syringomyelia and syringobulbia
- Tumours
- Abscesses
- Inflammatory diseases other than MS; myelitis caused by viruses, syphilis
- Epilepsy
- Parkinson's disease (?)

It is now clear that lesions at any level along the neuraxis can cause central pain. Thus lesions at the first synapse in the dorsal horn of the spinal cord or trigeminal nuclei, along the ascending pathways through the spinal cord and brainstem, in the thalamus, in the subcortical white matter, and probably in the cerebral cortex have all been reported to cause central pain (Pagni 1998, Tasker 2000). The highest prevalences have been noticed after lesions in the spinal cord, lower brainstem, and ventroposterior part of the thalamus (Tasker 2000).

The location of lesions that produce central pain has been best studied in central poststroke pain (CPSP). The role of thalamic lesions is one of the recurrent questions in this context. In one study using CT scans it was found that 9 of 27 patients had lesions involving the thalamus (33%), but the lesions were restricted to the thalamus in only 2 of these (Leijon et al 1989). In their prospective study, Andersen et al (1995) had 25% thalamic involvement among the CPSP patients (by CT scans), but in a recently published study of 70 patients using MRI it was found that about 60% had lesions engaging the thalamus (Bowsher et al 1998).

The importance of the location of the thalamic lesion within the thalamus was elucidated in a study of the clinical consequences of thalamic infarcts. The results showed that only patients with lesions including the ventroposterior thalamic region developed central pain (3 of 18 patients; Bogousslavsky et al 1988). In studies carried out by Bowsher et al (1998) and Leijon et al (1989) all thalamic lesions included part of the ventroposterior thalamic region. This region receives a particularly dense spinothalamic projection in primates (Boivie 1979).

Lesions affect somatic sensibility

The first requisite for a disease process to produce central pain seems to be that it affects structures involved in somatic sensibility, which is not surprising, because pain is part of somaesthesia. This notion is based on previous reviews, case reports, and recent studies in patients with central pain caused by stroke, multiple sclerosis, and syringomyelia, which indicate that central pain is independent of non-sensory symptoms and signs (Leijon et al 1989, Andersen et al 1995, Bowsher et al 1998, Pagni 1998, Tasker 2000). This excludes many lesion sites as possible causes of central pain. Fortunately, however, only a minority of the patients with lesions that carry a risk will develop central pain. The risk differs very much between diseases and locations of the lesion.

Most patients with central pain reported in the literature have had sensory abnormalities, and the dominating features have been abnormal sensibility to temperature and pain, and hyperaesthesia (Pagni 1998, Tasker 2000). Depending on the location of the lesion, the sensibility profiles differ, often in a predictable way.

These observations, and results from studies on patients with central pain as a result of cerebrovascular lesions, multiple sclerosis, traumatic spinal cord injuries, and syringomyelia employing quantitative methods to assess the sensory abnormalities, form the basis for the hypothesis that central pain only occurs after lesions that affect the spinothalamic pathways, i.e., the pathways most important for temperature and pain sensibility (Berić et al 1988, Boivie et al 1989, Bowsher et al 1998, Pagni 1998). If this hypothesis turns out to be correct it means that lesions of the dorsal column–medial lemniscal pathways are not a requisite for the occurrence of central pain. Such lesions were for many years thought to be essential in the mechanism of central pain (see below). This hypothesis states that central pain is the result of lesions of the lemniscal system, which remove the inhibition normally exerted on the spinothalamic projections. Undoubtedly the lemniscal projections are affected in many central pain patients, but the question is whether this part of the lesion is of importance for the pain. It certainly affects sensibility. No patients with central pain and lesions unequivocally restricted to the lemniscal pathways appear to have been published, whereas many cases of lesions strictly limited to the spinothalamic pathways have been reported, for instance in the Wallenberg syndrome and after cordotomy.

Epidemiology

The only prospective epidemiological study that has been carried out concerns central poststroke pain (Andersen et al 1995). In this study 191 patients were followed for 12 months after stroke onset with regard to sensory abnormalities and the development of spontaneous and evoked central pain. Sixteen of these developed central pain, i.e., 8.4%, which is a much higher incidence than had previously been predicted or suspected. Among patients with somatosensory deficits (42% of all stroke patients), the incidence of central pain was 18%. The corresponding figure in a mainly retrospective study of central pain in 63 patients with brainstem infarcts was 44% (MacGowan et al 1997). In this study the overall incidence for CPSP was 25%.

A recent study of the prevalence of central pain in 371 patients with multiple sclerosis has found that 28% of multiple sclerosis (MS) patients experience, or have experienced, central pain (Österberg and Boivie, in preparation; see below).

The highest prevalences are found with traumatic spinal cord injuries, multiple sclerosis, and syringomyelia. The latter is a rare disease with a very high incidence of central pain, probably the highest of any disease. In a recent survey of 22 patients it was found that most had central pain at some stage of the disease (Boivie and Rollsjö, unpublished observations).

Pathophysiology

The lesions that cause central pain vary enormously in location, size, and structure. There is no study indicating that a small lesion in the dorsal horn of the spinal cord carries less risk for central pain than a huge infarct involving much of the thalamus and large parts of the white matter lateral and superior to the thalamus. This raises the question whether the same pathophysiology underlies all central pain. The fact that the character of the pain also differs widely between patients with the same kind of lesion, and between groups, points in the same direction. However, this does not exclude the possibility that some common pathophysiological factors may be involved in central pain. The most important are:

1. The disease process, here called the lesion, involves the spinothalamic pathways, including the indirect spino-reticulo-thalamic and spino-mesencephalic projections, as indicated by abnormalities in the sensibility to pain and temperature.
2. The lesion probably does not have to involve the dorsal column–medial lemniscal pathways to invoke central pain.
3. The lesion can be located at any level of the neuraxis, from the dorsal horn to the cerebral cortex.
4. It is probable that all kinds of disease processes may cause central pain, but the probability of central pain occurring varies greatly between these diseases, from being rare to occurring in the majority of patients.
5. As yet no single region has been shown to be crucial in the processes underlying central pain, but three thalamic regions have been focused upon, namely the ventroposterior, reticular, and medial/intralaminar regions. The role of the cerebral cortex in central pain is unclear, but this issue has not been specifically studied.

6. The pain and hypersensitivity experienced by central pain patients are compatible with an increased burst activity at some level of the sensory pathways, including the cerebral cortex.
7. The cellular processes underlying central pain are still unknown, but processes involving excitatory amino acids, and particularly glutaminergic NMDA-receptors, have been implicated.

Clinical characteristics

Diagnosis of a CNS process

The definition of central pain states that it is caused by a lesion or dysfunction in the CNS. The first step in the diagnostic procedure is therefore to ensure that the patient has a CNS disorder. This is often obvious, as in many patients with stroke or multiple sclerosis (MS), but it is sometimes not clear that there is a CNS lesion, as in some patients with moderate spinal trauma or suspected minor stroke. A detailed history of the neurological symptoms and a neurological examination are important parts of the diagnostic procedure, but laboratory examinations are often necessary. These include computerized tomography with X-ray or magnetic resonance, i.e., a CT scan or MRI, assays of the cerebrospinal fluid (CSF), neurophysiological examinations, and other tests.

In addition to confirming the presence of a CNS process, one must also consider whether the patient has pain as a result of peripheral neuropathy. Polyneuropathy is not uncommon in, for instance, stroke patients, a group with a high incidence of diabetes. Neurography and electromyography are therefore indicated in some patients. Quantitative sensory tests are also valuable in the diagnosis of neuropathy. They include examination of sensibility to temperature and pain, as well as to vibration and touch (Lindblom 1994). Whereas neurography can only demonstrate abnormalties in large fibres, these tests can show dysfunction in both large and small sensory fibres.

Differential diagnosis of central versus nociceptive and psychogenic pain

Central pain can usually be distinguished from other forms of pain provided that one is familiar with the characteristics of central pain, but in some patients it is difficult to determine whether the pain is central, peripheral neuropathic, nociceptive, or psychogenic. Some patients have more than one kind of pain. A hemiplegic stroke patient, for instance, can have a nociceptive shoulder pain in addition to central pain. The examination of patients suspected of having central pain must be individually tailored in order to identify possible non-central causes of the pain. Diagnostic problems are particularly difficult in some patients with MS and spinal cord injury (SCI), because of the complex clinical picture, with a mixture of motor and sensory symptoms and pain. Paresis and dyscoordination may lead to abnormal strain in musculoskeletal structures and development of nociceptive pain. The diagnostic procedure often calls for consultations by specialists, particularly in orthopaedics.

Psychogenic factors are important in central pain, as in all pain, but with increasing knowledge of the characteristics of central pain it rarely turns out that pain suspected of being central is truly psychogenic. Psychiatric and psychological consultations may be indicated in some patients, even if there is certain central pain, because the patient may also be depressed, although patients with central pain do not appear to be more depressed than other pain patients.

Pain characteristics

The next step is to analyse the chacteristics of the pain, i.e., its location, quality, intensity, onset and development after onset, variation with time, and influence by external and internal events.

Pain location

It is usually stated with considerable emphasis that central pain is diffusely located. This notion appears to be largely derived from the fact that central pain often extends over large areas of the body, for instance the whole right or left side, or the lower half of the body. However, central pain can also involve one hand only, or just the ulnar or radial side of the hand, or one side of the face. Even patients with extensive central pain find it relatively easy to describe the extent of the painful regions, as shown in studies of patients with central pain after stroke and MS (Leijon et al 1989, Österberg and Boivie, unpublished). It is therefore more correct to state that most central pain is extensive than to describe it as diffuse.

The location of the lesion determines the location of the pain (Box 20.2). Thus large lesions in the ventroposterior thalamic region or the posterior limb of the internal capsule tend to cause hemibody pain, whereas large spinal cord lesions cause bilateral pain involving the body regions innervated by the segments caudal to the lesion. Even lesions that

> **BOX 20.2**
> **Common locations of central pain**
>
> **Stroke**
> All of one side
> All of one side except the face
> Arm and/or leg on one side
> Face on one side, extremities on the other side
> The face
>
> **Multiple sclerosis**
> Lower half of the body
> One or both legs
> Arm and leg on one side
> Trigeminal neuralgia
>
> **Spinal cord injury**
> Whole body below the neck
> Lower half of the body
> One leg
>
> **Syringomyelia**
> Arm and thorax on one side
> One arm
> Thorax on one side
> One leg in addition to one of the above

cause extensive loss of somatic sensibility may lead to central pain restricted to a small portion of the deafferented region. Examples of central pain engaging small regions were shown in patients with superficial cortical/subcortical vascular lesions by Michel et al (1990).

Cerebrovascular lesions in the medulla oblongata, i.e., mainly lesions caused by thrombosis in the posterior inferior cerebellar artery leading to Wallenberg syndromes, can induce central pain on both sides, the face and head being involved on the lesion side, and the rest of the body on the contralateral side (Leijon et al 1989, Bowsher et al 1998). This pattern is caused by injury to the ipsilateral spinal trigeminal nucleus and the crossed spinothalamic tract. Lesions affecting the spinothalamic tract in the spinal cord will lead to pain on the contralateral side, after cordotomy for example. In syringomyelia central pain may be restricted to part of one side of the thorax, but it may also be more extensive, including the arm too, and even the lower body regions.

Central pain is experienced as superficial or deep pain, or with both superficial and deep components, but the high incidence of cutaneous hyperaesthesias contribute to the impression that superficial pain dominates, although deep pain is common too. Among 27 CPSP patients, 8 described the pain as superficial, 8 as deep, and the remaining 11 as both superficial and deep (Leijon and Boivie 1989c).

Quality of pain

No pain quality is pathognomonic for central pain. Central pain is thus not always burning or 'dysaesthetic', as one might believe from reading some of the literature on the subject. In fact central pain can have any quality, and the variation between patients is great, although some qualities are more common than others.

Another basic feature is the presence of more than one pain quality in many patients. The different pains can coexist in a body region, or may be present in different parts of the body. A patient with CPSP, for instance, may have burning and aching pain in the leg and arm, and burning and stinging pain in the face. Other patients have a less complex pain condition, with aching pain in the arm or leg.

One would expect the location of the lesion to be a deciding factor regarding the quality of pain. This appears to be partly true, but it is also apparent that similar lesions can lead to different pain qualities, as illustrated by central pain caused by cerebrovascular lesions in the thalamus (Leijon et al 1989).

The most common central pain quality is probably burning pain, which has been found to be frequent in most central pain conditions (Boivie 1995, Bowsher 1996, Bowsher et al 1998, Pagni 1998, Tasker 2000). However, it was reported that burning pain is rare in patients with cortical/subcortical lesions (Michel et al 1990). As mentioned above, dysaesthetic pain has been reported to be common in some conditions, for instance in MS and incomplete SCI, and after cordotomy, which also is a form of incomplete SCI. However, the term has not been well defined, and evidently it has often been used to indicate a combination of dysaesthesias and spontaneous pain of differing qualities. This is indicated by the results of Davidoff and Roth (1991) where 19 SCI patients with 'dysaesthetic pain syndrome' experienced the following pain qualities: cutting (63%), burning (58%), piercing (47%), radiating (47%), and tight (37%). The descriptions 'cruel' and 'nagging' were each used by 37%. Since dysaesthesias are common in most central pain conditions, this results in high figures for 'dysaesthetic' pain.

Central pain caused by spinal cord processes commonly include a pressing belt-like pain (= a girdle pain) at the level of the upper border of the lesion, in addition to other pains. This pain occurs in patients with MS and traumatic SCI, and is similar to pain caused by lesions or inflammation affecting the spinal dorsal roots, which may present a diagnostic problem in SCI patients.

Intensity of pain

From much of the early literature one gets the impression that central pain is always excruciating. This is incorrect, because the intensity of central pain ranges from low to extremely high. However, even if the pain is of low or moderate intensity the patients assess the pain as severe because it causes much suffering due to its irritating character and constant presence. Thus a patient may indicate a pain intensity of 28 on a visual analogue scale (VAS 0–100), and yet may explain that the pain is a great burden making life very miserable. Interviews with patients show that many patients with central pain and severe motor handicap following strokes, MS, or SCI often rate the pain as their worst handicap (Britell and Mariano 1991).

Central pain may have a constant intensity or the intensity may vary. These variations seem to occur spontaneously or under the influence of external somatic or psychological stimuli, or as a result of internal events. In patients with more than one central pain quality, the variation in intensity may differ between pain forms.

Onset and other temporal aspects

Central pain may start almost immediately after occurrence of the lesion, or it may be delayed for up to several years. Delays are well known in poststroke central pain. This delay may be as long as 2–3 years, but in most patients the pain starts within a couple of weeks of the stroke (Mauguiere and Desmedt 1988, Michel et al 1990, Leijon and Boivie 1991, Andersen et al 1995, Bowsher 1996). Andersen et al noticed that 63% had pain onset within 1 month post stroke (Andersen et al 1995). When the onset is delayed it frequently coincides with changes in the subjective sensory abnormalities. For example, a patient with dense sensory loss may start to experience paraesthesias or dysaesthesias, and soon afterwards the pain starts.

Most spontaneous central pain is constantly present, with no pain-free intervals. In central poststroke pain 23 of 27 patients reported constant pain, whereas the other four patients had some pain-free intervals lasting at most a few hours each day (Leijon and Boivie 1989b). In addition to the spontaneous pain, many patients experience intermittent pain evoked by external and internal stimuli. Intermittent pain is well known in a minority of MS patients as part of tonic painful seizures and as trigeminal neuralgia. MS patients may also develop intermittent aching pain during physical activity, for instance during walking.

Unfortunately central pain is commonly permanent, but it may remit completely. This occurs spontaneously, or as a result of new lesions or other changes in the underlying disease. Some CPSPs successively cease completely, but most CPSP continues throughout life (Leijon and Boivie 1996). A few cases have been reported in which a new supratentorial stroke abolished the pain (Soria and Fine 1991). In SCI the central pain can be temporary lasting a few months only, but more commonly it is permanent (Berić et al 1988, Britell and Mariano 1991), which is similar to central pain in MS.

Stimuli affecting central pain

Many internal and external events influence central pain, such as cutaneous stimuli, body movements, visceral stimuli, emotions, and changes in mood. Allodynia, i.e., pain evoked by a stimulus that is normally not painful, for example touch, light pressure, or moderate heat or cold, is common in patients with central pain (Berić et al 1988, Boivie et al 1989, Pagni 1989, Boivie 1992, Hansson and Lindblom 1992, Bowsher 1996, Tasker 2000). Such stimuli often give prolonged aftereffects, and they may increase ongoing pain. Patients with central pain frequently experience an increase in pain associated with body movement, such as changes in body posture, non-strenuous walking, or movement of the extremities (Leijon and Boivie 1989c, Österberg and Boivie, unpublished observations in MS). Visceral stimuli, particularly from a full bladder or rectum, have long been thought to influence central pain.

It is also common that patients with central pain experience an immediate increase in pain after sudden fear, joy, loud noise, or bright light (Leijon and Boivie 1989b, Bowsher 1996, Tasker 2000). Experience from clinical practice indicates that central pain is as affected by psychological factors as other pain conditions; i.e., anxiety and depression aggravate central pain. On the other hand, there is no reason to believe that psychological factors per se are important in the development of central pain, which is clearly somatic organic pain caused by lesions in the CNS.

Neurological symptoms and signs

Because central pain is a neurological symptom emanating from processes in the CNS, it is of interest to know whether central pain is accompanied by any other particular neurological symptoms and signs, which should then be included in the criteria for diagnosis. All investigators agree that central pain is caused by perturbations of the somatosensory systems, usually a lesion. It is thus a somatosensory symptom, and it is therefore natural that abnormalities in somatic sensibility are the only symptoms and signs besides pain that are present in all patients with central pain. Several studies have shown that central pain is independent of abnormalities in muscle function, coordination, vision, hearing, vestibular functions, and higher cortical functions. In a study on CPSP all 27 patients had sensory abnormalities, whereas only 48% had paresis and 58% ataxia (Leijon et al 1989). Other neurological symptoms were present in a few patients. Similar results have been obtained in MS patients with central pain.

The important point is that the non-sensory symptoms are not necessary for the development of central pain. This is supported by the fact that many patients with central pain lack non-sensory symptoms.

Somatosensory abnormalities

Abnormalities in somatic sensibility are important in patients with central pain, both as criteria for diagnosis and as symptoms contributing to the patient's handicap. They may be subtle and may elude detection with clinical test methods which only provide a rough qualitative estimate. Thus one needs to use quantitative sensory tests (QSTs). The available devices for such tests are now available for clinical use. They include calibrated vibrameters, and sets of von Frey filaments for the analysis of touch, devices for quantitative testing of temperature and temperature pain sensibility with Peltier element stimulators, and devices for measuring mechanical pain (Lindblom 1994, Yarnitsky and Sprecher 1994).

There is a large variation in the spectrum of sensory abnormalities among patients with central pain. It ranges from a slightly raised threshold for one of the submodalities to complete loss of all somatic sensibility in the painful region. Hyperaesthesia also occurs often, as well as abnormal sensations. The most important sensory abnormalities include changes in detection thresholds and in stimulus–response function, spontaneous or evoked abnormal sensations, radiation of sensations from the stimulus site, prolonged response latency, and spatial and temporal summation. They represent both quantitative and qualitative abnormalities. The occurrence of these abnormalities in patients with central pain will be briefly summarized.

Hypoaesthesia

This term is usually used to denote a raised threshold, but it can also mean that the sensation evoked by a stimulus is weaker than normal. Raised thresholds or total loss of sensibility is common in central pain. It can affect some or all submodalities. In a study of CPSP, it was found that all patients had hypoaesthesia to temperature, whereas only about half of the patients had hypoaesthesia to touch, vibration, and kinaesthesia (Boivie et al 1989). Similar results, but less pronounced, were found in other CPSP patients (Bowsher et al 1998). Hypoaesthesia to noxious thermal and mechanical stimuli (heat, cold, pinprick, or pinching), i.e., hypoalgesia, was also found. In other studies using QSTs, similar observations were made in patients with MS (Boivie 1995) and SCI with central pain (Berić et al 1988), and in syringomyelia (Boivie and Rollsjö, unpublished observations). This is the basis for the hypothesis that central pain only occurs in patients who have dysfunctions in the spinothalamic systems, i.e., in the pathways most important for temperature and pain sensibility (Boivie et al 1989, Bowsher 1995).

Hyperaesthesia

Hyperaesthesia to touch, moderate cold and heat, allodynia to touch and cold, and hyperalgesia to cold, heat, or pinprick are common in many central pain conditions (Boivie et al 1989, Pagni 1989, Tasker 2000). Combinations of hypoaesthesia and allodynia to touch or cold are not uncommon.

Paraesthesias and dysaesthesias

These are common in central pain (Pagni 1989, Tasker 2000). In a study of CPSP 85 and 41% of the patients reported spontaneous and evoked dysaesthesia, respectively, whereas 41% experienced paraesthesia (Boivie et al 1989). Dysaesthesia is often evoked by touch and cold and is sometimes painful.

Numbness

Many central pain patients experience numbness, but it is not clear what underlies the perception of numbness. Is it primarily related to loss of tactile sensibility? Undoubtedly total sensory loss leads to numbness, but evidently it can also occur with normal threshold to touch, as shown in CPSP (Boivie et al 1989). Patients will sometimes use the term numbness when they experience paraesthesias or dysaesthesias.

Radiation, prolonged response latency, aftersensations, summation

These features are indicative of neuropathic pain and seem to be more common in central pain than in peripheral neuropathic pain. The term radiation means that the sensation spreads outside the site of stimulation, such as when touch with cotton wool or pinprick on the dorsum of the foot evokes a sensation in both the leg and foot. Radiation was demonstrated in 12 of 24 patients with CPSP (Boivie et al 1989), and is also found in other central pain conditions (Tasker et al 1991).

Prolonged latency between the stimulus and perception of the sensation can in some patients be demonstrated with tactile and pinprick stimulation. This appears to occur only when there is a hyperaesthetic/hyperalgesic response, which includes spatial and temporal summation. It is then that the delay in sensation is mostly prolonged, and it may also be of an explosive hyperpathic kind. Hyperalgesia is found in many, but not all central pain patients.

Neurophysiological examinations

The central somatosensory pathways can be examined with neurophysiological techniques, which offer objective information regarding the function of the pathways. The most commonly employed method is to study somatosensory evoked postentials (SEP) evoked by electrical stimulation of the median and tibial/sural nerves. This method tests the function of the dorsal column–medial lemniscal pathways, because the stimulation activates large primary afferent fibres innervating low-threshold mechanoreceptors.

As the sensory disturbances in central pain indicate that the lesions affect the spinothalamic pathways, it is of interest to study SEP evoked by peripheral stimulation of afferents that activate the spinothalamic pathways. This can be done by using lasers to stimulate cutaneous heat receptors (Bromm and Treede 1987, Pertovaara et al 1988, Treede et al 1988). A study with this technique on patients with CPSP showed that abnormalities in the laser-evoked cortical potentials, which have a long latency, correlate well with abnormalities in the sensibility to temperature and pain, but not to touch and vibration (Casey et al 1996).

Willer and collaborators have extensively studied the flexion reflex in patients with central pain and found that the latency of this reflex is prolonged in these patients. This reflex, the R III reflex, is dependent on activation of nociceptor afferents. Lesions in the CNS leading to decreased pain sensibility have been found to result in a delay of this reflex following electrical stimulation of the sural nerve (Dehen et al 1983).

Psychological factors

Central pain patients have CNS disease that is mostly chronic and, in many cases, causes severe handicap. It is therefore natural that these diseases per se can lead to depression, for example poststroke depression, and depression in MS and SCI patients. Because many investigations have shown that there are mutual correlations between pain and depression, one would expect to find a high incidence of depression in central pain patients. This has not been well studied and available data are incomplete and somewhat conflicting. In a group of SCI patients depression, anxiety, loneliness, and several other psychosocial factors correlated significantly with the degree of pain, but this study also included nociceptive pain (Umlauf et al 1992), whereas studies of 24 and 16 CPSP patients could not identify any signs of depression (Andersen et al 1995, Leijon and Boivie, unpublished observations). Nor were these CPSP patients different from a control group with regard to social situation or major life events.

Treatment

General aspects

Treating central pain is no easy task, because there is no universally effective treatment. This means that one often must try various treatment modalities to get the best results, which sometimes are achieved with combinations of treatments (Box 20.3). With each treatment it is important that the patient is well informed about possible adverse side effects, and how these should be regarded and when they should contact the doctor responsible. Treatment usually reduces the pain, rather than giving complete relief, and patients should be aware of this, so that they have realistic expectations. In this context it is interesting to note that relatively small decreases in pain intensity are often highly valued by the patients, with the result that they want to continue treatment even if the clinician responsible is doubtful about doing so.

Most treatment regimens for central pain are empirical and based on clinical experience. Many treatments have been claimed to be effective in the literature, mostly based on experience with small groups of patients. Few treatments have been tested in well-designed clinical trials. There is thus a great need for such trials on homogeneous patient groups. Furthermore, because it is conceivable that treatment affects some aspects of central pain but not others, it would be desirable to assess the effect of treatment on each pain modality separately. The practical problems in performing such studies are obvious.

An important but still largely unanswered question concerning treatment is whether the

BOX 20.3
Treatment modalities for central pain, including methods with unproven effect

Pharmacological
Antidepressant drugs (AD)
Antiepileptic drugs (AED)
Antiarrhythmic drugs, local anaesthetics
Analgesics
Other drugs
- Adrenergic drugs
- Cholinergic drugs
- GABA-ergic drugs
- Glutaminergic drugs
- Naloxone
- Neuroleptic drugs

Sensory stimulation
Transcutaneous electrical stimulation (TENS)
Dorsal column stimulation (DCS)
Brain stimulation

Neurosurgery
Cordotomy
Dorsal root entry zone (DREZ) lesions
Cordectomy
Mesencephalic tractotomy
Thalamotomy
Cortical and subcortical ablation

Sympathetic blockade

different central pain conditions respond differently to one particular treatment. This has not been systematically studied, but such differences appear to exist. From a study of the literature and from clinical experience one gets the impression that CPSP responds better to antidepressants than the central pain in SCI and MS. Conversely paroxysmal pain in MS responds much better to antiepileptic drugs than the other kinds of central pain.

One of the similarities between central pain and peripheral neuropathic pain is treatment. In both pain categories antidepressants and antiepileptic drugs are the most frequently used drugs. These are also the ones with the best documented effects, and virtually the only ones tested in well-conducted clinical trials. They are the first-line treatments, together with transcutaneous electrical nerve stimulation (TENS), which can only have a chance of giving relief, however, if the dorsal column–medial lemniscal pathways are not totally damaged. The other treatments listed in Box 20.3 have more of an experimental character, although some of them are used quite frequently by some pain specialists.

BOX 20.4
Antidepressant drugs used in central pain

Relatively unselective with regard to 5HT and NA
Amitriptyline
Doxepine
Nortriptyline

Some selectivity for 5HT
Clomipramine
Imipramine

High selectivity for 5HT
Citalopram
Fluoxetin
Fluvoxamine
Paroxetine
Trazodone

Some selectivity for NA
Desipramine
Maprotiline
Mianserine

Antidepressants

Documentation of effects, clinical aspects

Box 20.4 presents the first-line drugs for central pain. Controlled trials have been done only on CPSP and the central pain in SCI, with conflicting results. The CPSP study was a crossover study on 15 patients (mean age 66 years) in which the effects of amitriptyline (25 plus 50 mg), carbamazepine (400 mg b.i.d.), and placebo, given in randomized order, were assessed during three treatment periods, each 4 weeks long (Leijon and Boivie 1989a). Ten of the 15 patients were responders to amitriptyline, and there was a statistically significant reduction in pain as compared to placebo. No difference was noted between patients with thalamic (5 patients) and non-thalamic lesions, but the groups were small. The pain-relieving effect could not depend on an improvement of depression because none of the patients were depressed according to assessment and their depression scores did not decrease during treatment.

These results contrast with those from a controlled study of the effect of trazodone, a tricyclic antidepressant (AD) with specific action on serotonin reuptake, on central pain in 18 patients with SCI (Davidoff et al 1987a). No significant effects were found compared to placebo.

It is our impression that CPSP may be more amenable than the central pain in MS and SCI to relief by AD. The favourable responsiveness in CPSP has also been found by Bowsher and collaborators (Bowsher and Nurmikko 1996).

Mechanisms of action, adverse side effects

The mechanisms underlying the pain-relieving effect of AD are unclear. For a long time it has been believed that it depends on inhibition of the reuptake of serotonin, but this idea has been contested. Instead it has been argued that it depends on their effects on the noradrenergic systems (Lenz 1992). This conclusion is based on observations that AD, having major effects on noradrenaline (norepinephrine) function and minor or no effects on serotonin (e.g., desipramin, maprotilin, mianserin), appear to be more effective than the specific serotonin uptake inhibitors (SSRIs; including among others citalopram, fluoxetin, fluvoxamin, paroxetin, trazodone, zimelidin) in relieving neuropathic pain (Watson and Evans 1985). However, this issue has not been finally clarified yet, because results indicating a weak effect of SSRIs on peripheral neuropathic pain have been obtained (Sindrup et al 1990, Max et al 1992).

Amitriptyline, clomipramine, and doxepin have effects on both noradrenergic and serotonergic systems, in addition to rather strong anticholinergic and even some dopaminergic effects. It appears probable that it is an advantage to use drugs with mixed effects, because several of the transmitter systems that they affect are involved in pain and pain inhibition. However, there are undoubtedly problems in managing treatment with the first-generation tricyclics because of their side effects, mainly the anticholinergic ones. Thorough pre-treatment information, slow dose increases, the whole dose at bedtime, and close monitoring with frequent contacts are important steps to minimize the problems of treatment. In this way most patients can tolerate the drugs and test the effect. The SSRIs also have adverse effects that prevent their use in some patients, which is not surprising considering that they are potent drugs.

The new antidepressants with mixed serotinergic and noradrenergic effects have not yet been studied systematically with respect to their possible effects on central pain or other neuropathic pains.

Several studies on AD and neuropathic pain have shown that their pain-relieving effect is independent of their effect on depression (see Chap. 24).

Antiepileptic drugs

Documentation of effects, clinical aspects

These drugs are widely used for central and peripheral neuropathic pain. However, an effect on central pain has only been demonstrated for lamotrigine in central poststroke pain (Vestergaard et al, 2001). In Vestergaard et al´s study 27 patients with steady CPSP were included. A significant pain relief was found for lamotrigine compared to placebo. In two other controlled studies with carbamazepine an effect significantly better than placebo could not be demonstrated on CPSP (Leijon and Boivie 1989a), or in the three MS patients (Espir and Millac 1970). Clinical experience speaks strongly in favour of an effect by carbamazepine on tic douloureux and painful tonic seizures in MS.

A controlled trial with sodium valproate for the treatment of central pain following spinal cord injury showed no analgesic effect by the drug.

In recent years gabapentin has been widely recommended in the treatment of neuropathic pain, and two studies have shown a positive effect on postherpetic neuralgia and polyneuropathy pain (Backonja et al 1998, Rowbotham el al 1998), but so far no studies on central pain have been published. In clinical practice the results with gabapentin have differed from good to poor. The currently recommended daily doses are in the range of 1800–3600 mg.

Mechanism of action

The commonly used antiepileptic drugs (AED) are listed in Box 20.5. Carbamazepine and gabapentin are probably the most widely used drugs, but clonazepam gained popularity (Swerdlow 1986) and now lamotrigine is also an alternative. The rationale underlying the use of AED for central pain is their ability to suppress discharge in pathologically altered neurons, an effect that is also the basis for their use in epilepsy. Carbamazepine, lamotrigine, and phenytoin probably exert their effect by the inactivation of sodium channels (McLean and Macdonald 1986). Lamotrigine also suppresses the release of glutamate (see Vestergaard et al 2001). Clonazepam, like other benzodiazepines, binds to a

BOX 20.5
Antiepileptic drugs used in central pain

Carbamazepine
Lamotrigine
Gabapentin
Topiramate
Sodium valproate
Clonazepam
Phenytoin
Barbiturates

receptor associated with the GABA–chloride iontophoric complex, thus facilitating GABA-mediated inhibition, which is also thought to be the mechanism for sodium valproate (Budd 1989). The mechanisms of action underlying the pain-relieving effect of gabapentine is still not fully understood. It appears to modulate some Ca^{2+}, but it does not bind to glutamate receptor sites (Nicholson 2000).

Local anaesthetics, antiarrhythmic drugs

These substances have structural similarities and are thought to act on the same kind of pathophysiology as the antiepileptic drugs, i.e., to reduce pathological neuronal activity to a more normal level, mainly by acting on ion channels in the peripheral and central nervous systems (Wiesenfeld-Hallin and Lindblom 1985, Woolf and Wiesenfeld-Hallin 1985, Chabal et al 1989).

No controlled clinical trials on the use of these substances in central pain have been published, but according to results from a placebo-controlled study of intravenous lidocaine in 10 CPSP patients, 4 of the patients responded with short-term relief, 2 on placebo and 2 on lidocaine (lignocaine) (Coe et al, unpublished observations). A few patients with central pain have responded well in open-label treatment studies using lidocaine (lignocaine) (Boas et al 1982, Edwards et al 1985). Similar experiences were made with oral mexiletine in seven CPSP patients, of whom five responded well (Awerbuch 1990). Controlled clinical trials are evidently needed to establish the role of these substances in the treatment of central pain.

Analgesics

The question of whether neuropathic pain responds to analgesics is controversial. Some claim that their material indicates that neuropathic pain in general responds poorly or not at all. Others report experience to the contrary. Apparently most clinicians agree that neuropathic pain in general responds less well than most nociceptive pain to analgesics, and that many patients do not respond at all to opioids. Portenoy, Foley, and collaborators reason that neuropathic pain may respond to some but not to all opioids, in other words, that differences in pharmacological properties may be important, and that it is partly a matter of dosage (Portenoy and Foley 1986, Portenoy et al 1990). There may also be differences between different neuropathic pains in this respect, presumably because of differences in the pathophysiology involved. The positive effects of morphine on postherpetic neuralgia shown in a well-designed trial might be an illustration of this (Rowbotham et al 1991).

Most of the patients referred to specialists because of central pain have tried analgesics, often in relatively high doses, without experiencing relief, but a few have obtained some pain reduction, mostly with weak opioids such as codeine and dextropropoxyphene. The results from acute, single-blind tests of opioids on central pain also provide strong evidence for a low sensitivity to opioids (Arnér and Meyerson 1991, Kupers et al 1991, Kalman et al 2002). We tried doses in the order of 30–50 mg morphine over 2 h, i.e., close to doses causing the patient to sleep or develop confusion, and found analgesic effects only in a few patients with CPSP (unpublished observations) and central pain in MS (Kalman et al 2002). It is also common that patients with central pain who undergo operations and receive opioids postoperatively report that they have a good effect on the pain related to the operation, but no effect on the central pain. Portenoy et al, however, have reported good effects of long-term treatment with moderate doses of opioids in central pain (Portenoy and Foley 1986, Portenoy et al 1990).

A reasonable conclusion from the evidence available seems to be that a few central pain patients may benefit from analgesics, and that it is important to evaluate these effects carefully in each individual before prescribing them for long-term use. If the patient reports that the opioid clearly reduced the pain, and thereby the suffering significantly, then she should not be denied this relief.

Adrenergic, glutaminergic drugs, and naloxone

Adrenergic synapses play a role in the mechanisms of pain. It has therefore been postulated that adrenergic drugs may contribute to pain relief (Scadding et al 1982, Glynn et al 1986). For some years the interest focused on the α_2-agonist clonidine, which has been shown to block the release of transmitters and peptides in primary afferent terminals by presynaptic action. In a double-blind study, patients with pain induced by arachnoiditis responded equally well to 150 μg clonidine as to morphine, both given epidurally (Glynn et al 1988), as well as in an open trial in patients with MS/SCI and painful spasms (Glynn et al 1986). Clonidine gave fewer side effects and longer lasting relief.

Agents acting on β-adrenergic receptors have also been tried in neuropathic pain.

When administered intravenously ketamine, an NMDA-antagonist, has been found to reduce allodynia and painful dysaesthesia in patients with central pain (Backonja et al 1994, Wood and Sloan 1997), but presently available NMDA-antagonists have serious psychotropic effects that prevent their use in clinical practice.

Neuroleptic drugs

There is a long clinical tradition for the use of phenothiazines and other neuroleptic drugs in pain treatment. They are believed to increase the effect of analgesics and to have analgesic properties of their own. In neuropathic pain they are particularly used for dysaesthesia and hyperaesthesia. However, such effects have not been shown in controlled studies on any pain condition, or in any form of convincing study. Their potentially severe and partially irreversible adverse effects and the lack of documented effects are strong enough reasons to caution against the use of these drugs in the treatment of central pain. This is particularly so as many of these patients have brain lesions, which increase the risk for the occurrence of irreversible tardive dyskinesia, which is the most serious side effect of neuroleptics.

Sensory stimulation

Transcutaneous electrical nerve stimulation

This form of treatment provides relief for some central pains and has the advantage of few and mild adverse side effects, apart from possible effects on cardiac pacemakers (Sjölund 1991). It is applied in one of two modes: high-frequency stimulation (80–100 Hz; called conventional TENS by Sjölund), aiming at activation of myelinated cutaneous sensory fibres, or low-frequency stimulation (short trains of impulses with 1–4 Hz repetition rate; called acupunture-like TENS), aiming at activation of muscle efferents or muscle cells, thereby evoking muscle afferent inputs to the CNS. The mechanisms are believed to be mainly segmental, but suprasegmental mechanisms exist too (see Chap. 30). It is unclear how the effect of TENS in central pain is explained, but it appears that TENS can only reduce central pain if the dorsal column–medial lemniscal pathways are uninjured or only mildly injured.

This hypothesis is based on a study of TENS in CPSP. Three of 15 CPSP patients obtained long-term relief (Leijon and Boivie 1989c). All three had normal or almost normal thresholds to touch and vibration, indicating good function in the lemniscal pathways.

Spinal cord and brain stimulation

From a review of the literature and of his own patients Tasker and colleagues (Tasker et al 1991, Tasker 2000) concluded that spinal cord stimulation is not effective enough in central pain to be recommended, a view shared by Nashold and Bullitt (1981), Gybels and Sweet (1989), and Pagni (1998), although he and others have had patients with successful results from spinal cord stimulation in central pain due to SCI. Instead he favours brain stimulation. Richardsson et al observed good results at 1-year follow-up in 6 of 19 paraplegics, and Siegfried reported good to excellent relief at 1- to 4-year follow-up in about 70% of 84 patients with 'deafferentation' pain caused by various central and peripheral lesions (Richardsson et al 1980, Siegfried 1983).

Brain stimulation is an exclusive mode of treatment that should be reserved for particularly severe and treatment-resistant pain conditions. The exquisite pain suffered by many central pain patients fulfils these criteria. The periaqueductal and periventricular grey regions (PAG, PVG) are the primary targets for stimulation in the treatment of nociceptive pain, whereas stimulation for neuropathic pain is usually carried out along the lemniscal pathways in the ventroposterior thalamic region or the posterior limb of the internal capsule. In a recent review Tasker (2000) concludes that steady central pain may be relieved by stimulation in the ventroposterior thalamic region and that allodynia and hyperalgesia may respond to stimulation in PAG/PVG. Excellent results have also been reported following surface stimulation of the motor cortex in central pain (Peyron et al 1995, Tsubokawa 1995, Yamamoto et al 1997).

Neurosurgical ablative procedures

Many different surgical lesions have been tried to find relief for central pain, but no particular lesion has been found that reliably results in successful outcome (Sjölund 1991, Tasker et al 1991, Pagni 1998, Tasker 2000). Lesions have been made at almost all levels of the neuraxis from the spinal cord to the cerebral cortex. Even lesions of peripheral nerves, mainly rhizotomy, have been tried. It is interesting to note that such lesions have not had an effect on steady ongoing pain, but in some cases there has been improvement of hyperaesthesia (Tasker 2000). According to Tasker et al (1991), ablative procedures in the spinal cord and the brain have also given better results with the intermittent and evoked components of central pain.

Three main kinds of spinal cord lesion have been performed for the treatment of central pain, namely anterolateral cordotomy, dorsal root entry zone (DREZ) lesion, and cordectomy. The underlying lesion has usually been a traumatic cord lesion. A fair proportion of patients with sacrococcygeal lesions have been found to obtain relief from cordotomy, but there has been a tendency for the pain to recur, as after cordotomy for nociceptive pain (Tasker 2000). The more rostral the lesion, the lesser the chance that cordotomy will do anything for the patient.

DREZ lesions have gained interest over recent years for the treatment of central SCI pain (Nashold and Bullitt 1981, Edgar et al 1993). The procedure aims at destroying the Lissauer tract and the superficial part of the dorsal horn. One would thus expect the DREZ lesion to affect pain emanating from the segment where the original lesion is located, i.e., in the transitional zone of partially injured cord tissue. So far results have not been consistent, but some centres have reported a success rate of about 50% (Nashold and Bullitt 1981, Gybels and Sweet 1989, Sjölund 1991, Edgar et al 1993, Tasker 2000). Cordectomy is a more robust method for achieving a similar goal as the DREZ lesion, namely to interfere with the local pain-generating process. As with cordotomy, and probably also DREZ lesions, it appears that cordectomy rarely affects steady ongoing pain, but rather intermittent pain and hyperaesthesia, but has a low success-rate (Gybels and Sweet 1989, Tasker 2000).

Among the many intracranial ablative procedures that have been tried for central pain are mesencephalic tractotomy, medial and lateral thalamotomies, cingulotomy, and cortical ablation. None of these have turned out to produce successful long-term outcomes. Some operations have resulted in postoperative pain relief in some patients, but the overall results have not been good, because of unacceptably high complication rates or return to preoperative pain levels after some time. From a review of the literature and of his own material, Tasker concluded that the only procedures that can be recommended in selected cases are stereotactic mesencephalic tractotomy and/or medial thalamotomy (Tasker 2000). Of his own nine patients with central pain caused by brain lesions in whom such operations were performed, only three had 'modest' relief of steady pain, and another four had some effect on intermittent pain. Three had transient complications. It has been suggested that the pain-relieving effect of the mesencephalic lesion is obtained by interfering with the spino-reticulo-thalamic projections. Medial thalamotomy appears to affect the spinal and trigeminal projections to the intralaminar-submedius region. This kind of thalamotomy has been strongly advocated by Jeanmonod and collaborators (Jeanmonod et al 1996), but many neurosurgeons are sceptical about these lesions in the treatment of pain.

Sympathetic blockade

In the section on pathophysiology the idea that sympathetic dysfunction may be part of the mechanism underlying central pain was discussed. Oedema, decreased sweating, lowered skin temperature, change in skin colour, and trophic skin changes occur in regions affected by central pain (Bowsher 1996). Based on these observations sympathetic blockade has been tried in the treatment of central pain. Loh et al (1981) gave a detailed report of the results of sympathetic blockade in three patients with CPSP, one with a traumatic brainstem lesion, two with MS, one with a spinal cord tumour, and one with traumatic SCI. The short-term effects were remarkable. All patients experienced at least 50% reduction in pain and disappearance or improvement of hyperaesthesia, but the effects usually lasted only 1–24 h, apart from the patient with a traumatic brainstem lesion who experienced long-term relief.

Individual central pain conditions

Some features of particular interest regarding individual central pain conditions will be summarized in this section. Many of the features of individual central pain conditions have been discussed above. Much of this information will not be repeated in this section. For a more detailed presentation on central pain following SCI the reader is referred to Chap. 21.

Central poststroke pain

The lesions

All kinds of cerebrovascular lesion (CVL) can cause central poststroke pain (CPSP). There appears to be no difference between haemorrhages and infarcts as regards the tendency to induce central pain (Leijon et al 1989, Bowsher 1996, Bowsher et al 1998). The consequence of this is that there are many more patients with CPSP caused by infarct than haemorrhages, because approximately 85% of all strokes are caused by infarct.

Different principles can be used to classify CVL. One principle is according to the artery involved, giving two major groups, namely carotid and vertebrobasilar strokes. About 80% of all infarcts occur in the carotid territories. Infarcts in the territories of the thalamostriate and the posterior inferior cerebellar arteries (PICA) are particularly interesting, because they engage the ventroposterior part of the thalamus and the lower brainstem, respectively. These infarcts are probably among the most frequent causes of central pain.

Haemorrhages can only induce central pain when they damage the brain parenchyma. It is thus unusual that subarachnoid haemorrhage causes central pain, but it occurs when severe vasospasm develops and leads to an infarct and when the bleeding causes direct tissue injury (Bowsher et al 1989).

As regards central pain caused by vascular malformation, this mainly concerns arteriovenous malformations (AVM) and the result is similar to CVL. They can cause central pain in two ways, namely through rupture and haemorrhage, or if they increase in size and cause parenchymal damage. Patients with CPSP due to both these forms of lesion have been reported. The lesions were located cortically and subcortically in the parietal region and in the thalamus (Silver 1957, Waltz and Ehni 1966).

The location of the CVL, and not its size, is crucial as regards the probability that it will produce central pain (see 'Pathophysiology' above). The following major locations have been shown to be associated with central pain: lateral medulla oblongata (PICA), thalamus, posterior limb of the internal capsule, subcortical and cortical zones in the postcentral gyrus (i.e., in the regions of the first somatosensory area, SI), and the insular regions (second somatosensory area, SII).

A recent prospective study of 191 stroke patients followed for 12 months showed that the incidence of CPSP is 8% (Andersen et al 1995). The exact figures at 1, 6, and 12 months follow-up were 4.8, 6.0% and 8.4%, respectively. It appears that CVL in the lower brainstem and thalamus more often result in central pain than CVL in other locations, because these are not the most frequent locations of CVL and yet these locations are common in CPSP materials (Garcin 1968, Leijon et al 1989, Andersen et al 1995, Bowsher et al 1998). The incidence of central pain after lateral medullary infarcts may be as high as 25% (MacGowan et al 1997). In studies carried out by Leijon et al (1989) and by Andersen et al (1995), 33 and 25%, respectively, of the patients with CPSP had CVL involving the thalamus. These conclusions were based on X-ray CT scans. A later study using MRI indicated that about 60% of all CPSP patients have lesions engaging the thalamus (Bowsher et al 1998). It appears probable that about half of all CPSP patients have lesions that involve the thalamus.

Pain characteristics

The major problem in the diagnosis of CPSP is to distinguish central pain from nociceptive pains of various kinds, particularly hemiplegic shoulder pain, which is common in hemiplegic stroke patients. The development of shoulder pain can to a large extent be prevented by physiotherapy and information to everyone involved in the care of the patient.

The onset of CPSP is delayed in many patients. In one study, about half of the patients noticed the pain within a few days or during the first month, but in half of the patients the onset was delayed by more than 1 month (Leijon et al 1989). The longest delay was 34 months. In the Danish prospective study 63% had onset of pain within 1 month (Andersen et al 1995) and after brainstem infarcts the figure was 56% (MacGowan et al 1997).

CPSP is commonly experienced in a large part of the right or left side (Leijon et al 1989). However, some patients only have pain in a small region, such as the distal part of the arm and hand, or in the face. Two of the eight patients with brainstem infarcts had pain in the face on one side and in the rest of the body on the other side. The most common pain location after lateral medullary infarcts appears to be ipsilaterally around the eye (MacGowan et al 1997).

In our study two-thirds of the patients had left-sided pain, which was in accord with the material of Schott et al (1986) and a summary of published patients with thalamic stroke (Nasreddine and Saver 1997), but dominance of one side did not appear in a large study from one centre (Bowsher et al 1998).

Patients with CPSP report a large variety of pain qualities. Most patients experience two to four qualities. A burning sensation is the most frequent quality reported by about 60% of patients, with aching, pricking, and lacerating sensations being next in frequency. In another study 32 patients described the pain as principally burning and 30 patients described it as principally non-burning (Bowsher et al 1998). Bizarre pain qualities do occur, as mentioned in the first part of this chapter, but they are the exception rather than the rule.

Assessment of the intensity of CPSP reveals large individual variations. In a global sense most patients consider the pain to be severe, although some of them rate the pain intensity rather low on scales such as the VAS, but a few patients have a mild form of CPSP. There are also patients in whom it is difficult to determine whether the sensation experienced should be classified as pain or not. This for instance is true for some dysaesthesias, because there is no sharp transition from non-painful to painful dysaesthesias.

In many patients the pain is affected by internal and external stimuli. Such stimuli usually increase the pain, for instance body movements and cold (Leijon et al 1989, Michel et al 1990).

Neurological symptoms and signs

Somatosensory symptoms and signs regularly accompany CPSP, whereas other symptoms may or may not be present in patients with CPSP. Among 27 CPSP patients more than half had no paresis (Leijon et al 1989), and other non-sensory symptoms were much more uncommon.

Some of the sensory abnormalities are subtle, and are not noticed by the patients or revealed in the clinical sensory examination, but can be demonstrated by QSTs. However, in a few patients with CPSP, and other forms of central pain, it has not been possible even with quantitative methods to show any sensory disturbances.

Some of the sensory abnormalities are of a quantitative nature; others are more qualitative (Boivie et al 1989). The dominating features are abnormal temperature and pain sensibility, which was found in all of the patients examined, and hyperaesthesias and dysaesthesias, which were found in about 85% of the patients. The abnormalities in temperature sensibility were pronounced. Eighty-one percent could not identify temperatures between 0 and 50°C. About half of these patients had normal thresholds to touch and vibration. A similar but less pronounced tendency has been found in larger studies (Bowsher 1996, Bowsher et al 1998). These results are the basis for the hypothesis that CPSP only occurs in patients who have lesions affecting the spinothalamic pathways (see above).

Treatment

The reader is referred to the general section on treatment of central pain for details. In this section only a few comments will be made. It is recommended that TENS is tried as the primary treatment in patients who have not lost touch and vibration sensibility in the painful region, because this relatively inexpensive treatment with almost no adverse side effects will give some patients long-lasting relief.

Antidepressants have undoubtely been the most useful of the drugs. About 50–70% of CPSP patients have been found to benefit from these drugs. Next in order are antiepileptic drugs, which should not be restricted to patients with tic-like pain. Other drugs are not well documented, but may nevertheless be tried. The same is true for sympathetic blockade.

Multiple sclerosis

Epidemiology and pain characteristics

Multiple sclerosis is a severe chronic neurological disease that in many patients causes serious handicap and suffering. The disease process is of a neuroinflammatory nature and results in destruction of myelin, and eventually of the axons and cell bodies, in the CNS. The characteristic lesion is the plaque, which is a zone of demyelination. Such plaques may occur anywhere in the CNS, and in the optic nerves, but are most frequently found in the spinal cord, particularly in the dorsal columns, in the brainstem, and periventricularly in the forebrain. The two major clinical forms are the slowly progressive and remitting–relapsing forms. The cause of the inflammatory process is as yet unknown, but much is known about the various stages in the process in which different lymphatic T-cell populations play a crucial role.

In a comprehensive monograph on MS it was stated that pain is uncommon in MS (Tourtellotte and Baumhefner 1983). However, as soon as investigations were made on the prevalence of pain in MS it became evident that the majority of MS patients experience pain. Four studies obtained prevalence figures indicating that 42–65% of all MS patients have clinically significant pain. These results were based on interviews and examination of 723 patients. The figures include almost all forms of pain except headache. In one of the studies it was found that 45% had pain at the time of the investigation, and that 32% considered the pain to be one of their worst symptoms (Stenager et al 1991).

Not all MS pain is central. It is to be expected that MS patients with paresis, spasticity, and incoordination of movements will develop nociceptive musculoskeletal pain, and this is indeed the case. Vermote et al (1986) found that about 20% had such pain, including back pain, which is comparable to the 14% with back pain reported by Moulin et al (1988). It is also conceivable that peripheral neuropathic pain will be found in some MS patients. Primary psychogenic pain, i.e., pain as part of a major psychiatric disease, appears to be rare in MS. Vermote et al (1986) found only two such cases in their material of 83 patients.

It is important to carefully analyse the characteristics of the various pains experienced by MS patients to form a basis for the optimal management of the pain. According to the prevalence studies, the majority of MS patients with pain have central pain caused by the disease itself.

Idiopathic trigeminal neuralgia is usually considered to be peripherally induced, but it appears likely that in MS this pain is caused by demyelination in the brainstem, and it is therefore classified as central pain in this context. Its prevalence has now been shown to be 5%, which is higher than the previous estimates (Österberg and Boivie, in preparation).

In a retrospective study it was concluded that pain increases with age in MS (Clifford and Trotter 1984). A similar trend was found by Moulin et al (1988). No such trend was found regarding the age at onset of MS or disease duration, apart from the fact that pain was less common during the first 5 years of the disease than later (Clifford and Trotter 1984, Moulin et al 1988, Stenager et al 1991). These relationships were not analysed specifically for central pain, however.

Pain characteristics and neurological symptoms

The characteristics of trigeminal neuralgia is described in Chap. 14. Its character is similar in MS and idiopathic tic douloureux.

The Lhermitte sign is classical of MS. It consists of rapidly spreading paraesthesias or dysaesthesias, sometimes like an electric current, down the back and radiating to the extremities. It is mostly bilateral and sometimes painful. It is usually evoked by bending the head forward, and it has been proposed that it is produced when the cervical part of the inflamed dorsal columns are stretched.

Painful tonic seizures constitute another kind of paroxysmal pain in MS. A detailed description of these attacks is found in Shibasaki and Kuroiwa's (1974) report. They found 11 such cases among 64 patients with MS, which is higher than in our large material in which only 2% of the 100 patients with central pain have this component. The attacks consist of spreading paraesthesias, pain, and muscle spasm in the spinal segments involved. They are evoked by light touch or movement. No correlation was found between the pain and the degree of paresis or spasticity, but with sensory signs.

The most common form of central pain in MS is non-paroxysmal extremity pain, usually termed dysaesthetic pain. The quality of this pain shows a large interindividual variation and most patients experience more than one pain quality. Burning and aching pain are most frequent, occurring in about 40%, with pricking, stabbing, and squeezing being next in frequency. In Box 20.6 percentage figures for the location of central pain in MS are listed, showing that there is a large dominance for pain in the lower extremities.

BOX 20.6
Location of central pain in 86 patients with multiple sclerosis (Österberg and Boivie, in preparation)

Lower extremities	90%
Trunk	22%
Upper extremities	36%
Unilaterally	24%
Bilaterally	76%

The combination of different pain locations and qualities can be illustrated by one of our patients. He is a 53-year-old clerk with central pain of 4 years' duration. The pain started about 2 months after he rapidly developed signs of a transverse myelitis at T9, with total loss of voluntary motor and bladder control, and total sensory loss below the waist. He now has steady pain of three distinctly different kinds. The first is a burning pain from the waist down. The second is a tight belt-like pressing pain just above the waist; it feels like tight armour. The third pain is described as if he is sitting heavily on a tennis ball. It is interesting to know that the first symptom this patient noticed was hyperaesthesia to heat, i.e., an indication of dysfunction in the spinothalamic pathways.

Most investigators have found that MS patients with non-paroxysmal central pain have disturbed somatic sensibility. In our study of 63 patients using both clinical and quantitative sensory tests, only two patients were found to have completely normal sensibility (Österberg and Boivie, in preparation). The abnormalities found were dominated by abnormal temperature and pain sensibility, only two patients having normal pain and temperature sensibility, whereas more than one-third of the patients had normal threshold to touch. The vibration sense was also severely affected, but not to the same degree as temperature and pain. These results have similarities with the results from patients with central poststroke pain (see above).

As regards non-sensory symptoms and signs it appears that, at most, half of MS patients with non-paroxysmal central pain have paresis, ataxia, or bladder dysfunction (Österberg and Boivie, in preparation). Only 11 of 99 patients had severe paresis, whereas 29% had ataxia. This conforms with the results of other studies failing to find any covariation between central pain and disability (Vermote et al 1986, Moulin et al 1988, Stenager et al 1991). This also seems to be true for central pain and depression in MS (Stenager et al 1991, Österberg et al 1994). Stenager et al (1991) found no differences between MS patients with and without pain with respect to depressive symptoms.

Treatment

Antiepileptic drugs are the treatment of choice for trigeminal neuralgia and other paroxysmal pains in MS (Shibasaki and Kuroiwa 1974). These treatments are generally very successful. Carbamazepine is the first-line drug, but most other AED have a good effect too (see section on 'Antiepileptic drugs' above). The effects of treatment are dependent on the plasma concentration. It appears that many MS patients have difficulty in tolerating sufficiently high doses of carbamazepine, probably more so than other patient groups. One possible way around such problems is to try a combination of baclofen and an AED.

The AED have generally not been found effective against steady extremity pain (Clifford and Trotter 1984, Moulin et al 1988). In a controlled trial investigating the pain-relieving effects of carbamazepine and amitriptyline in 21 MS patients, it was found that carbamazepine did not have a significant effect, whereas amitriptyline had a weak effect on the spontaneous constant pain (Österberg and Boivie, in preparation). In this study it was noticed that MS patients do indeed have more problems with side effects than what has previously been found in patients with poststroke pain. A more recent alternative would be to try gabapentin, but no studies have been done in MS patients with this drug.

The outcome of treatment with antidepressants has varied. Thus Clifford and Trotter (1984) reported excellent results, while Moulin et al (1988) had a poor outcome with only 9 of 46 patients responding well to amitriptyline and imipramine.

TENS can be tried in patients with at least some preservation of dorsal column function. Electrical stimulation of the spinal cord (DCS) has been tried quite extensively, but the outcome has been poor (Rosen and Barsoum 1979, Young and Goodman 1979, Tasker 2000) and the method is not recommended. Intrathecal baclofen has been used successfully to treat severe spasticity, but the experience of its possible effect on central pain in MS is poorly known, although some centres have reported promising results (Herman et al 1992).

Spinal cord injury

The reader is referred to Chap. 21 for information about pain following spinal cord injury (SCI).

Syringomyelia and syringobulbia (also see Chap. 21)

Syringomyelia (in the spinal cord) and syringobulbia (in the lower brainstem) are rare diseases with a very high incidence of central pain. From a scientific point of view they are of particular interest for the understanding of the mechanisms that underlie central pain and sensory disturbances, because they illustrate the possible consequences of internal lesions in the spinal cord and brainstem. The lesion is a cystic cavity filled with a fluid that is similar to normal CSF. The size and extension of the cavity, i.e., the syrinx (from the Greek word for flute), varies enormously between patients, from a small lesion in the dorsal part of the spinal cord over a couple of segments to huge cavities extending from the most caudal part of the cord into the medulla oblongata, as illustrated by findings at autopsy, and in recent years by examination with MRI (Foster and Hudgson 1973, Schliep 1978, Milhorat et al 1996). The largest cavities leave only a thin layer of spinal cord tissue undamaged at the maximally cavitated regions.

Much is still unknown about how the cavities develop, and particularly about the cause of the disease. According to the most embraced theory hydromechanical forces are important for the expansion of the cavity. This theory states that the cavity develops as an enlargement of the central canal, which is where the spinothalamic fibres cross the midline to reach their position in the ventro-laterally located spinothalamic tract. A lesion with this location will affect the sensibility to temperature and pain; i.e., a dissociated sensory loss will appear. Studies have shown that this in fact happens, because this sensory abnormality was found in 248 of 250 patients with syringomyelia and syringobulbia (Foster and Hudgson 1973, Schliep 1978). Syringomyelia can also be post-traumatic and be caused by spinal cord haematomas.

Pain is common in syringomyelia (when this term is used in this chapter it also includes syringobulbia). In a recent survey of 22 patients it was found that all had pain, and that 16 (73%) had central pain (Boivie and Rollsjö, unpublished results). This pain, in most patients, was located in one of the upper extremities, seldom in both. The thorax was another rather common location, and a few had pain in the lower extremities. Burning, aching, and pressing were the most common pain qualities. Pain, often central pain, was a frequent initial symptom in this disease, which usually progresses slowly over decades.

The results from our study cast doubt on the notion that the somatosensory symptoms of syringomyelia, including central pain, are mainly caused by damage to the spinothalamic fibres as they cross the midline, because it has been found that the symptoms and signs are strictly unilateral in several patients who are probably in an early stage of the disease. Thus some patients have central pain and dissociated sensory loss in one arm and hand. This could be explained by either a lesion affecting the dorsal horn or one affecting the spinothalamic fibres on that side, before they cross.

Quantitative sensory tests show that all patients with syringomyelia have abnormal temperature and pain sensibility (Boivie 1984; Boivie and Rollsjö, unpublished results). These abnormalities are mostly pronounced with total loss of temperature sensibility.

The treatment of central pain in syringomyelia is similar to that of central pain after traumatic spinal cord injuries. In our clinical experience tricyclic antidepressants have been moderately successful.

Parkinson's disease

Parkinson's disease (PD) is rightfully considered to be a movement disorder. The dominating symptoms are rigidity, bradykinesia, tremor, and defective postural control. However, it is becoming increasingly clear that many patients with PD have pain and sensory symptoms (Snider et al 1976, Koller 1984, Goetz et al 1985, Schott 1985, Quinn et al 1986). In some patients these symptoms precede the onset of the motor symptoms. The mechanisms behind these symptoms are unknown. It is thus unclear to what extent the pain in PD should be classified as central pain, but it appears likely that at least part of it is of primarily central origin, i.e., central pain. A brief summary of published reports on this pain will be made.

In an investigation of 105 ambulatory PD patients it was found that 43% had sensory symptoms (pain, tingling, numbness; Snider et al 1976). Pain was the most common complaint, reported by 29%: 'It was usually described as an intermittent, poorly localized, cramp-like or aching sensation, not associated with increased muscle contraction and not affected by movement or pressure. It was often proximal and in the limb of greatest motor deficit.' Eleven percent had burning sensations and 12% had painful muscle spasm or cramps. In 7% the pain preceded the motor symptoms. In a similar study of 94 patients, 46% were found to have pain (Goetz et al 1985). The major pains were 'muscle cramps or tightness' (34% of all patients) and painful dystonias (13% of all patients).

A classification for the pain directly related to PD was proposed by Quinn et al (1986):

A. Pain preceding the diagnosis of PD.
B. Off-period pain (without dystonia) in patients with fluctuating response to levodopa (four subgroups).
C. Painful dystonic spasms (four subgroups).
D. Peak-dose pain.

Quinn et al (1986) did not give any prevalence figures for the four groups. They concluded that most of the pain is related to fluctuations in motor symptoms, which in turn are related to the response to the drug treatment. This idea was supported by observations in two patients in which the fluctuations in motor symptoms and pain were recorded (Nutt and Carter 1984). These observations are compatible with a modulatory influence of the basal ganglia on somatic sensibility, including pain. In all of the studies cited no significant abnormalities in the sensibility to cutaneous stimuli were found.

From the case reports of Quinn et al (1986), it appears that much of the pain in PD can be relieved by careful adjustment of the anti-Parkinson medication, but they also show that this is sometimes a difficult task.

Epilepsy, brain tumours and abscesses

In a survey of 858 patients with epilepsy it was found that 2.8% had pain as part of epileptic seizures (Young and Blume 1983). In several of the patients the cause of the epilepsy was unknown. Many were children. No patients with cerebrovascular lesions were included. The pain was either a symptom during the major part of the seizure or part of the aura.

Patients with cerebrovascular lesions that engage the cerebral cortex may develop epilepsy. Fine (1967) reported five such patients with epileptic seizures that included severe pain. This pain had qualities similar to those of CPSP, but it occurred spontaneously in short attacks, and disappeared completely when antiepileptic drugs were given.

In general brain tumours rarely induce central pain, but several patients with meningiomas and central pain have been reported (Bender and Jaffe 1958). Surprisingly not even thalamic tumours have a tendency to cause central pain. In a retrospective study only 1 of 49 patients with thalamic tumours had central pain (Tovi et al 1961).

Finally a late twentieth-century illustration of the fact that all kinds of lesion can result in central pain—two patients with brain abscesses in the thalamus and internal capsule and central pain were reported (Gonzales et al 1992). The cause of the abscesses was toxoplasma infection—the patients had AIDS!

Concluding comments

It is important to identify central pain when it is present because this is the basis for its rational management. An ad hoc committee in the Special Interest Group on Central Pain of the IASP has worked out an examination protocol for the diagnosis of central pain. This protocol can be recommended for clinical use. It has the following components:

Historical information

1. Is pain the major or primary complaint? If not, indicate the alternative.
2. Nature of primary neurological disability:
   a. Primary diagnosis (e.g., stroke, tumour, etc.)
   b. Location of disability (e.g., left hemiparesis).
3. Date of onset of neurological signs/symptoms.
4. Date of onset of pain.
5. Description of pain:
   a. Location:
      Body area—preferably use pain drawing
      Superficial (skin) and/or deep (muscle, viscera)
      Radiation or referral.
   b. Intensity (1–10 or VAS or categorical scaling):
      Most common intensity; at maximum; at minimum
   c. Temporal features:
      Steady, unchanging; intermittent
      Fluctuates over minutes, hours, days, weeks
      Paroxysmal features (shooting pain, tic-like).
   d. Quality:
      Thermal (burning, freezing, etc.)
      Mechanical (pressure, cramping, etc.)
      Chemical (stinging, etc.)
      Other (aching, etc.).
   e. Factors increasing the pain (cold, emotions, etc.).
   f. Factors decreasing the pain (rest, drugs, etc.).
6. Neurological symptoms besides pain:
   a. Motor (paresis, ataxia, involuntary movements)
   b. Sensory (hypo-, hyperaesthesia, paraesthesia, dysaesthesia, numbness, overreaction)
   c. Others (speech, visual, cognitive, mood, etc.).

Examination

1. Neurological disease—results of CT, MRI, SPECT, PET, CSF assays, neurophysiological examinations, etc.
2. Major neurological findings (e.g., spastic paraparesis).
3. Sensory examination—preferably use sensory chart with the dermatomes. Indicate whether modalities listed have normal, increased, or decreased threshold, and paraesthesias or dysaesthesias are evoked.
   a. Vibratory sense (tuning fork, Biothesiometer or Vibrameter)
   b. Tactile (cotton wool, hair movement)
   c. Skin direction sense, graphaesthesis
   d. Kinaesthesia
   e. Temperature (specify how tested; cold and warm, noxious and innocuous)
   f. Pinprick
   g. Deep pain (specify how tested)
   h. Allodynia to mechanical stimuli, cold, heat
   i. Hyperpathia (specify how tested)
   j. Other abnormalities like radiation, summation, prolonged aftersensation.

Criteria for the diagnosis of central pain

The examination protocol will in most patients lead to information that will enable the examiner to determine whether central pain is at hand. For this decision the following criteria for central pain may be used:

1. The presence of CNS disease. The lesion/dysfunction can be located at any level of the neuraxis from the dorsal horn grey matter of the spinal cord, and the trigeminal spinal nucleus, to the cerebral cortex, i.e., engaging either the ascending pathways and/or their brainstem or cortical relays.
2. Pain that started after the onset of this disease. The pain can be steady, intermittent, or paroxysmal, or be present in the form of painful hyperaesthesias such as allodynia or hyperpathia. Its onset can be immediate or delayed up to several years.

3. The pain can have virtually any quality, including trivial aching pain. More than one pain quality is often experienced, in the same region or in different regions.
4. The pain can engage large parts of the body (hemipain, one-quarter, lower body half, etc.) or be restricted to a small region such as one arm or the face.
5. The pain can be of high or low intensity. It is often increased, or evoked, by various internal or external stimuli, such as touch, cold, and sudden emotions.
6. The presence of abnormalities in somatic sensibility. The abnormalities can be subtle and in some patients it takes quantitative sensory tests to demonstrate their presence. However, in rare cases not even the quantitative methods can show such abnormalities. They are dominated by abnormal sensibility to temperature and pain, indicating involvement of the spinothalamic pathways. Abnormalities are common in touch, vibration, and kinaesthesia too, but their presence is not mandatory in central pain, and many patients with central pain have normal thresholds for these submodalities. Hyperaesthesias such as allodynia, hyperalgesia, and hyperpathia are common, but not demonstrable in all patients with central pain. Most patients with central pain experience paresthaesias or dysaesthesias that are sometimes painful, and thus themselves are a kind of central pain.
7. Non-sensory neurological symptoms and signs may or may not be present. There is thus no correlation between central pain and motor disturbances.
8. Psychological or psychiatric disturbances may or may not be present. A large majority of central pain patients are normal in these respects.
9. The pain should not appear to be of psychic origin.
10. The diagnosis of certain central pain should be ascertained on clinical grounds/criteria or with the help of laboratory examinations that show that the pain is not of nociceptive or peripheral neuropathic origin.

Treatment

Because no universally effective treatment is available for central pain it is important to try available modalities in a systematic way to find the best treatment for the individual patient. Therefore it is important to keep the patient well informed and to monitor treatment closely because of potential side effects. When drugs are used, increases in dosage should be gradual. It is also wise to inform the patient that the treatment may not relieve the pain completely, which it seldom does.

Central pain is truly chronic pain, often lasting for the rest of patients' lives, and it usually causes patients much suffering. It is therefore important that patients have a reliable long-lasting relationship with their physicians so that they know whom to contact when the pain brings them into despair when support by a psychotherapist may be indicated. Furthermore there is reason to include physiotherapy in the treatment programme, aiming at increased activity and rehabilitation.

The first-line specific treatments are TENS, antidepressants, and antiepileptic drugs. The reader is referred to the sections on these treatments or on the individual pain conditions for detailed information. In some patients the treatment of the central pain needs to be combined with other forms of treatment, because other pains may also be present.

References

Andersen G, Vestergaard K, Ingeman-Nielsen M, Jensen TS 1995 Incidence of central post-stroke pain. Pain 61: 187–193
Arnér S, Meyerson BA 1991 Genuine resistance to opioids—fact or fiction? Pain 47: 116–118
Awerbuch 1990 Treatment of thalamic pain syndrome with Mexiletine. Annals of Neurology 28: 233
Backonja M, Arndt G, Gombar KA, Check B, Zimmermann M 1994 Response of chronic neuropathic pain syndromes to ketamine: a preliminary study. Pain 56: 51–57
Backonja M, Beydon A, Edwards KR et al 1998 Gabapentin monotherapy for the treatment of painful neuropathy: a multicenter, double blind, placebo-controlled trial in patients with diabetes mellitus. Journal of American Medical Association 280: 1831–1836
Bender MB, Jaffe R 1958 Pain of central origin. Medical Clinics of North America 49: 691–700
Berić A, Dimitrijević MR, Lindblom U 1988 Central dysesthesia syndrome in spinal cord injury patients. Pain 34: 109–116
Boas RA, Covino BG, Shahnarian A 1982 Analgesic responses to i.v. lignocaine. British Journal of Anaesthesia 54: 501–505
Bogousslavsky J, Regli F, Uske A 1988 Thalamic infarcts: clinical syndromes, etiology, and prognosis. Neurology 38: 837–848
Boivie J 1979 An anatomic reinvestigation of the termination of the spinothalamic tract in the monkey. Journal of Comparative Neurology 168: 343–370
Boivie J 1984 Disturbances in cutaneous sensibility in patients with central pain caused by the spinal cord lesions of syringomyelia. Pain 2 (suppl): S82
Boivie J 1992 Hyperalgesia and allodynia in patients with CNS lesions. In: Willis WDJ (ed) Hyperalgesia and allodynia. Raven, New York, pp 363–373
Boivie J 1995 Pain syndromes in patients with CNS lesions and a comparison with nociceptive pain. In: Bromm B, Desmeth JE (eds) Advances in pain research and therapy. Raven, New York, pp 367–375

Boivie J, Leijon G 1991 Clinical findings in patients with central post-stroke pain. In: Casey KL (ed) Pain and central nervous system disease: the central pain syndromes. Raven, New York, pp 65–75

Boivie J, Leijon G 1996 Central post-stroke pain (CPSP)—long-term effects of amitryptiline. In: Abstracts 8th world congress on pain. IASP Press, Seattle, p 380

Boivie J, Leijon G, Johansson I 1989 Central post-stroke pain—a study of the mechanisms through analyses of the sensory abnormalities. Pain 37: 173–185

Bowsher D 1995 Central pain. Pain Reviews 2: 175–186

Bowsher D 1996 Central pain: clinical and physiological characteristics. Journal of Neurology, Neurosurgery and Psychiatry 61: 62–69

Bowsher D, Nurmikko T 1996 Central post-stroke pain. Drug treatment options. CNS Drugs 5: 160–165

Bowsher D, Foy PM, Shaw MDM 1989 Central pain complicating infarction following subarachnoid haemorrhage. British Journal of Neurosurgery 3: 435–442

Bowsher D, Leijon G, Thuomas K-Å 1998 Central post-stroke pain: correlation of magnetic resonance imaging with clinical pain characteristics and sensory abnormalities. Neurology 51: 1352–1358

Britell CW, Mariano AJ 1991 Chronic pain in spinal cord injury. Physical Medicine and Rehabilitation: State of Art Reviews 5: 71–82

Bromm B, Treede RD 1987 Human cerebral potentials evoked by CO_2 laser stimuli causing pain. Experimental Brain Research 67: 153–162

Budd K 1989 Sodium valproate in the treatment of pain. In: Chadwick D (ed) Fourth international symposium on sodium valproate and epilepsy. Royal Society of Medicine, London, pp 213–216

Casey KL, Beydoun A, Boivie J et al 1996 Laser-evoked cerebral potentials and sensory function in patients with central pain. Pain 64: 485–491

Chabal C, Russel LC, Burchiel KJ 1989 The effect of intravenous lidicaine, tocainide, and mexiletine on spontaneous active fibers originating in rat sciatic neuromas. Pain 38: 333–338

Clifford DB, Trotter JL 1984 Pain in multiple sclerosis. Archives of Neurology 41: 1270–1272

Davidoff G, Roth EJ 1991 Clinical characteristics of central (dysesthetic) pain in spinal cord injury patients. In: Casey KL (ed) Pain and central nervous disease: the central pain syndromes. Raven Press, New York, pp 77–83

Davidoff G, Guarrachini M, Roth E, Sliwa J, Yarkony G 1987a Trazodone hydrochloride in the treatment of dysesthetic pain in traumatic myelopathy: a randomized, double-blind, placebo-controlled study. Pain 29: 151–161

Davidoff G, Roth EJ, Guarracini M, Sliwa J, Yarkony G 1987b Function-limiting dysesthetic pain syndrome among traumatic spinal cord injury patients: a cross-sectional study. Pain 29: 39–48

Dehen H, Willer JC, Cambier J 1983 Pain in thalamic syndrome: electrophysiological findings in man. Advances in Pain Research and Therapy 5: 936–940

Edgar RE, Best LG, Quail PA, Obert AD 1993 Computer-assisted DREZ microcoagulation: posttraumatic spinal deafferentation pain. Journal of Spinal Disease 6: 48–56

Edwards WT, Habib F, Burney RG, Begin G 1985 Intravenous lidocaine in the management of various chronic pain states. Regional Anaesthesia 10: 1–6

Espir MLE, Millac P 1970 Treatment of paroxysmal disorders in multiple sclerosis with carbamazepine (Tegretol). Journal of Neurology, Neurosurgery and Psychiatry 33: 528–531

Fine W 1967 Post-hemiplegic epilepsy in the elderly. British Medical Journal 1: 199–201

Foster JB, Hudgson P 1973 Clinical features of syringomyelia. In: Barnett HJ, Foster JB, Hudgson P (eds) Syringomyelia. Saunders, London, pp 1–123

Garcin R 1968 Thalamic syndrome and pain central origin. In: Soulairac A, Cahn J, Charpentier J (eds) Pain. Academic, London, pp 521–541

Glynn CJ, Jamous MA, Teddy PJ, Moorem RA, Lloyd JW 1986 Role of spinal noradrenergic system in transmission of pain in patients with spinal cord injury. Lancet ii: 1249–1250

Glynn C, Dawson D, Sanders RA 1988 A double-blind comparison between epidural morphine and epidural clonidine in patients with chronic non-cancer pain. Pain 34: 123–128

Goetz CG, Tanner CM, Levy M, Wilson RS, Garron DG 1985 Pain in idiopathic Parkinson's disease. Neurology 35: 200

Gonzales GR, Herskovitz S, Rosenblum M et al 1992 Central pain from cerebral abscess: thalamic syndrome in AIDS patients with toxoplasmosis. Neurology 42: 1107–1109

Gybels JM, Sweet WH 1989 Neurosurgical treatment of persistent pain. Karger, Basel

Hansson P, Lindblom U 1992 Hyperalgesia assessed with quantitative sensory testing in patients with neuropathic pain. In: Willis WDJ (ed) Hyperalgesia and allodynia. Raven, New York, pp 335–343

Head H, Holmes G 1911 Sensory disturbances from cerebral lesions. Brain 34: 102–254

Herman RM, Luzansky SCD, Ippolito R 1992 Intrathecal baclofen suppresses central pain in patients with spinal lesions. Clinical Journal of Pain 8: 338–345

Jeanmonod D, Magnin M, Morel A 1996 Low-threshold calcium spike bursts in the human thalamus. Common physiopathology for sensory, motor and limbic positive symptoms. Brain 119: 363–375

Kalman S, Sörensen J, Österberg A, Boivie J, Bertler Å 2002 Morphine responsiveness in a group of well-defined multiple sclerosis patients. A study with i.v. morphine. European Journal of Pain 6: 69–80

Koller WC 1984 Sensory symptoms in Parkinson's disease. Neurology 34: 957–959

Kupers RC, Konings H, Adriasen H, Gybels JM 1991 Morphine differentially affects the sensory and affective ratings in neuropathic and ideopathic forms of pain. Pain 47: 5–12

Leijon G, Boivie J 1989a Central post-stroke pain—a controlled trial of amitriptyline and carbamazepine. Pain 36: 27–36

Leijon G, Boivie J 1989b Treatment of neuropathic pain with antidepressants. Nordisk Psykiatrisk Tidsskrift 43 (suppl 20): 83–87

Leijon G, Boivie J 1989c Central post-stroke pain—the effect of high and low frequency TENS. Pain 38: 187–191

Leijon G, Boivie J 1991 Pharmacological treatment of central pain. In: Casey KL (ed) Pain and central nervous system disease: the central pain syndromes. Raven, New York, pp 257–266

Leijon G, Boivie J 1996 Central post-stroke pain (CPSP)—A long-term follow-up. In: Abstracts 8th world congress on pain. IASP Press, Seattle, p 380

Leijon G, Boivie J, Johansson I 1989 Central post-stroke pain—neurological symptoms and pain characteristics. Pain 36: 13–25

Lenz FA 1992 Ascending modulation of thalamic function and pain; experimental and clinical data. In: Sicuteri F (ed) Advances in pain research and therapy. Raven, New York, pp 177–196

Lindblom U 1994 Analysis of abnormal touch, pain, and temperature sensation in patients. In: Boivie J, Hansson U, Lindblom U (ed) Touch, temperature, and pain in health and disease. IASP Press, Seattle, pp 63–84

Loh L, Nathan PW, Schott GD 1981 Pain due to lesions of central nervous system removed by sympathetic block. British Medical Journal 282: 1026–1028

MacGowan DJL, Janal MN, Clark WC et al 1997 Central post-stroke pain and Wallenberg's lateral medullary infarction: frequency, character, and determinants in 63 patients. Neurology 49: 120–125
Mauguiere F, Desmedt JE 1988 Thalamic pain syndrome of Dejérine–Roussy. Differentiation of four subtypes assisted by somatosensory evoked potentials data. Archives of Neurology 45: 1312–1320
Max MB, Lynch SA, Muir J, Shoaf SE, Smoller B, Dubner R 1992 Effects of desipramine, amitriptyline, and flouxetine on pain in diabetic neuropathy. New England Journal of Medicine 326: 1250–1256
McLean MJ, Macdonald RL 1986 Carbamazepine and 10,11-epoxycarbamazepine produce use- and voltage-dependent limitation of rapidly firing action potentials of mouse central neurons in cell culture. Journal of Pharmacology and Experimental Therapeutics 238: 727–738
Mersky H, Bogduk N 1994 Classification of chronic pain. IASP Press, Seattle, pp 1–222
Michel D, Laurent B, Convers P et al 1990 Douleurs corticales. Étude clinique, électrophysiologique et topographie de 12 cas. Revue Neurologique (Paris) 146: 405–414
Milhorat TH, Kotzen RM, Mu HTM, Copocelli AL, Milhorat RH 1996 Dysesthetic pain in patients with syringomyelia. Neurosurgery 38: 940–947
Moulin DE, Foley KM, Ebers GC 1988 Pain syndromes in multiple sclerosis. Neurology 38: 1830–1834
Nashold BS, Bullitt E 1981 Dorsal root entry zone lesions to control central pain in paraplegics. Journal of Neurosurgery 55: 414–419
Nasreddine ZS, Saver JL 1997 Pain after thalamic stroke: right diencephalic predominance and clinical features in 180 patients. Neurology 48: 1196–1199
Nicholson B 2000 Gabapentine use in neuropathic pain syndromes. Acta Neurologica Scandinavica 101: 359–371
Nutt JG, Carter JH 1984 Sensory symptoms in parkinsonism related to central dopaminergic function. Lancet 2: 456–457
Österberg A, Boivie J, Holmgren H, Thomas K-Å, Johansson I 1994 The clinical characteristics and sensory abnormalities of patients with central pain caused by multiple sclerosis. In: Gebhart GF, Hammond DL, Jensen TS (eds) Progress in pain research and management. IASP Press, Seattle, pp 789–796
Pagni CA 1989 Central pain due to spinal cord and brainstem damage. In: Wall PD, Melzack R (eds) Textbook of pain. Churchill Livingstone, Edinburgh, pp 634–655
Pagni C 1998 Central pain. A neurosurgical challenge. Edizioni Minerva Medica, Turin, p 211
Pertovaara A, Morrow TJ, Casey KL 1988 Cutaneous pain and detection thresholds to short CO_2 laser pulses in humans: evidence on afferent mechanisms and the influence of varying stimulus conditions. Pain 34: 261–269
Peyron R, Garcia-Larrea L, Deiber MP et al 1995 Electrical stimulation of precentral cortical area in the treatment of central pain: electrophysiological and PET study. Pain 62: 275–286
Portenoy RK, Foley KM 1986 Chronic use of opioid analgesics in non-malignant pain: report of 38 cases. Pain 25: 171–186
Portenoy RK, Foley KM, Inturrisi CE 1990 The nature of opioid responsiveness and its implications for neuropathic pain: new hypothesis derived from studies of opioid infusions. Pain 43: 273–286
Quinn NP, Koller WC, Lang AE, Marsden CD 1986 Painful Parkinson's disease. Lancet 1: 1366–1369
Richardsson RR, Meyer PR, Cerullo L 1980 Neurostimulation in the modulation of intractable paraplegic and traumatic neuroma pains. Pain 8: 75–84
Rosen JA, Barsoum AH 1979 Failure of chronic dorsal column stimulation in multiple sclerosis. Annals of Neurology 6: 66–67
Rowbotham MC, Reisner-Keller LA, Fields HL 1991 Both intravenous lidocaine and morphine reduce the pain of postherpetic neuralgia. Neurology 41: 1024–1028
Rowbotham MC, Harden N, Stacey B, Podolnick P, Magnus-Miller L 1998 Gabapentin for the treatment for post-herpetic neuralgia: a multicenter, double-blind, placebo-controlled study. Journal of the American Medical Association 280: 1837–1842
Scadding JW, Wall PD, Parry CBW, Brooks DM 1982 Clinical trial of propranolol in post-traumatic neuralgia. Pain 14: 283–292
Schliep G 1978 Syringomyelia and syringobulbia. In: Vinken G, Bruyn G (eds) Handbook of neurology. North-Holland, Amsterdam, pp 255–327
Schott B, Laurent B, Mauguière F 1986 Les douleurs thalamiques: étude critique de 43 cas. Revue Neurologique (Paris) 142: 308–315
Schott GD 1985 Pain in Parkinson's disease. Pain 22: 407–411
Shibasaki H, Kuroiwa Y 1974 Painful tonic seizure in multiple sclerosis. Archives of Neurology 30: 47–51
Siegfried J 1983 Long term results of electrical stimulation in the treatment of pain by means of implanted electrodes. In: Rizzi C, Visentin TA (eds) Pain therapy. Elsevier, Amsterdam, pp 463–475
Silver ML 1957 'Central pain' from cerebral arteriovenous aneurysm. Journal of Neurosurgery 14: 92–97
Sindrup SH, Gram LF, Brosen K, Eshöj O, Mogensen EF 1990 The selective serotonin reuptake inhibitor paroxetine is effective in the treatment of diabetic neuropathy symptoms. Pain 42: 135–144
Sjölund BH 1991 Role of transcutaneous electrical nerve stimulation, central nervous system stimulation, and ablative procedures in central pain syndromes. In: Casey KL (ed) Pain and central nervous disease: the central pain syndromes. Raven, New York, pp 267–274
Snider SR, Fahn S, Isgreen WP, Cote LJ 1976 Primary sensory symptoms in parkinsonism. Neurology 26: 423–429
Soria ED, Fine EJ 1991 Disappearance of thalamic pain after parietal subcortical stroke. Pain 44: 285–288
Stenager E, Knudsen L, Jensen K 1991 Acute and chronic pain syndromes in multiple sclerosis. Acta Neurologica Scandinavica 84: 197–200
Swerdlow M 1986 Anticonvulsants in the therapy of neuralgic pain. The Pain Clinic 1: 9–19
Tasker R 2000 Central pain states. In: Loeser J (ed) Bonica´s management of pain. Lippincott Williams & Wilkins, Philadelphia, pp 264–280
Tasker RR, de Carvalho G, Dostrovsky JO 1991 The history of central pain syndromes, with observations concerning pathophysiology and treatment. In: Casey KL (ed) Pain and central nervous disease: the central pain syndromes. Raven, New York, pp 31–58
Tourtellotte WW, Baumhefner WW 1983 Comprehensive management of multiple sclerosis. In: Hallpike JF, Adams CWM, Tourtellotte WW (eds) Multiple sclerosis. Williams & Wilkins, Baltimore, pp 513–578
Tovi D, Schisano G, Liljequist B 1961 Primary tumours of the region of the thalamus. Journal of Neurosurgery 18: 730–740
Treede RD, Kief S, Hölzer T, Bromm B 1988 Late somatosensory evoked cerebral potentials in response to cutaneous heat stimuli. Electroencephalography and Clinical Neurophysiology 70: 429–441
Tsubokawa T 1995 Motor cortex stimulation for deafferentation pain relief in various clinical syndromes and its possible mechanisms. In: Besson JM, Guildbaud G, Ollat H (eds) Forebrain areas involved in pain processing. John Libby Eurotext, Paris, pp 261–276
Umlauf RL, Moore JE, Britell CW 1992 Relevance and nature of the pain experience in spinal cord injured. Journal of Behavioural Medicine 37: 254–261

Vermote R, Ketelaer P, Carton H 1986 Pain in multiple sclerosis patients. Clinical Neurology and Neurosurgery 88: 87–93
Vestergard K, Andersen G, Gottrup H, Kristensen BT, Jensen TS 2001 Lamotrigine for central poststroke pain. A randomized controlled trial. Neurology 56: 184–190
Waltz TA, Ehni G 1966 The thalamic syndrome and its mechanism. Journal of Neurosurgery 24: 735–742
Watson C, Evans RJ 1985 A comparative trial of amitryptiline and zimilidine in post-herpetic neuralgia. Pain 23: 387–394
Wiesenfeld-Hallin Z, Lindblom U 1985 The effect of systemic tocaimide, lidocaine and bupivacaine on nociception in the rat. Pain 23: 357–360
Wood T, Sloan R 1997 Successful use of ketemine for central pain. Palliative Medicine 11: 57–58
Woolf CJ, Wiesenfeld-Hallin Z 1985 The systematic administration of local anesthetics produces a selective depression of C-afferent fibre evoked activity in the spinal cord. Pain 23: 361–374
Yamamoto T, Latayama Y, Hirayama T, Tsubokawa T 1997 Pharmacological classification of central post-stroke pain: comparison with the results of chronic motor cortex stimulation therapy. Pain 72: 5–12
Yarnitsky D, Sprecher E 1994 Different algorithms for thermal threshold measurement. In: Boivie J, Hansson P, Lindblom U (eds) Touch, temperature, and pain in health and disease: mechanisms and assessments. IASP Press, Seattle, pp 105–112
Young BG, Blume WT 1983 Painful epileptic seizures. Brain 106: 537–554
Young RF, Goodman SJ 1979 Dorsal spinal cord stimulation in the treatment of multiple sclerosis. Neurosurgery 5: 225–230

Chapter 21

Spinal cord injury

Aleksandar Berić

Introduction

Spinal cord injury (SCI) usually results from severe spinal column damage. Frequently, there is a concomitant ligamentous, joint, disc, and soft-tissue injury that contributes to an acute phase of pain (Berić 1997a). To a large extent, this pain usually subsides with general pain treatment and the management of acute SCI (Cairns et al 1996, Sved et al 1997). Usually SCI pains appear after a few months and not infrequently after several years, sometimes changing their characteristics as they appear or disappear. It is actually the chronic pain that may be so devastating that it may override any other motor, bladder and bowel, and functional disabilities in the postacute phase (Nepomuceno et al 1979). Fortunately, only a fraction of SCI patients suffer from such severe pain (Bonica 1991).

There are different pains present in different patients and also different pains present in the same patient at different times or simultaneously. There has been no consensus regarding classification. The International Association for the Study of Pain (IASP) has avoided SCI pain classification for years. Only recently have some more extensive attempts been made to classify SCI pains (Berić 1997a, b; Siddall et al 1997; Siddall and Loeser 2001).

The treatment of SCI is a very difficult task. There are no SCI pain-specific medications, reflecting our poor understanding of underlying pain mechanisms. Due to a variety of pain disorders, a practical classification would help in developing clinical therapeutic guidelines. However, this is only a part of the solution, as there is still no optimal therapy for some of the pains, for example central pains. Another complicating factor is the fragility of the SCI patient's medical condition regarding pain medication. Spasticity, bladder and bowel function, blood pressure regulation, etc., are all by different degrees influenced by our current pain medications and control measures.

Pain incidence in spinal cord injury

Pain is usually present in acute SCI and can take different courses. It may subside with or without treatment when early musculoskeletal abnormalities slowly subside. If it is caused by root injury or SCI, it may also subside if the injury is mild and does not trigger persistent central changes or may persist into the chronic stage. Incidence statistics are variable and, depending on the methodology, range from 10 to 90% (Lamid et al 1985, Rose et al 1988, Berić 1990, Levi et al 1995, Stormer et al 1997).

Recently, both inpatient and outpatient reports and telephone interviews estimate a 64–67% incidence of pain in the SCI population (Siddall et al 1999, Finnerup et al 2001). Intractable pain is present in about one-third of these patients. If SCI patients are asked historically whether they have ever experienced pain, the numbers rise to 90% and even higher (New et al 1997). Sometimes the cauda equina (CE) injuries are included because there are many overlapping features between CE injuries and SCI.

It would be advantageous to report the severity, distribution, quality, onset, and course of pain, together with the neurological condition of the patient, according to the American Spinal Injury Association (ASIA) criteria (Maynard et al 1997). Another parameter would be previous pain treatments, especially if destructive. As some treatments change the characteristics of pain, it would be useful to state these changes in relation to treatment.

Recognized pain conditions in spinal cord injury

Transitional zone pain

The cause of some pains in post-SCI is intuitively obvious based on the site and distribution of pain and its relationship to the primary injury. Among these types of pains are transitional zone segmental pains, which include root pains. They occur at the level of the SCI (Davis 1975, Burke and Woodward 1976). In our study one-third of patients with pain had a primary transitional zone-root pain associated with all levels of injury (Berić 1990). Chronic transitional pain was present more often in thoracic SCI patients with clinically complete sensory and motor dysfunction. The distribution was most often within a few contiguous segments and asymmetrical. Descriptions of pain sensation included aching, burning, and stinging. Frequently, there is an early allodynia to touch and hyperalgesia similar to reflex sympathetic dystrophy (RSD) that generally improves spontaneously. However, if severe, resolution of this pain may require a series of blocks or even DREZ surgery (Nashold and Bullitt 1981, Edgar et al 1993, Sampson et al 1995, Sindou et al 2001).

Transitional zone segmental pains may last for some time. However, they are frequently managed by pharmacological and local block treatments. Therefore, their natural course is usually modified in the relatively early stages due to a range of reasonably effective treatment modalities.

Cauda equina pain

When the spinal column lesion involves levels below L1, the CE is usually injured. The pain associated with this injury may involve the legs, feet, perineum, genitals, and rectum. The mechanism is similar to that of transitional zone pain in SCI. CE pain is considered a root neurogenic type of pain. In severe complete lesions of the lumbosacral segments, the upper- and mid-lumbar segments are partially injured and those dermatomes (anterior thigh) demonstrate hyperalgesia, allodynia to touch, and spontaneous pain. If the injury is lower at the L4 and L5 levels, hyperalgesia and pain affect the feet or perineum and rectum. The pain usually has a burning, causalgic quality. These pains are among the most severe in spinal injuries.

Central dysaesthesia syndrome

One of the most frequently described pain states in SCI is the diffuse burning sensation below the level of the lesion. Many terms have been used to describe this pain syndrome: burning dysaesthetic pain, function-limiting dysaesthesias, central pain, phantom pain, and more recently, central dysaesthesia syndrome (CDS) (Davis and Martin 1947, Pollock et al 1951, Davis 1975, Davidoff et al 1987, Berić et al 1988, Woodward and Vulpe 1991). The intriguing feature of this syndrome, almost invariably seen in these patients, is the relative dissociation between the anterolateral spinothalamic and dorsal column systems. Temperature, pinprick, and pain perception is severely impaired in these patients. However, in most cases light-touch sensitivity and discriminatory and vibratory senses are relatively spared, with some preserved motor function below the level of the lesion that is sufficient even to allow ambulation. The CDS represents a genuine central pain syndrome (CPS) (Berić 1998).

In our series, CDS was the second most frequent pain syndrome, which occurred in 29.4% of patients (Berić 1990). The pain was relatively symmetrical, with uniform diffuse burning below the level of the lesion. It was almost equally distributed between the lower cervical and thoracic segments of the primary SCI, with a slightly higher relative incidence in the upper cervical segments.

CDS is a rare entity in the general population, as it is present only in severe spinal cord pathology, usually in patients with incomplete SCI. Compared with poststroke pain, the evoked dysaesthesia component is less frequent; however, that does not mean that it is not the most prominent feature in some patients.

Similar to poststroke pain, CDS usually appears with some functional recovery in more severe cases and can appear months after the injury. This dysaesthesia usually increases slowly in intensity and can follow three possible courses. The first and most frequent is a stable course that can linger for an indefinite number of years, with some fluctuations in symptom intensity. The second more unusual possible course of pain is continuous escalation, requiring more aggressive treatment. The third and certainly the best possible course is the slow decrease in pain intensity within a few years.

It is more difficult to treat CDS in SCI than poststroke pain because some of the relatively minor nuisances of treatment can be disastrous in SCI. Dryness of mouth, for example, in quadriplegic patients is of different significance than in hemiparetic patients. Furthermore, constipation and bladder retention in quadriplegic or paraplegic patients can have dire consequences, including a major increase in intensity of their baseline pain.

Double-lesion syndrome

DLS represents dysfunction of the sacral and lumbosacral segments that are distant from the primary SCI, most frequently at the cervical or upper thoracic levels. In thoracic and cervical SCI patients, DLS consists of sacral dysfunction with amyotrophy and CE progressive degeneration, which is usually asymmetrical, along with bladder and sphincteric abnormalities (Berić et al 1987). DLS may be followed by a specific pain syndrome (Berić et al 1992). Approximately 25% had some clinically preserved sensation below the level of the lesion, whereas the other 75% were described as clinically complete.

In our series, 20% of patients complained of DLS type of pain (Berić 1990). The most frequent characteristic of pain was sharp pricking and electric shock sensations, with occasional burning, as well as aching and dull pain. The distribution was for the most part asymmetrical and localized to the leg, groin, thigh, or foot with frequent inclusion of the perineum, rectum, and genitals. These patients usually had progressive neurological syndrome with progressive muscle atrophy and conversion of the upper motor neuron (UMN) bladder to the lower motor neuron (LMN) bladder. Therefore, the diagnosis of this syndrome was based not only on the pain characteristics but also on the presence of neurological, neurophysiological, and urodynamic evidence of dysfunction of the lumbosacral segment along with cauda equina progressive dysfunction.

Patients with DLS pain tend to develop pain within a year after the time of injury. However, it is not uncommon for patients to develop pain later, along with a deterioration of function in the sacral and lumbosacral segments. Their pain condition often stabilizes within several months or several years but remains constant, with minimal fluctuation.

Anterior spinal artery syndrome

Anterior spinal artery syndrome (ASAS) can be considered a subsyndrome in SCI because it can be traumatic, although the pure syndrome is generally a vascular event and is also described as iatrogenic (Triggs and Berić 1992). It is the exaggeration of the CDS in SCI. There is profound anterolateral sensory system involvement, usually a complete absence of temperature and thermal pain perception, with a variable degree of motor paralysis and excellent preservation of the dorsal column modalities. It resembles a bilateral, deep, and extremely well-done surgical anterolateral cordotomy (Nathan and Smith 1979) with some additional motor deficit.

Syringomyelia

Syringomyelia is classified as a complication of SCI that generally appears much later in the post-SCI period (Williams et al 1981). Therefore, late appearance of pain in some SCI patients, for example, 5–10 years after the initial SCI, should alert us to the possibility of syringomyelia. Its hallmark is the development of an expanding post-traumatic cyst with ascension of the motor and sensory levels, increasing motor disability, and development of new pain (Vernon et al 1982, Dworkin and Staas 1985, Rossier et al 1985). Once the motor and sensory abnormalities are recognized and appropriate imaging studies obtained, it is not difficult to determine the cause of the new pain. However, if pain is one of the first symptoms of syringomyelia and superimposed on other post-SCI pain states, it becomes extremely difficult to diagnose initially. Patients with syringomyelia usually complain of an aching and burning pain at the level of the lesion, sometimes extending above and below the level of the lesion. The ascending cyst may increase the level of disability and even convert low cervical SCI, which is functionally considered as paraplegia, to quadriplegia. Rigorous and expedient assessment of sensory and motor functions coupled with magnetic resonance imaging (MRI) help determine the diagnosis (Wang et al 1996). If MRI is not possible due to prior surgical intervention–spinal stabilization, delayed computer tomography (CT) myelogram should be performed and intervention instituted as soon as possible.

There is another similar condition that can be sometimes differentiated from syringomyelia by MRI—progressive post-traumatic myelomalacic myelopathy. This subentity may lead to transitional zone pain and may be treated surgically by attempting to untether the abnormal spinal cord (Ragnarsson et al 1986, Lee et al 1997).

Other pains

Musculoskeletal pain most commonly occurs in patients with thoracic spine injuries. The pain is frequently localized around the level of the injury or just above the injury, due to stretching of the long muscles of the trunk. Shoulder pain in quadriplegics is an example of musculoskeletal pain (Silfverskiold and Waters 1991, Waring and Maynard 1991, Campbell and Koris 1996). It is most frequently triggered by a change in physical activity and aggravated by increased muscle activity and movement. A subgroup of these patients have RSD of the hand that is infrequently seen in patients with cervical SCI (Wainapel 1984, Davidoff and Roth 1991, Aisen and Aisen 1994). The pain, however, can also be present below the level of the lesion (Gallien et al 1995). Muscle, ligament, and joint pains in the lower extremities of patients with incomplete SCI are also musculoskeletal pains, including pains due to heterotopic ossification with muscle and soft-tissue calcification. These patients have ambulatory potential and asymmetrical corticospinal left/right leg deficits and asymmetrical spasticity, with more involvement in some muscle groups than in others.

Patients with absent voluntary activity below the level of the lesion can also have pain due to uncontrollable spasms. These pains are generally of the crescendo type, paralleling an increase in the intensity and spread of the spasm.

Musculoskeletal pain tends to appear when the patient becomes more active, with transfers, wheelchair activities, or ambulation in the case of incomplete SCI. The pain is usually proportional to the amount of offending activity. Rest alleviates or at least decreases pain. As treatment is instituted early, the pain generally subsides. In thoracic SCIs, however, sometimes sitting and abnormal positioning in the wheelchair cannot be easily modified. The long thoracic muscles can be stretched for an extended time, resulting in intractable pains that can resemble transitional zone or even CDS pain.

Carpal tunnel syndrome in paraplegics deserves a special consideration as it is a neurogenic pain syndrome triggered usually by overuse of hands, especially by propelling wheelchairs (Davidoff and Roth 1991, Sie et al 1992).

Visceral pain is deep abdominal pain usually related to urological procedures and concomitant bladder infections that are aggravated by bowel and bladder activity. The debate is far from resolved regarding the question of whether visceral pain warrants a separate classification.

In SCI patients, special consideration should be given to non-SCI-related pains including those due to urinary tract infections, bowel dysfunction with impaction, or abdominal infections such as acute abdomen due to appendicitis or cholecystitis. Typical physical signs of these conditions, such as localized muscle spasms, localized pain sensitivity, or even fever, may be absent. Often changes in bowel and bladder patterns and sometimes an increase or decrease in spasticity are the only indicators of infection. Such changes should alert physicians to perform a more complete clinical examination, especially in the event of new pain, for example visceral or abdominal pain. Due to SCI, the presentation of pains associated with bladder infection, bowel infection, or other abdominal causes is not typical of these conditions and may mimic genuine SCI pains. Therefore, with the appearance of new pain or exacerbation of otherwise stable pain in patients with SCI, evaluation of blood pressure, pulse, temperature, rectal examination, urinary analysis, and white blood cell count is necessary. In incomplete and especially ambulatory SCI patients, it is important to be aware of the possible appearance of other neurological conditions with manifestations that may be modified by the primary spinal cord lesion.

A separate condition in upper thoracic and cervical SCI is autonomic dysreflexia (Clinchot and Colachis 1996, Curt et al 1997). This can be brought on by a number of triggers: bladder distension, sphincter dyssynergia (concomitant contraction of the bladder and sphincter, with increasing pressure inside the bladder), bowel movements and impaction, and dysfunction due to severe spasms. This can be a life-threatening situation, causing an increase in blood pressure, the presence of headache, a possible increase in intracranial pressure, and the occurrence of a fatal intracranial haemorrhage. This is not a simple pain syndrome. The presence of discomfort, headache, and unpleasant internal sensations should be recognized. The cause of these symptoms should be determined and the condition treated appropriately. These episodes tend to be repetitive, short term, and acute.

Phantom sensations versus phantom pains

Phantom sensations should be distinguished from so-called phantom pains as described by Pollock et al (1957). In general, phantom sensations appear early, almost immediately after SCI, and vanish within hours or days of SCI. In about 25% these complex sensations persist for months or longer (Siddall and McClelland 1999). Furthermore, the quality and intensity of these sensations rarely interfere with activities of daily living. They are not painful or functionally limiting, although they are frequently bizarre in nature (Sweet 1975). On the other hand, pain in the paralysed and insensitive segment below the level of the lesion generally appears later in the post-SCI period, when phantom sensations fade.

Clinical classification

Classifications are plagued with uncertainty of either the aetiology of SCI pain or even which system is involved. There are some new classifications that try to take advantage of the triaxial system to better delineate different SCI pains (Siddall and Loeser 2001). However, only the site of the pain is non-disputable. The system, for example musculoskeletal, visceral, or neuropathic, is very much questionable in a large proportion of SCI pains, as it requires more than just a location and quality to be defined. The third axis, which is presumably a source of pain, is highly debatable as the aetiology remains in question.

Diagnostic approach

Clinical interview

Work-up of every SCI patient with pain should include a detailed history of pain in relation to SCI pain onset. An inventory of pain characteristics should be obtained: course; quality; distribution; factors affecting pain, especially spasms; transfers; and impact of physical therapy (PT). The relationship of pain onset to recovery or deterioration of sensory and motor function and overall functional status should also be determined. In addition, history of intercurrent episodes of infection, surgeries, new injuries, and pain treatments, followed by changes in pain character, are also important to the work-up for post-SCI pain. A standardized Pain Questionnaire (PQ) is usually useful in follow-up studies. The PQ should include the visual analogue scale, pain drawing, and the standard or modified McGill PQ.

Clinical examination

Neurological examination is mandatory and should include sensory, motor, and functional assessments and scales as recommended by the ASIA (Maynard et al 1997). The pain is localized within a region of a large sensory deficit. The presence of allodynia and hyperalgesia is helpful, if there are no local causes of irritation. Although the light-touch allodynia or proprioceptive allodynia can have bizarre clinical manifestations, intolerance of the skin to warm or cool is also frequently present as a more conventional continuous dull or burning pain.

Laboratory and electrodiagnostic tests

Laboratory tests are not useful in the diagnosis and classification of pain. However, they are extremely important in excluding urinary tract infections and other non-SCI pain-related conditions. Complete gastrointestinal and urological work-ups are recommended for visceral pains. Neurophysiological testing is useful for root and cauda equina as well as for conus medullaris lesion and is mandatory in DLS.

Imaging

MRI is invaluable for syringomyelia diagnosis. Sometimes, in addition to allowing observation of the level of the lesion, MRI can provide useful information regarding the cord below the level of the lesion. For example, it can provide evidence of suspected vascular extension of the lesion, i.e., an extended downward infarct with cord atrophy—spinal amyotrophy. MRI is not very useful, however, for the assessment of completeness of the lesion, except if the cord is totally separated at the injury level, which is rare.

Urodynamic testing

Urodynamic evaluation is important for differentiation of upper motor neuron (UMN) from lower motor neuron (LMN) bladder. Sometimes if pain and/or dysaesthesias are diffuse and located in lumbar and sacral segments, CDS and DLS can be differentiated based on the presence of UMN bladder in CDS and LMN bladder in DLS.

Quantitative sensory testing and other ancillary procedures

In CDS, quantitative sensory testing (QST) at the lesion level and at standard sites below the level of the lesion is necessary to document incompleteness as well as different degrees of dissociated sensory loss. In syringomyelia, QST may be used for follow-ups for assessment of progression.

Some pain syndromes can be better recognized by additional testing, while others are determined only through treatment trials and modification of PT and overall activity. In nociceptive musculoskeletal pains, PT and rehabilitation programme modifications are used as assessment tools in addition to their possible therapeutic effects. Psychological tests with a multiaxial approach have been recommended (Wegener and Elliott 1992). The Hamilton Depression Scale and Beck Inventory are useful, including both self-inventory and interview approaches, for the assessment of depression.

Nerve and spinal blocks

In transitional zone pain, anaesthetic blocks are employed diagnostically and repeatedly as a therapeutic option. Spinal blocks have been employed for all SCI pains and usually provide, as expected, temporary and frequently only a partial relief of pain (Loubser and Donovan 1991). Intrathecal baclofen is very useful in alleviating spasms. However, it has only at best a mixed effect on pain. Diagnostic anaesthetic blocks are of no prognostic value as further deafferentation is not a desired goal. Although there has been debate regarding sympathetic system dysfunction or its preservation as a pain ascending system, this has never been proven and sympathetic blocks are not routinely required. Nevertheless, some patients receive a significant temporary decrease of evoked pains with local, regional, and sympathetic blocks.

Management of spinal cord injury pains

General guidelines

The treatment of CPS follows the general rules of a stepwise conservative approach (Fenollosa et al 1993, Gonzales 1994). Antidepressants with antinor-adrenergic properties are first-line therapy, usually followed by membrane-stabilizing drugs and anticonvulsants. Narcotics should be used as adjuvants, especially at the peaks of pain or periods of increased intensity of pain. Stimulation techniques may follow, from simple non-invasive ones, such as TENS, to trials with spinal cord stimulation and possibly deep brain stimulation in very selected cases. Experimental drugs and experimental drug deliveries may follow, and finally surgical destructive modalities may be contemplated.

Antidepressants

Antidepressants with noradrenergic properties are first-line therapy for most SCI pains. Tricyclic antidepressant effectiveness has been shown in both non-controlled clinical trials and double-blind studies in CPS (Leijon and Boivie 1989, Sanford et al 1992). Amitriptyline appears to be most effective, but it also has the most side effects, which are mainly anticholinergic, including urinary retention, mouth dryness, drowsiness, and provoking glaucoma. Effective pain doses are below antidepressant doses. Due to frequent side effects, however, a very low starting dose is suggested. Increments should be gradual. If there is no response at approximately 2 weeks with an average daily dose, at least two different antidepressants from the same nor-adrenergic group should be tried.

Antiepileptics and membrane stabilizers

Second-line therapy includes antiepileptics and membrane-stabilizing drugs. Carbamazepine is probably most effective (Sanford et al 1992). The dosage is often above antiseizure recommendations. The blood level is irrelevant, unless there is an issue of non-compliance. Side effects are dose limiting and blood work-up is standard. Recently, a negative study on the effect of valproate on SCI pain was reported (Drewes et al 1994). There are a number of relatively new medications, such as gabapentine and lamotrigine, that have not undergone either rigorous double-blind studies or simply a test of time. Because of a relatively low side-effect profile, however, and some promising trials in neurogenic pains, they may be tried possibly in conjunction with other drugs. Mexiletine was tried in CPS; however, it was not beneficial in SCI (Chiou-Tan et al 1996).

Narcotics

Low-dose narcotics are useful in SCI as they are effective in nociceptive pains. They are, however, not effective in neurogenic pains (Arner and Meyerson 1988), especially CDS. High doses are limited because of side effects (Portenoy et al 1990). Narcotics should be used as adjuvants, especially at the peaks of pain or periods of increased intensity of pain, in addition to antidepressants and antiepileptics. Combinations with NSAIDs are useful for short courses, but the long-term use of NSAIDs may cause gastric disturbances or be renally toxic and therefore should be avoided. Sometimes intrathecal opioids can be a viable option (Winkelmuller and Winkelmuller 1996).

GABA agonists

GABA-A agonists have been used for a long time. Valium has both antispastic and analgesic effects; however, it is a non-specific sedative that impairs cognitive function and tolerance usually develops. GABA-B agonists, such as baclofen, in oral preparations are not effective for pain relief. Intrathecally administered in SCI patients, GABA-B agonists may occasionally have an analgesic effect (Herman et al 1992, Mertens et al 1995, Loubser and Akman 1996). It is, however, unclear whether they affect CPS or other neurogenic, spastic, and musculoskeletal pains in these patients, as they all can coexist.

Other medications

There is a potential beneficial effect of *N*-methyl-D-aspartate (NMDA) antagonists, although ketamine is limited by its adverse effects and only used for research trials (Eide et al 1995). Clonidine, neuroleptics, and even naloxone are sometimes tried (Middleton et al 1996).

Stimulation techniques

In some cases, stimulation techniques may also be useful such as low- and high-frequency TENS, and spinal cord and deep brain stimulation (Davis and Lentini 1975, Richardson et al 1980, Richardson 1995, Simpson 1999, and see Chap. 20).

Pain syndrome-specific treatments

Opiates alone or in combination with other analgesics and antidepressants are helpful in most of the transitional zone pains, with adjunctive use of intercostal and peripheral blocks. For conus medullaris and CE injuries, in addition to previously mentioned measures for transitional zone pain, DREZ surgery may be effective. It may, however, move the neurological levels for a few segments proximally with a consequent increase in disability.

CDS is unfortunately very difficult to treat and trials with antidepressants, anticonvulsants, and oral congeners of local anaesthetics are always warranted, probably in that order. There are anecdotal reports of the usefulness of intravenous lidocaine (lignocaine), deep brain stimulation, or even deafferentation. Syringomyelia pain resembles pain of CDS; therefore treatment should be similar to that for both CDS and CPS. However, surgical intervention is almost always necessary, including drainage and shunting of the cyst (Vernon et al 1983).

In some DLS patients, our own anecdotal reports demonstrate the efficacy of spinal cord stimulation below the level of the lesion, as well as TENS or a combination of spinal blocks and analgesics (Berić 1990, Berić et al 1992).

Musculoskeletal pain syndromes usually respond well to analgesics, local blocks, and trigger injections. The most effective treatment includes adjustment of activity level and use of certain muscle groups, as well as appropriate PT. Pain caused by spasms responds excellently to muscle relaxants, baclofen in particular, especially to intrathecal baclofen infusion (Loubser and Akman 1996).

Psychological interventions should also be employed (Umlauf 1992), as there are substantial psychosocial implications of pain and disability in SCI patients (Richards et al 1980, Lundquist et al 1991, Summers et al 1991, Mariano 1992, Stormer et al 1997). In general, destructive chemical and surgical procedures should be avoided as they further alter pre-existing abnormal function of the nervous system and broaden the gap between normal and abnormal nervous system function. Although some of these procedures may temporarily alleviate pain, in the long term they are detrimental. Furthermore, they may create conditions in these patients that disqualify them for procedures developed in the future.

References

Aisen PS, Aisen ML 1994 Shoulder–hand syndrome in cervical spinal cord injury. Paraplegia 32: 588–592

Arner S, Meyerson BA 1988 Lack of analgesic effect of opioids on neuropathic and idiopathic forms of pain. Pain 33: 11–23

Berić A 1990 Altered sensation and pain in spinal cord injury. In: Dimitrijevic MR, Wall PD, Lindblom U (eds) Recent achievements in restorative neurology, vol 3: altered sensation and pain. Karger, Basel, pp 27–36

Berić A 1997a Post-spinal cord injury pain states. Anesthesiology Clinics of North America 15: 445–463

Berić A 1997b Post-spinal cord injury pain states. Pain 72: 295–298

Berić A 1998 Central pain and dysesthesia syndrome. Neurology Clinics of North America 16: 899–918

Berić A, Dimitrijevic MR, Light JK 1987 A clinical syndrome of rostral and caudal spinal injury: neurologic, neurophysiologic and urodynamic evidence for occult sacral lesion. Journal of Neurology, Neurosurgery and Psychiatry 50: 600–606

Berić A, Dimitrijevic MR, Lindblom U 1988 Central dysesthesia syndrome in spinal cord injury patients. Pain 34: 109–116

Berić A, Dimitrijevic MR, Light JK 1992 Pain in spinal cord injury with occult caudal lesions. European Journal of Pain 13: 1–7
Bonica JJ 1991 Introduction: sematic, epidemiologic, and educational issues. In: Casey KL (ed) Pain and central nervous system disease: the central pain syndromes. Raven, New York, pp 13–29
Burke DC, Woodward JM 1976 Pain and phantom sensation in spinal paralysis. In: Vinken PJ, Bruyn GW (eds) Handbook of clinical neurology, vol 26: injuries of the spine and spinal cord, part II. North-Holland, Amsterdam, pp 489–499
Cairns DM, Adkins RH, Scott MD 1996 Pain and depression in acute traumatic spinal cord injury: origins of chronic problematic pain? Archives of Physical Medicine and Rehabilitation 77: 329–335
Campbell CC, Koris MJ 1996 Etiologies of shoulder pain in cervical spinal cord injury. Clinical Orthopedics and Related Research 322: 140–145
Chiou-Tan FY, Tuel SM, Johnson JC, Priebe MM et al 1996 Effect of mexiletine on spinal cord injury dysesthetic pain. American Journal of Physical Medicine and Rehabilitation 75: 84–87
Clinchot DM, Colachis SC 1996 Autonomic hyperreflexia associated with exacerbation of reflex sympathetic dystrophy. Journal of Spinal Cord Medicine 19: 225–257
Curt A, Nitsche B, Rodic B, Schurch B, Dietz V 1997 Assessment of autonomic dysreflexia in patients with spinal cord injury. Journal of Neurology, Neurosurgery and Psychiatry 62: 473–477
Davidoff G, Roth EJ 1991 Clinical characteristics of central (dysesthetic) pain in spinal cord injury patients. In: Casey KL (ed) Pain and central nervous system disease: the central pain syndromes. Raven, New York, pp 77–83
Davidoff G, Roth E, Guarracini M et al 1987 Function-limiting dysesthetic pain syndrome among traumatic spinal cord injury patients: a cross-sectional study. Pain 29: 39–48
Davis L, Martin J 1947 Studies upon spinal cord injuries II. The nature and treatment of pain. Journal of Neurosurgery 4: 483–491
Davis R 1975 Pain and suffering following spinal cord injury. Clinical Orthopedics 112: 76–80
Davis R, Lentini R 1975 Transcutaneous nerve stimulation for treatment of pain in patients with spinal cord injury. Surgical Neurology 4: 100–101
Drewes AM, Andreasen A, Poulsen LH 1994 Valproate for treatment of chronic pain after spinal cord injury. A double-blind cross-over study. Paraplegia 32: 565–569
Dworkin GE, Staas WE 1985 Posttraumatic syringomyelia. Archives of Physical Medicine and Rehabilitation 66: 329–331
Edgar RE, Best LG, Quail PA, Obert AD 1993 Computer-assisted DREZ microcoagulation: posttraumatic spinal deafferentation pain. Journal of Spinal Disorders 6: 48–56
Eide PK, Stubhaug A, Stenehjem AE 1995 Central dysesthesia pain after traumatic spinal cord injury is dependent on *N*-methyl-D-aspartate receptor activation. Neurosurgery 37: 1080–1087
Fenollosa P, Pallares J, Cervera J et al 1993 Chronic pain in the spinal cord injured: statistical approach and pharmacological treatment. Paraplegia 31: 722–729
Finnerup NB, Johannesen IL, Sindrup SH, Bach FW, Jensen TS 2001 Pain and dysesthesia in patients with spinal cord injury: A postal survey. Spinal Cord 39: 256–262
Gallien P, Nicolas B, Robineau S et al 1995 The reflex sympathetic dystrophy syndrome in patients who have had a spinal cord injury. Paraplegia 33: 715–720
Gonzales GR 1994 Central pain. Seminars in Neurology 14: 255–262
Herman RM, D'Luzansky SC, Ippolitio R 1992 Intrathecal baclofen suppresses central pain in patients with spinal lesions. Clinical Journal of Pain 8: 338–345
Lamid S, Chia JK, Kohli A, Cid E 1985 Chronic pain in spinal cord injury: comparison between inpatients and outpatients. Archives of Physical Medicine and Rehabilitation 66: 777–778
Lee TT, Arias JM, Andrus HL, Quencer RM, Falcone SF, Green BA 1997 Progressive posttraumatic myelomalacic myelopathy: treatment with untethering and expansive duraplasty. Journal of Neurosurgery 86: 624–628
Leijon G, Boivie J 1989 Central post-stroke pain—a controlled trial of amitriptyline and carbamazepine. Pain 36: 27–36
Levi R, Hultling C, Seiger A 1995 The Stockholm spinal cord injury study: 2. Associations between clinical patient characteristics and post-acute medical problems. Paraplegia 33: 585–594
Loubser PG, Akman NM 1996 Effects of intrathecal baclofen on chronic spinal cord injury pain. Journal of Pain and Symptom Management 12: 241–247
Loubser PG, Donovan WH 1991 Diagnostic spinal anaesthesia in chronic spinal cord injury pain. Paraplegia 29: 25–36
Lundquist C, Siosteen A, Blomstrand C, Lind B, Sullivan M 1991 Spinal cord injuries: clinical, functional and emotional status. Spine 16: 78–83
Mariano AJ 1992 Chronic pain and spinal cord injury. Clinical Journal of Pain 8: 87–92
Maynard FM, Bracken MB, Creasey G et al 1997 International standards for neurological and functional classification of spinal cord injury. Spinal Cord 35: 266–274
Mertens P, Parise M, Garcia-Larrea L et al 1995 Long-term clinical, electrophysiological and urodynamic effects of chronic intrathecal baclofen infusion for treatment of spinal spasticity. Acta Neurochirurgica 64 (suppl): 17–25
Middleton JW, Siddall PJ, Walker S, Molloy AR, Rutkowski SB 1996 Intrathecal clonidine and baclofen in the management of spasticity and neuropathic pain following spinal cord injury: a case study. Archives of Physical Medicine and Rehabilitation 77: 824–826
Nashold BS, Bullitt E 1981 Dorsal root entry zone lesions to control central pain in paraplegics. Journal of Neurosurgery 55: 414–419
Nathan PW, Smith MC 1979 Clinico-anatomical correlation in anterolateral cordotomy. In: Bonica JJ et al (eds) Advances in pain research and therapy, vol 3. Raven, New York, pp 921–926
Nepomuceno C, Fine PR, Richards JS et al 1979 Pain in patients with spinal cord injury. Archives of Physical Medicine and Rehabilitation 60: 605–609
New PW, Lim TC, Hill ST, Brown DJ 1997 A survey of pain during rehabilitation after acute spinal cord injury. Spinal Cord 35: 658–663
Pollock LJ, Brown M, Boshes B et al 1951 Pain below the level of injury of the spinal cord. Archives of Neurology and Psychiatry 65: 319–322
Pollock LJ, Boshes B, Arieff AJ et al 1957 Phantom limb in patients with injuries to the spinal cord and cauda equina. Surgery, Gynecology and Obstetrics 104: 407
Portenoy RK, Foley KM, Inturrisi CE 1990 The nature of opioid responsiveness and its implications for neuropathic pain: new hypotheses derived from studies of opioid infusions. Pain 43: 273–286
Ragnarsson TS, Durward QJ, Nordgren RE 1986 Spinal cord tethering after traumatic paraplegia with late neurological deterioration. Journal of Neurosurgery 64: 397–401
Richards JS, Meredith RL, Nepomuceno C et al 1980 Psycho-social aspects of chronic pain in spinal cord injury. Pain 8: 355–366
Richardson DE 1995 Deep brain stimulation for the relief of chronic pain. Neurosurgery Clinics 6: 135–143
Richardson RR, Meyer PR, Cerullo LJ 1980 Neurostimulation in the modulation of intractable paraplegic and traumatic neuroma pains. Pain 8: 75–84
Rose M, Robinson JE, Ells P et al 1988 Pain following spinal cord injury: results from a postal survey. Pain 34: 101–102
Rossier AB, Foo D, Shillito J et al 1985 Posttraumatic cervical syringomyelia. Incidence, clinical presentation,

electrophysiological studies, syrinx protein and results of conservative and operative treatment. Brain 108: 439–461
Sampson JH, Cashman RE, Nashold BS, Friedman AH 1995 Dorsal root entry zone lesions for intractable pain after trauma to the conus medullaris and cauda equina. Journal of Neurosurgery 82: 28–34
Sanford PR, Lindblom LB, Haddox JD 1992 Amitriptyline and carbamazepine in the treatment of dysesthesia pain in spinal cord injury. Archives of Physical Medicine and Rehabilitation 73: 300–301
Siddall PJ, Loeser JD 2001 Pain following spinal cord injury. Spinal Cord 39: 63–73
Siddall PJ, McClelland J 1999 Non-painful sensory phenomena after spinal cord injury. Journal of Neurology, Neurosurgery and Psychiatry 66: 617–622
Siddall PJ, Taylor DA, Cousins MJ 1997 Classification of pain following spinal cord injury. Spinal Cord 35: 69–75
Siddall PJ, Taylor DA, McClelland J, Rutkowski SB, Cousins MJ 1999 Pain report and the relationship of pain to physical factors in the first 6 months following spinal cord injury. Pain 81: 187–197
Sie IH, Waters RL, Adkins RH et al 1992 Upper extremity pain in the postrehabilitation spinal cord injured patient. Archives of Physical Medicine and Rehabilitation 73: 44–48
Silfverskiold J, Waters RL 1991 Shoulder pain and functional disability in spinal cord injury patients. Clinical Orthopedics and Related Research 272: 141–145
Simpson BA 1999 Spinal cord and brain stimulation. In: Wall PD, Melzack R (eds) Textbook of pain, 4th edn. Churchill Livingstone, Edinburgh, pp 1353–1381
Sindou M, Mertens P, Wael M 2001 Microsurgical DREZotomy for pain due to spinal cord and/or cauda equina injuries: long-term results in a series of 44 patients. Pain 92: 159–171
Stormer S, Gerner HJ, Gruninger W et al 1997 Chronic pain/dysaesthesiae in spinal cord injury patients: results of a multicentre study. Spinal Cord 35: 446–455
Summers JD, Rapoff MA, Verghese G et al 1991 Psychosocial factors in chronic spinal cord injury pain. Pain 47: 183–189
Sved P, Siddall PJ, McClelland J, Cousins MJ 1997 Relationship between surgery and pain following spinal cord injury. Spinal Cord 35: 526–530
Sweet WH 1975 Phantom sensations following intraspinal injury. Neurochirurgia 18: 139–154
Triggs W, Berić A 1992 Sensory abnormalities and dysaesthesia in the anterior spinal artery syndrome. Brain 115: 189–198
Umlauf RL 1992 Psychological interventions for chronic pain following spinal cord injury. Clinical Journal of Pain 8: 111–118
Vernon JD, Silver JR, Ohry A 1982 Post-traumatic syringomyelia. Paraplegia 20: 339–364
Vernon JD, Chir B, Silver JR et al 1983 Post-traumatic syringomyelia: the results of surgery. Paraplegia 21: 37–46
Wainapel SF 1984 Reflex sympathetic dystrophy following traumatic myelopathy. Pain 18: 345–349
Wang D, Bodley R, Sett P, Gardner B, Frankel H 1996 A clinical magnetic resonance imaging study of the traumatised spinal cord more than 20 years following injury. Paraplegia 34: 65–81
Waring WP, Maynard FM 1991 Shoulder pain in acute traumatic quadriplegia. Paraplegia 29: 37–42
Wegener ST, Elliott TR 1992 Pain assessment in spinal cord injury. Clinical Journal of Pain 8: 93–101
Williams B, Terry AF, Jones F et al 1981 Syringomyelia as a sequel to traumatic paraplegia. Paraplegia 19: 67–80
Winkelmuller M, Winkelmuller W 1996 Long-term effects of continuous intrathecal opioid treatment in chronic pain of nonmalignant etiology. Journal of Neurosurgery 85: 458–467
Woodward KG, Vulpe M 1991 The proximal tap or 'central Tinel' sign in central dysesthetic syndrome after spinal cord injury. Journal of the American Paraplegia Society 14: 136–138

Section 2

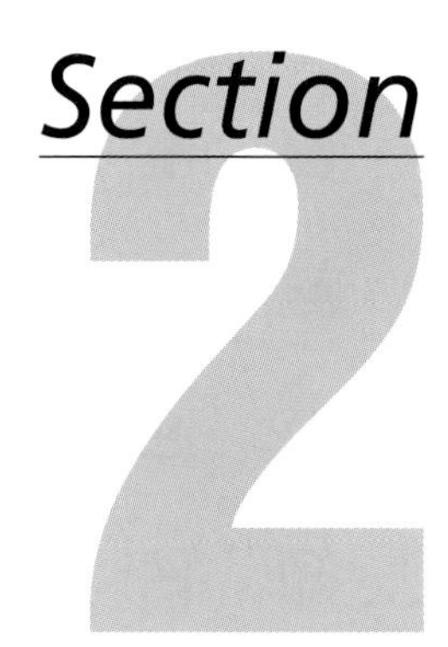

Therapeutic approaches

Pharmacology

Surgery

Physical therapies

Psychological therapies

Chapter 22

Antipyretic analgesics

Kay Brune and Hanns Ulrich Zeilhofer

Introduction

Fever was the cardinal symptom of disease in Hippocratic medicine. It was assumed to result from an imbalance of body fluids. Therefore it was the aim of Hippocratic medicine to correct the balances of fluids by either bloodletting, purging, sweating, or applying drugs to normalize body temperature. The leading compound for that purpose in the eighteenth and nineteenth centuries was quinine. The emerging drug industry concentrated on producing substances with similar antipyretic activity. These efforts led to the three prototypes of antipyretic non-narcotic analgesics: acetanilide (paracetamol, acetaminophen), antipyrine, and salicylic acid. They are still in use and consumed in millions of daily doses (for details see Brune 1997).

For more than a hundred years little was known about the mode of action of these compounds. Accumulating experimental and clinical findings within the past thirty years have now led to a coherent pharmacological picture, explaining most of the desired effects and also most of the side effects of these analgesics. Most effects are related to the blockade of prostaglandin production (Vane 1971). However, this simple monocausal explanation cannot reconcile all experimental findings (for review see McCormack and Brune 1991, Brune and McCormack 1994). For example, salicylic acid and paracetamol (acetaminophen) produce no inhibition of prostaglandin production in inflamed tissue at therapeutic concentrations.

The mode of action

Biodistribution of antipyretic analgesics—desired effects

The discovery of the inhibition of prostaglandin synthesis left the question unresolved as to why aspirin and its pharmacological relatives, the (acidic) non-steroidal anti-inflammatory drugs (NSAIDs, see Table 22.1), exert anti-inflammatory and analgesic effects while the non-acidic drugs, phenazone and acetaminophen, are analgesic only (Graf et al 1975). All acidic anti-inflammatory analgesics are highly bound to plasma proteins and show a similar degree of acidity (pK_a values between 3.5 and 5.5). Due to high protein binding and an open endothelial layer of the vasculature they achieve high concentrations in the liver, spleen, and bone marrow (Fig. 22.1), but also in body compartments with an acidic extracellular environment (Brune et al 1976), i.e., inflamed tissue, the wall of the upper GI tract, and the collecting ducts of the

Table 22.1 Acidic antipyretic analgesics (anti-inflammatory antipyretic analgesics, NSAIDs): chemical classes, structures, physico-chemical and pharmacological data, therapeutic dosage

Chemical/pharmacokinetic subclasses	Structure (prototype) Lipophil Hydrophil	pK_a (binding to plasma proteins)	t_{max}[a] time to peak plasma concentration	$t_{1/2}$[b] elimination half-life	Oral bioavailability (%)	Single dose (range) daily dose (max)
a) Low potency/fast elimination:	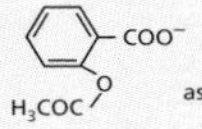 aspirin					
Salicylates:						
Aspirin[a]		3.5 (>80%)	~0.25 h[c]	~20 min[c]	20–70%	(0.05–0.1 g) ~6 g[b]
Salicylic acid	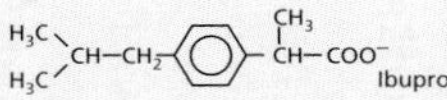 Ibuprofen	2.9 (>90%)	(0.5–2 h)[d]	2.5–7 h[e]	80–100%	(0.5–1 g) 6 g
Arylpropionic acids:						
Ibuprofen		4.4 (99%)	0.5–2 h	2–4 h	80–100%	(0.2–0.4) 3.2 g
Anthranilic acids:	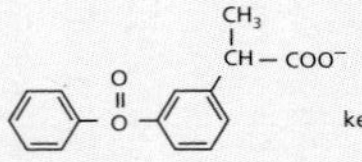 ketoprofen					
Mefenamic acid		4.2 (>90%)	2–4 h	1–2 h		(0.25–0.5) 1.25 g
b) High potency/fast elimination:						
Arylpropionic acids:	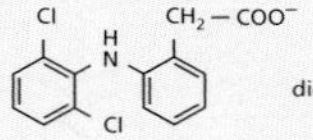 didofenac					
Flurbiprofen						
Ketoprofen		4.2 (99%)	0.5–2 h	1.1–4 h	~90%	(15–100 mg) 300 mg
Arylacetic acids:						
Diclofenac	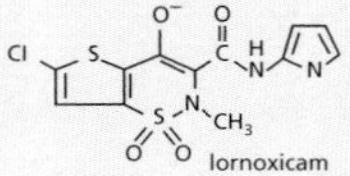 lornoxicam	4 (99%)	0.5–24 h[f]	1–2 h	30–80%[e]	(25–75 mg) 200 mg
Indomethacin		4.5 (99%)	0.5–2 h	2.6–(1.2) h[g]	90–100%	(25–75 mg) 200 mg
Ketorolac						
Oxicam:						
Lornoxicam		4.9 (99%)	0.5–2 h	4–10 h	~100%	(4–12 mg) 16 mg
c) Intermediate potency/ intermediate elimination speed:	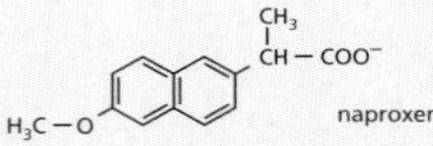 naproxen					
Salicylates:						
Diflunisal	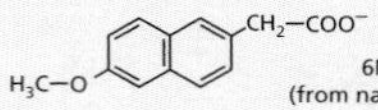 6MNA (from nabumetone)	3.8 (98–99%)	2–3 h	8–12 h	80–100%	(250–500 mg) 1 g
Arylpropionic acids:						
Naproxen		4.15 (99%)	2–4 h	13–15 h[g]	~95%	(0.5–1 g) 2 g
Arylacetic acids:						
6 MNA (from Nabumetone)[3]	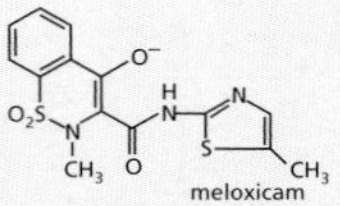 meloxicam	4.2	3–6 h	20–24 h	20–50 h	(0.5–1 g) 1.5 g
d) High potency/slow elimination						
Oxicams:						
Meloxicam	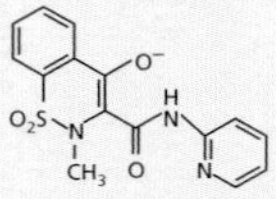 piroxicam	5.1 (>99%)	3–5 h	14–160 h[g]	~100%	(20–40 mg) initially: 40 mg
Piroxicam						
Tenoxicam		5.0 (>99%)	3–5 h	25–175 h[g]	~100%	(20-40 mg) initially: 40 mg

[a]Time to reach maximum plasma concentration after oral administration.
[b]Terminal half-life of elimination.
[c]Of aspirin the prodrug of salicylic acid.
[d]Depending on galenic formulation.
[e]Dose dependent.
[f]Monolithic acid resistant tablet or similar form.
[g]EHC, enterohepatic circulation.
Most data from Herzfeld and Kümmel (1983), Verbeck et al. (1983), Brune and Lanz (1985).

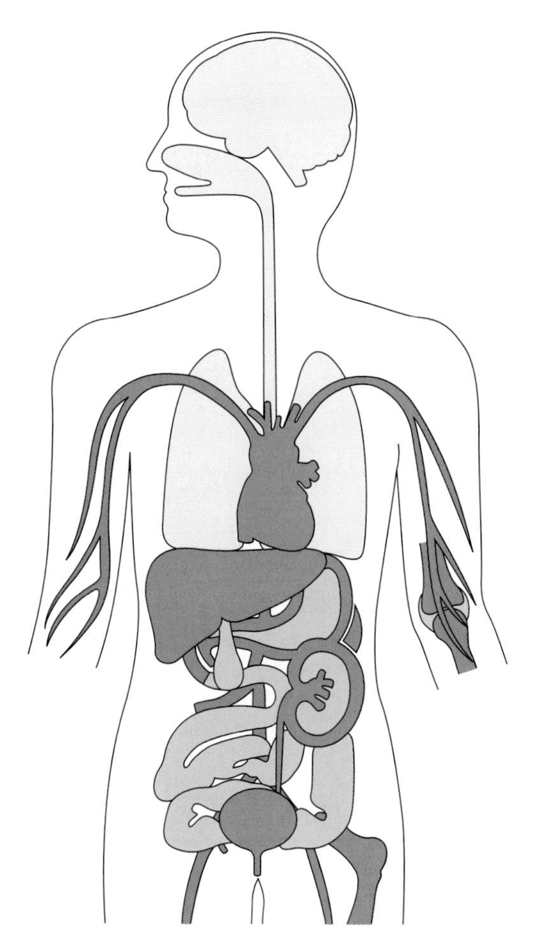

Fig. 22.1 Schematic representation of the distribution of acidic antipyretic analgesics in the human body (transposition of the data from animal experiments to human conditions). Dark areas indicate high concentrations of the acidic antipyretic analgesics, i.e., stomach and upper GI tract wall, blood, liver, bone marrow, and spleen (not shown) inflamed tissue (e.g., joints) as well as the kidney (cortex > medulla). Some acidic antipyretic analgesics are excreted in part unchanged in urine and achieve high concentration in this body fluid; others encounter enterohepatic circulation and are found in high concentrations as conjugates in the bile.

kidneys. By contrast (Fig. 22.1), acetaminophen and phenazone, compounds with neutral pK_a values and scarcely bound to plasma proteins, distribute almost homogeneously throughout the body (Brune et al 1980).

Biodistribution of antipyretic analgesics—side effects

Unequal drug distribution with accumulation in selective body compartments (NSAIDs) should lead to an almost complete inhibition of local cyclooxygenases. These observations and contentions explained the fact that only the acidic, antipyretic analgesics (NSAIDs) are anti-inflammatory and cause acute side effects in the GI tract (ulcerations), blood stream (inhibition of platelet aggregation), and the kidney (fluid and potassium retention), while the non-acidic drugs, e.g., phenazone (Table 22.2), should be devoid of both the anti-inflammatory activity and the gastric and the (acute) renal toxicity. Chronic inflammation of the upper respiratory tract as in asthma may lead to accumulation of NSAIDs in the mucosa. So-called 'aspirin asthma' in asthmatics comprises a well-defined risk (Hoigné and Szczeklik 1992).

Different cyclooxygenases

In 1991, molecular biologists discovered that two different genes code for cyclooxygenases (COX1 and COX2, Fig. 22.2). They were cloned, sequenced, expressed, and characterized (Kujubu et al 1991, O'Banion et al 1991). Selective inhibitors of either enzyme became available recently (Masferrer et al 1994, Patrignani et al 1994, Riendeau et al 1997, Tegeder et al 1999). The enzymes form a hydrophobic groove or channel opening through the membrane. The substrate (arachidonic acid) or an inhibitor inserts into this groove. Interestingly, the COX2 protein displays a slightly roomier channel than COX1, which makes a selective inhibition of COX2 possible (Kurumball et al 1996).

Both enzymes are differentially distributed throughout the body, regulated differently, and probably also serve different functions in health and disease (Vane 1994, Lipsky 1997). Summarizing these observations one may conclude that COX1 is constitutively present in most tissues. It appears to produce constant amounts of eicosanoids (prostaglandins and related substances), maintaining physiological homeostasis in many organs, e.g., the stomach, lung, kidney, and others. COX2 is expressed in macrophages and other cells of inflamed tissue (Harris et al 1994, Seibert et al 1994, Beiche et al 1996). The expression of this enzyme is suppressed by glucocorticoids (Masferrer et al 1992, Yamagata et al 1993). In some organs, COX2 appears to be expressed constitutively, e.g., in the central nervous system (Marcheselli and Bazan 1996, Maihöfner et al 2001) and the urogenital tract (Brater et al 2001). In other organs (e.g., the female genital tract) the activity of both COX1 and COX2 appears to be regulated by sex-steroids. From those results the concept arose that a selective inhibition of COX2

Table 22.2 Nonacidic antipyretic analgesics: chemical classes, structures, pharmacokinetic data, therapeutic dosage

Chemical/pharmacological class monosubstance	Structure	Fraction bound to plasma proteins	t_{max}[a]	$t_{1/2}$[b]	Oral bioavailability	Daily dose (single dose) in adults
Aniline derivative Paracetamol (acetaminophen)	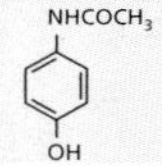 paracetamol	5–50% dose dependent	0.5–1.5 h	1.5–2.5 h	70–100%	1–6 g (0.5–1 g)
Phenazon derivatives (Pyrazolinone[c]) Phenazone (antipyrine)	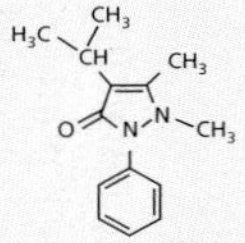 phenazone	<10%	0.5–2 h	5–24 h	~100%	1–6 g (0.5–2 g)
Propyphenazone (isopropylantipyrine)		~10%	0.5–1.5 h	1–2.5 h	~100%	1–6 g (0.5–1 g)
Metamizole-Na (dipyrone-Na)[d]	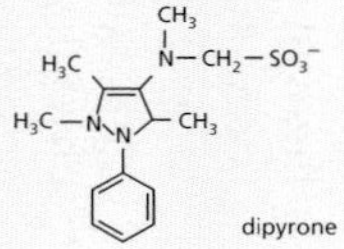 dipyrone	<20%	—	—	—	1–6 g (0.5–2 g)
4-MAP[e]		~50%	1–2 h	2–4 h	~100%	—
4-AP[f] (active metabolites)		~50%		4–5.5 h		—
Selective COX-inhibitors[g] Celecoxib (Celebrex)	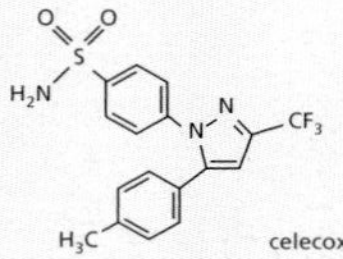 celecoxib	>90%	2–4 h	9–15 h	~100%	(40–200 mg) 400 mg
Rofecoxib (Vioxx)	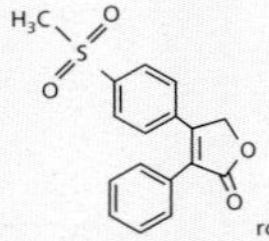 rofecoxib	~90%	2–4 h	~12 h	~100%	(12.5–25 mg) 50 mg

[a]Time to reach maximum plasma concentration after oral administration.
[b]Terminal half-life of elimination, dependent on liver function with phenazone.
[c]Terms like pyrazole and, incorrectly, pyrazolone are also in use.
[d]Noraminopyrinemethanosulfonate-Na.
[e]4-MAP, 4-methylaminophenazone.
[f]4-AP, 4-aminophenazone.
[g]Other antipyretic analgesics (exception: acetaminophen) block both COXs at therapeutic concentrations.

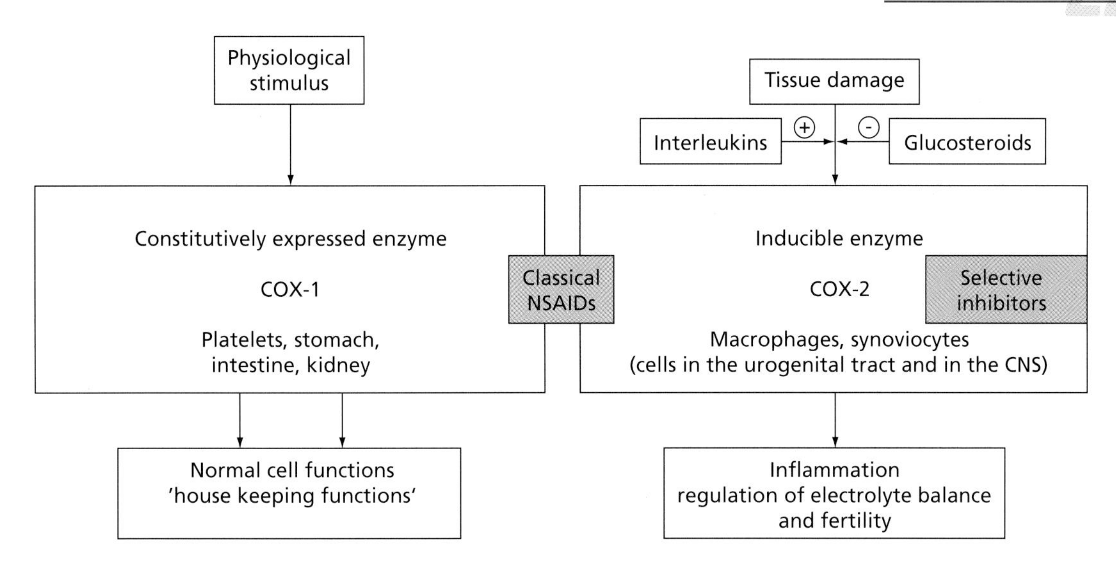

Fig. 22.2 Simplified description of the physiological and pathophysiological roles of COX1 and COX2. COX1 is expressed constitutively in most tissues and fulfils housekeeping functions by producing prostaglandins. COX2 is an inducible isoenzyme, which becomes expressed in inflammatory cells (e.g., macrophages and synoviocytes) after exposure to pro-inflammatory cytokines, and is down-regulated by glucocorticoids. In the kidney (*macula densa*) and other areas of the urogenital tract and in the CNS COX2 is already significantly expressed even in the absence of inflammation. The induction beyond baseline levels of COX2 in the peripheral nervous system and in the spinal cord appears to be most prominent in connection with inflammatory painful reactions. Both enzymes are blocked by classical acidic antipyretic analgesics (NSAIDs).

may be sufficient to achieve analgesic/anti-inflammatory effects but would spare the GI tract and most organ systems.

Animals lacking cyclooxygenases

Following the discovery of the COX genes, mice that were deficient in either enzyme (COX1 or COX2), so-called knockout mice, were generated. It was also possible to create double knockout cells (the corresponding animals did not survive outside the uterus): COX1 knockout mice show no major functional deficits. They show nociceptive reflexes and fever as well as inflammation. Interestingly, they get ulcers when treated with NSAIDs (Langenbach et al 1995). COX2 knockout mice are born with renal impairment; many die after birth due to an open ductus arteriosus Botalli (Lim et al 1997). Their nociceptive reflexes are impaired and they do not develop fever (Dinchuck et al 1995, Morham et al 1995, Morham, personal communication, 1998). Inflammatory responses are possible.

The possibility of blocking COX2 specifically has led to new drugs, which are currently in wide clinical use (see Table 22.2). They have definitely been shown to exert analgesic effects (Lane 1997), have less gastrointestinal toxicity, but impair renal function.

Prostaglandins in the generation of hyperalgesia

The antinociceptive (analgesic) action of antipyretic analgesics is due to inhibition of the production of prostaglandins at the site of inflammation and in the CNS. It has been believed for many years that inhibition at the site of an inflammation was the main mechanism. Prostaglandins sensitize certain primary afferent nerve fibres, so-called silent nociceptors, thereby causing primary hyperalgesia. Established molecular targets of prostaglandins in this process include, e.g., tetrodotoxin-resistant Na^+ channels.

Recently, it became apparent that prostaglandins produced in the spinal cord dorsal horn in response to peripheral inflammation contribute to the generation of so-called secondary hyperalgesia and allodynia. The underlying molecular mechanisms include a direct activation of deep dorsal horn neurons (Baba et al 2001) and a reduction in inhibitory glycinergic neurotransmission in the superficial layers of the dorsal horn (Ahmadi et al 2002).

Acidic antipyretic analgesics in clinical use

Aspirin at high doses (> 3 g/day) inhibits fever and pain, but also inflammation, i.e., swelling, redness, and warming. Within the past forty years many compounds with similar activity have been discovered (Table 22.1).

All these successors differ in two characteristics: the first is their potency, which ranges between a few milligrams (lornoxicam) and about 0.8 g (e.g., ibuprofen) as a single dose. The second is their pharmacokinetic characteristics, i.e., the speed of absorption (time to peak, t_{max}, which is influenced by the galenic formulation), the maximal plasma concentrations (c_{max}), the elimination halflife ($t_{1/2}$), and the oral bioavailability (AUC_{rel}). Interestingly, all these widely used drugs lack a relevant degree of COX2-selectivity, in other words, an inhibiton of COX2 at concentrations (doses) that do not block COX1. The key characteristics of the most important NSAIDs are compiled in Table 22.1.

This table also contains data on aspirin, which differs in many respects from the other NSAIDs. Otherwise the drugs can be categorized into four different groups:

a. NSAIDs with low potency and short elimination halflife
b. NSAIDs with high potency and short elimination halflife
c. NSAIDs with intermediate potency and elimination halflife
d. NSAIDs with high potency and long elimination halflife.

These differences have some bearing on the optimal clinical use (see Table 22.3).

NSAIDs with low potency and short elimination half-life

The prototype of a type (a) compound is ibuprofen. Depending on the galenic formulation, fast (salt) or slow absorption (encapsulated) may be achieved (Laska et al 1986, Geisslinger et al 1993). The bioavailability of ibuprofen is complete; the elimination is always fast even in patients with severe impairment of the liver or kidney function (Brune and Lanz 1985). Ibuprofen is used in single doses between 200 mg and 0.8 g. A maximum dose of 3.2 g per day (United States) or 2.4 g (Europe) for rheumatoid arthritis is possible. Ibuprofen (at low doses) appears particularly useful for treatment of acute inflammatory pain. It may also be used in chronic rheumatic diseases (high doses). At high doses the toxicity increases (Kaufman et al 1993). Ibuprofen is also used as a pure S-enantiomer. This enantiomer is a (direct) COX-inhibitor. The R-enantiomer, comprising 50% of the usual racemic mixture, is converted to the S-enantiomer in the human body (Rudy et al 1991). It has not been proven whether the use of the pure S-enantiomer offers any benefit (Mayer and Testa 1997). Other drugs of this group are salicylates and fenamates. The latter do not offer advantages. Salicylates and fenamates are more toxic than ibuprofen at overdosage (CNS).

NSAIDS with high potency and short elimination half-life

The drugs of group (b) are standard in the therapy of rheumatic (arthrotic) pain. The most widely used compound is diclofenac, which is less active on COX1 than on COX2 (Tegeder et al 1999). This is taken as a reason for the low incidence of gastrointestinal side effects (Henry et al 1996). The limitations of diclofenac result from the usual galenic formulation consisting of a monolythic acid-resistant encapsulation. This may cause retarded absorption of the active ingredient, due to retention of the tablet in the stomach (Brune and Lanz 1985). Moreover, diclofenac encounters first-pass metabolism, which limits oral bioavailability (about 50%). The lack of therapeutic effects may require adaptation of dosage or change of the drug. The higher incidents of liver toxicity with diclofenac may result from first-pass metabolization. Group (b) contains important drugs such as flubiprofen, indometacin, and ketoprofen. All of them show high oral bioavailability and good effectiveness but also unwanted drug effects (see Henry et al 1996).

NSAIDs with intermediate potency and intermediate elimination half-life

The third group (c) is intermediate in potency and speed of elimination. Some forms of migraine and menstrual cramps appear as adequate indications for diflunisal and, a drug that has been better investigated, naproxen.

NSAIDs with high potency and intermediate elimination half-life

The fourth group (d) consists of the oxicams (meloxicam, piroxicam, and tenoxicam). These compounds owe their slow elimination to slow

Table 22.3 Indications for antipyretic analgesics

Acidic antipyretic analgesics (antiinflammatory antipyretic analgesics, NSAIDs)[a]			
Acute and chronic pain, produced by inflammation of different etiology:	**High dose**	**Middle dose**	**Low dose**
Arthritis: chronic polyarthritis (rheumatoid arthritis ankylosing spondylitis (Morbus Bechterew) acute gout (gout attack)	Diclofenac, indometacin ibuprofen, piroxicam (phenylbutazone)[b]	Diclofenac, indometacin, ibuprofen, piroxicam (phenylbutazone)[b]	No
Cancer pain (e.g., bone metastasis)	(Indometacin[c]) diclofenac[c], ibuprofen[c], piroxicam[c]	(Indometacin[c]) diclofenac[c], ibuprofen[c], piroxicam[c]	Acetylsalicylic acid[d], ibuprofen[c]
Active arthrosis (acute pain-inflammatory analgesics are often prescribed but of limited value)	No	Diclofenac, indomethacin, ibuprofen	Ibuprofen, ketoprofen
Posttraumatic pain, swelling	No	(Indomethacin) diclofenac, ibuprofen	Acetylsalicylic acid, ibuprofen[c]
Postoperative pain, swelling	No	(Indometacin) diclofenac, ibuprofen	Ibuprofen
Non-acidic antipyretic analgesics			
Acute pain and fever	**Pyrazolinones (High dose)**	**Pyrazolinones (Low dose)**	**Anilines (High dose is toxic)**
Spastic pain (colics)	Yes	Yes	No
Conditions associated with high fever	Yes	Yes	No
Cancer pain	Yes	Yes	Yes
Headache, migraine	No	Yes	Yes[f]
General disturbances associated with viral infections	No	Yes[e]	Yes

[a]Dosage range of NSAIDs and example of monosubstances (but note dosage prescribed for each agent).
[b]Indicated only in gout attacks.
[c]Compare the sequence staged scheme of WHO for cancer pain.
[d]Blood coagulation and renal function must be normal.
[e]If other analgesics and antipyretics are contraindicated,e .g., gastroduodenal ulcer, blood coagulation disturbances, asthma.
[f]In particular patients.

metabolization together with a high degree of enterohepatic circulation (Brune and Lanz 1985, Schmid et al 1995). The long half-life (days) does not make these oxicam drugs of first choice for acute pain of (probably) short duration. Their main indication is inflammatory pain likely to persist for days, i.e., pain resulting from chronic polyarthritis or even cancer (bone metastases). The high potency and long persistence in the body may be the reason for the higher incidence of serious adverse effects in the gastrointestinal tract and the kidney (see Henry et al 1996).

Compounds of special interest

A few compounds deserve special discussion. Aspirin actually comprises two compounds: acetic acid, which is released before, during, and after absorption, and salicylic acid. Acetylsalicylic acid is about a hundred times more potent as an inhibitor of cyclooxygenases than salicylic acid, which is devoid of this effect at analgesic doses. The acetate released from aspirin acetylates a serine residue in the active centre(s) of COX1 and -2. Consequently, aspirin inactivates both cyclooxygenases permanently. Most cells compensate for the enzyme inactivation by the production of a new enzyme with the exception of platelets. A single dose of aspirin blocks the platelet COX1 and thromboxane synthesis for many days. When low doses are applied, aspirin acetylates the COX1 of platelets passing through the capillary bed of the gastrointestinal tract but not the cyclooxygenase of endothelial cells (prostacyclin synthetase) outside the abdomen. This is due to the rapid cleavage of aspirin leaving little if any unmetabolized aspirin after primary liver passage. Low-dose aspirin has its only indication in the prevention of thrombotic and embolic events. It may cause bleeding from existing ulcers and topical irritation of the gastrointestinal mucosa. Aspirin may have to be added to COX2 selective inhibitors when given to patients at cardiovascular risk (see Silverstein et al 2000).

Aspirin may be used as solution (effervescent) or as salt for very fast absorption, distribution, and pain relief. The inevitable irritation of the gastric mucosa may be acceptable in otherwise healthy patients. The old claim that aspirin is less toxic than salicylic acid to the GI tract is not based on scientific evidence. Aspirin should not be used in pregnant women (bleeding, closure of ductus arteriosus) or children before puberty (Reye's syndrome).

It has been claimed that nabumeton, etodolac, and meloxicam are particularly well tolerated by the GI tract because they inhibit predominantly COX2. These results are not generally accepted. The active metabolite of nabumeton shows no selectivity for COX2, and the selectivity of etodolac and meloxicam is not superior to that of diclofenac, when tested ex vivo in humans (Patrignani et al 1994, Riendeau et al 1997).

Two COX2 selective inhibitors are listed in Table 22.2. Their pharmacokinetic characteristics (slow absorption, slow elimination) make them poor candidates for acute pain of short duration. They have, however, both been shown to work in osteoarthritis pain (Lane 1997). As in all non acidic compounds, but also in line with the COX2 concept, these compounds are comparable to placebo with respect to GI toxicity. They interfere with water and salt excretion by the kidneys as standard drugs do. In addition, theoretical considerations and experimental (Fitzgerald et al 2000) and clinical evidence (Bombardier et al 2000) suggests that these compounds may increase the risk of cardiovascular events (CI) in patients at risk.

Non-acidic antipyretic analgesics

Aniline derivatives

The most widely used drug of this group, acetaminophen, was discovered at the same time as aspirin. The pharmacokinetic and pharmacodynamic data are compiled in Table 22.2. Acetaminophen is a very weak possibly indirect inhibitor of cyclooxygenases. Evidence that acetaminophen, which is clearly antipyretic and (weakly) analgesic, is indeed working through cyclooxygenase inhibition comes from COX2 knockout mice, which do not develop fever (Morham, personal communication). Induction of fever is clearly blocked by acetaminophen in several species. The major advantage of acetaminophen consists in its relative lack of (serious) side effects provided that the dose limits (approximately 1 g/10 kg body weight per day) are obeyed; yet serious liver toxicity was observed with lower doses in a few cases (Bridger et al 1998). Acetaminophen is metabolized to highly toxic nucleophilic benzoquinones, which bind covalently to DNA and structural proteins in parenchymal cells in the liver and kidney, where these reactive intermediates are produced (for review see Seeff et al 1986). The consequence often is fatal liver necrosis. At early detection overdosage can be remedied by administration of *N*-acetylcysteine or glutathion (Fig. 22.3). The predominant indication of paracetamol is fever and mild forms of pain, e.g., caused by viral infections. Many patients with recurrent headache also benefit from acetaminophen and its low toxicity. Acetaminophen is also used in children. Lethal overdosage is not uncommon.

Acetaminophen is often used in combination with aspirin and caffeine (Laska et al 1984). To what extent this combination is more potent in causing so-called analgesic nephropathy is unclear (Porter 1996). Such combinations are more frequently abused than single-entity analgesics. The reasons appear uncertain (Elseviers and DeBroe 1996). Acetanilide and phenacetine, the precursors of acetaminophen, have been banned because of their high toxicity. Acetaminophen should not be given to patients with seriously impaired liver function.

Phenazone and its derivatives

Following the discovery of phenazone 120 years ago the drug industry has tried to improve this compound in three aspects. It was chemically modified to obtain: (a) a more potent compound, (b) a water-soluble derivative to be given parenterally, and (c) to find a compound that is eliminated faster and more reliably than phenazone. The best known results of these attempts are aminophenazone, dipyrone, and propyphenazone (Table 22.3). Aminophenazone is not in use anymore. The other two compounds differ from phenazone in their potency and elimination half-life (Levy et al 1995), their water solubility (dipyrone is a water soluble prodrug of methylaminophenazone), and their general toxicity (propyphenazone and dipyrone do not produce nitrosamines in the acidic environment of the stomach).

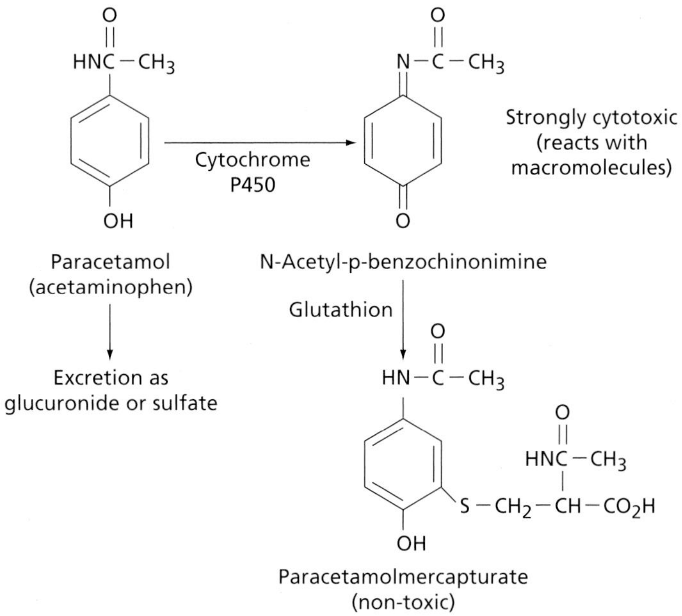

Cytochrome P450

Strongly cytotoxic (reacts with macromolecules)

Paracetamol (acetaminophen)

N-Acetyl-p-benzochinonimine

Glutathion

Excretion as glucuronide or sulfate

Paracetamolmercapturate (non-toxic)

Fig. 22.3 Schematic diagram of the metabolism of paracetamol (acetaminophen). At therapeutic doses most of the paracetamol (acetaminophen) is metabolized in the liver in a phase II reaction and excreted as glucuronide or sulfate. At higher doses the responsible enzymes become saturated and paracetamol is metabolized in the liver via a P450-dependent mechanism, which leads to the formation of *N*-acetyl-p-benzoquinoneimine, a highly cell toxic metabolite. This metabolite can initially be detoxified via a glutathion-dependent step to paracetamolmercapturate. At doses beyond 100 mg/kg glutathion become exhausted and *N*-acetyl-p-benzoquinoneimine now reacts with macromolecules in hepatocytes, leading to cell death and acute liver failure.

Phenazone, propyphenazone, and dipyrone are used in many countries worldwide as prevailing antipyretic analgesics (Latin America, many countries in Asia, Eastern Europe, and Central Europe). Dipyrone has been accused of causing agranulocytosis. Although there appears to be a statistically significant link, the incidence is rare (1 case per million treatment periods) (International Agranulocytosis and Aplastic Anemia Study 1986, Kaufman et al 1991).

All antipyretic analgesics have also been claimed to cause Stevens–Johnson's syndrome and Lyell's syndrome and shock reactions. New data indicate that the incidence of these events is in the same order of magnitude as with, e.g., penicillins (Roujeau et al 1995, Mockenhaupt et al 1996, International Collaborative Study of Severe Anaphylaxis 1998). All non-acidic phenazone derivatives lack anti-inflammatory activity and are devoid of gastrointestinal and (acute) renal toxicity. Dipyrone is safe at overdosage in contrast to paracetamol (Wolhoff et al 1983).

References

Ahmadi S, Lippross S, Neuhuber WL, Zeilhofer HU 2002 PGE_2 selectively blocks inhibitory glycinergic neurotransmission onto rat superficial dorsal horn neurons. Nature Neuroscience 5: 34–40

Baba H, Kohno T, Moore KA, Woolf CJ 2001 Direct activation of rat spinal dorsal horn neurons by prostaglandin E_2. Journal of Neuroscience 21: 1750–1756

Beiche F, Scheuerer S, Brune K, Geisslinger G, Goppelt-Struebe M 1996 Upregulation of cyclooxygenase-2 mRNA in the rat spinal cord following peripheral inflammation. FEBS Letters 390: 165–169

Bombardier C, Laine L, Reicin A, Shapiro D, Burgos-Vargas R, Davis B, Day R, Ferraz MB, Hawkey CJ, Hochberg MC, Kvien TK, Schnitzer TJ 2000 Comparison of upper gastrointestinal toxicity of rofecoxib and naproxen in patients with rheumatoid arthritis. VIGOR Study Group. New England Journal of Medicine 343: 1520–1528, 2 p following 1528

Brater DC, Harris C, Redfern JS, Gertz BJ 2001 Renal effects of Cox-2-selective inhibitors. American Journal of Nephrology 21: 1–15

Bridger S, Henderson K, Glucksman E, Ellis AJ, Henry JA, Williams R 1998 Deaths from low dose paracetamol poisoning. American Medical Journal 316: 1724–1725

Brune K 1997 The early history of non-opioid analgesics. Acute Pain 1: 33–40

Brune K, Lanz R 1985 Pharmacokinetics of non-steroidal anti-inflammatory drugs. In: Bonta I L, Bray M A, Parnham M J (eds) Handbook of inflammation, vol 5, The pharmacology of inflammation. Elsevier, Amsterdam, pp 413–449

Brune K, McCormack K 1994 The over-the-counter use of nonsteroidal anti-inflammatory drugs and other antipyretic analgesics. In: Lewis AJ, Furst DE (eds) Nonsteroidal anti-inflammatory drugs: mechanisms and clinical uses, 2nd ed. Marcel Dekker, New York, pp 97–126

Brune K, Glatt M, Graf P 1976 Mechanism of action of anti-inflammatory drugs. General Pharmacology 7: 27–33

Brune K, Rainsford K D, Schweitzer A 1980 Biodistribution of mild analgesics. British Journal of Clinical Pharmacology 10 (suppl 2): 279–284

Dinchuk JE, Car BD, Focht RJ, Johnston JJ, Jaffee BD, Covinton MB, Contel NR, Eng VM, Collins RJ, Czerniak PM, Gorry SA, Trzaskos JM 1995 Renal abnormalities and an altered inflammatory response in mice lacking cyclooxygenase II. Nature 378: 406–409

Elseviers MM, De Broe ME 1996 Combination analgesic involvement in the pathogenesis of analgesic nephropathy: the European perspective. American Journal of Kidney Diseases 28 (suppl 1): 48–55

Fitzgerald GA, Austin S, Egan K, Cheng Y, Pratico D 2000 Cyclo-oxygenase products and atherothrombosis. Annals of Medicine 32 (suppl 1): 21–26

Geisslinger G, Menzel S, Wissel K, Brune K 1993 Single dose pharmacokinetics of different formulations of ibuprofen and aspirin. Drug Investigation 5: 238–242

Graf P, Glatt M, Brune K 1975 Acidic nonsteroid anti-inflammatory drugs accumulating in inflamed tissue. Experientia 31: 951–954

Harris RC, McKanna JA, Aiai Y, Jacobson HR, DuBois RN, Breyer MD 1994 Cyclooxygenase-2 is associated with the macula densa of rat kidney and increases with salt restriction. Journal of Clinical Investigation 94: 2504–2510

Henry D, Lim LL, Garcia Rodriguez LA, Perez Gutthann S, Carson JL, Griffin M, Savage R, Logan R, Moride Y, Hawkey C, Hill S, Fries JT 1996 Variability in risk of gastrointestinal complications with individual non-steroidal anti-inflammatory drugs: results of a collaborative meta-analysis. British Medical Journal 312: 1563–1566

Herzfeldt CD, Kümmel R 1983 Dissociation constants, solubilities and dissolution rates of some selected nonsteroidal anti-inflammatories. Drug Development and Industrial Pharmacy 9: 767–793

Hoigné RV, Szczeklik A 1992 Allergic and pseudoallergic reactions associated with nonsteroidal anti-inflammatory drugs. In: Borda IT, Koff RS (eds), NSAIDs: a profile of adverse effects. Hanley & Belfus, Philadelphia and Mosby-Yearbook, St Louis, pp 57–184

International Agranulocytosis and Aplastic Anemia Study 1986 Risks of agranulocytosis and aplastic anemia: a first report of their relation to drug use with special reference to analgesics. Journal of the American Medical Association 256: 1749–1757

International Collaborative Study of Severe Anaphylaxis 1998 Epidemiology 9: 141–146

Kaufman DW, Kelly JP, Levy M, Shapiro S 1991 The drug etiology of agranulocytosis and aplastic anemia. Monographs in Epidemiology and Biostatistics 18. Oxford University Press, Oxford

Kaufman DW, Kelly JP, Sheehan JE, Laszlo A, Wiholm B-E, Alfredsson L, Koff RS, Shapiro S 1993 Nonsteroidal anti-inflammatory drug use in relation to major upper gastrointestinal bleeding. Clinical Pharmacology and Therapeutics 53: 485–494

Kujubu DA, Fletcher BS, Varnum BC, Lim RW, Herschman HR 1991 TIS 10, a phorbol ester tumor promoter-inducible mRNA from Swiss 3T3 cells, encodes a novel prostaglandin synthase/cyclooxygenase homologue. Journal of Biological Chemistry 266: 12866–12872

Kurumball RG, Stevens AM, Gierse JK et al 1996 Structural basis for the selective inhibition of cyclooxygenase-2 by anti-inflammatory agents. Nature 384: 644–648

Lane NE 1997 Pain management in osteoarthritis: the role of COX-2 inhibitors. Journal of Rheumatology 24 (suppl 49): 20–24

Langenbach R, Morham SG, Tiano HF, Loftin CD, Ghanayem BI, Chulada PC, Mahler JF, Lee CA, Goulding EH, Kluckman KD, Kim HS, Smithies O 1995 Prostaglandin synthase 1 gene disruption in mice reduces arachidonic acid-induced inflammation and indomethacin-induced gastric ulceration. Cell 83: 483–492

Laska EM, Sunshine A, Mueller F, Elvers WB, Siegel C, Rubin A 1984 Caffeine as an analgesic adjuvant. Journal of American Medical Association 251: 1711–1718

Laska EM, Sunshine A, Marrero I, Olson N, Siegel C, McCormick N 1986 The correlation between blood levels of ibuprofen and clinical analgesic response. Journal of American Medical Association 40: 1–7

Levy M, Zylber-Katz E, Rosenkranz B 1995 Clinical pharmacokinetics of dipyrone and its metabolites. Clinical Pharmacokinetics 28: 216–234

Lim H, Paria BC, Das SK, Dinchuk JE, Langenbach R, Trzaskos JM, Dey SK 1997 Multiple female reproductive failures in cyclooxygenase 2-deficient mice. Cell 91: 197–208

Lipsky PE 1997 Progress toward a new class of therapeutics: selective COX-2 inhibition: introduction and course description. Journal of Rheumatology 24 (suppl. 49): 1–5

Maihöfner C, Schlötzer-Schrehardt U, Gühring H, Zeilhofer HU, Naumann GOH, Pahl A, Mardin C, Tamm ER, Brune K 2001 Expression of cyclooxygenase-1 and -2 in normal and glaucomatous human eyes. Investigative Ophthalmology & Visual Science 42: 2616–2624

Marcheselli VL, Bazan NG 1996 Sustained induction of prostaglandin endoperoxide synthase-2 by seizures in hippocampus. Inhibition by a platelet-activating factor antagonist. Journal of Biological Chemistry 271: 24794–24799

Masferrer JL, Seibert K, Zweifel BS, Needleman P 1992 Endogenous glucocorticoids regulate an inducible cyclooxygenase enzyme. Proceedings of the National Academy of Science, USA 89: 3917–3921

Masferrer J, Zweifel B, Manning PT, Hauser SD, Leahy KM, Smith WG, Isakson PC, Seibert K 1994 Selective inhibition of inducible cyclooxygenase 2 in vivo is anti-inflammatory and non-ulcerogenic. Proceedings of the National Academy of Science, USA 91: 3228–3232

Mayer MM, Testa B 1997 Pharmacodynamics, pharmacokinetics and toxicity of ibuprofen enantiomers. Drugs of the Future 22: 1347–1366

McCormack K, Brune K 1991 Dissociation between the antinociceptive and anti-inflammatory effects of the nonsteroidal anti-inflammatory drugs. A survey of their analgesic efficacy. Drugs 41: 533–547

Mockenhaupt M, Schlingmann J, Schroeder W, Schoepf E 1996 Evaluation of non-steroidal anti-inflammatory drugs (NSAIDs) and muscle relaxants as risk factors for Stevens–Johnson syndrome (SJS) and toxic epidermal necrolysis (TEN). Pharmacoepidemiology and Drug Safety 5: 116

Morham SG, Langenbach R, Loftin CD, Tiano HF, Vouloumanos N, Jennette JC, Mahler JF, Kuckmann KD, Ledford A, Lee CA, Smithies O 1995 Prostaglandin synthase 2 gene disruption causes severe renal pathology in the mouse. Cell 83: 473–482

O'Banion MK, Sadowski HB, Winn V, Young DA 1991 A serum- and glucocorticoid regulated 4-kilobase mRNA encodes a cyclooxygenase-related protein. Journal of Biological Chemistry 266: 23261–23267

Patrignani P, Panara MR, Greco A, Fusco O, Natoli C, Iacobelli S, Cipollone F, Ganci A, Creminon C, Maclouf J, Patrono C 1994 Biochemical and pharmacological characterization of the cyclooxygenase activity of human blood prostaglandin endoperoxide synthase. Journal of Pharmacology and Experimental Therapeutics 271: 1705–1712

Porter GA 1996 Acetaminophen/aspirin mixtures: Experimental data. American Journal of Kidney Disease 28 (suppl 1): 30–33

Riendeau D, Charleson S, Cromslish W, Mancini JA, Wong E, Guay J 1997 Comparison of the cyclooxygenase-1 inhibitory properties of nonsteroidal anti-inflammatory drugs (NSAIDs) and selective COX-2 inhibitors, using sensitive microsomal and platelet assays. Canadian Journal of Physiology and Pharmacology 75: 1088–1095

Roujeau JC, Kelly JP, Naldi L, Rzany B, Stern RS, Anderson T, Auquier A, Bastuji-Garin S, Correia O, Locati F, Mockenhaupt M, Paoletti C, Shapiro S, Sheir N, Schöpf E, Kaufman D 1995 Drug etiology of Stevens–Johnson syndrome and toxic epidermal necrolysis, first results from an international case–control study. New England Journal of Medicine 333: 1600–1609

Rudy AC, Knight PM, Brater DC, Hall SD 1991 Stereoselective metabolism of ibuprofen in humans: administration of R-, S- and racemic ibuprofen. Journal of Pharmacology and Experimental Therapeutics 259: 1133–1139

Schmid J, Buisch U, Heinzel G, Bozler G, Kaschke S, Kummer M 1995 Meloxicam: pharmacokinetics and metabolic pattern after intravenous infusion and oral administration to healthy subjects. Drug Metabolism and Disposition 23: 1206–1213

Seeff LB, Cuccherini BA, Zimmerman HJ, Adler E, Benjamin SB 1986 Acetaminophen hepatotoxicity in alcoholics. Annals of Internal Medicine 104: 399–404

Seibert K, Zhang Y, Leahy K et al 1994 Pharmacological and biochemical demonstration of the role of cyclooxygenase (COX)-2 in inflammation and pain. Proceedings of the National Academy of Science USA 91: 12013–12017

Silverstein FE, Faich G, Goldstein JL, Simon LS, Pincus T, Whelton A, Makuch R, Eisen G, Agrawal NM, Stenson WF, Burr AM, Zhao WW, Kent JD, Lefkowith JB, Verburg KM, Geis GS 2000 Gastrointestinal toxicity with celecoxib vs nonsteroidal anti-inflammatory drugs for osteoarthritis and rheumatoid arthritis: the CLASS study: A randomized controlled trial. Celecoxib Long-term Arthritis Safety Study. Journal of the American Medical Association 284: 1247–1255

Tegeder I, Krebs S, Muth-Selbach U, Lötsch J, Brune K, Geisslinger G 1999 Comparison of inhibitory effects of meloxicam and diclofenac on human thromboxane biosynthesis after single doses and at steady state. Clinical Pharmacology and Therapeutics 65: 533–544

Vane JR 1971 Inhibition of prostaglandin synthesis as a mechanism of action of aspirin-like drugs. Nature New Biology 231: 232–235

Vane J 1994 Towards a better aspirin. Nature 367: 215–216

Verbeck RK, Blackburn JL, Loewen GR 1983 Clinical pharmacokinetics of non-steroidal anti-inflammatory drugs. Clinical Pharmacokinetics 8: 297–331

Wolhoff H, Altrogge G, Pola W, Sistovaris N 1983 Metamizol—akute Überdosierung in suizidaler Absicht. Deutsche Medizinische Wochenschrift 108: 1761–1764

Yamagata K, Andreasson KI, Kaufmann WE, Barnes CA, Worley PF 1993 Expression of a mitogen-inducible cyclooxygenase in brain neurons: regulation by synaptic activity and glucocorticoids. Neuron 11: 371–386

Chapter 23

Psychotropic drugs

Richard Monks and Harold Merskey

Introduction

The aim of this chapter is to describe the clinical use of various psychotropic drugs in the treatment of pain states, especially those of chronic duration. In this chapter the rationale and indications for use, effectiveness, and adverse effects of antidepressants, neuroleptics, lithium carbonate, and antianxiety drugs will be discussed.

Rationale for treatment

Antidepressants

A number of different but related mechanisms have been suggested to explain the presumed efficacy of tricyclic and heterocyclic antidepressants (TCAD), selective serotonin reuptake inhibitors (SSRI), serotonin-adrenaline (-epinephrine) reuptake inhibitors (SNRI), and monoamine oxidase inhibitors (MAOI) in pain conditions (Monks and Merskey 1999).

Analgesic effects of these drugs may result from their antidepressant action. A substantial minority of chronic pain patients are clinically depressed and, compared with non-depressed pain controls, show an increased incidence of familial affective disorders, biological markers of depression, and response to TCAD. In clinical trials with adequate data, the vast majority of patients with coexisting chronic pain and depression obtained relief from both disorders when responding to MAOI or TCAD.

There is also evidence to suggest the existence of an analgesic action of TCAD and MAOI that is not mediated by any measurable antidepressant action. The onset of analgesia with TCAD in chronic pain states is more rapid than the usual onset of an antidepressant effect in some clinically depressed patients (3–7 days vs 14–21 days). Moreover, chronic pain relief with TCAD, SSRI, and MAOI has been reported despite a lack of antidepressant response. Similar improvements have been obtained in patients without detectable depression.

It has been suggested that both the analgesic and antidepressant action of TCAD, SSRI, SNRI, and MAOI are caused by their action on central neurotransmitter functions including the catecholamine and indolamine systems, substance P, thyrotropin-releasing hormone-like peptides, and gamma amino-butyric acid (GABA). Drug trials comparing various TCAD used for patients with chronic pain tend to favour more serotonergic drugs. A recent meta-analysis of 39 placebo-controlled studies of antidepressant analgesia in chronic pain found that antidepressants with mixed serotonergic and noradrenergic properties had a larger effect size than that of drugs with more specific properties when other patient disorders and study variables were eliminated (Onghena and Van Houdenhove 1992).

The analgesic effect of the opiates, like TCAD and MAOI, appears to be modulated by central biogenic amines. TCAD, SSRI, and MAOI may enhance opiate analgesia. TCAD may also bind directly to opiate receptors.

Analgesic properties of antidepressants also have been attributed to effects such as sedation, diminished anxiety, muscle relaxation and restored sleep cycles, central or peripheral histamine receptor blockade, inhibition of prostaglandin synthetase, calcium-channel blockade effect, and anti-inflammatory effects.

Neuroleptics

Neuroleptics commonly used for pain include the phenothiazines, thioxanthenes, and butyrophenones (Monks and Merskey 1999). Of current interest are atypical neuroleptics such as clozapine and risperidone. Mechanisms of action responsible for any analgesic effects of these drugs are unknown. The vast majority of clinical pain syndromes relieved by neuroleptics are not delusional in nature and do not occur in the presence of a psychotic disorder.

Neuroleptic drugs show a wide range of actions on neurotransmitter systems centrally and peripherally. Based on results from acute animal pain studies, it has been suggested that neuroleptic analgesia might be mediated by inhibition of dopamine, noradrenaline (norepinephrine), serotonin, or histamine neurotransmission. Neuroleptic/opiate receptor interactions have also been cited to explain neuroleptic analgesia effects, synergistic action with narcotics and amelioration of narcotic withdrawal.

Sedation may explain single-dose analgesic effects of more sedating neuroleptics. However, high-potency alerting neuroleptics diminish chronic pain. Anxiolytic properties of neuroleptics in chronic pain patients have been reported.

Combined neuroleptic–antidepressant regimens might provide superior analgesic effectiveness because neuroleptics inhibit TCAD degradation and enhance TCAD plasma levels. Similarly, carbamazepine may augment TCAD levels in combined antidepressant–anticonvulsant regimens.

Lithium carbonate

Analgesic effects of lithium in cluster headache occur in the absence of depression or antidepressant effect and at lower serum levels than in bipolar affective disorders (Kudrow 1978). Lithium has complex acute and chronic effects on neurotransmission that may influence pain. It enhances serotonin availability in the brain, diminishes catecholamine neurone activity, alters central adrenergic, dopaminergic, GABA, and opiate receptor binding, and inhibits central and peripheral adenylate cyclase-mediated cyclic adenosine monophosphate production, including that induced by prostaglandin E.

Antianxiety drugs

The benzodiazepines (BDZ) and buspirone, a non-BDZ with D2 dopamine antagonist/agonist and 5-HT1A receptor agonist properties, are reported to have antinociceptive properties. BDZ usually are given to pain sufferers in an attempt to diminish anxiety, excessive muscle tension, and insomnia thought to worsen acute and chronic pain states. One benzodiazepine, alprazolam, has demonstrated antidepressant properties. Another, clonazepam, may achieve analgesic effects by its anticonvulsant properties. The stimulation of BDZ receptors affects noradrenaline (norepinephrine), serotonin, dopamine, and GABA neurotransmission. Possible long-term BDZ administration effects on serotonin turnover and BDZ receptor function are a concern (Monks and Merskey 1999).

Indications for use

The use of psychotropic drugs is only one of the adjunctive measures available in the comprehensive approach required for many pain problems, especially those of more chronic duration. A careful evaluation of psychological and social factors contributing to the pain complaint is necessary to prescribe these drugs rationally.

The antidepressants, neuroleptics, and benzodiazepines are often used for the initial control of target symptoms such as depression, anxiety, abnormal muscle tension, insomnia and fatigue. TCAD and occasionally neuroleptics are also used for withdrawal/detoxication from narcotics, other analgesics, minor tranquillizers, and alcohol (Khatami et al 1979, Halpern 1982). Combinations of TCAD and narcotics are used for some pain disorders refractory to either alone.

Treatment indications for each psychotropic group

Antidepressants (TCAD, SSRI, SNRI, and MAOI)

Depression

A trial of antidepressants is usually indicated if the patient with acute or chronic pain is clinically depressed. This is particularly so if the onset of depression preceded or coincided with the onset of pain (Bradley 1963) or if there is a past history of favourable response of depression or pain to antidepressants.

Tricyclic-type antidepressants

Chronic pain Table 23.1 lists trials of TCAD for chronic pain. Pain of 'psychological origin' refers to disorders in which structural damage was not found and in which anxiety and depression were obvious and antedated or coincided with the onset of atypical pain. 'Mixed' pain refers to various non-neoplastic chronic pain disorders. Unfortunately, most of the trials suffered from inadequacies of various sorts. However, in 46 out of 48 adequately controlled trials TCAD produced relief that was statistically and clinically superior to that obtained with placebo (Monks and Merskey 1999).

There were at least two adequately controlled trials supporting the use of amitriptyline and imipramine for chronic osteoarthritis and rheumatoid arthritis (McDonald Scott 1969, Gingras 1976, Frank et al 1988, Rani et al 1996), amitriptyline for fibromyalgia (Goldenberg et al 1986, 1996), amitriptyline and imipramine for diabetic neuropathy (Turkington 1980; Kvinesdal et al 1984; Max et al 1987; Sindrup et al 1989, 1990b; Vrethem et al 1997), amitriptyline for migraine (Gomersall and Stuart 1973, Couch et al 1976, Zeigler et al 1987), and amitriptyline and mianserin for chronic tension headaches (Lance and Curran 1964, Diamond and Baltes 1971, Martucci et al 1985, Loldrup et al 1989, Bendtsen et al 1996).

SSRI antidepressants

Table 23.1 lists trials of SSRI antidepressants given for chronic pain. Only 5 of 10 adequately controlled trials showed pain relief superior to placebo. No single SSRI drug had more than one trial supporting its use for a specific pain disorder (Monks and Merskey 1999).

Table 23.1 Chronic pain disorders treated with antidepressants

Disorder	Total trials	References (number of trials)
Tricyclic-type drugs		
Arthritis	13	Kuipers 1962 (3), McDonald Scott 1969, Thorpe and Marchant-Williams 1974, Gingras 1976, MacNeill and Dick 1976, Ganvir et al 1980, Macfarlane et al 1986, Frank et al 1988 (2), Puttini et al 1988, Rani et al 1996
Central poststroke	1	Leijon and Boivie 1989
Fibromyalgia	5	Carette et al 1986, Bibolotti et al 1986, Goldenberg et al 1986, Caruso et al 1987, Goldenberg et al 1996
Low back pain	6	Kuipers 1962, Jenkins et al 1976, Alcoff et al 1982, Ward et al 1984 (2)
Migraine	9	Gomersall and Stuart 1973, Couch and Hassanein 1976, Couch et al 1976, Noone 1977, Mørland et al 1979, Langohr et al 1985, Martucci et al 1985, Monro et al 1985, Zeigler et al 1987
Mixed	15	Rafinesque 1963, Adjan 1970, Desproges-Gotteron et al 1970, Radebold 1971, Evans et al 1973, Kocher 1976, Duthie 1977, Pilowsky et al 1982, Hameroff et al 1984, Zitman et al 1984, Edelbrock et al 1986, Sharav et al 1987 (2), Nappi et al 1990, Pilowsky et al 1995
Mixed neurological	6	Paoli et al 1960, Laine et al 1962, Merskey and Hester 1972, Castaigne et al 1979, Montastruc et al 1985, Ventafridda et al 1987
Myofascial dysfunction	2	Gessel 1975, Smoller 1984
Neoplastic	7	Hugues et al 1963, Parolin 1966, Fiorentino 1967, Gebhardt et al 1969, Adjan 1970, Bernard and Scheuer 1972, Bourhis et al 1978
Neuralgia postherpetic	9	Woodforde et al 1965, Taub 1973, Hatangdi et al 1976, Carasso 1979 (2), Watson et al 1982, Watson and Evans 1985, Max et al 1988, Kishore-Kumar et al 1990
Neuralgia trigeminal	2	Carasso 1979 (2)
Neurological perineal	1	Magni et al 1982

Table 23.1 Chronic pain disorders treated with antidepressants (*cont'd.*)

Disorder	Total trials	References (number of trials) (cont'd)
Tricyclic-type drugs		
Neuropathy		
Diabetic	16	Davis et al 1977, Gade et al 1980, Turkington 1980 (2), Mitas et al 1983, Kvinesdal et al 1984, Max et al 1987, Sindrup et al 1989, Lynch et al 1990 (2), Sindrup et al 1990a (2), 1990b, Max et al 1991, Vrethem et al 1997 (2)
Mononeuropathy	1	Langohr et al 1982
Postsurgical	1	Eija et al 1996
Painful shoulder syndrome	1	Tyber 1974
Phantom limb	1	Urban et al 1986
Psychological origin	13	Bradley 1963, Singh 1971 (2), Okasha et al 1973 (2), Ward et al 1979, Lindsay and Wyckoff 1981, Feinmann et al 1984, Magni et al 1982, Eberhard et al 1988 (2), Saran 1988, Valdes et al 1989
Tension headache	15	Lance and Curran 1964 (2), Diamond and Baltes 1971, Carasso 1979 (2), Kudrow 1980, Sjaastad 1983, Fogelholm and Morros 1985, Martucci et al 1985, Loldrup et al 1989 (2), Boline et al 1995, Bendtsen et al 1996, Mitsikostas et al 1997, Cohen 1997
SSRI-type drugs		
Arthritis	2	Frank et al 1988, Rani et al 1996
Fibromyalgia	2	Lynch et al 1990, Goldenberg et al 1996
Low back pain	1	Goodkin et al 1990
Migraine	3	Adly et al 1992, Saper et al 1994, Black and Sheline 1995
Mixed	3	Johansson and Von Knorring 1979, Gourlay et al 1986, Nappi et al 1990
Mixed neurological	2	Davidoff et al 1987, Ventafridda et al 1987
Neuralgia		
Diabetic	3	Khurana 1983, Theesen and Marsh 1989, Sindrup et al 1990b
Postherpetic	1	Watson and Evans 1985
Tension headache	3	Sjaastad 1983, Norregaard et al 1995, Bendtsen et al 1996
SNRI-type drugs		
Low back pain	1	Songer and Schulte 1996
Migraine	1	Adelman et al 2000
Mixed neurological	2	Taylor and Rowbotham 1996, Sumpton and Moulin 2001
Tension headache	1	Adelman et al 2000
MAOI-type drugs		
Chronic fatigue syndrome	1	Natelson et al 1996
Facial pain of psychological origin	2	Lascelles 1966 (2)
Fibromyalgia	1	Nicolodi and Sicuteri 1996
Migraine	2	Anthony and Lance 1969, Merikangas and Merikangas 1995
Psychological origin	3	Bradely 1963, Lindsay and Wyckoff 1981, Raskin 1982

SNRI antidepressants

Table 23.1 lists the trials of the SNRI-type antidepressant venlafaxine given for chronic pain. Although a number of case studies have reported pain relief similar to that with TCAD no adequately controlled trials were found.

Monoamine oxidase inhibitor

MAOI drugs, usually phenelzine, have been found to be successful in diminishing chronic pain in each of the trials listed in Table 23.1. Only two adequately controlled trials were found, both with phenelzine, one in chronic fatigue syndrome (Natelson et al 1996) and one in facial pain of psychological origin (Lascelles 1966). In one non-placebo-controlled trial, MAOI drugs with 5-hydroxytryptophan proved superior to MAOI and to amitriptyline for fibromyalgia (Nicolodi and Sicuteri 1996).

NEUROLEPTICS

Psychosis

Neuroleptics are indicated for those psychiatric disorders associated with delusional or hallucinatory

Table 23.2 Disorders treated with neuroleptics

Disorder	Total trials	References (number of trials)
Acute pain		
Mixed	1	Montilla et al 1963
Herpes zoster	3	Sigwald et al 1959 (2), Farber and Burks 1974
Postoperative	14	Jackson and Smith 1956 (3), Lasagna and DeKornfeld 1961 (3), Bronwell et al 1966, Stirman 1967, Taylor and Doku 1967, Fazio 1970, Minuck 1972 (2), Judkins and Harmer 1982 (2)
Migraine	2	Iserson 1983, Shrestha et al 1996
Myocardial infarction	1	Davidson et al 1979
Chronic pain		
Arthritis	1	Breivik and Slørdahl 1984
Migraine	1	Polliack 1979
Mixed	6	Sadove et al 1955, Bloomfield et al 1964, Kast 1966, Cavenar and Maltbie 1976, Kocher 1976, Langohr et al 1982
Mixed neurological	1	Merskey and Hester 1972
Myofascial dysfunction	1	Raft et al 1979
Neoplastic	10	Beaver et al 1966 (2), Maltbie and Cavenar 1977, Bourhis et al 1978, Schick et al 1979 (2), Breivik and Rennemo 1982, Hanks et al 1983 (2), Landa et al 1984
Neuralgia postherpetic	5	Sigwald et al 1959 (2), Nathan 1978 (2), Duke 1983
Neuropathy diabetic	2	Davis et al 1977, Mitas et al 1983
Radiation fibrosis	1	Daw and Cohen-Cole 1981
Tension headache (chronic)	2	Hakkarainen 1977, Hackett et al 1987
Thalamic pain	1	Margolis and Gianascol 1956

pain such as schizophrenia, delusional depressions, and monosymptomatic hypochondriacal psychosis (Munro and Chmara 1982).

Pain-associated problems

Overwhelming pain characterized by anxiety, psychomotor agitation, and insomnia, which does not respond to benzodiazepines in acute pain or TCAD in chronic pain, may be treated, at least on a short-term basis, by neuroleptics. In patients with neoplastic pain, neuroleptics are useful in managing nausea, vomiting, bladder or rectal tenesmus, and ureteral spasm.

Acute pain

In trials of neuroleptics given for acute pain (Table 23.2), the most common indication for use in the mixed and postoperative group was abdominal, dental, or postpartum pain. Only five of these trials were judged to be adequate. In two studies of acute postoperative pain (Taylor and Doku 1967, Fazio 1970) and one of acute myocardial infarction (Davidson et al 1979), levomepromazine (methotrimeprazine) 10–20 mg intramuscularly (IM) gave analgesic results equivalent to meperidine 50 mg intramuscularly. In one study chlorpromazine 25 mg intravenously (IV) was found to be as markedly successful as ketorolac 60 mg IM in acute migraine headache (Shrestha et al 1996). In the remaining trial, premedication with haloperidol 5 or 10 mg orally was no better than placebo (Judkins and Harmer 1982).

Chronic pain

In trials of neuroleptics for chronic pain (Table 23.2), the main indication was for patients with recognizable organic lesions not treatable by more conservative means. Because of their adverse effects, neuroleptics should only be given after transcutaneous electrical nerve stimulation, other benign local measures, and regular non-narcotic analgesics at fixed times have been tried. They may be used for thalamic or similar central pain that does not respond to antidepressants, carbamazepine, or clonazepam. They are often helpful in nerve lesions including causalgias, neuralgias, neuropathies, traumatic avulsion of the brachial plexus, and some instances of back pain, particularly if there is clear evidence of associated damage to nerves or nerve roots.

Only five adequate controlled trials were found. Single doses of levomepromazine (methotrimeprazine) 15 mg were found to have analgesic properties equal to 8–15 mg of morphine in patients with mixed sources of chronic pain (Bloomfield et al 1964, Kast 1966) and in patients with chronic pain of neoplastic origin (Beaver et al 1966). Fluphenazine and flupentixol each at 1 mg orally per day were both clinically and statistically superior to placebo in the treatment of chronic tension headache in trials of 2 months and 6 weeks respectively (Hakkarainen 1977, Hackett et al 1987).

Combined drug therapy

Antidepressant and anticonvulsant

A combination of TCAD and an anticonvulsant may be useful for neuralgias resistant to either drug alone. Three clinical trials were found describing the successful treatment of chronic postherpetic neuralgia with combinations of TCAD with carbamazepine or with diphenylhydantoin (Hatangdi et al 1976, Gerson et al 1977) or with valproic acid (Raferty 1979).

Antidepressant and neuroleptic

A TCAD neuroleptic combination was used for chronic pain in the trials listed in Table 23.3. Combined therapy is usually indicated when either drug group alone is indicated but has not proven efficacious and adverse effects are not a contra-indication. The best results seem to occur with arthritic pain, treatment-resistant headaches, neoplastic pain, and a variety of neurological pain disorders such as causalgias, deafferentation syndromes, neuralgias, and neuropathies.

Only two adequately controlled trials of TCAD–neuroleptic treatment were found. A nortriptyline and fluphenazine combination was found to be clearly superior to placebo in decreasing pain and paraesthesias in patients with diabetic polyneuropathy in one study (Gomez-Perez et al 1985), and equally efficacious and superior to placebo when compared to carbamazapine for diabetic poly-neuropathy pain (Gomez-Perez et al 1996).

Lithium

Lithium alone has been reported to be useful in episodic and chronic cluster headaches (Ekbom 1974, 1981; Kudrow 1977, 1978; Mathew 1978; Bussone et al 1979; Pearce 1980) and, when combined with amitriptyline, in the treatment of painful shoulder syndrome (Tyber 1974). Lithium alone or combined with TCAD or with neuroleptics may be useful for pain syndromes associated with bipolar affective disorders and some recurrent unipolar depressions. No controlled adequate trials of lithium therapy for acute or chronic pain were found.

Antianxiety drugs

Anxiety

The benzodiazepines may be useful in the short-term (4 weeks or less) management of anxiety, muscle spasm, and insomnia, which are frequently associated with acute pain and which may occur during acute exacerbations of chronic pain disorders. Non-drug psychological management techniques for these pain-related problems should be tried first where time and available resources permit.

Acute pain

There is suggestive evidence that short-term BDZ use may diminish the acute pain associated with myocardial infarction, anxiety-related gastrointestinal disorders, and acute and chronic intervertebral disc problems with skeletal muscle spasm. Only two adequately controlled trials were found. In the first, lorazepam was superior to placebo when added to opioids for procedural pain in major burn injuries but only for those persons with high baseline pain and high-state anxiety (Patterson et al 1997). In the second, alprazolam was superior to progesterone and to placebo in providing pain relief when used

Table 23.3 Disorders treated with antidepressant and neuroleptic combination

Disorder	Total trials	References
Head pain of psychological origin	1	Sherwin 1979
Mixed	3	Kocher 1976 (2), Duthie 1977
Mixed neurological	2	Merskey and Hester 1972, Langohr et al 1982
Neoplastic	3	Bernard and Scheuer 1972, Bourhis et al 1978, Breivik and Rennemo 1982
Neuralgia postherpetic	3	Taub 1973, Langohr et al 1982, Weis et al 1982
Neuropathy diabetic	6	Davis et al 1977; Gade et al 1980; Khurana 1983; Mitas et al 1983; Gomez-Perez et al 1985, 1996

cyclically in severe premenstrual syndrome (Freeman et al 1995).

Chronic pain

Although it may be necessary to continue established use of benzodiazepines for certain patients, initiation of their use in chronic pain is seldom indicated.

In two uncontrolled studies alprazolam was found to be very effective in relieving causalgic but not other types of neoplastic pain (Fernandez et al 1987), and clonazepam provided effective relief for more than 6 months in two patients with lancinating phantom limb pain (Bartusch et al 1996). Clonazepam also has shown some promise in the treatment of neuralgias (Swerdlow and Cundill 1981).

Only four of seven adequately controlled trials showed BDZ to be superior to placebo (Lance and Curran 1964, Okasha et al 1973, Hackett et al 1987, Shukla et al 1996) for chronic tension headache or pain of psychological origin. BDZ were inferior to TCAD controls in two of these four trials.

One controlled trial found buspirone to have analgesic effects comparable to amitriptyline in the treatment of chronic tension headache (Mitsikostas et al 1997).

Effectiveness

Antidepressants

Tricyclic antidepressants

Chronic pain The outcomes of adequate controlled TCAD trials for chronic pain listed in Table 23.1 have been summarized.

In three trials TCAD were compared with non-placebo control drugs. Amitriptyline and propranolol proved equally effective in decreasing the pain associated with high-frequency chronic migraine (Zeigler et al 1987). Low-dose amitriptyline was superior to naproxen in alleviating the pain and fatigue associated with fibromyalgia (Goldenberg et al 1986). Amitriptyline provided greater pain relief than carbamazepine and was better tolerated than carbamazepine in the treatment of persons with central poststroke pain (Leijon and Boivie 1989).

In one non-blinded trial amitriptyline was compared to spinal manipulation for chronic tension headache. While the amitriptyline was slightly more effective after 6 weeks of treatment, the drug group relapsed 4 weeks post-treatment while the non-drug group showed continued benefit (Boline et al 1995). In the other open trial patients with chronic non-neoplastic pain received amitriptyline with either cognitive behavioural therapy (CBT) or supportive therapy. There was no statistical difference between the groups despite a trend favouring the CBT group at 6 month follow-up (Pilowsky et al 1995).

In 59 of the 75 trials giving details, ≥50% of patients obtained moderate to total pain relief. Analgesic use was significantly diminished in those studies giving information. Dropout rates were <10%. Most TCAD trials lasted 3 months or less. In two longer trials of TCAD for chronic non-neoplastic pain two-thirds of patients were still improving or pain free at 9–16 months although one-third to one-half of patients still required the drug (Blumer and Heilbronn 1981, Feinmann et al 1984).

A number of clinical and laboratory factors may predict TCAD analgesic effect in chronic pain disorders. The presence of clinically important depression, a family history of depressive spectrum disorders, and an absence of previous analgesic use have been noted to correlate with TCAD-induced pain relief. Head pain, except that from closed head injury, is more likely to be associated with good outcome than that with other body sites. Blood levels of TCAD and their metabolites have been positively correlated with analgesic response in some studies but not others. Poorer outcomes with TCAD for chronic pain have been reported with certain Minnesota Multiphasic Personality Inventory profiles (Pheasant et al 1983), increased analgesic use, and a family history of pain disorders.

SSRI antidepressants

Twelve of the 20 chronic pain studies listed in Table 23.1 reported clinically important pain relief. Six of nine trials with relevant data showed >50% of patients with moderate to marked pain relief. Analgesic use was seldom documented. Compliance, as indicated by blood levels and a low dropout rate (average 4%), was excellent. About 70% of studies lasted ≤3 months. In four out of six adequate trials TCAD were superior to their SSRI controls (Sjaastad 1983, Frank et al 1988, Sindrup et al 1990b, Bendtsen et al 1996).

SNRI antidepressants

In the papers listed in Table 23.1, about one-half of those treated experienced >50% pain relief. The vast majority of those studied had inadequate pain relief or intolerable side effects with previous trials of at least one other antidepressant. The dropout rate was 23% overall. The treatment duration was 1–7 months.

Monoamine oxidase inhibitors

The majority of patients experienced ≥50% pain relief in those MAOI trials listed in Table 23.1. In most instances, depression and pain were alleviated at the same time. Substantial previous therapies had not been helpful for a majority of patients. The dropout rate averaged 4%. About 70% of the studies lasted less than 3 months.

Neuroleptics

Acute pain

Twenty of the 21 trials listed in Table 23.2 reported clinically important analgesic effects. In 15 of these trials, a single dose of levomepromazine (methotrimeprazine) was found to compare favourably with a narcotic control and/or to be superior to placebo in postoperative pain (see 'Indications for Use' above).

Three uncontrolled trials of ongoing regimens of neuroleptic therapy for acute herpes zoster neuralgia produced total relief in 92–100% of patients within 1–5 days if the therapy was started within 3 months of the onset of the disorder (Sigwald et al 1959, Farber and Burks 1974).

Chronic pain

Twenty-nine of the 31 trials listed in Table 23.2 reported clinically important analgesic effects of neuroleptics given for chronic pain. In 16 of the 20 trials with relevant data, the majority of patients experienced moderate to total pain relief.

Unfortunately, the majority of trials lasted less than 3 months. Two trials for postherpetic neuralgia lasting more than 6 months reported almost total failure after initial impressive relief (Nathan 1978). On the other hand, in another trial, 75% of patients with this disorder remained pain-free for 10–20 months on neuroleptic therapy (Duke 1983).

In herpes zoster neuralgia, less than 20% of patients obtained good or total pain relief if the condition was more than 3 months in duration (Sigwald et al 1959).

The evidence for neuroleptic-induced pain relief is supported by a series of anecdotal single-patient or uncontrolled group reports of patients with diabetic neuropathy, neoplastic pain, postherpetic neuralgia, and thalamic pain. Patients with very chronic stable baseline pain disorders, refractory to many interventions, responded rapidly (≤4 days), frequently had total pain relief, and suffered relapse rapidly with placebo substitution or stopping the neuroleptic.

Treatment acceptability in all but one trial was good (≤10% dropout).

In one trial, the addition of haloperidol to relaxation training led to important pain relief in a group of patients with chronic myofascial dysfunction who were previously unresponsive to this and other forms of behaviour therapy (Raft et al 1979).

Combined drug therapy

TCAD and anticonvulsant

In three trials 72–89% of patients with chronic postherpetic neuralgia experienced moderate to complete relief. Follow-up ranged from 1 to 18 months with a mean of 3 months. In two of the three trials dropout rates were similar to those noted for TCAD alone. In the third trial, patients were entered into a limited crossover non-blind study in which a regimen of clomipramine plus carbamazepine was compared with transcutaneous nerve stimulation, with each being given for 8 weeks. The dropout rate for the drug group was 50%, while that for transcutaneous nerve stimulation was 70%. Clearly superior analgesic results were reported for the drug group (Gerson et al 1977).

TCAD and neuroleptic

Seventeen of the 18 combined TCAD and neuroleptic trials for chronic pain listed in Table 23.3 reported good to total pain relief in the majority of patients. Follow-up was ≤3 months in six trials and 6–36 months in five further trials. The average dropout rate was 12%. Most patients had received extensive previous therapy. There is evidence to suggest that combined therapy may be more efficacious than TCAD or neuroleptic therapies alone. One controlled trial, comparing clomipramine plus neuroleptic to neuroleptic therapy alone for mixed neurological chronic pain, found 67% compared with 47% good to total relief in the combined and neuroleptic groups, respectively, with the dropout rate being lower in the combined therapy group (Langohr et al 1982). Another controlled trial found the TCAD–neuroleptic combination (nortriptyline with fluphenazine) equally markedly effective as carbamazepine for pain with diabetic polyneuropathy (Gomez-Perez et al 1996).

Lithium

Most evidence for the use of lithium in the management of pain is derived from studies with cluster headache. About one-third of patients treated with lithium for episodic cluster headache experienced good to total control of pain during a 1-month treatment period (Mathew 1978, Ekbom 1981). In chronic cluster headache, more than two-thirds of patients obtained good to total pain relief for periods of up to 6 months or longer (Ekbom

1974, 1981; Kudrow 1977; Mathew 1978; Bussone et al 1979; Pearce 1980). No adequate controlled trials were found. One open controlled trial reported lithium to be strikingly superior to methysergide and to prednisone in the treatment of this disorder (Kudrow 1978). Unfortunately no trials were found to compare lithium with verapamil treatment (Lewis and Solomon 1996).

Dropout rates were ≤3%.

Antianxiety drugs

Acute pain

The only two adequate controlled trials have been summarized under 'Indications for Use'. Three additional controlled trials reported clinically important analgesic effects during the first week postmyocardial infarction (Hackett and Cassem 1972, Melsom et al 1976, Dixon et al 1980). In these trials one-third to a majority of patients experienced moderate or good pain relief, and in one study analgesic use was diminished. Dropout rates were ≤2%.

Chronic pain

Of the seven adequate controlled trials and two uncontrolled BDZ trials presented in the section on 'Indications', only three reported >50% patients with moderate to marked relief. Analgesic use was diminished in one study reporting this data. Dropout rates averaged 5%.

Given the results it is not possible to recommend BDZ as first-line treatment for chronic pain.

In one controlled trial 54.4 and 60.7% of buspirone and amitriptyline patients, respectively, obtained >50% reduction in chronic tension headache pain, although patient opinion of treatment and analgesic use statistics favoured amitriptyline. Dropouts were comparable (15–16%) in this 12-week study (Mitsikostas et al 1997).

Adverse effects

Antidepressants

Tricyclic-type antidepressants

Adverse effects with TCAD are summarized below.

Anticholinergic autonomic effects are usually transient and irritating at worst (dry mouth, palpitations, decreased visual accommodation, constipation, and oedema) but may occasionally be more serious (postural hypotension, loss of consciousness, aggravation of narrow-angle glaucoma, urinary retention, and paralytic ileus). There is more risk in the elderly or those on other anticholinergic drugs (e.g., neuroleptics, antiparkinsonian drugs). Slowing initial administration, lowering TCAD doses, discontinuing other drugs, or using a less anticholinergic drug (Table 23.4) may be necessary. TCAD may cause sexual dysfunctions such as loss of libido, impotence, and ejaculatory problems. Trazodone may cause priapism and permanent impotence.

Allergic/hypersensitivity reactions such as cholestatic jaundice, skin reactions, and agranulocytosis are quite uncommon but require giving the patient adequate precautions. Anticholinergic and quinidine-like cardiac effects of tricyclic antidepressants cause serious reservations about their use in patients with pre-existing conduction defects and/or cardiac ischaemia, particularly postmyocardial infarction (Roose and Glassman 1994).

Orthostatic hypotension is common with TCAD, which block adrenergic receptors (Table 23.4). Imipramine is more hazardous for the elderly and others vulnerable to falls or hypotension. Those at risk require safer drugs and measurement of orthostatic change before and after an initial test dose. Possible interventions include patient education, use of a bedside commode and night light, surgical support stockings, and, in severe cases, 9-α-fluorohydrocortisone 0.025–0.05 mg orally twice a day.

Various central nervous system (CNS) adverse effects have been reported (sedation, tremor, seizures, insomnia, exacerbation of schizophrenia or mania, and atropine-like delirium). The elderly are at particular risk, especially if there is previous brain damage or when combinations of drugs with anticholinergic properties are used.

TCAD potentiate CNS depressants (alcohol, anxiolytics, narcotics), potentiate other anticholinergics, antagonize certain antihypertensives (α-methyldopa, guanethidine), and may produce lethal hypertensive episodes with MAOI.

Acute overdoses of TCAD in excess of 2000 mg can be fatal. Initial prescriptions of greater than 1 week's supply are unwise for the depressed patient.

The safety of TCAD during pregnancy and lactation has not been established. TCAD use during the first trimester of pregnancy is best avoided.

Mild withdrawal reactions have been observed after the abrupt cessation of TCAD. Gradual termination seems prudent.

In TCAD trials listed in Table 23.1, severe adverse effects were rare. Delirium (8–13% of patients) and drowsiness (3–28%) were the most common reasons for discontinuing therapy and were usually noted with high doses and drug combinations (TCAD with neuroleptics or with anticonvulsants), especially in the elderly. Adverse effects and dropout rates were correlated with higher plasma levels of TCAD and their metabolites in at least two studies (Gerson et al 1977, Kvinesdal et al 1984).

Although little is known about adverse effects of long-term TCAD administrations, one study reported on 46 depressed patients treated with doxepin for 2–10 years (Ayd 1979). No patients were noted to have any serious side effects or any drug-caused impairment of intellectual, social, or other functions.

SSRI antidepressants

Although SSRI antidepressants require further study to demonstrate any analgesic properties, they appear attractive for persons at risk of adverse effects from tricyclic antidepressants. Most are free of anticholinergic, adrenergic, and histaminergic receptor action and thus are relatively unlikely to produce anticholinergic autonomic, cardiac, orthostatic hypotension, sedation, or weight gain problems commonly seen with TCAD. Overdosage with these drugs are less dangerous than those with TCAD.

On the other hand, their use may be associated with increased insomnia, diarrhoea, nausea, agitation, anxiety, exacerbation of mania or psychosis, sexual disturbances, headache, and tremor. Akathisia, other extrapyramidal effects, anorgasmia, and a serum sickness-like illness have been reported with fluoxetine. A central hyperserotonergic syndrome, including autonomic instability, hyperthermia, rigidity, myoclonus, and delirium, may occur when these drugs are prescribed with other serotonergic drugs like lithium and/or monoamine oxidase inhibitors. Other more recently noted adverse effects include increased body sway and potential for falls, sinus node slowing, weight loss, and hyponatraemia.

The SSRI antidepressants are metabolized by and inhibit cytochrome 450 isoenzymes. Individual SSRI have widely differing drug interaction potential across isoenzyme systems. Important interactions can occur with other psychotropic agents, antiarrythmics, anticonvulsants, terfenadine, astemizole, cisapride, tolbutamide, and anticoagulants (Nemeroff et al 1996).

In the SSRI trials listed in Table 23.1 there were very few serious adverse effects, with the exception of one patient on zimelidine who developed increased levels of liver enzymes and fever. This drug has since been withdrawn from the market for similar problems. Gastrointestinal adverse effects were most common (46% of patients in studies with details). Dropout rates averaged 10% but varied widely (0–33%).

SNRI antidepressants

Venlafaxine blocks neuronal reuptake of serotonin and noradrenaline (norepinephrine) but is relatively free of muscarinic cholinergic, histaminic, and α-adrenergic receptor effects. It has little potential for drug interaction. However, venlafaxine may increase hypertensive problems, exacerbate existing seizure disorders, and trigger mania. More common complaints include nausea, asthenia, sweating, anorexia, somnolence, dizziness, and dry mouth. In the only clinical trials found, 2 out of 14 patients dropped out because of adverse effects, 1 for nausea and 1 for hypertension, ataxia, and drowsiness.

Monoamine oxidase inhibitors

Although relatively free of anticholinergic side effects, MAOI may cause urinary retention, orthostatic hypotension, severe parenchymal hepatotoxic reactions, CNS effects (insomnia, agitation, exacerbation of mania or schizophrenia), hypertensive crises, and drug interactions.

Fortunately, serious adverse effects are rare if medications, foods, and beverages with sympathomimetic activities are avoided. In pain patients, narcotics, especially meperidine, should be avoided and anaesthetics used with great caution (Janowski and Janowski 1985). Hypertensive crises resulting from enhanced sympathomimetic action are best treated with immediate but slow intravenous injection of phentolamine 5 mg or, in an emergency, chlorpromazine 50–100 mg intramuscularly.

In those trials in which MAOI were used to treat pain disorders, phenelzine was discontinued because of jaundice in 4%, impotence in 4%, and insomnia in 16% of patients in one study (Anthony and Lance 1969), while orthostatic hypotension was found in 6% and headache in 3% of patients in another (Lascelles 1966).

Long-term MAOI use in chronic pain is unreported, but efficacious and acceptably safe use has been described for up to several years in patients with anxiety disorders (Tyrer 1976).

A new class of compounds, the reversible inhibitors of MAO type A (RIMA), such as moclobemide, brofaromine, and toloxatone, appear to be effective antidepressants and are reported to be virtually free of the hepatotoxicity, hypertensive crises, and orthostatic hypotension encountered with the older irreversible mixed MAO-A and MAO-B inhibitors reported on in this chapter (Da Prada et al 1990). However, it is prudent to observe the same precautions for use, especially regarding drug–drug interactions, given mixed enzyme inhibition at higher RIMA doses. Unfortunately, it is not known whether RIMA have any analgesic properties.

Neuroleptics

Neuroleptics also may cause anticholinergic effects, orthostatic hypotension, quinidine-like cardiac effects, and sedation (Table 23.5). These side effects are more prominent with the low-potency phenothiazines and thiothixenes, particularly when they are combined with TCAD or carbamazepine.

CNS effects are a frequent source of patient non-compliance. Patients may note malaise, dysphoria (boring, 'unpleasant', or 'wretched' feelings), or overt depression. Acute extrapyramidal syndromes (parkinsonism, akathisia, and dystonia) usually occur early in treatment, especially with high-potency drugs. Other neurological syndromes include neuroleptic malignant syndrome, perioral tremor (relatively benign and responsive to anticholinergic drugs), and tardive dyskinesia (TD). Tardive dyskinesia may occur in up to 40% of those who have taken neuroleptics regularly over periods of 12 months or more. The likelihood of developing TD seems to be proportional to the total quantity of neuroleptic taken over time but occasionally may occur even with low doses taken over several months. It is more likely to occur in elderly females and in those with previous brain damage and may be more frequent in those who have also received antiparkinsonian drugs. TD is best managed by prevention (adequate indication for use, alternative regimen if possible), informed consent (patient and family adequately informed and vigilant regarding the emergence of TD), regular examination for TD by the physician at follow-up visits, and the use of low-dose, short-term therapy with regular attempts to decrease or discontinue the neuroleptic should it no longer be necessary. If neuroleptics are stopped at the first sign of TD, the symptoms become worse but gradually fade over a period of 2 or 3 months in most cases. Novel neuroleptics, such as clozapine and risperidone, have dopamine and serotonin receptor blocking activity and may have decreased risk for extrapyramidal symptoms (EPS) and TD. These newer drugs may offer a means to prevent TD or, where treatment with neuroleptics is essential, to continue their use for those with TD. Given their relatively better risk profile and their serotonergic activities the novel neuroleptics would seem of interest for use in chronic pain. Unfortunately no human clinical trials could be found.

Other adverse effects of neuroleptics include weight gain, sexual dysfunction, endocrine disorders, exacerbation of epileptic disorders, photosensitivity, blood dyscrasias (agranulocytosis, leucopenia), cholestatic jaundice, and ocular and skin pigmentation. The neuroleptics also increase the effects of CNS depressants and block the action of guanethidine.

In the trials of neuroleptics alone or in combination with TCAD, the commonest problems were somnolence and delirium, with a higher incidence of these problems occurring with high-dose chlorprothixene or levomepromazine (methotrimeprazine) therapy.

Lithium

Reported hazards of lithium administration include intoxication and the development of renal, thyroid, cardiac, neuromuscular, neurotoxic, dermatological, and birth abnormalities. With careful monitoring of clinical symptoms and blood levels of the drug, short-term lithium use is reasonably safe. The issue of renal morphological changes (interstitial fibrosis and nephron atrophy) with longer-term use is still a cause of concern and preventive measures should include using the lowest dose of lithium for the least time possible, using a single daily maintenance dose, and monitoring renal function. Lithium-induced goitre and hypothyroidism usually respond to thyroid hormone.

In studies of lithium use for cluster headaches, the drug had to be discontinued because of lithium headaches (3%), severe nausea and vomiting (6%), lethargy, general weakness (6%), or severe tremor (1%). The most common minor symptom was tremor, which was treatable by propranolol. Long-term lithium use in pain patients has yet to be reported.

Antianxiety drugs

Although physical dependency and withdrawal may occur with prolonged (≥6 weeks) moderate to high dosage use of BDZ, such problems are rarely encountered at therapeutic doses.

Daytime sedation, impaired coordination and judgement, and other forms of cognitive impairment have been reported to be common with prolonged steady use of these drugs for chronic pain. These adverse effects are more likely if the patient is elderly or brain damaged, if longer-acting BDZ are used, or if other central-depressant drugs are given at the same time. Other reported adverse effects include depression, suicidal thoughts, impulsivity, and rebound insomnia.

Studies of patients treated in pain centres suggest that global and specific neuropsychological test impairments and electroencephalogram abnormalities occur more often in patients on BDZ than in comparable controls (Hendler et al 1980, McNairy et al 1984). However, in one long-term study of patients with chronic pain and muscle pain 77% of patients felt that diazepam benefited them (Hollister et al 1981).

In those BDZ trials described under 'Indications for Use', initial sedation and dizziness were the commonest adverse effects. Acute depressive mood changes occurred in 18% of patients in one trial (Max et al 1988). Dropout rates due to BDZ effects were usually less than 5%.

Buspirone is usually well tolerated with dropout rates from non-pain trials averaging 10%. More frequent adverse effects include dizziness, headache, nausea, and, less frequently, insomnia. Dystonias and cogwheel rigidity have been reported.

Description of treatment

General considerations

Certain principles of psychotropic drug use are worth mentioning:

1. There must be adequate indications for the use of these drugs. Moreover, this symptomatic management must not delay the discovery of treatable causes of pain.
2. Every effort must be made to establish a working alliance with the patient and his support system (family, other health professionals). A clear explanation of indications, goals, methods, alternative management, and risk of intervention and non-intervention is essential in this regard.
3. Management should begin with the most benign efficacious intervention and a more hazardous regimen used only if treatment fails and informed consent is given (e.g., transcutaneous nerve stimulation then TCAD and neuroleptic therapy). Figures 23.1 and 23.2 depict one possible protocol based on this approach.
4. The therapeutic trial must be at an adequate dose for a sufficient length of time.
5. Other drugs should be reduced or eliminated, if at all feasible, as soon as possible. Detoxification from narcotics, alcohol, hypnotics, and antianxiety drugs is often necessary to obtain a therapeutic response (Halpern 1982, Buckley et al 1986).
6. The physician must be available during the initiation of the therapy and during changes in the regimen.
7. Elderly patients usually require only one-third to one-half of the usual adult dose. Cumulative increases in psychotropics and their metabolites occur over a much longer period and maximum adverse effects may not be seen for weeks.

Antidepressants

Tricyclic-type, SSRI, and SNRI antidepressants

Table 23.4 lists the generic names and approximate dosage ranges of some of the tricyclic-type antidepressants (bicyclic, tricyclic, tetracyclic, and similar drugs). Figures 23.1 and 23.2 illustrate the approach to antidepressant use outlined as follows.

Precautions Baseline blood studies (liver function, haemoglobin measurement, and blood count) are performed. An electrocardiogram is obtained in all elderly patients and those with cardiovascular problems. Patients at risk from possible hypotension may have lying and sitting blood pressure determination before and 1–2 h following an initial oral 10–50 mg test dose.

Choice of drugs There is little evidence to support the use of one TCAD over any other. However, a past positive response of pain or depression in the patient or his blood relative to a particular TCAD would favour its use. A history of therapeutic failure or adverse effects with a TCAD requires further information. These difficulties are usually a result of inadequate trials, non-compliance, or avoidable adverse effects. If the drug history is not helpful, patients with disorders should start one of the drugs proven effective in the adequately controlled trials summarized in the 'Treatment Indications' section. For most chronic pain disorders there appears to be an advantage to initiating therapy with a tricyclic antidepressant with mixed neurotransmitter properties (e.g., amitriptyline, imipramine, clomipramine, or doxepin) unless the potential side effects of these drugs dictate otherwise. Overall, amitriptyline is a reasonable choice for most younger persons.

Drug side effects may be exploited (e.g., by the use of a more sedating TCAD such as amitriptyline, doxepin, or trimipramine for patients with marked sleep disturbance or high daytime arousal). For example, a single dose of 50–75 mg of one of these TCAD at bedtime is often used in substitution–detoxification programmes during the initial 1–2 months of treatment to obtain rapid symptomatic relief, to prevent the exacerbation of anxiety and

Table 23.4 Antidepressant drugs used in the management of chronic pain

Drug	Oral dosage range (mg/day)	Anticholinergic potency	Orthostatic hypotension	Sedation
Tricyclic-type antidepressants				
Amitriptyline	10–300	High	Moderate	High
Clomipramine	20–300	Moderate	Moderate	Moderate
Desipramine	25–300	Low	Low	Low
Doxepin	30–300	Moderate	Moderate	High
Imipramine	20–300	High	High	Moderate
Maprotiline	50–300	Low	Low	High
Nortriptyline	50–150	Moderate	Low	Moderate
Ritanserin	10	Nil	Nil	Nil
Trazodone	50–600	Low	Moderate	High
Trimipramine	50–300	Moderate	?Moderate	High
SSRI-type antidepressants				
Fluoxetine	5–40	Nil	Nil	Nil
Paroxetine	20–40	Low	Nil	Nil
Ritanserin	10	Nil	Nil	Nil
Trazodone	50–600	Low	Moderate	High
SNRI antidepressant				
Venlafaxine	37.5–300	Nil	Nil	Nil
Monoamine oxidase inhibitors				
Phenelzine	30–90	Low	High	Nil
Tranylcypromine	10–40	Low	?Moderate	Nil

depression, and to facilitate optimal levels of function.

TCAD may be taken to minimize adverse effects. For example, there are fewer anticholinergic effects with desipramine or maprotiline (Table 23.4). Despite the preliminary nature of evidence supporting its use, venlafaxine may be a reasonable initial choice in patients at high risk of anticholinergic, hypotensive, or drug interaction adverse events.

Initial administration In dealing with chronic pain, schedules and doses of TCAD are best arranged to increase compliance and decrease adverse effects. For example, with amitriptyline, the patient is instructed to start with 10 mg orally 1–2 h before bedtime. The next day this dose is increased to 25 mg; subsequently, the dose is increased by 25 mg/day every several days as tolerated. This is continued until a therapeutic response is obtained or a total daily dose of 150 mg/day is reached. If undue side effects supervene, a dose lower than that at which these effects appeared should be employed. If there is no response after 150 mg/day for 1 week and there are no medical contraindications or serious adverse effects, the dose may be increased by 25 mg/day to the maximum dose indicated in Table 23.4. If there is no therapeutic effect after a further 3 weeks, a TCAD blood level should be performed (Fig. 23.1). If plasma levels are lower than usual antidepressant levels, i.e., amitriptyline plus nortriptyline metabolite >120 ng/ml, imipramine >225 ng/ml, or nortriptyline between 50 and 150 ng/ml (Perry et al 1987), check for non-compliance and attempt to achieve these plasma levels for at least 3–4 weeks. If there is no direct response despite adequate levels or if it is not possible to achieve these levels through discussion and regimen alterations to improve side effects and compliance, either discontinue the drug by 25 mg/day decrements or move to one of the alternative strategies outlined for non-response below.

In the majority of reported clinical trials and in clinical practice, the therapeutic dose of TCAD like amitriptyline, even in the initial phase, is between 50 and 150 mg/day orally (average 75 mg). There is some evidence that head pain (migraine, psychogenic head and face pain, and chronic tension headache) may respond at lower doses such as 25–75 mg/day.

Lower doses and slower rates of administration of TCAD are necessary in patients over 60 years old. Treatment is usually initiated at 20–30 mg/day

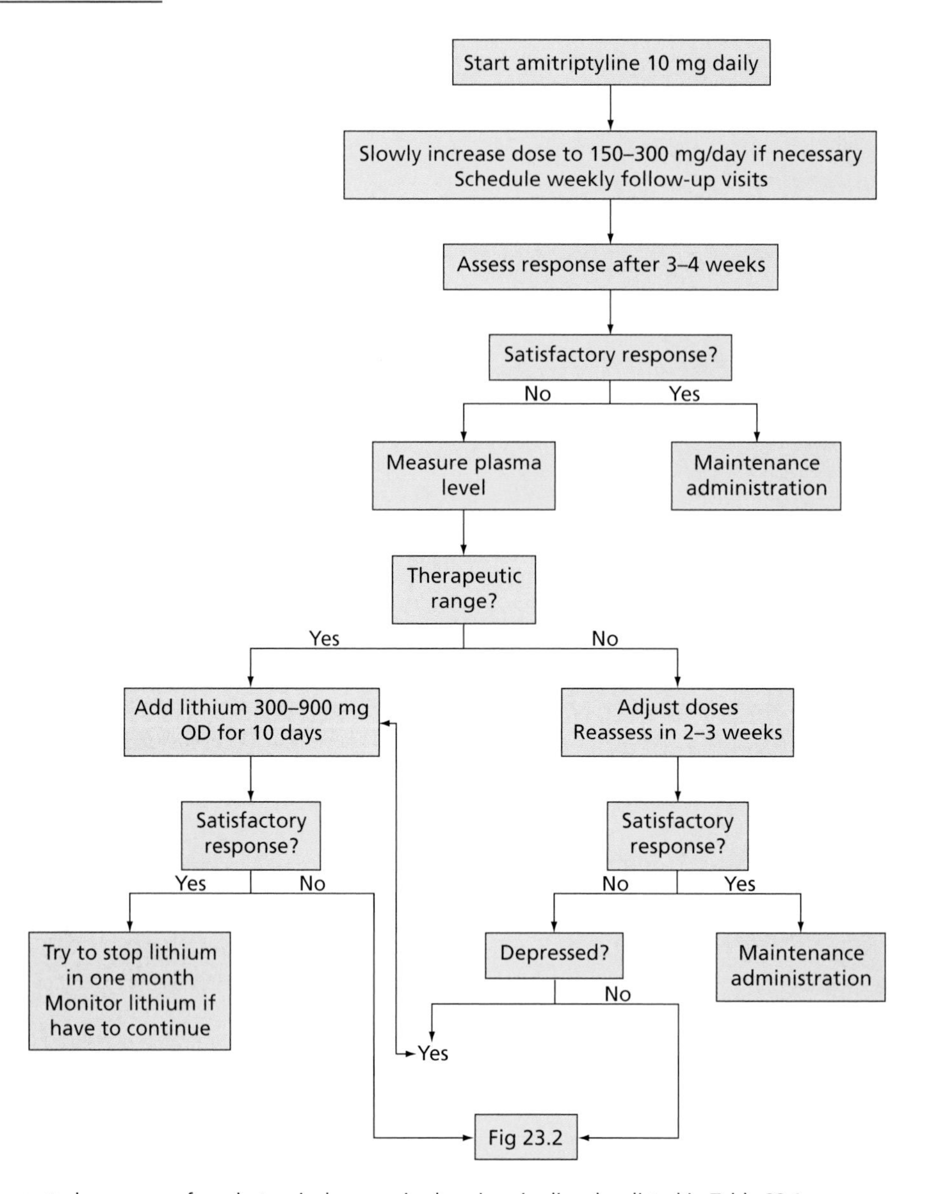

Fig 23.1 Suggested sequence of psychotropic drug use in chronic pain disorders listed in Table 23.1.

and increased by 10 mg, with total daily doses of 50–150 mg/day usually being adequate.

Initial parenteral TCAD administration for pain patients has been reported. A typical regimen would be clomipramine 25–50 mg/day intravenously for 3–5 days in hospital, then switching to usual oral doses.

Maintenance administration Certain patients require maintenance TCAD for months to years. In usual clinical practice, especially with higher initial doses, some slow reduction to lower maintenance levels may be possible 1 month after maximum therapeutic response has been obtained. After a further 3–6 months of remission, slow discontinuation of the drug may be tried as the patients are closely watched for relapse of pain and for depressive symptoms.

During maintenance therapy, a single daily evening dose of the more sedating TCAD may be used to improve compliance, decrease daytime adverse effects, and provide hypnotic effect. Patients vulnerable to nocturnal disorientation or postural hypotensive episodes may require continued divided doses.

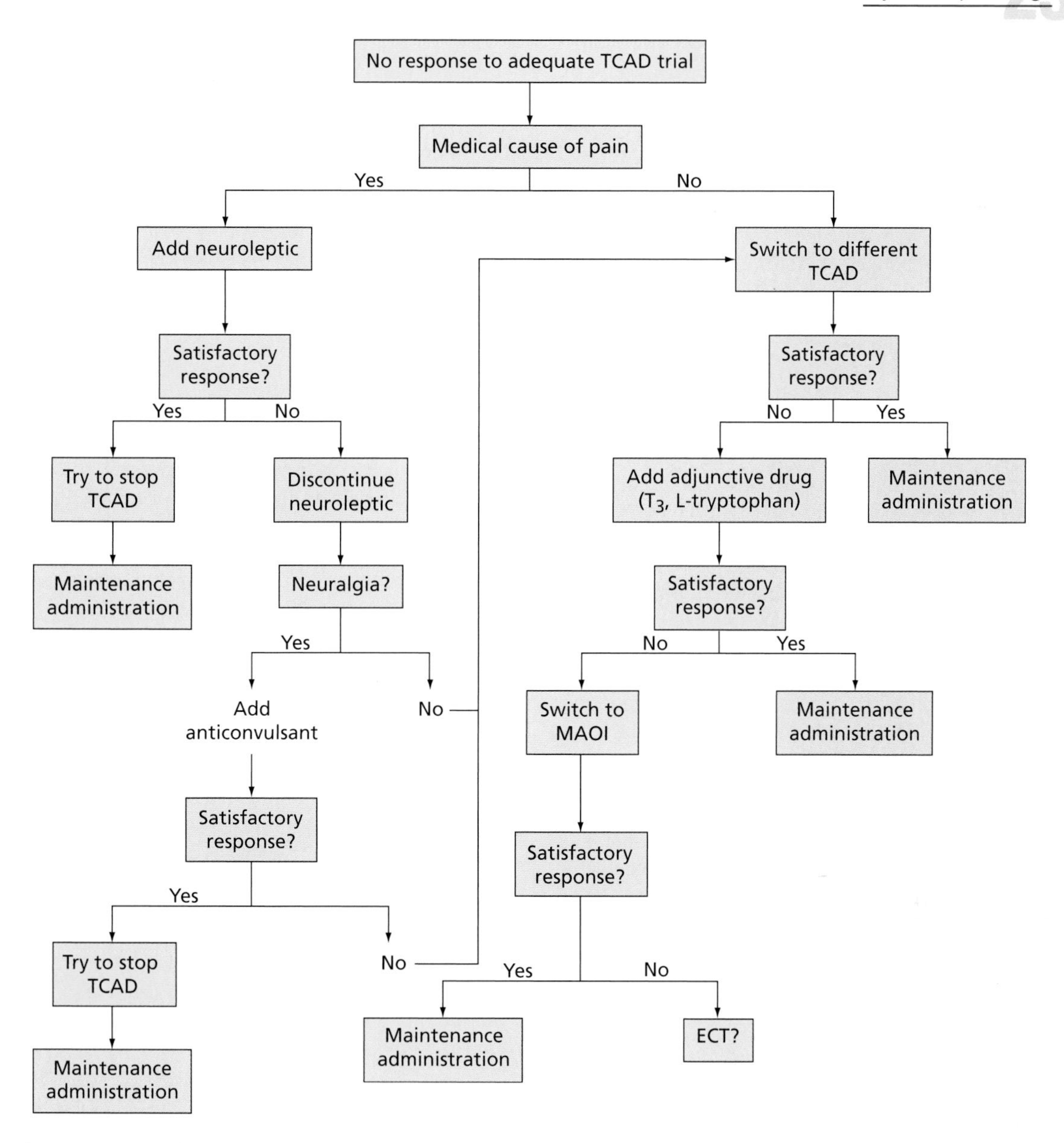

Fig 23.2 Suggested sequence of psychotropic drug use in chronic pain disorders listed in Table 23.1 (continued from Fig. 23.1).

Non-response or relapse Many instances of non-response are a result of poor compliance or an inadequate regimen. Careful preparation of patients, close initial follow-up, simplified, typed drug schedules, and the support of the family and or the primary physician are all important in increasing compliance.

In the case of non-response to an adequate trial of TCAD and where an alternative drug or non-drug therapy is unhelpful or unavailable, other strategies may be used:

1. Lithium potentiation If depression and chronic pain are present, lithium carbonate 300–900 mg/day may be added to the TCAD. If an antidepressant response is not seen within 10 days, lithium should be stopped and further alternatives considered (Fig. 23.2). If there is a satisfactory response, lithium may be discontinued after another month of therapy in a majority of persons (De Montigny et al 1981). Where there is an antidepressant but no analgesic response, additional therapy may be attempted (Fig. 23.2).

2. Alternate TCAD, SSRI, or other antidepressant In the obviously depressed patient, especially when depression is felt to be the primary disorder, a second therapeutic trial with a TCAD with different monoamine properties is initiated after tapering off the first TCAD over a period of 7–10 days. For example, if a more serotonergic drug was used first and failed, a drug with stronger noradrenergic effects (desipramine, imipramine, nortriptyline, or maprotiline) would be substituted and a second adequate trial instituted. If adverse effects prevent the use of the less selective TCAD, an SSRI (fluoxetine, paroxetine) or SNRI (venlafaxine) drug may be tried.

3. TCAD–neuroleptic combination For the patient with milder or no depressive symptoms, or where an obvious medical cause is present, an alternative approach would be to add a neuroleptic to the first TCAD regimen instead of switching to a second TCAD (Fig. 23.2, Table 23.5). In order to decrease adverse effects (Table 23.5), oral doses of fluphenazine 1–3 mg/day, haloperidol 0.5–5 mg/day, or perphenazine 4–16 mg/day are used. If one of these drugs is ineffective, if extrapyramidal adverse effects are a problem, or if more sedation is required, a low-potency neuroleptic such as levomepromazine (methotrimeprazine) 5–100 mg/day, chlorpromazine 25–100 mg/day, or pericyazine 5–100 mg/day may be used. The neuroleptic is started at the lowest dose listed above and stepped up by increments of this dose daily until a clear therapeutic effect or the maximum recommended dose is reached. If no therapeutic response is obvious by 2 weeks, the neuroleptic and then the TCAD are tapered off over 7–10 days each and discontinued. A different TCAD may then be tried (Fig. 23.2).

If the combination is effective, an attempt should be made to taper off the TCAD, as the neuroleptic alone may be adequate. If both drugs are necessary, it is worth trying to taper off the neuroleptic after 3 months of stable response as it may no longer be necessary. Otherwise, maintenance administration guidelines are those described for each drug group used alone.

4. TCAD–anticonvulsant combination Patients with neuralgias that are resistant to TCAD or a TCAD–neuroleptic combination may be aided by the addition of clonazepam 1.5–10 mg/day, carbamazepine 150–1000 mg/day, or valproic acid 200–600 mg/day to an adequate TCAD regimen. Because of frequent adverse effects, especially with TCAD–carbamazapine combinations, blood level monitoring of both drugs is advisable. Hospitalization of frail elderly patients during the initiation of therapy is advisable. If the combination is effective, attempt to taper off the TCAD after 3 months of stable response. Further maintenance administration guidelines are those for each drug group used alone. If there is no response, a different TCAD may be tried (Fig. 23.2).

5. Other alternatives The addition of an adjunctive drug, such as triiodothyronine (25–50 μg/day) to an adequate TCAD regimen, may produce an antidepressant response in a minority of depressives not responding to TCAD alone (Goodwin et al 1982). L-Tryptophan (2–4 g/day) may have some analgesic properties when used alone or with TCAD but further studies are needed (France and Krishnan 1988).

TCAD–SSRI combinations are occasionally used for the treatment of refractory depressions, and one pain trial found an amitriptyline–fluoxetine regimen superior to either drug alone for fibromyalgia (Goldenberg et al 1996). High plasma levels of the TCAD with increased risk for adverse effects may occur in such regimens.

For a patient with pain of psychological origin, especially in the presence of depressive symptoms, a trial with MAOI would be warranted following failed treatment with adequate trials of two different TCADs. Also, atypical depressive symptoms such as hypersomnia, increased appetite and weight, panics, phobias, and depersonalization may respond preferentially to MAOI (Liebowitz et al 1988). A washout period of 2 weeks between TCAD and MAOI trials is essential.

Finally, electroconvulsive therapy has been used successfully in a small number of drug-refractory pain patients with or without TCAD therapy (Lascelles 1966, Mandel 1975). It is likely this treatment is not indicated unless warranted by the clinical depression alone.

SSRI antidepressants

SSRI drugs and usual doses are listed in Table 23.4.

Precautions Baseline blood studies would include a haemogram and electrolytes. An electrocardiogram and liver function studies are prudent in patients with a history of cardiac or liver abnormalities. A baseline weight is advisable in the elderly.

Choice of drugs The same approach to choice as outlined under TCAD antidepressants is reasonable. Fluoxetine is helpful in lethargic patients, while paroxetine might offer some initial advantage in those with anxiety or psychomotor agitation.

Initial administration Fluoxetine is usually started at 10 mg (5 mg in the elderly) each morning to avoid insomnia. It is increased to 20 mg per day after 1–2 weeks if well tolerated and may be increased to 40 mg per day after a further 3 weeks if the results are inadequate and the drug is still tolerated. Higher doses often are required if obsessive–compulsive symptoms are prominent. Paroxetine doses and increases are similar, but the drug can be given any time of day. The speed of administration may have to be slowed if there is an increase in anxiety or jitteriness in the first 1–2 weeks. These usually diminish thereafter.

Non-response Alternative and augmentation strategies are outlined in the previous 'Antidepressants' section and in Figs. 23.1 and 23.2. SSRI should be tapered off over 1 week or so.

Maintenance The maintenance and initial doses are usually the same.

Monamine oxidase inhibitors

The characteristics of the irreversible mixed type MAO-A and MAO-B inhibitors, phenelzine and tranylcypromine, are listed in Table 23.4.

Precautions Because of potential adverse reactions and a narrower spectrum of antidepressant action, MAOI are usually reserved for TCAD-resistant chronic pain disorders. The MAOI should only be used with patients capable of following stringent restrictions of foods, beverages, and other medications, and not suffering from a variety of medical ailments (see 'Adverse Effects' above). The patient should be given a list of potentially dangerous items and a card to carry that details the drug and specific countermeasures for medical emergencies. Patients at risk of orthostatic hypotension should have lying and standing blood pressure monitored before and during initial treatment.

Maintenance administration Despite the absence of published data concerning MAOI and chronic pain, clinical experience suggests that the initial therapeutic and maintenance doses are of the same magnitude.

Non-response or relapse L-Tryptophan 0.5–1.0 g three times a day may be added to phenelzine in order to obtain improvement in patients with depression who have not responded sufficiently to the MAOI. There is evidence that this combination has a very potent antidepressant effect. One controlled trial found this combination superior to phenelzine or amitriptyline alone for fibromyalgia pain (Nicolodi and Sicuteri 1996). Once improvement appears, some side effects such as sluggish behaviour, slurred speech, and ataxia may also develop. These are easily dealt with by reduction of the dose of each drug (usually by about one-third).

Neuroleptics

Dosages for neuroleptics used in the treatment of chronic pain are listed in Table 23.5.

Table 23.5 Neuroleptic drugs used in the management of chronic pain

Drug	Oral dosage range (mg/day)	Anticholinergic potency	Orthostatic hypotension	Sedation potency	Extrapyramidal effects
Phenothiazines					
Chlorpromazine	25–500	High	High	High	Low
Fluphenazine	1–10	Low	Low	Low	High
Levomepromazine (methotrimeprazine)	15–100	High	High	High	Moderate
Pericyazine	5–200	High	High	High	Low
Perphenazine	8–64	Moderate	Moderate	Moderate	Moderate
Thioxanthenes					
Chlorprothixene	50–200	High	High	High	Low
Flupenthixol	0.5–2	Low	?None	Absent	High
Miscellaneous					
Haloperidol	0.5–10	Low	Low	Moderate	High

Precautions

As indicated, neuroleptics are best employed for pain associated with physical causes. In general, antidepressants should be considered before neuroleptics because, for the most part, they are better tolerated by patients and are much less prone to be associated with long-term complications such as TD. Baseline laboratory tests are identical to those for TCAD. A written informed consent is advisable, especially regarding the risk of TD.

Initial administration

The physician should familiarize herself with one or two of the neuroleptics and use them preferentially. There is no convincing evidence that one neuroleptic is more effective than another.

Among the low-potency neuroleptics, levomepromazine (methotrimeprazine) is a reasonable choice. This drug is started at 5–10 mg about 2–3 h before bedtime. This often enables a reduction to be made in the use of other night sedatives. If the medication is taken too near bedtime, the hypnotic effect will not occur for several hours and there may be morning drowsiness. If proven acceptable in the evening, enabling good sleep without waking from pain, the use of the medication may be extended to daytime with 2.5 mg taken three times a day. In general, it is not advisable to exceed 75–100 mg/day of levomepromazine (methotrimeprazine). Most adverse effects seem to occur above the 50-mg daily level. The same pattern of use may be applied with any of the other sedative phenothiazines, such as chlorpromazine or pericyazine, varying the dose with the potency of the individual medication.

High-potency neuroleptics are utilized for patients at risk from autonomic, anticholinergic, or sedative adverse effects, especially those on TCAD–neuroleptic combinations. Neuroleptics such as haloperidol or fluphenazine are started with a 1-mg oral test dose (0.25–0.5 mg in elderly) and, if tolerated, increased by 1 mg/day to the usual effective dose of 3–5 mg/day (0.5–2 mg/day in the elderly). If there is no response after 1 week, the drug is further increased by 1 mg/day, as tolerated, to effective or maximum dosage.

With either high- or low-potency neuroleptics, a therapeutic response should be seen within 2 weeks of maximum tolerable dosage; if not, the drug is tapered off and discontinued.

Maintenance administration

As with TCAD–neuroleptic combinations, intermittent (trimonthly) attempts should be made to lower and discontinue the neuroleptic in view of the risk of TD. A careful clinical examination and chart notation regarding involuntary movements should be made at each follow-up visit.

Lithium carbonate

Precautions

Lithium use for pain is contraindicated in the presence of certain medical conditions (renal tubular disease, myocardial infarction, myasthenia gravis, and cardiac conduction defects) and in early pregnancy. Patients must cooperate with regular blood tests and be capable of recognizing early signs of intoxication. Baseline investigations include serum creatinine and electrolytes, thyroid tests, haemogram, pregnancy test, urinalysis, 24-h urine volume, and creatinine clearance. Close monitoring of lithium blood levels is necessary for patients who are also taking drugs that may increase lithium levels, such as diuretics, carbamazepine, and various non-steroidal anti-inflammatory agents.

Initial administration

In studies reporting on the treatment of cluster headaches, lithium carbonate 300 mg was given orally on the first day and increased to 300 mg two or three times per day by the end of the first week (Ekbom 1974, Kudrow 1977, Mathew 1978). The dosage was adjusted according to clinical response, severity of side effects, and in order to keep weekly serum lithium levels between 0.5 and 1.2 mmol/l.

Maintenance therapy

Little data are available for episodic cluster headache beyond 2 weeks administration. In the chronic cluster group, maintenance periods of 16–32 weeks are reported with continuing improvement, despite lowered lithium dosages and mean serum levels (0.3–0.4 mmol/l).

Once maintenance dosage is achieved, lithium determinations may be performed less frequently (monthly, then trimonthly). Serum creatinine and thyroid stimulating hormone levels are repeated every 6 months. Creatinine clearance and 24-h urine volume are repeated each year. Other tests are undertaken if clinically indicated. After a 3- to 6-month symptom-free interval, lithium dosage may be tapered off and, if possible, discontinued.

Non-response or relapse

Most treatment failures were a result of intolerable adverse effects, despite serum lithium levels being less than 1.2 mmol/l. Some patients were able to continue with lower doses of lithium.

Table 23.6 Antianxiety drugs used in the management of chronic pain

Drug	Oral dosage range (mg/day)	Main indications
Alprazolam	0.75–6.0	Panics, anxiety, depression
Chlordiazepoxide	10–100	Generalized anxiety
Clonazepam	0.5–10	Panics, seizures, neuralgias, phantom pain
Clorazepate	7.5–60	Generalized anxiety
Diazepam	4–40	Generalized anxiety, muscle spasm
Lorazepam	1–6	Generalized anxiety
Oxazepam	30–120	Generalized anxiety

Antianxiety drugs

Benzodiazepine preparations used in the management of anxiety and pain are listed in Table 23.6.

Precautions

Patients should be educated to expect only short-term BDZ use. Alternative therapies for anxiety and muscle tension, such as behavioural cognitive techniques, should be started as soon as possible. Benzodiazepines should not be used for those subjects dependent on alcohol or other drugs. Baseline tests are only performed if clinically indicated, except for clonazepam, where a complete haemogram should be done.

Initial administration

Benzodiazepine choice, dose, and administration schedules are those used in the treatment of anxiety. Doses of BDZ in excess of diazepam 10–15 mg/day orally or its equivalent are seldom indicated.

After 3–4 weeks of therapy, BDZ are tapered off and withdrawn over 1–2 weeks. A longer period of withdrawal may be necessary for alprazolam, i.e., decrease by 0.125–0.25 mg every 4–7 days. Further brief, intermittent courses of BDZ may be used for exacerbations of the pain disorder.

In the rare instance where longer-term treatment is essential (e.g., phantom pain or chronic musculoskeletal pain unresponsive to other drug and non-drug approaches), BDZ use should be carefully monitored for the development of tolerance, cognitive disturbance, ataxia, depression, or unexpected escalation in pain complaints.

Conclusions

Antidepressants are indicated in most pain patients with clinically detectable depression. They may be useful in relieving pain-related problems such as anxiety, panics, and insomnia. They may help in the early stages of detoxification from narcotics and antianxiety–sedative drugs. They appear to have an analgesic effect in specific chronic pain states such as chronic osteo- and rheumatoid arthritis, diabetic neuropathy, fibromyalgia, migraine, head and face pain of psychological origin, postherpetic neuralgia, and chronic tension headaches. Further studies comparing antidepressants and anticonvulsants in neuropathic pain (McQuay et al 1996) and in chronic high-frequency migraine headache (Silberstein 1996) are needed. Tricyclic-type drugs remain the antidepressants of first choice for chronic pain. SSRI and MAOI may be useful where TCAD fail or are not advisable because of adverse effects. The SNRI antidepressant, venlafaxine, is a promising agent given some initial successes and a relatively benign adverse effect/drug interaction profile. More evidence is desirable.

Neuroleptics are the treatment of choice for delusional pain. They may be efficacious alone or in combination with TCAD for some types of chronic pain that are often resistant to other forms of therapy, i.e., arthritic pain, causalgias, neuralgias, neuropathies, phantom pain, and thalamic pain. Studies examining the use of novel neuroleptics in chronic pain are strongly recommended.

Lithium carbonate is effective in relieving chronic cluster headache and may prevent episodic cluster headache. Studies are needed to compare its use with calcium-channel blockers such as verapamil.

The benzodiazepines may be useful in the short-term management of acute or chronic pain, which is closely related to anxiety. Continuous benzodiazepine use for chronic pain is not recommended.

In general, with reasonable precautions, psychotropic regimens are well tolerated and acceptably free from important adverse effects.

References

Adelman LC, Adelman JU, Von Seggern R, Mannix LK 2000 Venlafaxine extended release (XR) for the prophylaxis of migraine and tension-type headache: a retrospective study in a clinical setting. Headache 40: 572–580

Adjan M 1970 Uber therapeutischen Beeinflussung des Schmerzsumptoms bei unheilbaren Tumorkranken. Therapie der Gegenwart 10: 1620–1627

Adly C, Straumanis J, Chesson A 1992 Fluoxetine prophylaxis of migraine. Headache 32: 101–104

Alcoff J, Jones E, Rust P, Newman R 1982 Controlled trial of imipramine for chronic low back pain. Journal of Family Practice 14: 841–846

Anthony M, Lance JW 1969 Monoamine oxidase inhibitors in the treatment of migraine. Archives of Neurology 21: 263–268

Ayd FJ 1979 Continuation and maintenance doxepin therapy: 10 years' experience. International Drug Therapy News 14: 9–16

Bartusch SL, Jernigan JR, D'Alessio JG, Sanders BJ 1996 Clonazepam for the treatment of lancinating phantom limb pain. Clinical Journal of Pain 12: 59–62

Beaver WT, Wallenstein SL, Houde RW et al 1966 A comparison of the analgesic effect of methotrimeprazine and morphine in patients with cancer. Clinical Pharmacology and Therapeutics 7: 436–446

Bendtsen L, Olesen J, Jensen R 1996 A non-selective (amitriptyline), but not a selective (citalopram), serotonin reuptake inhibitor is effective in the prophylactic treatment of chronic tension-type headache. Journal of Neurology, Neurosurgery and Psychiatry 61: 285–290

Bernard A, Scheuer H 1972 Action de la clomipramine (Anafranil) sur la douleur des cancers en pathologie cervico-faciale. Journal Francais d'Oto-rhino-laryngologie 21: 723–728

Bibolotti E, Borghi C, Pasculli E et al 1986 The management of fibrositis: a double blind comparison of maprotyline (Ludiomil chlorimipramine) and placebo. Clinical Trials Journal 23: 269–280

Black KJ, Sheline YI 1995 Paroxetine as migraine prophylaxis. Journal of Clinical Psychiatry 56: 330–331

Bloomfield S, Simard-Savoie S, Bernier J, Tétreault L 1964 Comparative analgesic activity of levomepromazine and morphine in patients with chronic pain. Canadian Medical Association Journal 90: 1156–1159

Blumer D, Heilbronn M 1981 Second-year follow-up study on systematic treatment of chronic pain with antidepressants. Henry Ford Hospital Medical Journal 29: 67–68

Boline PD, Anderson AV, Nelson C et al 1995 Spinal manipulation vs amitriptyline for the treatment of chronic tension-type headaches: a randomized clinical trial. Journal of Manipulative Physiological Therapeutics 18: 148–154

Bourhis A, Boudouresque G, Pellet W et al 1978 Pain infirmity and psychotropic drugs in oncology. Pain 5: 263–274

Bradley JJ 1963 Severe localized pain associated with the depressive syndrome. British Journal of Psychiatry 109: 741–745

Breivik H, Rennemo F 1982 Clinical evaluation of combined treatment with methadone and psychotropic drugs in cancer patients. Acta Anaesthetica Scandinavica 74: 135–140

Breivik H, Slørdahl J 1984 Beneficial effects of flupenthixol for osteoarthritic pain of the hip: a double blind cross-over comparison with placebo. Pain 2 (suppl): 52–54

Bronwell AW, Rutledge R, Dalton ML 1966 Analgesic effect of methotrimeprazine and morphine. Archives of Internal Medicine 111: 725–728

Buckley FP, Sizemore WA, Charlton JE 1986 Medication management in patients with chronic non-malignant pain: a review of the use of a drug withdrawal protocol. Pain 26: 153–165

Bussone G, Boiardi A, Merati B, Crenna P, Picco A 1979 Chronic cluster headache: response to lithium treatment. Journal of Neurology 221: 181–185

Carasso RL 1979 Clomipramine and amitriptyline in the treatment of severe pain. International Journal of Neuroscience 9: 191–194

Carette S, McCain GA, Bell DA, Fam AG 1986 Evaluation of amitriptyline in primary fibrositis: a double blind, placebo controlled trial. Arthritis and Rheumatism 29: 655–659

Caruso I, Sarzi Puttini PC, Boccassini L et al 1987 Double blind study of dothiepin versus placebo in the treatment of primary fibromyalgia syndrome. Journal of International Medical Research 15: 154–159

Castaigne P, Laplane D, Morales R 1979 Traitement par la clomipramine des douleurs des neuropathies périphériques. Nouvelle Presse Médicale 8: 843–845

Cavenar JO, Maltbie AA 1976 Another indication for haloperidol. Psychosomatics 17: 128–130

Cohen GL 1997 Protriptyline, chronic tension-type headaches, and weight loss in women. Headache 37: 433–436

Couch JR, Hassanein RS 1976 Migraine and depression; effect of amitriptyline prophylaxis. Transactions of the American Neurological Assocation 101: 1–4

Couch JR, Ziegler DK, Hassanein R 1976 Amitriptyline in the prophylaxis of migraine. Effectiveness and relationship of antimigraine and anti-depressant effects. Neurology 26: 121–127

Da Prada M, Kettler R, Burkard WP, Lorez HP, Haefely W 1990 Some basic aspects of reversible inhibitors of monoamine oxidase-A. Acta Psychiatrica Scandinavia (suppl 360): 7–12

Davidoff G, Guarracini M, Roth E, Sliwa J, Yarkony G 1987 Trazodone hydrochloride in the treatment of dysesthetic pain in traumatic myelopathy: a randomized double-blind placebo controlled study. Pain 29: 151–161

Davidson O, Lindeneg O, Walsh M 1979 Analgesic treatment with levomepromazine in acute myocardial infarction. Acta Medica Scandinavica 205: 191–194

Davis JL, Lewis SB, Gerich JE, Kaplan RA, Schultz TA, Wallin JD 1977 Peripheral diabetic neuropathy treated with amitriptyline and fluphenazine. Journal of the American Medical Association 238: 2291–2292

Daw JL, Cohen-Cole SA 1981 Haloperidol analgesia. Southern Medical Journal 74: 364–365

De Montigny C, Grunberg F, Mayer A, Deschenes JP 1981 Lithium induces rapid relief of depression in tricyclic antidepressant drug non-responders. British Journal of Psychiatry 138: 252–256

Desproges-Gotteron R, Abramon JY, Borderie J, Lathelize H 1970 Possibilités thérapeutiques actuelles dans les lombalgies d'origine névrotique. Rheumatologie 22: 45–48

Diamond S, Baltes BJ 1971 Chronic tension headache—treatment with amitriptyline—double blind study. Headache 11: 110–116

Dixon RA, Edwards RI, Pilcher J 1980 Diazepam in immediate post myocardial infarct period. A double blind trial. British Heart Journal 43: 535–540

Duke EE 1983 Clinical experience with pimozide: emphasis on its use in post herpetic neuralgia. Journal of the American Academy of Dermatology 8: 845–850

Duthie AM 1977 The use of phenothiazines and tricyclic antidepressants in the treatment of intractable pain. South African Medical Journal 51: 246–247

Eberhard G, Von Knorring L, Nilsson HL et al 1988 A double-blind randomized study of clomipramine versus maprotyline in patients with idiopathic pain syndromes. Neuropsychobiology 19: 25–34

Edelbroek PM, Linssen CG, Zitman FG et al 1986 Analgesic and antidepressant effects of amitryptyline in relation to its metabolism in patients with chronic pain. Clinical Pharmacology and Therapeutics 39: 156–162

Eija K, Pertti NJ, Tiina T 1996 Amitriptyline effectively relieves neuropathic pain following treatment of breast cancer. Pain 64: 293–302

Ekbom K 1974 Lithium vid kroniska symptom av cluster headache. Preliminart Meddelande Opuscula Medica (Stockholm) 19: 148–158

Ekbom K 1981 Lithium for cluster headache: review of the literature and preliminary results of long-term treatment. Headache 21: 132–139
Evans W, Gensler F, Blackwell B, Galbrecht C 1973 The effects of anti-depressant drugs on pain relief and mood in the chronically ill. Psychosomatics 14: 214–219
Farber GA, Burks JW 1974 Chlorprothixene therapy for herpes zoster neuralgia. Southern Medical Journal 67: 808–812
Fazio AN 1970 Control of postoperative pain: a comparison of the efficacy and safety of pentazocine, methotrimeprazine, meperidine and placebo. Current Therapeutic Research and Clinical Experimentation 12: 73–77
Feinmann C, Harris M, Cawley R 1984 Psychogenic facial pain: presentation and treatment. British Medical Journal 288: 436–438
Fernandez F, Frank A, Holmes VF 1987 Analgesic effect of alprazolam in patients with chronic organic pain of malignant origin. Journal of Clinical Psychopharmacology 7: 167–169
Fiorentino M 1967 Sperimentazione controllata dell'imipramina come analgesico maggiore in oncologia. Rivista Medica Trentina 5: 387–396
Fogelholm R, Murros K 1985 Maprotyline in chronic tension headaches: a double blind crossover study. Headache 25: 273–275
France RM, Krishnan KRR 1988 Psychotropic drugs in chronic pain. In: France RD, Krishnan KRR (eds) Chronic pain. American Psychiatric Press, Washington DC, pp 343–346
Frank RG, Kashani JH, Parker JC et al 1988 Antidepressant analgesia in rheumatoid arthritis. Journal of Rheumatology 15: 1632–1638
Freeman GW, Polansky M, Sondheimer SJ, Rickels K 1995 A double blind trial of oral progresterone, alprazolam, and placebo in the treatment of severe premenstrual syndrome. Journal of the American Medical Association 274: 51–57
Gade GN, Hofeldt FD, Treece GL 1980 Diabetic neuropathic cachexia. Journal of the American Medical Association 243: 1160–1161
Ganvir P, Beaumont G, Seldrup J 1980 A comparative trial of clomipramine and placebo as adjunctive therapy in arthralgia. Journal of International Medical Research 8 (suppl 3): 60–66
Gebhardt KH, Beller J, Nischik R 1969 Behandlung des Karzinomschmerzes mit Chlorimipramin (Anafranil). Medizinische Klinik 64: 751–756
Gerson GR, Jones RB, Luscombe DK 1977 Studies on the concomitant use of carbamazepine and clomipramine for the relief of post-herpetic neuralgia. Postgraduate Medical Journal 53 (suppl 4): 104–109
Gessel AH 1975 Electromyographic biofeedback and tricyclic anti-depressant in myofascial pain-dysfunction syndrome: psychological predictors of outcome. Journal of the American Dental Association 91: 1048–1052
Gingras M 1976 A clinical trial of Tofranil in rheumatic pain in general practice. Journal of International Medical Research 4 (suppl 2): 41–49
Goldenberg DL, Felson DT, Dinerman H 1986 A randomized controlled trial of amitriptyline and naproxen in the treatment of patients with fibromyalgia. Arthritis and Rheumatism 29: 1371–1377
Goldenberg D, Schmid C, Ruthazer R et al 1996 A randomized double-blind crossover trial of fluoxetine and amitriptyline in the treatment of fibromyalgia. Arthritis and Rheumatism 39: 1852–1859
Gomersall JD, Stuart A 1973 Amitriptyline in migraine prophylaxis. Changes in pattern of attacks during a controlled clinical trial. Journal of Neurology, Neurosurgery and Psychiatry 36: 684–690
Gomez-Perez FJ, Riell JA, Dies H et al 1985 Nortriptyline and fluphenazine in the symptomatic treatment of diabetic neuropathy. A double-blind cross-over study. Pain 23: 395–400
Gomez-Perez FJ, Rull JA, Aquilar CA et al 1996 Nortriptyline-fluphenazine vs carbamazepine in the symptomatic treatment of diabetic neuropathy. Archives of Medical Research 27: 525–529
Goodkin K, Gullion CM, Agras WS 1990 A randomized double-blind placebo controlled trial of trazodone hydrochloride in chronic low back pain syndrome. Journal of Clinical Psychopharmacology 10: 269–278
Goodwin RK, Prange AJ, Post RM, Muscettola G, Lipton MA 1982 Potentiation of antidepressant effect by L-triiodothyronine in tricyclic nonresponders. American Journal of Psychiatry 139: 34–38
Gourlay GK, Cherry DA, Cousins MF, Love BL, Graham JR, McLachlan MO 1986 A controlled study of a serotonin reuptake blocker, zimelidine, in the treatment of chronic pain. Pain 25: 35–52
Hackett G, Boddie HG, Harrison P 1987 Chronic muscle contraction headache: the importance of depression and anxiety. Journal of the Royal Society of Medicine 80: 689–691
Hackett TP, Cassem NH 1972 Reduction of anxiety in the coronary care unit: a controlled double blind comparison of chlordiazepoxide and amobarbital. Current Therapeutic Research 14: 649–656
Hakkarainen H 1977 Brief report, fluphenazine for tension headache; double blind study. Headache 17: 216–218
Halpern L 1982 Substitution-detoxification and the role in the management of chronic benign pain. Journal of Clinical Psychiatry 43: 10–14
Hameroff SR, Weiss JL, Lerman JC et al 1984 Doxepin effects on chronic pain and depression: a controlled study. Journal of Clinical Psychiatry 45: 45–52
Hanks GW, Thomas PJ, Trueman T, Weeks E 1983 The myth of haloperidol potentiation. Lancet ii: 523–524
Hatangdi VS, Boa RA, Richards EG 1976 Post herpetic neuralgia: management with antiepileptic and tricyclic drugs. In: Bonica JJ, Albe Fessard D (eds) Advances in pain research and therapy, vol 1. Raven, New York, pp 583–587
Hendler N, Cimini A, Terence MA, Long D 1980 A comparison of cognitive impairment due to benzodiazepines and to narcotics. American Journal of Psychiatry 137: 828–830
Hollister LE, Conley FK, Britt RH, Shuer L 1981 Long-term use of diazepam. Journal of the American Medical Association 246: 1568–1570
Hugues A, Chauvergne J, Lissilour T, Lagarde C 1963 L'imipramine utilisée comme antalgique majeur en carcinologie. Etude de 118 cas. Presse Médicale 71: 1073–1074
Iserson KV 1983 Parenteral chlorpromazine treatment of migraine. Annals of Emergency Medicine 12: 756–758
Jackson GL, Smith DA 1956 Analgesic properties of mixtures of chlorpromazine with morphine and meperidine. Annals of Internal Medicine 45: 640–652
Janowski EC, Janowski DS 1985 What precautions should be taken if a patient on an MAOI is scheduled to undergo anaesthesia? Journal of Clinical Psychopharmacology 5: 128–129
Jenkins DG, Ebbutt AF, Evans CD 1976 Imipramine in treatment of low back pain. Journal of International Medical Research 4 (suppl 2): 28–40
Johansson F, Von Knorring L 1979 A double-blind controlled study of a serotonin uptake inhibitor (zimelidine) versus placebo in chronic pain patients. Pain 7: 69–78
Judkins KC, Harmer M 1982 Haloperidol as an adjunct analgesic in the management of postoperative pain. Anaesthesia 37: 1118–1120
Kast EC 1966 An understanding of pain and its measurement. Medical Times 94: 1501–1513

Khatami M, Woody G, O'Brien C 1979 Chronic pain and narcotic addiction: a multitherapeutic approach—a pilot study. Comprehensive Psychiatry 20: 55–60
Khurana RC 1983 Treatment of painful diabetic neuropathy with trazodone. Journal of the American Medical Association 250: 1392
Kishore-Kumar R, Max MB, Schafer SC et al 1990 Desipramine relieves posherpetic neuralgia. Clinical Pharmacology and Therapeutics 47: 305–312
Kocher R 1976 Use of psychotropic drugs for treatment of chronic severe pain. In: Bonica JJ, Albe Fessard D (eds) Advances in pain research and therapy, vol 1. Raven, New York, pp 579–582
Kudrow L 1977 Lithium prophylaxis for chronic cluster headache. Headache 17: 15–18
Kudrow L 1978 Comparative results of prednisone, methylsergide and lithium therapy in cluster headache. In: Greene R (ed) Current concepts in migraine research. Raven, New York, pp 159–163
Kudrow L 1980 Analgesics and headache. In: The use of analgesics in the management of mild to moderate pain. Postgraduate Medical Communications, Riker Laboratories, Northridge, CA, pp 60–62
Kuipers RKW 1962 Imipramine in the treatment of rheumatic patients. Acta Rheumatologica Scandinavica 8: 45–51
Kvinesdal B, Molin J, Frøland A, Gram LF 1984 Imipramine treatment of painful diabetic neuropathy. Journal of the American Medical Association 251: 1727–1730
Laine E, Linguette M, Fossati P 1962 Action de l'imipramine injectable dans les symptômes douloureux. Lille Médicale 7: 711–716
Lance JW, Curran DA 1964 Treatment of chronic tension headache. Lancet i: 1236–1239
Landa L, Breivik H, Husebo S, Elgen A, Rennemo F 1984 Beneficial effects of flupenthixol on cancer pain patients. Pain 2 (suppl): S253
Langohr HD, Stöhr M, Petruch F 1982 An open and double-blind cross-over study on the efficacy of clomipramine (Anafranil) in patients with painful mono- and polyneuropathies. European Neurology 2: 309–317
Langohr HD, Gerber WD, Koletzki E, Mayer K, Schroth G 1985 Clomipramine and metoprolol in migraine prophylaxis: a double blind crossover study. Headache 25: 107–113
Lasagna RG, DeKornfeld TJ 1961 Methotrimeprazine. A new phenothiazine derivative with analgesic properties. Journal of the American Medical Association 178: 887–890
Lascelles RG 1966 Atypical facial pain and depression. British Journal of Psychiatry 122: 651–659
Leijon G, Boivie J 1989 Control post-stroke pain: a controlled trial of amitriptyline and carbamazepine. Pain 36: 27–36
Lewis TA, Solomon GD 1996 Advances in cluster headache management. Cleveland Clinic Journal of Medicine 63: 237–244
Liebowitz MR, Quitkin FM, Stewart JW et al 1988 Antidepressant specificity in atypical depression. Archives of General Psychiatry 45: 129–137
Lindsay PG, Wyckoff M 1981 The depression–pain syndrome and its response to antidepressants. Psychosomatics 22: 571–577
Loldrup D, Langemark M, Hansen HJ, Olesen J, Bech P 1989 Clomipramine and mianserin in chronic idiopathic pain syndrome. Psychopharmacology 99: 1–7
Lynch SA, Max MB, Muir J, Smoller B, Dubner R 1990 Efficacy of antidepressants in relieving diabetic neuropathy pain: amitriptyline vs desipramine, and fluoxetine vs placebo. Neurology 40 (suppl 1): 437
Macfarlane JG, Jalali S, Grace EM 1986 Trimipramine in rheumatoid arthritis: a randomized double-blind trial in relieving pain and joint tenderness. Current Medical Research and Opinion 10: 89–93
MacNeill AL, Dick WC 1976 Imipramine and rheumatoid factor. Journal of Internal Medicine Research 4 (suppl 2): 23–27
Magni G, Bertolini C, Dodi G 1982 Treatment of perineal neuralgia with antidepressants. Journal of the Royal Society of Medicine 75: 214–215
Maltbie AA, Cavenar JO 1977 Haloperidol and analgesia: case reports. Military Medicine 142: 946–948
Mandel MR 1975 Electroconvulsive therapy for chronic pain associated with depression. American Journal of Psychiatry 132: 632–636
Margolis LH, Gianascol AJ 1956 Chlorpromazine in thalamic pain syndrome. Neurology 6: 302–304
Martucci N, Manna V, Porto C, Agnoli A 1985 Migraine and the noradrenergic control of vasomotricity: a study with alpha-2 stimulated and alpha-2 blocker drugs. Headache 25: 95–100
Mathew NT 1978 Clinical subtypes of cluster headache and response to lithium therapy. Headache 18: 26–30
Max MB, Culnane M, Schafer SC et al 1987 Amitriptyline relieves diabetic neuropathy pain in patients with normal or depressed mood. Neurology 37: 589–596
Max MB, Schafer SC, Culnane M, Smoller B, Dubner R, Gracely RH 1988 Amitriptyline, but not lorazepam, relieves postherpetic neuralgia. Neurology 38: 1427–1432
Max MB, Kishore-Kumar R, Schafer SC et al 1991 Efficacy of desipramine in painful diabetic neuropathy: a placebo-controlled trial. Pain 45: 3–9
McDonald Scott WA 1969 The relief of pain with an antidepressant in arthritis. Practitioner 202: 802–807
McNairy SL, Maruta T, Ivnik RJ, Swanson DW, Ilstrup DM 1984 Prescription medication dependence and neuropsychologic function. Pain 18: 169–178
McQuay HJ, Moore RA, Wissen PJ et al 1996 A systematic review of antidepressants in neuropathic pain. Pain 68: 217–227
Melsom M, Andreassen P, Melsom H 1976 Diazepam in acute myocardial infarction: clinical effects and effects on catecholamine, free fatty acids and cortisol. British Heart Journal 38: 804–810
Merikangas KR, Merikangas JR 1995 Combination monoamine oxidase inhibitor and beta blocker treatment of migraine, with anxiety and depression. Biological Psychiatry 38: 603–610
Merskey H, Hester RN 1972 The treatment of chronic pain with psychotropic drugs. Postgraduate Medical Journal 48: 594–598
Minuck R 1972 Postoperative analgesia—combination of methotrimeprazine and meperidine as postoperative analgesic agents. Canadian Medical Association Journal 90: 1156–1159
Mitas JA, Mosley CA, Drager AM 1983 Diabetic neuropathic pain: control by amitriptyline and fluphenazine in renal insufficiency. Southern Medical Journal 76: 462–467
Mitsikostas DD, Ilias A, Thomas A, Gatzonis S 1997 Buspirone vs amitriptyline in the treatment of chronic tension-type headache. Acta Neurologica Scandinavica 96: 247–251
Monks, RC, Merskey H 1999 Psychotropic drugs. In: Wall P, Melzack R (eds) Textbook of pain, 4th ed. Churchill Livingstone, Edinburgh, pp 1155–1186
Monro D, Swade C, Coppen A 1985 Mianserin in the prophylaxis of migraine: a double-blind study. Acta Psychiatrica Scandinavica S320: 98–103
Montastruc JL, Tran MA, Blanc M et al 1985 Measurement of plasma levels of clomipramine in the treatment of chronic pain. Clinical Neuropharmacology 8: 78–82
Montilla E, Fredrik WS, Cass LJ 1963 Analgesic effect of methotrimeprazine and morphine. Archives of Internal Medicine 111: 91–94
Mørland TJ, Storli OV, Mogstead TE 1979 Doxepin in the prophylactic treatment of mixed 'vascular' and tension headache. Headache 19: 382–383

Munro A, Chmara J 1982 Monosymptomatic hypochondriacal psychoses. A diagnostic checklist based on 50 cases of the disorder. Canadian Journal of Psychiatry 27: 374–376
Nappi G, Sandrini G, Granella F et al 1990 A new 5-HT_2 antagonist (ritanserin) in the treatment of chronic headache with depression. A double-blind study vs amitriptyline. Headache 30: 439–444
Natelson BH, Findley TW, Policastro T et al 1996 Randomized double blind, controlled placebo-phase in trial of low dose phenelzine in the chronic fatigue syndrome. Psychopharmacology (Berlin) 124: 226–230
Nathan PW 1978 Chlorprothixene (Taractan) in post herpetic neuralgia and other severe chronic pain. Pain 5: 367–371
Nemeroff CB, DeVane CL, Pollack BG 1996 Newer antidepressants and the cytochrome P450 system. American Journal of Psychiatry 153: 331–320
Nicolodi M, Sicuteri F 1996 Fibromyalgia and migraine, two faces of the same mechanism, serotonin as the common clue for pathogenesis and therapy. Advances in Experimental Medicine and Biology 398: 373–379
Noone JF 1977 Psychotropic drugs and migraine. Journal of International Medical Research 5 (suppl 1): 66–71
Norregaard J, Danneskiold-Samsoe B, Volkmann H 1995 A randomized controlled trial of citalopram in the treatment of fibromyalgia. Pain 61: 445–449
Okasha A, Ghaleb HA, Sadek A 1973 A double-blind trial for the clinical management of psychogenic headache. British Journal of Psychiatry 122: 181–183
Onghena P, van Houdenhove B 1992 Antidepressant-induced analgesia in chronic non-malignant pain: a meta-analysis of 39 placebo controlled studies. Pain 49: 205–219
Paoli F, Darcourt G, Cossa P 1960 Note préliminaire sur l'action de l'imipramine dans les états douloureux. Revue Neurologique 102: 503–504
Parolin AR 1966 El tratamiento del dolor y la ansiedad en el carcinoma avanzado. El Medico Practico 21: 3–4
Patterson DR, Sharar SR, Carrougher GJ, Ptaceck JT 1997 Lorazepam as an adjunct to opioid analgesics in the treatment of burn pain. Pain 72: 367–374
Pearce JMS 1980 Chronic migraneous neuralgia, a variant of cluster headache. Brain 103: 149–159
Perry PJ, Pfohl BM, Holstad G 1987 The relationship between antidepressant response and tricyclic antidepressant plasma concentration. A retrospective analysis of the literature using logistic regression analysis. Clinical Pharmacokinetics 13: 381–392
Pheasant H, Bursk A, Goldfarb J et al 1983 Amitriptyline and chronic low back pain: a randomized double blind cross over study. Spine 8: 552–557
Pilowsky I, Hallett EC, Bassett DL, Thomas PG, Penhall RK 1982 A controlled study of amitriptyline in the treatment of chronic pain. Pain 14: 169–179
Pilowsky I, Soda J, Forsten C et al 1995 Out-patient cognitive-behavioural therapy with amitriptyline for chronic non-malignant pain: a comparative study with 6-month follow-up. Pain 60: 49–54
Polliack J 1979 Chronic recurrent headaches. South African Medical Journal 56: 980
Puttini PS, Cazzola M, Boccasini L et al 1988 A comparison of dothiepin versus placebo in the treatment of pain in rheumatoid arthritis and the association of pain with depression. Journal of International Medical Research 16: 331–337
Radebold H 1971 Behandlung chronischer Schmerzzustande mit Anafranil. Medizinische Welt 22: 337–339
Raferty H 1979 The management of post herpetic pain using sodium valproate and amitriptyline. Journal of the Irish Medical Association 72: 399–401
Rafinesque J 1963 Emploi du Tofranil à titre antalgique dans les syndromes douloureux de diverses origines. Gazette Médicale de France 1: 2075–2077
Raft D, Toomey T, Gregg JM 1979 Behavior modification and haloperidol in chronic facial pain. Southern Medical Journal 72: 155–159
Rani PU, Shobha JC, Rao TR et al 1996 An evaluation of antidepressants in rheumatic pain conditions. Anesthesia and Analgesia 83: 371–375
Raskin DE 1982 MAO inhibitors in chronic pain and depression. Journal of Clinical Psychiatry 43: 122
Roose SP, Glassman AH 1994 Antidepressant choice in the patient with cardiac disease: lessons from the Cardiac Arrhythmia Suppression Trial (CAST) Studies. Journal of Clinical Psychiatry (suppl A): 83–87
Sadove MS, Rose RF, Balagot RC, Reyes R 1955 Chlorpromazine in the management of pain. Modern Medicine 23: 117–120
Saper JR, Silberstein SD, Lake AE III, Winters ME 1994 Double-blind trial of fluxetine: chronic daily headache and migraine. Headache 34: 497–502
Saran A 1988 Antidepressants not effective in headache associated with minor closed head injury. International Journal of Psychiatry in Medicine 18: 75–83
Schick E, Wolpert E, Reichert A, Queisser W 1979 Neuroleptanalgesie mit einen hechpotenten Depotneuroleptikum zur Schmerztherapie bei metastasierenden Malignomen. Verhandlungen der Deutschen Gesellschaft fur Innere Medizin 85: 1113–1114
Sharav Y, Singer E, Schmidt E, Dionne RA, Dubner R 1987 The analgesic effect of amitriptyline on chronic facial pain. Pain 31: 199–209
Sherwin D 1979 A new method for treating 'headaches'. American Journal of Psychiatry 136: 1181–1183
Shrestha M, Hayes TE, Moreden J, Singh R 1996 Ketorolac vs chlorpromazine in the treatment of acute migraine without aura—a prospective randomized, double-blind trial. Archives of Internal Medicine 156: 1725–1728
Shukla R, Ahuja RC, Nag D 1996 Alprazolam in chronic tension type headache. Journal of the Association of Physicians of India 44: 641–644
Sigwald J, Bouttier D, Caille F 1959 Le traitement du zona et des algies zostériennes. Etude des résultats obtenus avec la levomepromazine. Thérapie 14: 818–824
Silberstein SD 1996 Divalproex sodium in headache: literature review and clinical guidelines. Headache 36: 547–555
Sindrup SH, Ejlertsen B, Frøland A, Sindrup EH, Brøsen K, Gram LF 1989 Imipramine treatment in diabetic neuropathy: relief of subjective symptoms without changes in peripheral and autonomic nerve function. European Journal of Clinical Pharmacology 37: 151–153
Sindrup SH, Gram CF, Skjold T et al 1990a Clomipramine vs desipramine vs placebo in the treatment of diabetic neuropathy symptoms: a double-blind crossover study. British Journal of Clinical Pharmacology 30: 683–691
Sindrup SH, Gram LF, Brosen K, Eshoj O, Mogensen EF 1990b. The selective serotonin reuptake inhibitor paroxetine is effective in the treatment of diabetic neuropathy symptoms. Pain 42: 135–144
Singh G 1971 Drug treatment of chronic intractable pain in patients referred to a psychiatry clinic. Journal of the Indian Medical Association 56: 341–345
Sjaastad O 1983 So-called 'tension headache'—the response to a 5-HT uptake inhibitor: femoxetine. Cephalgia 3: 53–60
Smoller B 1984 The use of dexamethasone suppression test as a marker of efficacy in the treatment of a myofascial syndrome with amitriptyline. Pain 2 (suppl): S250
Songer DA, Schulte H 1996 Venlafaxine for the treatment of chronic pain. American Journal of Psychiatry 153: 737

Stirman J 1967 A comparison of methomeprazine and meperidine as analgesic agents. Anesthesia and Analgesia 46: 176–180

Sumpton JE, Moulin DE 2001 Treatment of neuropathic pain with venlafaxine. Annals of Pharmacotherapy 35: 557–559

Swerdlow M, Cundill JG 1981 Anticonvulsant drugs used in the treatment of lancinating pain. A comparison. Anaesthesia 36: 1129–1132

Taub A 1973 Relief of post herpetic neuralgia with psychotropic drugs. Journal of Neurosurgery 39: 235–239

Taylor K, Rowbotham MC 1996 Venlafaxine hydrochloride and chronic pain. Western Journal of Medicine 165: 147–148

Taylor RG, Doku HC 1967 Methotrimeprazine: evaluated as an analgesic following oral surgery. Journal of Oral Medicine 22: 141–144

Theesen KA, Marsh WR 1989 Relief of diabetic neuropathy with fluoxetine. DICP. Annals of Pharmacotherapy 23: 572–574

Thorpe P, Marchant-Williams R 1974 The role of an antidepressant, dibenzepin (Noveril), in the relief of pain in chronic arthritic states. Medical Journal of Australia 1: 264–266

Turkington RW 1980 Depression masquerading as diabetic neuropathy. Journal of the American Medical Association 243: 1147–1150

Tyber MA 1974 Treatment of the painful shoulder syndrome with amitriptyline and lithium carbonate. Canadian Medical Association Journal 111: 137–140

Tyrer P 1976 Towards rational therapy with monoamine oxidase inhibitors. British Journal of Psychiatry 128: 354–360

Valdes M, Garcia L, Treserra J, De Pablo J, De Flores T 1989 Psychogenic pain and depressive disorders: an empirical study. Journal of Affective Disorders 16: 21–25

Ventafridda V, Bonezzi C, Caraceni A et al 1987 Antidepressants for cancer pain and other painful syndromes with deafferentation component: comparison of amitriptyline and trazodone. Italian Journal of Neurological Sciences 8: 579–587

Vrethem M, Thorell LH, Lindstrom T et al 1997 A comparison of amitriptyline and maprotiline in the treatment of painful polyneuropathy in diabetics and nondiabetics. Clinical Journal of Pain 13: 313–323

Ward NG, Bloom VL, Friedel RO 1979 The effectiveness of tricyclic antidepressants in the treatment of coexisting pain and depression. Pain 7: 331–341

Ward N, Bokan JA, Phillips M, Benedetti C, Butler S, Spengler D 1984 Antidepressants in concomitant chronic back pain and depression: doxepin and desipramine compared. Journal of Clinical Psychiatry 45: 54–59

Watson CPN, Evans RJ 1985 A comparative trial of amitriptyline and zimelidine in post-herpetic neuralgia. Pain 23: 387–394

Watson CPN, Evans RJ, Reed K, Merskey H, Goldsmith L, Warsh J 1982 Amitriptyline versus placebo in postherpetic neuralgia. Neurology 32: 671–673

Weis O, Sriwatanakul K, Weintraub M 1982 Treatment of post-herpetic neuralgia and acute herpetic pain with amitriptyline and perphenazine. South African Medical Journal 62: 274–275

Woodforde JM, Dwyer B, McEwen BW et al 1965 Treatment of post-herpetic neuralgia. Medical Journal of Australia 2: 869–872

Zeigler DK, Hurwitz A, Hassanein RS, Kodanaz HA, Preskorn SH, Mason J 1987 Migraine prophylaxis. A comparison of popranolol and amitriptyline. Archives of Neurology 44: 486–489

Zitman FG, Linssen ACG, Edelbroek PM 1984 Amitriptyline versus placebo in chronic benign pain: a double blind study. Pain 2 (suppl): S250

Chapter 24

Opioids

Catherine Sweeney and Eduardo Bruera

Introduction

Opioids are highly effective analgesics and they continue to be the mainstay in the management of pain for most patients with cancer. However, opioids are underutilized in the management of patients with moderate to severe cancer pain (Bruera et al 1989a, World Health Organization 1990, Cleeland et al 1994). Many factors contribute to the underuse of opioids (Table 24.1). Lack of education and inappropriate beliefs held by physicians and healthcare professionals have been identified as major factors limiting adequate pain management and opioid use (Von Roenn et al 1993, Cherny et al 1994).

In recent years there has been limited development of new opioids. However, significant progress has been made in understanding the mechanisms of action of opioids as well as in the development of slow release preparations, new routes of administration, and identification and management of side effects. This chapter addresses concepts of clinical pharmacology of these agents and their use in patients with pain.

Pharmacological aspects

Receptors

Endogenous opioid systems are complex (Herz et al 1993) and not fully understood. Three main distinct types of opioid receptors have been identified: μ,κ, and δ receptors. These are sometimes referred to as MOP, KOP, and DOP receptors (Pasternak 2001). Recently a new opioid-like receptor ORL-1 has been identified (Meunier et al 1995). Several opioid receptor subtypes have been proposed (Paul et al 1989, Traynor and Elliott 1993, Makman 1994). Recent work has identified a number of μ (MOP) receptor subtypes at a molecular level (Pasternak 2001). Incomplete tolerance between opioids could reflect relative selectivity of specific opioids for receptor subtypes.

Opioid receptors are glycoproteins and are found in cell membranes at multiple sites in the central nervous system and the periphery. Opioid receptors exist in many organ systems including the gastrointestinal tract, lungs, cardiovascular system, and the bladder (Lipman and Gautier 1997,

Table 24.1 Factors that contribute to under use of opioids

Physician factors	Patient factors	Other factors
Inadequate pain assessment	Under reporting of pain	Legal restrictions
Fear of addiction potential	Fear of addiction	Limited availability of preparations in some countries
Fear of side effects especially respiratory depression	Fear of side effects such as sedation	
Lack of education in the management of side effects such as technique of opioid rotation	Fear of loss of analgesic effects	
Lack of knowledge of appropriate dosing regimens	Cost of some preparations	
Fear of legal consequences		

Stein et al 1999). When an opioid binds to a receptor, an excitatory or inhibitory response may occur. This may be mediated by a change in the conformation of the receptor ion channel, and/or via a secondary messenger such as adenylyl cyclase (Grudt and Williams 1995).

Mechanisms of action

The activation of opioid receptors can inhibit transmission of pain impulses in the brain and spinal cord (Cesselin et al 1999, Stein et al 1999). Opioid receptors have also been demonstrated on peripheral sensory nerves, and endogenous opioid peptides have been shown to produce analgesia at a peripheral level (Stein et al 1993), with growing evidence that exogenous opioids may also work at this level (Kalso et al 1997, Stein et al 1997). In addition to direct effects, opioids can indirectly produce analgesia by modulating noxious stimuli via the descending inhibitory pathway (Lipman and Gautier 1997).

Classification of opioids

Over 20 different opioids are used in clinical settings. Some are naturally occurring (e.g., morphine, codeine), some are semisynthetic (e.g., diamorphine, buprenorphine), and some are synthetic (e.g., methadone, pethidine). Various systems have been used for the classification of opioids. Table 24.2 outlines a classification system that utilizes drug effect on the opioid receptor. From a practical point of view it is useful to categorize opioids as those used for mild to moderate pain (weak opioid) and those used for moderate to strong pain (strong opioid). In 1984 the World Health Organization first proposed a simple analgesic ladder for cancer pain that used this concept (Fig. 24.1) (World Health Organization 1996). Experience with this ladder in many countries around the world has demonstrated that the principle of escalating from non-opioid analgesia to opioids for use in moderate to severe pain is safe and effective.

Table 24.2 Drug effect on opioid receptors

Agonist	Agonist–antagonist	Partial agonist	antagonist
Morphine	Pentazocine	Buprenorphine	Naloxone
Diamorphine	Butorphanol	Naltrexone	
Hydromorphone	Nalbuphine		
Oxymorphone	Dezocine		
Oxycodone			
Hydrocodone			
Codeine			
Levorphanol			
Pethidine			
Fentanyl			
Sufentanil			
Alfentanil			
Methadone			
Proxyphene			
Loperamide			
Diphenoxylate			

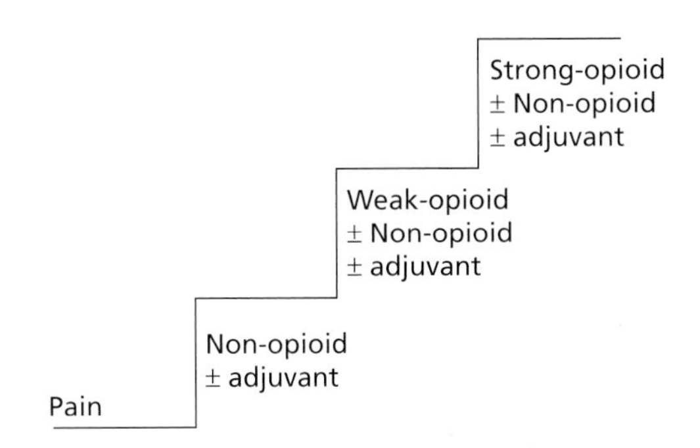

Fig. 24.1 Summary of WHO analgesic ladder.

Pharmacology of individual agents

Various opioid agents exhibit important pharmacological differences. These differences can be of clinical importance and convey advantages in certain situations and in individual patients. Table 24.3 summarizes some of the pharmacological properties of weak opioids. In the following paragraphs we will describe some key pharmacological aspects of some commonly used strong opioids.

Morphine

Morphine is a potent μ agonist. It is available in formulations for oral, rectal, parenteral, and spinal administration. It has good oral bioavailability but undergoes considerable first-pass metabolism in the liver. There is marked interindividual variation in bioavailability. The liver is the main site of morphine metabolism (Hasselstrom et al 1990), but metabolism also occurs in other organs (Mazoit et al 1987). The plasma half-life is approximately 2–3 h if renal function is normal. The duration of analgesia is usually 4–6 h. In patients on chronic therapy oral morphine is approximately 2–3 times less potent than parenteral morphine. The main metabolites of morphine are morphine-3-glucuronide (M3G) and morphine-6-glucuronide (M6G). Glucuronidation of morphine is not usually affected in patients with hepatic impairment; however, with severe hepatic failure the dose may need to be reduced or the interval between doses lengthened. Animal studies suggest that M3G may play a role in the development of opioid-induced neurotoxicity (OIN) (Labella et al 1979, Smith et al 1990). A recent analysis in patients on long-term morphine treatment indicates that elevated concentrations of morphine-3-glucuronide in plasma, as well as plasma and cerebrospinal fluid morphine-3-glucuronide/morphine-6-glucuronide ratios, may have a role in the development of OIN (Sjogren et al 1998). M6G is a potent opioid agonist and has significant opioid effects including analgesia in humans (Osborne et al 1986, 1988). M6G is excreted by the kidney and can accumulate in patients with renal impairment (Osborne et al 1986, D'Honneur et al 1994). High M6G concentrations have been associated with toxicity (Osborne et al 1986, Lehmann and Zech 1993). Other metabolites with central excitatory properties such as normorphone are produced in smaller proportions (approximately 4%). However, these metabolites can accumulate in patients receiving high doses of morphine or in those with renal impairment.

Hydromorphone

Hydromorphone is approximately 5 times more potent than morphine. It has similar pharmacokinetic and pharmacodynamic properties to morphine and can also be administered by the oral, rectal, parenteral, and spinal routes. There is wide interindividual variation in bioavailability. Single-dose studies suggest that the potency of parenteral hydromorphone is 5 times that of the oral preparation (Houde 1986). However, in patients on chronic therapy the equianalgesic oral dose is approximately twice that of the parenteral compound. Hydromorphone is available in preparations for oral and parenteral administration. Its good water solubility together with its high potency makes it particularly suitable for subcutaneous infusion.

Oxycodone

Oxycodone is a semisynthetic opioid agonist. It has high oral bioavailability. Its half-life is approximately 2–4 h and it is primarily excreted by the kidney. Maximum plasma concentrations increase in renal failure and can cause toxicity. Its principal metabolites are noroxycodone and oxymorphone. Oxymorphone has some analgesic activity but is present in low plasma concentrations, and the parent compound is considered to be the main analgesic (Heiskanen and Kalso 1997). Its analgesic effect is about the same as morphine but its higher oral bioavailability means that its oral potency is approximately 1.5–2 times that of oral morphine. Oral controlled release oxycodone is available in some countries.

Diamorphine

Diamorphine (heroin) is only available in the UK and Canada. It is a semisynthetic analogue of morphine and is a prodrug (Inturrisi et al 1984). Its metabolites monoacetylmorphine and morphine are the active analgesics. Orally it is approximately equipotent with morphine, however parentally it is approximately twice as potent (Kaiko et al 1981).

Table 24.3 Summary of pharmacological properties of weak opioids

Opioid	Potency	Analgesic effect	Main clinical uses	Main metabolites	Comments
Codeine phosphate	Approximately one-tenth that of morphine. Oral to parenteral potency 2:3.	μ agonist (low affinity). Metabolites may contribute to analgesic effect (Findlay et al 1978, Vree et al 2000).	Analgesia mild to moderate pain. Antitussive. Anti-diarrhoeal	Codeine-6-glucuronide. Lesser amounts of norcodeine, morphine and morphine-6-glucuronide. Morphine-3-glucuronide	Usually combined with a non-opioid analgesic. Usual dosing interval 4–6 h. Biotransformation to morphine impaired by drugs that interfere with microsomal P450 2D6 system or in slow metabolizers.
Hydrocodone	Potency approximately 6 times that of oral codeine.	codeine. Usual dosing active metabolites (Cone et al 1978)	Analgesia mild to moderate pain, Antitussive.	Hydromorphone, norcodeine, 6-β-hydrocodol, 6-α-hydrocodol.	Semisynthetic analogue of codeine. Usual dosing interval 4–6 h. Several active metabolites (Cone et al 1978)
Dextropropoxyphene	Potency half to two-thirds that of codeine.	μ agonist. NMDA agonist (Hewitt 2000).	Analgesia mild to moderate pain.	Norpropoxyphene	Synthetic derivative of methadone. Usual dosing interval 6–8 h. Extensive dose-dependent first-pass effect. Half-life may be >50 h in elderly patients (Crome et al 1984).
Tramadol	Parenterally one-tenth as potent as morphine. Orally one-fifth as potent as morphine.	Opioid effects. Non-opioid effects (Raffa et al 1993) stimulates serotonin release and inhibits presynaptic reuptake of serotonin and noradrenaline (norepinephrine).	Analgesia mild to moderate pain.	O-desmethyltramadol	Synthetic centrally acting. Less opioid side effects than morphine and less addiction potential. Usual dosing interval 4–6 h.

Diamorphine is more soluble than morphine and is favoured for subcutaneous use in the UK. Diamorphine does not have advantages over morphine when administered orally.

Fentanyl

Fentanyl is a semisynthetic opioid. It is a potent μ agonist and is used mainly intravenously as a perioperative analgesic agent and transdermally for the treatment of cancer pain. An oral transmucosal preparation also exists and is gaining popularity for use in the treatment of breakthrough pain. Transdermal fentanyl usually takes 12–24 h to produce an analgesic effect after its initiation; hence alternative breakthrough analgesia such as immediate release morphine is needed to cover this period. Patches are designed to provide analgesia for 72 h. If analgesia wears off before the end of a 72-h period the dose should be increased. In a small number of patients new patches need to be reapplied every 48 h. After discontinuation of transdermal fentanyl, serum concentrations gradually fall by approximately 50% in the first 17 h. The system is best suited to those patients with stable pain. Apart from the convenience afforded by the use of a patch, fentanyl is also potentially less constipating than other opioids (Hunt et al 1999). Transdermal fentanyl is not suitable for patients with unstable pain who need rapid titration of their analgesia. The rate of absorption of transdermal fentanyl increases in febrile patients and this can lead to toxicity. Patches should be applied to non-irritated, non-irradiated skin in a non-hairy area. The torso and upper arms are preferred areas and sites should be rotated. The patch may need to be secured in place with additional tape. The use of transdermal fentanyl is discussed further under principles of opioid use in cancer pain.

Meperidine (Pethidine)

Meperidine is a synthetic opioid agonist. Potential side effects limit its suitability for the treatment of cancer pain. Parenteral meperidine is 7–8 times less potent than parenteral morphine. The parenteral form is approximately 4 times more potent than the oral form. The duration of analgesia following a single dose is 2–4 hours. Meperidine is metabolized to normeperidine. Normeperidine is a CNS stimulant and can cause agitation, myoclonus, and convulsions (Szeto et al 1977, Eisendrath et al 1987). Accumulation occurs with repeated dosing, making these adverse effects more likely. In addition, meperidine can interact with MAO inhibitors to cause the potentially fatal serotonin syndrome (Inturrisi 1990).

Methadone

Methadone is a synthetic opioid agonist. In addition to opioid agonist activity, methadone has been found to be a relatively potent *N*-methyl-D-aspartate (NMDA) receptor antagonist (Ebert et al 1995, Gorman et al 1997). It is subject to considerable tissue distribution (Sawe 1986). The resulting peripheral reservoir sustains plasma concentrations during chronic treatment (Dole and Kreek 1973). Methadone is extensively metabolized in the liver to inactive metabolites via *N*-demethylation (Inturrisi et al 1987). In the United States methadone is available as methadone hydrochloride powder, which can be used for the preparation of oral, rectal, and parenteral solutions. In many countries methadone is commercially available in these formulations. It is generally available as a mixture of D-methadone and L-methadone (racemic form). In some countries such as Germany, L-methadone is available and its analgesic effect is approximately twice that of the racemic form (Nauck et al 2001). The oral bioavailability of methadone is generally high (Nilsson et al 1982, Gourlay et al 1986). Clearance is not significantly affected by renal impairment. It has a long unpredictable half-life. Administration every 8 h provides adequate analgesia for the majority of patients and extended dosing intervals of 12–24 h may be possible in a proportion of patients (Daeninck et al 1998). Although it has no active metabolites accumulation and toxicity can occur as a result of the long half-life in some patients.

Methadone is generally used as a second-line opioid in patients who have had poor analgesic response or experienced toxicity with other opioids (Bruera and Neumann 1999). It may offer additional benefit in patients with neuropathic pain due to its NMDA receptor activity.

Levorphanol

Levorphanol is a synthetic opioid agonist that is approximately 5 times more potent than morphine. It is well absorbed after oral administration. The parenteral form is twice as potent as the oral form. The half-life is 12–16 h and the duration of analgesia it produces is 4–8 h. Like methadone, accumulation can be a problem and it is usually used as a second-line opioid.

Naloxone

Naloxone is an opioid antagonist. It reverses the effect of opioid agonists and is used for treating opioid-induced respiratory depression. When given by the oral route it is rapidly metabolized in the liver and its oral-to-parenteral potency ratio is approximately 1:15. Oral naloxone can reverse opioid-induced constipation without antagonizing opioid analgesia (Kreek et al 1983, Culpepper-Morgan et al 1992, Sykes 1996, Meissner et al 2000). However some patients experience opioid withdrawal symptoms with this treatment.

Drug interactions

Interactions involving opioids are important and can result in either toxicity or undertreatment of pain. Table 24.4 outlines some potential interactions involving opioids.

Principles of opioid use in cancer pain

Over the past 15 years a number of organizations have focused on education of physicians regarding pain management and the use of opioids. Several bodies including the World Health Organization, the International Association for the Study of Pain, and the American Pain Society have produced excellent guidelines that use similar approaches for the management of cancer pain (American Pain Society 1992, International Association for the Study of Pain 1992, World Health Organization 1996).

Opioids are the most effective treatment for pain in cancer patients and should be considered for all cancer patients with moderate or severe pain. Pain syndromes in cancer patients are unique in their duration and intensity. There is no maximum recommended dose of morphine in cancer pain management. The individual patient's needs determine the appropriate dose. Side effects determine the maximum dose. Frequently, recommended doses of opioids are derived from single-dose studies and are not applicable in cancer pain (Brescia et al 1992). Pure opioid agonists used as a single agent are preferred for treating pain in cancer patients. Partial agonists and mixed agonist–antagonists have limited use in the management of cancer pain due to mixed receptor activity, side effects, and dose-related ceiling effects.

Choice of opioid

The selection of an opioid depends on patient and drug factors. The intensity of pain influences the initial opioid prescribed. Moderate pain is usually treated with a weak opioid and severe pain with a strong opioid according to steps 2 and 3 of the WHO ladder (Fig. 24.1). Weak opioids are often combined with non-opioid analgesics such as acetaminophen (paracetamol) or NSAIDs that may also influence the choice of compound to be used. In addition, prior exposure and response to opioids should help to determine the choice of opioid. Boxes 24.1 and 24.2 summarize approaches to the management of moderate and severe pain in cancer patients who are opioid naïve. If a weak opioid has not provided adequate analgesia a strong opioid should be prescribed rather than another weak opioid or a combination of weak opioids. If side effects or toxicity do not limit the dose of the current opioid the dose should be increased. Box 24.3 summarizes an approach to management of opioid tolerant patients with poorly controlled pain.

Table 24.4 Potential interactions involving opioids

Opioid	Drug	Interaction	Reference
All opioids	Alcohol, CNS depressants	Sedative effects	(Inturrisi 1990)
Morphine	Benzodiazepines	Antagonize analgesic effects Sedation	(Gear et al 1997) (Bernard and Bruera 2000)
	Antidepressants	Increased bioavailability	
	Rifampacin	Increased metabolism—reduced effect	
Methadone	Fluvoxamine, ketoconazole	Inhibition of clearance—increased effect	(Iribarne et al 1998, Bernard and Bruera 2000)
	Macrolides, ciprofloxacin		(Herrlin et al 2000)
	Rifampacin, corticosteroids	Increased metabolism—reduced effect	(Bernard and Bruera 2000)
	Phentytoin, carbamazepine		(Schlatter et al 1999)
Fentanyl	Macrolides, cimetidine	Inhibition of clearance—increased effect	(Bernard and Bruera 2000)
Meperidine	MAO inhibitors	Serotonin syndrome	(Bernard and Bruera 2000)
	Phenytoin, phenobarbital	Increased metabolism—accumulation of normeperidine	(Stambaugh et al 1977)

BOX 24.1
Opioid treatment of mild to moderate pain in opioid naïve patients

1. A combination of a non-opioid with a weak opioid can be used, such as acetaminophen (paracetamol) 500 mg 1–2 tablets q4h around the clock (atc) (maximum 4 g/day) and codeine 30 mg 1–2 tablets q4h atc with 1 tablet q2h prn for breakthrough pain. Where a compound formulation is available this can be more convenient for the patient as it reduces the number of tablets that have to be taken.
2. Antiemetic and laxative regimens should be commenced. A prokinetic agent such as metoclopramide is usually effective when given regularly around the clock with breakthrough doses as needed for the first 3 days and prn thereafter. A combination of two contact (stimulant) laxatives such as sennoside (senna) and docusate is commonly used in cancer patients.
3. The patient should be frequently assessed for response and side effects.

BOX 24.2
Opioid treatment of moderate to severe pain in opioid naïve patients

1. Commence a strong opioid such as:

Morphine 10 mg po (5 mg IV/sc) q4h atc and 5 mg po (2.5 mg IV/sc q2h prn for breakthrough pain

or

Hydromorphone 2 mg po (1 mg IV/sc) q4h atc and 1 mg po (0.5 mg IV/sc) q2h for breakthrough pain

or

Oxycodone 5 mg po q4h atc and 5 mg po q2h for breakthrough pain.

2. Commence antiemetic and laxative regimen as above.
3. Assess frequently for response and side effects.
4. After 24–48 h assess opioid use and increase the q4h dose as necessary so that the new daily total in regular medication is equivalent to the regular and prn dose for the previous 24 h. Continue to provide prn medication for breakthrough pain.
5. Continue the regimen as long as it is needed and effective.
6. Add adjuvant or non-opioid analgesic as needed

Coexisting disease such as renal impairment will influence the choice of opioid. Patients with renal impairment are at risk of accumulating the active metabolites of a number of opioids including morphine, meperidine (pethidine), and dextropropoxyphene (Chan and Matzke 1987, Portenoy et al 1991). There is evidence to suggest that these active metabolites may lead to toxicity (Hagen et al 1991, Ashby et al 1997).

BOX 24.3
Management of opioid tolerant patient with poorly controlled pain

1. Assess patient; is there a new source of pain or worsening of pre-existing pain?
2. Find out the patient's previous response to and side effects with opioids (avoid those that have not been effective or produced troublesome side effects).
3. Determine total opioid daily dose (atc + prn) and increase by 30%. Divide the increased dose over the q4h dose and q2h prn breakthrough dose.
4. Continue antiemetic and laxative regimens, titrating or changing as needed.
5. Continue adjuvant or non-opioid analgesic as needed.
6. Assess response and side effects frequently.
7. Increase opioid dose (as described above) if necessary until satisfactory pain relief is obtained or side effects or toxicity prevent further increases.
8. Treat side effects or toxicity and consider dose change or rotation to another opioid.

Choice of administration route

Oral administration is a convenient and effective way of delivering most opioids. It is the route of choice in cancer patients unless there is a contraindication to oral intake. The parenteral route produces a shorter time to onset of activity and peak levels in the serum. However, this should not be an issue when oral doses are delivered regularly around the clock and opioid levels are kept above the threshold needed for pain control. Rectal route should be considered when the oral route is not appropriate. Routes of administration are discussed later in the chapter.

Administer around the clock

In patients with ongoing nociceptive input regular around-the-clock (atc) dosing allows the maintenance of effective serum concentrations of opioids. The aim is to prevent recurrence of pain by maintaining adequate analgesia. Long-acting and slow release (SR) opioids offer the advantage of extended dose intervals. Long-acting opioids such as methadone

Table 24.5 Potential advantages and disadvantages of SR opioids as compared to immediate release (IR) preparations

Potential advantages	Potential disadvantages
Convenient extended dosing intervals	In opioid naïve patients initial dosing with IR opioid allows more rapid and safer titration
Improved compliance	Unstable pain may be difficult to manage and change to IR opioids may be necessary Patients with renal insufficiency at greater risk of accumulation Significantly more expensive

and levorphanol can be given at 8- to 12-h intervals in the majority of patients, but they carry the risk of accumulation and patients should be monitored for signs of increasing sedation and respiratory depression. Table 24.5 summarizes the advantages and disadvantages of SR opioid preparations. Patients with good pain control and stable opioid dose with minimal breakthrough dosing are generally suitable candidates for a change from an immediate release (IR) to a sustained release (SR) opioid preparation (Box 24.4). Patients who are on a SR preparation and are experiencing unstable pain or opioid toxicity or develop renal insufficiency may need to be changed to an IR preparation. This can be done by calculating the 24-h dose of the SR opioid and basing the q4h atc and q2h prn doses on this daily total. The IR is started when the next SR dose would have been due (12 or 24 h). Availability of adequate breakthrough dosing is particularly important during the change-over. Transdermal fentanyl is a slow-onset long-lasting opioid delivery system. It offers convenience but is not suitable for patients with uncontrolled pain. An approach for change from another opioid to transdermal fentanyl is outlined in Box 24.5.

Titrate the dose to the individual's needs

Individualized care involving titration of the opioid according to response is the best way to ensure optimal treatment for each patient. Patients may also require rescue doses of opioid for breakthrough pain. This is especially important in those who are commencing opioids or rotating from one opioid to another. It is important when using compound preparations of weak opioids with

BOX 24.4

Changing from an immediate release (IR) opioid to a sustained release (SR) preparation

1. Calculate the total 24-h opioid dose (i.e., atc +prn).
2. The same equivalent daily dose of SR opioid is prescribed. This is divided into 2 doses for q12h medication or the total is given as a single dose for q24h preparations.
3. The first dose is given 4 h after the last IR dose
4. If available, an immediate release preparation of the same opioid should be prescribed for breakthrough pain at 10% of the total daily opioid dose.
5. Continue antiemetic and laxative regimens.
6. Assess for response and side effects frequently.

BOX 24.5

Changing from another opioid to transdermal fentanyl q72h

1. Calculate the 24-h dose of the current opioid (atc+prn).
2. Calculate the equianalgesic parenteral morphine dose using Tables 24.6 and 24.7.
3. Calculate the equivalent transdermal fentanyl dose (Table 24.8).
4. Continue the previous opioid for the first 12–18 h after initiation of treatment
5. Prescribe breakthrough dosing of an immediate release opioid. For oral morphine the dose should be half the patch strength in mg (e.g., fentanyl 100 μg use morphine IR 50 mg)
6. Increase the patch strength depending on the additional amount of opioid needed during the first 72 h.

Changing from transdermal fentanyl to an immediate release opioid

1. Calculate the 24-h parenteral morphine dose equivalent of Fentanyl and prn medication using.
2. Calculate the equivalent 24-h dose of the new opioid.
3. Calculate the scheduled atc dose and breakthrough dose of the new opioid.
4. Start the new opioid 12 h after removal of the fentanyl patch as there is a reservoir in the skin that results in significant blood levels persisting for at least 12–24 h.

acetaminophen or NSAIDs to not exceed the maximum daily dose of the non-opioid component. Rescue doses of morphine are usually calculated as one-half of the scheduled 4-h dose and are given every 2 h as needed. For patients on a sustained release opioid an immediate release opioid at 10% of the daily opioid SR dose is prescribed for use every 2 h as needed. Recent research using transmucosal fentanyl for breakthrough pain has found that effective rescue doses can range from 5 to 20% of the daily dose and may need titration by a process similar to that used for the regular opioid dose (Christie et al 1998). In general it is recommended that the same opioid be used for both atc and breakthrough dosing, although this is not always possible. Box 24.3 summarizes an approach to upwards titration of an opioid dose. If the patient's pain does not improve with progressive escalation of opioid medication other confounding factors, such as pain syndromes less responsive to opioids, psychological distress, somatization, and chemical coping, should be considered.

Adjuvant drugs

Adjuvant drugs should be considered for managing specific pain syndromes that have an incomplete response to opioids. In addition, adjuvant drugs can allow for a reduction in opioid dose in patients with troublesome side effects. Table 24.9 summarizes adjuvant drugs commonly used in the management of patients with pain (see Chaps. 23, 42–45). Other treatment modalities that produce analgesia such as radiation therapy, radioisotope administration, and orthopedic surgery should be considered in suitable cancer patients.

Opioid rotation

In patients with uncontrolled pain despite high opioid doses, in those where escalation to very high doses makes administration difficult, or when tolerance or toxicity develops, rotation to an alternative opioid may be indicated (Mercadante 1999). Several studies have shown that opioid rotation is a safe and effective method for reducing toxicity and at the same time retaining analgesia (MacDonald et al 1993, Sjogren et al 1994a, Bruera et al 1995a, de Stoutz et al 1995, Mercadante et al 2001). Differences in analgesic and adverse effects following opioid rotation are thought to be the result of a number of mechanisms, including receptor activity, asymmetry in cross-tolerance among different opioids, different opioid efficacies, and accumulation of toxic metabolites (Mercadante 1999). Box 24.6 outlines the principles of opioid rotation.

BOX 24.6
Principles of opioid rotation

1. Calculate the total daily dose of the opioid.
2. Calculate the equivalent daily dose of the new opioid using equianalgesic dose ratios such as those in Table 24.6.
3. Reduce the new opioid dose by 30–50% to allow for incomplete cross-tolerance between opioids.
4. Calculate the regular atc dose of the new opioid using the appropriate dosing interval.
5. Prescribe dose for breakthrough pain.
6. Assess for response and side effects frequently.

Opioid rotation to methadone

Methadone has unique advantages when compared to other opioids including combined opioid and NMDA antagonistic analgesic effects, excellent oral bioavailability (50–100%), extremely low cost (20–30 times lower than other opioids), and absence of active metabolites. However, it presents a unique situation with regard to opioid rotation. Large interindividual variations exist in the equianalgesic ratio of methadone to other opioids The equianalgesic dose ratio varies dramatically depending on the extent of previous exposure to opioids (Lawlor et al 1998, Ripamonti et al 1998, Pereira et al 2001). Methadone becomes relatively more powerful with increasing prior exposure to other opioids and can be up to 10 times more potent in patients given greater than 500 mg per day of morphine than in patients given less than 100 mg per day (Ripamonti et al 1998). This large variation prevents the use of simple equianalgesic tables to calculate the required dose of methadone. The process of switching from another opioid agonist to methadone is complex and should be attempted only by physicians who are experienced in cancer pain management. Even when methadone is administered by experienced physicians serious toxicity can occasionally occur (Oneschuk and Bruera 2000). Contrary to what would be expected with other opioids, toxicity appears to occur more frequently in patients previously exposed to high doses of opioids than in patients who have received low doses. A number of strategies for rotating to methadone from other opioids have been employed by various groups (Mercadante et al 1999, 2001; Bruera et al 2000a; Nauck et al 2001). The best method for rotation to methadone has not yet been determined.

Educate the patient regarding addiction, tolerance, and side effects

Many patients and their families have fears that being exposed to opioids will cause addiction.

Patients should be reassured that development of addiction is very rare in patients treated with opioids for pain (World Health Organization 1990, American Pain Society 1992). Patients should also be reassured that opioids will not lose their effect and that doses can be increased in the future should their pain worsen. Education regarding common side effects and their management should be given to patients. If appropriate counselling is not given to patients and their families compliance may be limited.

Consider opioids as only one part of the overall management plan

Prior to commencing a patient on an opioid or to changing the type or dose of opioid for poor pain control an evaluation of the patient with respect to physical, social, and psychological factors is of great importance (see Chap. 46). Assessing the pain and putting it in the context of the patient allows for appropriate management of the patient. A multidimensional assessment allows identification of factors prognostic for poor pain control, including neuropathic pain, incidental pain, psychological distress, cognitive impairment, and history of alcohol or drug abuse.

Ongoing assessment should take place at regular intervals, when pain changes (worsens or new pain develops) and when treatment is changed. Good pain assessment allows the factors contributing to pain in an individual patient to be identified and addressed. Prescribing may be rationalized, pain syndromes may be identified and appropriate adjuvant medication commenced, and confounding factors such as depression or anxiety may be identified, allowing appropriate treatment. This approach is important in maximizing analgesia and preventing toxicity from opioids.

Chronic non-malignant pain

In patients with non-malignant chronic pain the use of opioids is not as clearly defined and is somewhat controversial. Fear of side effects, opioid abuse, and addiction has prevented systematic research of opioid use in chronic non-malignant pain. There is evidence to support the use of opioids in some chronic pain patients (France et al 1984, Portenoy and Foley 1986, Zenz et al 1992).

Failure of non-opioid and other analgesic approaches should be carefully documented before proceeding to an opioid trial. Prior to commencing a patient with chronic non-malignant pain on opioid medication, a detailed assessment of the patient should be performed. This includes detailed pain and psychosocial history and physical examination. Opioids should be prescribed with great caution in patients with a history of substance abuse, personality disorder, or psychiatric conditions. Goals of treatment such as improved function or level of pain reduction should be agreed prior to commencing treatment. An initial trial of opioid for a predetermined period of the time should be agreed with the patient. Unacceptable behaviour such as drug-seeking behaviour should be discussed. A written contract is used by some groups to document agreed terms for treatment. Ideally a single physician should prescribe opioids for the patient. Continuation of opioid treatment after the initial period should only be considered if predetermined goals have been met. Regular ongoing review of the patient is important.

Acute pain

Use of opioids in the acute pain situation such as postoperative pain, pain after injuries, or pain in acute medical conditions differs from that in cancer patients and in those with chronic pain. In patients with acute pain, opioids are often administered parenterally and the duration of use is frequently limited to days as the cause of pain usually resolves. Consequently, the approach to opioid use outlined above does not apply in these situations. In patients with postoperative pain, patient-controlled analgesia is commonly used. This treatment modality is less suitable for the long-term treatment of chronic pain.

Routes of administration

In addition to oral administration, opioids can be effectively delivered by several other routes. Table 24.10 summarizes traditional and emerging routes of opioid administration. In most patients with cancer pain or chronic non-malignant pain the oral route is appropriate. However, approximately 70% of cancer patients will require an alternative route for opioid delivery before death (Coyle et al 1986, Bruera 1990). In patients with acute pain, parenteral administration is most commonly used. Opioids vary in potency depending on whether oral or parenteral route is used. Table 24.7 summarizes the oral to parenteral conversion ratios of some commonly used opioids.

Table 24.6 Equianalgesic ratios of various opioids to morphine[a]

Opioid	Parenteral opioid to parenteral morphine	Parenteral morphine to parenteral opioid	Oral opioid to oral morphine	Oral morphine to oral opioid
Hydromorphone	5	0.2	5	0.2
Pethidine (meperidine)	0.13	8	0.1	10
Levorphanol	5	0.2	5	0.2
Oxycodone	–	–	1.5	0.7
Codeine	–	–	0.15	7
Hydrocodone	–	–	0.15	7

[a]To get equivalent dose multiply by conversion factor in table.

Table 24.7 Conversion between oral and parenteral opioids[a]

Opioid	From parenteral to oral	From oral to parenteral
Morphine	2.5	0.4
Hydromorphone	2	0.5
Meperidine (pethidine)	4	0.25
Levorphanol	2	0.5

[a]Calculate the total amount of opioid used in 24 h, multiply by appropriate conversion factor, and divide into the number of doses/day.

Table 24.8 Recommended transdermal fentanyl dose based on daily parenteral morphine dose

Daily parenteral morphine dose (mg)	Transdermal fentanyl dose (μg/h)
8–22	25
23–37	50
38–52	75
53–67	100
68–82	125
83–97	150

Oral route

Oral administration of opioids is preferred in cancer patients and in those with chronic non-malignant pain. The onset of action is slower following oral than parenteral administration. This is not usually a problem in patients who are taking opioids at appropriate regular intervals as opioid

Table 24.9 Adjuvant drugs used in the management of cancer pain

Drugs	Etiology of pain/Indication
Tricyclic antidepressants	Neuropathic pain
Anticonvulsants	Neuropathic pain
Selective serotonin reuptake inhibitors	Neuropathic pain
Oral local anaesthetic drugs	Neuropathic pain
Corticosteroids	Multiple
NMDA receptor antagonists	Multiple
Psychostimulants	Multiple/opioid-induced sedation
Bisphosphonates	Bone pain
Antibiotics	Tissue damage due to infection
Muscle relaxants	Muscle spasm

Table 24.10 Routes of opioid administration

Traditional routes	Emerging routes
Oral	Sublingual
Rectal	Transmucosal
Subcutaneous	Inhalational
Transdermal	Nasal
Intravenous	
Intrathecal/epidural	

plasma concentrations should not fall below the threshold needed for analgesia. Oral administration is not suitable for patients who cannot swallow or have gastrointestinal obstruction. In some patients with severe pain who require rapid onset of analgesia parenteral administration may be more appropriate.

Rectal route

A number of opioids are effectively absorbed when administered rectally as suppositories or in liquid solution (Ripamonti and Bruera 1991, Bruera and Ripamonti 1992, Bruera et al 1995b, De Conno et al 1995, Ripamonti et al 1995). The bioavailability of rectally administered opioids can vary depending on how much of the drug is absorbed into the portal or systemic circulation. The same dose is usually given rectally as orally but may need some subsequent adjustment. The need for frequent rectal administration of immediate release opioids is a disadvantage. In addition, the insufficient strength of commercially available preparations is a limitation of the rectal route. Custom-made suppositories of methadone are a cheap and simple technique for the administration of a wide range of doses of methadone (Bruera et al 1995b). In countries where suppositories are not available methadone hydrochloride solution can be administered as a microenema (Ripamonti et al 1995). Sustained release morphine suppositories have also been found to be comparable to subcutaneous morphine for analgesia in patients with cancer pain (Bruera et al 1995c, d). Patients with diarrhea or rectal pain are not suitable for rectal administration of opioids.

Subcutaneous route

The subcutaneous route is commonly used in cancer patients in whom the oral route is no longer suitable. Most opioid agonists including morphine, hydromorphone, oxycodone, diamorphine, fentanyl, and meperidine are suitable for subcutaneous administration. Methadone is generally not considered to be suitable for subcutaneous administration as it tends to cause local irritation (Bruera et al 1991). A subcutaneous injection site usually lasts for around 5–7 days. The subcutaneous route can be used for continuous infusions, patient-controlled analgesia, or intermittent injections (Bruera and Ripamonti 1992). Some other drugs such as metoclopramide can be combined with opioids in continuous subcutaneous infusions, resulting in added convenience. A number of different portable devices are available for the delivery of subcutaneous infusions ranging from electronic devices to simple low-cost injection systems (Bruera et al 1993). Patients with severe edema or coagulopathies may not be suitable for subcutaneous administration of medication.

Intravenous route

The intravenous route usually limits patient mobility and is generally reserved for those patients who require an intravenous route for another reason. The intravenous route can be used for continuous infusions or intermittent injections.

Transdermal route

Transdermal fentanyl is well absorbed. It offers convenience and is particularly effective in patients with excellent pain control on relatively low doses of opioids. The main limitations of this route are the length of time taken to reach steady state and the slow elimination of drug following removal of the patch, both of which prevent rapid titration of the drug for pain control.

Transmucosal route

The transmucosal route appears to offer the possibility of rapid relief from pain. The onset of meaningful pain relief in postoperative patients has been shown to occur within 5 min of administration of oral transmucosal fentanyl citrate (OTFC; Lichtor et al 1999). OTFC is presented in a lollipop that dissolves in the mouth. Approximately 25% of the total available dose is absorbed transmucosally over the initial 15 min and a further 25% is absorbed from the stomach over the next 90 min. The analgesic effect of this preparation is relatively short acting. Two recent randomized controlled trials have studied OTFC for breakthrough pain in cancer patients and have found it to be effective in most patients (Christie et al 1998, Farrar et al 1998).

Epidural and intrathecal routes

The use of spinal routes for analgesia is discussed in Chap. 26. Epidural and intrathecal routes involve potentially higher morbidity than other routes and are usually reserved for patients in whom adequate analgesia is not achieved or in whom side effects are very troublesome using conventional routes.

Other routes

Sublingual, inhalational, and nasal routes are currently under investigation.

Side effects and their management

Opioids have several common and well-known side effects. A highly desirable increase in the use of opioids in many countries over the past 15 years, combined with increased vigilance, has resulted in increased detection of other side effects, most notably neurotoxicity. Patients who are on high doses of opioids, require opioids for a prolonged time, or develop renal impairment are at increased risk of developing toxicity (Sjogren and Eriksen 1994, Daeninck and Bruera 1999). In addition, patients taking longer-acting opioids such as methadone are at a greater risk for accumulation of the drug and developing side effects due to the longer half-life (Oneschuk and Bruera 2000). Table 24.11 summarizes both well-known and more recently identified opioid side effects.

Respiratory depression

Respiratory depression is a dose-dependent side effect of opioid use. It generally occurs after administration of high doses of opioids in opioid-naïve individuals.

In cancer patients who are on long-term opioid treatment tolerance to the respiratory depressant effects develops with repeated administration of the drugs (Walsh 1984). In these patients respiratory depression does not occur in the absence of other concurrent side effects such as sedation. Patients who ignore sedation and continue to take regular opioid medication may develop respiratory depression. In renal impairment the build-up of renally excreted morphine metabolites such as morphine-6-glucuronide can lead to respiratory depression (Osborne et al 1986). Rotation from another opioid to methadone has been associated in occasional case reports with respiratory depression (Hunt and Bruera 1995, Oneschuk and Bruera 2000). Problems with dose ratios and reduced cross-tolerance are believed to be responsible.

Pain is an effective antagonist to the respiratory depressant effects of opioids. Abolition of pain in patients on opioid medication has resulted in respiratory depression (Hanks et al 1981, Wells et al 1984).

Naloxone should not be used unless there is respiratory depression (sedation alone is not an indication for the use of naloxone). When indicated it should be administered in a diluted solution and titrated in small increments to avoid precipitating severe pain and withdrawal symptoms. In the postoperative situation this approach can allow maintenance of analgesia. It is usually possible to start with 0.1 mg every 2–5 min until reversal of the symptoms occur. In patients with an ongoing need for analgesia the opioid involved should be reduced or temporarily discontinued and treatment changed to a different opioid if necessary. The patient should be monitored as naloxone has an elimination half-life of 30 min and respiratory depression may recur. Repeat administration or a continuous intravenous or subcutaneous infusion may be required.

Table 24.11 Opioid side effects

Traditional view	Emerging view
Sedation	Non-cardiogenic pulmonary oedema
Nausea and vomiting	Opioid-induced neurotoxicity (OIN)
Constipation	Severe sedation
Respiratory depression	Cognitive failure
Less commonly; pruritus, anaphylaxis, sweating, urinary retention	Hallucinosis/delirium Myoclonus/grand mal seizures Hyperalgesia/allodynia Immune system effects Endocrine function effects (hypopituitarism, hypogonadism)

Sedation

Sedation is a common adverse effect when patients initially receive opioid analgesics or after a significant increase in dose (Bruera et al 1989b, Banning and Sjogren 1990, Banning et al 1992, Sjogren et al 1994b, Vainio et al 1995). This usually improves over the first few days. In cancer patients who are taking opioid medication there are often other possible causes or contributors to sedation such as infection, metabolic disturbance, renal impairment, dehydration, CNS involvement, or concomitant use of other sedative drugs (tricyclic antidepressants). Underlying contributing factors should be addressed.

Approximately 7–10% of patients receiving strong opioids for cancer pain have persistent sedation related to their opioid medication (Bruera and Watanabe 1994). These patients have a very narrow or non-existing therapeutic window. In cancer patients who present with sedation related to opioid use the administration of naloxone is not indicated in the absence of signs of respiratory depression. Naloxone use can precipitate an unnecessary opioid withdrawal syndrome and severe pain (Manfredi et al 1996). In patients where there is persistent sedation at opioid doses necessary to achieve pain control, adjuvant sparing measures should be considered as these may allow reduction in the opioid dose. A trial of psychostimulants may be useful in patients who are sedated at opioid doses needed for adequate pain control.

Psychostimulants have multiple effects as adjuvant drugs in pain management. They potentiate opioid-induced analgesia, counteract opioid-related sedation and cognitive dysfunction, and allow an escalation of opioid dose in patients with pain syndromes difficult to treat (Bruera and Watanabe 1994). Psychostimulants are contraindicated in patients with a history of hallucinations, delirium, or paranoid disorders. They are also relatively contraindicated with a history of substance abuse or hypertension. In clinical practice the usual starting doses of psychostimulants are methylphenidate 10 mg/day, dextroamphetamine 2.5 mg/day, or pemoline 20 mg/day. The dose can be increased if no adverse effects are observed. The therapeutic effect is evident within 2 days of treatment. Morning and noon administration are advised so as not to disturb sleep (Wilens and Biederman 1992). In patients who do not qualify for traditional psychostimulants, donepezil or modafinil may be tried (Lin et al 1996, Slatkin et al 2001). In patients with persistent sedation a change of opioid may be helpful.

When somnolence is encountered in the presence of residual pain it is necessary to re-examine the possibility that previously unsuspected anxiety, depression, or other unresolved psychological distress is augmenting the patient's expression of pain, and that the opioid dose is excessive in relation to the nociceptive component of the pain. In these cases, the opioid dose should be reduced and other symptoms should be appropriately treated.

Nausea and vomiting

Opioid analgesia can cause nausea and vomiting in patients after initiation or increase in dose. This usually responds well to antiemetics and disappears spontaneously within the first 3 or 4 days of treatment (Clarke 1984, Allan 1993). Some patients, particularly those receiving high doses of opioids, experience chronic and severe nausea. In cancer patients there are often other factors that may contribute to nausea and vomiting such as constipation, metabolic abnormalities, bowel obstruction chemotherapeutic agents, autonomic failure, and raised intracranial pressure. Accumulation of opioid metabolites such as morphine-6-glucuronide has been associated with chronic nausea (Hagen et al 1991).

Underlying causes should if possible be identified and corrected.

Those patients starting on opioids or those who undergo a significant dose increase should have universal access to antiemetics. Prokinetic agents such as metoclopramide are usually effective (Bruera et al 1994a, 1996, 2000b). A commonly used regimen is metoclopramide 10 mg 4 h atc and 10 mg 2 h as needed. In cancer patients who do not initially respond to antiemetics the addition of corticosteroids can dramatically improve the effects of prokinetic drugs (Bruera et al 1983, 1996). There have been no randomized controlled trials comparing different agents in the management of opioid-induced emesis. Other antiemetic agents such as haloperidol and dimenhydrinate can be effective in some patients. Dimenhydrinate should be considered in patients where there appears to be a vestibular component with movement-induced vomiting. In patients with persistent vomiting a change of opioid may be effective in reducing symptoms.

Constipation

Constipation occurs in approximately 90% of patients treated with opioids (Twycross and Lack 1986). Tolerance to this symptom develops very slowly, and many patients require laxative therapy for as long as they take opioids. In cancer patients, coexisting conditions may contribute to constipation. Dehydration, reduced oral intake, immobility, electrolyte abnormalities (hypercalcaemia, hypokalaemia), autonomic failure, and abdominal involvement can all contribute to constipation.

Patients who are starting on opioid medication should be prescribed laxatives concomitantly and the dose titrated to effect. All patients on regular opioid medication should be assessed for constipation because of its prevalence in this group. Assessment of constipation is often inadequate (Bruera et al 1994b).

Coexisting contributing factors should be corrected if possible. Therapeutic interventions involve the use of laxatives, rectal suppositories, enemas, and manual disimpaction. Oral laxatives include bulk agents, osmotic agents, contact cathartics, lubricants, prokinetic drugs, and oral naloxone. Contact cathartics (senna, cascara, dantron, phenophthalein, bisacodyl, docusates, and castor oil) are the most commonly administered laxatives for opioid-induced constipation. A combination of contact cathartics is commonly used. Combined laxative treatment is not universally effective; 40% of advanced cancer patients also require the use of enemas and/or rectal manipulation (Twycross and Lack 1986).

Prokinetic agents such as metoclopramide can be given as an infusion in particularly resistant cases (Bruera et al 1987). Opioid antagonists naloxone and methylnaltrexone have been given orally with effect (Kreek et al 1983, Yuan et al 2000, Yuan and Foss 2000). There is some evidence suggesting that fentanyl and methadone have less constipation-inducing potential than morphine (Hunt et al 1999, Mancini et al 2000). If a change of opioid is planned for a patient who has troublesome constipation, one of these opioids could be tried.

Opioid-induced neurotoxicity

Opioid-induced neurotoxicity is a recently recognized syndrome of neuropsychiatric consequences of opioid administration (Bruera and Pereira 1997). The features of OIN include cognitive impairment, severe sedation, hallucinosis, delirium, myoclonus, seizures, hyperalgesia, and allodynia. Patients exhibiting some or all of these features are suffering from opioid-induced neurotoxicity. OIN is most often seen in patients receiving high doses of opioid analgesics for prolonged periods, often in association with psychoactive medications. Fluid depletion and renal failure are also often present. Risk factors for OIN include high opioid dose and prolonged opioid exposure, pre-existing borderline cognition/delirium, dehydration, renal failure, the use of opioids with mixed agonist/antagonist activity (e.g., pentazocine, butorphanol, and nalbuphine), and the use of other psychoactive drugs (e.g., tricyclic antidepressants, hypnotics).

An approach to the management of OIN includes:

- Hydrate if dehydrated
- Reduce or discontinue opioid dose
- Rotate opioid
- Stop other contributing drugs (e.g., psychoactive drugs, NSAIDS, etc.)
- Treat symptoms with haloperidol or other medications as needed.

Prevention of OIN is best achieved by an awareness and assessment of risk factors and avoidance where possible of opioid dose escalation. Opioid escalation is more likely to occur in certain patient populations such as those with neuropathic pain, incident pain, rapid development of tolerance, somatization, and substance abuse.

Pruritus

Pruritus is more common with neuraxial (epidural and intrathecal) administration of opioids (Cousins and Mather 1984) and has been reported to occur in 8.5 and 46% of patients receiving epidural and intrathecal opioids, respectively (Ballantyne et al 1988). It is rare in patients on systemic opioid therapy. The aetiology is unknown but may be related to histamine release or a central effect. An antihistamine or a change of opioid are possible treatment options.

Urinary retention

Urinary retention like pruritus is also more common with neuraxial administration of opioids (Cousins and Mather 1984). It is more likely to occur in opioid naïve patients and in the first days of treatment with opioids. Low-dose intravenous naloxone may be useful but care must be taken not to induce withdrawal; alternatively a programme of intermittent catheterization can be used but is rarely needed.

Non-cardiogenic pulmonary oedema

This side effect has been well documented with street use of narcotics. In recent years with use of high doses of opioids for management of cancer pain this phenomenon has been described in cancer patients (Bruera and Miller 1989). It is usually related to a large increase in opioid dose in the days prior to its onset. In cancer patients with a non-intensive management approach it has a high mortality, whereas in drug addicts the incidence has been described as less than 1% (Cooper et al 1986).

The apparent relationship between recent large increases in opioid dose and the development of non-cardiogenic pulmonary oedema indicates that it should be anticipated in patients who have required massive dose increases of their opioids. In these patients consideration should be given to the use of adjuvant analgesic measures with other pharmacologic and non-pharmacologic agents in order to try to prevent the need for rapid opioid dose escalation. Opioid rotation may be helpful in reducing dose increases because of incomplete cross-tolerance between different opioids (Foley 1985).

Endocrine and immune system effects

Opioid administration has been shown to inhibit ACTH (Grossman and Besser 1982) and cortisol levels, and naloxone stimulates the release of ACTH (Morley et al 1980, Volavka et al 1980, Allolio et al 1982). Opioids have also been shown to inhibit vasopressin and oxytocin release at posterior pituitary level, to elevate insulin and glucagon, and to inhibit somatostatin (Pfeiffer and Herz 1984). A study of 73 patients receiving long-term intrathecal opioid administration for intractable non-malignant pain showed hypogonadotrophic hypogonadism in a large majority of patients. In addition, 15% were shown to have developed hypocorticism and approximately the same percentage had developed growth hormone deficiency.

There is also emerging evidence that opiates have an effect on host defense and are associated with the pathogenesis of infection among intravenous drug users (Risdahl et al 1998). The importance of these findings for patients receiving opioids for cancer pain or chronic pain is as yet unknown. Future research is needed to look at these two important areas.

Tolerance, physical dependence, and addiction issues

These three issues are often confused and fear of tolerance and dependence often lead to undertreatment of cancer pain.

Tolerance

Tolerance to the analgesic effect of opioids may develop. It is a normal physiological effect and may represent alteration at the opioid receptor level or changes in metabolism of the opioid. The development of tolerance varies considerably between patients and opioids. It tends to occur in the first few weeks of opioid therapy. Tolerance has been well documented for some opioid effects in humans including sedation and respiratory depression. While tolerance to nociception has been well documented in animal models there is still controversy about the level of this phenomenon in humans. With continued opioid use, dose requirements tend to remain stable over time unless there is disease progression (Twycross 1974, Collin et al 1993). Tolerance should not be mistaken for progression of underlying disease in advanced cancer patients; careful ongoing assessments are needed in patients who require increasing opioid doses for analgesia. If tolerance develops, opioid doses can be increased to achieve analgesia. Cross-tolerance between opioids is incomplete. If tolerance is becoming a problem, or increases in the opioid dose results in side effects, an alternative opioid can be used. Many patients worry that if opioids are started too soon tolerance will develop and that analgesia will not be available when pain worsens. It is important to reassure patients that this is not a problem and that it is not necessary to reserve opioids for later in the progression of the disease.

Physical dependence

Physical dependence is a normal and common physiological effect of chronic opioid use (it also occurs with the use of beta-blockers and corticosteroids). Abrupt discontinuation of the medication results in physical symptoms. With opioid withdrawal the patient may develop agitation, tremulousness, fever, diaphoresis, tachycardia, mydriasis, and abdominal and muscle cramps. Use of an opioid antagonist can lead to the same syndrome. If cessation of opioids is indicated the opioid dose can be reduced initially by 50–75% without risk of withdrawal. Further dose reduction should take place at a rate of approximately 20% per day until a total dose of 15 mg/day or less is reached. At this point the opioid can be discontinued.

Addiction

Addiction is characterized by psychological dependence and implies compulsion to use a substance for its psychological effect. This leads to compulsive drug-seeking behaviour. Persons who have psychological dependence are likely to have physical dependence. However, physical dependence without psychological dependence does not indicate addiction. Fear of addiction is an important cause of underprescription of opioids for analgesia (Hill 1993). There is evidence that addiction to opioids is very rare in medical patients (Porter and Jick 1980, Kanner and Foley 1981). Important risk factors for addiction include a history of abuse of street drugs, prescription drugs, or alcoholism. It is important for all patients exposed to opioids to undergo careful screening for all these major risk factors.

In some cancer patients drug-seeking behaviour is seen because of unrelieved pain and not psychological dependence. This can be the result of prn prescription of opioids rather than regular administration of adequate analgesia. This behaviour usually responds to escalation of the opioid dose, resulting in adequate analgesia. Improved assessment and rational pain management should help to eliminate this problem.

Management of cancer pain in patients with a history of substance abuse

The basic principles of cancer pain management also apply to patients with a history of substance abuse. Early identification of patients with a history of substance abuse is important as there are additional factors that should be considered in their management. Request for dose increases by the patient may be the result of primarily psychological rather than physical distress and will not be addressed by increases in opioid dose. Drug-seeking behaviour including unauthorized dose escalation and acquisition of opioids from other sources should be openly addressed with the patient. It is important that one physician should be responsible for the patient's pain management as this provides continuity of care and helps to prevent misunderstandings. A supportive setting should be established in which the patient can have pain effectively treated (Passik and Theobald 2000).

References

Allan SG 1993 Nausea and vomiting. In: Doyle D, Hanks GW, MacDonald N (eds) Oxford Textbook of palliative medicine, 1st edn. Oxford Medical Press, Oxford, pp 282–290

Allolio B, Winkelmann W, Hipp FX et al. 1982 Effects of a met-enkephalin analog on adrenocorticotropin (ACTH), growth hormone, and prolactin in patients with ACTH hypersecretion. Journal of Clinical Endocrinology and Metabolism 55: 1–7

American Pain Society 1992 Principles of analgesic use in the treatment of acute pain and chronic cancer pain, 3rd edn. Skokie, American Pain Society

Ashby M, Fleming B, Wood M et al 1997 Plasma morphine and glucuronide (M3G and M6G) concentrations in hospice inpatients. Journal of Pain and Symptom Management 14: 157–167

Ballantyne JC, Loach AB, Carr DB 1988 Itching after epidural and spinal opiates. Pain 33: 149–160

Banning A, Sjogren P 1990 Cerebral effects of long-term oral opioids in cancer patients measured by continuous reaction time. Clinical Journal of Pain 6: 91–95

Banning A, Sjogren P, Kaiser F 1992 Reaction time in cancer patients receiving peripherally acting analgesics alone or in combination with opioids. Acta Anaesthesiologica Scandinavica 36: 480–482

Bernard SA, Bruera E 2000 Drug interactions in palliative care. Journal of Clinical Oncology 18: 1780–1799

Brescia FJ, Portenoy RK, Ryan M et al. 1992 Pain, opioid use, and survival in hospitalized patients with advanced cancer. Journal of Clinical Oncology 10: 149–155

Bruera E 1990 Subcutaneous administration of opioids in the management of cancer pain. In: Foley K, Ventafridda V (eds) Advances in pain research and therapy, vol 16. Raven Press, New York, pp 203–218

Bruera E, Miller MJ 1989 Non-cardiogenic pulmonary edema after narcotic treatment for cancer pain. Pain 39: 297–300

Bruera E, Neumann CM 1999 Role of methadone in the management of pain in cancer patients. Oncology 13: 1275–1282

Bruera E, Pereira J 1997 Acute neuropsychiatric findings in a patient receiving fentanyl for cancer pain. Pain 69: 199–201

Bruera E, Ripamonti C 1992 Alternate routes of administration of opioids for the management of cancer pain. In: Patt R (ed) Cancer pain. Lippincott, Philadelphia, pp 161–184

Bruera E, Watanabe S 1994 Psychostimulants as adjuvant analgesics. Journal of Pain and Symptom Management 9: 412–415

Bruera ED, Roca E, Cedaro L et al 1983 Improved control of chemotherapy-induced emesis by the addition of dexamethasone to metoclopramide in patients resistant to metoclopramide. Cancer Treatment Reports 67: 381–383

Bruera E, Brenneis C, Michaud M et al 1987 Continuous Sc infusion of metoclopramide for treatment of narcotic bowel syndrome [letter]. Cancer Treatment Reports 71: 1121–1122

Bruera E, Macmillan K, Hanson J et al 1989a The cognitive effects of the administration of narcotic analgesics in patients with cancer pain. Pain 39: 13–16

Bruera E, Brenneis C, Michaud M et al 1989b Influence of the pain and symptom control team (PSCT) on the patterns of treatment of pain and other symptoms in a cancer center. Journal of Pain and Symptom Management 4: 112–116

Bruera E, Fainsinger R, Moore M et al 1991 Local toxicity with subcutaneous methadone. Experience of two centers. Pain 45: 141–143

Bruera E, Velasco-Leiva A, Spachynski K et al 1993 Use of the Edmonton Injector for parenteral opioid management of cancer pain: a study of 100 consecutive patients. Journal of Pain and Symptom Management 8: 525–528

Bruera ED, MacEachern TJ, Spachynski KA et al 1994a Comparison of the efficacy, safety, and pharmacokinetics of controlled release and immediate release metoclopramide for the management of chronic nausea in patients with advanced cancer. Cancer 74: 3204–3211

Bruera E, Suarez-Almazor M, Velasco A et al 1994b The assessment of constipation in terminal cancer patients admitted to a palliative care unit: a retrospective review. Journal of Pain Symptom Management 9: 515–519

Bruera E, Franco JJ, Maltoni M et al 1995a Changing pattern of agitated impaired mental status in patients with advanced cancer: association with cognitive monitoring, hydration, and opioid rotation. Journal of Pain and Symptom Management 10: 287–291

Bruera E, Watanabe S, Fainsinger RL et al 1995b Custom-made capsules and suppositories of methadone for patients on high-dose opioids for cancer pain. Pain 62: 141–146

Bruera E, Fainsinger R, Spachynski K et al 1995c Clinical efficacy and safety of a novel controlled-release morphine suppository and subcutaneous morphine in cancer pain: a randomized evaluation. Journal of Clinical Oncology 13: 1520–1527

Bruera E, Fainsinger R, Spachynski K et al 1995d Steady-state pharmacokinetic evaluation of a novel, controlled-release morphine suppository and subcutaneous morphine in cancer pain. Journal of Clinical Pharmacology 35: 666–672

Bruera E, Seifert L, Watanabe S et al 1996 Chronic nausea in advanced cancer patients: a retrospective assessment of a metoclopramide-based antiemetic regimen. Journal of Pain and Symptom Management 11: 147–153

Bruera E, Rico MA, Bertolino M et al 2000a A prospective, open study of oral methadone in the treatment of cancer pain. In: Devor M, Rowbotham MC, Weisenfeld-Hallin Z (eds) Proceedings of the 9th world congress on pain. IASP Press, Seattle, pp 957–963

Bruera E, Belzile M, Neumann C et al 2000b A double-blind, crossover study of controlled-release metoclopramide and placebo for the chronic nausea and dyspepsia of advanced cancer. Journal of Pain and Symptom Management 19: 427–435

Cesselin F, Benoliel J-J, Bourgoin S et al 1999 Spinal mechanisms of opioid analgesia. In: Stein C (ed) Opioids in pain control: basic and clinical aspects. Cambridge University Press, Cambridge, pp 70–95
Chan GL, Matzke GR 1987 Effects of renal insufficiency on the pharmacokinetics and pharmacodynamics of opioid analgesics. Drug Intelligence and Clinical Pharmacy 21: 773–783
Cherny NJ, Ho MN, Bookbinder M et al 1994 Cancer pain: knowledge and attitudes of physicians at a cancer center. Proceedings of the American Society of Clinical Oncology 12: 434
Christie JM, Simmonds M, Patt R et al 1998 Dose-titration, multicenter study of oral transmucosal fentanyl citrate for the treatment of breakthrough pain in cancer patients using transdermal fentanyl for persistent pain. Journal of Clinical Oncology 16: 3238–3245
Clarke RS 1984 Nausea and vomiting. British Journal of Anaesthesia 56: 19–27
Cleeland CS, Gonin R, Hatfield AK et al 1994 Pain and its treatment in outpatients with metastatic cancer. New England Journal of Medicine 330: 592–596
Collin E, Poulain P, Gauvain-Piquard A et al 1993 Is disease progression the major factor in morphine 'tolerance' in cancer pain treatment? Pain 55: 319–326
Cone EJ, Darwin WD, Gorodetsky CW et al 1978 Comparative metabolism of hydrocodone in man, rat, guinea pig, rabbit and dog. Drug Metabolism and Disposition 6: 488–493
Cooper A, White D, Matthay R 1986 Drug-induced pulmonary disease. American Review of Respiratory Diseases 133: 488–505
Cousins MJ , Mather LE 1984 Intrathecal and epidural administration of opioids. Anesthesiology 61: 276–310
Coyle N, Mauskop A, Maggard J et al 1986 Continuous subcutaneous infusions of opiates in cancer patients with pain. Oncology Nursing Forum 13: 53–57
Crome P, Gain R, Ghurye R et al 1984 Pharmacokinetics of dextropropoxyphene and nordextropropoxyphene in elderly hospital patients after single and multiple doses of distalgesic. Preliminary analysis of results. Human Toxicology 3 (Suppl): 41S–48S
Culpepper-Morgan JA, Inturrisi CE, Portenoy RK et al 1992 Treatment of opioid-induced constipation with oral naloxone: a pilot study. Clinical Pharmacology and Therapeutics 52: 90–95
D'Honneur G, Gilton A, Sandouk P et al 1994 Plasma and cerebrospinal fluid concentrations of morphine and morphine glucuronides after oral morphine. The influence of renal failure. Anesthesiology 81: 87–93
Daeninck PJ, Bruera E 1999 Opioid use in cancer pain. Is a more liberal approach enhancing toxicity? Acta Anaesthesiologica Scandinavica 43: 924–938
Daeninck P, Watanabe S, Walker P et al 1998 Effective pain relief in cancer patients using methadone at extended dosing intervals. Journal of Palliative Care 13: 117
De Conno F, Ripamonti C, Saita L et al 1995 Role of rectal route in treating cancer pain: a randomized crossover clinical trial of oral versus rectal morphine administration in opioid-naive cancer patients with pain. Journal of Clinical Oncology 13: 1004–1008
De Stoutz ND, Bruera E, Suarez-Almazor M 1995 Opioid rotation for toxicity reduction in terminal cancer patients. Journal of Pain and Symptom Management 10: 378–384
Dole VP, Kreek MJ 1973 Methadone plasma level: sustained by a reservoir of drug in tissue. Proceedings of the National Academy of Science USA 70: 10
Ebert B, Andersen S, Krogsgaard-Larsen P 1995 Ketobemidone, methadone and pethidine are non-competitive N-methyl-D-aspartate (NMDA) antagonists in the rat cortex and spinal cord. Neuroscience Letters 187: 165–168
Eisendrath SJ, Goldman B, Douglas J et al 1987 Meperidine-induced delirium. American Journal of Psychiatry 144: 1062–1065
Farrar JT, Cleary J, Rauck R et al 1998 Oral transmucosal fentanyl citrate: randomized, double-blinded, placebo-controlled trial for treatment of breakthrough pain in cancer patients. Journal of National Cancer Institute 90: 611–616
Findlay JW, Jones EC, Butz RF et al 1978 Plasma codeine and morphine concentrations after therapeutic oral doses of codeine-containing analgesics. Clinical Pharmacology and Therapeutics 24: 60–68
Foley K 1985 The treatment of cancer pain. New England Journal of Medicine 313: 84–95
France RD, Urban BJ, Keefe FJ 1984 Long-term use of narcotic analgesics in chronic pain. Social Science Medicine 19: 1379–1382
Gear RW, Miaskowski C, Heller PH et al 1997 Benzodiazepine mediated antagonism of opioid analgesia. Pain 71: 25–29
Gorman AL, Elliott KJ, Inturrisi CE 1997 The d- and l-isomers of methadone bind to the non-competitive site on the N-methyl-D-aspartate (NMDA) receptor in rat forebrain and spinal cord. Neuroscience Letters 223: 5–8
Gourlay GK, Cherry DA, Cousins MJ 1986 A comparative study of the efficacy and pharmacokinetics of oral methadone and morphine in the treatment of severe pain in patients with cancer. Pain 25: 297–312
Grossman A, Besser GM 1982 Opiates control ACTH through a noradrenergic mechanism. Clinical Endocrinology 17: 287–290
Grudt TJ, Williams JT 1995 Opioid receptors and the regulation of ion conductances. Review of Neuroscience 6: 279–286
Hagen NA, Foley KM, Cerbone DJ et al 1991 Chronic nausea and morphine-6-glucuronide. Journal of Pain and Symptom Management 6: 125–128
Hanks GW, Twycross RG, Lloyd JW 1981 Unexpected complication of successful nerve block. Morphine induced respiratory depression precipitated by removal of severe pain. Anaesthesia 36: 37–39
Hasselstrom J, Eriksson S, Persson A et al 1990 The metabolism and bioavailability of morphine in patients with severe liver cirrhosis. British Journal of Clinical Pharmacology 29: 289–297
Heiskanen T, Kalso E 1997 Controlled-release oxycodone and morphine in cancer related pain. Pain 73: 37–45
Herrlin K, Segerdahl M, Gustafsson LL et al 2000 Methadone, ciprofloxacin, and adverse drug reactions. Lancet 356: 2069–2070
Herz A, Akil H, Simon EJ 1993 Handbook of experimental pharmacology. Springer-Verlag, New York
Hewitt DJ 2000 The use of NMDA-receptor antagonists in the treatment of chronic pain. Clinical Journal of Pain 16: S73–S79
Hill CS 1993 The barriers to adequate pain management with opioid analgesics. Seminars in Oncology 20: 1–5
Houde RW 1986 Clinical studies of hydromorphone. In: Foley K, Inturrisi C (eds) Advances in pain research and therapy, vol 8. Raven Press, New York, pp 129–136
Hunt G, Bruera E 1995 Respiratory depression in a patient receiving oral methadone for cancer pain. Journal of Pain and Symptom Management 10: 401–404
Hunt R, Fazekas B, Thorne D et al 1999 A comparison of subcutaneous morphine and fentanyl in hospice cancer patients. Journal of Pain and Symptom Management 18: 111–119
International Association for the Study of Pain 1992 Management of acute pain: A practical guide. IASP, Seattle
Inturrisi CE 1990 Effects of other drugs and pathologic states on opioid disposition and response. In: Benedetti C, Giron G, Chapman C (eds) Advances in pain research and therapy, vol 14. Raven Press, New York, pp 171–180
Inturrisi CE, Max MB, Foley KM et al 1984 The pharmacokinetics of

heroin in patients with chronic pain. New England Journal of Medicine 310: 1213–1217
Inturrisi CE, Colburn WA, Kaiko RF et al 1987 Pharmacokinetics and pharmacodynamics of methadone in patients with chronic pain. Clinical Pharmacology and Therapeutics 41: 392–401
Iribarne C, Picart D, Dreano Y et al 1998 In vitro interactions between fluoxetine or fluvoxamine and methadone or buprenorphine. Fundamental Clinical Pharmacology 12: 194–199
Kaiko RF, Wallenstein SL, Rogers A et al 1981 Relative analgesic potency of intramuscular heroin and morphine in cancer patients with postoperative pain and chronic pain due to cancer. NIDA Research Monograph 34: 213–219
Kalso E, Tramer MR, Carroll D et al 1997 Pain relief from intra-articular morphine after knee surgery: a qualitative systematic review. Pain 71: 127–134
Kanner RM, Foley KM 1981 Patterns of narcotic drug use in a cancer pain clinic. Annals of the New York Academy of Science 362: 161–172
Kreek MJ, Schaefer RA, Hahn EF et al 1983 Naloxone, a specific opioid antagonist, reverses chronic idiopathic constipation. Lancet 1: 261–262
Labella FS, Pinsky C, Havlicek V 1979 Morphine derivatives with diminished opiate receptor potency show enhanced central excitatory activity. Brain Research 174: 263–271
Lawlor PG, Turner KS, Hanson J et al 1998 Dose ratio between morphine and methadone in patients with cancer pain: a retrospective study. Cancer 82: 1167–1173
Lehmann KA, Zech D 1993 Morphine-6-glucuronide a pharmacologically active morphine metabolite: a review of the literature. European Journal of Pain 12: 28–35
Lichtor JL, Sevarino FB, Joshi GP et al 1999 The relative potency of oral transmucosal fentanyl citrate compared with intravenous morphine in the treatment of moderate to severe postoperative pain. Anesthesia and Analgesia 89: 732–738
Lin JS, Hou Y, Jouvet M 1996 Potential brain neuronal targets for amphetamine-, methylphenidate-, and modafinil-induced wakefulness, evidenced by c-fos immunocytochemistry in the cat. Proceedings of the National Academy of Science of the USA 93: 14128–14133
Lipman AG, Gautier GM 1997 Pharmacology of opioid drugs: basic principles. In: Portenoy RK, Bruera E (eds) Topics in palliative care, vol 1. Oxford University Press, New York, pp 137–161
MacDonald N, Der L, Allan S et al 1993 Opioid hyperexcitability: the application of alternate opioid therapy. Pain 53: 353–355
Makman MH 1994 Morphine receptors in immunocytes and neurons. Advances in Neuroimmunology 4: 69–82
Mancini I, Hanson J, Neumann C et al 2000 Opioid type and other clinical predictors of laxative dose in advanced cancer patients: A retrospective study. Journal of Palliative Medicine 3: 49–56
Manfredi PL, Ribeiro S, Chandler SW et al 1996 Inappropriate use of naloxone in cancer patients with pain. Journal of Pain and Symptom Management 11: 131–134
Mazoit JX, Sandouk P, Zetlaoui P et al 1987 Pharmacokinetics of unchanged morphine in normal and cirrhotic subjects. Anesthesia and Analgesia 66: 293–298
Meissner W, Schmidt U, Hartmann M et al 2000 Oral naloxone reverses opioid-associated constipation. Pain 84: 105–109
Mercadante S 1999 Opioid rotation for cancer pain: rationale and clinical aspects. Cancer 86: 1856–1866
Mercadante S, Casuccio A, Calderone L 1999 Rapid switching from morphine to methadone in cancer patients with poor response to morphine. Journal of Clinical Oncology 17: 3307–3312
Mercadante S, Casuccio A, Groff L et al 2001 Switching from morphine to methadone to improve analgesia and tolerability in cancer patients: A prospective study. Journal of Clinical Oncology 19: 2898–2904
Meunier JC, Mollereau C, Toll L et al 1995 Isolation and structure of the endogenous agonist of opioid receptor-like ORL1 receptor. Nature 377: 532–535
Morley JE, Baranetsky NG, Wingert TD et al 1980 Endocrine effects of naloxone-induced opiate receptor blockade. Journal of Clinical Endocrinology and Metabolism 50: 251–257
Nauck F, Ostgathe C, Dickerson ED 2001 A German model for methadone conversion. American Journal of Hospice Palliative Care 18: 200–202
Nilsson MI, Meresaar U, Anggard E 1982 Clinical pharmacokinetics of methadone. Acta Anaesthesiologica Scandinavica 74 (Suppl): 66–69
Oneschuk D, Bruera E 2000 Respiratory depression during methadone rotation in a patient with advanced cancer. Journal of Palliative Care 16: 50–54
Osborne RJ, Joel SP, Slevin ML 1986 Morphine intoxication in renal failure: the role of morphine-6-glucuronide. British Medical Journal (Clin Res Ed) 292: 1548–1549
Osborne R, Joel S, Trew D et al 1988 Analgesic activity of morphine-6-glucuronide [letter]. Lancet 1: 828
Passik SD, Theobald DE 2000 Managing addiction in advanced cancer patients: why bother? Journal of Pain and Symptom Management 19: 229–234
Pasternak GW 2001 Incomplete cross-tolerance and multiple mu opioid peptide receptors. Trends in Pharmacological Science 22: 67–70
Paul D, Bodnar RJ, Gistrak MA et al 1989 Different mu receptor subtypes mediate spinal and supraspinal analgesia in mice. European Journal of Pharmacology 168: 307–314
Pereira J, Lawlor P, Vigano A et al 2001 Equianalgesic dose ratios for opioids: A critical review and proposals for long-term dosing. Journal of Pain and Symptom Management 22: 672–687
Pfeiffer A, Herz A 1984 Endocrine actions of opioids. Hormone and Metabolic Research 16: 386–397
Portenoy RK, Foley KM 1986 Chronic use of opioid analgesics in non-malignant pain: report of 38 cases. Pain 25: 171–186
Portenoy RK, Foley KM, Stulman J et al 1991 Plasma morphine and morphine-6-glucuronide during chronic morphine therapy for cancer pain: plasma profiles, steady-state concentrations and the consequences of renal failure. Pain 47: 13–19
Porter J, Jick H 1980 Addiction rare in patients treated with narcotics. New England Journal of Medicine 302: 123
Raffa RB, Friderichs E, Reimann W et al 1993 Complementary and synergistic antinociceptive interaction between the enantiomers of tramadol. Journal of Pharmacol Exp Ther 267: 331–340
Ripamonti C, Bruera E 1991 Rectal, buccal, and sublingual narcotics for the management of cancer pain. Journal of Palliative Care 7: 30–35
Ripamonti C, Zecca E, Brunelli C et al 1995 Rectal methadone in cancer patients with pain. A preliminary clinical and pharmacokinetic study. Annals of Oncology 6: 841–843
Ripamonti C, De Conno F, Groff L et al 1998 Equianalgesic dose/ratio between methadone and other opioid agonists in cancer pain: comparison of two clinical experiences. Annals of Oncology 9: 79–83
Risdahl JM, Khanna KV, Peterson PK et al 1998 Opiates and infection. Journal of Neuroimmunology 83: 4–18
Sawe J 1986 High-dose morphine and methadone in cancer patients. Clinical pharmacokinetic considerations of oral treatment. Clinical Pharmacokinetics 11: 87–106
Schlatter J, Madras JL, Saulnier JL et al 1999 [Drug interactions with methadone]. Presse Medicale 28: 1381–1384
Sjogren P, Eriksen J 1994 Opioid toxicity. Current Opinions in Anaesthesia 7: 465–469
Sjogren P, Jensen NH, Jensen TS 1994a Disappearance of morphine-induced hyperalgesia after discontinuing or substituting morphine with other opioid agonists. Pain 59: 313–316

Sjogren P, Banning AM, Christensen CB et al 1994b Continuous reaction time after single dose, long-term oral and epidural opioid administration. European Journal of Anaesthesiology 11: 95–100

Sjogren P, Thunedborg LP, Christrup L et al 1998 Is development of hyperalgesia, allodynia and myoclonus related to morphine metabolism during long-term administration? Six case histories. Acta Anaesthesiologica Scandinavica 42: 1070–1075

Slatkin NE, Rhiner M, Bolton TM 2001 Donepezil in the treatment of opioid-induced sedation: report of six cases. Journal of Pain and Symptom Management 21: 425–438

Smith MT, Watt JA, Cramond T 1990 Morphine-3-glucuronide—a potent antagonist of morphine analgesia. Life Science 47: 579–585

Stambaugh JE, Wainer IW, Hemhill DM et al 1977 A potentially toxic drug interaction between pethidine (meperidine) and phenobarbitone. Lancet 1: 398–399

Stein C, Hassan AH, Lehrberger K et al. 1993 Local analgesic effect of endogenous opioid peptides. Lancet 342: 321–324

Stein C, Schafer M, Cabot PJ 1997 Peripheral opioid analgesia. Pain Review 4: 171–185

Stein C, Cabot PJ, Schafer M 1999 Peripheral opioid analgesia: Mechanisms and clinical implications. In Stein C (ed) Opioids in pain control: basic and clinical aspects. Cambridge University Press, Cambridge, pp 96–108

Sykes NP 1996 An investigation of the ability of oral naloxone to correct opioid-related constipation in patients with advanced cancer. Palliative Medicine 10: 135–144

Szeto HH, Inturrisi CE, Houde R et al 1977 Accumulation of normeperidine, an active metabolite of meperidine, in patients with renal failure of cancer. Annals of Internal Medicine 86: 738–741

Traynor JR, Elliott J 1993 δ-Opioid receptor subtypes and cross-talk with mu-receptors. Trends in Pharmacological Science 14: 84–86

Twycross RG 1974 Clinical experience with diamorphine in advanced malignant disease. International Journal of Clinical Pharmacology 7: 184–198

Twycross RG , Lack SA 1986 Control of alimentary symptoms in far advanced cancer. Churchill Livingstone, London, pp 166–207

Vainio A, Ollila J, Matikainen E et al 1995 Driving ability in cancer patients receiving long-term morphine analgesia. Lancet 346: 667–670

Volavka J, Bauman J, Pevnick J et al 1980 Short-term hormonal effects of naloxone in man. Psychoneuroendocrinology 5: 225–234

Von Roenn JH, Cleeland CS, Gonin R et al 1993 Physician attitudes and practice in cancer pain management. A survey from the Eastern Cooperative Oncology Group. Annals of Internal Medicine 119: 121–126

Vree TB, van Dongen RT, Koopman-Kimenai PM 2000 Codeine analgesia is due to codeine-6-glucuronide, not morphine. International Journal of Clinical Practice 54: 395–398

Walsh TD 1984 Opiates and respiratory function in advanced cancer. Recent Results in Cancer Research 89: 115–117

Wells CJ, Lipton S, Lahuerta J 1984 Respiratory depression after percutaneous cervical anterolateral cordotomy in patients on slow-release oral morphine [letter]. Lancet 1: 739

Wilens TE, Biederman J 1992 The stimulants. Psychiatric Clinics of North America 15: 191–222

World Health Organization 1990 Expert Committee report, cancer pain relief and palliative care. Technical Series 804

World Health Organization 1996 Cancer pain relief, 2nd edn. Report of a WHO Expert Committee. World Health Organization, Geneva

Yuan CS, Foss JF 2000 Oral methylnaltrexone for opioid-induced constipation [letter]. Journal of the American Medical Association 284: 1383–1384

Yuan CS, Foss JF, O'Connor M et al 2000 Methylnaltrexone for reversal of constipation due to chronic methadone use: a randomized controlled trial. Journal of the American Medical Association 283: 367–372

Zenz M, Strumpf M, Tryba M 1992 Long-term oral opioid therapy in patients with chronic nonmalignant pain. Journal of Pain and Symptom Management 7: 69–77

Chapter 25

Local anaesthetics and epidurals

H J McQuay and R A Moore

Introduction

Local anaesthetics are amazing drugs. Injected into tissue, around a nerve, or for a regional block they produce reversible block. Asking radical questions about acute postoperative management, such as 'Why are all operations not ambulatory, pain-free, and risk-free?' or, more familiar, 'Why is this patient still in hospital?', is forcing a reconsideration of the role of combined (local or regional plus general anaesthesia) approaches. Instead of asking questions such as 'Is regional better than general anaesthesia' we need to look at the whole episode before, during, and after surgery, not just the operative period (Kehlet 1994, 1997). Costs of any care episode should fall if the hospital stay is reduced, and a healthy patient returned home will cost the community less than a sick patient requiring considerable input from the primary care team. The chapter considers three main topics: these radical changes, which depend on the use of nerve blocks or regional techniques using local anaesthetics; one of the conundrums of local anaesthetic use in chronic pain, which is why pain relief from local anaesthetics can far outlast the duration of action of the local anaesthetic (Arnér et al 1990); and the epidural use of opioids alone and in combination with local anaesthetics. The aim is not to cover the mechanics of particular blocks, but to ask which areas need greater research focus.

Acute pain

A simple operation

The first example is of a common operation, inguinal hernia repair, which can be done under local anaesthetic alone. Outcomes that need to be considered include the choice of anaesthesia and analgesia, post-herniorrhaphy pain and convalescence, postoperative morbidity (predominantly urinary retention), and choice of surgical technique and recurrence rate. In a randomized double-blind double-dummy study (Nehra et al 1995) of 200 men Nehra and colleagues compared 0.5% bupivacaine ilioinguinal field block plus oral papaveretum-aspirin tablets with bupivacaine plus oral placebo, saline plus papaveretum-aspirin, or saline plus oral placebo to assess pain relief after hernia surgery. Patients were prescribed postoperative opioids to be given on demand. Pain levels and mobility were assessed 6 and 24 h after operation. The combination of bupivacaine plus papaveretum-aspirin provided the best results, producing (not surprisingly) significantly less pain, and requiring less additional opioid and with better mobility than saline plus oral placebo. A similar trial over 20 years ago (Teasdale et al 1982) randomized 103 patients to either local or general anaesthesia; those patients having local anaesthesia were able to walk, eat, and pass urine significantly earlier than those having general anaesthesia, who experienced more nausea, vomiting, sore throat, and headache.

An audit of inguinal hernia repair under local anaesthesia in an ambulatory setup provides confirmation that these results may be generalized. Prospective data were collected from 400 consecutive elective ambulatory operations for inguinal hernia (29 operations in ASA group III patients) under unmonitored local anaesthesia (Callesen et al 1998). Median postoperative hospital stay was 85 min. Two patients needed general anaesthesia, and nine patients (2%) needed overnight admission. One-week postoperative morbidity was low with one patient with transient cerebral ischaemia and one with pneumonia, but none with urinary retention. The high satisfaction (88%) on follow-up makes this a triumph for local anaesthesia, but the variation in general practitioners' recommendations for convalescence, such as between 1 and 12 weeks off work, may need to be changed if the full benefit to the individual and to the society is to be harnessed (Kehlet and Callesen 1998).

A complex operation—what is the question? Is it still general versus regional?

Our old question was whether regional or regional-supplemented general anaesthesia could produce major reductions in morbidity and mortality—the general versus regional anaesthesia question. An example is vascular surgery. The Yeager study (Yeager et al 1987) did suggest improvement in patients with regional anaesthesia in patients undergoing abdominal aortic aneurysm or lower extremity vascular surgery. A feature of subsequent studies that showed no difference between regional and general anaesthesia was an increasing extent of control over all aspects of postoperative care (Christopherson et al 1993, Bode et al 1996). The effect of the detailed protocols was that bad outcomes were reduced in all groups (Beattie et al 1996). The implication is that even if there was a difference it would take a really huge study to show it using the morbidity and mortality outcomes (Rigg and Jamrozik 1998). However, the suggestion is that it is only if the postoperative protocols allow any advantage to be expressed, such as advantage in time to feeding or time to walking, that we will see a difference between regional and general anaesthesia. Epidural local anaesthetic may well allow bowel function to return earlier (Liu et al 1995), but only if protocol allows it will we see patients going home two days after major surgery (Bardram et al 1995). The point is that this radical change is only possible if the procedure is done under an epidural, because the epidural makes it possible for the patient to mobilize early and for bowel function to return earlier.

For some operations there is proven advantage of regional over general anaesthesia. For hip (Sharrock and Salvati 1996) and knee (Williams-Russo et al 1996) replacements 'solid' epidural anaesthesia with sedation during surgery followed by postoperative epidural can produce reduced blood loss, faster surgery, reduced morbidity, and faster rehabilitation. In this context change has been gradual rather than radical, but again the key is the epidural, for both the operation and afterwards.

Returning to the old question, general versus regional anaesthesia, a recent set of meta-analyses looked at randomized, controlled trials (RCTs) to assess the effects of seven different interventions on postoperative pulmonary function after a variety of procedures (Ballantyne et al 1998). The seven were epidural opioid, epidural local anaesthetic, epidural opioid with local anaesthetic, thoracic versus lumbar epidural opioid, intercostal nerve block, wound infiltration with local anaesthetic, and intrapleural local anaesthetic. Compared with systemic opioids, epidural opioids decreased the incidence of atelectasis significantly. Epidural local anaesthetics compared with systemic opioids increased PaO_2 significantly and decreased the incidence of pulmonary infections and pulmonary complications overall. Intercostal nerve blockade did not produce significant improvement in pulmonary outcome measures. On the surrogate measures of pulmonary function (FEV1, FVC, and PEFR), there were no clinically or statistically significant differences, showing again the importance of choice of outcome measure. The results do confirm that postoperative epidural pain control can significantly decrease the incidence of pulmonary morbidity (Ballantyne et al 1998).

A recent meta-analysis purported to show that mortality was reduced when regional anaesthesia was used in conjunction with general anaesthesia (Rodgers et al 2000). The analysis was probably faulty, because 75% of the deaths occurred in just 25% of the papers, and the credibility of these papers should be questioned. Few of us work in contexts with an operative mortality of 25% or more.

What are the implications for local anaesthetics?

The so-called multimodal approach to the post-operative period uses local anaesthetics together with NSAIDs and paracetamol (Kehlet 1997, McQuay et al 1997). Slow release or very-long-acting local anaesthetics may deliver further radical improvement by improving the postoperative period. Long-acting local anaesthetics are not a new thought (Scurlock and Curtis 1981, King 1984), and the problem is to be sure that the block is indeed reversible and that the extended duration is not due to a toxic effect (Lipfert et al 1987).

Comparing blocks for a particular procedure

Many comparisons of one type of block against another are designed as A versus B comparisons. Unless the trials are very large, which most are not, one ends up concluding that the trial showed no difference, and we do not know whether the trial was capable of revealing a difference if in fact there was one (McQuay and Moore 1998). Choice of block also involves comparing the morbidity of the contenders. Again size of trial is crucial. Rare events will not be picked up in small trials.

Problems with local blocks

One important question is whether using nerve blocks or powerful epidural techniques has deleterious consequences. For most nerve blocks, for instance axillary brachial plexus block, we just do not know the incidence of long-term nerve problems. In all likelihood it is vanishingly small. In a one-year prospective survey of the French-Language Society of Pediatric Anesthesiologists Giaufre et al (1996) reported that 38% of the 24 409 local anaesthetic procedures were peripheral nerve blocks and local anaesthesia techniques. These were reported as 'generally safe'.

In the same survey 'central blocks' (15 013), most of which were caudals, accounted for more than 60% of all local anaesthetic procedures. Their complication rate for central blocks works out at 15 per 10 000 (25 incidents involving 24 patients). These were rated as minor, and did not result in any sequelae or medicolegal action.

In adults a report from Finland (Aromaa et al 1997) reviewed all claims (1987–1993) about severe complications associated with epidural and spinal anaesthesia. Eighty-six claims were associated with spinal and/or epidural anaesthesia. There were 550 000 spinals and 170 000 epidurals. With spinals there were 25 serious complications: cardiac arrests (2), paraplegia (5), permanent cauda equina syndrome (1), peroneal nerve paresis (6), neurological deficits (7), and bacterial infections (4). With epidurals there were 9 serious complications: paraparesis (1), permanent cauda equina syndrome (1), peroneal nerve paresis (1), neurological deficit (1), bacterial infections (2), acute toxic reactions related to the anaesthetic solution (2), and overdose of epidural opioid (1). This gives an overall incidence of serious complications of 0.45 per 10 000 for spinal and 0.52 per 10 000 for epidural.

Again in adults a French survey (Auroy et al 1997) reported on 40 640 spinals and 30 413 epidurals. Of the 98 severe complications 89 were attributed fully or partially to the regional anaesthesia. There were 26 cardiac arrests with spinals (6.4 ± 1.2 per 10 000 patients), and 6 were fatal. There were 3 arrests with epidurals. Of 34 neurological complications (radiculopathy, cauda equina syndrome, paraplegia), 21 were associated either with paraesthesiae during puncture (n = 19) or with pain during injection (n = 2), suggesting nerve trauma or intraneural injection. Neurological sequelae were significantly commoner after spinal anaesthesia (6 ± 1 per 10 000) than after each of the other types of regional procedures (1.6 ± 0.5 per 10 000).

Yuen et al (1995) described 12 patients (out of an estimated 13 000) with complications after lumbar epidurals. Eleven patients had lumbosacral radiculopathy or polyradiculopathy, 10 after epidural and 1 after subarachnoid injection of medication during the intended epidural. One patient had a thoracic myelopathy after an unintended spinal. From their data one may estimate the incidence of short-term (persisting less than one year) neurological sequelae after an epidural as 9 per 10 000, and for longer term (persisting more than one year) 2 per 10 000. As the authors point out these incidences appear to have changed little from previous case series.

An important RCT looked at the question of whether there was any difference in long-term cognitive dysfunction after total knee replacement surgery in 262 older adults (median age 69 years; 70% women) after epidural or general anaesthesia (Williams-Russo et al 1995). The importance is that it was the largest trial to date of the effects of general versus regional anaesthesia on cerebral function, with more than 99% power to detect a clinically significant difference on any of the neuropsychological tests. Preoperative neuropsychological assessment was repeated postoperatively at 1 week and 6 months. Cognitive outcome was assessed by within-patient change on 10 tests of memory, psychomotor, and language skills. There were no significant differences between the epidural and general anaesthesia groups on any of the 10 cognitive tests at either 1 week or 6 months. Overall, 5% of patients showed a long-term clinically significant deterioration in cognitive function.

Chronic pain; why can blocks last a long time?

Many of us do peripheral nerve blocks with local anaesthetic for pain due to trauma or surgery, and the dogma is that the local anaesthetic block alone can occasionally produce a cure and more often reduce pain for a duration that far exceeds the pharmacological action of the local anaesthetic. In a descriptive study Arnér et al (1990) reported on 38 consecutive patients with neuralgia after peripheral nerve injury, treated with one or two series of peripheral local anaesthetic blocks. The blocks were technically successful, with all patients experiencing an initial total relief of ongoing pain between 4 and 12 h. In the 17 patients who had evoked pain (hyperalgesia or allodynia) it was blocked together with the spontaneous pain. In 18 patients the analgesia outlasted the conduction block. Thirteen patients had complete pain relief for 12 to 48 h, and in 5 pain relief was complete for 2 to 6 days. Eight patients had a second phase of analgesia, varying from 4 h to 6 days, and coming on within 12 h of the pain recurring.

Arnér et al chose to concentrate on complete pain relief, and using this yardstick mono- or biphasic prolonged complete analgesia occurred in 25 out of 38 patients. A tantalizing further result is that for 15 of the 20 patients who had initial complete analgesia, but lasting less than 12 h, partial improvement lasting weeks to months was noted. Conversely only 1 of the 18 patients who had more than 12 h initial relief reported prolonged partial improvement. Their paper provides some empirical support for the (common) clinical use of local anaesthetic blocks in this context, and also reopens the interesting question of why a block can reduce pain for far longer than the local anaesthetic should work.

Arnér et al discuss systemic uptake and axoplasmic transport of local anaesthetic as putative mechanisms, but their experiments showed little evidence of transport. The explanation may lie in 'breaking the cycle'. The peripheral pain input is blocked, and the system can then reset itself. This begs many questions. For how long must the input be blocked to allow the system to reset? For which types of pain is this true? Their study provides clinical legitimacy for further investigation.

More on epidurals—local anaesthetic and opioid

For over 20 years we have known that opioids applied to the spinal cord have an analgesic effect. It has proved surprisingly difficult to define a clinical role for spinal (epidural and intrathecal) opioids, maximizing the analgesic benefit while minimizing the risk. The original question addressed was the advantage of spinal opioids over spinal local anaesthetics. The next question was the advantage of spinal opioids over intramuscular, oral, or subcutaneous opioids. Now we have come full circle because it is the use of spinal combinations of local anaesthetic and opioid that promises the greatest clinical benefit.

It is ironic that these questions are being addressed for spinal opioids while our ignorance about the conventional routes of administration for opioids, whether oral, subcutaneous, intramuscular, or intravenous, remains profound. The single most important point is to distinguish between the phenomenon 'it can be done' and the clinical questions 'should it be done?' and if so when and to whom? New routes often have a high profile such that it may be very difficult to determine their real clinical role. The ultimate arbiter of the clinical role is the risk:benefit ratio. The aim is better analgesia with fewer adverse effects and with no increase in morbidity. For instance in chronic pain oral opioids can provide good relief with manageable adverse effects for the majority of patients. New routes must be considered as replacements, adjuncts, or alternatives to the oral route.

Well-designed randomized controlled trials that compared the new route with the established routes would give us the answers. There are still few such trials available. They are hard to do well, particularly in chronic and cancer pain.

The underlying issues for new routes are kinetic and clinical logic. The spinal routes have the kinetic logic of applying the opioid directly to opioid receptors in the cord. The clinical advantage sought is better analgesia without the problems of systemic opioid use, or even the same analgesia with fewer adverse effects. Proposed alternatives must provide an improved risk:benefit ratio and be logistically feasible.

Underlying issues

The epidural space

The spinal epidural space extends from the sacral hiatus to the base of the skull. Drugs injected into the epidural space can then block or modulate afferent impulses and cord processing of those impulses. The way in which they block and modulate impulses and processing is probably the same as the mechanism that operates when the same drugs are injected intrathecally. The fact that the epidural space is a relatively indirect method of access compared with the intrathecal provides potential clinical advantage compared with the intrathecal route, but also complicates matters.

The potential clinical advantage of an epidural is the fact that the meninges are not physically breached, so that a headache from cerebrospinal fluid (CSF) leakage does not occur, and the danger of meningitis is also reduced. Chronic administration through catheters should therefore be safer by the epidural route than by the subarachnoid route. The first disadvantage is that the epidural space is vascular and contains fat. A large proportion of the epidural dose is taken up by extradural fat and by vascular absorption and so less drug is immediately available for neural-blocking action. The second disadvantage is that the epidural tissues react to foreign bodies more than the sheltered subarachnoid space. Epidural catheters often become walled off by fibrous tissue within days to weeks, whereas intrathecal catheters are much less prone to blockage (Durant and Yaksh 1986); this problem is in part overcome by using continuous epidural infusion rather than intermittent bolus.

Reaching the site of action

It used to be thought that the dura mater was impermeable to local anaesthetics and that epidural block with local anaesthetic occurred at the mixed nerve and dorsal root ganglia beyond the dural sleeves surrounding each pair of anterior and posterior spinal roots. Radioactive tracer studies showed that the dura mater is not impermeable, and that subarachnoid and epidural local anaesthetics act at precisely the same sites, the spinal roots, mixed spinal nerves, and the surface of the spinal cord to a depth of 1 mm or more, depending on the lipid solubility of the anaesthetic (Bromage et al 1963). With both epidural and subarachnoid injection the local anaesthetic drug enters the CSF and remains there until taken up by the lipids of the cord and spinal roots, or until 'washed out' by vascular uptake into the blood vessels of the region.

Opioids must reach the opioid receptors in the substantia gelatinosa of the cord in order to have spinal effect. Some of the opioid injected into the epidural space will reach the CSF and then the cord. Some will be absorbed into the blood stream, and some will be bound by fatty tissue in the epidural space. The proportion of the dose injected that goes in each of these directions depends on lipid solubility and on molecular weight (Moore et al 1982). Lipid-soluble opioids will be subject to greater vascular uptake from the epidural space than lipid insoluble opioids. High-molecular-weight drugs diffuse across the dura with less ease than drugs of low molecular weight. Once across the dura drugs that have low lipid solubility may maintain high concentrations in the CSF for long periods of time, and so can spread rostrally. Sampling at the cisternal level after lumbar intrathecal injection of morphine confirmed that high concentrations are found within an hour (Moulin et al 1986). Drugs with high lipid solubility will be bound much faster in the cord, leaving lower concentrations of drug in the CSF available to spread rostrally.

There is a similar range of lipophilicity and molecular size for the two drug classes, local anaesthetics and opioids, so that the journey from the place of injection to the target sites is likely to be accomplished in roughly the same time span for both classes of drug, and proportional losses by vascular absorption and uptake into neighbouring fat depots are also likely to be similar. With both local anaesthetics (Burm et al 1986) and opioids (Jamous et al 1986), vascular uptake is slowed and neural blockade increased by adding a dilute concentration of adrenaline (epinephrine; 3–5 μg/ml) to the injected agent.

Lipophilicity and potency

Within each class of drug, however, there is a wide range of lipophilicity, and this may have considerable influence on the relative potencies of the drugs within a class. Using an electrophysiological model, single-unit recordings were made in the lumbar dorsal horn in the intact anaesthetized rat from convergent, multireceptive neurones. Activity was evoked by Aβ and C fibre transcutaneous electrical stimulation of hindpaw receptive fields. With intrathecal application of opioids the effect of lipid solubility in determining relative intrathecal potency was measured. Initially four μ opioid receptor agonists were used, morphine, pethidine, methadone, and normorphine, because all four drugs had relatively high affinity for μ and little for δ and κ, precluding receptor affinity to other receptor subtypes as a complicating factor. The ED_{50} values from the dose–response curves were expressed against the partition coefficients. A significant correlation was found between the log ED_{50} and lipophilicity, but this was an inverse relationship, so that the least lipid-soluble agonists, morphine and normorphine, were the most potent, and the highly lipid-soluble methadone was considerably the least potent.

The same approximate order of potency, morphine = normorphine > pethidine > methadone, was seen in behavioural hot plate and tail flick tests, although the cutoff maxima necessary in those tests made it difficult to determine an ED_{50} for the more lipophilic and hence less potent compounds (Yaksh and Noueihed 1985). In a second study (Dickenson et al 1990) three opioids, fentanyl, etorphine, and buprenorphine, all highly potent by the systemic route in man and animals, were applied either intrathecally or intravenously. Figure 25.1 shows the relationship between intrathecal potency and lipophilicity for the 7 opioids tested. For fentanyl and buprenorphine potency correlated well with lipophilicity. The potency of etorphine, however, was considerably greater than would be expected if lipophilicity was the only determinant.

Non-specific binding is the probable explanation of the inverse correlation between intrathecal potency and lipid solubility. When radiolabelled opioid distribution was visualized by autoradiography (Herz and Teschemacher 1971) the highly lipid-soluble opioids were found to be restricted largely to fibre tracts, and penetrated the grey matter poorly. The thickly myelinated large A fibres cap the spinal cord grey matter. They pass medially over the dorsal horn before penetrating the grey matter. This means that the lipid-rich A fibres come between the injection site and the opioid receptors in the grey matter. Lipid-soluble opioids will be taken up rapidly but preferentially in this lipid-rich tissue. Drug bound in this non-specific way cannot then go on to bind to the receptors.

Systemic potency ratios in man are thus unlikely to be accurate guides to spinal effectiveness, which makes it difficult to choose the dose of intrathecal (or extradural) opioid necessary to produce the same analgesia as a given dose of morphine. Many of the epidural opioid studies that used opioids other than morphine have used the systemic potency ratio to morphine as the guide for spinal potency. Extrapolation from the animal data suggests that for drugs with high lipophilicity the intrathecal dose required to give analgesia equivalent to that produced by a 0.5-mg bolus dose of intrathecal morphine is likely to be on the order of 5 mg for pethidine and close to 8.5 mg for methadone.

Clinical studies support this argument. Systemically, methadone is equipotent to morphine. From the animal work intrathecal methadone was approximately 18-fold less potent than intrathecal morphine (McQuay et al 1989). An intrathecal dose of 0.5 mg of morphine provided significantly superior analgesia to 20 mg of methadone (Jacobson et al 1990).

For extradural use life is even less straightforward. Previous calculations showed that the

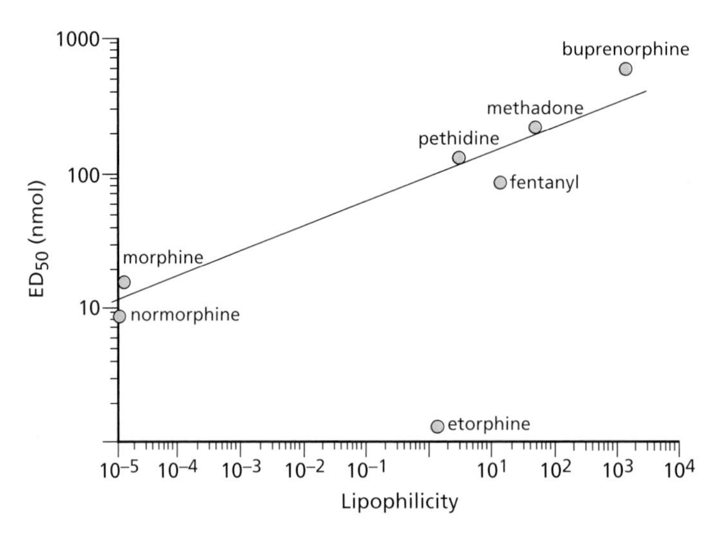

Fig. 25.1 Redrawn from Dickenson et al (1990). The relationship between lipophilicity (heptane/water partition coefficient) and potency (ED_{50} nmol) for morphine, normorphine, pethidine, methadone, buprenorphine, etorphine, and fentanyl.

proportion of an extradural dose transferred across the dura could vary from up to 20% for morphine (low lipid solubility) to 0.2% for buprenorphine (high lipid solubility) (Moore et al 1982). Because of the significant inverse correlation between lipid solubility and potency shown for the drug once in the cerebrospinal fluid, the extradural dose of highly lipid-soluble drugs may have to be surprisingly high to give effect equianalgesic to that of 5 mg of extradural morphine.

This theory means that no clinical advantage should be seen with extradural fentanyl (lipophilic) compared with intravenous injection of the same dose, as in either postoperative orthopaedic pain (Loper et al 1990) or after caesarean section (Ellis et al 1990). After laparotomy intravenous alfentanil (0.36 mg/h), combined with epidural bupivacaine 0.125%, was as effective as epidural alfentanil (0.36 mg/h; van den Nieuwenhuyzen et al 1998). The classic danger of course is that these are A versus B trial designs often with small numbers of patients. The trials may be insensitive to real differences. Others have found epidural fentanyl to provide superior analgesia to intravenous fentanyl, after thoracotomy (Salomäki et al 1991), during childbirth (D'Angelo et al 1998), and after caesarean section (Cooper et al 1995). These trials are also small, with maximum group size of 20. The trials in childbirth and after caesarean section really investigated epidural fentanyl plus local anaesthetic rather than fentanyl alone. We would conclude that this controversy shows the necessity of systemic controls in extradural studies, because the vascular uptake of a lipophilic drug from the epidural space will in itself result in analgesia and is similar in its time course and extent to the uptake seen after the same dose given parenterally.

We would also contend that lipophilic opioids on their own (not combined with local anaesthetic) are a poor choice for epidural use; non-specific binding means that they have low spinal potency, and substantial systemic analgesic effect makes it difficult to determine any spinal action. In practice bolus injection of epidural opioid often is given with, or soon after, injection of epidural local anaesthetic. Clinical impressions of good analgesia after epidural injection of lipophilic opioid may reflect synergism between the opioid and the local anaesthetic and systemic effect of the opioid.

Combinations of local anaesthetic and opioid

Epidural opioids on their own did not provide reliable analgesia in several pain contexts (Husemeyer et al 1980, Hogan et al 1991). Empirically combinations of local anaesthetic and opioid were found to work well, and extradural infusions of these combinations are used widely now for postoperative pain. The benefit is analgesia with minimal motor block and hypotension.

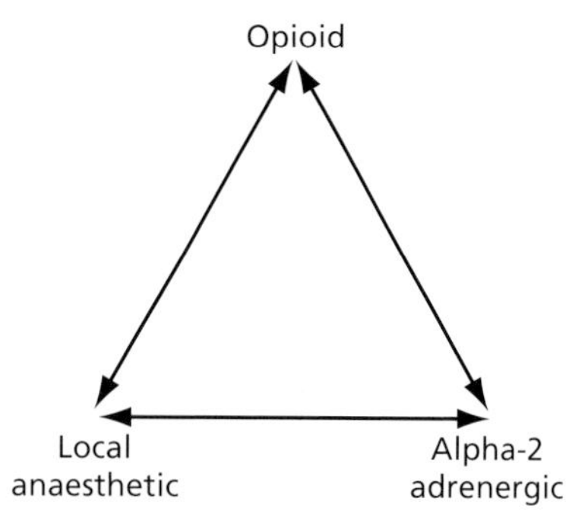

Fig. 25.2 Diagram of interactions between epidural local anaesthetic, opioid, and α_2-adrenergic agonists. The relationships with midazolam are not clear.

Two experimental studies have confirmed synergism between local anaesthetic and opioid (Fig. 25.2). Using visceral as well as conventional behavioural tests Maves and Gebhart did an isobolographic analysis for morphine and lignocaine (Maves and Gebhart 1992). They showed that the analgesic effect of the intrathecal combination was greater than would be expected for a simply additive relationship. Using an electrophysiological model Fraser et al (1992) compared the dose–response curve for lidocaine (lignocaine) combined with a dose of morphine with the dose–response curve for lidocaine (lignocaine) alone. Adding morphine, at a dose well below the ED_{50}, produced a 10-fold leftward shift in the lidocaine (lignocaine) dose–response curve.

These studies support what has been observed clinically, that doses of local anaesthetic and opioid, doses that might be regarded as homeopathic for either drug independently, can produce good analgesia. Neither study was designed to answer the important question of the minimal effective doses of the combination components. While the minimum effective doses will vary with pain context, studies answering the question for one type of pain may tell us which component is the prime mover. The mechanism of the synergy is not known. It may be that the local anaesthetic, by reducing the afferent input, is moving the opioid dose–response to the right. Such explanations, however, only account for one direction of synergy, and the evidence suggests that the synergy is bidirectional (Fig. 25.2). Clinical observations suggest that chronic infusion of the combination can produce selective blockade, blocking pain fibres while leaving other sensory input (and motor function) intact. These contradict the observation that blocking pain by epidural opioid alone is associated with blunting sensitivity to cold and pin-scratch sufficient for a segmental effect on cutaneous sensation to be detectable (Bromage et al 1982b). Such selectivity may of course be dose-dependent.

Other drugs

Many drugs have been given as analgesics via the epidural route. Caveats about toxicity are necessary.

α_2-Adrenergic agonists

In both electrophysiological (Jacobsen et al 1995) and behavioural studies α_2-adrenergic agonists have antinociceptive effect. Much of the early work was with clonidine, and this may have been misleading in terms of the properties of purer α_2-adrenergic agonists. Intrathecal clonidine showed a plateau at 50% of maximum effect. The newer drug, dexmedetomidine, is considerably more potent than clonidine and did not show such a ceiling to antinociception (Sullivan et al 1992a).

α_2-Adrenergic agonists have synergistic effect with both spinal opioid (Ossipov et al 1989, Sullivan et al 1992b, Jacobsen et al 1995) and spinal local anaesthetic (Fig. 25.2). The evidence for the local anaesthetic interaction comes mainly from clinical studies (Racle et al 1988; Bonnet et al 1989b, 1990; Carabine et al 1992; Huntoon et al 1992; Eisenach et al 1995).

Midazolam

Midazolam on its own has very limited antinociceptive effect in standard behavioural or electrophysiological models (Clavier et al 1992, Dirig and Yaksh 1995), although effects have been found in other models (Niv et al 1983, Goodchild and Serrao 1987). Midazolam may have effects on Aδ fibres (Clavier et al 1992), and may interact when combined with opioid (Moreau and Pieri 1988).

Therapeutic aspects

Both epidural local anaesthetics and epidural opioids can produce analgesia. The adverse effects of the two drug classes are different. Epidural local anaesthetics can produce hypotension because of sympathetic blockade, and carry the risks of local anaesthetic toxicity for which there is no specific antagonist. Epidural local anaesthetics produce motor block in a dose-dependent way. Epidural opioids can produce delayed respiratory depression, urinary retention, pruritus, and nausea and vomiting, particularly in the opioid naïve patient. Naloxone is a specific antagonist. Epidural opioids do not produce a motor block. The combination of epidural local anaesthetic and opioid can also produce pain relief, and the synergism between the drug classes offers the potential of effective analgesia at low doses of the components, minimizing the adverse effects of both.

Analgesic effect of epidural analgesics can be measured by a number of techniques, directly by measuring decrease in intensity or increase in pain relief, or indirectly via decreased need for other (parenteral) analgesics. Comparison with other, non-epidural, methods of pain relief has also involved indirect measures, such as the relative effects on respiration, time for patients to recover, and effects on stress hormones. The ultimate arbiter must be analgesic effect, because indirect measures, such as reduction of the expected rise of stress hormones, do not have a direct relationship with analgesia.

For many years randomized controlled trials that compared the analgesia and adverse effects of oral or parenteral analgesics used the rule that sensible comparisons of adverse effect incidence can only be made when the study drugs are compared at equianalgesic dosage. Very few randomized controlled trials that compare the adverse effects of different epidural opioids (or indeed epidural opioids with other techniques) have made equianalgesia the key criterion. Pronouncements about relative incidence of adverse effects can carry little weight unless the disparity in incidence or severity is measured at doses that produce equivalent analgesic effect.

The clinical decision to use epidural analgesia for pain relief is just that, a clinical decision. It presupposes that the analgesia is as good or better than analgesia from lower technology methods, that the potentially higher risk of adverse effects is worthwhile, and that the facilities exist to deliver the epidural analgesia effectively and safely. Combination techniques are superseding the use of epidural opioids on their own, and the randomized controlled trials to define the clinical role are still emerging.

Acute pain

Analgesia

Although both epidural local anaesthetics and epidural opioids can produce analgesia there is some doubt about the ability of epidural opioids to produce as good analgesia (Husemeyer et al 1980) as epidural local anaesthetics in severe pain states. In childbirth the degree of analgesia was inadequate to relieve the pain of second-stage labour (Husemeyer et al 1980, Hughes et al 1984), although satisfactory relief of first-stage pain could be achieved. No such doubt is seen with the epidural combination of local anaesthetics and opioids. The difference between the pain severity of different pain states should be emphasized, because it also means that categoric prescriptions for the doses to be used in combination infusions are likely to be valid only for a particular pain state or set of circumstances. Indeed the dynamic nature of postoperative pain means that the dosage required on the day of surgery may be much higher than the dosage required on subsequent days.

A clear demonstration of the advantage of the combination of local anaesthetic and opioid was seen in a comparison of 0.125% bupivacaine in saline, diamorphine 0.5 mg in 15 ml, and diamorphine mixed with 0.125% bupivacaine (0.5 mg in 15 ml) infused at a rate of 15 ml/h for pain after major gynaecological surgery. The combination produced significantly superior analgesia to either of its components alone, without major adverse effects (Lee et al 1988). Giving the diamorphine intravenously with epidural bupivacaine was significantly less effective than giving the same dose epidurally in combination with epidural bupivacaine (Lee et al 1991).

Many important questions are still to be answered. One practical issue is the ability of combination infusions to control pain remote from the catheter site, as with thoracic pain and a lumbar catheter. Another is whether there is any difference in efficacy or adverse effects if the drugs are given continuously rather than intermittently. For local anaesthetic alone there was little difference (Duncan et al 1998).

Combination dosage Three strategies in dosage are discernible, the low (Cullen et al 1985, Logas et al 1987, Lee et al 1988), the intermediate (Bigler et al 1989, Seeling et al 1990), and the high (Hjortso et al 1985, Schulze et al 1988, Scott et al 1989). High doses (bupivacaine 0.5% 25 mg/h and morphine 0.5 mg/h) were used to produce analgesia immediately after upper abdominal surgery but at some risk (Scott et al 1989). The stress response was not blocked. Lower doses (bupivacaine 0.1% 4 mg/h and morphine 0.4 mg/h) did not provide total pain relief after thoracotomy (Logas et al 1987). The issue of the minimum effective dose is of great importance, and unfortunately may have to be defined for particular circumstances.

Other analgesics

α_2-Adrenergic agonists The role of these drugs as analgesics on their own remains unclear. It is very difficult to preserve the double blinding in studies of α_2-adrenergic agonists because of the hypotensive and sedative effects of the drugs. Comparisons of epidural clonidine with epidural placebo for postoperative pain relief are all marred by this fault because significant hypotension was a feature (Gordh 1988, Bonnet et al 1989a, Bernard et al 1991). No analgesic dose–response curve could be defined for clonidine (Mendez et al 1990).

There is clear evidence, however, for both enhancement of the effect of local anaesthetics (Racle et al 1988; Bonnet et al 1989b, 1990; Carabine et al 1992; Huntoon et al 1992) and enhancement of the effect of opioids. With fentanyl (Rostaing et al 1991) and sufentanil (Vercauteren et al 1990) duration of effect was extended; with morphine Motsch et al (1990) found that adding clonidine produced significantly better pain scores. There may thus be an adjuvant rôle for α_2-adrenergic agonists.

Midazolam Midazolam is reported to have analgesic effect in postoperative pain (see Serrao et al 1992) but this is hard to understand in view of the drug's failure in animal nociceptive pain models.

Adverse effects

Toxicity Epidural delivery necessarily places drugs at the neuraxis. Toxicity is therefore a real risk. Standard epidural analgesics, specifically local anaesthetics and opioids, have not produced toxicity to date, and clonidine was tested before it was used. Perhaps the major worry is that new analgesics without toxicology will be introduced.

Motor block Techniques of epidural local anaesthesia have been refined to a point where the neural pathways conducting pain can be blocked with a high degree of anatomical selectivity, but motor block is an inevitable accompaniment if large doses of local anaesthetic are needed to stop the pain. In labour pain the motor block may result in a higher incidence of instrumental delivery than with non-epidural pain relief. This motor block is not seen with epidural opioids alone or when low doses of local anaesthetic are combined with opioid.

Vasodilatation and hypotension Vasodilatation in the lower parts of the body from blockade of sympathetic vasomotor nerves in the segments involved is another inevitable accompaniment of epidural local anaesthetic. In labour this requires prophylaxis. Hypotension also occurs with α_2-adrenergic agonists, and their use in combination with local anaesthetics could accentuate the risk. Again the risk is minimized with epidural opioids alone or with the low doses of local anaesthetic used when combined with opioid.

Respiratory depression Epidural block with local anaesthetics of intercostal and abdominal muscles is unlikely to cause significant impairment of respiratory function unless the phrenic segments (C3, C4, and C5) are also blocked. Respiratory depression after epidural opioids in opioid-naïve subjects is much more subtle, more delayed in onset, and longer lasting. The epidural opioids all reach the CSF by diffusion through the meninges, and variable degrees of cephalad spread occur within the CSF. Morphine, being relatively less lipid-soluble, will maintain substantial CSF concentrations to a greater extent than more lipid-soluble drugs, increasing the chance of drug reaching opioid receptors in the brain and so increasing the chance of respiratory depression. In volunteers 10 mg of epidural morphine produced a depression of the CO_2-response curve far greater than that seen after intravenous administration, with the nadir of depression between the 6th and 12th hours after administration (Camporesi et al 1983).

Profound respiratory depression may be precipitated if other opioids are given parenterally during this danger period. Precautions must be taken to see that this mixed type of medication is avoided, and that patients are under appropriate surveillance, so that any case of delayed respiratory depression can be treated promptly (Ready et al 1988). Life-threatening apnoeic intervals can also arise abruptly after small doses of epidural opioids alone, with little warning. Theoretically highly lipid-soluble opioids such as fentanyl and sufentanil should be less prone to rostral spread in the CSF. In practice volunteer studies suggest that although apnoeic intervals after epidural sufentanil were less frequent and less prolonged than after morphine (Klepper et al 1987), at equianalgesic doses of the drugs the CO_2-response curve was depressed and displaced equally severely.

Epidural opioids given on their own for relief of acute pain in opioid-naïve subjects are only as safe as the quality of surveillance that is given. Whether the lower doses used in combination with local anaesthetics reduce the risk still must be established.

Systemic effects With epidural opioids systemic effects of the opioid are to be expected. Vascular uptake from the epidural space is appreciable, with blood concentration curves of opioid almost indistinguishable from those after intramuscular or intravenous administration (see for morphine Bromage et al 1982b, Chauvin et al 1982, Nordberg et al 1983). All the adverse effects of systemic opioids should therefore be expected. Placental transfer of opioid to the fetus and subsequent neonatal respiratory depression are thus not prevented by changing from parenteral opioid to epidural opioid.

Bladder function Urinary retention is a common complication of epidural analgesic techniques after either local anaesthetics or opioids. The incidence appears to be dose-related, and in the case of local anaesthetics retention is probably due to bladder deafferentation because the distended bladder does not give rise to discomfort. With epidural opioids the mechanism seems to be more complicated, because retention and bladder distension to volumes above 800 ml in volunteers gave rise to marked discomfort and distress (Bromage et al 1982a).

Urodynamic and electromyographic studies in male volunteers indicated that the cause was detrusor muscle relaxation and not increased motor activity in the pelvic floor muscles (Rawal et al 1983). The origin of this detrusor relaxation is unclear, but the time sequence mirrors that of antinociception, beginning within 15 min but taking about 60 min to reach peak effect, and then lasting 14–16 h. The overall intensity and duration of bladder relaxation appears to be independent of dose within the range of 2–10 mg. Retention with epidural opioids, like all the other adverse effects of epidural opioids, can be relieved by naloxone, although repeated doses may be needed to ensure complete evacuation of the bladder (Bromage et al 1982a).

The high incidence of retention from either local anaesthetic or opioid blockade is a factor in the clinical decision to use epidural analgesia.

Pruritus Pruritus is not seen after epidural local anaesthetics, but it is a frequent adverse effect of epidural opioids in the opioid-naïve patient. The itching is usually generalized but can be in the analgesic segments. The cause of the pruritus is unclear. The onset is often hours after analgesic effect is established, perhaps suggesting modulation of cutaneous sensation in the cord. Pruritus can be a major problem in acute pain management with epidural opioids, severe enough to cause distress. It can be reversed by naloxone, but then the analgesia is likely to be reversed.

Long-term risks The incidence of severe infective complications is low but finite.

Chronic pain

Epidural analgesics have roles in both chronic non-malignant pain and cancer pain.

Chronic non-malignant pain

In chronic non-malignant pain the primary role for epidural local anaesthetics is their injection sometimes combined with steroid for the management of back pain with the object of reducing local oedema and nerve-root compression (Koes et al 1995, Watts and Silagy 1995).

Epidural opioids alone have little place in the long-term management of on-going non-malignant pain (but see Plummer et al 1991), although acute exacerbations may be handled on a one-off basis.

The role of epidural clonidine is contentious. Apart from its ability to extend the duration of local anaesthetics it may have the ability to relieve some forms of neuropathic or deafferentation pain. Glynn et al (1988) found epidural clonidine to be as effective as epidural morphine in 20 chronic pain patients using a crossover design. As in earlier studies there was a suggestion that clonidine was more effective than morphine for neuropathic pain. α_2-Adrenergic drugs have a place as adjuvants in local anaesthetic and opioid combinations for resistant neuropathic pain (Eisenach et al 1995).

Epidural midazolam was found in one randomized controlled trial to be as effective as epidural steroid in the management of chronic back pain (Serrao et al 1992). Experience is limited, so that more studies are needed to clarify whether there is a clinical role.

Cancer pain

Epidural opioids are used in chronic cancer pain as an alternative to other (oral or subcutaneous) routes (Plummer et al 1991). There has been little evidence from randomized controlled trials to support the argument that better analgesia is provided at lower incidence of adverse effects. Indeed one trial found that subcutaneous opioid was just as good as epidural opioid alone (Kalso et al 1996).

Long-term administration, either as intermittent bolus or by infusion, is technically feasible. The choice of delivery system lies between the low technology percutaneous exterior epidural catheter and micropore filter, tunnelled subcutaneous catheter with external injection port and micropore filter, and high technology totally implanted system with small subcutaneous reservoir and injection port, totally implanted system with large internal reservoir and automatic metered or manually controlled dosing device. Implanted systems are more likely to maintain hygiene and convenience, in theory protecting from infection and mechanical displacement. Implanted devices have high initial costs compared with simple percutaneous approaches, but over a period of months this may even out because of the higher costs of maintaining or replacing percutaneous catheters.

These technical approaches for administering small metered doses of spinal morphine over periods of weeks or months have proved to be well suited to home management, and highly appreciated by the patients and their families. The problems include blockage, infection, pain on injection, and leaks (Plummer et al 1991). It is important to be sure that the patient's pain cannot be controlled by simpler routes and that it can indeed be controlled by this method before embarking on what is a substantial undertaking (Jadad et al 1991). Preliminary trials with a percutaneous catheter to assess the effectiveness and the acceptability of adverse effects are necessary.

The main argument against the use of the epidural route as (merely) an alternative way to deliver opioid is that the opioid, whether given orally or spinally, must in the end be working at the opioid receptor. Failed management with oral opioid, failed because the pain was not responsive (Arnér and Meyerson 1988, Jadad et al 1992) rather than failed because the opioid was not absorbed, is thus a questionable indication for epidural opioid. The protagonists can point to many thousands of patients treated. Epidural opioids alone, however, are not a universal panacea in cancer pain (Hogan et al 1991); if conventional routes for opioids do not relieve the pain, combinations of local anaesthetic and opioid appear to have a higher success rate than opioid alone.

A systematic review (Ballantyne et al 1996) compared the efficacy of epidural, subarachnoid, and intracerebroventricular opioids in cancer. Intracerebroventricular therapy appeared at least as effective against pain as other approaches, and was the only fixed system associated with fewer technical problems than the use of simple percutaneous epidural catheters.

Combination of local anaesthetic and opioid
The situation is changing with the advent of

epidural infusion of combination of local anaesthetics and opioid. Intrathecal use of such combinations in cancer pain is described by Sjöberg et al (1991). Most cancer pain, some 80%, responds to simple management with oral opioid and other analgesics. The two kinds of cancer pain which respond badly to simple management are movement-related pain and neuropathic pain.

Movement-related pain can theoretically be controlled with oral opioid. In practice the dose of opioid required to control the patient's pain on movement is such that the patient is soundly sedated when not moving (not in pain). Conventional wisdom is that NSAIDs should be added if they have been omitted. In practice this often has little impact in established severe pain. Some such pains, for instance due to vertebral metastases, can be helped by extradural steroid. The final resort is to use continuous epidural infusion of a combination of local anaesthetic and opioid. The synergy between the local anaesthetic and the opioid means that low doses can provide analgesia with little loss of mobility. There are few randomized controlled trials of this usage. The need for greater volume means that few of the devices available for implanted infusion of opioid alone are suitable, so that percutaneous catheters and external syringe drivers may be necessary. This method appears to produce analgesia for pains poorly responsive to opioids alone. The logic then is that pains poorly responsive to opioid orally are unlikely to improve simply by changing the route by which the opioid is given. Epidural use of local anaesthetic and opioid can produce the necessary analgesia.

The management of neuropathic cancer pain is often not straightforward. If such pain cannot be controlled by opioid, antidepressant or anticonvulsant, and steroids are inappropriate, then again epidural infusion of a combination of local anaesthetic and opioid should be considered. An RCT of 85 patients comparing 30 μg per hour epidural clonidine with placebo for 14 days showed successful analgesia was commoner with epidural clonidine (45%) than with placebo (21%), and more so in neuropathic pain (56 vs 5%) (Eisenach et al 1995).

Conclusion

Epidural local anaesthetics have been used for many years in the management of acute pain in trauma, surgery, and obstetrics, as well as in chronic pain, and their limitations and capabilities are well understood in these clinical areas. Opioids by this route are a new departure, and our short experience in human subjects dates from as recently as 1979. Early enthusiasm in this field has been tempered by randomized controlled trials, and the field remains dynamic, with a switch from the use of either local anaesthetics or opioids on their own to the combination of the two. The α_2-adrenergic agonists in existing forms may also have a limited role on their own but may interact with local anaesthetics and opioids to provide a clinical advantage. Their importance is that they suggest that other beneficial interactions may emerge.

The fact that the field is dynamic, with a recent switch to the combination of local anaesthetics and opioids, means that we do not yet have the necessary information as to minimal effective dose. Randomized controlled trials are then required to define the clinical role of epidural combinations versus non-epidural pain relief in all the various pain contexts. There is still major concern that these powerful analgesic tools should be used effectively, safely, and economically. The dream of attaining prolonged and powerful analgesia without adverse effects has not yet been realized, and as far as these epidural techniques are concerned, pain relief must still be bought at the cost of some risk. In some areas of pain management, however, these techniques are changing radically the quality of the service we deliver.

References

Arnér S, Meyerson BA 1988 Lack of analgesic effect of opioids on neuropathic and idiopathic forms of pain. Pain 33: 11–23

Arnér S, Lindblom U, Meyerson BA, Molander C 1990 Prolonged relief of neuralgia after regional anesthetic blocks. A call for further experimental and systematic clinical studies. Pain 43: 287–297

Aromaa U, Lahdensuu M, Cozanitis DA 1997 Severe complications associated with epidural and spinal anaesthesias in Finland 1987–1993. A study based on patient insurance claims. Acta Anaesthesiologica Scandinavica 41: 445–452

Auroy Y, Narchi P, Messiah A, Litt L, Rouvier B, Samii K 1997 Serious complications related to regional anesthesia: results of a prospective survey in France. Anesthesiology 87: 479–486

Ballantyne JC, Carr DB, Berkey CS, Chalmers TC, Mosteller F 1996 Comparative efficacy of epidural, subarachnoid, and intracerebroventricular opioids in patients with pain due to cancer. Regional Anesthesia 21: 542–556

Ballantyne JC, Carr DB, deFerranti S, Suarez T, Lau J, Chalmers TC, Angelillo IF, Mosteller F 1998 The comparative effects of postoperative analgesic therapies on pulmonary outcome: cumulative meta-analyses of randomized, controlled trials. Anesthesia and Analgesia 86: 598–612

Bardram L, Funch-Jensen P, Jensen P, Crawford ME, Kehlet H 1995 Recovery after laparoscopic colonic surgery with epidural analgesia, and early oral nutrition and mobilisation. Lancet 345: 763–764

Beattie C, Roizen MF, Downing JW 1996 Cardiac outcomes after regional or general anesthesia: do we know the question? Anesthesiology 85: 1207–1209

Bernard J-M, Hommeril J-L, Passuti N, Pinaud M 1991 Postoperative analgesia by intravenous clonidine. Anesthesiology 75: 577–582

Bigler D, Dirkes W, Hansen R, Rosenberg J, Kehlet H 1989 Effects of thoracic paravertebral block with bupivacaine versus combined thoracic epidural block with bupivacaine and morphine on pain and pulmonary function after cholecystectomy. Acta Anaesthesiologica Scandinavica 33: 561–564

Bode RJ, Lewis KP, Zarich SW, Pierce ET, Roberts M, Kowalchuk GJ, Satwicz PR, Gibbons GW, Hunter JA, Espanola CC 1996 Cardiac outcome after peripheral vascular surgery. Comparison of general and regional anesthesia. Anesthesiology 84: 3–13

Bonnet F, Boico O, Rostaing S, Saada M, Loriferne J, Touboul C, Abhay K, Ghignone M 1989 Postoperative analgesia with extradural clonidine. British Journal of Anaesthesia 63: 465–469

Bonnet F, Diallo A, Saada M, Belon M, Guilbaud M, Boico O 1989 Prevention of tourniquet pain by spinal isobaric bupivacaine with clonidine. British Journal of Anaesthesia 63: 93–96

Bonnet F, Buisson V, Francois Y, Catoire P, Saada M 1990 Effects of oral and subarachnoid clonidine on spinal anesthesia with bupivacaine. Regional Anesthesia 15: 211–214

Bromage P, Joyal A, Binney J 1963 Local anaesthetic drugs: penetration from the spinal extradural space into the neuraxis. Science 140: 392–393

Bromage PR, Camporesi EM, Durant PAC, Nielson CH 1982a Nonrespiratory side effects of epidural morphine. Anesthesia and Analgesia 61: 490–495

Bromage PR, Camporesi EM, Durant PAC, Nielson CH 1982b Rostral spread of epidural morphine. Anesthesiology 56: 431–436

Burm A, van Kleef JW, Gladines M, Olthof G, Spierdijk J 1986 Epidural anesthesia with lidocaine and bupivacaine: effects of epinephrine on the plasma concentration profiles. Anesthesia and Analgesia 65: 1281–1284

Callesen T, Bech K, Kehlet H 1998 The feasibility, safety and cost of infiltration anaesthesia for hernia repair. Hvidovre Hospital Hernia Group. Anaesthesia 53: 31–35

Camporesi E, Nielson C, Bromage P, Durant P 1983 Ventilatory CO_2 sensitivity following intravenous and epidural morphine in volunteers. Anesthesia and Analgesia 62: 633–640

Carabine U, Milligan K, Moore J 1992 Extradural clonidine and bupivacaine for postoperative analgesia. British Journal of Anaesthesia 68: 132–135

Chauvin M, Samii K, Schermann J, Sandouk P, Bourdon R, Viars P 1982 Plasma pharmacokinetics of morphine after i.m. extradural and intrathecal administration. British Journal of Anaesthesia 54: 843–847

Christopherson R, Beattie C, Frank SM, Norris EJ, Meinert CL, Gottlieb SO, Yates H, Rock P, Parker SD, Perler BA et al 1993 Perioperative morbidity in patients randomized to epidural or general anesthesia for lower extremity vascular surgery. Perioperative Ischemia Randomized Anesthesia Trial Study Group. Anesthesiology 79: 422–434

Clavier N, Lombard M-C, Besson J-M 1992 Benzodiazepines and pain: effects of midazolam on the activities of nociceptive non-specific dorsal horn neurons in the rat spinal cord. Pain 48: 61–71

Cooper DW, Ryall DM, Desira WR 1995 Extradural fentanyl for postoperative analgesia: predominant spinal or systemic action? British Journal of Anaesthesia 74: 184–187

Cullen M, Staren E, El-Ganzouri A, Logas W, Ivankovich D, Economou S 1985 Continuous epidural infusion for analgesia after major abdominal operations: A randomised, prospective, double-blind study. Surgery 10: 718–728

D'Angelo R, Gerancher JC, Eisenach JC, Raphael BL 1998 Epidural fentanyl produces labor analgesia by a spinal mechanism. Anesthesiology 88: 1519–1523

Dickenson AH, Sullivan AF, McQuay HJ 1990 Intrathecal etorphine, fentanyl and buprenorphine on spinal nociceptive neurones in the rat. Pain 42: 227–234

Dirig DM, Yaksh TL 1995 Intrathecal baclofen and muscimol, but not midazolam, are antinociceptive using the rat-formalin model. Journal of Pharmacology and Experimental Therapeutics 275: 219–227

Duncan LA, Fried MJ, Lee A, Wildsmith JA 1998 Comparison of continuous and intermittent administration of extradural bupivacaine for analgesia after lower abdominal surgery. British Journal of Anaesthesia 80: 7–10

Durant P, Yaksh T 1986 Distribution in cerebrospinal fluid, blood, and lymph of epidurally injected morphine and inulin in dogs. Anesthesia and Analgesia 65: 583–592

Eisenach JC, DuPen S, Dubois M, Miguel R, Allin D 1995 Epidural clonidine analgesia for intractable cancer pain. The Epidural Clonidine Study Group. Pain 61: 391–399

Ellis D, Millar W, Reisner L 1990 A randomised double-blind comparison of epidural versus intravenous fentanyl infusion for analgesia after Cesarian section. Anesthesiology 72: 981–986

Fraser H, Chapman V, Dickenson A 1992 Spinal local anaesthetic actions on afferent evoked responses and wind-up of nociceptive neurones in the rat spinal cord: combination with morphine produces marked potentiation of nociception. Pain 49: 33–41

Giaufre E, Dalens B, Gombert A 1996 Epidemiology and morbidity of regional anesthesia in children: a one-year prospective survey of the French-Language Society of Pediatric Anesthesiologists. Anesthesia and Analgesia 83: 904–912

Glynn C, Dawson D, Sanders R 1988 A double blind comparison between epidural morphine and epidural clonidine in patients with chronic non cancer pain. Pain 34: 123–128

Goodchild C, Serrao J 1987 Intrathecal midazolam in the rat: evidence for spinally-mediated analgesia. British Journal of Anaesthesia 59: 1563–1570

Gordh TJ 1988 Epidural clonidine for treatment of postoperative pain after thoracotomy. A double blind placebo controlled study. Acta Anaesthesiologica Scandinavica 32: 702–709

Herz A, Teschemacher H 1971 Activities and sites of antinociceptive action of morphine like analgesics. Advances in Drug Research 6: 79–119

Hjortso NC, Neumann P, Frosig F, Andersen T, Lindhard A, Rogon E, Kehlet H 1985 A controlled study on the effect of epidural analgesia with local anaesthetics and morphine on morbidity after abdominal surgery. Acta Anaesthesiologica Scandinavica 29: 790–796

Hogan Q, Haddox J, Abram S, Weissman D, Taylor M, Janjan N 1991 Epidural opiates and local anaesthetics for the management of cancer pain. Pain 46: 271–279

Hughes SC, Rosen MA, Shnider SM, Abboud TK, Stefani SJ, Norton M 1984 Maternal and neonatal effects of epidural morphine for labor and delivery. Anesthesia and Analgesia 63: 319–324

Huntoon M, Eisenach J, Boese P 1992 Epidural clonidine after cesarian section. Anesthesiology 76: 187–193

Husemeyer R, O'Connor M, Davenport H 1980 Failure of epidural morphine to relieve pain in labour. Anaesthesia 35: 161–163

Jacobsen SJ, Oesterling JE, Lieber MM 1995 Community-based population studies on the natural history of prostatism. Current Opinion in Urology 5: 13–17

Jacobson L, Chabal C, Brody MC, Ward RJ, Wasse L 1990 Intrathecal methadone: a dose-response study and comparison with intrathecal morphine 0.5 mg. Pain 43: 141–148

Jadad AR, Popat MT, Glynn CJ, McQuay HJ 1991 Double-blind testing fails to confirm analgesic response to extradural morphine. Anaesthesia 46: 935–937

Jadad AR, Carroll D, Glynn CJ, Moore RA, McQuay HJ 1992 Morphine responsiveness of chronic pain: double-blind randomised crossover study with patient-controlled analgesia. Lancet 339: 1367–1371

Jamous MA, Hand CW, Moore RA, Teddy PJ, McQuay HJ 1986 Epinephrine reduces systemic absorption of extradural diacetylmorphine. Anesthesia and Analgesia 65: 1290–1294
Kalso E, Heiskanen T, Rantio M, Rosenberg PH, Vainio A 1996 Epidural and subcutaneous morphine in the management of cancer pain: a double-blind cross-over study. Pain 67: 443–449
Kehlet H 1994 Postoperative pain relief—what is the issue? British Journal of Anaesthesia 72: 375–378
Kehlet H 1997 Multimodal approach to control postoperative pathophysiology and rehabilitation. British Journal of Anaesthesia 78: 606–617
Kehlet H, Callesen T 1998 Recommendations for convalescence after hernia surgery. A questionnaire study. Ugeskr Laeger 160: 1008–1009
King J 1984 Dexamethasone—a helpful adjunct in management after lumbar discectomy. Neurosurgery 14: 697–700
Klepper I, Sherrill D, Boetger C, Bromage P 1987 The analgesic and respiratory effects of epidural sufentanil and the influence of adrenaline as an adjuvant. Anesthesiology 59: 1147–1159
Koes BW, Scholten RPM, Mens JMA, Bouter LM 1995 Efficacy of epidural steroid injections for low-back pain and sciatica: a systematic review of randomized clinical trials. Pain 63: 279–288
Lee A, Simpson D, Whitfield A, Scott D 1988 Postoperative analgesia by continuous extradural infusion of bupivacaine and diamorphine. British Journal of Anaesthesia 60: 845–850
Lee A, McKeown D, Brockway M, Bannister J, Wildsmith JAW 1991 Comparison of extradural and intravenous diamorphine as a supplement to extradural bupivacaine. Anaesthesia 46: 447–450
Lipfert P, Seitz R, Arndt J 1987 Ultralong-lasting nerve block: triethyldodectyl ammonium bromide is probably a neurotoxin rather than a local anesthetic. Anesthesiology 67: 896–904
Liu SS, Carpenter RL, Mackey DC, Thirlby RC, Rupp SM, Shine TS, Feinglass NG, Metzger PP, Fulmer JT, Smith SL 1995 Effects of perioperative analgesic technique on rate of recovery after colon surgery. Anesthesiology 83: 757–765
Logas W, El Baz N, El Ganzouri A, Cullen M, Staren E, Faber L, Ivankovich A 1987 Continuous thoracic epidural analgesia for postoperative pain relief following thoracotomy: a randomized prospective study. Anesthesiology 67: 787–791
Loper K, Ready B, Downey M, Sandler A, Nessly M, Rapp S, Badner N 1990 Epidural and intravenous fentanyl infusions are clinically equivalent after knee surgery. Anesthesia and Analgesia 70: 72–75
Maves TJ, Gebhart GF 1992 Antinociceptive synergy between intrathecal morphine and lidocaine during visceral and somatic nociception in the rat. Anesthesiology 76: 91–99
McQuay HJ, Moore RA 1998 An evidence-based resource for pain relief. Oxford University Press, Oxford
McQuay HJ, Sullivan AF, Smallman K, Dickenson AH 1989 Intrathecal opioids, potency and lipophilicity. Pain 36: 111–115
McQuay HJ, Justins D, Moore RA 1997 Treating acute pain in hospital. British Medical Journal 314: 1531–1535
Mendez R, Eisenach J, Kashtan K 1990 Epidural clonidine analgesia after cesarean section. Anesthesiology 73: 848–852
Moore RA, Bullingham RE, McQuay HJ, Hand CW, Aspel JB, Allen MC, Thomas D 1982 Dural permeability to narcotics: in vitro determination and application to extradural administration. British Journal of Anaesthesia 54: 1117–1128
Moreau J-L, Pieri L 1988 Effects of an intrathecally administered benzodiazepine receptor agonist, antagonist and inverse agonist on morphine-induced inhibition of a spinal nociceptive reflex. British Journal of Pharmacology 93: 964–968
Motsch J, Graber E, Ludwig K 1990 Addition of clonidine enhances postoperative analgesia from epidural morphine: a double blind study. Anesthesiology 73: 1067–1073
Moulin D, Inturrisi C, Foley K 1986 Epidural and intrathecal opioids: cerebrospinal fluid and plasma pharmacokinetics in cancer pain patients. Foley K, Inturrisi C (eds) Advances in pain research and therapy, vol 8. Raven Press, New York, pp 369–383
Nehra D, Gemmell L, Pye JK 1995 Pain relief after inguinal hernia repair: a randomized double-blind study. British Journal of Surgery 82: 1245–1247
Niv D, Whitwam J, Loh L 1983 Depression of nociceptive sympathetic reflexes by the intrathecal administration of midazolam. British Journal of Anaesthesia 55: 541–547
Nordberg G, Hedner T, Mellstrand T, Dahlstrom B 1983 Pharmacokinetic aspects of epidural morphine analgesia. Anesthesiology **58**: 545–551
Ossipov M, Suarez L, Spaulding T 1989 Antinociceptive interactions between alpha2-adrenergic and opiate agonists at the spinal level in rodents. Anesthesia and Analgesia 68: 194–200
Plummer J, Cherry D, Cousins M, Gourlay G, Onley M, Evans H 1991 Long term spinal administration of morphine in cancer and non-cancer pain: a retrospective study. Pain 44: 215–220
Racle J, Poy J, Benkhadra A, Jourdren L, Fockenier F 1988 Prolongation of spinal anesthesia with hyperbaric bupivacaine by adrenaline and clonidine in the elderly. Annales Francaises d'Anesthesie Reanimation 7: 139–144
Rawal N, Möllefors K, Axelsson K, Lingårdh G, Widman B 1983 An experimental study of urodynamic effects of epidural morphine and naloxone reversal. Anesthesia and Analgesia 62: 641–647
Ready LB, Oden R, Chadwick HS, Benedetti C, Rooke GA, Caplan R, Wild LM 1988 Development of an anaesthesiology based postoperative pain management service. Anesthesiology 68: 100–106
Rigg JRA, Jamrozik K 1998 Outcome after general or regional anaesthesia in high-risk patients. Current Opinion in Anaesthesiology 11: 327–331
Rodgers A, Walker N, Schug S, McKee A, Kehlet H, van Zundert A, Sage D, Futter M, Saville G, Clark T, MacMahon S 2000 Reduction of postoperative mortality and morbidity with epidural or spinal anaesthesia: results from overview of randomised trials. British Medical Journal 321: 1493
Rostaing S, Bonnet F, Levron J, Vodinh J, Pluskwa F, Saada M 1991 Effect of epidural clonidine on analgesia and pharmacokinetics of epidural fentanyl in postoperative patients. Anesthesiology 75: 420–425
Salomäki T, Laitinen J, Nuutinen L 1991 A randomised double-blind comparison of epidural versus intravenous fentanyl infusion for analgesia after thoracotomy. Anesthesiology 75: 790–795
Schulze S, Roikjaer O, Hasselstrom L, Jensen N, Kehlet H 1988 Epidural bupivacaine and morphine plus systemic indomethacin eliminates pain but not systemic response and convalescence after cholecystectomy. Surgery 103: 321–327
Scott N, Mogensen T, Bigler D, Lund C, Kehlet H 1989 Continuous thoracic extradural 0.5% bupivacaine with or without morphine: effect on quality of blockade, lung function and the surgical stress response. British Journal of Anaesthesia 62: 253–257
Scurlock J, Curtis B 1981 Tetraethylammonium derivatives: ultralong-acting local anesthetics. Anesthesiology 54: 265–269
Seeling W, Bruckmooser K, Hufner C, Kneitinger E, Rigg C, Rockemann M 1990 No reduction in postoperative complications by the use of catheterized epidural analgesia following major abdominal surgery. Anaesthesist 39: 33–40
Serrao J, Marks R, Morley S, Goodchild C 1992 Intrathecal midazolam for the treatment of chronic mechanical low back pain: a conrolled comparison with epidural steroid in a pilot study. Pain 48: 5–12
Sharrock NE, Salvati EA 1996 Hypotensive epidural anesthesia for total hip arthroplasty: a review [see comments]. Acta Orthopaedica Scandinavica 67: 91–107

Sjöberg M, Applegren L, Einarsson S, Hultman E, Linder L, Nitescu P, Curelaru C 1991 Long-term intrathecal morphine and bupivacaine in 'refractory' cancer pain. I. Results from the first series of 52 patients. Acta Anaesthesiologica Scandinavica 35: 30–43

Sullivan AF, Kalso EA, McQuay HJ, Dickenson AH 1992a The antinociceptive actions of dexmedetomidine on dorsal horn neuronal responses in the anaesthetized rat. European Journal of Pharmacology 215: 127–133

Sullivan AF, Kalso EA, McQuay HJ, Dickenson AH 1992b Evidence for the involvement of the mu but not delta opioid receptor subtype in the synergistic interaction between opioid and alpha 2 adrenergic antinociception in the rat spinal cord. Neuroscience Letters 139: 65–68

Teasdale C, McCrum AM, Williams NB, Horton RE 1982 A randomised controlled trial to compare local with general anaesthesia for short-stay inguinal hernia repair. Annals of the Royal College of Surgeons of England 64: 238–242

van den Nieuwenhuyzen M, Stienstra R, Burm AG, Vletter AA, van Kleef J 1998 Alfentanil as an adjuvant to epidural bupivacaine in the management of postoperative pain after laparotomies: lack of evidence of spinal action. Anesthesia and Analgesia 86: 574–578

Vercauteren M, Lauwers E, Meert T, De Hert S, Adriaensen H 1990 Comparison of epidural sufentanil plus clonidine with sufentanil alone for postoperative pain relief. Anaesthesia 45: 531–534

Watts RW, Silagy CA 1995 A meta-analysis on the efficacy of epidural corticosteroids in the treatment of sciatica. Anaesthesia and Intensive Care 23: 564–569

Williams-Russo P, Sharrock NE, Mattis S, Szatrowski TP, Charlson ME 1995 Cognitive effects after epidural vs general anesthesia in older adults. A randomized trial. Journal of the American Medical Association 274: 44–50

Williams-Russo P, Sharrock NE, Haas SB, Insall J, Windsor RE, Laskin RS, Ranawat CS, Go G, Ganz SB 1996 Randomized trial of epidural versus general anesthesia: outcomes after primary total knee replacement. Clinical Orthopaedics and Related Research 331: 199–208

Yaksh T, Noueihed R 1985 The physiology and pharmacology of spinal opiates. Annual Review of Pharmacology and Toxicology 25: 433–462

Yeager M, Glass D, Neff R, Brinck-Johnsen T 1987 Epidural anaesthesia and analgesia in high risk surgical patients. Anesthesiology 66: 729–736

Yuen EC, Layzer RB, Weitz SR, Olney RK 1995 Neurologic complications of lumbar epidural anesthesia and analgesia. Neurology 45: 1795–1801

Chapter 26

Atypical analgesic drugs and sympathetic blockers

C A Chong, R Munglani, R G Hill

Introduction

This chapter describes recent developments in the physiology and pharmacology of pain and also deals with the utility of drugs introduced for other therapeutic targets but found empirically to have a place in the treatment of pain. We also try to put the established techniques of sympathetic block in their proper context following the lead set by Hannington-Kiff (1994). Although there is overlap with other chapters dealing with the preclinical pharmacology of analgesia, the emphasis here is on drugs that have been evaluated in the clinic or are in routine clinical use but do not yet have a completely explained mechanism of action.

Atypical analgesic drugs

Adrenoceptor agonists for spinal analgesia

The α_2 adrenoceptor agonist clonidine has distinct analgesic properties, when given either systemically or spinally, which are separable from its other pharmacology. The use of this drug as an analgesic is limited by its sedative and vasodepressor properties. The ratio of unwanted to wanted effects can be maximized by giving clonidine intrathecally and it also works well when given epidurally. It has been claimed to be effective against acute and chronic pains, including cancer pain (Coombs et al 1985; Eisenach et al 1989, 1995) and may be effective in patients who have become tolerant to opioids or are suffering neuropathic pain. In a multicentre double-blind trial, epidural clonidine given concomittantly with epidural morphine improved pain relief in patients with severe cancer pain (Eisenach et al 1995). Only those patients with neuropathic pain benefited from this treatment. Falls in systemic blood pressure after epidural clonidine were rated as severe in only two patients out of 38 studied and the incidence of dry mouth and sedation was similar to that seen on morphine alone.

Clonidine has been shown to potentiate the action of opioids and local anaesthetics. Related drugs have similar properties, e.g., xylazine, dexmedetomidine and tizanidine. Tizanidine, although initially introduced for the treatment of spasticity (e.g., Gelber et al 2001), has been suggested to be useful in treating a range of painful conditions including myofascial and neuropathic pain (Gosy 2001). The postsynaptic mechanism of action of α_2 agonists is similar to that of morphine and is exerted via activation of postsynaptic receptors coupled to an increasing outward $K+$ conductance, which reduces cellular excitability.

Recent studies using selective antibodies to identify the localization of the A, B, and C subtypes of α_2 receptor within the dorsal horn of the spinal cord suggest that the α_{2A} receptor is responsible for the analgesic properties (Stone et al 1998). An extensive review of the role of monoamines and their receptors in the control of nociception can be found in Millan (1997).

Serotonin receptor ligands and uptake blockers

Serotonin or 5-hydroxytryptamine (5HT) has been implicated in the control of pain sensation as a result of physiological studies on the descending inhibition of dorsal horn nociception by stimulation of 5HT-containing pathways originating in the vicinity of the midbrain raphe nuclei. The use of 5HT receptor agonists as analgesics has been very limited to date due to the lack of agents that are selective for the different receptor subtypes (14 to date) and also to limiting side effects (nausea, sedation, decreased blood pressure) that have been seen with the agents that have been evaluated in man. It is unlikely that the analgesic properties of tricyclic antidepressants are due to effects on 5HT because the selective 5HT uptake blockers such as fluoxetine and paroxetine appear less useful for the treatment of pain than the non-selective agents such as amitriptyline (see McQuay et al 1996).

The $5HT_{1B/D}$ agonists such as sumatriptan, zolmitriptan, naratriptan, and rizatriptan are extremely effective in the treatment of migraine headache but do not appear to be generally analgesic. This is likely to be attributable to a selective regional distribution of these receptors such that, for example, sensory input within the dorsal horn of the spinal cord originating in the occipital division of the trigeminal nerve can be attenuated by agents of this class (Storer and Goadsby 1997) but that from lumbar dorsal roots cannot (Cumberbatch et al 1998).

Excitatory amino acid receptor antagonists

Glutamate is the most widely distributed excitatory neurotransmitter in the central nervous system and is released by all primary afferent fibres synapsing with secondary sensory neurons in the dorsal horn of the spinal cord (see Salt and Hill 1983 for historical review). It is now known that glutamate can act at two families of ionotropic receptors, for convenience referred to as NMDA and non-NMDA receptors, and at a group of G-protein coupled receptors known as the metabotropic glutamate receptors. The majority of studies in man have used agents that act at NMDA receptors.

NMDA receptors

The dissociative anaesthetics phencyclidine and ketamine have analgesic actions at subanaesthetic doses, recently explained by blockade of glutamate action at NMDA receptors. These agents produce hallucinations and ataxia at doses only slightly higher than those needed to produce analgesia, but nevertheless ketamine in particular has been shown to have an application in controlling pain that may not be sensitive to other analgesic agents. Post-surgically it has been shown that ketamine will suppress the central sensitization expressed as punctate hyperalgesia around a surgical incision (Stubhaug et al 1997) and the secondary hyperalgesia in man following an experimental burn (Warnke et al 1997). Interestingly, in this latter study, the wind-up of pain caused by repeated stimulation with a Von Frey hair in the region of secondary analgesia was suppressed by ketamine but not by morphine. In patients with the usually intractable pain of postherpetic neuralgia, subcutaneous ketamine was found to give relief (Eide et al 1995). Ketamine, although usually administered by injection as part of anaesthetic practice, has reasonable oral bio-availability and will relieve the pain of glossopharyngeal neuralgia (Eide and Stubhaug 1997) or postamputation stump pain (Nikolajsen et al 1997) when given by this route.

Drugs with the same mechanism of action as ketamine (i.e., use-dependent block of the NMDA receptor ion channel) are in clinical trial. Amantidine, better known as an antiviral and dopamine receptor ligand, in a double-blind trial was found to give pain relief in cancer patients suffering from neuropathic pain (Pud et al 1998). Cambridge Neuroscience have reported that CNS-5161 was effective at reducing pain in volunteers and Neurobiological Technologies have reported that diabetic patients treated with memantine experienced a 30% reduction of night-time pain and an 18% reduction in daytime pain and a variety of studies with dextromethorphan indicate that this compound has weak but reproducible analgesic effects (company communications, 1998).

Antagonists of the action of substance P

There has been interest in the role of substance P in nociception since the suggestion that this peptide was concentrated in dorsal roots (see Salt and Hill 1983 for historical review). Mice in which the gene for the NK_1 receptor had been deleted showed deficiencies in spinal wind-up and intensity coding of spinal reflexes, although baseline nociception was unaffected (De Felipe et al 1998). In mice where the gene encoding the precursor for substance P, preprotachykinin, had been deleted, responses to mildly painful stimuli were intact but the response to more intense stimuli was attenuated (Cao et al 1998, Zimmer et al 1998). The discovery of non-peptide antagonists of the NK_1 (substance P) receptor (for review, see Longmore et al 1995) allowed testing of the hypothesis that antagonism of the effects of substance P might lead to analgesia. In animal experiments, convincing evidence has been obtained for antinociceptive effects with these compounds, especially in inflammatory hyperalgesia (Rupniak et al 1995) or hypersensitivity induced by experimental diabetes (Field et al 1998). However, investigations in man have failed to demonstrate convincing analgesic properties in most studies so far published (see, for example, Block et al 1998, Reinhardt et al 1998).

Ion channel blockers

Ever since the introduction of local anaesthetics, it has been common for clinicians to use drugs that block ion channels in order to control pain. This approach has expanded recently with the use of membrane-stabilizing anticonvulsant drugs to treat various intractable pain conditions. The molecular biology of ion channels is now sufficiently well understood to allow the rational design of blockers for a single channel subtype. Many established drugs, such as morphine, exert their effects by influencing the activity of ion channels indirectly by activating receptors coupled to ion channels by second messenger systems. This section is not concerned with such drugs but rather with those that directly influence the activity of voltage-gated ion channels. Recent reviews of this area can be found in McClure and Wildsmith (1991) and Fields et al (1997).

Na channels

Na channels are overexpressed in biopsies taken from painful neuromas (England et al 1996). It has been suggested that the slow, tetrodotoxin-resistant Na current is the best target for a drug that will relieve pain but have minimal side effects (Rizzo et al 1996). This channel is overexpressed in the presence of inflammation and is found on the NGF-dependent unmyelinated nociceptive afferent fibres (Akopian et al 1996, Friedel et al 1997). It has also been found in unmyelinated fibres of biopsied human sural nerve (Quasthoff et al 1995). No compound that will block the TTX-resistant Na current in a selective way is available at present but the recent cloning and expression of the channel (Akopian et al 1997) should make this an achievable objective.

Those agents currently available, although widely used, are suboptimal. For example, lidocaine (lignocaine) does not select between Na channels in neurons and those in other tissues, and in molar terms it is a rather weak blocker. It has a higher affinity for the TTX-sensitive current in myelinated fibres than for the TTX-resistant current in nociceptors (Scholz et al 1998). Only its use-dependent mechanism of action has allowed its safe application as a local anaesthetic (see Murdoch Ritchie 1994). When given intravenously, it has been found to be effective in the treatment of a number of neuropathic pain states, whereas efficacy against other pains is the subject of debate, with positive and negative studies being reported. If infusion rate is limited to 5 mg/kg/h (Fields at al 1997) then side effects are mild with minimal cardiovascular changes. Pain relief after a 1-h infusion lasts several hours and on occasion very much longer than this. It has also been found to be effective against migraine headache when given intranasally (Maizels et al 1996).

The anticonvulsants phenytoin and carbamazepine also inhibit both TTX-resistant and TTX-sensitive currents in rat dorsal root ganglion (DRG) cells (Rush and Elliot 1997) and this may explain the clinical effectiveness of these agents in treating pain (McQuay et al 1995). Lamotrigine is also proving useful in the treatment of neuropathic pain, and the recent demonstration that it reduces cold-induced pain in volunteer subjects may indicate a wider utility in treating other pains (Webb and Kamali 1998). The more recently introduced anticonvulsant topiramate has shown efficacy in animal experiments that suggest that it should be useful against neuropathic pain (Tremont-Lukats et al 2000) and there are some clinical reports appearing suggesting it may be effective against trigeminal neuralgia (e.g., Zvartau-Hind et al 2000). It is also relevant to note that tricyclic antidepressants have been shown to block neuronal Na channels and this may account for some of the analgesic activity of this class of compound (Pancrazio et al 1998).

Ca channels

The neuronal Ca channels are now a large, complex family with L-, N-, P-, Q-, R-, and T-type currents being found in brain and other neuronal tissues

(Birnbaumer et al 1994, Perez-Reyes et al 1998). This diversity, although confusing, provides a number of alternative targets for the design of new analgesic drugs. Blockers of L-type Ca currents are the most accessible, having been used to treat cardiovascular disorders for many years. Although the cardiovascular effects may limit their utility it has recently been shown that nimodipine will reduce the daily dose of morphine needed to provide pain relief in a group of cancer patients (Santillan et al 1998), and that this effect is not due to a pharmacokinetic interaction of the drugs. Epidural verapamil has been shown to reduce analgesic consumption in patients after lower abdominal surgery (Choe et al 1998). In animal experiments it is readily demonstrable that L-channel blockers (such as nimodipine, verapamil, and diltiazem) have antinociceptive properties (Rupniak et al 1993, Neugebauer et al 1996), and it is important to consider the presence of this type of activity when evaluating a novel agent as an analgesic (Rupniak et al 1993).

N-, P-, and Q-type Ca currents have all been implicated in pain perception on the basis of anatomical location and animal experiments with invertebrate toxins that show some blockade specificity for the individual channels (Bowersox et al 1994, Malmberg and Yaksh 1995, Miljanich and Ramachandran 1995, Neugebauer et al 1996, Nebe et al 1998). Peptide blockers of P-type channels have also been studied for their antinociceptive effects in animals. They appear to be most effective in the presence of inflammation (Nebe et al 1997) and have a different effect on N-channel blockers in that they attenuate the late but not the early phase of the formalin response (Diaz and Dickenson 1997). No information is yet available about the action of P-channel blockers in man but it is relevant to note that mutation of P/Q-type calcium channels has been associated with the occurrence of familial hemiplegic migraine (Ophoff et al 1996), suggesting one logical therapeutic use for blockers of this channel.

Gabapentin is a novel anticonvulsant agent that is proving useful for the treatment of neuropathic pain (Rosner et al 1996, Rosenberg et al 1997), especially for postherpetic neuralgia (Rice et al 2001). It is rapidly becoming the drug of choice for neuropathic pain due to its improved separation between wanted and unwanted effects compared with other anticonvulsants and tricyclics (Rice et al 2001, Tremont-Lukats et al 2000). It has also been suggested to be useful in treating the pain of multiple sclerosis (Houtchens et al 1997). The precise mode of action of this drug is obscure but it binds with high affinity to the $\alpha 2\delta$ subunit of calcium channels (Gee et al 1996), although this may not be its only mechanism. It will reduce transmitter release and is active in a number of animal nociception assays (Taylor 1998). A more potent analogue (pregabalin, S-(+)-3-isobutylgaba), is currently in development for the treatment of pain (Field et al 1997). It has been shown to be effective in a randomized double-blind study in patients with postoperative dental pain (Hill et al 2001) and in a variety of animal tests has a profile similar to that of gabapentin (Bryans and Wustrow 1999).

Nicotinic agonists

Cholinergic agonists are antinociceptive in animals but clinical exploitation has been limited by severe side effects produced by non-specific activation of cholinergic systems. Recent detailed knowledge of the molecular biology of cholinoceptors makes it possible to design agents that are receptor subtype selective and thus may have an improved ratio of wanted to unwanted effects.

The cholinergic analgesia story was revived following the discovery (Spande et al 1992) that epibatidine, an alkaloid extracted from the skin of an Ecuadorean frog, was a more potent analgesic than morphine. This compound was subsequently shown to be a potent nicotinic agonist (Badio and Daley 1994) but was too toxic to be developed as a clinical analgesic (Rupniak et al 1994). An analogue of epibatidine, ABT-594, has recently been reported as an analgesic development candidate with an improved therapeutic ratio. This agent, in contrast to epibatidine, does not act at neuromuscular junction nicotinic receptors and has low affinity at some CNS nicotinic sites ($\alpha 7$) but high affinity at others ($\alpha 4\beta 2$). It has moderate affinity at autonomic and sensory ganglion ($\alpha 3$-containing) receptors (Donelly-Roberts et al 1998). In vivo, ABT-594 showed antinociceptive activity in thermal and chemical (formalin) tests that was reversed by the brain penetrant nicotinic antagonist mecamylamine and analgesia persisted after chronic dosing of drug (Bannon et al 1998). Acute dosing caused a decrease in locomotor activity, a decrease in body temperature, and loss of balance but these effects, unlike the antinociception, showed tolerance on repeated dosing. A part of the analgesia produced by ABT-594 may be due to activation of descending inhibitory pathways originating in the nucleus raphe magnus (Bitner et al 1998). It remains to be demonstrated whether agents of this type will be clinically useful. One limitation may be the ability of such drugs to interact with brain reward systems and thus produce dependence (Epping-Jordan et al 1998).

Capsaicin (VR-1) receptor activators and blockers

The use of capsaicin as a rubefacient in treatment of painful disorders is traditional but it is only in the past 20 years that the pharmacology of the active principle, capsaicin, has become well understood. The early work of the Janscos in Hungary (see Salt and Hill 1983 for background) showed that systemic administration to rodents would deplete peptides from small primary afferent fibres without affecting CNS neurons, large sensory fibres, or autonomic fibres. Such administration produced initial nociceptive behaviour, consistent with the pain seen when capsaicin is injected or applied topically in man, followed by prolonged elevation of nociceptive thresholds.

Preparations containing capsaicin for topical application are now widely available and are sometimes effective in painful conditions involving unmyelinated fibre dysfunction. These include postherpetic neuralgia, postmastectomy pain, and diabetic neuropathy (Szallasi 1997). Commercial preparations generally contain only low concentrations of capsaicin (<1%) and even at this dose compliance can be low because of the burning sensation experienced on application. Recently a trial has been made of high-dose (5–10%) topical capsaicin applied under regional anaesthetic cover in patients with refractory pain (Robbins et al 1998). Even with regional anaesthesia, burning pain due to the capsaicin was experienced by some patients and had to be treated with IV fentanyl. Marked temporary pain relief was obtained in 9 out of 10 patients, with 7 of these achieving significant and prolonged pain relief on repeated application. Capsaicin is not suitable for oral administration to man as it is poorly absorbed from and highly irritant to the GI tract. It is not yet clear whether it is necessary to first stimulate the receptor to desensitize it (causing the patient discomfort) or whether it might be possible to block the receptor painlessly with a silent antagonist or partial agonist yet still provide clinical pain relief.

Workers at Novartis have produced analogues of capsaicin that are not pain producing yet still have antinociceptive properties in animals and are free of unwanted bronchoconstrictor activity. One of these drugs has entered clinical development as a potential analgesic (Wrigglesworth et al 1996). Recently a specific receptor (VR-1) for capsaicin-like compounds has been expression cloned (Caterina et al 1997) from a DRG library. It is likely that this discovery will rapidly lead to further novel agonists and antagonists of this receptor which can be clinically evaluated for treatment of pain.

Sympathetic blocks: present and future roles

The past 15 years have seen major advances in the understanding of the role of the sympathetic nervous system in pain states. However, the benefits of sympathetic blockade for these various conditions have been subject to some controversy. More importantly, the complex regional pain syndrome (CRPS) classification (Chap. 18) has little value in predicting response to sympathetic blockade or prognosis. Several papers and editorials have questioned the concept of the role of the sympathetic system in pain states and dismissed the short- and long-term results of sympathetic blockade in clinical practice (Ochoa and Verdugo 1993; Verdugo and Ochoa 1994; Schott 1994, 1995, 1998; Baron 1999; Max and Gilron 1999). The sympathetic system interacts with the patient's pain state at several neuro-anatomical locations; therefore it is likely that an apparently clinically uniform group of patients in a study will have a range of pathophysiology on presentation. The sensitivity of a pain state to sympathetic block changes with time. Thus, it is understandable that there is a wide range of response to sympathetic blockade in different pain states. The complexity of the system we are dealing with and its lack of predictive clinical signs, symptoms, and investigations makes it challenging to determine the appropriate treatment for an individual patient.

In this section we will briefly outline the pathophysiology of sympathetically related pain disorders and attempt to relate this to clinical pain conditions. Commonly used techniques, their indications, and possible side effects are presented in Table 26.1

Basic scientific evidence for the role of the sympathetic nervous system in pain

The sympathetic nervous system has very little effect on the function of normal nociceptors. However, in the presence of injury, it can interact with the sensory system at several levels: (1) dorsal root ganglion, (2) distal segments of regenerating nerves, and (3) undamaged fibres in partially injured nerves. Furthermore, cross-excitation occurs between nerves of all sizes after injury, and experimentally these sensory nerve endings have been shown to be exquisitely sensitive to mechanical and thermal stimuli, to local or systemic cathecholamines, and to electrical stimulation of postganglionic sympathetic neurons. This sympathetic facilitation

Table 26.1 Summary of sympathetic block, indications and side effects

Areas of blockade	Indications	Side effects
Sphenopalatine ganglion	Sluder's neuralgia Cluster headache Migraine Atypical facial pain	Epistaxis Paraesthesia of teeth and hard palate
Stellate ganglion	**Pain** SMP of CRPS 1 or 2 Herpes zoster Early postherpetic neuralgia Neoplastic Paget's disease Postradiation neuritis Intractable angina pectoris Pain from CNS lesions **Vascular insufficiency** Raynaud's disease Frostbite Vasospasm Occlusive or embolic vascular disease Scleroderma **Other** Hyperhydrosis Meniere's disease Shoulder–hand syndrome Stroke Vascular headaches Sudden blindness	Horner's syndrome Miosis Ptosis Enopthalmos Anhydrosis Conjunctival injection Nasal congestion Nerve injury Brachial plexus Recurrent laryngeal Phrenic Perforated trachea Perforated oesophagus Inadvertent vascular injection Inadvertent intrathecal injection
Thoracic sympathetic chain including splanchnic nerves	Non-malignant and malignant pain of abdomen, thorax, neck and head	Pneumothorax (4% incidence). Bleeding from vascular trauma
Coeliac plexus	Pain Upper abdominal malignancy: pancreas, liver, gallbladder Non malignant Chronic pancreatitis	Procedure Bleeding Retroperitoneal haematoma Intravascular injection Intrapsoas injection Intrathecal or epidural injection Nerve root injury Perforated viscera: kidney, liver Pneumothorax Chylothorax Infection, peritonitis, abscess Local anaesthetic/neurolytic related Hypotension Diarrhoea Lower extremity warmness Thrombosis or embolism Impotence (3%) Paraplegia (0.15%) possibly from damage to artery of Adamkiewicz Metabolic and chemical complications from alcohol (in patients with aldehyde dehydrogenase deficiency) or phenol intravascularly.
Lumbar sympathetic	Vascular insufficiency SMP of CRPS 1 or 2 Post herpetic neuralgia Neuropathic pain in lower limbs Phantom limb pain Malignant pain Intractable back pain	Bleeding/haemorrhage Trauma to viscera Intravascular injection Epidural/intrathecal injection Nerve trauma Genitofemoral—leads to groin pain

Table 26.1 Summary of sympathetic block, indications and side effects (*cont'd*)

Areas of blockade	Indications	Side effects
Superior hypogastric plexus	Pelvic pain both malignant and non malignant	Trauma to viscera Bleeding, haemorrhage Bladder, rectal and erectile dysfunction
Ganglion of Impar (ganglion of Walther)	Perineal pain Usually neoplastic Benign coccidynia	As above

appears to be working via cathecholamines on α_1 and α_2 receptors and via neuropeptide Y (NPY) that works via Y_1 and Y_2 receptors (Tracey et al 1995). See also Coughnon et al (1997) and Munglani et al (1998) for reviews.

The dorsal root ganglion is important because after injury, there is spontaneous discharge within days of injury (Devor and Wall 1990). Cross-excitation occurs between DRG and myelinated neurons (Utzschneider et al 1992) and there is profuse growth of sympathetic fibres into the dorsal root ganglion and around large myelinated afferent nerves (McLachlan et al 1993). The mechanism may be due to nerve growth factor (NGF) (Davis et al 1994, McMahon and Bennett 1997).

Although there is much evidence for sympathetic nervous system effects on somatosensory nerves, the sympathetic system itself may show decreased activity after damage. Arnold et al (1993) have shown that the symptomatic limb has reduced circulating adrenaline (epinephrine) in the venous outflow and this may be due to denervation supersensitivity. The affected limb may have thermoregulatory disturbances, and animal experiments have shown that the sympathetic cell bodies and fibres atrophy after nerve injury. This atrophy could predispose to denervation supersensitivity of receptors on blood vessels, which could account for a 'cooler' affected limb. Cooling of the limb may be consistent with the phenomenon of cold allodynia (Janig 1988, Magerl et al 1996)

The sympathetic system may also contribute to inflammation-related pain. There are anecdotal reports of patients with rheumatoid arthritis responding to IVRB with guanethidine (Hannington-Kiff 1994, Levine et al 1986a). Capsaicin-induced hyperalgesia can be slightly enhanced by coadministration of noradrenaline (norepinephrine) whilst phentolamine slightly decreases it (Meyer et al 1992, Drummond 1995, Liu et al 1996). However, this is not the case when a subject's sympathetic system is stimulated naturally by heating or cooling with a thermal suit (Baron et al 1999).

There is evidence that the sympathetic system can mediate inflammation per se. Clinical reports of IVRB with ketorolac for sympathetically maintained pain (SMP) have been effective. Activation of α_2 receptors may release prostaglandins and sympathectomy diminishes the effects of interleukin-8 (IL8), NGF, IL1, and TNFα (Cunha et al 1992a, b; Safieh-Garabedian et al 1995; Andreev et al 1995; Woolf et al 1996). However, sympathectomy does not abolish hyperalgesia in man (Meyer et al 1992).

Diagnosis and treatment of sympathetically maintained pain

The diagnosis of SMP is simple: if at any stage of the pain history, a placebo-controlled block of the sympathetic system causes relief of symptoms then that patient has SMP. Failure to relieve symptoms leads to diagnosis of SIP (sympathetically independent pain). Unfortunately, history, symptoms, and signs are no predictors of whether a case is likely to be a SMP, although a few conditions are more likely to be associated with it (Table 26.2). It has been reported that cold allodynia is a feature of all SMP and 50% of SIP patients (Frost et al 1988, Campbell et al 1994).

Table 26.2 Conditions associated with sympathetically mediated pain (SMP)

Acute shingles
Neuralgias including postherpetic neuralgia
Painful metabolic neuropathies
Phantom pain
Traumatic nerve injuries
Soft tissue injury

The CRPS taxonomy (see Chap. 18) introduced in Orlando in 1993 recognizes that there may be a SIP component of a pain state. It also recognized that with time a pain state, which was SMP, could become SIP. Therefore, the rationale for diagnostic and therapeutic sympatholytic procedures is not automatic when a diagnosis of CRPS is made. The CRPS complex has many components, of which the sympathetic system is only one; they include sympathetic, sensory, autonomic, inflammatory, psychological, and motor components (Boas 1996).

In practice, an intravenous phentolamine infusion (dose of 0.5 to 1 mg/kg) is used as a diagnostic tool because it can be placebo controlled. Phentolamine is an α-adrenergic antagonist that blocks the α receptors that may be involved in SMP. The use of IVRB with guanethidine as a diagnostic tool is not recommended. Various other tests exist for sympathetic dysfunction. These are summarized in Table 26.3.

It is possible also to use local anaesthetic blocks of the sympathetic chain for diagnosis but there may be a false positive response from diffusion onto somatosensory nerve roots or absorption resulting in systemic action (Charlton 1986, Stolker et al 1994, Hogan 1997).

Sympathetic blocks

The indications and possible complications of sympathetic blocks are described in Table 26.1. It is important to note that very few randomized controlled trials to evaluate their usefulness in SMP have been done. This chapter will not attempt to explain the techniques due to lack of space and the availability of some excellent books on neural blockade (Hahn et al 1996, Prithvi Raj et al 1996, Waldman and Winnie 1996, Cousins and Bridenbaugh 1998). A list of common sympathetic blocks is given in Table 26.1.

Table 26.3 Interventional techniques for therapeutic sympatholysis[a]

Percutaneous techniques
Sympathetic ganglion block
Epidural nerve block with or without clonidine
Peripheral nerve block
Phenol or alcohol block of the sympathetic chain
Pulsed or continuous radiofrequency sympathectomy
Intravenous techniques
IVRB (e.g., guanethidine, bretylium, ketorolac, phentolamine, clonidine, reserpine, ketanserin with or without local anaesthetic)
Systemic (e.g., phentolamine, pamidronate)
Surgery
Oral
Prazosin, phenoxybenzamine, nifedipine, clonidine
Topical
Clonidine

[a]Adapted from Campbell et al (1994).

Sphenopalatine ganglion block

This is located posterior to the middle turbinate and these cells communicate with the trigeminal and facial nerves as well as carotid plexus. This can be blocked with topical cocaine or local anaesthetic or by a lateral approach under the zygoma using fluoroscopy. Radiofrequency of this ganglion has also been described and may be useful for the treatment of atypical facial pain.

Stellate ganglion block

This ganglion receives sympathetic fibres from T1–T2 (head and neck) and T8–T9 (upper limb). The stellate ganglion is often fused with first thoracic ganglion and lies over C7 to T1. There are two common techniques to block the stellate ganglion. The first uses Chaussignac's tubercle (transverse process of C6) and the second is a more medial approach to the anterolateral border of C7.

This block is achieved with 5 to 10 ml of local anaesthetic. A rise in temperature of the upper limb was thought to indicate successful sympathicolysis. However it has been shown that 48% of patients who show a temperature rise have an undisturbed sympathetic nervous function when this is assessed with laser Doppler flowmetry (Schurmann et al 2001). The success rate even with experienced operators is 75% (Stanton-Hicks et al 1996). Neurolytic blockade runs the risk of permanent side effects.

Radiofrequency lesioning of the stellate ganglion has been described and a retrospective analysis has shown its efficacy is similar to other ways of blocking the stellate ganglion (Forouszanfar et al 2000).

Thoracic sympathetic block

The thoracic sympathetic chain lies near the somatic nerves as they emanate from the intravertebral foramen. There is a 4% incidence of pneumothorax during blockade even in experienced hands (Prithvi Raj et al 1996). Though historically having few indications, one of the authors has found discogenic cervical pain does respond to T2 sympathetic blockade or radiofrequency.

Coeliac plexus block

The coeliac plexus lies anterolateral to the aorta and receives fibres from T5 to T12 that pass through splanchnic nerves. It innervates all abdominal viscera except for part of the transverse colon, descending colon, rectum, and pelvic viscera (Prithvi Raj et al 1996). Blockade is achieved using local anaesthetic with or without steroid and also neurolytic agents such as phenol or alcohol. Neurolytic coeliac blocks work for 6–12 months before the nerves regenerate.

Prithvi Raj et al (1999) has described successful splanchnic nerve radiofrequency lesioning as an alternative to coeliac plexus blockade for abdominal pain.

Lumbar sympathetic block

Preganglionic sympathetic neurons arise from the anterolateral dorsal horn from T10 to L2–L3 and pass through the white rami and sympathetic trunk to the sympathetic and sacral ganglia and then usually join the L1–L5 and S1–S3 spinal nerves by way of the grey rami or form a diffuse plexus around the iliac arteries. Preganglionic fibres for the visceral structures synapse commonly in T10–T12 and L1 ganglia and then join the aortic and hypogastric plexus to supply the kidney, ureter, bladder, distal transverse colon, rectum, prostate, testicle, cervix, and uterus.

Patients often respond to a diagnostic local block but only 30% respond to the subsequent neurolytic blockade, with duration of action of 6–12 months. One explanation is that LSB using local anaesthetic may spread to the somatosensory nerves and there may be some systemic absorption that leads to a false-positive result (Stanton-Hicks et al 1996).

Several approaches to the lumbar sympathetic plexus have been described but the lateral approach is more direct and causes less discomfort. Bonica recommended blockade at T12–L1 level to achieve total interruption of sympathetic outflow to the lower limb but this may carry more risk to the genitofemoral nerve. The block is usually made at L3 (Stanton-Hicks et al 1996).

Hypogastric plexus block (presacral sympathetic block)

The superior hypogastric plexus lies anterior to L5 and just inferior to the aortic bifurcation. It may be useful as a treatment for pelvic malignant and non-malignant pain (Plancarte et al 1989, De Leon-Casasola et al 1993, Prithvi Raj et al 1996).

Ganglion of Impar (Walther) block

Plancarte et al (1996) has described this for the treatment of intractable neoplastic perineal pain of sympathetic origin. The ganglion of Impar is a solitary retroperitoneal structure at the level of the sacrococcygeal junction. It is reached by a bent needle around the coccyx or through the sacro-coccygeal membrane. In a pilot study, 16 patients with advanced cancer of the cervix, colon, bladder, or rectum experienced symptomatic relief with a diagnostic local block. Eight of these patients experienced 100% relief with 4–6 ml of phenol and the rest experienced at least 50% relief.

Intravenous regional anaesthesia

Pharmacological end-organ manipulation can be used to both diagnose (now controversially) and treat SMP. The technique was introduced by Hannington-Kiff (1977) using guanethidine, which depletes nerve endings of noradrenaline (norepinephrine) stores and prevents reuptake. Other drugs that have been used include bretylium, ketorolac, phentolamine, reserpine, and ketanserin. This technique has advantages because it is easy to perform and can be done in an anticoagulated patient. Possible complications include hypotension and neuropraxia from the cuff. Ramamurthy et al (1995) and Wahren et al (1995) have reported very good results with IVRB using guanethidine. However, recent randomized, controlled trials (Jadad et al 1995, Kaplan et al 1996) have failed to show any benefit, suggesting (1) a placebo response, (2) an effect of the inflated cuff itself, or (3) failure to understand the complex nature of CRPS in patients.

Sympathetic blocks: defining a future role in therapy

Whilst there may be little doubt as to the role of sympathetic (especially neurolytic) blocks in the management of vascular insufficiency and malignant pains (Plancarte et al 1996, Boas 1998), randomized controlled trials have cast doubt on the benefits of such autonomic blocks (and IVRB with guanethidine) for conditions such as postherpetic neuralgia, low back pain, and CRPS of limbs.

Boas (1999) points out that although autonomic blocks may produce dramatic changes when first performed, there is little evidence that early treatment changes outcome. Pain states such as postherpetic neuralgia can evolve from being a SMP initially to a SIP. Treatment of mechanisms that maintain a pain initially may not delay or prevent the development of subsequent alternative neurobiological mechanisms maintaining the pain over a longer period (Munglani et al 1996, Munglani 1997). CRPS itself has many contributing factors and its management should include adjuvant drugs such as antidepressants, anticonvulsants, physiotherapy, and addressing psychological issues. Established therapies as well as new techniques such as epidural clonidine (Rauck et al 1993) and radiofrequency of the sympathetic ganglions, will have to run the imperfect gauntlet of our changing understanding of SMP within the taxonomy of CRPS and randomized controlled trials to gain a place in our clinical armamentarium.

References

Akopian AN, Sivlotti L, Wood JN 1996 A tetrodotoxin resistant voltage gated sodium channel expressed by sensory neurones. Nature 379: 257–262

Andreev NY, Dimitrieva N, Koltzenburg M, McMahon SB 1995 Peripheral administration of nerve growth factor in the adult rat produces a thermal hyperalgesia that requires the presence of sympathetic post-ganglionic neurones. Pain 63: 109–115

Arnold J, Teasell RW, Macleod AP, Brown JE, Carruthers SG 1993 Increased venous alpha-adrenoreceptor responsiveness in patients with reflex sympathetic dystrophy. Annals of Internal Medicine 118: 619–621

Badio B, Daley JW 1994 Epibatidine, a potent analgesic and nicotinic agonist. Molecular Pharmacology 45: 563–569

Bannon AW, Decker MW, Curzon P et al 1998 ABT-594 [(R)-5-(2-azetidinylmethoxy)-2-chloropyridine]: a novel, orally effective antinociceptive agent acting via neuronal nicotinic acetylcholine receptors: II. In vivo characterisation. Journal of Pharmacology and Experimental Therapeutics 285: 787–794

Baron R et al 1999 Effect of sympathetic activity on capsaicin-evoked pain, hyperalgesia and vasodilatation. Neurology 52: 923–932

Birnbaumer L, Campbell KP, Catterall WA et al 1994 The naming of voltage gated calcium channels. Cell 13: 505–506

Bitner RS, Nikkel AL, Curzon P, Arneric SP, Bannon AW, Decker MW 1998 Role of the nucleus raphe magnus in antinociception produced by ABT-594: immediate early gene responses possibly linked to neuronal nicotinic acetylcholine receptors on serotoninergic neurons. Journal of Neuroscience 18: 5426–5432

Block G, Rue D, Panebianco D, Reines S 1998 The substance P antagonist L-754,030 is ineffective in the treatment of postherpetic neuralgia. American Academy of Neurology, Annual Meeting, Minneapolis, April

Boas RA 1996 Complex regional pain syndromes: symptoms, signs, differential diagnosis. In: Janig W, Stanton-Hicks M (eds) Reflex sympathetic dystrophy: a reappraisal. IASP Press, Seattle, pp 93–105

Boas RA 1998 Sympathetic nerve blocks: in search of a role. Regional Anaesthesia and Pain Management 23: 292–305

Bowersox SS, Valentino KL, Luther RR 1994 Neuronal voltage-sensitive calcium channels. Drug News and Perspectives 7: 261–268

Bryans JS, Wustrow DJ 1999 3-substituted GABA analogs with central nervous system activity: a review. Medicinal Research Reviews 19: 149–177

Campbell JN, Raja SN, Selig DK, Belzberg AJ, Meyer RA 1994 Diagnosis and management of sympathetically maintained pain. In: Fields HL, Liebskind JC (eds) Pharmacological approaches to the treatment of chronic pain: new concepts and critical issues. IASP Press, Seattle, pp 85–100

Cao YQ, Mantyh PW, Carlsson EJ, Gillespie A-M, Epstein CJ, Basbaum AI 1998 Primary afferent tachykinins are required to experience moderate to intense pain. Nature 392: 390–394

Caterina MJ, Schumacher MA, Tominaga M, Rosen TA, Levine JD, Julius D 1997 The capsaicin receptor: a heat activated ion channel in the pain pathway. Nature 389: 816–824

Charlton JE 1986 Current views on the use of nerve blocking in the relief of chronic pain. In: Swerdlow M (ed) The therapy of pain. MTP, Lancaster, pp 133–164

Choe H, Kim J-S, Ko S-H, Kim D-C, Han Y-J, Song H-S 1998 Epidural verapamil reduces analgesic consumption after lower abdominal surgery. Anesthesia and Analgesia 86: 786–790

Coombs DW, Saunders RL, LaChance D, Savage S, Ragnarsson TS, Jensen LE 1985 Intrathecal morphine tolerance: use of intrathecal clonidine, DADLE and intraventricular morphine. Anesthesiology 62: 357–363

Coughnon N, Hudspith M, Munglani R 1997 The therapeutic potential of NPY in central nervous system disorders with special reference to pain and sympathetically maintained pain. Expert Opinion in Investigational Drugs 6: 759–769

Cousins MJ, Bridenbaugh PO 1998 Neural blockade. Lippincott-Raven, Philadelphia

Cuhna FQ, Lorenzetti BB, Ferreira SH 1992a Interleukin-8 as a mediator of sympathetic pain. British Journal of Pharmacology 107: 660–664

Cuhna FQ, Poole S, Lorenzetti BB, Ferreira SH 1992b The pivotal role of tumour necrosis factor alpha in the development of inflammatory hyperalgesia. British Journal of Pharmacology 107: 660–664

Cumberbatch MJ, Hill RG and Hargreaves RJ 1998. Differential effects of the 5-HT ID/IB receptor agonist naratriptan on trigeminal versus spinal nociceptive responses. Cephalalgia 18: 659–663

Davis BM, Albers KM, Seroogy KB, Katz DM 1994 Over expression of nerve growth factor in transgenic mice induces novel sympathetic projections to primary sensory neurones. Journal of Comparative Neurology 349: 464–474

De Felipe C, Herrero JF, O'Brien JA et al 1998 Altered nociception, analgesia and aggression in mice lacking the receptor for substance P. Nature 329: 394–397

De Leon-Casasola OA, Kent E, Lema MJ 1993 Neurolytic superior hypogastric plexus block for chronic pelvic pain associated with cancer. Pain 64: 145–151

Devor M, Wall PD 1990 Cross-excitation in dorsal root ganglia of nerve-injured and intact rats. Journal of Neurophysiology 64: 1733–1746

Diaz A, Dickenson AH 1997 Blockade of spinal N- and P-type, but not L-type, calcium channels inhibits the excitability of rat dorsal horn neurones produced by subcutaneous formalin inflammation. Pain 69: 93–100

Donelly-Roberts DL, Puttfarken PS, Kuntzweiler TA et al 1998 ABT-594 [(R)-5-(2-azetidinylmethoxy)-2-chloropyridine]: a novel, orally effective antinociceptive agent acting via neuronal nicotinic acetylcholine receptors: I in vitro characterisation. Journal of Pharmacology and Experimental Therapeutics 285: 777–786

Drummond PD 1995 Noradrenaline increases hyperalgesia to heat in skin sensitized by capsaicin. Pain 60: 311–315

Eide PK, Stubhaug A 1997 Relief of glossopharyngeal neuralgia by ketamine-induced N-methyl aspartate receptor blockade. Neurosurgery 41: 505–508

Eide PK, Stubhaug A, Oye I, Breivik H 1995 Cutaneous subcutaneous administration of the N-methyl-D-aspartic acid (NMDA) receptor antagonist ketamine in the treatment of post-herpetic neuralgia. Pain 61: 221–228

Eisenach JC, Rauck RL, Buzzanell C, Lysak SZ 1989 Epidural clonidine analgesia for intractable cancer pain: phase I. Anesthesiology 71: 647–652

Eisenach JC, DuPen S, Dubois M, Miguel R, Allin D, Epidural Clonidine Study Group 1995 Epidural clonidine analgesia for intractable cancer pain. Pain 61: 391–399

England JD, Happel LT, Kline DG et al 1996 Sodium channel accumulation in humans with painful neuromas. Neurology 47: 272–276

Epping-Jordan MP, Watkins SS, Koob GF, Markou A 1998 Dramatic decreases in brain reward function during nicotine withdrawal. Nature 393: 76–79

Field MJ, Oles RJ, Lewis AS, McCleary S, Singh L 1997 Gabapentin (neurontin) and 3-(+)-isobutylgaba represent a novel class of selective antihyperalgesic agent. British Journal of Pharmacology 121: 1513–1522

Field MJ, McLeary S, Boden P, Suman-Chauhan N, Hughes J, Singh L 1998 Involvement of the central tachykinin NK_1 receptor during maintenance of mechanical hypersensitivity induced by diabetes in the rat. Journal of Pharmacology and Experimental Therapeutics 285: 1226–1232

Fields HL, Rowbotham MC, Devor M 1997 Excitability blockers: anticonvulsants and low concentration local anaesthetics in the treatment of chronic pain. In: Dickenson A, Besson J-M (eds) The pharmacology of pain. Springer-Verlag, Berlin, pp 93–116

Forouszanfar T et al 2000 Radiofrequency lesions of the stellate ganglion in chronic pain syndromes: retrospective analysis of clinical efficacy in 86 patients. Clinical Journal of Pain 16: 164–168

Friedel RH, Schnurch H, Stubbusch J, Barde Y-A 1997 Identification of genes differentially expressed by nerve growth factor- and neurotrophin-3-dependent sensory neurons. Proceedings of the National Academy of Sciences of the USA 94: 12670–12675

Frost SA, Raja SN, Campbell JN, Meyer RA, Khan AA 1988 Does hyperalgesia to cooling stimuli characterise patients with sympathetically maintained pain? In: Dubner GF, Gebhart J, Bond MR (eds) Proceedings of the 5th world congress on pain. Elsevier, Amsterdam, pp 151–156

Gee NS, Brown JP, Dissanayake VUK, Offord J, Thurlow R, Woodruff GN 1996 The novel anticonvulsant drug, gabapentin (neurontin), binds to the $\alpha 2\delta$ subunit of a calcium channel. Journal of Biological Chemistry 271: 5768–5776

Gelber DA, Good DC, Dromerick A, Sergay S, Richardson M 2001 Open-label dose-titration safety and efficacy study of tizanidine hydrochloride in the treatment of spasticity associated with chronic stroke. Stroke 32: 1841–1846

Gosy E 2001 Spectrum of the clinical use of Zanaflex (tizanidine) in pain management. In: Krames E, Reig E (eds) Practice of neurology and pain management. Monduzzi Editore, Bologna, pp 385–389

Hahn MB, McQuillan PM, Sheplock GJ 1996 Regional anesthesia. Mosby, St Louis

Hannington-Kiff JG 1977 Relief of Sudeck's atrophy by regional intravenous guanethidine. Lancet 1: 1132–1133

Hannington-Kiff JG 1994 Sympathetic nerve blocks in painful limb disorders. In: Wall PD, Melzack R (eds) Textbook of pain, 3rd edn. Churchill Livingstone, Edinburgh, pp 1035–1052

Hill CM, Balkenohl M, Thomas DW, Walker R, Mathe H, Murray G 2001 Pregabalin in patients with postoperative dental pain. European Journal of Pain 5: 119–224

Hogan QH 1997 Neural blockade for diagnosis and prognosis. Anesthesiology 86: 216–241

Houtchens MK, Richert JR, Sami A, Rose JW 1997 Open label gabapentin treatment for pain in multiple sclerosis. Multiple Sclerosis 3: 250–253

Jadad AR, Carroll D, Glynn CJ, McQuay HJ 1995 Intravenous sympathetic blockade for pain relief in reflex sympathetic dystrophy: a review and a randomized double blind crossover study. Journal of Pain and Symptom Management 10: 13–20

Janig W 1988 Pathophysiology following nerve injury. In: Dubner GF, Gebhart J, Bono MR (eds) Proceedings of the 5th world congress on pain. Elsevier, Amsterdam, p 89

Janig W, Stanton-Hicks M 1996 Reflex sympathetic dystrophy: a reappraisal. IASP Press, Seattle

Kaplan R, Claudio M, Kepes E, Gu XF 1996 Intravenous guanethidine in patients with reflex sympathetic dystrophy. Acta Anaesthesiologica Scandinavica 40: 1216–1222

Levine JD, Fye K, Heller P, Basbaum AI, Whiting OK 1986a Clinical response to regional intravenous guanethidine in patients with rheumatoid arthritis. Journal of Rheumatology 13: 1040–1043

Liu M, Max MB, Parada S, Robinovitz E, Bennett GJ 1996 Sympathetic blockade with intravenous phentolamine inhibits capsaicin evoked allodynia in humans. Abstracts of the 8th world congress on pain, Vancouver

Longmore J, Swain CJ, Hill RG 1995 Neurokinin receptors. Drug News and Perspectives 8: 5–23

Magerl W, Koltzenburg M, Schmitz J, Handwerker HO 1996 Asymmetry and time course of cutaneous sympathetic reflex responses following sustained excitation of the chemosensitive nociceptors in humans. Journal of the Autonomic Nervous System 57: 63–72

Maizels M, Scott B, Cohen W, Chen W 1996 Intranasal lidocaine for treatment of migraine. Journal of the American Medical Association 276: 319–321

Malmberg AB, Yaksh TL 1995 Effect of continuous intrathecal infusion of ω-conopeptides, N-type calcium channel blockers, on behaviour and antinociception in the formalin and hotplate tests in rats. Pain 60: 83–90

Max M, Gilron I 1999 Sympathetically maintained pain: has the emperor no clothes? Neurology 52: 905–907

McClure JH, Wildsmith JAW 1991 Conduction blockade for postoperative analgesia. Edward Arnold, London, p 230

McLachlan EM, Janig W, Devor M, Michaelis M 1993 Peripheral nerve injury triggers noradrenergic sprouting within dorsal root ganglia. Nature 363: 543–545

McMahon SB, Bennett DHL 1997 Growth factors and pain. In: Dickenson A, Besson J-M (eds) The pharmacology of pain. Springer-Verlag, Berlin, pp 135–165

McQuay H, Carroll D, Jadad AR, Wiffen P, Moore A 1995 Anticonvulsant drugs for management of pain: a systematic review. British Medical Journal 311: 1047–1052

McQuay HJ, Tramer M, Nye BA, Carroll D, Wiffen PJ, Moore RAA 1996 Systematic review of antidepressants in neuropathic pain. Pain 68: 217–227

Meyer RA, Davis KD, Raja SN, Campbell JN 1992 Sympathectomy does not abolish bradykinin induced cutaneous hyperalgesia in man. Pain 51: 323–327

Miljanich GP, Ramachandran J 1995 Antagonists of neuronal calcium channels: structure, function and therapeutic implications. Annual Review of Pharmacology and Toxicology 35: 707–734

Millan MJ 1997 The role of descending noradrenergic and serotoninergic pathways in the modulation of nociception: focus on receptor multiplicity. In: Dickenson A, Besson J-M (eds) The pharmacology of pain. Springer-Verlag, Berlin, pp 385–446

Munglani R 1997 Advances in chronic pain therapy with special reference to back pain. In: Ginsburg R, Kaufmann L (eds)

Anaesthesia review, vol 14. Churchill Livingstone, Edinburgh, pp 153–174
Munglani R, Fleming B, Hunt SP 1996 Remembrance of times past: the role of c-fos in pain. British Journal of Anaesthesia 76: 1–4
Munglani R, Hudspith M, Hunt SP 1998 Therapeutic potential of NPY. Drugs 52: 371–389
Murdoch Ritchie JM 1994 Mechanism of action of local anaesthetics. In: Fields HL, Liebeskind JC (eds) Progress in pain research and management. IASP Press, Seattle, pp 189–204
Nakamura SI, Takahashi K, Takahashi Y, Yamagata M, Moriya H 1996 The afferent pathways of discogenic low-back pain. Evaluation of L2 spinal nerve infiltration. Journal of Bone and Joint Surgery 78: 606–612
Nebe J, Vanegas H, Neugebauer V, Schaible H-G 1997 ω-agatoxin IVA, a P-type calcium channel antagonist, reduces nociceptive processing in spinal cord neurons with input from the inflamed but not from the normal knee joint—an electrophysiological study in the rat in vivo. European Journal of Neuroscience 9: 2193–2201
Nebe J, Vanegas H, Scaible H-G 1998 Spinal application of ω-conotoxin GIVA, an N-type calcium channel antagonist, attenuates enhancement of dorsal spinal neuronal responses caused by intra-articular injection of mustard oil in the rat. Experimental Brain Research 120: 61–69
Neugebauer V, Vanegas H, Nebe J, Rumenapp P, Schaible H-G 1996 Effects of N-, L-type calcium channel antagonists on the responses of spinal cord neurons to mechanical stimulation of the normal and the inflamed knee joint. Journal of Neurophysiology 76: 3740–3749
Nikolajsen L, Hansen PO, Jensen TS 1997 Oral ketamine therapy in the treatment of postamputation stump pain. Acta Anaesthesiologica Scandinavica 41: 427–429
Ochoa JL, Verdugo RJ 1993 Reflex sympathetic dystrophy: definitions and history of ideas with critical review of human studies. In: Low P (ed) Clinical autonomic disorders. Little, Brown, Boston, p 473
Ophoff RA, Terwindt GM, Vergouwe MN et al 1996 Familial hemiplegic migraine and episodic ataxia type-2 are caused by mutations in the Ca++ channel gene CACNL1A4. Cell 87: 543–552
Pancrazio JJ, Kamatchi GL, Roscoe AK, Lynch C 1998 Inhibition of neuronal Na+ channels by antidepressant drugs? Journal of Pharmacology and Experimental Therapeutics 284: 208–214
Perez-Reyes E, Cribbs LL, Daud A et al 1998 Molecular characterisation of a neuronal low-voltage-activated T-type calcium channel. Nature 391: 896–900
Plancarte R 1989 Hypogastric block: retroperitoneal approach. Anaesthesiology 71: A739
Plancarte R, Velazquez R, Patt RB 1996 Neurolytic blocks of the sympathetic axis. In: Patt RB (ed) Cancer pain. Lippincott, Philadelphia, pp 384–420
Prithvi Raj P, Rauck RL, Racz GB 1996 Autonomic blocks. In: Prithvi Raj P (ed) Pain medicine. Mosby, St Louis, pp 227–258
Prithvi Raj P et al 1999 The development of a technique for radiofrequency lesioning of splanchnic nerves. Current Review of Pain 3: 377–387
Pud D, Eisenberg E, Spitzer A, Adler R, Fried G, Yarnitsky D 1998 The NMDA receptor antagonist amantadine reduces surgical neuropathic pain in cancer patients: a double blind, randomized, placebo controlled trial. Pain 75: 349–354
Quasthoff S, Grosskreutz J, Schroder JM, Schneider U, Grafe P 1995 Calcium potentials and tetrodotoxin resistant sodium potentials in unmyelinated C fibres of biopsied human sural nerve. Neuroscience 69: 955–965
Raja SN, Treede RD, Davis KD, Campbell JN 1991 Systemic alpha adrenergic blockade with phentolamine: a diagnostic test for sympathethetically maintained pain. Anesthesiology 74: 691–698
Ramamurthy S, Hoffman J, Guanethidine Study Group 1995 Intravenous regional guanethidine in the treatment of reflex sympathetic dystrophy/causalgia: a randomised double blind study. Anaesthesia and Analgesia 81: 718–723
Rauck R, Eisenach JC, Young LD 1993 Epidural clonidine treatment for refractory reflex sympathetic dystrophy. Anesthesiology 79: 1163–1169
Reinhardt RR, Laub JB, Fricke J, Polis AB, Gertz BJ 1998 Comparison of a neurokinin-1 antagonist, L-754,030, to placebo, acetaminophen and ibuprofen in the dental pain model. American Society of Clinical Pharmacology and Therapeutics, New Orleans
Rice ASC, Maton S, Postherpetic Neuralgia Study Group 2001 Gabapentin in postherpetic neuralgia: a randomised, double blind, placebo controlled study. Pain 94: 215–224
Rizzo MA, Kocsis JD, Waxman SG 1996 Mechanisms of paresthesiae, dysesthesiae and hyperesthesiae: role of Na+ channel heterogeneity. European Neurology 36: 3–12
Robbins WR, Staats PS, Levine J et al 1998 Treatment of intractable pain with topical large-dose capsaicin; preliminary report. Anesthesia and Analgesia 86: 579–583
Rosenberg JM, Harrell C, Ristic H, Werner RA, De Rosayro AM 1997 The effect of gabapentin on neuropathic pain. Clinical Journal of Pain 13: 251–255
Rosner H, Rubin L, Kestenbaum A 1996 Gabapentin adjunctive therapy in neuropathic pain states. Clinical Journal of Pain 12: 56–58
Rupniak NMJ, Boyce S, Williams AR et al 1993 Antinociceptive activity of NK1 receptor antagonists: non-specific effects of racemic RP-67580. British Journal of Pharmacology 110: 1607–1613
Rupniak NMJ, Patel S, Marwood R et al 1994 Antinociceptive and toxic effects of (+) epibatidine oxalate attributable to nicotinic agonist activity. British Journal of Pharmacology 113: 1487–1493
Rupniak NMJ, Carlson E, Boyce S, Webb JK, Hill RG 1995 Enantioselective inhibition of the formalin paw late phase by the NK1 receptor antagonist L-733,060 in gerbils. Pain 67: 188–195
Rush AM, Elliot JR 1997 Phenytoin and carbamazepine: differential inhibition of sodium currents in small cells from adult rat dorsal root ganglia. Neuroscience Letters 226: 95–98
Safieh-Garabedian B, Poole S, Allchorne A, Winter J, Woolf CJ 1995 Contribution of interleukin-1 beta to the inflammation-induced increase in nerve growth factor levels and inflammatory hyperalgesia. British Journal of Pharmacology 115: 1265–1275
Salt TE, Hill RG 1983 Transmitter candidates of somatosensory primary afferent fibres. Neuroscience 10: 1083–1103
Santillan R, Hurle MA, Armijo JA, De Los Mozos R, Florez J 1998 Nimodipine-enhanced opiate analgesia in cancer patients requiring morphine dose escalation: a double blind placebo-controlled study. Pain 76: 17–26
Scholz A, Kuboyama N, Hempelmann G, Vogel W 1998 Complex block of TTX-resistant Na+ currents by lidocaine and bupivicaine reduce firing frequency in DRG neurons. Journal of Neurophysiology 79: 1746–1754
Schott GD 1994 Visceral afferents and their contribution to 'sympathetic dependent' pain. Brain 117: 397–413
Schott GD 1995 An unsympathetic view of pain. Lancet 345: 634–635
Schott GD 1998 Interrupting the sympathetic outflow in causalgia and reflex sympathetic dystrophy. British Medical Journal 316: 1
Schurmann M, Gradl G, Wizgal I 2001 Clinical and physiologic evaluation of stellate ganglion blockade for complex regional pain syndrome type 1. Clinical Journal of Pain 17: 94–100

Spande TF, Garraffo HM, Edwards MW, Yeh HJC, Pannell L, Daley JW 1992 Epibatidine: a novel (chloropyridyl) azabicycloheptane with potent analgesic activity from an Ecuadorian poison frog. Journal of the American Chemical Society 114: 3475–3478

Stanton-Hicks M 1986 Blocks of the sympathetic nervous system. In: Prithvi Raj P (ed) Practical management of pain. Year Book Medical, Chicago, pp 661–681

Stanton-Hicks M, Janig W, Hassenbusch S, Haddox JD, Boas R, Wilson P 1995 Reflex sympathetic dystrophy: changing concepts and taxonomy. Pain 63: 127–133

Stanton-Hicks M, Prithvi Raj P, Racz GB 1996 Use of regional anaesthetics in the diagnosis of reflex sympathetic dystrophy and sympathetically maintained pain. In: Janig W, Stanton-Hicks M (eds) Reflex sympathetic dystrophy: a reappraisal. IASP Press, Seattle, pp 217–237

Stolker RJ, Vervest ACM, Groen GJ 1994 The management of chronic spinal pain by blockades: a review. Pain 58: 1–20

Stone LS, Broberger C, Vulchanova L et al 1998 Differential distribution of α_{2A} and α_{2C} adrenergic receptor immunoreactivity in the rat spinal cord. Journal of Neuroscience 18: 5928–5937

Storer RJ, Goadsby PJ 1997 Microiontophoretic application of serotonin 5-$HT_{1B/1D}$ agonists inhibits trigeminal cell firing in the cat. Brain 120: 2171–2177

Stubhaug A, Breivik H, Eide PK, Kreunen M, Foss A 1997 Mapping of punctate hyperalgesia around a surgical incision demonstrates that ketamine is a powerful suppressor of central sensitization to pain following surgery. Acta Anaesthesiologica Scandinavica 41: 1124–1132

Szallasi A 1997 Perspectives on vanilloids in clinical practice. Drug News and Perspectives 10: 522–527

Taylor CP 1998 Mechanisms of action of gabapentin. Drugs of Today 34: 3–11

Tracey DJ, Romm MA, Yao NNL 1995 Peripheral hyperalgesia in experimental neuropathy: exacerbation by neuropeptide Y. Brain Research 669: 245–254

Tremont-Lukats LW, Megeff C, Backonja MM 2000 Anticonvulsants for neuropathic pain syndromes: mechanism od action and place in therapy. Drugs 60: 1029–1052

Utzschneider D, Kocsis J, Devor M 1992 Mutual excitation among dorsal root ganglion neurons in the rat. Neuroscience Letters 146: 53–56

Verdugo RJ, Ochoa JL 1994 Sympathetically mediated pain. Phentolamine block questions the concept. Neurology 44: 1003–1009

Wahren LK, Gordh T, Torebjork E 1995 Effects of regional intravenous guanethidine in patients with neuralgias in the hand: a follow up study over a decade. Pain 62: 379–385

Waldman SD, Winnie AP 1996 Interventional pain management. Saunders, Philadelphia

Warnke T, Stubhaug A, Jorum E 1997 Ketamine, an NMDA receptor antagonist, suppresses spatial and temporal properties of burn-induced hyperalgesia in man: a double blind, cross over comparison with morphine and placebo. Pain 72: 99–106

Webb J, Kamali F 1998 Analgesic effects of lamotrigine and phenytoin on cold induced pain: a cross over, placebo controlled study in healthy volunteers. Pain 76: 357–363

Woolf CJ, Ma QP, Allchorne A, Poole S 1996 Peripheral cell types contributing to the hyperalgesic action of nerve growth factor in inflammation. Journal of Neuroscience 16: 2716–2723

Wrigglesworth R, Walpole CSJ, Bevan S et al 1996 Analogues of capsaicin with agonist activity as novel analgesic agents: structure activity studies. 4. Potent, orally active analgesics. Journal of Medicinal Chemistry 39: 4942–4951

Zimmer A, Zimmer AM, Baffi J et al 1998 Hypoalgesia in mice with a targeted deletion of the tachykinin I gene. Proceedings of the National Academy Science of the USA 95: 2630–2635

Zvartau-Hind M, Din MU, Gilani A, Lisak RP, Khan OA 2000 Topiramate relieves refractory trigeminal neuralgia in MS patients. Neurology 55: 1587–1588

Chapter 27

Disc surgery

Bo Salén and Erik Spangfort

Introduction

There is a growing awareness among low back specialists that the damage caused by a disc herniation depends not only on the volume of disc tissue protruding or extruding into the spinal canal, but also on the space available for herniated disc tissue in the individual spinal canal. Recently evidence has indicated a more complex process, with a combination of mechanical and inflammatory/immunologic factors causing sciatic pain (Brisby 2000). Disc herniation is only one of several pathomechanisms causing lumbar pain and sciatica. Reduction of the space available for the neural elements, generally called spinal stenosis, is recognized as a nosological entity which, alone or in combination with disc herniation, may produce disabling symptoms from the spine. It is also recognized that when stenosis is involved in a disc syndrome, the results of surgical treatment with traditional discectomy are usually unsatisfactory. Spinal stenosis requires a radical change in surgical technique. Despite impressive development of technological investigative methods as computed tomography (CT) and magnetic resonance imaging (MRI), it may still be extremely difficult to supply the necessary diagnostic foundation for decisions about proper surgical treatment in individual cases of lumbar pain syndromes. Surgical management of these conditions cannot be satisfactorily improved without a better clinical analysis and interpretation of the main symptom, i.e., pain.

Disc operation

Surgical technique

In 1939, Love described the unilateral interlaminar approach, which is still the routine technique in most quarters. The laminae of the two vertebrae between which the herniation has occurred are exposed by subperiosteal dissection and the strong ligamentum flavum is resected, if necessary together with some part of the adjacent lamina. In most cases this exposure allows identification of the underlying nerve root, inspection of the surface of the intervertebral disc after medial retraction of the root, and removal of the possible herniation. Occasionally more bone must be removed and in some cases a hemilaminectomy and/or a partial resection of the posterior facet joint is performed to obtain an adequate exposure. Bilateral exposure is usually not necessary in typical cases of disc herniation.

Extent of exposure

It is, of course, desirable to minimize surgical damage to the anatomical structures as much as possible, even if it is still unproven that the extent of exposure has any major effect on the results of disc operation (Busch et al 1950, Eyre-Brook 1952, Naylor 1974, Fager and Freidberg 1980, Weber 1983). Inadequate exposure, on the other hand, increases the risk of surgical injuries to the nerve roots, the dura, and the vessels and also the risk of failure to locate displaced and migrating fragments extruded from a ruptured disc.

The development of microsurgical technique facilitates the procedure and implies less surgical trauma, but early expectations of considerably better results by microsurgery have not been confirmed (Tullberg et al 1993, McCulloch 1996). It is possible that percutaneous lumbar discectomy is useful in a small group of strictly selected patients, but the proper indications are not yet established (Onik et al 1997). The method is not suitable for patients with rupture of the annulus (complete herniations).

Volume of tissue removed

In several reports the specimens of disc tissue removed by operation are measured by weight and the reported mean values range from 0.79 g (Boemke 1951) to 9.88 g (Hanraets 1959). O'Connell (1951) found a mean weight of 1.95 g; he also reported that the mean weight of lumbar discs excised at autopsy was 24.6 g.

In an extensive study of the lumbar disc operation (Spangfort 1972), the volume of disc tissue removed was analysed in 645 cases (unpublished). The mean volume in this series was 2.14 (s.d. 1.04) ml, with no single specimen larger than 7 ml. The mean volume was correlated with the degree of herniation and increased from 1.25 ml in negative explorations to 1.52 ml in 'bulging discs', 2.01 ml in incomplete herniations, and 2.36 ml in ruptured discs. In 90 reoperations, where a disc herniation was found, the mean volume was almost the same (2.09 ml). These studies indicate that the average volume of disc tissue removed by discectomy represents only 6–8% of the total disc volume.

The 'combined operation'

Concomitant discectomy and some type of fusion operation as a standard procedure in an attempt to improve the results of disc surgery are used. The dominating conclusion has been that the advantage of the 'combined operation' is too small to warrant the use of this method as a routine in patients with typical lumbar disc herniations. The surgical indications for discectomy and spine fusion are different. The special indications for fusion should be considered separately in each individual case when disc surgery is planned (Symposium 1981).

Reoperation after discectomy

The rate of reoperations after a first disc operation is usually reported as 10–15%, but rarely within the first year after a discectomy. The pathological process, which in some patients results in a true disc herniation, tends to begin at the lumbosacral level and proceed in the cranial direction with age. The mean age at operation for verified ruptures at the level L5–S1 was found to be 38 years, at the level L4–L5 42 years, and in the unusual herniations at the three higher levels, 47 years (Spangfort 1972).

The results of reoperations are generally less favourable than those of first operations. This is partly due to a higher rate of surgical complications at reoperation, but the main reason is diagnostic difficulties in patients assessed for repeat surgery, which results in high rates of negative explorations in this group. When the degree of herniation found by reoperation is considered, the results are, however, almost as good.

In Spangfort's study of disc operations, the rate of excellent results (i.e., complete relief of both low back pain and sciatica) decreased from 62.0% after first operations to 43.1% after second operations and 28.6% after third operations. If a disc herniation was found by reoperation (161 cases) the rate of excellent results was still 53.4%, but if the reoperation was a negative exploration (69 cases) the rate was as low as 14.5%. Again, preoperative diagnosis is crucial for the result of operation.

The multioperated low back patient with a 'failed back surgery syndrome' should be carefully examined by a qualified investigation before further 'salvage surgery' is attempted: 'No matter how severe or how intractable the pain, it can always be made worse by surgery' (Finneson 1978).

Epidural scar formation

The prevalent pathological condition found in reoperations for recurrent pain after disc surgery is often a dense fibrous scar formation strangling the dura and nerve roots. This scar formation is considered a major cause of recurrent symptoms after discectomy; it also complicates correct diagnosis and reoperation of a true recurrent disc herniation.

Excision of the scar tissue (neurolysis) is difficult and the results are usually poor.

Langenskiöld and Kiviluoto (1976) reported efficient prevention of epidural scar formation by the use of free grafts of subcutaneous fat tissue placed outside the spinal canal. It has been confirmed that covering raw bone, muscles, and nerve roots with free fat grafts effectively prevents epidural scar formation (Yong-Hing et al 1980, Quist et al 1998).

Urgent disc surgery

The only indication for immediate disc surgery is acute compression of the cauda equina by a large herniation causing a sacral syndrome with neurological signs from the second and lower sacral roots, i.e., dysfunction of the bladder and bowel with loss of sphincter control, impairment of sexual function, and saddle-shaped loss of sensation in the sacral dermatomes. In most cases the herniation is large, situated in the midline and ruptured. The condition is rare, probably less than one case per year in a population of 200 000.

In patients with symptoms of acute cauda equina compression a qualified examination and CT or MRI is urgent. Bladder dysfunction is, however, a common symptom in patients with severe low back pain and not necessarily caused by a large disc herniation. Immediate surgical decompression is generally considered mandatory when an acute disc herniation is identified as the cause of the syndrome. Severe impairment of bladder function, bilateral saddle anaesthesia, and a preoperative duration of more than 2 days appear to imply a poor prognosis for satisfactory neurological recovery after surgical decompression (Aho et al 1969).

Surgical indications and selection of patients

Except for the rare cases of acute cauda equina syndrome, the purpose of discectomy is relief of pain, in particular severe sciatic pain, caused by a disc herniation. The disc herniation is a special lesion occurring sometimes in the course of disc degeneration.

Complete relief of sciatic pain after discectomy is correlated primarily with the degree of herniation (Fig. 27.1). The rate of complete relief is excellent in patients with high-grade herniations and the ideal indications for discectomy are recently ruptured herniations and large incomplete herniations in the process of rupturing or dissecting beneath the posterior longitudinal ligament. Only by meticulous selection of patients with high-grade herniations is it possible to improve the results of discectomy and avoid a growing number of disastrous failures (Spangfort 1972, Vucetic 1997).

Disc surgery is pain surgery: the first condition for considering the possibility of discectomy is that the pain is severe enough to motivate surgical treatment. The next condition is that the pain is caused predominantly by a high-grade herniation. These conditions must be strictly respected. The point is to establish the presence and location of an offending disc herniation and, unfortunately, surgical exposure is still the only way to do so with complete certainty.

The decision to advise discectomy must be based on a systematic and comprehensive diagnostic investigation, comprising a detailed history and an adequate analysis of the pain syndrome, disentangling in each case debut and duration of pain, temporal pattern, activities and circumstances affecting the pain, anatomical and topographical patterns, sensory modalities, and an assessment of the intensity of the pain. Furthermore, a complete physical examination is necessary, including the recording of posture and gait, degree of lordosis, range and pattern of spinal motion, pattern of pain by rest, motion and weight bearing, and a neurological examination, as well as psychological assessment, routine laboratory tests, and plain radiographs of the spine and pelvis.

To achieve detailed analyses of the pain syndrome, in our experience, a pain-drawing method

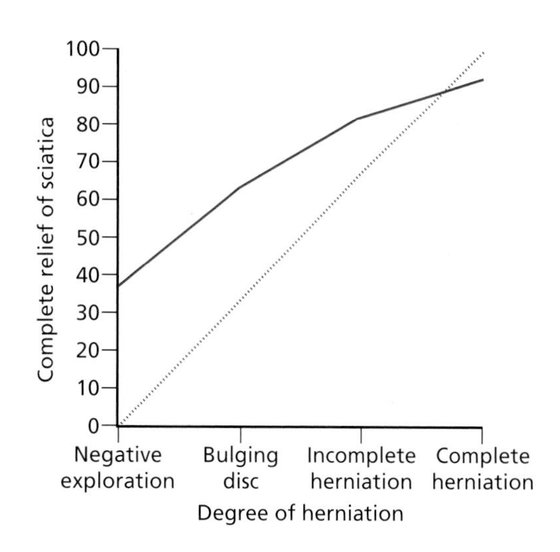

Fig. 27.1 The correlation between complete relief of sciatica and the degree of herniation in 2503 operations (from Spangfort 1972).

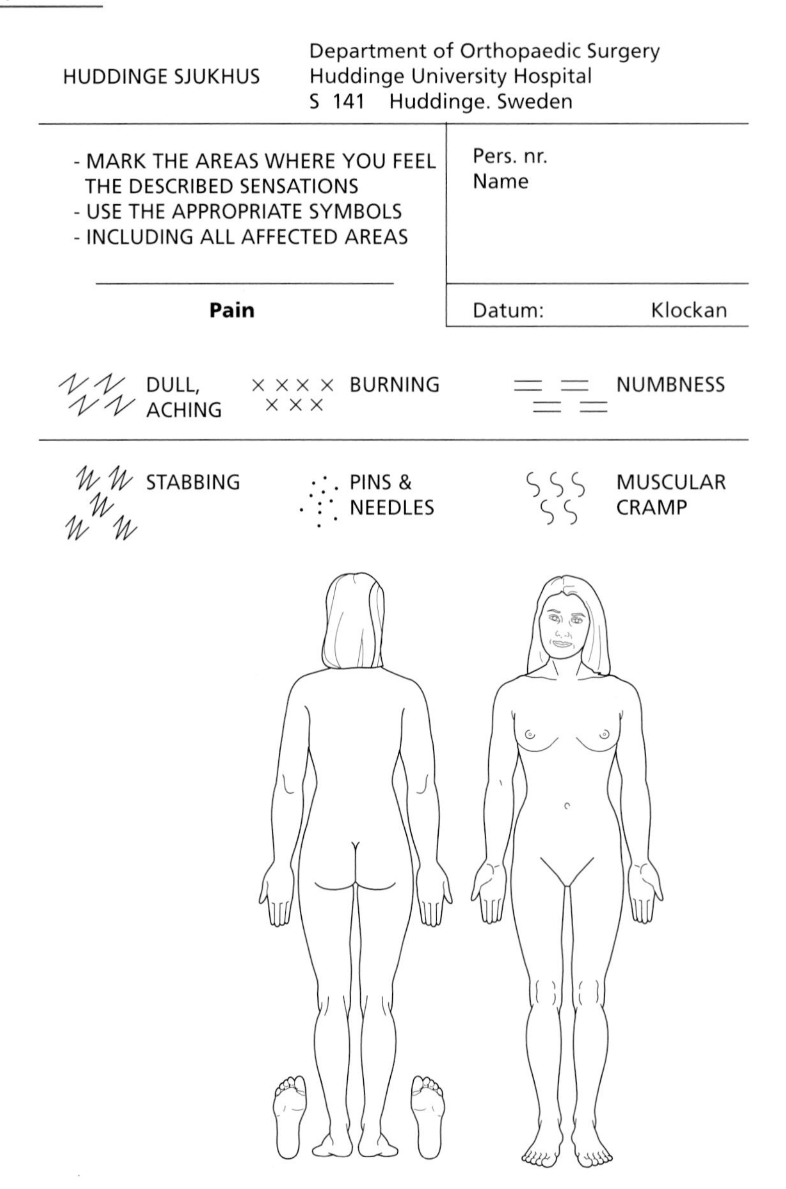
HUDDINGE SJUKHUS

Department of Orthopaedic Surgery
Huddinge University Hospital
S 141 Huddinge. Sweden

- MARK THE AREAS WHERE YOU FEEL THE DESCRIBED SENSATIONS
- USE THE APPROPRIATE SYMBOLS
- INCLUDING ALL AFFECTED AREAS

Pers. nr.
Name

Pain

Datum: Klockan

DULL, ACHING

× × × × × × × BURNING

NUMBNESS

STABBING

PINS & NEEDLES

MUSCULAR CRAMP

Fig. 27.2 Main form for pain drawing used for patients with low back pain (modified from Ransford et al 1976).

is definitely superior, as well as being cheap and convenient. Our present pain-drawing system (Fig. 27.2) was developed from the model published by Ransford et al (1976) and has become indispensable in our preoperative investigation (Brismar et al 1996).

We consider neurological deficits important diagnostic signs but not an independent indication for discectomy, as surgical treatment has not been shown to improve the average prognosis of peripheral neurological deficits. If surgical treatment of a disc herniation cures neurological deficits, which is most likely in some cases, we still cannot identify the subgroup of patients who will benefit from discectomy in this respect.

The rupture of a disc herniation into the spinal canal is an anatomical disaster and surgical measures against it are independent of the patient's general psychological status. In the case of an unequivocal diagnosis of disabling disc herniation we do not deny the patient surgical relief for psychological reasons. The emotionally unstable patient may, indeed, be in greater need of immediate pain relief than the stable one.

It is generally recognized that, with the exceptions already mentioned, surgical treatment of a disc herniation should be advised only if non-surgical treatment fails. A reasonable trial period is 1–3 months in many cases, but we hesitate to accept rigid rules, as a wide variety of circumstances necessitates individual evaluation and decision in every case.

Non-surgical versus surgical treatment

So far, it has not been possible to design a clinical trial of the differences between non-surgical and surgical treatment that completely fulfils scientific criteria. A major problem is that a disc herniation can be definitely confirmed and classified only by surgical exposure.

A few studies from which it is possible to draw tentative conclusions (e.g., Hakelius 1970, Nashold and Hrubec 1971, Hasue and Fujiwara 1979) do, however, indicate that surgical treatment does not necessarily improve the prognosis in the long term, as regards either pain or the risk of persistent neurological deficits. Weber (1983) allocated 126 patients to either operation or physiotherapy and then compared the groups for 10 years. After 1 year the results were significantly better after surgical treatment than after non-surgical treatment. After 4 years the operated patients still showed better results, but the difference was no longer significant. After 10 years no patients in the two groups complained of sciatic pain and the rates of persistent low back pain were equal in the groups. The severity of low back pain decreased over the last 6 years in both groups.

If the clinical situation allows a choice between non-surgical and surgical treatment, the patient should be informed that the benefit expected from the operation is immediate relief of sciatic pain and not necessarily an improvement of the long-range prognosis, which is fairly good anyway.

Nucleolysis

The efficacy of chemonucleolysis has now been shown in controlled trials and the method is recommended subject to strict selection of patients (Brown 1996, Nordby et al 1996). Still, in some countries the method is seldom or never used.

Nucleolysis has also been achieved by percutaneous laser disc decompression, by which a portion of the nucleus is vaporized by laser energy. The method is still at an experimental stage (Quigley and Maroon 1994).

Drug treatment

There are ongoing attempts to develop and evaluate new treatment modalities for sciatic pain including substances that inhibit factors in the inflammatory response (Brisby 2000).

Complications of disc surgery

Mortality rate

In a survey of 54 reports from the period 1937–1972 with a total of 25 392 operations, the mean rate of mortality was 0.3% and constantly decreasing over the years. Pulmonary embolism and postoperative infections were the most frequent causes of death (Spangfort 1972).

Injury to vessels and viscera

Injury to abdominal vessels occurs when the instrument used for evacuating tissue from the interior of the disc space accidentally and without the surgeon being aware of it passes through the anterior wall of the disc is an uncommon but extremely dangerous complication in disc surgery. An estimated incidence of this complication is less than one case in 2000 operations (DeSaussure 1959, Birkeland and Taylor 1969). Injuries to the bowel, the ureter, and the sympathetic trunk may occur by the same mechanism, but are less commonly reported in the literature.

In 95% of all disc operations the total loss of blood is less than 500 ml. The bleeding may cause troublesome difficulties, at least in the narrow field exposed by the interlaminar approach.

Injuries to neural structures

Surgical damage to nerve roots is reported by surgeons in 0.5–3% of all operations; in reoperations the rate is two or three times higher. Verified damage to a nerve root is not always followed by significant clinical symptoms. Motor weakness in the leg, obviously caused by the operation, occurs in at least 5% of all operations, but in the majority the paresis is partial and recovers satisfactorily with time.

Dura lesions

Minor surgical lesions to the dura are not uncommon and are often revealed by leakage of cerebrospinal fluid during the operation. If the lesion is located and closed with fine sutures, the complication is usually harmless.

Thromboembolism

Postoperative thromboembolism is reported to average 2% in the literature. The complication is usually diagnosed between the 4th and 12th day after the operation and is rare in patients below 40 years. A period of immobilization before surgery is probably a pathogenetic factor.

Postoperative infections

With modern surgical technique and facilities, the mean rate of postoperative wound infections after discectomy should not exceed a total of 2–3%, with severe infections accounting for less than 0.5%.

Postoperative discitis

Most cases are caused by a low-grade infection of the disc space, but an aseptic or 'mechanical' type of postoperative discitis also seems to occur (Fouquet et al 1992). The true incidence does probably not exceed 1–2%. The most typical symptom, almost pathognomonic, is violent, spasmodic pain in the back precipitated by the slightest movement and in most cases appearing during the first or second week in the postoperative course. The pain is referred to the lower abdomen, the groins, hips, or upper thighs.

Systemic reactions are scarce. Some patients have a moderate fever and/or infection of the surgical wound. The sedimentation rate (ESR) is usually elevated and a second rise of the postoperative ESR, which normally reaches its peak 3–4 days after the operation, is a significant warning. Early radiological changes as fuzziness and irregular defects of the endplates occur 3–4 weeks after the onset of pain. MRI is considered the best method for diagnosing the condition. Adequate treatment with antibiotics until the ESR is normal is recommended. The complication seems to increase the risk of chronic low back pain and vocational disability, but otherwise many studies indicate a fairly good long-term prognosis (Iversen et al 1992, Rohde et al 1998).

Spinal arachnoiditis

An association between lumbar disc disease and arachnoiditis, a progressive inflammatory reaction of the pia arachnoid, was suspected long ago (French 1946). Recent studies indicate, however, that some degree of arachnoiditis is common, at least in patients with severe pain and disability secondary to disc surgery.

Symptoms vary considerably and mild cases are probably often overlooked. In severe cases, the condition is extremely distressing. The pain is constant in the back and radiates to one or both legs, often in a well-defined distribution of more than one root. The pain is described as burning or cramping—painful muscle cramps and violent spasms of the legs are usual. The cauda equina may be involved. Pain is unrelieved by rest and poorly correlated to weight bearing and motion.

Treatment of this neuralgic pain syndrome is extremely difficult, but the condition is not inevitably progressive—a slow recovery over the years occurs in some patients. Severe psychological complications in response to the constant torturing pain are, however, the rule.

References

Aho AJ, Auranen A, Pesonen K 1969 Analysis of cauda equina symptoms in patients with lumbar disc prolapse. Acta Chirurgica Scandinavica 135: 413–420

Birkeland IW Jr, Taylor TKF 1969 Major vascular injuries in lumbar disc surgery. Journal of Bone and Joint Surgery 51B: 4–19

Boemke F 1951 Feingewebliche Befunde beim Bandscheibenvorfall. Langenbecks Archiv 267: 484–492

Brisby H 2000 Nerve tissue injury markers, inflammatory mechanisms and immunologic factors in lumbar disc herniation. Thesis, Göteborg University, Göteborg

Brismar H, Vucetic N, Svensson O 1996 Pain patterns in lumbar disc hernia. Drawings compared to surgical findings in 159 patients. Acta Orthopaedica Scandinavica 67: 470–472

Brown MD 1996 Update on chemonucleolysis. Spine 21 (suppl 24S): 62S–68S

Busch E, Andersen A, Broager B et al 1950 Le prolapsus discal lombaire. Acta Psychiatrica et Neurologica 25: 443–500

DeSaussure RL 1959 Vascular injury coincident to disc surgery. Journal of Neurosurgery 16: 222–229

Eyre-Brook AL 1952 A study of late results from disc operations. British Journal of Surgery 39: 289–296

Fager CA, Freidberg SR 1980 Analysis of failures and poor results of lumbar spine surgery. Spine 5: 87–94

Finneson BE 1978 A lumbar disc surgery predictive score card. Spine 3: 186–188

Fouquet B, Goupille P, Jattiot F et al 1992 Discitis after lumbar disc surgery. Features of 'aseptic' and 'septic' forms. Spine 17: 356–358

French JD 1946 Clinical manifestations of lumbar spinal arachnoiditis. Surgery 20: 718–729

Hakelius A 1970 Prognosis in sciatica. Acta Orthopaedica Scandinavica 129 (suppl): 1–76

Hanraets PRMJ 1959 The degenerative back and its differential diagnosis. Elsevier, Amsterdam

Hasue M, Fujiwara M 1979 Epidemiologic and clinical studies of long-term prognosis of low-back pain and sciatica. Spine 4: 150–155

Iversen E, Herss Nielsen VA, Gadegaard Hansen L 1992 Prognosis in postoperative discitis. A retrospective study of 111 cases. Acta Orthopaedica Scandinavica 63: 305–309

Langenskiöld A, Kiviluoto O 1976 Prevention of epidural scar formation after operations on the lumbar spine by means of free fat transplants. Clinical Orthopaedics and Related Research 115: 92–95

Love JG 1939 Removal of protruded intervertebral disks without laminectomy. Proceedings of the Staff Meetings of the Mayo Clinic 14: 800 (1940, 15: 4)

McCulloch JA 1996 Focus issue on lumbar disc herniation: macro- and microdiscectomy. Spine 21 (suppl 24S) 45S–56S

Nashold BS, Hrubec Z 1971 Lumbar disc disease. A 20-year clinical follow-up study. Mosby, St Louis

Naylor A 1974 The late results of laminectomy for lumbar disc prolapse. Journal of Bone and Joint Surgery 56B: 17–29

Nordby EJ, Fraser RD, Javid MJ 1996 Spine update. Chemonucleolysis. Spine 21: 1102–1105

O'Connell JEA 1951 Protrusions of the lumbar intervertebral discs. Journal of Bone and Joint Surgery 33B: 8–30

Onik GM, Kambin P, Chang MK 1997 Controversy. Minimally invasive disc surgery. Nucleotomy *versus* fragmentectomy. Spine 22: 827–830

Quigley MR, Maroon JC 1994 Laser discectomy: A review. Spine 19: 53–56

Quist JJ, Dhert WJA, Meij BP et al 1998 The prevention of peridural adhesions. A comparative long-term histomorphometric study using a biodegradable barrier and a fat graft. Journal of Bone and Joint Surgery 80B: 520–526

Ransford AO, Cairns D, Mooney V 1976 The pain drawing as an aid to the psychologic evaluation of patients with low back pain. Spine 1: 127–134

Rohde V, Meyer B, Schaller C, Hassler WE 1998 Spondylodiscitis after lumbar discectomy. Incidence and a proposal for prophylaxis. Spine 23: 615–620

Spangfort EV 1972 The lumbar disc herniation. A computer-aided analysis of 2504 operations. Acta Orthopaedica Scandinavica 142 (suppl): 1–95

Symposium 1981 The role of spine fusion for low-back pain. Spine 6: 277–314

Tullberg T, Isacson J, Weidenhielm L 1993 Does microscopic removal of lumbar disc herniation lead to better results than the standard procedure? Spine 18: 24–27

Vucetic N 1997 Clinical diagnosis of lumbar disc herniation. Outcome predictors for surgical treatment. Thesis, Karolinska Institute, Stockholm

Weber H 1983 Lumbar disc herniation—a controlled, prospective study with 10 years of observation. Spine 8: 131–140

Yong-Hing K, Reilly J, de Korompay V, Kirkaldy-Willis WH 1980 Prevention of nerve root adhesions after laminectomy. Spine 5: 59–64

Chapter 28

Orthopaedic surgery

Robert F McLain and James N Weinstein

Introduction

The orthopaedist is called on to treat neoplastic, inflammatory, developmental, metabolic, degenerative, and traumatic conditions, among which pain is often the common denominator. Pain is a non-specific symptom and provides little insight, by itself, into the serious or benign nature of the underlying malady. It is, however, the symptom that most often drives the patient to seek treatment. Whether the pain source is a life-threatening tumour or an ankle sprain, it is the physician's responsibility to formulate a plan that best treats the underlying disease while effectively reducing the patient's pain.

The physician's initial task is to identify the true nature of the patient's problem: is the pain severe and debilitating or does it simply trigger the patient's fear of an underlying disease? Is it a manifestation of underlying psychological turmoil or is it physiologically normal pain interfering with an active, functioning patient? The next task is to identify the source and cause of the pain, and to exclude an underlying systemic or malignant process that may threaten the patient's life. Finally, the orthopaedic surgeon formulates a treatment plan suited to the individual patient and the specific disorder.

Mechanisms of musculoskeletal pain

The musculoskeletal system consists of the bones and articulations of the skeleton and the ligaments, muscles, and tendons that connect and mobilize them. Injuries or disorders of the musculoskeletal system may affect muscle, bone, tendon, ligament, articular cartilage, periosteum, synovium, or articular capsule. These tissues are richly innervated by a variety of neural receptors.

Joint pain

The joints of the human skeleton are specialized to bear loads and allow motion through specific, prescribed arcs of excursion. In the extremities and in the posterior elements of the spine, these are synovial joints. The components of these joints are specialized to meet specific demands of function: articular cartilage absorbs and distributes loads; subchondral bone resists deformation and supports and nourishes the cartilage; ligaments maintain alignment and constrain joint excursion; musculotendinous units flex, extend, and stabilize the joint. Derangement of the joint may result in destruction of the articular cartilage, fracture of the subchondral bone, attenuation or disruption of the ligaments, and excessive strains and inflammation of the muscles. Nerve endings in these or other tissues may signal the presence of ongoing or incipient tissue damage, producing the sensation of pain.

Synovial joints enjoy a dual pattern of innervation: primary articular nerves are independent branches from larger peripheral nerves, which specifically supply the joint capsule and ligaments; accessory articular nerves reach the joint after passing through muscular or cutaneous tissues to which they provide primary innervation (Wyke 1972). Both primary and accessory articular nerves are mixed afferent nerves, containing proprioceptive and nociceptive fibres. These fibres supply innervation to virtually all of the periarticular soft tissues.

Freeman and Wyke (1967) described four basic types of afferent nerve endings in articular tissues and documented their presence in a wide variety of joints. While the Type 4 receptors (free nerve endings) are the only ones thought to be exclusively nociceptive, it is known that the proprioceptive endings of Types 1–3 are capable of responding to excessive joint excursion as a noxious stimulus and that they play an important role in maintaining joint stability (Palmer 1958, Eckholm et al 1960). Deandrade et al (1965) and Kennedy et al (1982) have both demonstrated that the presence of a joint effusion can produce reflex inhibition of the quadriceps mechanism. Histological studies have demonstrated receptors in ligaments (Gardner 1948, O'Connor and Gonzales 1979, De Avila et al 1989), capsule (Freeman and Wyke 1967, Grigg et al 1982), and meniscal tissues (O'Connor and McConnaughey 1978), as well as periarticular fat and muscle (Freeman and Wyke 1967, Dee 1978). Giles and Harvey (1987) have demonstrated nociceptive free nerve endings in capsular tissue from human facets and reported similar endings in the apophyseal synovium. McLain has identified all four receptor types in capsular and pericapsular tissues of the cervical, and to a lesser extent, the thoracic and lumbar facet joints (McLain 1994, McLain and Pickar 1998).

While capsule, fat, and muscle are richly supplied with nociceptive free nerve endings, investigators have previously reported a relative paucity of these receptors in the synovium, ligaments, and menisci. The stimuli that these periarticular receptors respond to may be either mechanical (capsular distension, ligamentous instability, direct trauma) or chemical (Wyke 1981).

Synovial tissues may produce joint pain by both direct and indirect mechanisms. Using antisera against specific neuronal markers, investigators re-examining synovial innervation have found vastly greater numbers of small-diameter nerve fibres than were previously reported using standard histological methods (Gronblad et al 1988, 1991; Weinstein et al 1988a; Kidd et al 1990). Substance P (sP) has been shown to accumulate in articular fluid following capsaicin injection and is known to produce plasma extravasation and vasodilatation (Yaksh 1988; Lam and Ferrell 1989, 1991). Levels of sP are higher in joints with more severe arthritis, and infusion of the neuropeptide into joints with mild disease has been shown to accelerate the degenerative process (Levine et al 1984). Calcitonin gene-related peptide (CGRP) has also been implicated as a mediator in the early stages of arthritis (Konttinen et al 1990). Whether sP plays a direct role in the stimulation or sensitization of intra-articular pain receptors is not established, but sensitization is important and several mechanisms have been confirmed experimentally. Grigg et al (1986) have shown that induction of experimental arthritis results in sensitization of free nerve endings in the joint capsule. When acute inflammation is induced, afferent receptors that are normally silent during joint motion become responsive to previously innocuous stimuli, including motion in the normal range. A similar sensitizing effect is produced by intra-articular infusion of prostaglandins or bradykinin (Schaible et al 1987, Neugebauer et al 1989), providing further evidence that local sensitization is at least partly responsible for the pain felt in arthritic or inflamed joints. There is also strong evidence of a central nervous system component further amplifying the nociceptive discharges from the joint (Neugebauer and Schaible 1990).

Bone and periosteum

Bone is a dynamic composite tissue involved in a variety of physiological processes. It is the only tissue in the body able to repair itself after injury without forming scar. It responds to minute piezoelectric currents generated by stresses by increasing its mass in areas of increased load and by removing support from areas seeing little load. It is sensitive to pressure internally and to direct injury externally.

The external covering of the bone is the periosteum. This tough fibrous sheath is highly vascular and copiously supplied with both free nerve endings and encapsulated endings; the complex free nerve endings are thought to generate painful discharges, while the encapsulated endings are thought to be sensitive to pressure (Cooper 1968,

Hill and Elde 1991). Gronblad et al (1984) have demonstrated an extensive ramification of sP-reactive nerve fibres in both the superficial and deep layers of the periosteal sheath.

Bjurholm et al (1988) have demonstrated both sP- and CGRP-containing nerves in the marrow, periosteum, and cortex of long bones, as well as the associated muscles and ligaments. These two neuropeptides, sP and CGRP, have been associated with nociceptor transmission (Skofitsch and Jacobowitz 1985, Badalamente et al 1987) as well as an acceleration of experimental arthritis and an increase in its severity following local infusion (Colpaert et al 1983, Levine et al 1984).

The vasodilatory effect of vasoactive intestinal peptide (VIP) has been clearly demonstrated (Said and Mutt 1970), while neuropeptide Y (NPY) has been shown to be a powerful vasoconstrictor (Lundberg et al 1982). Fibres containing these neuropeptides tend to congregate at the osteochondral junction of the epiphyseal plate. Although the primary role of these peptides is likely to be related to the regulation of growth, it is possible that they might also play a role in the production or prevention of intraosseous hypertension, a proposed cause of bone and joint pain.

Musculotendinous pain

The nociceptive innervation of muscle has been discussed previously. The primary nociceptive endings in muscle are unencapsulated free nerve endings. Intramuscular mechanoreceptors may also produce pain impulses when exposed to noxious stimuli. Muscular pain receptors may be either chemonociceptive or mechanonociceptive and may respond to stimuli as either specific or polymodal receptors. Chemonociceptive endings may respond to metabolites that accumulate during anaerobic metabolism, to products of cell injury produced by trauma or ischaemia, or to chemical irritants such as bradykinin, serotonin, or potassium. Mechanonociceptive units may respond to stretch, pressure, or disruption. Some receptors may also respond to thermal stimuli (Kumazawa and Mizumura 1977, Mense and Schmidt 1977). It is thought that the neurogenic inflammatory response produced by CGRP, which results in persistent vasodilatation, erythema, and oedema formation, may also serve to sensitize nociceptors to the presence of other pain-related neuropeptides (Piotrowski and Foreman 1986, Fuller et al 1987). This receptor sensitization, as well as the increase in intramuscular blood flow and interstitial oedema, may represent a primary mechanism of muscular pain.

Muscular pain may be the result of a direct injury, such as a blow or puncture, which disrupts or damages the muscle tissue and its intrafascicular nerve fibres, or the distension and pressure produced by the ensuing haematoma and oedema. Inflammation and oedema, components of the normal healing process, play a role in the mediation of pain symptoms. In major musculoskeletal injuries persistent spasm may occur, resulting in severe muscle pain as well as further trauma to the muscle and other tissues of the soft tissue envelope.

A more ominous type of muscle pain occurs when excessive pressure in or around the muscle results in ischaemia. Compartment syndromes occur in patients with bleeding disorders, vascular injuries, musculoskeletal trauma, and systemic infections and can result from constrictive dressings or casts. They are also a common finding in patients with stroke, intoxication, metabolic disorders, or head injuries; patients with these conditions are often 'found down' and have lain in one position for so long that the blood supply to an extremity has been compromised. Pain in compartment syndrome is severe and unremitting and out of proportion to the injury sustained. The clinical condition mimics the symptoms produced by experimental tourniquet pain, and it is likely that the pathophysiology of the two conditions is the same (Smith et al 1966, Sternbach et al 1974). Like tourniquet pain, compartment syndrome pain is progressive in intensity and rapidly resolves if pressure is released in a timely fashion, either by removing the constricting dressing or by performing a surgical release of the compartment fascia (Mubarak and Owen 1977).

Neural elements

Nerves are subject to injury and irritation as they pass through the muscular compartments and around the bony articulations of the extremities. Several recent studies have shown that environmental stimuli can produce histological changes in dorsal root ganglion neurons similar to those seen following injury and can induce marked changes in the levels of pain-related neuropeptides contained within the ganglion (Weinstein 1986; Weinstein et al 1988b; McLain and Weinstein 1991, 1992). Compression and injury to the spinal nerves and dorsal root ganglion are discussed in Chap. 19.

Treatment modalities—principles and application

The goals of orthopaedic treatment are to reduce pain, correct deformity, and improve function. To accomplish these goals, the surgeon may employ any of a number of different treatment modalities, both surgical and non-surgical. These modalities can be roughly segregated into four different levels:

1. immobilization
2. fusion
3. resection
4. reconstruction.

The orthopaedist uses a number of tools—injections, physical therapy, non-steroidal anti-inflammatory medications, and oral analgesics—to further supplement pain relief.

Immobilization

Immobilization of injured extremities is among the oldest and most effective means of controlling musculoskeletal pain. It can be accomplished by either direct or indirect means, using internal splints, external splints, or traction. Splinting effectively reduces pain by preventing joint motion, muscle contraction, and displacement of bony fractures. It ensures rest of the injured tissues, eliminating stimuli that trigger local nociceptors.

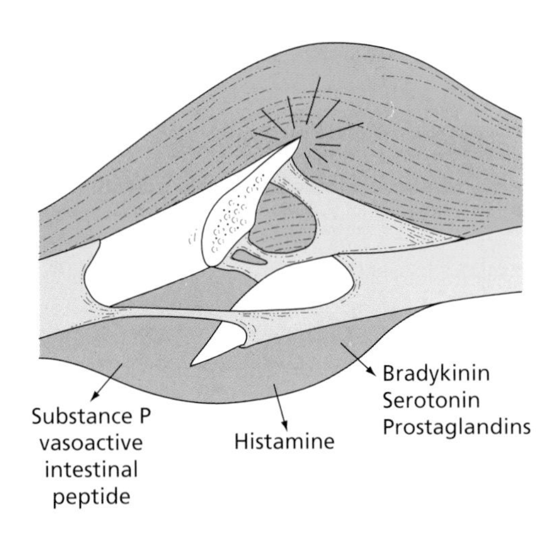

Fig. 28.1 Pain in musculoskeletal trauma. Fractures, dislocations, and sprains elicit pain through a variety of inter-related and independent mechanisms that act locally and systemically to generate and mediate the pain sensation: fine nerve endings in the cancellous bone and periosteal lining are triggered by the physical disruption of the bone and the tearing and stretching of the periosteum; nerve endings in the surrounding muscle and soft tissue may be damaged directly or subjected to pressure or stretch by the displaced fracture fragments or the expanding haematoma; inflamed muscle may be triggered to spasm, producing pain and further distortion of tissues; damaged cells, nerve endings, and inflammatory cells elaborate a variety of neurochemical mediators, including neuropeptides, algesic chemicals, and inflammatory components.

In the fractured limb, pain is initially produced by the distortion of intramedullary nerve fibres in the broken bone, by stretched or disrupted receptors in the torn periosteum, and by injury or pressure on receptors in the soft tissue overlying the fracture (Fig. 28.1). A haematoma rapidly accumulates and expands until the pressure within the compartment is significantly elevated; distension of the fascia and soft tissue triggers further pain receptors. Damaged tissues release bradykinin, histamine, potassium, and neurotransmitters which sensitize local nociceptors, alter vascular permeability, and mediate the influx of inflammatory cells. The result is oedema, inflammation, and irritation of the injured muscle, triggering muscle spasms and involuntary contractions. These produce further tissue damage and increasing deformity, as well as uncontrolled pain. In a patient with multiple fractures this may lead to life-threatening haemorrhage and systemic shock (Chapman 1989). A variety of splinting techniques may be needed to manage such a patient through the course from initial resuscitation to definitive fixation (Fig. 28.2).

In conditions of joint inflammation, haemarthrosis, or pyarthrosis, pain is produced by the distension of the joint capsule. Chemical pain mediators directly stimulate chemonociceptors (Heppelmann et al 1985, 1986). Irritation of the synovium results in secondary oedema, synovial hypertrophy, and an effusion, which stretch and distort the capsule. Any motion of the joint serves to increase the tension on the capsule and mechanically distorts the inflamed tissues, resulting in increased pain. Joint motion in this inflamed state causes further release of noxious neuropeptides, kinins, and inflammatory agents that act to stimulate receptors in the capsule and surrounding periosteum. Inflammation results in an increase in sensitivity to movement (Schaible and Schmidt 1985). By immobilizing the joint in a splint, these mechanisms can be attenuated. The period of immobilization depends on the aetiology of the problem: Bony injuries heal well with 6–12 weeks of rigid immobilization, while ligamentous injuries often heal better with earlier motion, despite pain.

Traction has long been recognized as an effective means of obtaining and maintaining a reduction in fractures of long bones (Charnley 1961a). By applying persistent longitudinal traction, muscle spasm can often be overcome and bony alignment restored. This prevents further tissue damage and reduces pain caused by distortion of soft tissues and movement of the ends of the fractured bone. Once

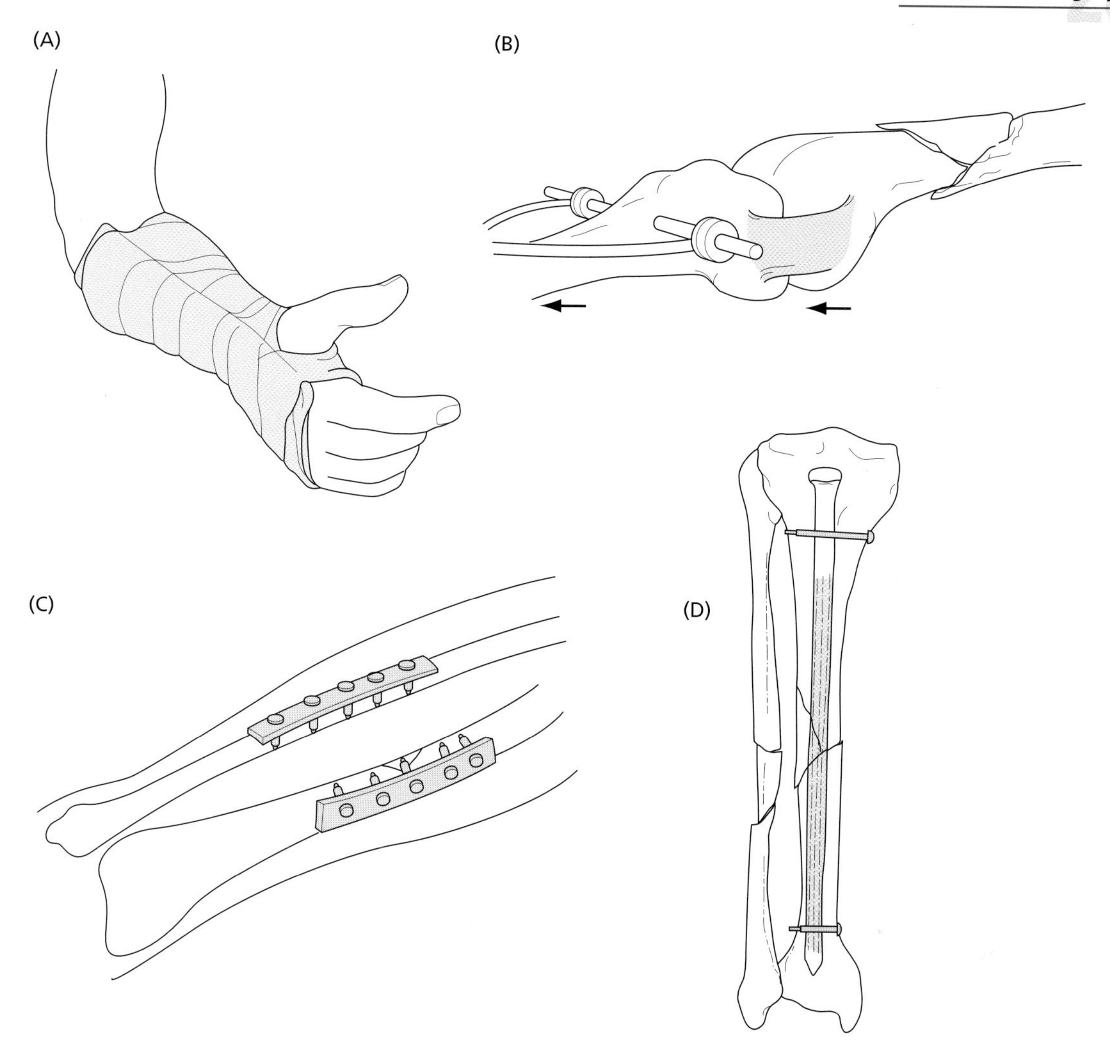

Fig. 28.2 Immobilization of musculoskeletal injuries: methods of immobilizing injured limbs range from passive, non-invasive techniques to sophisticated methods of internal fixation. (A) Splint immobilization can be applied to any extremity. The external splint is easy to apply, prevents excessive motion of joints and stabilizes soft tissues, and allows the patient to return to limited function. (B) Skeletal traction is applied primarily in fractures of the femur, but can be used in any long bone fracture. The longitudinal traction overcomes powerful muscle spasm and controls alignment in injuries that cannot be splinted. (C) Internal fixation, using plates and screws, allows the surgeon to reduce anatomically the fracture fragments and rigidly fix the fracture. This ensures the best possible result in terms of alignment, joint congruency, and anatomical relationships and also permits the patient to start range-of-motion exercises before the fracture has healed. (D) Intramedullary fixation restores alignment without exposing the fractures site, thereby reducing the risk of infection. By sharing the load applied to the limb, the intramedullary device minimizes the risk of non-union and allows early mobilization.

the muscle fatigues and the spasm is overcome, muscle pain quickly subsides. In patients who cannot tolerate surgery, skeletal traction remains a viable method of treating fractures. The complications of traction and prolonged immobilization (deep venous thrombosis, pulmonary embolus, pneumonia, infection) must be weighed against the risk of operative treatment.

Internal fixation provides all the benefits of fracture reduction, tissue immobilization, and protection from additional injury, but offers the additional benefit of early functional return. Because the bone is fixed internally, the adjacent joints can be left free for early range of motion. Rigid fixation of fractures eliminates motion at the injured bone ends and the pain caused by the abrading fracture surfaces. Immobilization limits the extent of subsequent muscle damage, reducing the quantity of noxious metabolites, kinins, and debris produced at the site of injury.

Depending on the location and the comminution of a fracture, the surgeon may elect to stabilize it using either plates and screws or an intramedullary device. In applying a plate to the fracture, the surgeon opens the fracture site and reduces the fragments under direct vision. The plate is then applied so that it compresses the fracture fragments and promotes healing. Additional screws may be used to reduce and fix additional fragments that have broken off from the main segments of bone (Fig. 28.2). This is particularly important in fractures of the upper extremity where malalignments are poorly tolerated. In fractures of the forearm, for instance, cast treatment requires prolonged immobilization of the elbow, the wrist, and the hand. This form of treatment is rarely adequate to control the position of the broken bones, and results in stiffness and pain in the joints, adhesions of the finger flexor muscles, and loss of forearm rotation because of bony malalignment. Open reduction and internal fixation of this injury are universally preferred; the patient is able to begin elbow motion the day after surgery and begins active finger motion and grip within a few days. Range of motion is restored to nearly normal and pain is a rare complication.

Intramedullary fixation of long bone fractures involves opening a portal into the medullary canal at a site remote to the actual fracture. A rod is then passed down the medullary canal, across the fracture, and into the canal of the far fragment. Locking screws can be placed proximally and distally to

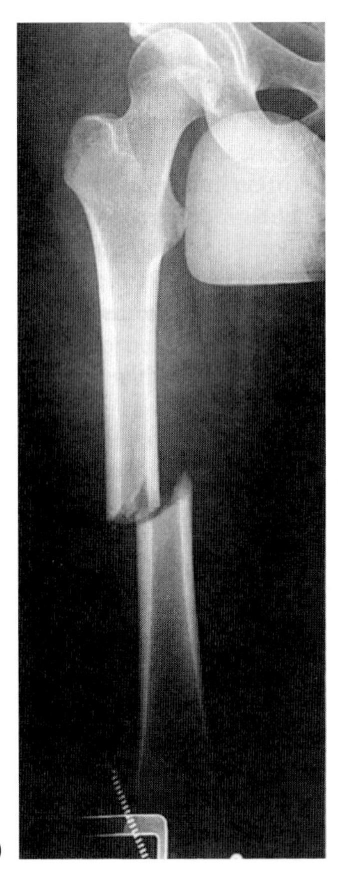
(A)

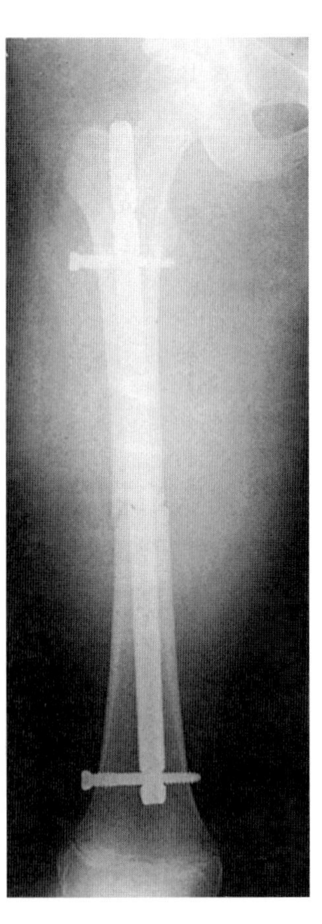
(B)

Fig. 28.3 Intramedullary fixation of a femur fracture. Intramedullary rodding allows the surgeon to restore length and axial alignment of this long bone fracture without opening the fracture site or damaging the massive muscular sheath that surrounds the femur. (A) AP radiograph of transverse femur fracture sustained in a road traffic accident; alignment and length are being maintained by longitudinal skeletal traction. (B) Same extremity after intramedullary fixation. Locking screws have been placed proximally and distally to prevent rotational or angular displacement. This patient was able to walk with crutches within 48 h of surgery and was fully weight bearing at 3 weeks.

control shortening and rotation (Küntscher 1968, Winquist and Hanson 1978). The use of intramedullary rods has two advantages over plate fixation. Firstly, the surgeon does not open the fracture site to fix the fracture, thus reducing the risk of infection. Secondly, the device allows gravity and muscle contraction to compress the fracture, stimulating the healing process. Intramedullary fixation is most commonly used in femur fractures, but can be applied to injuries of the tibia, humerus, and ulna as well (Fig. 28.3).

Specialized fixation devices have been developed for injuries such as hip fractures, for example, which have proven particularly difficult to treat by closed means. In 1931 Smith-Peterson demonstrated a reduction in mortality from 75 to 25% and an increase in union rate from 30 to 70% when femoral neck fractures were internally fixed (Smith-Peterson et al 1931). Intertrochanteric hip fractures are particularly serious injuries and even as late as 1966, Horowitz reported a 35% mortality rate in patients treated non-operatively. Open treatment of intertrochanteric fractures is the treatment of choice for most patients. The sliding hip screw and side plate has provided reliable fracture healing (Fig. 28.4), while allowing the patient to bear weight on the injured limb immediately post-operatively, permitting rehabilitation of muscles and avoiding recumbency and contractures. Failure rates have been reduced and 70% of patients regain good to excellent function (Miller 1978).

Fusion

Joint fusion represents a permanent form of musculoskeletal immobilization. Fusions are carried out in patients with pain secondary to joint infections, severe degenerative disease, severe

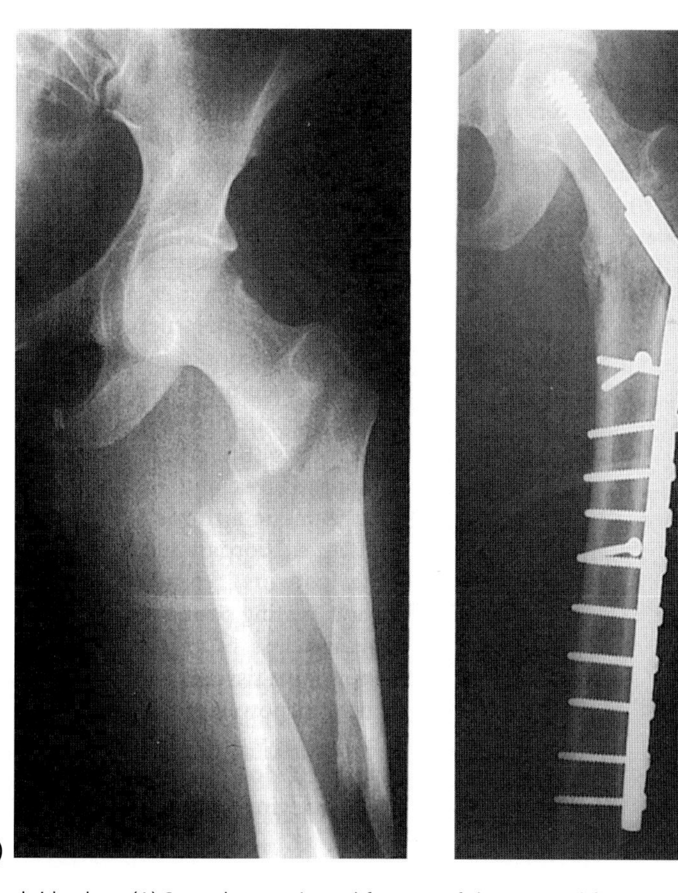

Fig. 28.4 Hip screw and side plate. (A) Severely comminuted fracture of the proximal femur in a middle-aged patient. Non-operative management is likely to result in non-union, deformity, and pain. (B) Specially designed hip screw provides fixation of long spiral fracture of the femoral shaft while maintaining alignment of the femoral head and neck. The screw placed in the femoral head is designed to slide through the barrel of the side plate, allowing this fragment to collapse down on the shaft fragments during weight bearing while maintaining an appropriate angle between the neck and the shaft.

articular trauma, or disabling ligament instability, with the goal of restoring maximum function while eliminating pain. Although unglamorous, joint arthrodesis is still a highly successful operation for selected patients with rugged functional demands. Patients younger than 40 years, weighing in excess of 200 lbs, with excessive activity requirements, are at high risk for failure when treated with a conventional total joint prosthesis. In these patients a hip or knee fusion may be the right choice. Callaghan et al (1985) reviewed 28 patients with hip fusions, followed up for an average of 35 years. Although most patients eventually developed some degree of pain in the ipsilateral knee or low back, these patients had enjoyed years of physical activity before developing symptoms. Symptomatic patients underwent a late conversion to a total hip arthroplasty, with subsequent relief of their pain.

Fusion is often the best choice for pain relief and improved function in the wrist. Wrist arthrodesis has long enjoyed a reputation for reliable and satisfactory reconstruction among patients suffering from trauma, infection, inflammatory disease, or tumour. Steindler recommended the procedure for patients with polio or spastic hemiparesis (Steindler 1918) and later for tuberculosis (Steindler 1921), and others have described the procedures and outcomes for rheumatoid arthritis, post-traumatic arthritis, and infections (Abbott et al 1942, Haddad and Riordan 1967, Millender and Nalebuff 1973). Arthrodesis removes the painful joint tissues, eliminates motion, and restores alignment and power grip. For patients with limited areas of joint disease within the wrist, a variety of intercarpal fusions that maintain some joint motion while relieving pain and instability have been described (Watson and Hempton 1980).

Arthrodesis is performed by removing the articular cartilage and preparing the bone ends so that broad areas of bleeding, cancellous bone can be approximated and held firmly in place. Either internal or external fixation may be applied to ensure compression of the surfaces until fusion occurs. The positioning of the limb at the time of surgery is critical to the patient's ability to use the extremity productively and painlessly. A patient with a solid arthrodesis in a position of function will consistently demonstrate greater function and satisfaction than a patient with a mobile but painful joint.

Resection

The ability to surgically remove the pathological tissue, segment, or limb from a patient provides the orthopaedist with a variety of options in palliating painful musculoskeletal conditions. The simplest resections may require only the removal of a small piece of tissue, as in the patient with a torn meniscal cartilage, while the most complex of procedures may result in the internal resection of an entire long bone and its muscular envelope, for the patient with a primary bone tumour. Modern techniques allow us to consider limb-salvaging operations where terminal amputations were once the principle option, and modern prosthetics provide excellent function and cosmesis when amputation is the logical and preferred choice.

Removal of pathological tissue from within a joint is a commonly performed procedure in patients with post-traumatic or inflammatory problems involving the articular cartilage, menisci, or synovium. Arthroscopic surgery now allows surgeons to perform many of these procedures without opening the joint and can be used in the knee, shoulder, hip, wrist, or ankle.

Osteochondral loose bodies are most common within the knee. These fragments usually result from previous cartilage injuries and may produce pain by impinging between the joint surfaces, compressing the synovial lining or irritating the capsular tissues (O'Connor and Shahriaree 1984). Simply removing the loose bodies and lavaging the joint can significantly relieve pain, particularly if there is associated synovitis (O'Connor 1973). Meniscal tears are common in the most active segment of our population. Depending on the size and pattern of a tear, patients may present with persistent, nagging pain; occasional, severe pain; or an acutely 'locked' knee, in which the torn meniscal tissue is found incarcerated within the joint, preventing flexion or extension. Through the arthroscope the orthopaedist is able to partially or completely resect the torn meniscus or repair it when possible. Since total meniscectomy has been shown to precipitate degenerative changes in the knee, partial meniscectomy or repair is widely recommended (Dandy and Jackson 1975, Jackson and Rouse 1982).

Synovial inflammation and hypertrophy may occur with any chronic inflammatory process, but are particularly prominent in rheumatoid and tuberculous arthritis, in haemophilic arthritis, and in pigmented villonodular synovitis (Wilkinson 1969, Montane et al 1986).

Synovectomy, either open or arthroscopic, has been shown to be effective in reducing pain and disability in patients with persistent synovitis. Montane et al (1986) demonstrated that open synovectomy was able to eliminate recurrent haemarthroses due to haemophilia, reduce pain, and arrest the progressive arthrosis. Although some studies have questioned the efficacy of synovectomy in treating clinical symptoms of rheumatoid arthritis (Arthritis Foundation 1977), others have shown significant benefit to function and pain relief when carried out in early stages of the disease (Ishikawa et al 1986).

Resection of tumours of bone or soft tissue, and of destructive infections of bone, is often necessary for patient welfare as well as pain relief. Tumours produce pain as they displace normal tissues during growth. Expansile lesions, whether tumour or infection, may elevate the periosteum away from the bone, producing local pressure and disrupting nerve endings. Destructive lesions may weaken bone to the point of fracture or impending fracture. Compression of vascular structures may produce ischaemia or venous congestion, and of nerves, paralysis, paraesthesias, or pain. Some neoplastic lesions, such as osteoid osteomas and osteoblastomas, may elaborate factors that produce pain directly (Sherman and McFarland 1965, Marsh et al 1975). Pain relief can be obtained by any means that reduces the pressure on the soft tissues or neurovascular structures. In cases of soft tissue infection, simple drainage of the abscess provides prompt and dramatic pain relief. Pain due to expanding tumour mass can be reduced by radiotherapy or chemotherapy; necrosis and shrinkage of the tumour relieves pressure on surrounding structures. While medical management is often able to control pain or slow the progress of disease, in many cases surgery is needed to ensure the best chance of curing the patient. In infections, debridement or resection of infected bone is necessary to prevent recurrence, and in tumours, removal of the tumour, the surrounding soft tissues, and sometimes all of the associated musculature may be necessary to provide local tumour control, depending on the tumour type. In any case, the type of resection chosen is determined on the basis of the location and nature of the lesion involved and the health and prognosis of the patient.

The oldest and most straightforward form of resection is amputation. Until the twentieth century this was the only effective treatment of tumours, infections, open fractures, or other severely painful or potentially lethal lesions of the extremities. Amputation is still indicated in a number of clinical situations. Diabetic patients, with poor sensation, poor circulation, and impaired healing potential, often require amputation to cure chronic infections, non-healing wounds, and neuropathic pain (Ecker and Jacobs 1970, Wagner 1986). Vascular insufficiency, due to atherosclerosis or diabetes mellitus, is the cause of nearly 80% of all lower extremity amputations. Tumours requiring a wide resection distal to the mid-tibia are still best treated by amputation, as reconstruction of this area is very difficult and the results somewhat unreliable.

Amputation remains an appropriate alternative in the care of some traumatic injuries. Advances in surgical technique, microvascular repair, and soft tissue transfers have made it possible to 'save' almost any extremity; the decision to do so may be a disservice to some patients, however (Lange et al 1985). Patients with severe injuries to the hand or lower leg often require multiple surgeries to repair the damage. Patients with prolonged ischaemia of the limb, disruption of major nerves, or mangling injuries of hand or foot are often left with a marginally viable, functionless extremity, prone to infection and often painful. In these patients primary amputation offers a better likelihood of painless activity and function (Caudle and Stern 1987, Hansen 1987).

Limb salvage resections amount to 'internal amputations' and their success depends on the surgeon's ability to replace adequately the resected tissue elements with something that will function in an acceptably similar way. Likewise, the segment of the limb being salvaged must be of enough importance to warrant a highly technical and demanding operation and extensive rehabilitation. Because below-knee prostheses provide excellent, pain-free function with few problems or activity restrictions, and reconstructions of the foot and ankle often function poorly, salvage of the foot and ankle is rarely warranted. On the other hand, patients with above-knee amputations expend significantly more energy in walking than do those with below-knee amputations. When the amputation is performed high up on the thigh, the fit becomes difficult and the function poorer, and these patients have a greater tendency to become wheelchair bound (Volpicelli et al 1983). For this reason, a tumour of the femur or knee is one of the most common indications for limb salvage surgery (Fig. 28.5).

Reconstruction

Of all procedures performed by the orthopaedic surgeon, joint reconstruction can have the most dramatic impact on the patient's function and satisfaction with life.

The fundamental problem in end-stage joint disease is the erosion or destruction of the articular surfaces. Operative treatment seeks to accomplish one or more of the following.

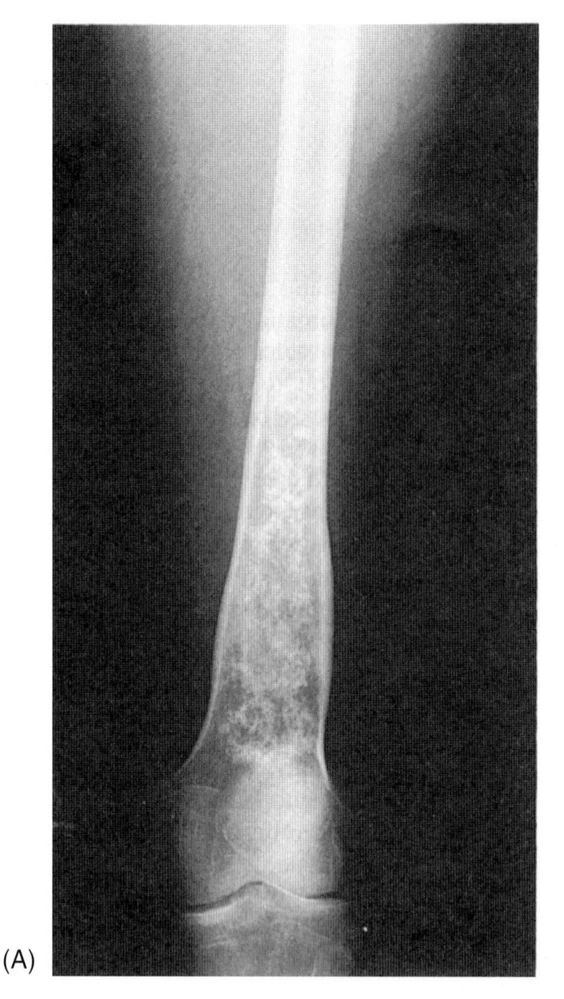

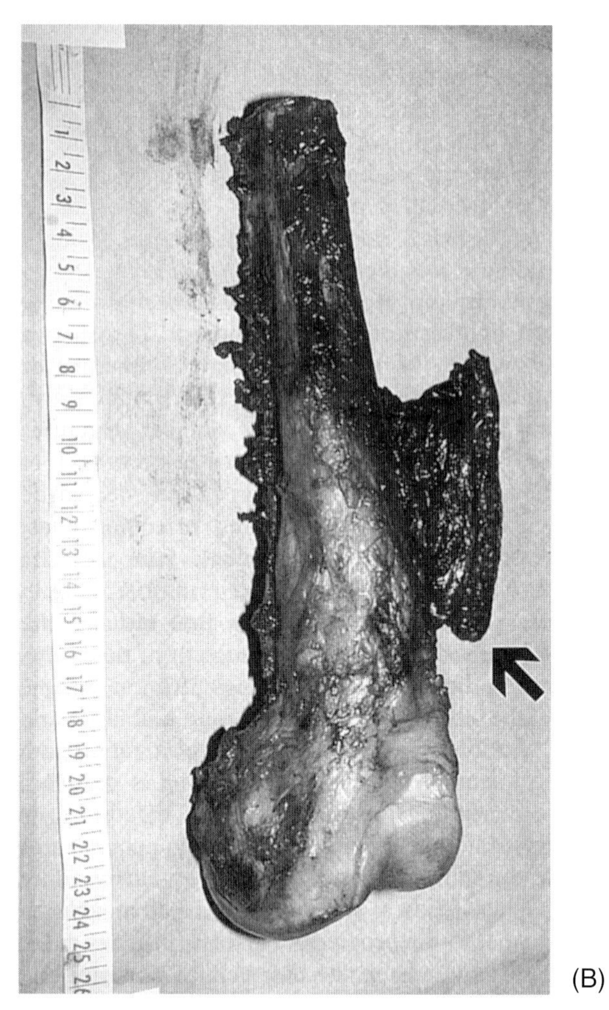

(A) (B)

Fig. 28.5 Limb salvage surgery. (A) Grade I chondrosarcoma of the distal femur in a 40-year-old man; the tumour is confined to the medullary canal but has extended well up the shaft. The prognosis for this lesion, which has a tendency to recur locally, is good if local control can be obtained. Traditional treatment would have been a high thigh amputation. (B) Resection of the tumour involves removal of the entire distal femur, with a suitable margin of normal bone at the proximal end. The biopsy tract has also been excised en bloc with the specimen to limit the chances of local recurrence (arrow).

1. Reduce the contact between the two damaged joint surfaces. Excisional arthroplasty and interpositional arthroplasty either remove the damaged joint surfaces or place tissue between them to reduce contact.
2. Transfer contact from damaged cartilage to areas of healthy cartilage. Osteotomies alter joint contact by changing the alignment of the limb or the orientation of the joint surfaces.
3. Replace the joint surfaces. Total joint arthroplasty has had its most profound effect on disorders of the hip, knee, and shoulder.

Excisional arthroplasty

One of the earliest forms of joint reconstruction was the excisional arthroplasty, performed by excising the joint surfaces and allowing a pseudarthrosis to form. This allowed reasonable motion and function with tolerable pain.

The Girdlestone excision of the hip remains a viable treatment of hip fractures or infections in elderly or ill patients whose primary need is to sit or transfer comfortably (Girdlestone 1943). It may be the only option in patients with infections of the hip joint or those who have failed previous total

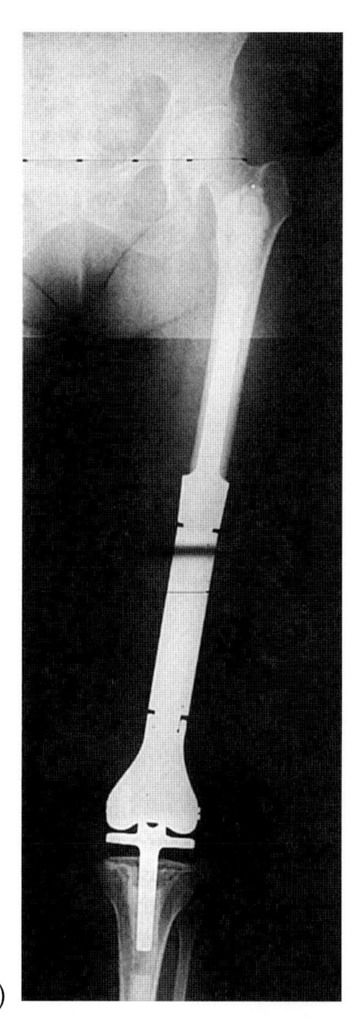

Fig. 28.5, *cont'd* Limb salvage surgery. (C) A custom endoprosthesis was implanted to salvage the limb. This prosthesis has a long proximal stem cemented into the amputated end of the femur and an artificial knee joint that replaces both the femoral and tibial side of the articulation. Pain relief is excellent with this implant and the patient has near-normal function despite the wide resection of this tumour.

joint arthroplasty. Patients are able to walk on a Girdlestone hip, but usually have a significant limp and require some assistive device. The quality of the outcome depends on the formation of a tough scar around the proximal end of the femur. Prolonged traction and bracing may be required to allow scar to mature between the femur and acetabulum, providing enough stability to walk on. Few patients are very satisfied with the long-term results of resection arthroplasty (Petty and Goldsmith 1980).

Interpositional arthroplasty

Soft tissue arthroplasties are performed by interposing adjoining soft tissues between the joint's ends to provide a resilient, gliding surface where the original articular surface has been worn away. Interposition has been tried in large weight-bearing joints, and has largely been abandoned in favour of fusion or joint replacement. In smaller joints, however, fascial interposition remains a successful operation, providing excellent symptomatic relief and good function in the joints of the elbow, wrist, and thumb (Smith-Peterson et al 1943, Froimson 1970, Beckenbaugh and Linscheid 1982).

Osteotomy

Osteotomy is primarily used in one of two scenarios: cases in which deformity or malalignment result in poor function and predispose to early joint degeneration, and cases in which degenerative disease has damaged one area of weight-bearing cartilage while sparing the rest. Congenital and acquired deformities of the lower extremity may sufficiently derange the weight-bearing axis of the limb so as to assure progressive deformity and early joint destruction (Langenskiold and Riska 1964, Schoenecker et al 1985). In these patients, corrective osteotomies, performed at the right age, may restore alignment, height, and function, with relatively little risk (Deitz and Weinstein 1988). In children with congenital dislocation of the hip, osteotomy may be necessary to correct the rotational deformity of the proximal femur and to allow reduction of the coxa-femoral joint.

Osteotomies are sometimes needed for post-traumatic malunion. Injuries resulting in a varus or valgus deformity of the lower extremity force the weight-bearing joints to be loaded eccentrically, causing pain and early joint destruction. Corrective osteotomies are designed to return the limb to its natural alignment and restore normal joint mechanics. For instance, malunion of a distal radius fracture (Colles' fracture) can be satisfactorily corrected with a distal radius osteotomy to restore joint alignment and stability, grip strength, and pain-free function (Fernandez 1988) (Fig. 28.6).

Proximal tibial osteotomy (Fig. 28.7) remains the most successful operation for osteoarthritis of the knee, short of joint replacement (Jackson and Waugh 1961). In younger patients with greater functional demands this procedure is the treatment of choice, allowing the patient unrestricted activity without lifting limits or restrictions of sports or recreation. By transferring contact forces from the side of the joint with advanced degenerative

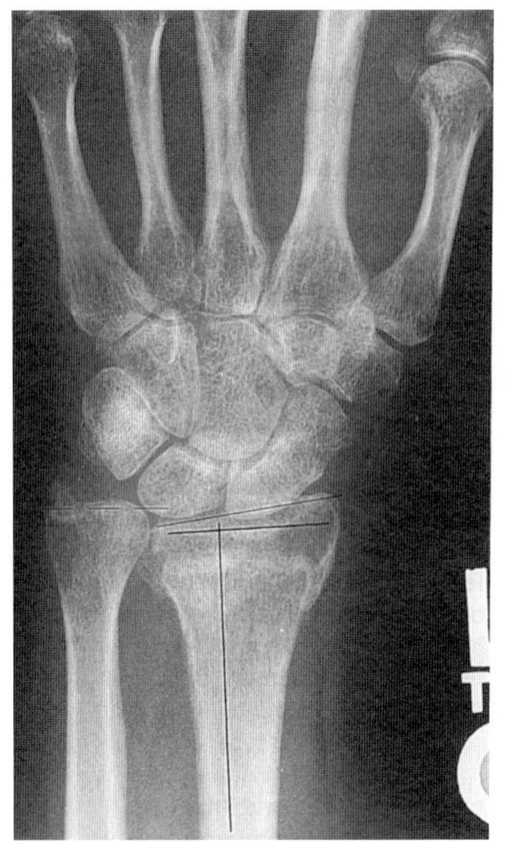

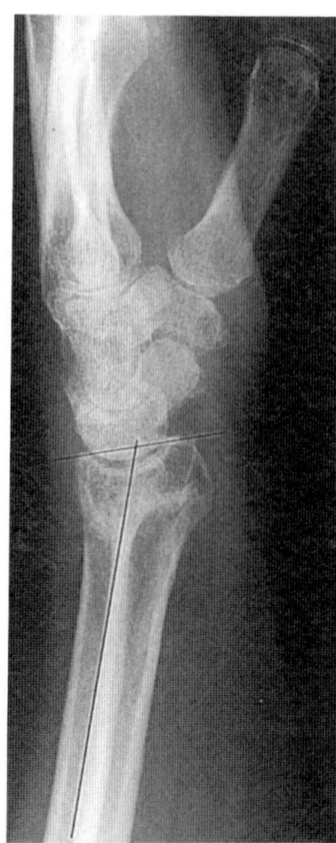

(A)

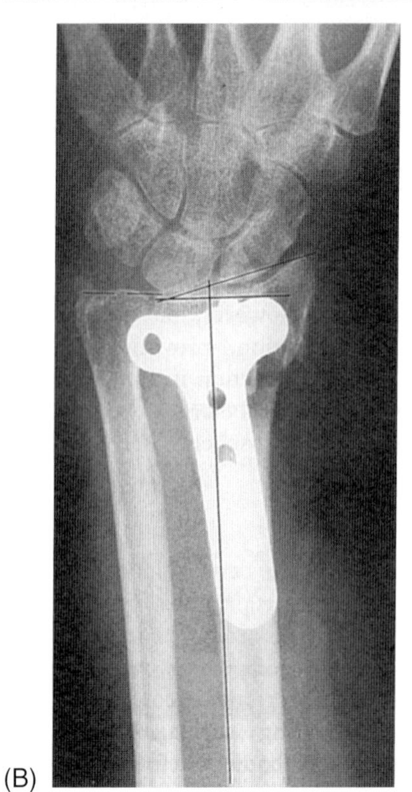

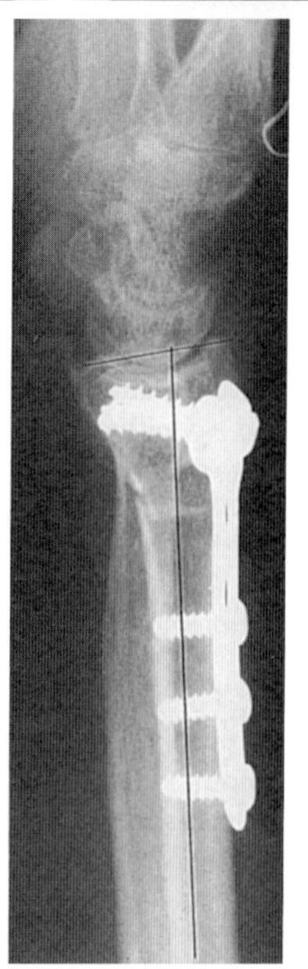

(B)

Fig. 28.6 Distal radial osteotomy. (A) AP and lateral views show malunion of wrist. Note on the AP view that radial inclination is reduced to 5° (normal, 20°–25°) and that the radius is considerably shortened relative to the ulna. On the lateral view, the wrist is dorsally angulated 18°, compared to a normal palmar tilt of 10°–25°, resulting in derangement of the radiocarpal articulation. This patient has chronic pain, weakness, and a predisposition to severe degenerative disease. (B) A distal radial osteotomy was performed using an iliac crest bone graft to restore the normal orientation of the radiocarpal joint. Following the corrective osteotomy, the radial inclination is improved and length restored. The normal volar tilt has also been restored.

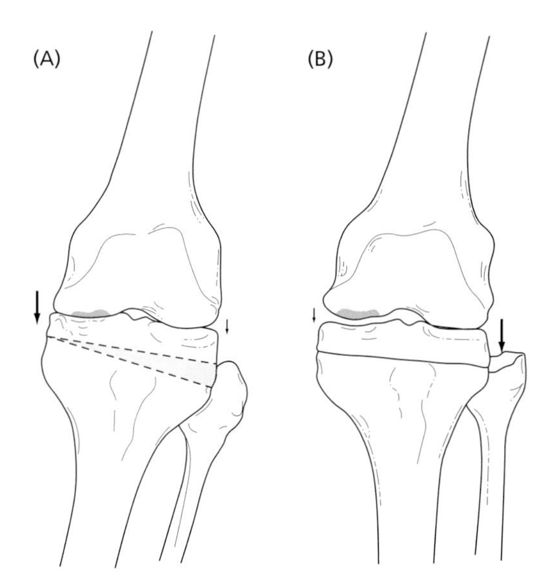

Fig. 28.7 Proximal tibial osteotomy. Osteotomy to correct deformity of the knee and reduce stress on a joint compartment with severe arthritis is an effective and commonly used operation. (A) Patients with severe medial compartment osteoarthritis develop genu valgum, which result in a progressive shift of loads onto the injured side (large arrow). As weight is shifted to the diseased compartment, the healthy cartilage in the lateral compartment sees less load and remains intact. A corrective osteotomy performed through the cancellous bone of the proximal tibia (cross-hatched area) corrects the valgus deformity, shifting weight away from the damaged medial cartilage and on to the healthy lateral cartilage. (B) By restoring the normal alignment of the knee, ligament and muscle stresses are normalized. An osteotomy performed through the vascular cancellous bone of the tibial metaphysis heals reliably.

disease to the side with residual healthy cartilage, tibial osteotomy may provide the patient with years of unrestricted function (Holden et al 1988). Total hip arthroplasty has largely replaced hip osteotomy as a treatment of osteoarthritis. A proximal femoral osteotomy requires a longer convalescence than a total hip arthroplasty and greater patient compliance is required for success. Also, since the range of motion of the hip is not improved by osteotomy, patients with contractures or limited motion are poor candidates. Nonetheless, in young, active patients at risk for early total joint failure, osteotomies of the hip provide a valuable treatment alternative (Fortune 1990).

Total joint arthroplasty

There are few, if any, operations as successful for managing pain and restoring function as joint replacement arthroplasty. Since Charnley first reported his hip replacement procedure (Charnley 1961b), total joint arthroplasty has become the most frequently performed reconstructive procedure in orthopaedic surgery. Total hip arthroplasty can provide dramatic and long-lasting pain relief in patients with osteoarthritis, rheumatoid arthritis, avascular necrosis, non-unions of the femoral neck, post-traumatic degenerative disease, and a number of other congenital or acquired maladies of the hip joint. Total hip arthroplasty can also be performed in patients with previous fusions or osteotomies and in patients with previous arthroplasties that have loosened. Relative contraindications to arthroplasty include obesity, youth, high functional demands, and active or chronic infection in the joint (Salvati et al 1991). The use of bone ingrowth (cementless) prostheses promises improved success even in these difficult patients.

Although modern implants are the product of significant technological evolution, the basic concept behind the original plastic and metal prosthesis still pertains: a small-diameter, polished metal head, mounted on a femoral stem, articulates with a metal-backed high-density polyethylene socket embedded in the acetabulum, with both components fixed so as to restore anatomical alignment and range of motion (Fig. 28.8). Because the longevity of the device is determined, in part, by the positioning and fixation of the components, attention to surgical technique is critical to the survival of the implant and the duration of symptomatic relief. Failure of the arthroplasty usually occurs because of loosening or infection or a combination of the two.

In performing a total hip arthroplasty, the capsule of the joint is excised and the femoral head dislocated from the acetabulum. The femoral neck is transected and the femoral head discarded. The acetabulum is prepared by removing the remaining articular cartilage with a domed reamer, and the femoral shaft by inserting a broach contoured to match the femoral implant being used. The implant is then inserted and either fixed in place with polymethylmethacrylate (PMMA) cement or press-fitted in the case of bone ingrowth components. The patient is usually out of bed on the first post-operative day and ambulating independently within the week. In patients with severe degenerative disease pain relief is often immediate and range of motion improved. A review of Charnley low-friction arthroplasties at 15- to 21-year follow-up showed that less than 4% had become painful, 11% produced occasional discomfort, and 85% were still functioning painlessly (Wroblewski 1986). McCoy et al (1988) reported good to excellent results in 88% of hips followed for 15 years or more. Improve-

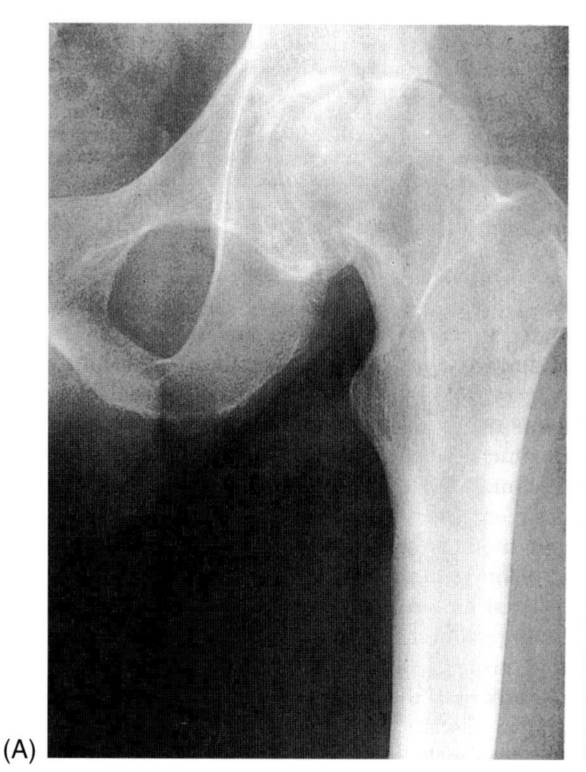

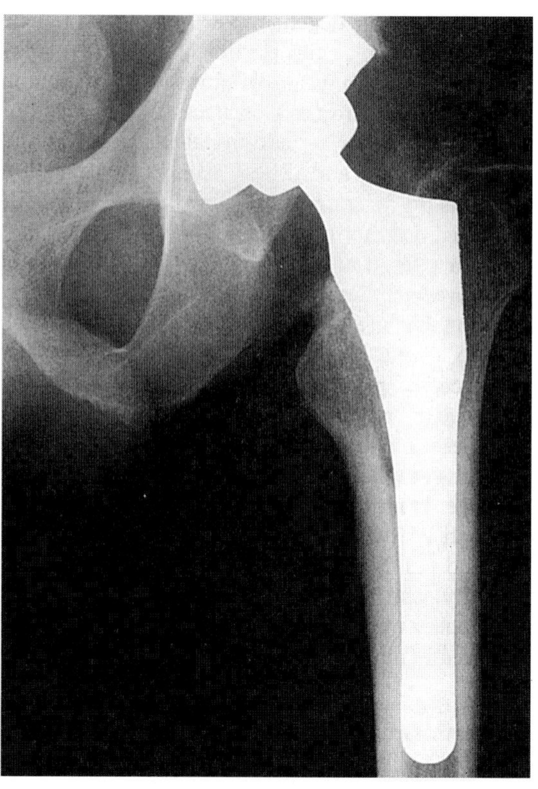

Fig. 28.8 Total hip arthroplasty. (A) AP view of the pelvis, showing severe, unilateral degenerative disease of the hip. Loss of the joint space is apparent, while several signs of DJD (sclerosis of the subchondral bone, formation of subchondral cysts, osteophyte formation) are also seen. (B) A total hip arthroplasty, with a metal-backed acetabular cup and an uncemented femoral component. Pain relief is reliably excellent.

ments in cement technique promise even greater longevity for the hips currently being implanted.

Total knee arthroplasty has enjoyed a similar rise in popularity as implant technology has been refined; the clinical success of knee arthroplasty now equals or exceeds that of total hip arthroplasty with respect to pain relief, functional restoration, and survival of the implant at 10 years (Insall et al 1983, Ewald et al 1984). Currently, most knee implants are cemented in place with PMMA, as bone ingrowth implants have proven less reliable in knee surgery than in the hip.

Summary

The orthopaedic surgeon has a vast array of techniques and technology available for treating musculoskeletal disorders. The surgeon must match the treatment to the disease and promote options in the order of their invasiveness and potential risk. As many interventions cannot provide permanent pain relief, the patient may require a series of procedures over the course of his or her lifetime, and the physician must use good judgement early on to avoid 'burning bridges' with respect to later procedures. The majority of patients will be well cared for with a judicious combination of medical management and an occasional surgical intervention, well timed and tailored to the patient's needs. The injudicious application of technology to orthopaedic problems can lead to unmanageable problems in later life; cementing a total hip implant into a young, non-compliant patient is bound to lead to early failure, repeated revisions, and, in the end, an excisional arthroplasty before the patient reaches middle age. On the other hand, a patient with a traumatic injury to the knee might undergo an acute ligament or meniscal repair as a young man, arthroscopic debridement or synovectomy to control symptoms in middle age, a high tibial osteotomy for unicompartmental degenerative disease at 50, a hemiarthroplasty at 60, and a total condylar knee replacement at the age of 70, at which time that arthroplasty could be expected to provide excellent function for another 15–20 years. The goal of such a treatment hierarchy, as aggressive as it may appear, is to keep the patient functioning at the highest possible level throughout his life, with a minimal level of pain; such a patient is pleased with his care and an asset to his family and community rather than a burden. The orthopaedist's challenge is to maintain the patient as an independent, productive member of society, capable of enjoying and participating in life; if this can be accomplished both the physician and the patient will be well satisfied.

References

Abbott LC, Saunders JB de CM, Bost FC 1942 Arthrodesis of the wrist with the use of grafts of cancellous bone. Journal of Bone and Joint Surgery 24: 883–898

Arthritis Foundation Committee on Evaluation of Synovectomy 1977 Multicenter evaluation of synovectomy in the treatment of rheumatoid arthritis. Report of results at the end of three years. Arthritis and Rheumatology 20: 765–771

Badalamente MA, Dee R, Ghillani R, Chien PF, Daniels K 1987 Mechanical stimulation of dorsal root ganglia induces increased production of substance P: a mechanism of pain following nerve root compromise? Spine 12: 552–555

Beckenbaugh RD, Linscheid RL 1982 Arthroplasty in the hand and wrist. In: Green DP (ed) Operative hand surgery. Churchill Livingstone, New York, pp 141–184

Bjurholm A, Kreicbergs A, Brodin E, Schultzberg M 1988 Substance P and CGRP immunoreactive nerves in bone. Peptides 9: 165–171

Callaghan JJ, Brand RA, Petersen DR 1985 Hip arthrodesis. Journal of Bone and Joint Surgery 67A: 1328–1335

Caudle RJ, Stern PJ 1987 Severe open fractures of the tibia. Journal of Bone and Joint Surgery 69A: 801–807

Chapman MW 1989 Orthopaedic management of the multiply injured patient. In: Evarts CM (ed) Surgery of the musculoskeletal system, 2nd edn. Churchill Livingstone, New York, pp 19–35

Charnley J 1961a The closed treatment of common fractures. Churchill Livingstone, Edinburgh, pp 1–67

Charnley J 1961b Arthroplasty of the hip. Lancet 1: 1129–1132

Colpaert FC, Donnerer J, Lembeck F 1983 Effects of capsaicin on inflammation and on the substance P content of nervous tissues in rats with adjuvant arthritis. Life Sciences 32: 1827–1834

Cooper RR 1968 Nerves in cortical bone. Science 160: 327–328

Dandy DJ, Jackson RW 1975 The diagnosis of problems after meniscectomy. Journal of Bone and Joint Surgery 57B: 349–352

Deandrade JR, Grant C, Dixon A 1965 Joint distension and reflex muscle inhibition in the knee. Journal of Bone and Joint Surgery 47A: 313–332

De Avila GA, O'Connor BL, Visco DM, Sisk TD 1989 The mechanoreceptor innervation of the human fibular collateral ligament. Journal of Anatomy 162: 1–7

Dee RM 1978 The innervation of joints. In: Sokoloff L (ed) Joints and synovial fluid. Academic Press, New York

Dietz FR, Weinstein SL 1988 Spike osteotomy for angular deformities of the long bones. Journal of Bone and Joint Surgery 70A: 848–852

Ecker MD, Jacobs BS 1970 Lower extremity amputations in diabetic patients. Diabetes 19: 189–195

Eckholm J, Eklund G, Skoglund S 1960 On the reflex effects from the knee joint of the cat. Acta Physiologica Scandinavica 50: 167–174

Ewald FC, Jacobs MA, Miegel RE, Walker PS, Poss R, Sledge CB 1984 Kinematic total knee replacement. Journal of Bone and Joint Surgery 66A: 1032–1040

Fernandez DL 1988 Radial osteotomy and Bowers arthroplasty for malunited fractures of the distal end of the radius. Journal of Bone and Joint Surgery 70A: 1538–1551

Fortune WP 1990 Hip osteotomies. In: Evarts CM (ed) Surgery of the musculoskeletal system, vol 3. Churchill Livingstone, New York, pp 2795–2832

Freeman MAR, Wyke BD 1967 The innervation of the knee joint. An anatomical and histological study in the cat. Journal of Anatomy 101: 505–532

Froimson AI 1970 Tendon arthroplasty of the trapeziometacarpal joint. Clinical Orthopaedics and Related Research 70: 191–199

Fuller RW, Conradson TB, Dixon CMS, Crossman DC, Barnes PJ 1987 Sensory neuropeptide effects in human skin. British Journal of Pharmacology 92: 781–788

Gardner E 1948 The innervation of the knee joint. Anatomical Record 101: 109–130

Giles LGF, Harvey AR 1987 Immunohistochemical demonstration of nociceptors in the capsule and synovial folds of human zygapophyseal joints. British Journal of Rheumatology 26: 362–364

Girdlestone GR 1943 Acute pyogenic arthritis of the hip. An operation giving free access and effective drainage. Lancet 1: 419–421

Grigg P, Hoffman AH, Fogarty KE 1982 Properties of Golgi–Mazzoni afferents in cat knee joint capsule as revealed by mechanical studies in isolated joint capsule. Journal of Neurophysiology 47: 31–40

Grigg P, Schaible HG, Schmidt RF 1986 Mechanical sensitivity of group III and IV afferents from posterior articular nerve in normal and inflamed cat knee. Journal of Neurophysiology 55: 635–643

Gronblad M, Liesi P, Korkala O, Karaharju E, Polak J 1984 Innervation of human bone periosteum by peptidergic nerves. Anatomical Record 209: 297–299

Gronblad M, Konttinen Y, Korkala O, Liesi P, Hukkanen M, Polak J 1988 Neuropeptides in synovium of patients with rheumatoid arthritis and osteoarthritis. Journal of Rheumatology 15: 1807–1810

Gronblad M, Weinstein JN, Santavirta S 1991 Immunohistochemical observations on spinal tissue innervation. Acta Orthopaedica Scandinavica 62: 614

Haddad RJ, Riordan DC 1967 Arthrodesis of the wrist. A surgical technique. Journal of Bone and Joint Surgery 49A: 950–954

Hansen ST 1987 The type-IIIC tibial fracture. Salvage or amputation? Journal of Bone and Joint Surgery 69A: 799–800

Heppelmann B, Schaible HG, Schmidt RF 1985 Effects of prostaglandin E1 and E2 on the mechanosensitivity of group III afferents from normal and inflamed cat knee joints. In: Fields HL, Dubner R, Cervero F (eds) Advances in pain research and therapy. Raven Press, New York, pp 91–101

Heppelmann B, Pfeffer A, Schaible HG, Schmidt RF 1986 Effects of acetylsalicylic acid and indomethacin on single group III and IV sensory units from acutely inflamed joints. Pain 26: 337–351

Hill EL, Elde R 1991 Distribution of CGRP-, VIP-, DβH-, SP-, and NPY-immunoreactive nerves in the periosteum of the rat. Cell and Tissue Research 264: 469–480

Holden DL, Stanley LJ, Larson RL, Slocum DB 1988 Proximal tibial osteotomy in patients who are fifty years old or less. Journal of Bone and Joint Surgery 70A: 977–982

Horowitz BG 1966 Retrospective analysis of hip fractures. Surgery, Gynecology and Obstetrics 123: 565–570

Insall JN, Hood RW, Flawn LB, Sullivan DJ 1983 The total condylar knee prosthesis in gonarthrosis. A five to nine year follow-up of the first one hundred consecutive replacements. Journal of Bone and Joint Surgery 65A: 619–628

Ishikawa H, Ohno O, Hirohata K 1986 Long-term results of synovectomy in rheumatoid patients. Journal of Bone and Joint Surgery 68A: 198–205

Jackson RW, Rouse DW 1982 The results of partial arthroscopic meniscectomy in patients over 40 years of age. Journal of Bone and Joint Surgery 64B: 481–486

Jackson JP, Waugh W 1961 Tibial osteotomy for osteoarthritis of the knee. Journal of Bone and Joint Surgery 43B: 746–751

Kennedy JC, Alexander IJ, Hayes KC 1982 Nerve supply of the human knee and its functional importance. American Journal of Sports Medicine 10: 329–335

Kidd BL, Mapp PI, Blake DR, Gibson SJ, Polak JM 1990 Neurogenic influences in arthritis. Annals of the Rheumatic Diseases 49: 649–652

Konttinen Y, Rees R, Hukkanen M et al 1990 Nerves in inflammatory synovium: immunohistochemical observations on the adjuvant arthritic rat model. Journal of Rheumatology 17: 1586–1591

Kumazawa T, Mizumura K 1977 Thin fiber receptors responding to mechanical, chemical and thermal stimulation in the skeletal muscle of the dog. Journal of Physiology 273: 179–194

Küntscher G 1968 The intramedullary nailing of fractures. Clinical Orthopaedics and Related Research 60: 5–12

Lam FY, Ferrell WR 1989 Inhibition of carrageenan-induced inflammation in the rat knee joint. Annals of the Rheumatic Diseases 48: 928–932

Lam FY, Ferrell WR 1991 Neurogenic component of different models of acute inflammation in the rat knee model. Annals of the Rheumatic Diseases 50: 747–751

Lange RH, Bach AW, Hansen ST, Johansen KH 1985 Open tibial fractures with associated vascular injuries. Prognosis for limb salvage. Journal of Trauma 25: 203–208

Langenskiold A, Riska EB 1964 Tibia vara (osteochondrosis deformans tibia). A survey of seventy-one cases. Journal of Bone and Joint Surgery 46A: 1405–1420

Levine JD, Clark R, Devor M, Helms C, Moskowitz M, Basbaum AI 1984 Interneuronal substance P contributes to the severity of experimental arthritis. Science 226: 547–549

Lundberg JM, Terenius L, Hokfelt T et al 1982 Neuropeptide Y (NPY)-like immunoreactivity in peripheral noradrenergic neurons and effects of NPY on sympathetic function. Acta Physiologica Scandinavica 116: 477–480

Marsh BW, Bonfiglio M, Brady LP, Enneking WF 1975 Benign osteoblastoma: range of manifestations. Journal of Bone and Joint Surgery 57A: 1–9

McCoy TH, Salvati EA, Ranawat CS 1988 A fifteen year follow-up study of one hundred Charnley low-friction arthroplasties. Orthopedic Clinics of North America 19: 467–476

McLain RF 1994 Mechanoreceptor endings in human cervical facet joints. Spine 19: 495–501

McLain RF, Pickar JG 1998 Mechanoreceptor endings in human thoracic and lumbar facet joints. Spine 23: 168–173

McLain RF, Weinstein JN 1991 Ultrastructural changes in the dorsal root ganglion associated with whole body vibration. Journal of Spinal Disorders 4: 142–148

McLain RF, Weinstein JN 1992 Nuclear clefting in dorsal root ganglion neurons. A response to whole body vibration. Journal of Comparative Neurology 322: 538–547

Mense S, Schmidt RF 1977 Muscle pain. Which receptors are responsible for the transmission of noxious stimuli? In: Clifford Rose (ed) Physiological aspects of clinical neurology. Blackwell, Oxford, pp 265–278

Millender LH, Nalebuff EA 1973 Arthrodesis of the rheumatoid wrist. An evaluation of sixty patients and a description of a different surgical technique. Journal of Bone and Joint Surgery 55A: 1026–1034

Miller CW 1978 Survival and ambulation following hip fracture. Journal of Bone and Joint Surgery 60A: 930–934

Montane I, McCollough NC, Lian EC-Y 1986 Synovectomy of the knee for hemophilic arthropathy. Journal of Bone and Joint Surgery 68A: 210–216

Mubarak SJ, Owen CA 1977 Double incision fasciotomy of the leg for decompression of compartment syndromes. Journal of Bone and Joint Surgery 59A: 184–187

Neugebauer V, Schaible HG 1990 Evidence for a central component in the sensitization of spinal neurons with joint input during development of acute arthritis in cat's knee. Journal of Neurophysiology 64: 299–311

Neugebauer V, Schaible HG, Schmidt RF 1989 Sensitization of articular afferents to mechanical stimuli by bradykinin. Pflügers Archiv 415: 330–335

O'Connor BL, Gonzales J 1979 Mechanoreceptors of the medial collateral ligament of the cat knee joint. Journal of Anatomy 129: 719–729

O'Connor BL, McConnaughey JS 1978 The structure and innervation of the cat knee menisci and their relation to a 'sensory hypothesis' of meniscal function. American Journal of Anatomy 153: 431–442

O'Connor RL 1973 The arthroscope in the management of crystal-induced synovitis of the knee. Journal of Bone and Joint Surgery 55A: 1443–1449

O'Connor RL, Shahriaree H 1984 Arthroscopic technique and normal anatomy of the knee. In: Shahriaree H, O'Connor RL (eds) O'Connor's textbook of arthroscopic surgery. Lippincott, Philadelphia

Palmer I 1958 Pathophysiology of the medial ligament of the knee joint. Acta Chirurgica Scandinavica 115: 312–318

Petty W, Goldsmith S 1980 Resection arthroplasty following infected total hip arthoplasty. Journal of Bone and Joint Surgery 62A: 889–896

Piotrowski W, Foreman JC 1986 Some effects of calcitonin gene-related peptide in human skin and on histamine release. British Journal of Dermatology 114: 37–46

Said SI, Mutt V 1970 Polypeptide with broad biological activity isolation from small intestine. Science 169: 1217–1218

Salvati EA, Huo MH, Buly RL 1991 Cemented total hip replacement: long-term results and future outlook. In: Tullos HS (ed) Instructional course lectures, vol 40. AAOS, pp 121–134

Schaible HG, Schmidt RF 1985 Effects of an experimental arthritis on the sensory properties of fine articular afferent nerves. Journal of Physiology 54: 1109–1122

Schaible HG, Schmidt RF, Willis WD 1987 Spinal mechanisms in arthritis pain. In: Schaible HG, Schmidt RF, Vahle-Hinz C (eds) Fine afferent nerve fibers and pain. VCH, Weinheim, pp 399–409

Schoenecker PL, Meade WC, Pierron RL, Sheridan JJ, Capelli AM 1985 Blount's disease. A retrospective review and recommendations for treatment. Journal of Pediatric Orthopedics 5: 181–186

Sherman MS, McFarland G 1965 Mechanism of pain in osteoid osteomas. Southern Medical Journal 58: 163

Skofitsch G, Jacobowitz DM 1985 Calcitonin gene-related peptide co-exists with substance P in capsaicin sensitive neurons and sensory ganglia of the rat. Peptides 6: 747–754

Smith GM, Egbert LD, Markowitz RA, Mosteller F, Beecher HK 1966 An experimental pain method sensitive to morphine in man. The submaximal effort tourniquet technique. Journal of Pharmacology and Experimental Therapeutics 154: 324–332

Smith-Peterson MN, Cave EF, Vangorder GW 1931 Intracapsular fractures of the femoral neck—treatment by internal fixation. Archives of Surgery 23: 715–759

Smith-Peterson MN, Aufranc OE, Larson CB 1943 Useful surgical procedures for rheumatoid arthritis involving joints of the upper extremity. Archives of Surgery 46: 764–770

Steindler A 1918 Orthopaedic operations on the hand. Journal of the American Medical Association 71: 1288–1291
Steindler A 1921 Operative methods and end-results of disabilities of the shoulder and arm. Journal of Orthopaedic Surgery 3: 652–658
Sternbach RA, Murphy RW, Zimmermans G, Greenhoot JH, Akeson WH 1974 Measuring the severity of clinical pain. In: Bonica JJ (ed) Advances in neurology, vol 4. Raven Press, New York
Volpicelli LJ, Chambers RB, Wagner FW 1983 Ambulation levels of bilateral lower extremity amputees. Journal of Bone and Joint Surgery 65A: 599–604
Wagner FW Jr 1986 Amputations of the foot. In: Chapman MW (ed) Operative orthopaedics. Lippincott, Philadelphia, pp 1777–1797
Watson HK, Hempton RF 1980 Limited wrist arthrodeses I: the triscaphoid joint. Journal of Hand Surgery 5: 320–327
Weinstein JN 1986 Mechanisms of spinal pain. The dorsal root ganglion and its role as a mediator of low-back pain. Spine 11: 999–1001
Weinstein JN, Claverie J, Gibson S 1988a The pain of discography. Spine 13: 1444–1448
Weinstein JN, Pope M, Schmidt R, Serroussi R 1988b Neuropharmacological effects of vibration on the dorsal root ganglion. An animal model. Spine 13: 521–525
Wilkinson MC 1969 Tuberculosis of the hip and knee treated by chemotherapy, synovectomy, and debridement. Journal of Bone and Joint Surgery 51A: 1343–1359
Winquist RA, Hanson ST 1978 Segmental fractures of the femur treated by closed intramedullary nailing. Journal of Bone and Joint Surgery 60A: 934–993
Wroblewski BM 1986 15–21 year results of the Charnley low-friction arthroplasty. Clinical Orthopaedics and Related Research 211: 30–35
Wyke B 1972 Articular neurology—a review. Physiotherapy 58: 94–99
Wyke B 1981 The neurology of joints. A review of general principles. Clinics in Rheumatology 7: 233–239
Yaksh TL 1988 Substance P release from knee joint afferent terminals: modulation by opioids. Brain Research 458: 319–324

Chapter 29

Central neurosurgery

Jan M Gybels and Ron R Tasker

Introduction

In this chapter we will address the various surgical procedures performed on the spinal cord and brain for the relief of chronic pain, citing available outcome data. With few exceptions these will not have been obtained using the placebo-controlled approach; we will be forced to make do with what data we have in defining the overall usefulness of each procedure.

Procedures on the spinal cord

Cordotomy

Indications

Percutaneous cordotomy should be considered for the relief of pain dependent upon transmission of signals from below the level of the intervention such as that caused by cancer, particularly through invasion of the lumbosacral plexus by cervical and colorectal disease. In cancer patients midline truncal pain responds less well than limb pain (Meyerson et al 1984), for which low midline 'commissurotomy' may be preferred (Nauta et al 1997).

The myth that cordotomy is more effective for 'malignant' than 'benign' pain probably arises from the fact that 'benign pain' is often neuropathic in origin where the commonest type is steady burning pain, which in our opinion responds poorly to pain tract interruption (Tasker and Dostrovsky 1989). Because spinothalamic fibres decussate over several dermatomes before entering the spinothalamic tract the highest level of persistently attainable analgesia with percutaneous cordotomy at the C1, C2 level is about C5.

Neuropathic pain may have at least three components (Tasker et al 1980, 1992; Tasker and Dostrovsky 1989): a steady, often dysaesthetic causalgic, a neuralgic, and an evoked element, the latter including allodynia and hyperpathia. Our experience suggests that only the latter two components respond to cordotomy (Tasker 1987, Tasker and De Carvalho 1990, Tasker et al 1992). Possibly the neuralgic element depends upon ectopic impulse generation at a lesion site in the nervous system discharging into the spinothalamic tract while allodynia and hyperpathia result from garbled programming in the dorsal horn (Woolf 1992), leading to transmission in the spinothalamic tract.

Indications for percutaneous cordotomy in the author's series (Tasker 1995) were cancer of the cervix (22%), cancer of the rectum (16%), cancer of the colon (10%), cancer of the lung (7%), cancer of the breast (4%), cancer at other sites (29%), central pain caused by cord lesions (7%), and other non-cancerous disorders (5%).

The target of cordotomy

Noordenbos and Wall (1976) concluded that the effective cordotomy divided spinothalamic, spinotectal, spinoreticular, and dorsal and ventral spinocerebellar pathways, leading to degeneration in nucleus ventralis posterior lateralis, parafascicularis, centralis lateralis, and cuneiformis, as well as in periaqueductal grey and lower brainstem reticular nuclei. Lahuerta et al (1990, 1994) carefully documented the sensory deficits incurred by successful cordotomy implicating both Aδ and C fibres although the modalities involved in the sensory loss were rather variable. They concluded that the effective lesion need only encompass the anterolateral funiculus between the level of the dentate ligament and a line drawn perpendicularly from the medial angle of the ventral grey matter or the dorsal horn to the surface of the cord destroying 20% of the hemicord. Such lesions do not necessarily abolish the flexion reflex in response to pain (Garcià-Larrea et al 1993), which appears to depend on descending reticulospinal pathways. Di Piero et al (1991) using PET scanning demonstrated that the reduced blood flow in hemithalamus contralateral to cancer pain was restored by successful cordotomy.

Results

Published data suggest 63–77% complete, 68–96% significant pain relief after unilateral percutaneous cordotomy (Tasker 1982a, 1988, 1993, 1995). Rosomoff et al (1990) found complete pain relief in 90% of patients immediately after surgery, 84% at 3 months, 61% at 1 year, 43% between 1 and 5 years, and 37% between 5 and 10 years, clearly documenting pain recurrence with time. In our own experience with 244 percutaneous cordotomies, nearly all done in patients with cancer, significant pain relief occurred in 94.4% immediately postoperatively, 82.3% at latest follow-up (1–3 months). In eight patients with neuropathic pain caused by spinal cord injury and one with cerebral palsy, pain recurred after 1, 1.2, 4, 4, 5, 6, 7, 13, and 21 years respectively. Repetition of cordotomy in six patients after 4, 4, 5, 6, 7, and 21 years respectively restored the level of analgesia in all, but pain relief in only three.

Complications

The chief complications of unilateral cordotomy (Tasker 1982a, 1988, 1993, 1995) are death (nearly always from respiratory complications) (0–5%), significant reversible respiratory complications (up to 10%), significant persistent paresis or ataxia (up to 10%), significant worsening of control of micturition (up to 15%), and significant post-cordotomy dysaesthesia (less than 10%). Respiratory complications can be avoided by attention to the factors mentioned under 'Indications'. Paresis and ataxia can be minimized by careful attention to physiological monitoring of the lesion site. However, postcordotomy dysaesthesia cannot be anticipated or avoided, being an example of idiosyncratic central pain caused by an iatrogenic spinal cord lesion. The pathways for control of micturition lie adjacent to the spinothalamic tract where they are vulnerable to damage with a correctly placed cordotomy lesion. However, if the pathway on the opposite side of the cord to that on which the cordotomy is being done is intact and micturition is not grossly defective to start with, damage to the pathway by unilateral cordotomy usually does not worsen bladder control.

'Mirror pain' (Nathan 1956; Bowsher 1988; Nagaro et al 1987, 1993a, b; Ischia and Ischia 1988) is a curious complication of cordotomy seen in about 40% of the author's patients and reported in 9–63.3% of patients in series in the literature (Tasker 1982a, 1988, 1993, 1995). Essentially, the patient develops new pain or aggravation of pre-existing but minor pain in much the same location somatotopographically as that of the pain for which the cordotomy was done but on the other side of the body. This may be associated with allochria, the induction of mirror image pain by application of, say, pinch below the level of the analgesia induced by the cordotomy. These phenomena are thought to be the result of opening up, after the cordotomy, of previously inactive synapses since they may appear immediately postoperatively and are abolished by epidural blockade below the level of the analgesia (Nagaro et al 1993a).

Bilateral cordotomy

When bilateral procedures must be considered, it is best to separate them by at least 1 week. It must be remembered that if the expected rate of significant pain relief with unilateral cordotomy is, say, 80%, that after bilateral surgery is 80% × 80% or 64%. Moreover, it the first cordotomy has produced high levels of analgesia into the cervical dermatomes, then a second procedure must not do so for fear of death from respiratory insufficiency. Although it is unusual to have micturitional complications from unilateral cordotomy, they are very likely after the bilateral procedure (20% of patients, Tasker 1993, 1995).

Some authors have however minimized the risks of the bilateral operation. Amano et al (1991) have suggested that the bilateral operation is not only more effective than the unilateral for pain relief but also carries little added risk, although Sanders and Zuurmond (1995), in a recent review, found the bilateral procedure exposed the patient to too great a risk for them to recommend it. Eighty percent of 44 patients undergoing unilateral and 50% of 18 bilateral surgery for cancer had 'satisfactory' results. Urinary retention occurred in 6.5% of the unilateral, 11.1% of the bilateral group, hemiparesis in 8.1 and 11.1% respectively, and mirror pain in 6.5 and 5.6% respectively. There were no respiratory complications.

CT-guided percutaneous cordotomy

Izumi et al (1992) and particularly Kanpolat et al (1993, 1995) have pioneered the use of CT guidance for cordotomy: Kanpolat et al (1995) report 97% complete pain control in a series of 67 patients with cancer, operated on between 1987 and 1995. In 45 cases analgesia was tailored so as to affect only the painful portion of the body. Complications may be reduced using CT guidance for they reported only one case of transient hemiparesis and one of ataxia in a series of 54 procedures.

Lesions of the dorsal root entry zone

Introduction

Capitalizing on the anatomical segregation of pain-conducting fibres from other somatosensory fibres in the dorsal root entry zone (DREZ) area into Lissauer's tract (Hyndman 1942, Denny-Brown et al 1973), Hyndman advocated sectioning of Lissauer's tract during open cordotomy to raise the level of the analgesia. In more recent times Sindou demonstrated convergence of the fine group III and IV afferents in the ventrolateral part of the DREZ (Sindou 1972, Sindou et al 1974b) and developed a microsurgical procedure in which the pain-related, small myelinated, and unmyelinated afferent fibres and the median pain-activating part of Lissauer's tract were severed with a blade for relief of chronic pain in the dermatomes related to the section (Sindou et al 1974a, 1976, 1986, 1991, Sindou and Groutelle 1983, Sindou and Daher 1988, Sindou and Jeanmonod 1989, Sindou 1995). At the same time, Nashold and Ostdahl (1979) and Nashold et al (1976) developed a related procedure in which multiple radiofrequency lesions were made under direct vision in the DREZ.

Sindou's procedure appears to have been used initially to treat nociceptive pain, having the advantage of inducing analgesia in the cervical as well as lower dermatomes without risk to the respiratory fibres in the reticulospinal tract while Nashold's procedure was directed towards the control of neuropathic pain syndromes, possibly stimulated by the notion that it destroyed bursting cells in the dorsal horn (Loeser et al 1968), which Albe-Fessard and Lombard (1983) had demonstrated in the laboratory to be related to denervation and which were candidate generators of neuropathic pain. Although we are unaware of any comparative study of the two procedures, they appear similar except for the method of lesion making. The Nashold DREZ operation appears to have been much more widely adopted, particularly for controlling the pain associated with brachial plexus avulsion. Unlike cordotomy, the DREZ procedure continues to occupy an important role in current neurosurgery.

Indications

Sindou and his colleagues (Sindou and Goutelle 1983, Sindou and Daher 1988, Sindou and Jeanmonod 1989, Sindou 1995, Emery et al 1997) used his procedure to treat the pain of cancer, pain and spasticity in patients with central nervous lesions and neuropathic pain. The Nashold procedure (Nashold et al 1976, 1990; Bronec and Nashold 1990; Sampson et al 1995; Roth et al 1997) was advocated for a variety of neuropathic syndromes such as the pain of brachial plexus avulsion, the rarely encountered lumbosacral plexus avulsion, postherpetic neuralgia, pain associated with amputations, and central pain of the spinal cord origin. The efficacy in postherpetic neuralgia now appears questionable, while for patients with cord central pain, the operation appears most effective in 'end-zone pain' according to the Nashold group.

Results

The Sindou procedure Sindou (1995) reports 83% good results with the DREZ procedure in cancer pain. Whereas in neuropathic pain allodynia was relieved in 88.2%, spontaneous steady pain responded less well unless it was lancinating. Jeanmonod and Sindou (1991) found muscle tone and stretch reflexes were reduced at sites somatotopographically related to the lesion and their operation produced analgesia or severe hypalgesia, moderate hypaesthesia, but only slight diminution of proprioception and cutaneous spatial discrimination in affected dermatomes. Their lesioning was guided by electrodiagnostic studies.

In a series of 20 patients undergoing electrophysiologically guided procedures (Jeanmonod and Sindou 1991), 3 patients developed minimal and 2 reversible lower limb weakness, and 1 urinary retention. In a review of 220 patients with pain (139 neuropathic, 81 cancerous), operated on over 20 years, Sindou (1995) found that the best results occurred in well-localized cancer pain, brachial plexus avulsion, pain caused by injury to the cauda equina and cord, peripheral nerve injury, amputation-related pain, and herpes zoster, especially when the pain was neuralgic, allodynic, or hyperpathic.

Emery et al (1997), using the Sindou technique, reported that 79% of their 37 patients enjoyed over 75% pain relief, while 22% had 50–75% relief. In the patients followed longer term (1–10 years), 70% still reported over 50% pain relief, with 13% under 50% pain relief.

The Nashold procedure

Brachial plexus avulsion An extensive literature attests to the importance of the operation in the treatment of pain of brachial plexus avulsion (Friedman et al 1988, 1996; Nashold and El-Naggar 1992; Roth et al 1997) and the much rarer lumbosacral avulsions (Moossy et al 1987), making it one of the few destructive procedures still in regular use for the relief of chronic pain. According to Gybels and Sweet (1989), Nashold operated on 39 cases of pain from brachial plexus avulsion with 54% good and 13% fair results, a result that improved to 82% good as further technical refinements were introduced. Thomas and Jones (1984) reported 59% of patients with 75–100% pain relief; 12% of patients suffered new neurological deficits. Gybels and Sweet (1989) summarized the results of 98 other DREZ operations for pain from brachial plexus avulsion from the literature, with 67% giving more than 70% of pain relief.

Friedman et al (1996) noted a variation in published results from 29–100% pain relief in a total of 341 cases. In their own series, there were 59% good, 12% fair results; 40% suffered increased neurological deficit postoperatively including 25% with sensory changes and 27% clumsiness, fatigue, or hyperreflexia in the ipsilateral lower limb. Roth et al (1997) reported 68% good or fair results in 22 patients over a mean 52-month follow-up. In their whole series of 63 patients, which included patients with other than brachial plexus avulsion, there were three deaths from pulmonary embolism and myocardial infarction, a 9% incidence of permanent ataxia, and 14% of minor neurological deficits; 22% of procedures had to be repeated.

Pain from spinal cord lesions The DREZ procedure has also been used extensively to treat cord central pain (Nashold 1991, Nashold and El-Naggar 1992, Sampson et al 1995, Friedman et al 1996, Roth et al 1997), but is effective only for certain elements of cord central pain, which seem similar to those responding to cordotomy (discussed above) and cordectomy (reviewed below).

Sampson et al (1995) reviewed 39 patients with a mean 3-year follow-up, 12 suffering from steady burning pain, 12 from electrical intermittent pain, 7 from both types. In 16 patients pain was diffuse below the level, and in 23 it was present only in a hyperaesthetic end zone just above their level. Fifty-four percent of these patients enjoyed a good result, 20% fair. Patients with incomplete lesions and end-zone and electrical pain and those injured by blunt trauma did best. Friedman and Bullitt (1988) found, in a review of 31 cases, that end-zone pain, whether it was burning or neuralgic in nature, was relieved in 80% of cases, diffuse pain in 32%; 3 patients suffered new weakness postoperatively. Wiegand and Winkelmüller (1985) reported that 45% of 20 patients gained 100% pain relief and 5% had 80% relief with 1 patient developing additional paresis. Friedman et al (1996) reported pain relief in 54% of patients with cord central pain, relief being most readily achieved when the pain extended into dermatomes immediately caudal to the injury (described as root, radicular, or end-zone pain), rather than into remotely distal dermatomes when it tended to be diffuse and burning. Roth et al (1997) reported 52% good or fair pain relief in 23 patients with cord central pain over a mean 53-month follow-up, noting that diffuse distal pain was poorly relieved.

Postherpetic neuralgia The DREZ operation was used initially for the relief of postherpetic neuralgia (Friedman and Bullitt 1988, Gybels and Sweet 1989, Friedman et all 1996, Roth et al 1997) but results have been disappointing. Gybels and Sweet's review (1989) of the Duke experience (32 patients) records 90% early pain relief, 50% after 6 months, and eventual recurrence in 66%. Only 25% of patients enjoy excellent extended relief. Ten of those with recurrent pain postoperatively developed pain different from that present preoperatively and 69% developed significant gait disturbance. Roth et al (1997) reported 20% of 10 patients with post-herpetic neuralgia relieved. Friedman et al (1996) noted 24% relief with gradual recurrence.

Amputation-related pain The usefulness of the DREZ operation in amputation-related pain appears restricted to amputations carried out after brachial or lumbosacral plexus avulsion (Nashold et al 1976; Saris et al 1985, 1988a, b; Sindou 1995). Saris et al (1988a), reviewing 22 Duke patients, found results better in phantom pain than in stump or combined stump/phantom pain. Six out of nine of their cases of phantom pain enjoyed good pain relief but five of these six had had their amputations because of brachial plexus avulsion. Stump pain was not relieved in any of their nine cases and results were poor (two out of seven relieved) in combinations of stump and phantom pain together. Miscellaneous authors quoted by Gybels and Sweet (1989) contributed 17 cases with amputation-related pain, 25% of whom enjoyed total relief, 12% more than 50% relief. Saris et al (1988b) found 14% of patients with amputation-related pain did well if the amputation was unrelated to brachial plexus avulsion.

Miscellaneous neuropathic pain The Nashold DREZ procedure has little success in conditions other than plexus avulsion and cord injury (Saris et al 1988b, Gybels and Sweet 1989, Roth et al 1997).

Complications Fazl et al (1995), in a literature review, found a 0–60% (mean 38%) reported complication rate after the Nashold DREZ procedure. In the series of patients with cord central pain described by Nashold's group (Nashold and Ostdahl 1979), 10% suffered from permanent weakness, 8% bladder or sexual dysfunction, and 3% paraesthesiae.

Commissural myelotomy, stereotactic C_1, central myelotomy and limited (punctate) midline myelotomy

The first commissural myelotomy (Armour 1927) intended to cut the decussation of the spinothalamic tract. A series of surgical variations subsequently evolved (see Gybels and Tasker 1999). It is difficult to estimate the real success of these interventions but in eight articles reporting on 175 cases of complete commissural myelotomy, early complete relief of pain was achieved in an average of 92% of the cases, but with time the outcome decays. In the cases where follow-up was longer (up to 11 years), 59% of 63 patients with malignant tumours and 48% of 21 patients with other than malignant causes had a 'good' outcome at the latest follow-up.

Summary of destructive procedures in the spinal cord for the relief of chronic pain

Percutaneous cordotomy is one of the most effective surgical procedures for the relief of nociceptive pain, and still ought to be employed, as the DREZ operation still is, in properly selected patients. Unfortunately, many pain patients are indiscriminately treated with morphine infusions, some of whom would be more effectively managed by percutaneous cordotomy (Sweet et al 1994). The DREZ procedure is admirably effective in patients with pain from brachial plexus avulsion and neuralgic or end-zone pain associated with lesions of the conus and cauda equina. It is one of the great recent contributions to pain surgery. The extent to which both commissural and central myelotomy should be utilized at present is unclear (Gybels 1997).

Operations on the brain

Introduction

After the introduction of cordotomy, it seemed logical to extend the principle of pain tract interruption cephalad, first by open means (section of the medullary and mesencephalic spinothalamic tracts and of the trigeminal thalamic pathways). With the advent of stereotactic techniques (Spiegel and Wycis 1949), it became possible to perform the same procedures more precisely with less impact on the patient, and to address a greater range of targets than had been possible by open means. An unexplained bonus in the case of mesencephalic tractotomy was the unexplained lower incidence of neuropathic pain after the stereotactic procedure than had been seen when the operation was done by open means.

Indications

Gybels and Nuttin (1995) sent 215 questionnaires to the members of the European Society for Stereotactic and Functional Neurosurgery in 1994, 54 of which were completed. For cancer pain, 63 supraspinal destructive lesions were done in 1993, 51 for neuropathic pain, compared with 836 spinal procedures. Overall, they concluded that 'for the time being there are only very few indications for destructive neurosurgery at supraspinal levels for the relief of pain'.

However, the field of stereotactic surgery is constantly evolving. Just as stereotactic lesion making replaced open surgery, the use of radiosurgery has the potential to make lesion making non-invasive once functional imaging becomes sufficiently accurate. Although many functional procedures have already been done with the gamma-knife (Leksell et al 1972, Steiner et al 1980,

Young et al 1995) there is still concern that physiological corroboration is necessary for optimal results requiring invasive studies.

The indications for destructive surgery on the brain for pain relief are pain syndromes caused by cancer that cannot be managed by more peripheral procedures (Gybels 1991, Hassenbusch 1995) and central pain syndromes caused by spinal cord injury and stroke that are usually refractory to simpler measures, as well as difficult neuropathic pains such as phantom and stump pain, postherpetic neuralgia, and anaesthesia dolorosa. Like more peripheral surgery these central procedures are more useful for the relief of nociceptive pain caused by cancer and the allodynia, hyperpathia, and neuralgic elements of neuropathic syndromes, while the diffuse, steady, burning dysaesthetic pain of neuropathic syndromes responds better to chronic stimulation that induces paraesthesia in the area of pain. In four patients (Parrent et al 1992) periventricular grey stimulation, which is thought to act by blocking entry of nociceptive impulses into the spinothalamic tract, also suppressed allodynia and hyperpathia in stroke-induced pain while Nashold and Wilson (1966) have documented the relief of intermittent lancinating bouts of neuropathic pain caused by stroke by mesencephalic lesions. Bendok and Levy (1998) found that paraesthesiae-producing DBS was more effective for the relief of neuropathic pain of unspecified type, steady, diffuse pain being commonest, while DBS in periventricular or periaqueductal grey was more effective for relieving nociceptive pain.

Lesions in the brainstem and diencephalon

Multiple lesions of descending cephalic pain tract and nucleus caudalis DREZ lesions

Nashold (Bernard et al 1987) performed the first nucleus caudalis DREZ in 1982 by making a row of lesions in the axis of the spinal grey column and Lissauer's tract extending from the uppermost C2 dorsal root up to or slightly above the level of the obex. The lesions are of course distant from the entry zones of the roots V, VII, IX, and X and referring to them as DREZ lesions perhaps obscures the difference between them and the truly DREZ lesions in the spinal cord. The Duke experience, with 46 nucleus caudalis DREZ coagulations performed during the preceding 5 years with a mean follow-up of 32 months, was reviewed retrospectively (Gorecki et al 1995). It turned out that: fewer than half of the patients who underwent nucleus caudalis DREZ coagulation indicated that they had obtained enough benefits to do it again. A similar number described improved quality of life. Complications affect nearly half of the patients.

Bulbar and pontine spinothalamic tractotomy

Only a limited number of open bulbar spinothalamic tractotomies have been reported (White and Sweet 1969). Cassinari and Pagni (1969) collected about 60 cases in the literature, mostly cancer cases with a short life expectancy, and commented that it was rare for central pain to occur after bulbar spinothalamic tractotomy possibly because the surgical incision interrupts the spinoreticular fibres, which run intermingled with the spinothalamic fibres before the spinoreticular fibres reach the nucleus gigantocellularis of Olszewski in the bulbar reticular formation.

Stereotactic mesencephalic tractotomy and thalamotomy

Most published experience about destructive brain operations relates to mesencephalic tractotomy and medial thalamotomy. Frank et al (1987) compared the two procedures for the relief of cancer pain. In their hands, mesencephalotomy achieved 83.5% relief at the expense of a 1.8% mortality and a 10.1% complication rate, while medial thalamotomy yielded 57.9% pain relief, with a tendency towards pain recurrence, with no mortality and a lower morbidity mainly in the form of transient cognitive problems.

Mesencephalic tractotomy Published outcome data for mesencephalic tractotomy report 80–85% relief of nociceptive (mostly cancer) pain compared with 27–36% of neuropathic pain at the expense of a 5–10% mortality and a 15–20% incidence of dysaesthesiae and oculomotor deficits. A report by Amano et al (1992) underlines the safety of the procedure in their hands, as does the report of Frank et al (1987) and Frank and Fabrizi (1997) listing 40 cases operated on between 1990 and 1996, 6 bilaterally, in whom only five incidences of Parinaud's syndrome and two of mild dysaesthesia occurred.

In contrast to our poorer results and those of others in the treatment of neuropathic pain, Amano et al (1986) found 64% good long-term results in 28 patients with this type of pain while Shieff and Nashold (1987) were successful in relieving 67% of 27 patients with stroke-induced pain with an 8% mortality. We do not have descriptions of the types of pain syndromes involved in these patients and the explanation for the discrepancy is unclear. We must await further evidence supporting this encouraging experience in a most refractory condition.

Medial thalamotomy Medial thalamotomy presumably interrupts pain transmission in the non-specific spinoreticulothalamic tract and would therefore be expected to relieve nociceptive pain, particularly that caused by cancer, but not the diffuse, steady, burning dysaesthetic element of neuropathic pain. There is a 46% incidence of useful relief of nociceptive pain compared with 29% of neuropathic pain.

Against these older sobering data, Jeanmonod et al (1993, 1994) have recently reported that 67% of patients in two series of 45 and 69 individuals, respectively, suffering from neuropathic pain enjoyed 50–100% relief after lesioning of the centrolateral nucleus, apparently attributing success to destruction of bursting cells, which are seen as possible pain generators (Jeanmonod et al 1994, 1996; Rinaldi et al 1991). Discussion with Jeanmonod suggests that the types of neuropathic pain relieved in his experience are similar to those in our experience, particularly neuralgic-like and evoked pain. However, we have been unable to find any correlation between bursting cells and pain.

Gamma-knife medial thalamotomy Young et al (1995) report 24 gamma-knife thalamotomies for intractable pain, 15 of whom have been followed for an average of 12 months; 27% were virtually pain free at follow-up and 33% enjoyed more than 50% relief. In another publication (Young et al 1994) concerning 10 patients, 4 of whom suffered from pain caused by spinal disorders, 2 from postherpetic neuralgia, 1 spinal cord injury, 1 with 'thalamic syndrome', 1 with facial anaesthesia dolorosa, and 1 with brainstem infarction, 3 enjoyed excellent and 4 good pain relief without complications. Particularly careful evaluations of radio thalamotomy will be necessary in order to compare efficacy and safety with that of conventional techniques in view of the current inadequacies of imaging studies.

Basal thalamotomy The tactile relay of the thalamus in the ventrocaudal nucleus, readily identified physiologically, which also relays nociceptive information, is no longer lesioned in attempts to relieve pain because of the associated high complication rate (Tasker et al 1987, Lenz et al 1988). However, lesions in the posteroinferior rim region (Tasker 1976) produce contralateral dissociated sensory loss and may be effective for the relief of chronic pain (Hitchcock and Teixeira 1981, Tasker et al 1982). Although the results of basal thalamotomy are encouraging, numbers of patients treated are small so that conclusions concerning the usefulness of this procedure are difficult to make.

Pulvinarotomy

The pulvinar is an enigmatic nucleus whose involvement in pain perception is unclear. Willis (1985) does not include it in his monograph reviewing the pathophysiology of pain. Limited reported experience (Tasker 1982b, Gybels and Sweet 1989, Yoshii et al 1990, Whittle and Jenkinson 1995) suggests that pulvinarotomy is more effective for the relief of cancer than of neuropathic pain and that the pain relief tends to be short-lived. Autopsy studies (Tasker 1982b) suggest that the supranucleus of the pulvinar is the preferable target choice. A personal literature review suggests 81% of patients with cancer pain enjoyed short-term relief whereas only 22% of those with neuropathic pain did so.

Hypothalamotomy

Spiegel et al (1954) suggested that the hypothalamus plays a role in pain processing. The hypothalamic target is located 2–5 mm lateral to the third ventricle wall in the triangle defined by the mid-point of the anterior commissure–posterior commissure line, mamillary body, and posterior commissure where stimulation causes elevation of the blood pressure and pulse rate, dilatation of pupils, and possibly neck tilting and EEG desynchronization (Sano 1977, 1979).

Fairman (1976) reported relief of pain in 76% of 54 patients with cancer following hypothalamotomy with only 10% transient complications. Sano (1977) operated on 20 patients. None of the seven with neuropathic pain did well, but 9 of the 13 with cancer pain (69%) did so. Other published experience is similar (Sano 1979, Moser et al 1980, Tasker 1982b, Mayanagi and Sano 1988, Levin 1993). A personal literature review suggests a two-thirds chance of relief of cancer pain but a tendency for postoperative pain recurrence. Sano's target was thought to be the projection site of δ fibres, and subsequent studies have confirmed a spinohypothalamic pain pathway.

Pituitary ablation

Hypophyseal ablation has long been used in the treatment of hormone-dependent cancer and the pain that accompanies it. The introduction of alcohol into the pituitary gland (Moricca 1976) has greatly simplified the procedure and reduced its impact on sick patients. A cannula is introduced through one nasal passage across the sphenoid sinus and through the anterior wall or floor of the sella turcica until it is confirmed radiologically to lie in the hypophysis. The procedure can also be done stereotactically (Levin 1988). Increments of 0.1 ml of absolute alcohol to a total of 2.0 ml are injected at one or multiple sites while neurological responses are monitored. Not only is the pain of hormone-dependent cancer relieved (41–95% short-term) but also that of non-hormone-dependent cancer (69%). Pain tends to recur after 3–4 months and complications include mortality (2–6.5%), CSF rhinorrhoea (3–20%), meningitis (0.3–1%), visual and oculomotor deficits (2–10%), and diabetes insipidus (5–60%). Levin (1888) found a 75–94% incidence of relief of cancer pain in a literature review while in his own 100 patients, 73–97% were relieved depending on the type of cancer treated. Pain tended to recur and even in those patients enjoying relief, pain exacerbations occurred frequently postoperatively. There was only one incidence of CSF rhinorrhea in his series, and six of oculomotor palsies with or without visual field defects. Various studies have failed to reveal a mechanism of pain relief from the procedure.

Lesions in the telencephalon

Pre- and postcentral gyrectomy

White and Sweet summarized results of postcentral gyrectomy up to 1969 in their classical treatise on pain. Of 30 early successes in 38 cases from 23 centres, only 7 persisted with pain relief at 10 or more months. Since that time, only few cases have been reported and with this limited evidence pre- and postcentral gyrectomy must be considered as experimental neurosurgery. However, stimulation of the motor cortex for pain control is actually a subject of intense clinical and experimental research (Garcia–Larrea et al 1999).

Limbic surgery

In this section, the emphasis will be placed on cingulotomy because long-term follow-up and quantitative outcome data are available and the procedure is actually being used. In the 23 years ending September 1987, Ballantine et al (1987) carried out their bilateral cingulotomy in 139 patients for the treatment of chronic pain.

Severe persistent, disabling pain refractory to all commonly accepted treatments was the primary indication for the operation, with the presence of clinical depression as a factor also favouring its choice. Of the 95 patients with non-malignant pain followed for 1–21 years and an average of 7 years after operation, the pain in 61 was related to the 'failed low back syndrome'. Complete or marked pain relief was sustained in 26% and moderate relief continued in another 36% of this difficult group.

Judging from postoperative MRI scans (Ballantine et al 1995) the bilateral lesions were situated in the cingulum in front of area 24. This is of interest in view of recent functional imaging studies with PET or MRI showing multiple regions of the human cerebral cortex being activated by noxious stimuli and in persistent pain (Talbot et al 1991). In one such study (Rainville et al 1997), in order to differentiate cortical areas involved in pain affect, hypnotic suggestions were used to alter selectively the unpleasantness of noxious stimuli, which showed changes in the perceived intensity. PET revealed significant changes in pain-evoked activity within the anterior cingulate cortex, consistent with the encoding of perceived unpleasantness, whereas primary somatosensory cortex activation was unaltered. These findings provide direct experimental evidence linking frontal lobe limbic activity with pain affect, as was strongly suggested by the careful clinical studies. In another PET study, Hsieh et al (1995) showed that the posterior section of the right anterior cingulate cortex (ACC), corresponding to Brodmann area 24, was activated in ungoing neuropathic pain, and this regardless of the side of the painful mononeuropathy; the experiments confirmed that the ACC participates in the sensorial/affectional aspect of the pain experience but there was also a strong suggestion, and this is the new exciting finding, that there is a possible right hemispheric lateralization of the ACC for affective processing in chronic ungoing neuropathic pain.

As far as we are aware of, limbic surgery for persistent pain must be performed at a very limited scale. If a parallel can be drawn between results of stereotactic lesions in the limbic system for psychiatric disorders and persistent pain, there is a good argument to explore stimulation of the same areas instead of making lesions since it has recently been shown that acute stimulation of the crus anterior of the capsula interna can induce relevant beneficial effects in obsessive-compulsive disorder, suggesting that long-term stimulation may be useful in the management of treatment-resistant forms of this disease (Nuttin et al 1999).

Conclusion

The formulation of the gate control theory (Melzack and Wall 1965), together with the possibility of selectively activating pain-inhibitory pathways with electrical current or blocking transmission pathways by intrathecal drug administration without destruction of nervous tissue, have had a profound impact on the neurosurgical treatment of pain. The effects of these procedures are reversible and unwanted side effects can be avoided. Furthermore, test treatment and placebo control are often possible and reliable hardware is available. Major goals remain to be pursued, such as the search for more rigorous selection criteria and the reporting of results in a way that is accepted by the scientific community at large. Boivie (Chap. 20) and Simpson (1999) have reviewed and evaluated the growing field of spinal cord and brain stimulation.

References

Albe-Fessard D, Lombard MC 1983 Use of an animal model to evaluate the origin of and protection against deafferentation pain. In: Bonica JJ et al (eds) Advances in pain research and therapy, vol 5. Raven, New York, pp 691–700

Amano K, Kawamura H, Tanikawa T, Kawabatake H, Nolan M, Iseki H, Shiwaku T, Nagao T, Iwata Y, Taira T, Umezawa Y, Simizu T, Kitamura K 1986 Long-term follow-up study of rostral mesencephalic reticulotomy and pain relief—report of 34 cases. Applied Neurophysiology 49: 105–111

Amano K, Kawamura H, Tanikawa T et al 1991 Bilateral versus unilateral percutaneous high cervical cordotomy as a surgical method of pain relief. Acta Neurochirurgica (Wien) 52 (suppl): 143–145

Amano K, Kawamura H, Tanikawa T, Kawabatake H, Iseki H, Taira T 1992 Stereotactic mesencephalotomy for pain relief. A plea for stereotactic surgery. Stereotactic and Functional Neurosurgery 59: 25–32

Armour D 1927 Surgery of the spinal cord and its membranes. Lancet 1: 691–697

Ballantine HT, Bouckoms AJ, Thomas EK et al 1987 Treatment of psychiatric illness by stereotactic cingulotomy. Biological Psychiatry 22: 807–819

Ballantine HT, Cosgrove R, Giriunas I 1995 Surgical treatment of intractable psychiatric illness and chronic pain by stereotactic cingulotomy. In: Schmidek H, Sweet W (eds) Operative neurosurgical techniques: indications, methods and results, 3rd edn. Saunders, Philadelphia, pp 1423–1430

Bendok B, Levy RM 1998 Brain stimulation for persistent pain management. In: Gildenberg PL, Tasker RR (eds) Textbook of stereotactic and functional neurosurgery. McGraw–Hill, New York, pp 1539–1546

Bernard EJ, Nashold BS, Caputi F et al 1987 Nucleus caudalis DREZ lesions for facial plain. British Journal of Neurosurgery 1: 81–92

Bowsher D 1988 Contralateral mirror-image pain following anterolateral cordotomy. Pain 33: 63–65

Bronec PR, Nashold BS Jr 1990 Dorsal root entry zone lesions for pain. In: Youmans JR (ed) Neurological surgery. A comprehensive reference guide to the diagnosis and management of neurosurgical problems. Saunders, Philadelphia, pp 4036–4044

Cassinari V, Pagni CA 1969 Central pain: a neurosurgical survey. Harvard University Press, Cambridge

Denny-Brown D, Kirk EJ, Yanagisawa N 1973 The tract of Lissauer in relation to sensory transmission in the dorsal horn of spinal cord in the macaque monkey. Journal of Comparative Neurology 151: 175–200

Di Piero V, Jones AKP, Iannotti et al 1991 Chronic pain: a PET study of the central effects of percutaneous high cervical cordotomy. Pain 46: 9–12

Emery E, Blondet E, Mertens P, Sindou M 1997 Microsurgical DREZ-otomy for chronic pain due to brachial plexus avulsion: long-term results in a series of 37 patients. In: Abstracts of oral presentations at the XII meeting of the World Society for Stereotactic and Functional Neurosurgery, Lyon, July 1–4

Fairman D 1976 Neurophysiological bases for the hypothalamic lesion and stimulation by chronic implanted electrodes for the relief of intractable pain in cancer. In: Bonica JJ, Albe-Fessard D (eds) Advances in pain research and therapy, vol 1. Raven Press, New York, pp 843–847

Fazl M, Houlden DA, Kiss Z 1995 Spinal cord mapping with evoked responses for accurate localization of the dorsal root entry zone. Journal of Neurosurgery 82: 587–591

Frank F, Fabrizi AP 1997 Stereotactic mesencephalic tractotomy for cancer pain. In: Abstracts of oral presentations XII meeting of the World Society for Stereotactic and Functional Neurosurgery, Lyon, July 1–4

Frank F, Fabrizi AP, Gaist G, Weigel K, Mundinger F 1987 Stereotactic lesions in the treatment of chronic cancer pain syndromes: mesencephalotomy or multiple thalamotomies. Applied Neurophysiology 50: 314–318

Friedman AH, Bullitt E 1988 Dorsal root entry zone lesions in the treatment of pain following brachial plexus avulsion, spinal cord injury, and herpes zoster. Applied Neurophysiology 51: 164–169

Friedman AH, Nashold BS Jr 1986 DREZ lesions for relief of pain related to spinal cord injury. Journal of Neurosurgery 65: 465–469

Friedman AH, Nashold BS Jr, Bronec PR 1988 Dorsal root entry zone lesions for the treatment of brachial plexus avulsion injuries: a follow-up study. Neurosurgery 22: 369–373

Friedman AH, Nashold JRB, Nashold BS Jr 1996 DREZ lesions for treatment of pain. In: North RB, Levy RM (eds) Neurosurgical management of pain. Springer-Verlag, New York, pp 176–190

García-Larrea L, Charles N, Sindou M, Mauguière F 1993 Flexion reflexes following anterolateral cordotomy in man: dissociation between pain sensation and nociceptive reflex RIII. Pain 55: 139–149

García-Larrea L, Peyron R, Mertens P, Grégoire R, Lavenne F, Le Bars D, Convers P, Maugiere F, Sindou M, Laurent B 1999 Electrical stimulation of motor cortex for pain control: a combined PET scan and electrophysiological study. Pain 83: 259–273

Gorecki JP, Nashold BS Jr, Rubin L, Ovelmen-Levitt J 1995 The Duke experience with nucleus caudalis DREZ coagulation. Proceedings of the Meeting of the American Society for Stereotactic and Functional Neurosurgery 65: 111–116

Gybels JM 1991 Indications for the use of neurosurgical techniques in pain control. In: Bond, MR, Charlton JE, Woolf, J (eds) Proceedings of the sixth world congress on pain. Elsevier, Amsterdam, pp 475–482

Gybels J 1997 Commissural myelotomy revisited. Pain 70: 1–2

Gybels J, Nuttin B 1995 Are there still indications for destructive neurosurgery at supra-spinal levels for the relief of painful syndromes? In: Besson JM, Guilbaud G, Ollat H (eds) Forebrain areas involved in pain processing. John Libbey Eurotext, Paris, pp 253–259

Gybels JM, Sweet WH 1989 Neurosurgical treatment of persistent pain. Physiological and pathological mechanisms of human pain. In: Gildenberg PG (ed) Pain and headache, vol. II. Karger, Basel, pp 141–145

Gybels JM, Tasker RR 1999 Central neurosurgery. In: Wall PD, Melzack R (eds) Textbook of pain, 4th edn. Churchill Livingstone, Edinburgh, pp 1307–1339

Hassenbusch SJ 1995 Surgical management of cancer pain. Neurosurgery Clinics of North America 6(1): 127–134

Hitchcock ER, Teixeira MJA 1981 A comparison of results from center-median and basal thalamotomies for pain. Surgical Neurology 15: 341–351

Hsieh JC, Belfrage M, Stone-Elander S et al 1995 Central representation of chronic ongoing neuropathic pain studied by positron emission tomography. Pain 63: 225–236

Hyndman OR 1942 Lissauer's tract section. A contribution to chordotomy for the relief of pain (preliminary report). Journal of the International College of Surgeons 5: 314–400

Ischia S, Ischia A 1988 A mechanism of new pain following cordotomy (Letter). Pain 32: 383–384

Izumi J, Hirose Y, Yazaki T 1992 Percutaneous trigeminal rhizotomy and percutaneous cordotomy under general anesthesia. Stereotactic and Functional Neurosurgery 59: 62–68

Jeanmonod D, Sindou M 1991 Somatosensory function following dorsal root entry zone lesions in patients with neurogenic pain or spasticity. Journal of Neurosurgery 74(6): 916–932

Jeanmonod D, Sindou M, Magnin M, Baudet M 1989 Intraoperative unit recordings in the human dorsal horn with a simplified floating microelectrode. EEG Clinical Neurophysiology 72: 450–454

Jeanmonod D, Magnin M, Morel A 1993 Thalamus and neurogenic pain: physiological, anatomical and clinical data. Neuroreport 4(5): 475–478

Jeanmonod D, Magnin M, Morel A 1994 Chronic neurogenic pain and the medial thalamotomy. Schweizerische Rundschau fur Medizin Praxis 83(23): 702–707

Jeanmonod D, Magnin M, Morel A 1996 Low-threshold calcium spike bursts in the human thalamus. Common physiopathology for sensory, motor and limbic positive symptoms. Brain 119: 363–375

Kanpolat Y, Akyar S, Caglar S, Unlu A, Bilgic S 1993 CT-guided percutaneous selective cordotomy. Acta Neurochirurgica 123: 92–96

Kanpolat Y, Caglar S, Akyar S, Temiz C 1995 CT-guided pain procedures for intractable pain in malignancy. Acta Neurochirurgica 64 (suppl): 88–91

Lahuerta J, Bowsher D, Lipton S 1990 Clinical and instrumental evaluation of sensory function before and after percutaneous anterolateral cordotomy at cervical level in man. Pain 42: 23–30

Lahuerta J, Bowsher D, Lipton S, Buxton PH 1994 Percutaneous cervical cordotomy: a review of 181 operations on 146 patients with a study in the location of 'pain fibers' in the C2 spinal cord segment of 29 cases. Journal of Neurosurgery 80: 975–985

Leksell L, Meyerson BA, Forster DMC 1972 Radiosurgical thalamotomy for intractable pain. Confinia Neurologica 34: 264 (abstract)

Lenz FA, Dostrovsky JO, Kwan HC, Tasker RR, Yamashiro K, Murphy JT 1988 Methods for microstimulation and recording of single neurons and evoked potentials in the human central nervous system. Journal of Neurosurgery 68: 630–634

Levin AB 1988 Stereotactic chemical hypophysectomy. In: Lunsford LD (ed) Modern stereotactic neurosurgery. Nijhoff, Boston, pp 365–375

Levin AB 1993 Hypophysectomy in the treatment of cancer pain. In: Arbit E (ed) Management of cancer-related pain. Futura, Mt Kisko, NY, pp 281–295

Loeser JD, Ward AA Jr, White LE Jr 1968 Chronic deafferentation of human spinal cord neurons. Journal of Neurosurgery 29: 48–50

Mayanagi Y, Sano K 1988 Posteromedial hypothalamotomy for behavioural disturbances and intractable pain. In: Lunsford LD (ed) Modern stereotactic neurosurgery. Nijhoff, Boston, pp 377–388

Melzack R, Wall PD 1965 Pain mechanisms: a new theory. Science 150: 971–979

Meyerson BA, Arnér S, Linderoth B 1984 Pelvic cancer pain (somatogenic pain): pros and cons of different approaches to the management of pelvic cancer pain. Acta Neurochirurgica (Wien) 33 (suppl): 407–419

Moossy JJ, Nashold BS Jr, Osborne D et al 1987 Conus medullaris nerve root avulsions. Journal of Neurosurgery 66: 835–841

Moricca G 1976 Neuroadenolysis for diffuse unbearable cancer pain. In: Bonica JJ, Albe-Fessard D (eds) Advances in pain research and therapy, vol. 1. Raven, New York, pp 863–866

Moser RP, Yap JC, Fraley EE 1980 Stereotactic hypophysectomy for intractable pain secondary to metastatic prostate carcinoma. Applied Neurophysiology 43: 145–149

Nagaro T, Kumura S, Arai T 1987 A mechanism of new pain following cordotomy: reference of sensation. Pain 30: 89–91

Nagaro T, Amakawa K, Arai T, Ohi G 1993a Ipsilateral referral of pain following cordotomy. Pain 55: 275–276

Nagaro T, Amakawa K, Kimura S et al 1993b Reference of pain following percutaneous cervical cordotomy. Pain 53: 205–211

Nashold BS Jr 1991 Paraplegia and pain. In: Nashold BS Jr, Ovelmen-Levitt J (eds) Deafferentation pain syndromes: pathophysiology and treatment. Raven, New York, pp 301–309

Nashold BS Jr, El-Naggar AO 1992 Dorsal root entry zone (DREZ) lesioning. In: Rengachary SS, Wilkins RH (eds) Neurosurgical operative atlas. Williams & Wilkins, Baltimore, pp 9–24

Nashold BS Jr, Ostdahl RH 1979 Dorsal root entry zone lesions for pain relief. Journal of Neurosurgery 51: 59–69

Nashold BS Jr, Wilson WP 1966 Central pain. Observations in man with chronic implanted electrodes in the midbrain tegmentum. Confinia Neurologica 27: 30–44

Nashold BS Jr, Urban B, Zorub DS 1976 Phantom pain relief by focal destruction of the substantia gelatinosa of Rolando. In: Bonica JJ, Albe-Fessard D (eds) Advances in pain research and therapy, vol 1. Raven, New York, pp 959–963

Nashold BS Jr, Vieira J, El-Naggar AC 1990 Pain and spinal cysts in paraplegia: treatment by drainage and DREZ operation. British Journal of Neurosurgery 4: 327–336

Nathan PW 1956 Reference of sensation at the spinal level. Journal of Neurology, Neurosurgery and Psychiatry 19: 88–100

Nauta HJW, Hewitt E, Westlund KN, Willis WD 1997 Surgical interruption of a midline dorsal column visceral pathway. Journal of Neurosurgery 86: 538–542

Noordenbos W, Wall PD 1976 Diverse sensory functions with an almost totally divided spinal cord: a case of spinal cord transection with preservation of one anterolateral quadrant. Pain 2: 185–195

Nuttin B, Cosyns P, Demeulemeester H, Gybels J, Meyerson B 1999 Electrical stimulation in anterior limbs of internal capsules in patients with obsessive-compulsive disorder. Lancet 354: 1526

Parrent A, Lozano A, Tasker RR, Dostrovsky J 1992 Periventricular gray stimulation suppresses allodynia and hyperpathia in man. Stereotactic and Functional Neurosurgery 59: 82

Rainville P, Duncan GH, Price DD et al 1997 Pain affect encoded in human anterior singulate but not somatosensory cortex. Science 277: 968–971

Rinaldi PC, Young RF, Albe-Fessard D, Chodakiewitz J 1991 Spontaneous neuronal hyperactivity in the medial intralaminar thalamic nuclei of patients with deafferentation pain. Journal of Neurosurgery 74: 415–521

Rosomoff HL, Papo I, Loeser JD 1990 Neurosurgical operations on the spinal cord. In: Bonica JJ (ed) The management of pain, 2nd edn. Lea & Febiger, Philadelphia, pp 2067–2081

Roth SA, Seitz K, Soliman N, Rahamba JF, Antoniadis G, Richter H-P 1997 DREZ coagulation for deafferentation pain related to spinal and peripheral nerve lesions: indications and results of 72 consecutive procedures. In: Abstracts of oral presentations XII meeting of the World Society for Stereotactic and Functional Neurosurgery, Lyon, July 1–4

Sampson JH, Chasman RE, Nashold BS, Friedman AH 1995 Dorsal root entry zone lesions for intractable pain after trauma to the conus medularis and cauda equina. Journal of Neurosurgery 82: 28–34
Sanders M, Zuurmond W 1995 Safety of unilateral and bilateral percutaneous cervical cordotomy in 80 terminally ill cancer patients. Journal of Clinical Oncology 13(6): 1509–1512
Sano K 1977 Intralaminar thalamotomy (thalamolaminotomy) and posterior hypothalamotomy in the treatment of intractable pain. In: Krayenbühl H, Maspes PE, Sweet WH (eds) Progress in neurological surgery, vol. 8. Karger, Basel, pp 50–103
Sano K 1979 Stereotaxic thalamolaminotomy and posteromedial hypothalamotomy for the relief of intractable pain. In: Bonica JJ, Ventrafridda V (eds) Advances in pain research and therapy, vol. 2. Raven Press, New York, pp 475–485
Saris SC, Iacono RP, Nashold BS 1985 Dorsal root entry zone lesions for post-amputation pain. Journal of Neurosurgery 62: 72–76
Saris SC, Iacono RP, Nashold BS Jr 1988a Successful treatment of phantom pain with dorsal root entry zone coagulation. Applied Neurophysiology 51: 188–197
Saris SC, Vieira JFS, Nashold BS Jr 1988b Dorsal root entry zone coagulation for intractable sciatica. Applied Neurophysiology 51: 206–211
Shieff C, Nashold BS 1987 Stereotactic mesencephalotomy for thalamic pain. Neurological Research 9: 101–104
Simpson BA 1999 Spinal cord and brain stimulation. In: Wall PD, Melzack R (eds) Textbook of pain. Churchill Livingstone, Edinburgh, pp 1353–1381
Sindou M 1972 Study of the dorsal root–spinal cord junction. A target for pain surgery. These Doctorat Médecine, Lyon
Sindou M 1995 Microsurgical DREZotomy (MDT) for pain, spasticity, and hyperactive bladder: a 20-year experience. Acta Neurochirurgica 137(1–2): 1–5
Sindou M, Daher A 1988 Spinal cord ablation procedures for pain. In: Dubner R, Gebhart GF, Bond MR (eds) Proceedings of the fifth world congress on pain. Pain research and clinical management, vol. 3. Elsevier, Amsterdam, pp 477–495
Sindou M, Goutelle A 1983 Surgical posterior rhizotomies for the treatment of pain. In: Krayenbühl H (ed) Advances and technical standards in neurosurgery, vol. 10. Springer-Verlag, New York, pp 147–185
Sindou M, Jeanmonod D 1989 Microsurgical DREZ-otomy for the treatment of spasticity and pain in the lower limbs. Neurosurgery 24: 655–670
Sindou M, Fischer G, Goutelle A et al 1974a La radicellotomie postérieure sélective: premiers résultats dans la chirurgie de la douleur. Neurochirurgie 20: 391–408
Sindou M, Quoex C, Baleydier C 1974b Fiber organization at the posterior spinal cord–rootlet junction in man. Journal of Comparative Neurology 153: 15–26
Sindou M, Fischer G, Mansuy L 1976 Posterior spinal rhizotomy and selective posterior rhizidiotomy. In: Krayenbühl H, Maspes PE, Sweet WH (eds) Progress in neurological surgery, vol. 7. Karger, Basel, pp 201–250
Sindou M, Mifsud JJ, Boisson D et al 1986 Selective posterior rhizotomy in the dorsal root entry zone for treatment of hyperspasticity and pain in the hemiplegic upper limb. Neurosurgery 18: 587–595
Sindou M, Jeanmonod D, Mertens P 1991 Surgery in the dorsal root entry zone: microsurgical drez-otomy (MDT) for treatment of spasticity. In: Sindou M, Abbott R, Keravel Y (eds) Neurosurgery for spasticity. Springer-Verlag, New York, pp 165–182
Spiegel EA, Wycis HT 1949 Pallidothalamotomy in chorea. Presented at Philadelphia Neurological Society, April 22
Spiegel EA, Kletzkin M, Szekely EG, Wycis HT 1954 Role of hypothalamic mechanisms in thalamic pain. Neurology 4: 739–751
Steiner L, Forster D, Leksell L, Meyerson BA, Boethius J 1980 Gammathalamotomy in intractable pain. Acta Neurochirurgica 52: 173–184
Sweet WH, Poletti CE, Gybels JM 1994 Operations in the brainstem and spinal canal, with an appendix on the relationship of open to percutaneous cordotomy. In: Wall PD, Melzack R (eds) Textbook of pain, 3rd edn. Churchill Livingstone, Edinburgh, pp 1113–1135
Talbot JD, Marrett S, Evans AC, Meyer E, Bushnell C, Duncan GH 1991 Multiple representations of pain in human cerebral cortex. Science 251: 1355–1358
Tasker RR 1976 The human spinothalamic tract. Stimulation mapping in spinal cord and brainstem. In: Bonica JJ, Albe-Fessard D (eds) Advances in pain research and therapy, vol. 1. Raven, New York, pp 251–257
Tasker RR 1982a Percutaneous cordotomy: the lateral high cervical technique. In: Schmidek HH, Sweet WH (eds) Operative neurosurgical techniques: indications, methods and results. Grune & Stratton, New York, pp 1137–1153
Tasker RR 1982b Pain. Thalamic procedures. In: Schaltenbrand G, Walker AE (eds) Textbook of stereotaxy of the human brain. Thieme, Stuttgart, pp 484–497
Tasker RR 1987 The problem of deafferentation pain in the management of the patient with cancer. Journal of Palliative Care 2: 8–12
Tasker RR 1988 Percutaneous cordotomy: the lateral high cervical technique. In: Schmidek HH, Sweet WH (eds) Operative neurosurgical techniques: indications, methods and results, 2nd edn. Grune & Stratton, Orlando, pp 1191–1205
Tasker RR 1993 Ablative central nervous system lesions for control of cancer pain. In: Arbit E (ed) Management of cancer-related pain. Futura, Mt. Kisko, NY, pp 231–255
Tasker RR 1995 Percutaneous cordotomy. In: Schmidek HH, Sweet WH (eds) Operative neurosurgical techniques: indications, methods, and results, 3rd edn. Saunders, Philadelphia, pp 1595–1611
Tasker RR, De Carvalho GTC 1990 Pain in thalamic stroke. In: Pain and ethical and social issues in stroke rehabilitation. Inter-urban Stroke Academic Association, July, pp 1–25
Tasker RR, Dostrovsky JO 1989 Deafferentation and central pain. In: Wall PD, Melzack R (eds) Textbook of pain, 2nd edn. Churchill Livingstone, Edinburgh, pp 154–180
Tasker RR, Dostrovsky JO 1992 Computers in functional stereotactic surgery. In: Kelly PJ, Kall BA (eds) Computers in stereotactic neurosurgery: contemporary issues in neurological surgery. Blackwell, Boston, pp 155–164
Tasker RR, Organ LW, Hawrylyshyn PE 1980 Deafferentation and causalgia. In: Bonica JJ (ed) Pain research publications, Association for Research in Nervous and Mental Diseases, vol. 58. Raven Press, New York, pp 305–329
Tasker RR, Organ LW, Hawrylyshyn PE 1982 The thalamus and midbrain of man. A physiological atlas using electrical stimulation. Thomas, Springfield, IL
Tasker RR, Lenz F, Yamashiro K, Gorecki J, Hirayma T, Dostrovsky JO 1987 Microelectrode techniques in localization of stereotactic targets. Neurosurgical Research 9(2): 105–112
Tasker RR, de Carvalho GTC, Dolan EJ 1992 Intractable pain of spinal cord origin: clinical features and implications for surgery. Journal of Neurosurgery 77: 373–378
Thomas DGT, Jones SJ 1984 Dorsal root entry zone lesions (Nashold's procedure) in brachial plexus avulsion. Neurosurgery 15: 966–968
White JC, Sweet WH 1969 Pain and the neurosurgeon. A forty-year experience. Thomas, Springfield, IL
Whittle IR, Jenkinson JT 1995 CT-guided stereotactic antero-medial pulvinotomy and centromedian-parafascicular thalamotomy for intractable malignant plain. British Journal of Neurosurgery 9(2): 195–200

Wiegand H, Winkelmüller W 1985 Behandlung des Deafferentierumgsschmerzes durch Hochfrequenzläsion der Hunterwurzel-Eintrittszone. Deutsche Medizinische Wochenschrift 110: 216–220

Willis WD 1985 The pain system: the neural bases of nociceptive transmission in the mammalian nervous system. In: Gildenberg PL (ed) Pain and headache, vol. 8. Karger, Basel

Woolf CJ 1992 Excitability changes in central neurons following peripheral damage: Role of central sensitization in the pathogenesis of pain. In: Willis W (ed) Hyperalgesia and allodynia. Raven, New York, pp 221–243

Yoshii N, Mizokami T, Usikubo Y, Samejima H, Adachi K 1990 Postmortem study of stereotactic pulvinarotomy for relief of intractable pain. Stereotactic and Functional Neurosurgery 54, 55: 103

Young RF, Jacques DS, Rand RW, Copcutt BR 1994 Medial thalamotomy with the Leksell Gamma Knife for treatment of chronic pain. Acta Neurochirurgica 62 (suppl): 105–110

Young RF, Jacques DS, Rand RW, Copcutt BC, Vermeulen SS, Posewitz AE 1995 Technique of stereotactic medial thalamotomy with the Leksell Gamma Knife for treatment of chronic pain. Neurological Research 17(1): 59–65

Chapter 30

Transcutaneous electrical nerve stimulation

Per Hansson and Thomas Lundeberg

Introduction

The introduction of the gate control theory concept in 1965 (Melzack and Wall 1965) has facilitated the global proliferation of different afferent stimulation techniques for pain alleviation, such as transcutaneous electrical nerve stimulation and vibration. The quality of the scientific documentation of transcutaneous electrical nerve stimulation (TENS) as a pain-relieving measure does not, however, correspond to its widespread and uncritical application in a multitude of painful conditions by different health care providers. This chapter highlights part of the scientific literature on the pain-alleviating effect of TENS in a number of acute and chronic painful conditions and briefly addresses technical issues and tentative mechanisms of action. Important methodological considerations for the critical evaluation of existing studies or the performance of future studies on the pain-relieving potential of TENS are suggested.

Transcutaneous electrical nerve stimulation

Numerous physiological studies since the late 1950s (Kolmodin and Skoglund 1960, Wall 1964, Woolf and Wall 1982, Chung et al 1984, Garrison and Foreman 1996) support the notion that activity in large-diameter afferents may alter transmission in central pathways conveying messages ultimately experienced as pain. Such interaction may take place in the dorsal horn (Garrison and Foreman 1996) and in the thalamus (Olausson et al 1994). Although challenged in some of its original aspects (Schmidt 1972, Nathan and Rudge 1974), the gate control theory concept (Melzack and Wall 1965) has facilitated the global proliferation of different afferent stimulation techniques for pain alleviation, such as transcutaneous electrical nerve stimulation. TENS is by far the most extensively used biomedical technique in this area and was embraced early on by health professionals despite a severely limited scientific documentation. Thirty years after the appearance of the first report in the field (Wall and Sweet 1967), the number of randomized controlled clinical trials in well-diagnosed patients is still conspicuously low. Despite the continuous shortage of high-quality studies, the method has gained footing as a technique for pain alleviation in a variety of conditions, possibly as a result of an uncritical and insatiable need for therapeutic measures. The continuing survival of TENS for pain relief may also in part be explained by the fact that experienced clinicians have witnessed its efficacy in subgroups of patients and that the technique has been favourably presented in previous reviews by clinical authorities (Meyerson 1983, Long 1991).

The starting point of the launching of TENS for clinical pain relief was a study by Wall and Sweet (1967) of a small group of patients with 'chronic cutaneous pain', reporting pain relief after acute exposure to TENS or percutaneous electrical stimulation. Initially, TENS was mainly used to screen for patients suitable for spinal cord stimulation. The predictive value of TENS effects for the outcome of spinal cord stimulation has, however, never been documented, and clinical experience certainly does not point to any clear relationship between the two methods in terms of efficacy.

The strength of conclusions that may be drawn regarding the clinical efficacy of TENS for pain alleviation critically depends on the quality of the evidence contained in the scientific literature. Lack of proper randomization and blinding in TENS studies have been demonstrated to heavily influence study results, with overoptimistic efficacy outcome (Carroll et al 1996). Due to the nature of the method, realistic placebo and blinding are inherent problems in TENS trials, both notoriously difficult to solve adequately. The survey presented in the following, based on a selection of available data from the literature, does not claim to be complete but rather has focused on some clinically important aspects of TENS and conditions where TENS has been applied.

Technical and practical aspects

Commercial TENS machines offer at least three different pulse patterns: high frequency (HF, usually 50–120 Hz), low frequency (LF, 1–4 Hz), and bursts of high frequency delivered at low frequency (2 Hz), i.e., acupuncture-like (AKU) TENS. In addition, pulse width and stimulus amplitude can be controlled. Some stimulators also offer adjustable pulse configuration. Leads are used to connect the machine with electrodes that are usually made of carbon rubber. No compelling evidence to support increased therapeutic efficacy as a result of refining the electrical parameters of TENS machines has been presented. Further, no recommendation can be provided on the choice of stimulus parameters in different painful conditions.

In general, HF stimulation in the centre of the pain area is recommended as the first choice of stimulation, with an intensity just below the pain threshold so that paraesthesias are felt in the painful region. It is mandatory to start the TENS trial by examining tactile sensibility in the area to be stimulated to ensure a substrate for stimulation. A pronounced loss of large-fibre function offsets the use of TENS within the denervated area. If HF stimulation fails or is inconvenient, e.g., due to aggravation of pain in an area of tactile allodynia, LF or AKU TENS may be tried in an anatomically related area with normal sensibility. It is a general conception among TENS advocates that to increase the efficacy of LF and AKU TENS the stimulation should be intense enough to produce visible muscle contractions. Scientific evidence to support this notion is lacking. Regardless of the mode of TENS, a duration of stimulation of at least 30–45 min is recommended. In optimal situations a TENS trial may relieve ongoing and/or stimulus-evoked pain for several hours after termination of stimulation. Patients who report pain alleviation during stimulation only, with no post-stimulatory effect, will sometimes still volunteer to have a machine prescribed if other pain-relieving measures have proven ineffective for their pain. Frequent initial follow-ups are crucial to reinstruct the patients if necessary and to carefully extract the possible benefits of stimulation. Importantly, a fraction of patients with different pain diagnoses report increased pain intensity during TENS. For further details on technical and practical aspects, the reader is referred to handbooks on TENS.

Acute nociceptive/inflammatory pain

Different painful conditions have been screened and some of the better explored areas are presented in the following.

Orofacial pain

From randomized and placebo-controlled trials in patients with different acute painful dental conditions, including pulpitis, apical periodontitis, and postoperative intraoral pain, there is evidence that HF and AKU TENS have a pain-relieving potential during single-trial exposure (Hansson and Ekblom 1983). The effect of extrasegmental TENS, including AKU TENS, on the HoKu point (between the thumb and index finger) was comparable to the effect of placebo TENS applied within the painful area (Ekblom and Hansson 1985). These findings therefore suggest that TENS is more effective when applied within the painful area and also point to the potential of TENS in the treatment of pain from deep somatic tissue. A study aiming to use HF or

AKU TENS to provide surgical analgesia for intraoral operative procedures such as endodontic surgery, tooth extraction, or abscess incision demonstrated their failure in all included patients (Hansson and Ekblom 1984). This finding parallels the clinical impression that phasic intense pain is rarely diminished by TENS treatment.

Postoperative pain

Short-term effects of TENS have been monitored after a variety of operative procedures. Outcome measures have included visual analogue scale ratings of spontaneous pain intensity and stimulus-evoked pain, time to request for analgesics, total medication intake, tolerance to physical therapy, expiratory peak flow rate, arterial blood gas determinations, and duration of stay in the recovery room. Positive results for several outcome measures have been reported in randomized and placebo-controlled trials, e.g., using HF TENS after thoracic (Bennedetti et al 1997) and abdominal/thoracic surgery (VanderArk and McGrath 1975). Negative outcome was demonstrated, e.g., after herniorrhaphy (Gilbert et al 1986) and appendicectomy (Conn et al 1986), both randomized and placebo-controlled studies of HF TENS. A systematic review of TENS effects in acute postoperative pain concluded that non-randomized trials usually overestimate treatment effects and that randomized controlled studies usually report a negative outcome (Carroll et al 1996).

Labour pain

Early on, non-randomized and non-placebo-controlled trials (Augustinsson et al 1977, Bundsen et al 1981) indicated a pain-relieving effect of HF TENS primarily during the first stage of labour, i.e., when the nociceptive system presumably is activated by nociceptors in the contracting uterus and the dilating cervix. Later, Harrison and co-workers (1986) reported no difference between TENS (HF or AKU) and placebo TENS regarding pain relief. Another randomized, placebo-controlled clinical trial, monitoring the first stage of labour, reported TENS to be no more effective than placebo TENS (Van der Ploeg et al 1996). In that study, AKU TENS was used between uterine contractions and HF TENS during contractions. A systematic review of the efficacy of TENS for pain relief in labour found that randomized controlled trials provided no compelling evidence for TENS having any analgesic effect during labour (Carroll et al 1997). Several studies have reported TENS to be safe for the infant during delivery (Augustinsson et al 1977, Bundsen et al 1981, Van der Ploeg et al 1996).

Dysmenorrhoea

Dysmenorrhoea affects a large proportion of females and is a challenging entity from a pain relief perspective. Studies claiming a pain-relieving effect of TENS in this condition are available. A randomized, placebo-controlled study (Dawood and Ramos 1990) reported favourable effects of HF TENS compared to placebo TENS or ibuprofen. Significantly more TENS-treated patients reported substantial pain relief than patients treated with placebo TENS. The group receiving TENS also needed less rescue medication than the groups receiving placebo TENS or ibuprofen. An open, crossover study comparing high-intensity HF TENS and naproxen reported significantly reduced pain intensity from both interventions (Milsom et al 1994). Treatment with naproxen but not TENS was associated with a significant change in uterine activity. In a randomized, placebo-controlled single-trial study HF TENS was argued to be superior to LF and placebo TENS (Lundeberg et al 1985). LF TENS seemed to be no more effective than placebo TENS.

Angina pectoris

There is evidence to suggest that TENS is effective in the treatment of angina pectoris. Mannheimer and colleagues (1985) demonstrated that HF TENS favourably influenced pacing-induced angina compared to controls. Pacing was better tolerated, lactate metabolism improved, and ST segment depression was less pronounced with than without TENS. Results from the same study of a 10-week follow-up period, during which the patients were instructed to self-administer at least three 1-h HF TENS treatments a day, demonstrated increased work capacity as measured with bicycle ergometer tests, decreased ST segment depression, reduced frequency of anginal attacks, and reduced consumption of short-acting nitroglycerine per week compared with a control group not receiving TENS. Recent results indicate that at least part of the beneficial effect of TENS for pain relief in angina is secondary to decreased myocardial ischaemia (Chauhan et al 1994, Borjesson et al 1997). Chauhan and co-workers (1994) demonstrated HF TENS to significantly increase coronary blood flow velocity in patients with syndrome X and coronary artery disease but not in heart transplant patients. Borjesson et al (1997), in a randomized, placebo-controlled trial, demonstrated HF TENS treatment (30 min three times a day and during angina attacks) to be a safe additional treatment in unstable angina pectoris and to reduce the number and duration of silent ischaemic events. Interestingly, the number of painful events was unaltered, as was the number of episodes of pain leading to stimulation or consumption of analgesics.

Chronic nociceptive/inflammatory pain

This area suffers from too few systematic studies of conditions with a homogeneous aetiology. Rheumatoid arthritis is an exception. A substantial fraction of patients included in studies of other conditions suffer from painful syndromes that, from a diagnostic point of view, are ill defined, e.g., low back pain (Deyo et al 1990, Herman et al 1994), due to the lack of strict diagnostic criteria for painful conditions in certain body regions. A number of patients with pain of unknown origin/aetiology are likely to have been included in many of these studies, which seriously affects their conclusions.

Rheumatoid arthritis

Studies aiming at elucidating the efficacy of TENS for pain relief in rheumatoid arthritis have included a number of different outcome measures such as resting pain, joint tenderness, grip strength, grip pain, and loading tests. Studies lacking placebo control (Mannheimer et al 1978, Mannheimer and Carlsson 1979) reported relief from HF TENS of spontaneous pain and pain during a loading test. Abelson and colleagues (1983), in a randomized placebo-controlled study, examined the therapeutic effect of once-weekly HF TENS, lasting three weeks, in a group of patients with wrist involvement. Compared to placebo TENS, significant relief of resting pain and pain while gripping was reported. The same group later reported results from a similar study where suggestion and focused attention were added to the placebo treatment (Langley et al 1984). In this scenario HF, AKU, and placebo TENS were equally effective in producing analgesia of similar degree and trend over time. The latter study casts serious doubt on the specific efficacy of TENS in rheumatoid arthritis but at the same time also points to the complexity and power of the placebo effect. The prominent effect of placebo was also highlighted in a study on pain from temporomandibular joint involvement of rheumatoid arthritis (Moystad et al 1990). HF TENS in the painful area and LF TENS of the hand was no more effective than placebo TENS in either region.

Chronic neuropathic pain

Peripheral neuropathic pain

It seems to be a general opinion among experienced clinicians within the field of neurological pain that subgroups of patients with peripheral neuropathic pain are among the best TENS-responding groups, although the scientific documentation is weak. Numerous studies, all with some methodological drawbacks and several of them including only small groups of patients diagnosed with neuropathic pain of different aetiology, have hinted at the usefulness of different modes of TENS in different peripheral neuropathic pain conditions (Nathan and Wall 1974, Loeser et al 1975, Thorsteinsson et al 1977, Eriksson et al 1979, Bates and Nathan 1980, Johnson et al 1991a, Meyler and De Jongste 1994, Fishbain et al 1996). There are no known predictors as to which patients may benefit from TENS. In this group of patients it is especially important to survey the somatosensory status of the region to be treated. Tactile allodynia is a relative contraindication for HF TENS since the activation of myelinated mechanoreceptive fibres is painful in this subset of patients. It is our clinical impression, however, that in a subgroup of patients with neuropathic pain and allodynia to touch the method still has a potential to relieve ongoing as well as stimulus-evoked pain. Due to the pain initially induced when turning on the TENS machine, it is important that the patient is thoroughly informed before such a trial is commenced. If aggravation of pain is tolerated for up to a few minutes, there is a possibility of obtaining pain relief. Patients with tactile allodynia accompanied by autonomic reactions such as nausea, palpitation, and syncope should not be treated by TENS.

Central neuropathic pain

Only a few non-randomized, non-placebo-controlled studies that focus on central neuropathic pain exist. Leijon and Boivie (1989) studied central post-stroke pain patients and Davis and Lentini (1975) studied a subgroup of patients with central pain after spinal cord injury. Minor pain-relieving effects were reported. Still, a TENS trial may be recommended in patients with central neuropathic pain since only a few alternative pain-relieving measures exist, all with a major risk of failure.

The field of neuropathic pain and TENS would certainly benefit from randomized, controlled trials of diagnostic entities where detailed clinical examination is performed to try to unravel possible pathophysiological mechanisms underlying the painful condition. A multitude of possible mechanisms, not universally sensitive to TENS treatment, is to be expected.

Contraindications

The following issues should be considered.

- To avoid any possible influence on the uterus or fetus, TENS should not be applied over the pregnant uterus or in the proximity of that region. Other regions of the body may well be suited for TENS trials.
- Cardiac pacemakers of the on-demand type may malfunction if disturbed by electrical output from a TENS machine. This is not the case with pacemakers of fixed frequencies.
- Stimulation within the anterior/lateral part of the neck is hazardous since spasm of the intrinsic muscles of the larynx may be induced as well as activation of cells in the carotid sinus involved in blood pressure regulation, risking a fall in pressure due to reflex bradycardia. Stimulation of the vagus nerve may also contribute to the latter.

Appropriate steps should be taken to avoid complications. Mandatory for the first and second conditions is discussion of the suggested treatment with the patient's care-giving specialist.

Tentative mechanisms of action of TENS

The detailed antinociceptive mechanisms of action of TENS are still largely unknown. A number of physiological studies have contributed to the notion that afferent activity set up by TENS blocks nociceptive transmission in the spinal cord (Kolmodin and Skoglund 1960, Wall 1964, Woolf and Wall 1982, Chung et al 1984, Garrison and Foreman 1996). Pre- as well as postsynaptic inhibitory mechanisms have been implicated. As stated earlier, not only the spinal cord needs necessarily to be involved but also thalamic regions (Olausson et al 1994). The most effective block of projecting neurons of the cord is achieved by activation not only of large myelinated fibres (Aα, Aβ) but also of Aδ and C fibres (Chung et al 1984, Lee et al 1985, Sjölund 1985). In a clinical setting this implies that painful TENS would be more effective for pain alleviation, an inconceivable option from a practical standpoint.

Of interest in the context of optimal stimulation intensity is a number of experimental studies, with some conflicting results, where different TENS techniques and different pain-inducing measures have been used. Woolf (1979), in a placebo-controlled study, demonstrated the need of high-intensity (i.e., painful) HF TENS to significantly alter the heat pain threshold and the tolerance to heat. TENS at non-painful intensities failed to alter the sensitivity to heat and noxious mechanical stimuli but modified ischaemic pain after a submaximal effort tourniquet test. To explain pain-relieving effects of painful afferent stimulation, it seems appropriate also to consider the theoretical concept of DNIC (diffuse noxious inhibitory control) (LeBars et al 1979a, b, 1991). More recently, HF non-painful TENS was reported to significantly reduce subjects' ratings of painful and near-painful heat stimuli and to increase the heat pain threshold (Marchand et al 1991). The perception threshold to cold pressor-induced pain and tolerance to ice pain were demonstrated to be significantly increased by a variety of stimulation patterns using TENS (Johnson et al 1991b). Failure of LF or HF non-painful TENS in altering pain induced by the submaximal effort tourniquet test and the cold pressor test were significant findings in a study by Foster and colleagues (1996). A reasonable conclusion from these studies is that the message conveyed in the nociceptive system set up by different painful stimuli, resulting in different temporospatial patterns of ascending activity, is differentially susceptible to alteration by different modes of TENS. A differential sensitivity to different modes of TENS may well, for the same reason, be the case in clinical pain states.

A peripheral mechanism of action contributing to pain alleviation by TENS has been suggested (Ignelzi and Nyquist 1976). Based on work employing microneurographic techniques, this hypothesis seems less likely. Janko and Trontelj (1980) were unable to demonstrate impulse transmission failure in Aδ fibres during TENS.

The neurochemical events set up by TENS are largely unknown. Somewhat conflicting results have been reported from studies in healthy subjects (Chapman and Benedetti 1977, Pertovaara and Kemppainen 1981, Salar et al 1981) and in patients with different acute (Woolf et al 1978, Hansson et al 1986) and chronic (Sjölund and Eriksson 1979, Abrams et al 1981, Freeman et al 1983) painful conditions, addressing the question of whether endogenous opioids mediate at least part of the pain-relieving effect of TENS. Such studies have been performed either by injecting the non-specific opioid antagonist naloxone to try to counteract TENS-induced pain relief or by analysing endogenous opioid compounds in the cerebrospinal fluid or plasma. Importantly, naloxone in physiological doses predominantly blocks μ-receptors. The contribution of other opioid receptors needs to be studied further when specific antagonists become available. Summarizing these data, it seems that pain relief by HF TENS is not mediated by an opioid link counteracted by naloxone. The literature provides some data, however, supporting an opioid link for pain alleviation by LF TENS.

Conclusions

A number of acute and chronic painful conditions have been reported to respond favourably to TENS. A substantial fraction of reports suffer, however, from serious methodological shortcomings. Most studies provide short-term outcome/single-trial results, and long-term follow-up studies of chronic pain conditions are needed. Studies of optimal stimulation parameters, including pulse pattern characteristics, site of electrode placement, duration of stimulation, and optimal number of treatments per day, in well-diagnosed patients should be done. The inherent problem of a realistic placebo and blinding remain substantial obstacles in TENS trials. If available, a gold standard may be used for comparison, i.e., the best available measure for relief in different pain conditions. It is important to present detailed descriptions of stimulus parameters and outcome measures. Further, it is crucial to describe patient populations meticulously, not only labelling them diagnostically but also, if possible, subgrouping patient populations with regard to plausible underlying pathophysiological mechanisms of the specific condition. In neuropathic pain, it seems reasonable to include data on presence or absence of, for example, dynamic mechanical allodynia and cold allodynia. This may give clues as to susceptibility to pain alleviation by TENS in subgroups of patients with different diagnostic entities. It seems appropriate to conclude that despite being around for three decades, rigorous clinical scientific evidence to support the widespread use of TENS is still lacking.

Vibration and acupuncture

An analysis of studies of the effectiveness of these procedures by Hansson and Lundeberg (1999) has led to the following conclusions.

Vibration

Although the literature hints at a pain-relieving potential for vibration in a small number of painful conditions, the use of vibratory stimulation in clinical practice has been hampered by the lack of commercially available, convenient stimulation units. The area needs further exploration.

Acupuncture

The bulk of studies on pain relief from acupuncture suffer from methodological shortcomings. Results from randomized, controlled studies do not accord with the more enthusiastic conclusions from studies without appropriate controls.

References

Abelson K, Langley GB, Sheppeard H, Vlieg M, Wigley RD 1983 Transcutaneous electrical nerve stimulation in rheumatoid arthritis. New Zealand Medical Journal 727: 156–158

Abrams SE, Reynold AC, Cusick JF 1981 Failure of naloxone to reverse analgesia from transcutaneous electrical stimulation in patients with chronic pain. Anesthesia and Analgesia 60: 81–84

Augustinsson L-E, Bohlin P, Bundsen P et al 1977 Pain relief during delivery by transcutaneous electrical nerve stimulation. Pain 4: 59–65

Bates JA, Nathan PW 1980 Transcutaneous electrical nerve stimulation for chronic pain. Anaesthesia 8: 817–822

Bennedetti F, Amanzio M, Casadio C et al 1997 Control of postoperative pain by transcutaneous electrical nerve stimulation after thoracic operations. Annals of Thoracic Surgery 3: 773–776

Borjesson M, Eriksson P, Dellborg M, Eliasson T, Mannheimer C 1997 Transcutaneous electrical nerve stimulation in unstable angina pectoris. Coronary Artery Disease 8–9: 543–550

Bundsen P, Peterson L-E, Selstam U 1981 Pain relief in labor by transcutaneous electrical nerve stimulation. Acta Obstetrica et Gynaecologica Scandinavica 60: 459–468

Carroll D, Tramer M, McQuay H, Nye B, Moore A 1996 Randomization is important in studies with pain outcomes: systematic review of transcutaneous electrical nerve stimulation in acute postoperative pain. British Journal of Anaesthesia 6: 798–803

Carroll D, Tramer M, McQuay H, Nye B, Moore A 1997 Transcutaneous electrical nerve stimulation in labour pain: a systematic review. British Journal of Obstetrics and Gynaecology 104: 169–175

Chapman CR, Benedetti C 1977 Analgesia following transcutaneous electrical stimulation and its partial reversal by a narcotic antagonist. Life Sciences 11: 1645–1648

Chauhan A, Mullins PA, Thuraisingham SI, Taylor G, Petch MC, Schofield PM 1994 Effect of transcutaneous electrical nerve stimulation on coronary blood flow. Circulation 2: 694–702

Chung JM, Lee KH, Hori Y, Endo K, Willis WD 1984 Factors influencing peripheral nerve stimulation produced inhibition of primate spinothalamic tract cells. Pain 19: 277–293

Conn IG, Marshall AH, Yadav SN, Daly JC, Jaffer M 1986 Transcutaneous electrical nerve stimulation following appendicectomy. Annals of the Royal College of Surgeons of England 4: 191–192

Davis R, Lentini R 1975 Transcutaneous nerve stimulation for treatment of pain in patients with spinal cord injury. Surgical Neurology 1: 100–101

Dawood MY, Ramos J 1990 Transcutaneous electrical nerve stimulation (TENS) for the treatment of primary dysmenorrhea: a randomized crossover comparison with placebo TENS. Obstetrics and Gynecology 4: 656–660

Deyo RA, Walsh NE, Martin DC, Schoenfeld LS, Ramamurthy S 1990 A controlled trial of transcutaneous electrical nerve stimulation (TENS) and exercise for chronic low back pain. New England Journal of Medicine 23: 1627–1634

Ekblom A, Hansson P 1985 Extrasegmental transcutaneous electrical nerve stimulation and mechanical vibratory stimulation as compared to placebo for the relief of acute oro-facial pain. Pain 23: 223–229

Eriksson MBE, Sjölund BH, Nielzen S 1979 Long term results of peripheral conditioning stimulation as an analgesic measure in chronic pain. Pain 6: 335–347

Fishbain DA, Chabal C, Abbott A, Heine LW, Cutler R 1996 Transcutaneous electrical nerve stimulation (TENS) treatment outcome in long-term users. Clinical Journal of Pain 3: 201–214

Foster NE, Baxter F, Walsh DM, Baxter GD, Allen JM 1996 Manipulation of transcutaneous electrical nerve stimulation variables has no effect on two models of experimental pain in humans. Clinical Journal of Pain 4: 301–310

Freeman TB, Campbell JN, Long DM 1983 Naloxone does not affect pain relief induced by electrical stimulation in man. Pain 17: 189–195

Garrison DW, Foreman RD 1996 Effects of transcutaneous electrical nerve stimulation (TENS) on spontaneous and noxiously evoked dorsal horn cell activity in cats with transected spinal cords. Neuroscience Letters 216: 125–128

Gilbert JM, Gledhill T, Law N, George C 1986 Controlled trial of transcutaneous electrical nerve stimulation (TENS) for postoperative pain relief following inguinal herniorrhaphy. British Journal of Surgery 9: 749–751

Hansson P, Ekblom A 1983 Transcutaneous electrical nerve stimulation (TENS) as compared to placebo TENS for the relief of acute oro-facial pain. Pain 15: 157–165

Hansson P, Ekblom A 1984 Afferent stimulation induced pain relief in acute orofacial pain and its failure to induce sufficient pain reduction in dental and oral surgery. Pain 20: 273–278

Hansson P, Lundeberg T 1999 Transcutaneous electrical nerve stimulation, vibration and acupuncture as pain-relieving measures. In: Wall PD, Melzack R (eds) Textbook of pain, 4th edn. Churchill Livingstone, Edinburgh, pp 1341–1351

Hansson P, Ekblom A, Thomsson M, Fjellner B 1986 Influence of naloxone on relief of acute oro-facial pain by transcutaneous electrical nerve stimulation (TENS) or vibration. Pain 24: 323–329

Harrison RF, Woods T, Shore M, Mathews G, Unwin A 1986 Pain relief in labour using transcutaneous electrical nerve stimulation (TENS). A TENS/TENS placebo controlled study in two parity groups. British Journal of Obstetrics and Gynaecology 93: 739–746

Herman E, Williams R, Stratford P, Fargas-Babjak A, Trott M 1994 A randomized controlled trial of transcutaneous electrical nerve stimulation (CODETRON) to determine its benefits in a rehabilitation program for acute occupational low back pain. Spine 5: 561–568

Ignelzi RJ, Nyquist JK 1976 Direct effect of electrical stimulation on peripheral nerve evoked activity: implications in pain relief. Journal of Neurosurgery 45: 159–166

Janko M, Trontelj JV 1980 Transcutaneous electrical nerve stimulation: a microneurographic and perceptual study. Pain 9: 219–230

Johnson MI, Ashton CH, Thompson JW 1991a An in-depth study of long-term users of transcutaneous electrical nerve stimulation (TENS). Implications for clinical use of TENS. Pain 44: 221–229

Johnson MI, Ashton CH, Bousfield DR, Thompson JW 1991b Analgesic effects of different pulse patterns of transcutaneous electrical nerve stimulation on cold-induced pain in normal subjects. Journal of Psychosomatic Research 35: 313–321

Kolmodin GM, Skoglund CR 1960 Analysis of spinal interneurons activated by tactile and nociceptive stimulation. Acta Physiologica Scandinavica 50: 337–355

Langley GB, Sheppeard H, Johnson M, Wigley RD 1984 The analgesic effects of transcutaneous electrical nerve stimulation and placebo in chronic pain patients. Rheumatology International 4: 119–123

LeBars D, Dickenson AH, Besson JM 1979a Diffuse noxious inhibitory controls. II. Lack of effect on non convergent neurons, supraspinal involvement and theoretical implications. Pain 6: 305–327

LeBars D, Dickenson AH, Besson JM 1979b Diffuse noxious inhibitory controls. I. Effect on dorsal horn convergent neurons in the rat. Pain 6: 283–304

LeBars D, Villanueva L, Willer JC, Bouhassira D 1991 Diffuse noxious inhibitory controls (DNIC) in animals and in man. Acupuncture in Medicine 9: 47–56

Lee KH, Chung JM, Willis WDJ 1985 Inhibition of primate spinothalamic tract cells by TENS. Journal of Neurosurgery 62: 276–287

Leijon G, Boivie J 1989 Central post stroke pain—the effect of high and low frequency TENS. Pain 38: 187–191

Loeser JD, Black RG, Christmas A 1975 Relief of pain by transcutaneous stimulation. Journal of Neurosurgery 42: 308–314

Long DM 1991 Fifteen years of transcutaneous electrical stimulation for pain control. Stereotactic and Functional Neurosurgery 56: 2–19

Lundeberg T, Bondesson L, Lundstöm V 1985 Relief of primary dysmenorrhea by transcutaneous electrical nerve stimulation. Acta Obstetrica Gynaecologica Scandinavica 64: 491–497

Mannheimer C, Carlsson CA 1979 The analgesic effect of transcutaneous electrical nerve stimulation (TNS) in patients with rheumatoid arthritis. A comparative study of different pulse patterns. Pain 6: 329–334

Mannheimer C, Lund S, Carlsson CA 1978 The effect of transcutaneous electrical nerve stimulation (TNS) on joint pain in patients with rheumatoid arthritis. Scandinavian Journal of Rheumatology 7: 13–16

Mannheimer C, Carlsson CA, Emanuelsson H, Vedin A, Waagstein F 1985 The effects of transcutaneous electrical nerve stimulation in patients with severe angina pectoris. Circulation 2: 308–316

Marchand S, Bushnell MC, Duncan GH 1991 Modulation of heat pain perception by high frequency transcutanous electrical nerve stimulation (TENS). Clinical Journal of Pain 2: 122–129

Melzack R, Wall PD 1965 Pain mechanisms: a new theory. Science 150: 971–978

Meyerson B 1983 Electrostimulation procedures: effects, presumed rationale, and possible mechanisms. In: Bonica JJ, Lindblom U, Iggo A (eds) Advances in pain research and therapy. Raven Press, New York, pp 495–534

Meyler WJ, De Jongste MJL 1994 Clinical evaluation of pain treatment with electrostimulation: a study on TENS in patients with different pain syndromes. Clinical Journal of Pain 10: 22–27

Milsom I, Hedner N, Mannheimer C 1994 A comparative study of the effect of high-intensity transcutaneous nerve stimulation and oral naproxen on intrauterine pressure and menstrual pain. American Journal of Obstetrics and Gynecology 1: 123–129

Moystad A, Krogstad BS, Larheim TA 1990 Transcutaneous nerve stimulation in a group of patients with rheumatic disease involving the temporomandibular joint. Journal of Prosthetic Dentistry 5: 596–600

Nathan PW, Rudge P 1974 Testing the gate-control theory of pain in man. Journal of Neurology, Neurosurgery and Psychiatry 37: 1366–1372

Nathan PW, Wall PD 1974 Treatment of post-herpetic neuralgia by prolonged electric stimulation. British Medical Journal 3: 645–647
Olausson B, Xu Z Q, Shyu BC 1994 Dorsal column inhibition of nociceptive thalamic cells mediated by gamma-aminobutyric acid mechanisms in the cat. Acta Physiologica Scandinavica 152: 239–247
Pertovaara A, Kemppainen P 1981 The influence of naloxone on dental pain threshold elevation produced by peripheral conditioning stimulation at high frequency. Brain Research 215: 426–429
Salar G, Job I, Mingrino S, Bosio A, Trabucci M 1981 Effect of transcutaneous electrotherapy on CSF B-endorphin content in patients without pain problems. Pain 10: 169–172
Schmidt RF 1972 The gate control theory of pain. A critical hypothesis. In: Janzen R, Kreidel W D, Herz A, Steichele C (eds) Pain. Churchill Livingstone, London, pp 124–127
Sjölund BH 1985 Peripheral nerve stimulation suppression of C-fiber-evoked flexion reflex in rats. Part 1: parameters of continuous stimulation. Journal of Neurosurgery 63: 612–616
Sjölund BH, Eriksson MBE 1979 The influence of naloxone on analgesia by peripheral conditioning stimulation. Brain Research 173: 295–301
Thorsteinsson G, Stonnington HH, Stillwell GK, Elveback LR 1977 Transcutaneous electrical stimulation: a double-blind trial of its efficacy for pain. Archives of Physical Medicine and Rehabilitation 58: 8–13
VanderArk GD, McGrath KA 1975 Transcutaneous electrical stimulation in treatment of postoperative pain. American Journal of Surgery 130: 338–340
Van der Ploeg JM, Vervest HAM, Liem AL, Van Leeuwen JHS 1996 Transcutaneous nerve stimulation (TENS) during the first stage of labour: a randomized clinical trial. Pain 68: 75–78
Wall PD 1964 Presynaptic control of impulses at the first central synapse in the cutaneous pathway. In: Eccles JC, Schade JP (eds) Physiology of spinal neurons. Elsevier, New York, pp 92–115
Wall PD, Sweet WH 1967 Temporary abolition of pain in man. Science 155: 108–109
Woolf CJ 1979 Transcutaneous electrical nerve stimulation and the reaction to experimental pain in human subjects. Pain 7: 115–127
Woolf CJ, Wall PD 1982 Chronic peripheral nerve section diminishes the primary afferent A-fibre mediated inhibition of rat dorsal horn neurones. Brain Research 1: 77–85
Woolf CJ, Mitchell D, Myers RA, Barrett GD 1978 Failure of naloxone to reverse peripheral transcutaneous electro-analgesia in patients suffering from acute trauma. South African Medical Journal 53: 179–180

Chapter 31

Ultrasound, shortwave, microwave, laser, superficial heat and cold in the treatment of pain

Justus F Lehmann and Barbara J de Lateur

Introduction

This chapter discusses the use of common physical modalities to produce pain relief directly and indirectly. The modalities include cold application and heat in the forms of radiant heat, ultrasound, shortwave diathermy, microwave, and laser. To maximize the effectiveness of the modalities, it is important to understand how they work and when and how to use each technique properly.

Reduction of pain by relieving painful conditions

Both cold and heat are commonly used to reduce painful muscle spasms secondary to underlying skeletal or neurological pathology. For example, painful muscle spasm is associated with low back pain of various causes such as degenerative joint disease or intervertebral disc disease, with or without resultant nerve root irritation. Lehmann and de Lateur (1999) recently reviewed physiological studies on the effects of cold on muscle spasm and concluded that, to decrease muscle tone, i.e., spasticity, cooling should be applied in such a way that the muscle temperature is lowered. As a result, reflex muscle activity is diminished and the therapeutic effect on spasticity is achieved and maintained for a meaningful period of time.

Another condition that creates a great deal of discomfort to the patient is joint or 'morning' stiffness as it is encountered in collagen diseases, most commonly in rheumatoid arthritis. Wright and Johns (1960) and Bäcklund and Tiselius (1967) showed that the complaint correlated closely with physical measurements of the viscoelastic properties of the joints. Specifically they measured maximal elasticity in extension and flexion, as well as resistance to motion due to viscous properties and to friction. There was a 20% decrease in stiffness at 45°C as compared with 33°C when a superficial joint was treated with infrared radiation (Wright and Johns 1961).

A well-documented physiological response to heat application is the increase in blood flow with a corresponding decrease when cold is applied. In an active organ, local temperature elevation will lead to a marked increase in blood flow (Guy et al 1974; Lehmann et al 1979; Sekins et al 1980, 1984; Lehmann and De Lateur 1990b). Reflexly induced changes usually consist of an increase in blood flow to the skin and superficial tissues and a decrease in blood flow to an inactive organ. Thus, when heat is applied to the skin, blood flow to the underlying musculature is reduced. When the skin is heated, blood flow to the skin is increased not only in the area heated but also in other areas of the skin not heated (consensual reaction; Fischer and Solomon 1965). On the other hand, cooling produces vasoconstriction. Vasodilatation in response to cold occurs only if the temperatures are low enough to be potentially destructive to the tissues. The increase in vascularity and blood flow due to heating may play a role in obtaining relief from painful conditions.

Pain in trauma, as it is commonly encountered in sports injuries, can be alleviated and to a degree prevented by early cold application, often in combination with application of pressure, for instance via an elastic bandage. In these cases cold reduces not only pain perception but also bleeding and oedema formation as a result of vasoconstriction (Nilsson 1983, Derscheid and Brown 1985, Kay 1985). At a later date, heat application with vasodilatation may help with the healing and haematoma resolution (Schmidt et al 1979, Lehmann et al 1983, Lehmann and De Lateur 1990b).

Heat and cold applications to the skin of the abdominal wall have a profound effect on pain resulting from spasm of the smooth musculature in the gastrointestinal tract or in the uterus. This pain is commonly associated with gastrointestinal upset or menstrual cramps. It has been shown (Fischer and Solomon 1965) that there is a marked reduction of peristalsis of the gastrointestinal tract with heat application and an increase of peristalsis with cold application. This is associated with a decrease in acid production of the stomach and blanching of the mucous membrane when heat is applied to the abdominal skin. Acid production and blood flow to the mucous membrane are increased with cold application to the abdominal skin.

'Counterirritant' effects

Parsons and Goetzl (1945) showed that cold applied with ethyl chloride spray for 20 s to the skin covering the tibia increased the pain threshold of the tooth pulp as measured by electrical stimulation. Similarly, Melzack et al (1980a) reduced dental pain by ice massage applied to the web of the thumb and index finger of the hand on the same side as the painful region. Melzack et al (1980b) also showed that ice massage and transcutaneous electrical stimulation are equally effective in relieving low back pain. Murray and Weaver (1975) showed that counterirritation (consisting of 10-s immersion of the finger into a 28°C water bath) reduced itching significantly more than a control procedure. Melzack et al (1980a) suggested that the observations could be explained on the basis of the gate theory (Melzack and Wall 1965). Studies of morphine receptors in the central nervous system and of the role of enkephalins and endorphins (Field and Basbaum 1978) suggested that this mechanism could play a role in explaining the counterirritant effect, especially when the stimulus is applied distant from the site of the pain-producing process (Kerr and Casey 1976). Gammon and Starr (1941) also showed that heat producing a significant temperature elevation resulted in the same analgesic effect as cold application. The effects produced by this mechanism seem to be on the same order of magnitude as those obtained by transcutaneous electrical nerve stimulation (Melzack et al 1980b). Benson and Copp (1974) also found that heat and cold both raised the normal pain threshold significantly. Ice therapy was more effective than heat but following either form of treatment, the effect declined within 30 min.

Effects on nerve and nerve endings

Goodgold and Eberstein (1977) and De Jong et al (1966) showed that, in general, nerve conduction drops with decreasing temperature and that finally (Li 1958) nerve fibres cease conducting. It is assumed that pain sensation may be reduced by local cooling due to an indirect effect on nerve fibres and free endings. There is also evidence that heat applied to the peripheral nerve or free nerve endings reduces pain sensation (Lehmann et al 1958).

In a study by Barker et al (1991), administration of cold saline prior to injection of propofol (2,6-di-isopropylphenol) anaesthetic increased the amount of pain relief obtained as compared with propofol injection alone. Recently, it has been shown (Hong 1991) that ultrasound therapy may cause a reversible nerve conduction block and pain relief in patients with polyneuropathy.

Lasers

In laser therapy, except for surgical purposes, lower level intensities are used. Unfortunately, most studies on the use of laser for the relief of pain do not have suitable controls.

A few studies with control groups found a significant effect of laser stimulation on pain (Walker 1983, Walker et al 1988, Ceccherelli et al 1989, Johannsen et al 1994) but most found no effect on pain (Lundeberg et al 1987; Seibert et al 1987; Waylonis 1988; Haker and Lundeberg 1990, 1991a; Klein and Eck 1990; Taube et al 1990).

Differences in the effects of heat and cold application

A review of the literature reveals that the effect of heat and cold may be similar in many cases. In others, cold produces effects in the opposite direction of heat. Both heat and cold reduce muscle spasm secondary to underlying joint and skeletal pathology and nerve root irritation, as in low back syndromes, and therefore relieve the associated pain. A vicious cycle consisting of muscle spasm, ischaemia, pain, and more muscle spasm is interrupted. In the case of upper motor neuron lesions with painful spasticity, the effect of heat is short-lived because the temperature in the muscle is rapidly restored to its pretreatment level by the increase in blood flow. If the reduction in spasticity with reduction in pain relief is produced by muscle cooling, this effect lasts much longer. Rewarming from the outside is slow because of the insulating subcutaneous fat layer and rewarming from the inside is retarded because of the vasoconstriction in the muscle. However, neither heat nor cold has a permanent effect on spasticity.

In the presence of an acute deep-seated inflammatory reaction, vigorous heat application is contraindicated. It usually increases hyperaemia and oedema with pain and acceleration of abscess formation. This does not contradict the fact that such heat application is used in superficial boils to bring the abscess to a head with subsequent easy evacuation. Mild heat application is used in superficial thrombophlebitis. In contrast, in an inflammatory reaction it is generally agreed that cold may reduce oedema, hyperaemia, and pain.

In acute rheumatoid arthritis, vigorous deep heat application is likely to aggravate the pain and discomfort. On the other hand, painful joint stiffness is improved by heat and aggravated by cold application (Wright and Johns 1960, 1961; Bäcklund and Tiselius 1967). However, an intensive cooling may numb pain despite the increase in stiffness. In acute trauma with aggravation of pain resulting from oedema and bleeding, cold application will reduce both because of vasoconstriction. Heat will increase both oedema and bleeding tendency.

A review by Chapman (1991) cites several studies showing that heat and cold were each effective in relieving pain in conditions such as frozen shoulder, chronic low back pain, and rheumatoid arthritic knees and shoulders. In contrast, Finan et al (1993) studied the effect of cold therapy on postoperative pain in gynaecologic patients in a randomized prospective study and concluded that cold pack application does not improve postoperative pain.

The use of heat for pain relief

Dosimetry and technique of heat application

Local temperature elevation at the site of the pathology can produce a large number of different responses, including changes in neuromuscular activity, blood flow, capillary permeability, enzymatic activity, and pain threshold. These reactions can be produced to varying degrees depending on the condition of heating.

If the site of temperature elevation is distant from the painful pathology to be treated, only a limited number of physiological responses, reflexogenic in nature, can be obtained at the site of the pathology. These reactions are always milder than those produced locally at the site of the temperature elevation. These distant reactions include blood flow changes in skin and in the mucous membranes of the gastrointestinal tract; reflexogenic changes in muscle activity, relaxation of both voluntary striated muscle and smooth muscle of the gastrointestinal tract and uterus; and reflex reduction of gastric acidity. When vigorous responses are desired, local heat is strongly preferred. The factors that determine the intensity of the physiological reaction locally are, first, the level of tissue temperature elevation (approximately 40–45°C) and, second, the duration of tissue temperature elevation (5–30 min).

Mild versus vigorous effects

In order to obtain vigorous responses to heat therapy, it is necessary to attain the highest temperature at the site of the tissue pathology to be treated and to elevate this temperature close to the maximally tolerated level. Dosimetry and proper technique of application of the modalities are essential, since the therapeutic range for a given effect extends only over a few degrees. If a mild, limited response is desired, one can select a modality that produces the highest temperature at the site of the pathology, but then limit the output of the modality so that only a moderate temperature rise occurs; this in turn produces a mild effect. The alternative to this procedure is to heat the superficial tissues and rely on mild limited reflexogenic responses at the site of the pathology in the depth of the tissues.

Selection of modality according to temperature distribution

If vigorous heating is indicated, one must select that type of heating modality that produces the highest temperature in the distribution at the site of the treatable pathology. Since the temperature at this site is brought to tolerance level, this method avoids burns elsewhere. This represents the rationale for the various deep-heating devices: shortwave diathermy, a high-frequency electromagnetic current operating at the frequency of 27.12 MHz; microwaves, an electromagnetic radiation at the frequency of 2456 and 915 MHz; and ultrasound, a high-frequency acoustic vibration at a frequency of 0.8–1.0 MHz. The approach to using these modalities primarily as deep-heating agents is justified in the light of overwhelming experimental evidence that most of the therapeutically desirable effects are due to heating and not due to non-thermal reactions (Lehmann and De Lateur 1982, 1990a, b; Kramer 1985).

The superficial heating agents such as hot packs, paraffin bath, Fluidotherapy, hydrotherapy, and radiant heat produce temperature distributions similar to one another, with the highest temperature in the most superficial tissues. Some of these modalities have non-thermal effects of therapeutic advantage; for instance, hydrotherapy allows exercise of painful joints with reduced stress because the buoyancy of the water reduces the gravitational forces. Also, the cleansing action of a whirlpool bath can be beneficial in wound treatments and the drying action of radiant heat may be desirable in weeping lesions.

In order to select the appropriate modality for a given site of a treatable pathology, one must take into account the propagation and absorption characteristics of the tissues for each form of energy used for heating. In general, skin and superficial subcutaneous tissues are selectively heated by infrared, visible light, hot packs, paraffin bath, Fluidotherapy, and hydrotherapy. Subcutaneous tissues and superficial musculature are selectively heated by shortwave diathermy with condenser application and by microwaves at a frequency of 2456 MHz. Superficial musculature is heated preferentially by shortwave diathermy using induction coil applicators. Deep-seated joints and fibrous scars within soft tissues are selectively heated by ultrasound, as are myofascial interfaces, tendon and tendon sheath, and nerve trunks. Pelvic organs are selectively heated by shortwave diathermy using internal vaginal or rectal electrodes.

In addition, it is most important to realize that the desirable temperature distribution can be achieved only if proper technique of application and proper dosimetry are used. Nykanen (1995) used ultrasound in the treatment of painful shoulders of various aetiologies. Thirty-five subjects were treated with pulsed ultrasound 1.0 W/cm^2 intensity in a 1:4 on–off ratio and 37 were treated with ultrasound placebo in this 'double-blind' study, which also used massage and group gymnastics aimed at improving range of motion. No benefit was found by adding the ultrasound. Unfortunately, the *average* intensity of the ultrasound was so low (0.2 W/cm^2) that no therapeutic benefit could have been anticipated. The use of a randomized, double-blind design does not, in and of itself, ensure a valid study if the dosage of the intervention is not appropriate. Also, it is difficult to blind the subject to ultrasound usage if the intensity is appropriate, since the ultrasound will be perceived (although the evaluator could be blinded). Several of these modalities are very powerful and, if inappropriately used, can do severe tissue damage in a short period of time.

Non-thermal effects of the diathermy modalities, i.e., shortwave, microwave, and ultrasound, have been well documented (Lehmann and De Lateur 1990a, b, c). However, none of them is essential for therapeutic effectiveness. Some non-thermal effects may represent potential hazards, but few of them have been documented as being destructive. These can be avoided by use of proper equipment and proper technique of application (see review by Lehmann and de Lateur 1999).

Techniques of cold application

Melting ice, together with water, is commonly used for cryotherapy since it ensures a steady temperature of 0°C. Most commonly, a rubber bag containing ice cubes with water is applied as a compress. A layer of terry cloth between the ice bag and the skin may slow down cooling. Other methods use terry cloth dipped into a mixture of ice shavings with water. The cloth is wrung out and then applied to the body part. This application has to be repeated frequently. Finally, a hand or foot may be treated by immersion in ice water; this, however, is a potentially more dangerous method because of the possible development of necrosis of fingers or toes. If the objective is to cool musculature to relieve muscle spasm or spasticity, it is necessary to apply the ice for a significant period of time. Even in a relatively slender individual with a subcutaneous fat layer of less than 1 cm, more than 10 min of ice application is necessary to achieve significant cooling of the underlying musculature. In many cases 20–30 min may be necessary to achieve the desired result, which can be gauged by clinical observation of the resolution of the muscle spasm, the reduction of spasticity, clonus, and the spindle reflexes (Bierman and Friedlander 1940, Hartviksen 1962).

Ice massage, in which a block of ice is rubbed over the skin surface, is also used for the same purpose. However, it must be remembered that short-term ice massage is more likely just to cool the skin, with a subsequent increase in muscle tone (Hartviksen 1962).

Evaporative cooling with ethyl chloride spray is done by spraying the skin from a distance of about 1 m with a stroking motion. Bierman (1955) suggested a movement of the spray of 4 in./s. Each area should be exposed only for a few seconds, followed by a pause. More recently, chlorofluoromethanes have been used since they are less flammable than ethyl chloride (Traherne 1962). This method is more frequently used as a 'counterirritant'. It is doubtful whether it is suitable for cooling a large muscle covered by a significant fat layer.

Common therapeutic applications of heat and cold for pain relief

It is essential for successful therapeutic application of heat and cold that the correct diagnosis be made first. The local condition to be treated is assessed and a judgement is made as to whether or not it is treatable with heat or cold. The location of the pathological process is clearly identified and the proper modality is selected. It is equally important that the application should be done with appropriate technique. Painful skeletal muscle spasms, which frequently occur in the back as a result of nerve root irritation or spinal pathology, may be successfully treated with heat or cold to achieve muscle relaxation and thus abolition of pain. Shortwave diathermy may be applied with either induction coil applicators or condenser pads. Treatment should occur once or twice daily for 20–30 min. Relaxation may be achieved by direct muscle heating and an effect on the spindle mechanism as well as reflexly by surface heating. Microwave direct contact applicators can be used for this purpose. Also helpful are superficial heating agents, including hot packs such as Hydrocollator packs or radiant heat with heat lamp or cradle. Treatment should be for 20–30 min. In this case, reflexogenic relaxation is achieved.

As an alternative mode of treatment, ice pack or ice massage may be applied to cool the muscle and thus reduce spindle sensitivity. Therefore, applications for a minimum of 10 min (although 20 min would be better) would be required. Landen (1967) showed in 117 patients with back pain that heat and cold applications were equally effective. In acute conditions heat was found to reduce hospital stay more effectively than ice applications, while in chronic conditions, ice was more effective than heat application. All these treatments are for symptomatic relief and produce their effects by reduction of the painful muscle spasm.

In myofibrositis in the presence of so-called trigger points, both cold application, often with ethyl chloride spray, and local application of heat have been used successfully. Ultrasound in low or medium dose applied to the painful area has also been found to be effective. In this condition heat application is often followed by deep sedative massage. In cases of mild fibrositis more vigorous friction massage may also be used.

In tension states with increased EMG activity, discomfort can be relieved by heat application; commonly shortwave or superficial heat are used. These forms of heat application are often followed by deep sedative massage. This treatment is usually combined with relaxation training with biofeedback to reduce the muscle tension. In any one of these conditions, but specifically in myofibrositis, there is also evidence that these modalities represent a 'counterirritant' and reduce pain as explained by the gate theory (Parsons and Goetzl 1945, Melzack and Wall 1965).

In gastrointestinal upset, cramping of the smooth musculature of the tract produces pain. The peristalsis and discomfort can be reduced by superficial heat application to the abdomen in the form of hot packs (Bisgard and Nye 1940, Molander 1941, Fischer and Solomon 1965). This reduction of cramps is associated with reduction of blood flow to the mucous membranes and hydrochloric acid secretion in the stomach. Cold application aggravates the discomfort. Menstrual cramps seem to respond in the same fashion.

The common complaint of joint stiffness and pain in rheumatic diseases such as rheumatoid arthritis is alleviated measurably by heat application (Wright and Johns 1960, 1961; Johns and Wright 1962; Bäcklund and Tiselius 1967). Cold application aggravates the objective signs. Clinically, superficial heat such as radiant heat and a hot tub bath is commonly used for this purpose. Also, the secondary muscle spasms can be treated in this fashion. Modalities that selectively heat the joints, such as ultrasound, are not used in this condition because the vigorous heating of the inflamed synovium may produce exacerbation. The whirlpool bath or the dip method of paraffin may be used for mild heating of hands and feet. If the Hubbard tank is used, exercise of the joints can occur at the same time with elimination of the force of gravity by buoyancy. Furthermore, contrast baths, according to Martin et al (1946), may be used to relieve stiffness.

Contrast baths are often recommended for the treatment of stiffness associated with Heberden's nodes. If many joints of the upper and lower extremity are involved in the rheumatic process, radiant heat applied with a double baker is a method of heat application. It has been suggested that ice should be used to numb the pain of the joint, and this application has been advocated on the basis that Harris and McCroskery (1974) found that the activity of destructive enzymes such as collagenase is reduced at lower temperatures. These same experiments have been quoted to indicate that heating of the joint itself is contraindicated. This conclusion exceeds the parameters of the experiment, which investigated the effects on the collagenase of temperatures only up to 36°C, whereas therapeutic temperatures reach or exceed 43°C. At these therapeutic temperatures other enzyme systems have shown a markedly reduced activity (Harris and Krane 1973, Harris and McCroskery 1974).

Joint contractures due to capsular tightness or synovial scarring are frequently painful when mobilized by range of motion exercises and stretch. The effectiveness of the treatment can be increased and the associated pain markedly reduced by using ultrasound in high dosage, which has been shown selectively to raise the temperature in the tight structures, which in turn show an increase in extensibility, rendering the treatment programme less painful and more effective (Friedland 1975). Depending on the soft tissue covering of the joint, ultrasound applied with the multiple-field method is used at intensities between 2 and 4 W/cm^2 with a total output between 20 and 40 W. The application is with a stroking technique.

In acute calcific bursitis of the subdeltoid and subacromial bursae, the acute pain is due to swelling and pressure within the content of the bursa, resulting in an inflammatory reaction. Ice application may alleviate the acute pain, especially if used in conjunction with removal of bursal content and hydrocortisone injection combined with local anaesthetic. At the later stage, the limitation of the range of motion of the shoulder joint, which is frequently associated with calcific tendinitis, should be appropriately treated with ultrasound in combination with range of motion exercises and stretch (Lehmann and De Lateur 1990b).

In the shoulder–hand syndrome or reflex sympathetic dystrophy, superficial heat and ultrasound treatment in combination with a programme to increase range of motion may be used as an adjunct to other therapy, including stellate ganglion block.

In painful lateral epicondylitis or 'tennis elbow', the primary treatment should consist of rest, splinting, ice application, and possibly also an injection of hydrocortisone and local anaesthetic. During the later stage of resolution, superficial heat may be used. Also, ultrasound in low dosage to produce mild effects could be used at this stage since ultrasound selectively raises the temperature at the common tendon of origin and the extensor aponeurosis. The dosage should be approximately 0.5 W/cm^2. Binder et al (1985) treated 76 patients with lateral epicondylitis. The patients were randomly allocated to groups such that 38 received ultrasound and 38 received placebo treatment. A total of 63% of the patients treated with ultrasound were improved, compared with 29% of those given placebo treatment.

Steinberg and Callies (1992) treated epicondylitis with ultrasound and with ultrasound in combination with prednisolone ointment (phonophoresis). They found that ultrasound significantly reduced the pain. However, there was no difference between the ultrasound application alone or with phonophoresis; Haker and Lundeberg (1991b) did not find pulsed application of ultrasound effective in this condition.

Jan and Lai (1991) treated 94 knees in female patients with osteoarthritis of the knees. They randomly assigned subjects to treatment with ultrasound, shortwave diathermy, ultrasound and exercise, or shortwave diathermy and exercise. They found increased functional capacity and torque after all four treatments. More improvement was obtained when exercise was added to the ultrasound or shortwave. There was no significant difference between the shortwave or ultrasound.

In a retrospective analysis of medical records of acute surgical trauma patients, Schaubel (1946) found that cold application reduced the need for recasting due to swelling from 42.3 to only 5.3% of the cases. Also, he found a marked reduction in the requirement for narcotics for pain relief. Cohen et al (1989) found that cooling after surgical repair of the anterior cruciate ligament reduced the need for pain medication. Seino et al (1985) used an intercostal nerve probe to produce cryoanalgesia—a nerve-freezing technique—to control pain after thoracotomy. The cryoanalgesia group had lower postoperative pain scores and required less than half the analgesia compared with the control group. Scarcella and Cohn (1995) assessed the effect of cold (50°F) versus normal temperature (70°F) in total hip arthroplasty (THA) and total knee arthroplasty (TKA). The shortening of hospital stay of 1.4 days for cold-treated THA patients was statistically significant but the 1.5-day shortening of the cold-treated TKA group was not. Cold-treated patients did not differ significantly in narcotic use, post-operative range of motion (ROM), or rate of progression of ROM.

Moore and Cardea (1977) found that the combination of intermittent pressure and ice application promptly reduced the compartmental pressures in the calf that were markedly increased as a result of tibial and fibular fractures, but Matsen et al (1975) found in animal experiments that swelling after fracture was not reduced and perhaps even increased when cold was applied. In the case of minor sports injuries, cryotherapy in combination with compression, for instance using an elastic bandage, is usually used (Basur et al 1976). Also, elevation of the limb and immobilization are recommended. It must be remembered, however, that ice should be applied just long enough to prevent swelling and bleeding since prolonged ice application may unnecessarily retard healing (Vinger and Hoerner 1981). At a later date resolution can be assisted by heat application. In superficial thrombophlebitis, one adjunct of therapy may be application of moist hot packs or the heat cradle to reduce discomfort.

Contraindications and precautions

In general, there are conditions when heat should be used with special precautions. These include heat application to anaesthetic areas or to an obtunded patient. Dosimetry, especially in the deep-heating modalities, is not developed to the point where the tissue temperatures can be safely controlled and destructive temperatures can be reliably avoided. Therefore pain is an essential signal that safe temperature limits are exceeded, and it has been documented that if the signal is heeded, tissue destruction does not occur. Also, tissues with inadequate vascular supply should not be heated, since the temperature elevation increases metabolic demand without associated vascular adaptations. As a result, ischaemic necrosis may occur. Heat should not be applied if there is a haemophagic diathesis, since the increase in blood flow and vascularity will produce more bleeding. Heat should not be applied to malignancies without exact tissue temperature monitoring since otherwise therapeutic temperatures may accelerate tumour growth. Heat should not be applied to the gonads or the developing fetus because of the possible development of congenital malformations (Dietzel and Kern 1971a, b; Dietzel et al 1972; Edwards 1972; Edwards et al 1974; Menser 1978; Smith et al 1978; Hendrickx et al 1979; Harvey et al 1981).

Some specific contraindications also exist for specific diathermy modalities. Shortwave diathermy is contraindicated if an appreciable amount of energy can reach the site of a metal implant (Lehmann et al 1979). The dangers involved are caused by shunting of current through the metal implant or by increasing the current density surrounding the implant. In either case, excessively high temperatures are produced. This contraindication includes intrauterine devices containing copper or other metals until proven otherwise. However, these devices would be reached by significant amounts of current only with application with internal vaginal or rectal electrodes (Sandler 1973). Also, electronic implants such as cardiac pacemakers and electrophysiological orthoses represent contraindications. Contact lenses may lead to excessive heating of the eye (Scott 1956). Some clinicians have suggested that shortwave diathermy applied to the low back may result in increased menstrual flow (Lehmann and De Lateur 1990c). The use of pelvic diathermy in pregnant women is contraindicated for the reasons given under general contraindications. Safe levels of stray radiation have not been worked out for shortwave diathermy.

Sensitive organs that should not be exposed to any significant amount of microwave radiation include the eyes, since in experimental animals (Carpenter and Van Ummerson 1968, Guy et al 1975), cataracts were produced due to a selective heating effect. The testicles should not be exposed because of the great sensitivity of these reproductive organs to temperature elevation. Exposure of the skull and the brain could lead to focusing of the intensity inside the skull and produce higher levels of exposure than anticipated from measurement outside the body (Johnson and Guy 1972). In the USA, safety standards proposed by the Food and Drug Administration for therapeutic application specify a level of 5 mW/cm^2 at a distance of 5 cm from the applicator. Damage during therapeutic exposure, however, has not been observed under 100–150 mW/cm^2 (Michaelson 1990) and is clearly related to the heating effect. Precautions should be used when microwaves are applied over bony prominences, since the reflection of the wave at the bone interface may produce increased absorption in the tissues superficial to the bone. Burns have been observed in these circumstances.

In the case of ultrasound, as mentioned previously, proper equipment and technique of application must be used to avoid the occurrence and destructive effects of gaseous cavitation. Also, exposure of the fluid media of the eye, of the cerebrospinal fluid, and of effusions should be avoided because in these media with low cellular content and low viscosity, gaseous cavitation can occur even at therapeutic intensities. For the same reason, the amniotic fluid of the pregnant uterus should not be exposed and the heating effect of ultrasound would represent a contraindication when ultrasound is applied to the fetus. However, due to the excellent beaming properties of ultrasound, exposure of the pregnant uterus can easily be avoided. These precautions do not include imaging of the fetus with ultrasound since the intensities are far below the therapeutic level and therefore cannot produce any harmful effects. Thus, ultrasound can be used for other indications. Also, it can be applied to the intervertebral joints without significant exposure of cerebrospinal fluid and spinal cord because of the intervening tissues such as bone, ligaments, and muscles and because the beam can be aimed at the joint facets.

If superficial heat is applied by means of a Hubbard tank or hot tub and the entire body is submerged, the body temperature should be monitored. In this situation, the heat regulatory mechanisms are disabled and therefore an artificial fever is easily produced. Oral temperatures should be taken at water temperatures over 100°F (37.8°C).

There are also contraindications to the use of cold. Severe adverse effects to local cold application are rare and are usually due to hypersensitivity to cold. Four groups of hypersensitivity may be distinguished (Juhlin and Shelley 1961). The first group of hypersensitivity syndromes is a result of release of histamine or histamine-like substances, presenting frequently as classic cold urticaria. The pathogenesis is primarily due to an effect of histamine on capillary vessels and smooth musculature with skin manifestations of urticaria, erythema, itching, and sweating. There may be facial flush, puffiness of the eyelids, and laryngeal oedema with respiratory impairment. In severe cases there is shock or so-called anaphylaxis with syncope, hypotension, and tachycardia. Gastrointestinal symptoms are associated with gastric hyperacidity and include dysphagia, abdominal pain, diarrhoea, and vomiting. Horton et al (1936) demonstrated that this type of sensitivity is treatable by a programme of careful desensitization. The second group of hypersensitivity is due to the presence of cold haemolysins and agglutinins. Renal haemoglobinuria and skin manifestations of urticaria and Raynaud's phenomenon are part of the symptomatology. The third group of syndromes is due to the presence of cryoglobulins. There are severe manifestations such as reduced vision, impairment of hearing, conjunctival haemorrhages, epistaxis, cold urticaria, Raynaud's phenomenon, and ulceration and necrosis. Also, gastrointestinal upset with melaena and gingival bleeding have been observed. Finally, a marked cold pressor response may be observed in some patients with submersion of limbs in ice water (Wolf and Hardy 1941, Wolff 1951, Boyer et al 1960, Larson 1961, Shelley and Caro 1962).

Some of these responses are severe. Prominent vasospasm can produce a necrosis of fingers and toes in submersion of the limbs. Therefore, careful medical evaluation of the patients is essential, and also a trial of localized ice application over a small area—for instance, on the thigh—may produce skin manifestations of sensitivity as a warning sign.

References

Bäcklund L, Tiselius P 1967 Objective measurement of joint stiffness in rheumatoid arthritis. Acta Rheumatologica Scandinavica 13: 275–288

Barker P, Langton JA, Murphy P, Rowbotham DJ 1991 Effect of prior administration of cold saline on pain during propofol injection. Anaesthesia 46: 1069–1070

Basford JR 1995 Low intensity laser therapy: still not an established clinical tool. Lasers in Surgery and Medicine 16: 331–342

Basford JR, Sheffield CG, Mair SD, Ilstrup DM 1987 Low-energy helium-neon laser treatment of thumb osteoarthritis. Archives of Physical Medicine and Rehabilitation 68: 794–797

Basur RL, Shephard E, Mouzas GL 1976 A cooling method in the treatment of ankle sprains. Practitioner 216: 708–711

Benson TB, Copp EP 1974 The effects of therapeutic forms of heat and ice on the pain threshold of the normal shoulder. Rheumatology and Rehabilitation 13: 101–104

Bierman W 1955 Therapeutic use of cold. Journal of the American Medical Association 157: 1189–1192

Bierman W, Friedlander M 1940 The penetrative effect of cold. Archives of Physical Therapy 21: 585–591

Binder A, Hodge G, Greenwood AM, Hazleman BL, Page Thomas DP 1985 Is therapeutic ultrasound effective in treating soft tissue lesions? British Medical Journal 290: 512–514

Bisgard JD, Nye D 1940 The influence of hot and cold application upon gastric and intestinal motor activity. Surgery, Gynecology and Obstetrics 71: 172–180

Bliddal H, Hellesen C, Ditlevsen P, Asselberghs J, Lyager L 1987 Soft-laser therapy of rheumatoid arthritis. Scandinavian Journal of Rheumatology 16: 225–228

Boyer JT, Fraser JRE, Doyle AE 1960 The haemodynamic effects of cold immersion. Clinical Science 19: 539–550

Carpenter RL, Van Ummerson CA 1968 The action of microwave power on the eye. Journal of Microwave Power 3: 3–19

Ceccherelli F, Altafini L, Lo Castro G et al 1989 Diode laser in cervical myofascial pain: a double-blind study versus placebo. Clinical Journal of Pain 5: 301–304

Chapman CE 1991 Can the use of physical modalities for pain control be rationalized by the research evidence? Canadian Journal of Physiology and Pharmacology 69: 704–712
Cohen BT, Draeger RI, Jackson DW 1989 The effects of cold therapy in the postoperative management of pain in patients undergoing anterior cruciate ligament reconstruction. American Journal of Sports Medicine 17: 344–349
De Jong RH, Hershey WN, Wagman IH 1966 Nerve conduction velocity during hypothermia in man. Anesthesiology 27: 805–810
Derscheid GL, Brown WC 1985 Rehabilitation of the ankle. Clinics in Sports Medicine 4: 527–544
Dietzel F, Kern W 1971a Kann hohes mutterliches Fieber beim Kind auslÿsen? Originalmitteilungen ist ausschliesslich der Verfasser verantwortlich. Naturwissenschaften 2: 24–26
Dietzel F, Kern W 1971b Kann hohes mutterliches Fieber Missbildungen beim Kind auslÿsen? Geburtshilfe und Frauenheilkunde 31: 1074–1079
Dietzel F, Kern W, Steckenmesser R 1972 Missbildungen und intrauterines Absterben nach Kurzwellenbehandlung in der Fruschwangerschaft. Munchener Medizinische Wochesschrift 114: 228–230
Edwards MJ 1972 Influenza, hyperthermia, and congenital malformation. Lancet i: 320–321
Edwards MJ, Mulley R, Ring S, Wanner RA 1974 Mitotic cell death and delay of mitotic activity in guinea-pig embryos following brief maternal hyperthermia. Journal of Embryology and Experimental Morphology 32: 593–602
Field HL, Basbaum AI 1978 Brainstem control of spinal pain-transmission neurons. Annual Review of Physiology 40: 217–248
Finan MA, Roberts WS, Hoffman MS, Fiorica JV, Cavanagh D, Dudney BJ 1993 The effects of cold therapy on postoperative pain in gynecologic patients: a prospective, randomized study. American Journal of Obstetrics and Gynecology 168(2): 542–544
Fischer E, Solomon S 1965 Physiological responses to heat and cold. In: Licht S (ed) Therapeutic heat and cold, 2nd edn. E Licht, New Haven, pp 126–129
Friedland F 1975 Ultrasonic therapy in rheumatic diseases. Journal of the American Medical Association 163: 799
Gammon GD, Starr I 1941 Studies on the relief of pain by counterirritation. Journal of Clinical Investigation 20: 13–20
Gerschman JA, Ruben J, Gebart-Eaglemont J 1994 Low level laser therapy for dentinal tooth hypersensitivity. Australian Dental Journal 39(6): 353–357
Goldman JA, Chiapella J, Casey H et al 1980 Laser therapy for rheumatoid arthritis. Lasers in Surgery and Medicine 1: 93–101
Goodgold J, Eberstein A 1977 Electrodiagnosis of neuromuscular diseases, 2nd edn. Williams & Wilkins, Baltimore
Guy AW, Lehmann JF, Stonebridge JB 1974 Therapeutic applications of electromagnetic power. Proceedings of the Institute of Electrical and Electronic Engineers 62: 55–75
Guy AW, Lin JC, Kramer PO, Emery AF 1975 Effect of 2450-MHz radiation on the rabbit eye. Institute of Electrical and Electronic Engineers, Transactions on Microwave Theory and Techniques MTT 23: 492–498
Haker E, Lundeberg T 1990 Laser treatment applied to acupuncture points in lateral humeral epicondylalgia. A double-blind study. Pain 43: 243–247
Haker EHK, Lundeberg TCM 1991a Lateral epicondylalgia: report of non-effective midlaser treatment. Archives of Physical Medicine and Rehabilitation 72: 984–988
Haker EHK, Lundeberg TCM 1991b Pulsed ultrasound treatment in lateral epicondylalgia. Scandinavian Journal of Rehabilitation Medicine 23: 115–118
Hall J, Clarke AK, Elvins DM, Ring EFJ 1994 Low level laser therapy is ineffective in the management of rheumatoid arthritic finger joints. British Journal of Rheumatology 33: 142–147
Hansen HJ, Thoroe U 1990 Low power laser biostimulation of chronic oro-facial pain. A double-blind placebo controlled cross-over study in 40 patients. Pain 43: 169–179
Harris ED Jr, Krane SM 1973 Cartilage collagen: substrate in soluble and fibrillar form for rheumatoid collagenase. Transactions of the Association of American Physicians 86: 82–94
Harris ED Jr, McCroskery PA 1974 The influence of temperature and fibril stability on degradation of cartilage collagen by rheumatoid synovial collagenase. New England Journal of Medicine 290: 1–6
Hartviksen K 1962 Ice therapy in spasticity. Acta Neurlogica Scandinavica 38 (suppl 3): 79–84
Harvey MAS, McRorie MM, Smith DW 1981 Suggested limits of exposure in the hot tub and sauna for the pregnant woman. Canadian Medical Association Journal 125: 50–53
Hendrickx AG, Stone GW, Henrickson RV, Matayoshi K 1979 Teratogenic effects of hyperthermia on the bonnet monkey (*Macaca radiata*). Teratology 19: 177–182
Hong C-Z 1991 Reversible nerve conduction block in patients with polyneuropathy after ultrasound thermotherapy at therapeutic dosage. Archives of Physical Medicine and Rehabilitation 72: 132–137
Horton BT, Browne GE, Roth GM 1936 Hypersensitiveness to cold. Journal of the American Medical Association 107: 1263–1268
Jan MH, Lai JS 1991 The effects of physiotherapy on osteoarthritic knees of females. Journal of the Formosan Medical Association 90(10): 1008–1013
Johannsen F, Hauschild B, Remvig L, Johnsen V, Petersen M, Bieler T 1994 Low energy laser therapy in rheumatoid arthritis. Scandinavian Journal of Rheumatology 23(3): 45–147
Johns RJ, Wright V 1962 Relative importance of various tissues in joint stiffness. Journal of Applied Physiology 17: 824–828
Johnson CC, Guy AW 1972 Nonionizing electromagnetic wave-effects in biological materials and systems. Proceedings of the Institute of Electrical and Electronic Engineers 66: 692–718
Juhlin L, Shelley WB 1961 Role of mast cell and basophil in cold urticaria with associated systemic reactions. Journal of the American Medical Association 117: 371–377
Kay DB 1985 The sprained ankle: current therapy. Foot and Ankle 6: 22–28
Kerr FWL, Casey KL 1976 Pain. Neurosciences Research Program Bulletin 16: 1–207
Klein RG, Eck BC 1990 Low-energy laser treatment and exercise for chronic low-back pain: double-blind controlled trial. Archives of Physical Medicine and Rehabilitation 71: 34–37
Kramer JF 1985 Effect of therapeutic ultrasound intensity on subcutaneous tissue temperature and ulnar nerve conduction velocity. American Journal of Physical Medicine 64: 1–9
Landen BR 1967 Heat or cold for the relief of low back pain? Physical Therapy 47: 1126–1128
Larson DL 1961 Systemic lupus erythematosus. Little, Brown, Boston
Lehmann JF, De Lateur BJ 1982 Therapeutic heat. In: Lehmann JF (ed) Therpeutic heat and cold, 3rd edn. Williams & Wilkins, Baltmore
Lehmann JF, De Lateur BJ 1990a Cryotherapy. In: Lehmann JF (ed) Therapeutic heat and cold, 4th edn. Williams & Wilkins, Baltimore
Lehmann JF, De Lateur BJ 1990b Therapeutic heat. In: Lehmann JF (ed) Therapeutic heat and cold, 4th edn. Williams & Wilkins, Baltimore
Lehmann JF, De Lateur BJ 1990c Diathermy, superficial heat, laser and cold therapy. In: Kottke FJ, Lehmann JF (eds) Handbook of physical medicine and rehabilitation, 4th edn. Saunders, Philadelphia

Lehmann JF, De Lateur BJ 1999 Ultrasound, shortwave, microwave, laser, superficial heat and cold in the treatment of pain. In: Wall PD, Melzack R (eds) Textbook of pain, 4th edn. Churchill Livingstone, Edinburgh, pp 1383–1397
Lehmann JF, Brunner GD, Stow RW 1958 Pain threshold measurements after therapeutic application of ultrasound, microwaves, and infrared. Archives of Physical Medicine and Rehabilitation 39: 560–565
Lehmann JF, Stonebridge JB, Guy AW 1979 A comparison of patterns of stray radiation from therapeutic microwave applicators measured near tissue-substitute models and human subjects. Radio Science 14: 271–283
Lehmann JF, Dundore DE, Esselman PC, Nelp WB 1983 Microwave diathermy: effects on experimental muscle hematoma resolution. Archives of Physical Medicine and Rehabilitation 64: 127–129
Li C-L 1958 Effect of cooling on neuromuscular transmission in the rat. American Journal of Physiology 194: 200–206
Lim HM, Lew K, Tay D 1995 A clinical investigation of the efficacy of low level laser therapy in reducing orthodontic postadjustment pain. American Journal of Orthodontics and Dentofacial Orthopedics 108(6): 614–622
Lowe AS, McDowell BC, Walsh DM, Baxter GD, Allen JM 1997 Failure to demonstrate any hypoalgesic effect of low intensity laser irradiation (830nm) of Erb's point upon experimental ischaemic pain in humans. Lasers in Surgery and Medicine 20: 69–76
Lundeberg T, Haker E, Thomas M 1987 Effect of laser versus placebo in tennis elbow. Scandinavian Journal of Rehabilitation Medicine 19: 135–138
Martin GM, Roth GM, Elkins EC, Krusen FH 1946 Cutaneous temperature of the extremities of normal subjects and of patients with rheumatoid arthritis. Archives of Physical Medicine 27: 665–682
Matsen FA III, Questad K, Matsen AL 1975 The effect of local cooling on post fracture swelling. Clinical Orthopedics and Related Research 109: 201–206
Melzack R, Wall PD 1965 Pain mechanisms: a new theory. Science 150: 971–979
Melzack R, Guite S, Gonshor A 1980a Relief of dental pain by ice massage of the hand. Canadian Medical Association Journal 122: 189–191
Melzack R, Jeans ME, Stratford JG, Monks RC 1980b Ice massage and transcutaneous electrical stimulation: comparison of treatment for low-back pain. Pain 9: 209–217
Menser M 1978 Does hyperthermia affect the human fetus? Medical Journal of Australia 2: 550
Michaelson SM 1990 Bioeffects of high frequency currents and electromagnetic radiation. In: Lehmann JF (ed) Therapeutic heat and cold, 4th edn. Williams & Wilkins, Baltimore
Moktar B, Baxter GD, Walsh DM, Bell AJ, Allen JM 1995 Double-blind, placebo-controlled investigation of the effect of combined phototherapy/low intensity laser therapy upon experimental ischaemic pain in humans. Lasers in Surgery and Medicine 17: 74–81
Molander CO 1941 Physiologic basis of heat. Archives of Physical Therapy 22: 335–340
Moore CD, Cardea JA 1977 Vascular changes in leg trauma. Southern Medical Journal 70: 1285–1286
Murray FS, Weaver MM 1975 Effects of ipsilateral and contralateral counter-irritation on experimentally produced itch in human beings. Journal of Comparative and Physiological Psychology 89: 819–826
Nilsson S 1983 Sprains of the lateral ankle ligaments, an epidemiological and clinical study with special reference to different forms of conservative treatment. Part II, a controlled trial of different forms of conservative treatment. Journal of the Oslo City Hospitals 33: 13–36
Nykanen M 1995 Pulsed ultrasound treatment of the painful shoulder: a randomized, double-blind, placebo-controlled study. Scandinavian Journal of Rehabilitation Medicine 27: 105–108
Parsons CM, Goetzl FR 1945 Effect of induced pain on pain threshold. Proceedings of the Society for Experimental Biology and Medicine 60: 327–329
Reid R, Omoto KH, Precop SL et al 1995 Flashlamp-excited dye laser therapy of idiopathic vulvodynia is safe and efficacious. American Journal of Obstetrics and Gynecology 172(6): 1684–1696
Sandler B 1973 Heat and the ICUCD. British Medical Journal 25: 458
Scarcella JB, Cohn BT 1995 The effect of cold therapy on the postoperative course of total hip and knee arthroplasty patients. American Journal of Orthopedics 24(11): 847–852
Schaubel HJ 1946 The local use of ice after orthopedic procedures. American Journal of Surgery 72: 711–714
Schmidt KL, Ott VR, Röcher G, Schaller H 1979 Heat, cold and inflammation. Rheumatology 38: 391–404
Scott BO 1956 Effect of contact lenses on short wave field distribution. British Journal of Ophthalmology 40: 696–697
Seino H, Watanabe S, Tanaka J et al 1985 Cryoanalgesia for postthoracotomy pain. Masui 34: 842–845
Sekins KM, Dundore D, Emery AF, Lehmann JF, McGrath PW, Nelp WB 1980 Muscle blood flow changes in response to 915 MHz diathermy with surface cooling as measured by Xe133 clearance. Archives of Physical Medicine and Rehabilitation 61: 105–113
Sekins KM, Lehman JF, Esselman P et al 1984 Local muscle blood flow and temperature responses to 915 MHz diathermy as simultaneously measured and numerically predicted. Archives of Physical Medicine and Rehabilitation 65: 1–7
Shelley WB, Caro WB 1962 Cold erythema. Journal of the American Medical Association 180: 639–642
Siebert W, Seichert N, Siebert B, Wirth CJ 1987 What is the efficacy of 'soft' and 'mid' lasers in therapy of tendinopathies? Archives of Orthopaedic and Trauma Surgery 106: 358–363
Smith DW, Clarren SK, Harvey MAS 1978 Hyperthermia as a possible teratogenic agent. Journal of Pediatrics 92: 878–883
Steinberg R, Callies R 1992 Vergleichsstudie Ultraschall und Prednisolonphonophorese bei Patienten mit Epicondylopathia humeri. Physikalische Medizin Rehabilitationsmedizin Kurortmedizin 2: 84–87
Taube S, Piironen J, Ylipaavalniemi P 1990 Helium-neon laser therapy in the prevention of postoperative swelling and pain after wisdom tooth extraction. Proceedings of the Finnish Dental Society 86: 23–27
Traherne JB 1962 Evaluation of the cold spray technique in the treatment of muscle pain in general practice. Practitioner 189: 210–212
Vinger PF, Hoerner EF (eds) 1981 Sports injuries, the unthwarted epidemic. PSG Publishing, Littleton, MA
Walker J 1983 Relief from chronic pain by lower power laser irradiation. Neuroscience Letters 43: 339–344
Walker JB, Akhanjee LK, Cooney MM et al 1988 Laser therapy for pain of trigeminal neuralgia. Clinical Journal of Pain 3: 183–187
Waterworth RF, Hunter IA 1985 An open study of diflunisal, conservative and manipulative therapy in the management of acute mechanical low back pain. New Zealand Medical Journal 98(779): 372–375
Waylonis GW, Wilke S, O'Toole D, Waylonis DA, Waylonis DB 1988 Chronic myofascial pain: management by low-output helium-neon laser therapy. Archives of Physical Medicine and Rehabilitation 69: 1017–1020
Wolf S, Hardy JD 1941 Studies on pain. Observations on pain due to local cooling and on factors involved in the 'cold pressor' effect. Journal of Clinical Investigation 20: 521–533

Wolff HH 1951 The mechanism and significance of the cold pressor response. Quarterly Journal of Medicine 20: 261–273

Wright V, Johns RJ 1960 Physical factors concerned with the stiffness of normal and diseased joints. Bulletin of the Johns Hopkins Hospital 106: 215–231

Wright V, Johns RJ 1961 Quantitative and qualitative analysis of joint stiffness in normal subjects and in patients with connective tissue diseases. Annals of the Rheumatic Diseases 20: 36–46

Chapter 32

Mobilization, manipulation, massage, and exercise for the relief of musculoskeletal pain

Paul D Hooper and Scott Haldeman

Introduction

Humans are dependent upon the integrity of their locomotor system for movement, which is essential for work, entertainment, adventure, and most activities of daily living. If the integrity of this system is compromised through disease, trauma, or the consequences of ageing, the resulting pain and restricted function can have devastating effects on the quality of life of an individual.

The primary approach to patients with musculoskeletal pain that results in restricted function, therefore, is the restoration of movement and the soothing of pain. Any attempt at relieving pain without simultaneously improving movement and mobility will have limited success. The tools to achieve these ends include massage, active/passive mobilization of joints, manipulation, and exercise. These approaches have the additional advantages of being relatively inexpensive and free of any drug or medication effects or the necessity for surgery. Despite recent medical advances, manual therapies and exercise remain the most widely utilized method of treating musculoskeletal pain and disability.

Massage and manipulation techniques

Massage and manipulation fall into the larger field referred to as manual medicine, manual therapy or manipulative therapy, where the hands are used to touch, massage, or manipulate tissue therapeutically. The diversity of methods and techniques of massage and manipulation is too great to include in a short chapter on the topic. There are, however, a number of principles that allow for a classification of the various manual therapeutic approaches. The most common classification of manual techniques is based on a differentiation between massage, passive movement, mobilization, and the manipulative or adjustive techniques. These techniques are applied at different positions within a specific range of motion of a joint, as shown in Fig. 32.1.

Massage

Massage is the application of touch or force to soft tissues, usually muscles, tendons, or ligaments, without causing movement or change in a position of a joint. Each massage technique is performed

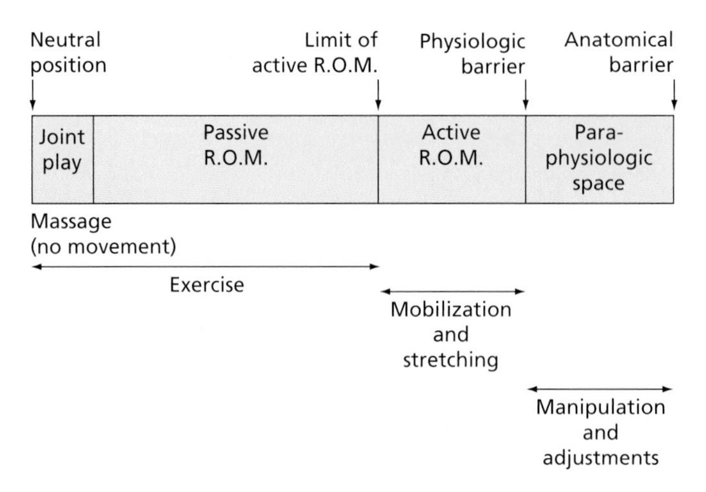

Fig. 32.1 The presumed barriers to motion in a joint and the position or range of motion where the various forms of manual therapy are performed.

with a specific goal in mind. The most commonly applied techniques are as follows.

Stroking or effleurage

This is the light movement of the hands over the skin in a slow, rhythmic fashion. The hands mould to the contour of the area being massaged and are in constant contact with the skin. The hands may gently stroke the skin or influence deeper tissues depending on the amount of pressure exerted. Light stroking tends to be non-painful and soothing and can be either centripetal or centrifugal. Deeper pressure techniques can be slightly uncomfortable and are administered in the direction of venous or lymph flow with the stated goal of reducing oedema.

Connective tissue massage

This technique uses deeper stroking motions and is presumed to free subcutaneous connective tissue adhesions. This deep stroking in specifically defined patterns results in a sensation of warmth and hyperaemia of the skin.

Kneading and petrissage

These techniques require the clinician to grasp, lift, squeeze, or push the tissues being massaged. The skin moves with the hands over the underlying tissues. This differs from stroking, where the hands move over the skin. Commonly these techniques are applied to muscles.

Friction and deep massage

The theoretical goal of these techniques is the loosening of scars or adhesions between deeper structures (Cyriax 1971, Wood 1974). These procedures are presumed to aid in the absorption of local effusion within these tissues. The direction of movement of the fingers may be circular, or transverse across the fibres of the structure being massaged. It may require several sessions to achieve this result and the massage should be followed by exercise to maintain mobility.

Tapotement, percussion, or clapping

These techniques consist of a series of gentle taps or blows applied to the patient (Hofkosh 1985). These methods have been described as hacking, clapping or cupping, tapping, or beating. These percussive movements have been used primarily in postural draining of the lungs, to obtain muscle contraction and relaxation or to increase circulation. They are generally not recommended for the treatment of pathological tissues (Wood 1974) and are commonly used on athletes to tone and relax muscles.

Shaking and vibration

These massage methods require the clinician to take hold of a portion of the patient's body and apply either a coarse shaking or a fine vibrating motion. They are not widely used except in postural drainage of the lungs.

Passive movement

The use of the hands to maintain passive motion in a joint falls into the category of manual therapy. The clinician systematically moves the joint through each of its normal motions, from the neutral point to the point of resistance or pain. No attempt is made to force the joint but the entire length of the range of motion must be traversed and each direction of potential motion must be included. The goal is to prevent stiffening or shortening of the ligamentous structures as well as to maintain motion and lubrication in the joint and surrounding tissues.

The natural progression from passive motion is to active motion or exercise. Exercise is performed within the same boundaries of joint motion as is passive motion, although not all directions of motion that can be achieved passively can be reproduced by exercise. Exercise has the additional advantage of including muscle activity and developing strength and coordination. Passive movement is usually discontinued, where possible, in favour of active exercise.

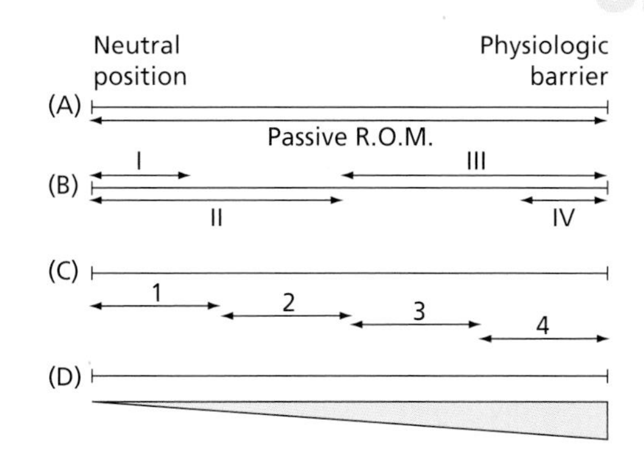

Fig. 32.2 The different forms of mobilization. Active and passive ranges of motion are included under 'passive range of motion' as all of these mobilizations are performed passively. (A) Continuous passive range of motion; (B) graded oscillations; (C) progressive stretch mobilization; and (D) sustained progressive stretching.

Mobilization and stretching

Mobilization includes those manual procedures that attempt to increase the range of motion beyond the resistance barrier (Fig. 32.1). Certain mobilization methods include stretching of muscles and ligaments while others include movement of joints in non-physiologic directions of motion. Mobilization differs from manipulation or adjustment by the absence of a forceful thrust or jerking motion.

Graded oscillation or mobilization

These techniques were popularized by Maitland (1973), who proposed four levels or grades of mobilization. Grade I mobilization is a fine oscillation with very little force or depth. Grade II uses a greater depth but remains within the first half of the range of motion (ROM). Grade III is a deeper mobilization at the limits of motion, whereas Grade IV is a deep, fine oscillation at the limits of potential motion. The clinician tends to start at grade I and increase to grade IV as greater motion becomes possible. Each of these grades is illustrated in Fig. 32.2B.

Progressive stretch mobilization

These techniques require the application of successive short-amplitude stretching movements to the joint. The depth of the stretching is increased as permitted by the joint. Again, four grades or depths are described (Nyberg 1985) but in this situation the grades refer to each quarter of the potential motion of the joint as illustrated in Fig. 32.2C. These techniques are used primarily to overcome soft tissue restriction to joint motion.

Sustained progressive stretch

This is a sustained stretching motion with progressively increasing pressure. This technique is recommended to stretch shortened periarticular soft tissues and is performed slowly and carefully to avoid tearing (Fig. 32.2D).

Spray and stretch

These techniques have been taught widely for the treatment of painful myofascial trigger points (Mennel 1960, Travell 1976). The muscle being treated is placed in a light stretch and a fluoromethane spray is applied to the muscle in a specific pattern. This results in a cooling of the skin as the fluoromethane evaporates. The muscle can then be stretched further, allowing increased ROM and, theoretically, the elimination of the trigger point.

Muscle energy

These methods (hold–relaxation technique) require the use of muscle activity and subsequent relaxation to set the stage for increasing motion. The clinician places the muscle in light stretch. The patient then contracts the muscle against resistance applied by the clinician. The contraction is held for a brief period and the patient then relaxes, at which point the muscle is stretched. Certain osteopathic physicians (Kimberly 1979, Goodridge 1981) have modified these techniques to allow for specific directional mobilization or manipulation of vertebrae.

Manipulation

The difference between mobilization and manipulation or adjustment is the application of a high-velocity, low-amplitude thrust to the joint. Many chiropractors feel that there is a difference between non-specific manipulation and the classic adjustment which has specific direction, force, and presumed physiologic effects. Others include the various mobilization and muscle-energy techniques under the heading of manipulation. There is, however, fairly clear differentiation between the previously described non-thrust procedures and the thrusting techniques described here. These techniques force the joint beyond the physiologic ROM, through the paraphysiological space, to the anatomical limits of motion (Fig. 32.1). The thrust is commonly followed by a 'click' or 'pop', which is felt to be related to release of gases within the joint space.

Non-specific long-lever manipulation

These techniques are becoming less popular because of the potential to exert large, possibly harmful forces. Force is applied via a long bone as a lever (e.g., shoulder or leg) to exert force into the spine (Cyriax 1971, Coplans 1978). These techniques, in the past, were commonly used under anaesthesia, allowing for the exertion of strenuous forces to a joint. In large patients treated by small clinicians, the utilization of such long levers with directed force may be helpful.

Specific spinal adjustment

The application of high-velocity, small-amplitude thrusting techniques to short levers of the spine such as a spinous or transverse process has been the mainstay of traditional chiropractic practice. The goal has been variously described as correcting misalignments or subluxations, eliminating fixations in intersegmental motion, and bringing about a variety of neural and muscular reflex changes. Numerous techniques have been described (Logan 1950; Greco 1953; States 1968; Haldeman 1980, 1992). Each vertebra can be adjusted in a number of different directions and the patient can be placed in very specific positions prior to the administration of an adjustment to allow for control of the depth and direction of the force to be applied. It has yet to be established, however, that such precise application of force does in fact bring about specific vertebral movements as claimed.

Toggle–recoil

Certain chiropractic techniques (Thompson 1973) require the patient to be placed on a table that is constructed so that one vertebral segment is locked or blocked while a rapidly controlled force is applied to the adjacent vertebra. The portion of the table supporting the vertebra being adjusted then drops approximately 1 cm, allowing for a concussion or recoil effect. Properly performed, high-velocity forces can be applied very specifically to a vertebra without the clinician exerting much force or effort.

Joint play

Most joints have some degree of play at rest because of ligamentous elasticity. When joints cease to have this play due to tightening of the ligaments and especially if the joint is locked in a slightly abnormal position, the joint can be manipulated in specific directions to increase the play.

Traction and distraction

Manual traction and the combination of mechanical traction or distraction with manipulation techniques are commonly accompanied by pulling or thrusting methods while the patient is in traction (Cox 1980) and are widely used by chiropractors under the term 'adjustments'. Manual traction without thrusting is also used as a standard physiotherapeutic technique and could be included under mobilization methods.

Mechanically assisted manipulation

Over the years, a number of mechanical devices have been developed to assist in the delivery of the manipulative thrust. These include special tables with drop-away pieces; manual and motorized tables that move up, down, and sideways; and small, hand-held instruments such as the Activator Adjusting Instrument (AAI). Some of these are promoted as assistive devices that aid the clinician with the delivery of the necessary force. Others have been suggested as potential replacements to manual manipulation (Polkinghorn 1998).

The effectiveness of massage and manipulation

By far the majority of people who request massage or manipulation do so for relief of pain, muscle spasm, tension, or stiffness. Surveys reveal that 80–90% of patients do so for the relief of spinal pain or headaches (Vear 1972, Breen 1977, Nyiendo and Haldeman 1987). A recent study in Sweden demonstrated that most patients sought chiropractic care for low back pain of less than 1 month duration and received 2–3 spinal manipulation treatments (SMT) (Leboeuf-Yde et al 1997). The anecdotal surveys and descriptive studies demonstrate a very high success or patient satisfaction rate. The success rates reported for manipulation in uncontrolled trials and in various comparative trials are between 60 and 100% (Haldeman 1978, Brunarski 1984, Bronfort 1992). However, this type of study ignores the problems of spontaneous recovery, placebo effect, difficulty in quantitating pain, and natural prejudice of practitioners reporting on the success of their own treatment. In the case of spinal pain, the problem of different populations of patients and pathological causes of pain also makes it difficult to compare studies. The fact that the majority of patients visiting a practitioner of manipulation feel better while undergoing treatment is undoubtedly the primary reason for its popularity.

Despite its universal usage, there have not been many serious controlled trials. There are, however, few clinicians or patients who would deny that rubbing or massaging sore muscles or stiff joints produces a soothing feeling and pain relief. It can be argued that even if the relief described after massage and manipulation is due to placebo or psychological effects, such treatments should not be discarded. Pope et al (1994) found that satisfaction rates in patients receiving massage were significantly higher than in those being treated with corsets or transcutaneous muscle stimulation (TMS). These rates increased with repeated treatments, thus demonstrating the high acceptance of this procedure.

Manipulation, on the other hand, has been the subject of increasing clinical research, and the number of published controlled clinical trials has grown rapidly during the past few years. Shekelle et al (1992) lists 29 controlled clinical trials on low back pain, and Bronfort (1992) reviewed 47 randomized, comparative trials on the treatment of back pain, neck pain, and headaches using manipulation. In a review of criteria-based meta-analyses, Koes et al (1995) identified 69 different randomized, controlled clinical trials (RCTs), and in a systematic review, Van Tulder et al (1997) reported 28 high-quality RCTs on acute and 20 on chronic low back pain. Many of these studies have shown favourable results for manipulation (Koes et al 1996).

In one of the more publicized RCTs, Meade et al (1990) demonstrated a short-term favourable outcome for chiropractic care when compared to hospital-based outpatient treatment. A 3-year follow-up study (Meade et al 1995) confirmed the earlier findings that patients treated by chiropractors derive more benefit and long-term satisfaction than those treated in hospital. This later study also suggested some potential long-term benefit to the patients treated by chiropractors.

There are now sufficient numbers of well-designed trials to perform meta-analyses and to sort the trials into different subgroups of patients (Ottenbacher and DiFabio 1985). This has made it possible to discuss the effectiveness of manipulation in more specific forms, such as condition or diagnosis, and expected outcome measures.

Acute uncomplicated low back pain

The majority of the controlled clinical trials on manipulation have been performed on patients with recent onset of symptoms (within 2–4 weeks). These studies tended to exclude patients with complicating factors such as systemic or metabolic diseases, sciatica or disc herniation, workers' compensation, or other psychosocial factors. There are many difficulties in reviewing these papers. For example, Jayson (1986) found that manipulation was superior to controls when given in an outpatient clinic, but was ineffective in hospitalized patients with back pain who presumably had more severe pathology. Berquist-Ullman and Larsson (1977) found manipulation to be more effective than placebo but no better than a comprehensive education programme. Glover et al (1974, 1977) found that manipulation had a significant positive effect in patients with acute pain when assessed immediately after treatment but not in more chronic cases. Doran and Newell (1975), Coxhead et al (1981), and Sloop et al (1982) each showed non-statistically significant trends towards improvement in their manipulation groups when compared to controls. Greenland et al (1979) suggest that a different statistical analysis of Doran and Newell's data would find manipulation significantly more effective than controls.

Even in the trials where manipulation was reported as clearly more effective than controls, the picture is not clear. The studies by Coyer and Curwen (1955) and Lewith and Turner (1982) were not blinded or statistically analysed. The studies by Sims-Williams et al (1978, 1979), Buerger (1978, 1979), and Hoehler et al (1981) were well controlled but showed only short-term changes with no long-lasting results from manipulation. However, one point is clear: the multiple comparative trials have shown that no other conservative treatment is superior to manipulation. Additionally, none of the trials reported any complications from the application of manipulation.

Shekelle et al (1992) analysed all the controlled trials on manipulation and assigned quality scores. They selected seven papers that had used single-outcome measures or assessed outcome measures

Table 32.1 Outcome measures combined in meta-analysis of acute low back pain studies[a]

Author (reference)	Outcome measure	When assessed	Number of patients recovered	
			Manipulated group	Comparison group
Coyer and Curwen 1955	'Well' (relief of symptoms)	3 wk	58 of 76	36 of 60
Bergquist-Ullman and Larsson 1977	Return to work	3 wk	30 of 61	25 of 56
Farrell and Twomey 1982	'Symptom-free', very low pain score, can do all functional activity without difficulty, and objective lumbar movements are without pain	3 wk	22 of 24	15 of 24
Godfrey et al 1984	1–5-point scale of 'general symptomatology' dichotomized by the original authors into 'marked improvement' or not	Mean, 2 wk	14 of 39	7 of 33
Rasmussen 1979	'Fully restored', no pain, normal function, no sign of disease, fit to work	2 wk	11 of 12	3 of 12
Matthews et al 1987	6-point pain scale divided into 'recovered' and 'not recovered'	2 wk	116 of 152	73 of 108
Waterworth and Hunder 1985	'Excellent overall improvement' by patient self-report	12 days	23 of 38	15 of 36

[a]From Shekelle et al (1992).

independently (see Table 32.1). They then developed differences in probability of recovery from back pain for each of the studies (Fig. 32.3). The results show that manipulation increased the probability of recovery at 2 or 3 weeks, indicating that manipulation hastens recovery from acute uncomplicated low back pain.

A prospective randomized trial compared the effect of SMT, transcutaneous muscle stimulation, massage, and corset use in patients with subacute low back pain (Pope et al 1994). After 3 weeks, the manipulation group scored the greatest improvement in flexion and pain. In addition, patient confidence was greatest in the manipulation group. In a randomized study of manual therapy (i.e., manipulation, specific mobilization, and muscle stretching) compared with steroid injections for patients with acute and subacute low back pain, patients receiving manual therapy had significantly less pain and disability both in the early phase as well as at 90 days follow-up. The manual therapy group also had a faster rate of recovery and lower drug consumption (Blomberg et al 1994). Andersson et al (1999) also found less medication use in manual therapy patients. Koes et al (1996) identified 36 RCTs comparing SMT with other treatments for patients with low back pain. Twelve of these included only patients with acute pain. Of these, 5 reported positive results, 4 reported negative results, and 3 reported positive results in a subgroup of the population only.

Two studies have recently attempted to look at long-term effects. Meade et al (1990) compared the effects of hospital-based, outpatient, physical therapy department treatment with office-based chiropractic treatment and noted a small but detectable (7%) long-term effect on Oswestry scores over a 2-year period. Waagen et al (1990) also demonstrated a long-term (2 year) higher satisfaction rate with chiropractic care compared with care received from a family physician's office. The significance of these studies, however, is not clear but at least they raise the possibility that manipulation is of greater benefit than simple acute pain relief.

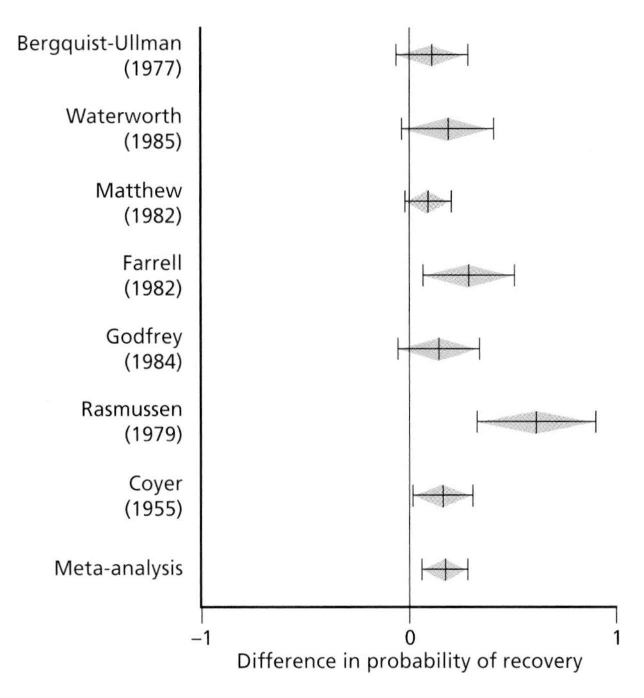

Fig. 32.3 Difference in probability of recovery in seven trials of manipulation. A difference in probability of greater than 0 represents a beneficial effect of manipulation. For individual studies, 95% confidence intervals are shown; for the meta-analysis, the 95% probability limits are shown. (From Shekelle et al 1992.)

Chronic low back pain (CLBP)

Until recently there have been only a few studies on the effect of spinal manipulation therapy in patients with chronic low back pain (CLBP) and these are more difficult to interpret. Waagen et al (1986), for example, showed a statistical benefit from manipulation in patients with recurrent or chronic low back pain at 2 weeks, whereas Gibson et al (1985) failed to show such an effect. Evans et al (1978) showed diminished codeine use in patients undergoing manipulation, and Ongley et al (1987) demonstrated that a group that received both rotational manipulation and proliferent injections showed significant improvement. It may be that, in patients with chronic back pain, the support of a physician and the relief, even if temporary, following manipulation serves to make the patients tolerate their pain and thereby reduce pain scores.

In a blinded randomized trial of patients with chronic back and neck complaints, Koes et al (1992a) found that manual therapy showed a faster and larger improvement in physical functioning than physiotherapy, treatment by a general practitioner, and a placebo therapy. They also note that manipulative therapy was slightly better than physiotherapy after 12 months. And in a comparison of manipulation and mobilization of the spine with physiotherapy (i.e., exercises, massage, heat, electrotherapy, ultrasound, and shortwave diathermy), Koes et al (1993) demonstrated that, for patients with chronic conditions (i.e., duration of 1 year or longer), improvement was greater in those treated with manual therapy.

Triano et al (1995) compared SMT with education programmes for patients with CLBP. Greater improvement was noted in pain and activity tolerance in the manipulation group. Bronfort et al (1996) compared trunk exercise combined with SMT or non-steroidal anti-inflammatory drug therapy. Each of the three therapeutic regimens was associated with similar and clinically important improvement over time that was considered superior to the expected natural history. In separate reviews of the literature, Koes et al (1996) and Van Tulder et al (1997) have identified a number of RCTs of sufficiently high quality to demonstrate a positive effect of SMT. Stig et al (2001) investigated the recovery pattern in chiropractic patients with chronic or recurrent low back pain. They stated that 50% of patients reported improvement at the 4th visit (within 2 weeks), and 75% improved by the 12th visit. Nyiendo et al (2000) showed that patients with CLBP treated by chiropractors showed greater improvement and satisfaction at 1 month than patients treated by family physicians. Giles and Muller (1999) compared needle acupuncture, NSAIDs, and chiropractic spinal manipulation for patients with CLBP. SMT was the only intervention that achieved statistically significant improvement after 30 days. These studies suggest that spinal manipulation can now be considered a reasonable approach to patients with CLBP and that the effect might be greater if combined with exercise.

Sciatica

A growing number of studies looked specifically at patients with sciatica. Although Nwuga (1982), Coxhead et al (1981), and Edwards (1969) all report improvement in certain outcome measures following manipulation in patients with sciatica, the significance of these studies is not clear. It appears, however, that patients with demonstrated disc herniation and sciatica do less well following manipulation than patients with back pain alone (Chrisman et al 1964, Cassidy and Kirkaldy-Willis 1985).

Several recent case studies have described successful treatment of patients with low back pain and sciatica in the presence of a confirmed disc herniation (Cox et al 1993, Hession and Donald 1993, Zhao and Feng 1997, Bergmann and Jongeward 1998, Polkinghorn and Colloca 1998). In a RCT for patients with low-back-related sciatica, Bronfort et al (2000) compared medical care, chiropractic care, and epidural steroid injections. All 3 groups showed substantial improvement at 12 weeks, with bothersomeness of leg symptoms the most responsive outcome.

In a prospective study of 27 patients with MRI-documented, symptomatic disc herniations of either the cervical or lumbar spine, 80% (22) of the patients reported a good clinical outcome and in 63% (17), there was either a reduction or complete resorption of the disc (Ben Eliyahu 1996). In a case series of consecutive patients, 71 patients presented with low back pain and radiating leg pain clinically diagnosed as lumbar disc herniations. Subjective improvement reported by the patient, ROM, and nerve root tension signs were used to assess improvement. Of the 59 patients who received a course of treatment, 90% reported improvement. The authors conclude that non-operative treatment including manipulation may be effective and safe for the treatment of back and radiating leg pain (Stern et al 1995).

In studies on the use of manipulation in the presence of an intervertebral disc herniation, many of the authors indicate preference for the use of a modified manipulation procedure (Cox et al 1993, Polkinghorn and Colloca 1998, Polkinghorn 1998). However, others conclude that side posture manipulation is both safe and effective for lumbar disc herniation (Cassidy et al 1993). Burton et al (2000) compared manipulation with chemonucleolysis for symptomatic lumbar disc hernation. Manipulation produced a statistically significant greater improvement in the early weeks, but by 12 months there was no significant difference between the groups.

Based on the available evidence, it is not yet possible to unequivocally state that spinal manipulation is an effective treatment for disc herniation and sciatica. It is, however, a reasonable option that can be considered in the conservative management of such conditions.

Neck pain

After low back pain, neck pain and headaches are the most common complaints for which SMT has been recommended. This has primarily been based on descriptive clinical studies and large case series (see Bronfort 1992). These case series cover an extremely broad and often poorly defined group of patients with cervical and thoracic pain and cervicogenic and migraine headaches. These reports have been universally enthusiastic but without controls or even proper research protocols. There are, in addition, isolated case reports of patients with confirmed cervical disc herniation that responded to cervical manipulation (Ben Eliyahu 1994, Polkinghorn 1998).

The few prospective controlled clinical trials performed have covered a wide variety of conditions and outcome parameters. Parker et al (1978) and Hoyt et al (1979) reported significant improvement in headache severity and frequency when compared to controls but not in all parameters. Brodin (1982) and Howe et al (1983) reported decreased neck pain following manipulation when compared with analgesics or no treatment. In addition, Howe et al (1983) described increased cervical rotation following manipulation. Bitterli (1977), on the other hand, did not show a change in headache following mobilization, and Sloop et al (1982) failed to show improvement in neck pain following a single manipulation.

Several literature reviews have evaluated the efficacy and complications of cervical spine manual therapy. Hurwitz et al (1996) concluded that cervical SMT and mobilization probably provide at least some short-term benefits for some patients with neck pain and headaches. Aker et al (1996) concluded that there had not been sufficient studies to adequately prove the effectiveness of any treatment approach. Gross et al (1996) conclude that the best available evidence supports the use of manual therapies in combination with other treatments for short-term relief of neck pain.

Cassidy et al (1992) compared the immediate results of SMT to mobilization in 100 consecutive outpatients suffering from unilateral neck pain with referral to the trapezius muscles. The patients received either a single high-velocity, low-amplitude, rotational manipulation (n=52) or mobilization in the form of muscle-energy technique (n=48). The results show that both treatments increase range of motion, but manipulation has a significantly greater effect on pain intensity. Eighty-five percent of the patients receiving SMT and 69% of the mobilized patients reported pain relief immediately after treatment. However, the decrease in pain intensity was greater (1.5 times) in the manipulated group. A randomized, prospective clinical trial by Jordan et al (1998) included 119 patients with neck pain of greater than 3 months' duration. All three treatment interventions (intensive training of the cervical musculature, a physiotherapy regimen, and chiropractic treatment) demonstrated meaningful improvement in all primary effect parameters.

Polkinghorn (1998) also describes the use of the Activator Adjusting Instrument (AAI) in the case of a cervical disc herniation that had failed to respond to manual manipulation of the spine. The author suggests that instrument-delivered adjustments may provide benefit in cases in which manual manipulation causes an exacerbation of the symptoms. Ben Eliyahu (1994) reports on three cases of patients with documented cervical disc herniations who responded to chiropractic management and manipulative therapy.

Headaches

Several recent studies have looked at the efficacy of SMT in the treatment of headaches. In a RCT, 53 patients suffering from frequent headaches were randomized into two groups (Nilsson et al 1997). Twenty-eight received high-velocity, low-amplitude cervical manipulation and 25 received low-level laser in the upper cervical region and deep friction massage in the lower cervical/upper thoracic region. Results showed a statistically significant decrease in the use of analgesics (36%) in the manipulation groups, with no change in the soft tissue group. In addition, the number of headache hours per day decreased by 69% in the manipulation group, compared with 37% in the soft tissue group. Finally, headache intensity per episode decreased by 36% in the manipulation group, compared with 17% in the soft tissue group. The authors conclude that SMT has a significant positive effect in cases of cervicogenic headache. In a similar earlier study, Nilsson (1995) demonstrated a reduction in symptoms in all outcome measures following manipulation. However, no statistically significant difference was seen between groups.

Vernon (1995) identified nine studies of manipulation for tension-type headaches reporting quantitative outcomes. Of these, four were RCTs and five were case series designs. Outcomes ranged from good to excellent. The studies cited indicate that manipulation seems to be better than no treatment and/or some types of mobilization and ice. It also seems to be equivalent to amitryptiline but with greater durability of effect. Only three studies on migraine headaches were identified, of which only one was an RCT. Outcomes ranged from fair to very good. The author states that, although there is a limited number of studies regarding the efficacy of SMT in the treatment of headache, the overall results are encouraging.

Boline et al (1995) reported on a RCT comparing SMT to amitryptiline for the treatment of chronic tension-type headaches. A total of 150 patients with a diagnosis of tension-type headaches of at least 3 months' duration and a frequency of at least once per week were randomized into two groups: 6 weeks of SMT provided by a chiropractor, and 6 weeks of amitriptyline administered by a medical physician. During the treatment period, both groups improved at very similar rates in all primary outcomes. Amitryptiline was slightly more effective in reducing pain at the end of the treatment period but was associated with more side effects. Four weeks after the cessation of treatment, however, the patients who received SMT experienced a sustained therapeutic benefit in all major outcomes in contrast to the patients who received amitryptiline, who reverted to baseline values.

Mechanisms of pain relief by massage and manipulation

The exact mechanism by which massage and manipulation relieve pain has been the subject of a great deal of debate but relatively little experimentation. The problem, in part, has been the difficulty of isolating the primary cause of spinal pain. For virtually every theory on the cause of spinal pain, there has been a corresponding theory as to how manipulation might help. The following are the more prominent theories under debate.

Change in pain threshold

Since many of the effects of manipulation are immediate (Glover et al 1974, Hoehler et al 1981), some investigators feel that manipulation may increase the pain threshold. Terrett and Vernon (1984) measured tolerance to electrically induced pain in paraspinal tissues before and after spinal manipulation and before and after inducing joint play. Both groups showed increases in pain tolerance but the increase was significantly higher in the manipulation group. Vernon et al (1985) reported a small but significant increase in subjects undergoing spinal manipulation. Christian et al (1988) and Sanders et al (1990), however, were not able to confirm these results.

Relief of muscle pain or spasm

Both manipulation and massage are thought to reduce muscle spasms. Cyriax (1971) has stated that deep friction separates adhesions and restores movement between individual muscle fibres. Wakim (1980) describes the effects of massage as relieving muscle fatigue from overexertion by improving circulation and removing waste products.

It has been proposed that manipulation results in stretch of the muscle and a subsequent reflex relaxation of the muscle. A number of studies (Diebert and England 1972, Grice 1974, Grice and Tschumi 1985, Shambaugh 1987) report decreased muscle activity following manipulation, however, these studies all suffer from small sample size and methodological problems and are not conclusive. A recent study by Zhu et al (1993) reports normalization of magnetically induced muscle contraction cortical-evoked responses following manipulation and suggests that this may reflect changes in muscle spindle activity. Keller and Colloca (2000) suggest that altered muscle function may be a short-term therapeutic effect of SMT.

Improved circulation

The erythema that follows massage is presumed to be due to an increase in blood flow, which has been extrapolated to suggest that massage removes waste products and promotes healing. A number of individuals have reported measuring increased circulation from various massage techniques (Skull 1945, Wakim et al 1949).

The early research of Starling (1894), in which the role of muscle contraction on lymph flow was demonstrated, is often quoted to suggest that massage, passive motion, and exercise may have their primary effect on lymphatic drainage. A few researchers (Elkins et al 1953, Wakim et al 1955) have demonstrated that massage and compression of an oedematous extremity can increase lymph flow and reduce oedema. Extrapolation of these theories to the massage of areas of tenderness in muscles and ligaments, however, has yet to be demonstrated.

Reduction in disc protrusion

This theory, proposed by Cyriax (1971), was based partially on the observations of Matthews and Yates (1969). Many of the traction–distraction techniques have also been proposed on the basis of a presumed effect on the intervertebral disc (Cox 1980). There remains, however, considerable controversy concerning this theory. Clinical studies by Chrisman et al (1964) and Cassidy and Kirkaldy-Willis (1985) have demonstrated that patients with demonstrated disc herniation respond less favourably to manipulation. In contrast, several recent studies have provided support for the practice of using SMT in cases of intervertebral disc herniation (Cox et al 1993, Hession and Donald 1993, Ben Eliyahu 1994, Stern et al 1995, Bergmann and Jongeward 1998).

Changes in posterior joint function

Pathology of the posterior facets and its relationship to posture and leg length have been studied intensively by Giles and Taylor (1982, 1984, 1985). The discovery of intra-articular synovial protrusions with nerve endings containing substance P has led to the suggestion that protrusions may become entrapped within the joint, resulting in pain. Giles (1986) has suggested that manipulation may relieve this entrapment and any resulting muscle spasm. Other anatomists (Bogduk and Jell 1985), however, are not as yet convinced that such entrapment occurs. Cramer et al (2000) demonstrated separation (gapping) of the zygapophyseal joints with lumbar side-posture spinal manipulation.

Increased range of motion

By far the most popular theory regarding the effect of manipulation is that it increases range of motion (see Fig. 32.1). According to this theory, spinal or peripheral joint motion can become restricted, and such restrictions (fixations or blockage) can be detected by palpation and other examination techniques. In a relationship between pain and ROM in the cervical spine, 100 consecutive patients with unilateral neck pain without neurological deficits were studied (Cassidy et al 1992). Fifty-two patients received a single cervical manipulation, while 48 received mobilization. The results showed an increase in all planes of post-treatment ROM and a decrease in post-treatment pain scores. The study suggests a significant relationship between a decrease in pain and an increase in cervical motion.

One mechanism by which joint motion may be restricted is the shortening of ligamentous structures. The goal of treatment in this situation is the stretching of these tissues. In another mechanism, joints can be restricted through pathology in the bony elements themselves (e.g., degenerative spondylosis). It is generally assumed that manipulation will not result in any change in this form of restriction but instead is aimed at any concomitant ligamentous or muscular changes. Next, limitation of joint play in the neutral position or at some point in the ROM may restrict movement. Such joint play is usually associated with accessory movements felt to be essential for smooth motion of a joint. Treatment is directed at restoring the joint play. Combinations of these methods of restricting ROM of a joint are also thought to occur.

The exact mechanism through which restricted motion can cause pain is not clear and is probably multifactorial. Movement in the joint can stretch strained ligaments or pull on contracted muscles, resulting in pain. Restricted motion may also reduce nutrition to the intervertebral disc or joint cartilage, resulting in breakdown of these tissues and inflammation (Akeson et al 1980, Holm and Nachemson 1982).

There is a growing body of evidence that manipulation can increase spinal ROM (Evans et al 1978, Rasmussen 1979, Nwuga 1982, Waagen et al 1986). Howe et al (1983) demonstrated increased rotation and lateral flexion of the neck when compared to controls. It appears, however, that only certain directions of movement show increased range after manipulation. Jirout (1972a, b) reported changes in ROM. Several authors have noted an increase in straight leg raising following manipulation (Fisk 1979; Buerger 1978, 1979), and Lehman and McGill (1999) demonstrated changes in spine kinematics following manipulation.

Psychological effects of manipulation

The growing recognition of the close relationship between psychosocial and psychological factors and back pain with its related disability has resulted in a closer look at the psychological effects of manipulation. Most patients and their physicians who offer this modality have a strong, enthusiastic belief in the effectiveness of manipulation. Furthermore, there is confidence in a physician who uses his or her hands to 'find' the pain and then apply a treatment directly to the painful area. In addition, there is the soothing effect of laying on of hands and the natural empathy and concern commonly found in practitioners of manipulation.

There are now some data that actually document these changes. Kane et al (1974) were the first to demonstrate that patients were more satisfied when chiropractors took time to explain their opinions and make patients feel welcome. Hsieh et al (1992) have furthermore shown that not only are patients' confidence levels for massage and manipulation higher than for TMS and corsets, but also that the confidence levels increase with ongoing treatment. Lehman and McGill (2001) suggest that the response to manipulation is variable and dependent upon the individual, with the largest changes seen in those patients in the most pain.

Exercise

Exercise has long been a fundamental tool in the treatment of musculoskeletal pain. While a number of different exercise approaches are utilized, in general they all target the following objectives: decreasing pain, strengthening weak muscles, decreasing mechanical stress on spinal structures, improving fitness levels, stabilizing hypermobile segments, improving posture, improving mobility, and 'when all else fails' (Jackson and Brown 1983). Another reason for using exercise, perhaps the most important of all, is to provide patients with some control over their situation.

Exercise techniques

There are a number of different schools of thought regarding the most appropriate technique or exercise method. Unfortunately, there are very few studies comparing the techniques and they are often recommended for their theoretical effect. The most divisive opinions surround the use of exercise for low back pain. A discussion of the different exercise approaches to this condition is therefore of interest.

Flexion vs extension exercises

While the precise mechanism remains unclear, it has long been assumed that there is a relationship between posture and back pain. Both Fahrni (1976) and Williams (1974) felt that back pain was largely due to the lordotic curve in the lumbar spine. Consequently, Williams developed a series of exercises to reduce the lumbar lordosis and thereby eliminate back pain. This was accomplished by increasing the strength of the abdominal and gluteal muscles. In contrast, McKenzie (1985) attributed the development of back pain to a loss of lumbar extension and to frequency of flexion. He introduced a treatment protocol that involved the use of exercises that employed extending the back. These exercises initially were targeted at producing extension of the lumbar spine. However, the ultimate goal of the McKenzie programme was a full ROM in all directions.

Stabilization exercises

In the past few years, the use of stabilization exercises has become popular (Saal 1992, Robison 1992). The goal of stabilization exercises (also known as 'stabilization training' and 'sensory motor stimulation') is to increase the role of the trunk musculature in protecting the spine. Hyman and Liebenson (1996) state that stabilization exercises train a patient to control posturally destabilizing forces. Examples of such basic exercises include pelvic tilts, bridges, trunk curls, and lunges.

Strength training

While there is not much agreement on which muscles need to be strengthened, or which training method is best, the use of exercises to strengthen weak muscles is a common approach in the treatment of patients with back pain. In recent years, the introduction of sophisticated strength-training devices using computer-assisted technology has become popular (Mooney 1979, Manniche et al 1991, Timm 1994). Dynamic, strength-training exercises use a variety of tools including isotonic progressive resistance exercise (PRE), isometric training, and isokinetic training. While there may be no clear winner in terms of the most effective form of strength training, it would appear that these programmes enable patients to regain strength and function while providing sufficient feedback to encourage compliance.

Aerobic exercise

Patients with back pain and other complaints often find that aerobic activities such as walking, cycling, or swimming improve their conditions and overall health. In a randomized, controlled study of the use of walking versus other physical methods (heat, cold, massage, relaxation, and distraction), Ferrell et al (1997) demonstrated that fitness walking can improve overall pain management in elderly patients with chronic musculoskeletal problems.

Effectiveness

Recently, a number of studies have attempted to evaluate the effectiveness of various exercise regimens for specific conditions. The results of this research have been conflicting, certain studies showing exercise to be effective while others have not demonstrated any significant effect.

In a blinded review of RCTs, Koes et al (1992b) state that no conclusion can be drawn about whether exercise therapy is any better than any other form of therapy for back pain or whether any specific form of exercise therapy is more effective. A recent study of patients with acute back pain compared the use of bedrest (2 days), back-mobilizing exercises, and a control group consisting of the continuation of ordinary activities as tolerated (Malmivera et al 1995). Contrary to expectations, continuing with ordinary activities within the limits permitted by the pain led to a more rapid recovery.

The effect of exercise appears to vary with the chronicity of the symptoms. In a systematic review of RCTs, Van Tulder et al (1997) concluded that there was strong evidence of the ineffectiveness of exercise therapy for acute low back pain and for its effectiveness in chronic low back pain. Similarly, in a criteria-based review, Faas (1996) concluded that exercise therapy is ineffective for acute back pain, whereas exercise with a graded activity programme may benefit those with subacute back pain and intensive exercising may be of benefit for those with chronic pain.

A number of studies have looked at the value of specific exercise programmes. A recent study to evaluate the effectiveness of extension in the treatment of acute low back pain showed no significant benefit over conventional care (Underwood and Morgan 1998). Dettori et al (1995) concluded that there was no difference for any outcomes between flexion or extension exercises, but that either was more effective than no exercise at all. Similarly, Elnaggar et al (1991) concluded that both flexion and extension exercises were equally effective in relieving back pain severity, but the flexion exercises had an advantage in increasing mobility in the sagittal plane.

Several investigators have attempted to evaluate the usefulness of stabilization exercises. O'Sullivan et al (1998) demonstrated a beneficial effect from a 10-week programme of specific stabilizing exercises in the treatment of chronic back pain. The benefits were maintained at 30 months. In a study of stabilization exercises, Nelson et al (1995) demonstrated that 76% of patients completing the programme had excellent or good results. At 1-year follow-up, 94% reported maintaining their improvement. Results in the control group were significantly poorer in all areas surveyed except employment.

Several studies have attempted to evaluate the use of dynamic strength-training programmes. Manniche (1996) claims that the most important factor that influences the effect of exercise in chronic low back patients is the administration of a high training stimulus (number of repetitions of the exercise, exercise resistance, and the total number of sessions). He states that the poor results seen in many studies may be due to the low dosage or short duration of the exercise programme. In a study of exercise following first-time lumbar disc surgery, Manniche (1995) also noted that, while exercise programmes are generally free of side effects, high-dosage exercises with training periods lasting at least 12–16 sessions are of critical importance for success. Johannsen et al (1995) compared the use of two training models: intensive training of muscle endurance; and muscle training, including coordination. Pain score, disability score, and spinal mobility improved in both training groups without differences between the groups.

Hansen et al (1993) showed that subgroups of patients responded favourably to different treatments. Physiotherapy appeared superior for the male participants, whereas the female patients responded best to exercises. Exercises also appeared more beneficial for those patients with sedentary or light job functions. Whether these observations represent anatomical or physiologic differences or simply show patient preferences is not clear. The use of high-intensity, dynamic back extension and abdominal exercises was compared with a more traditional programme of mild, general mobility-improving exercises (Manniche et al 1993). Patients who did the high-intensity exercises experienced greater results with regard to disability index and work capabilities. However, no significant differences were seen in pain or any objective measurements.

Manniche et al (1991) looked at the effect of dynamic back extensor exercises over a 3-month intensive training programme. A total of 105 patients were divided into three groups: an intensive training programme of dynamic back extensor exercises; a group that underwent one-fifth of the treatment group's exercise programme; and a control group in which treatment consisted of heat, massage, and mild exercise. A statistically significant difference was found in favour of the treatment group at 3 months follow-up, and those patients in the treatment group for at least once a week for the entire 1-year follow-up period were the only patients with any significant improvement.

The use of exercise in patients with low back pain requires further study. The literature, so far, suggests that: (1) there is a short-term positive effect from a variety of exercises; (2) those who exercise regularly have a better chance of maintaining any derived benefit; (3) there does not appear to be one particular form of exercise that is clearly superior to any other form; (4) intensity and frequency of exercise are probably more important than the type of exercise performed; and (5) maintaining normal daily work and play activities by avoiding debility may be as effective as a formal exercise programme.

References

Aker PD, Gross AR, Goldsmith CH, Peloso P 1996 Conservative management of mechanical neck pain: Systematic overview and meta-analysis. British Medical Journal 313: 1291–1296

Akeson WH, Amiel D, Woo S 1980 Immobility effects on synovial joints. The pathomechanics of joint contracture. Biorheology 17: 95–110

Andersson GB, Lucente T, Davis AM, Kappler RE, Lipton JA, Leurgans S 1999 A comparison of osteopathic spinal manipulation with standard care for patients with low back pain. New England Journal of Medicine 341(19): 1426–1431

Ben Eliyahu DJ 1994 Chiropractic management and manipulative therapy for MRI documented cervical disk herniation. Journal of Manipulative and Physiological Therapeutics 17(3): 177–185

Ben Eliyahu DJ 1996 Magnetic resonance imaging and clinical follow-up: study of 27 patients receiving chiropractic care for cervical and lumbar disc herniations. Journal of Manipulative and Physiological Therapeutics 19(9): 597–606

Bergmann TF, Jongeward BV 1998 Manipulative therapy in lower back pain with leg pain and neurological deficit. Journal of Manipulative and Physiological Therapeutics 21(4): 288–294

Berquist-Ullman M, Larsson U 1977 Acute low back pain in industry. Acta Orthopaedica Scandinavica 170(suppl): 11–117

Bitterli J 1977 Zur Objektivierung der manual therapeutischen. Beeinflussbarkeit des spondylogenen Kopfschmerzes. Nervenarzt 48: 259–262

Blomberg S, Svardsudd K, Tibblin G 1994 A randomized study of manual therapy with steroid injections in low-back pain. Telephone interview follow-up of pain, disability, recovery and drug consumption. European Spine Journal 3(5): 246–254

Bogduk N, Jell G 1985 The theoretical pathology of acute locked back: a basis for manipulation. Manual Medicine 1: 78–82

Boline PD, Kassak K, Bronfort G, Nelson C, Anderson AV 1995 Spinal manipulation vs amitriptyline for the treatment of chronic tension-type headaches: a randomized clinical trial. Journal of Manipulative and Physiological Therapeutics 18(3): 148–154

Breen AC 1977 Chiropractors and the treatment of back pain. Rheumatology and Rehabilitation 16: 46–53

Brodin H 1982 Cervical pain and mobilization. Manual Medicine 20: 90–94

Bronfort G 1992 Effectiveness of spinal manipulation and adjustment. In: Haldeman S (ed) Principles and practice of chiropractic. Appleton and Lange, Norwalk, CT, pp 415–441
Bronfort G, Evans RL, Anderson AV, Schellhas KP, Garvey TA, Marks RA, Bittell S 2000 Nonoperative treatments for sciatica: a pilot for a randomized clinical trial. Journal of Manipulative and Physiological Therapeutics 23(8): 536–544
Brunarski DJ 1984 Clinical trials of spinal manipulation: a critical appraisal and review of the literature. Journal of Manipulative and Physiological Therapeutics 7: 243–249
Buerger AA 1978 A clinical trial of rotational manipulation. International Association for the Study of Pain, Second World Congress on Pain, Montreal, Canada. Pain Abstracts 1: 248
Buerger AA 1979 A clinical trial of spinal manipulation. Federation Proceedings 38: 1250
Burton AK, Tillotson KM, Cleary J 2000 Single-blind randomized controlled trial of chemonucleolysis and manipulation in the treatment of symptomatic lumbar disc herniation. European Spine Journal 9(3): 202–207
Cassidy JD, Kirkaldy-Willis WH 1985 Spinal manipulation for the treatment of chronic low back and leg pain: an observational study. In: Buerger AA, Greenman PE (eds) Empirical approaches to the validation of spinal manipulation. Thomas, Springfield, IL, pp 119–148
Cassidy JD, Lopes AA, Yong-Hing K 1992 The immediate effect of manipulation versus mobilization on pain and range of motion in the cervical spine: a randomized controlled trial. Journal of Manipulative and Physiological Therapeutics 15(9): 570–575
Cassidy JD, Thiel HW, Kirkaldy-Willis WH 1993 Side posture manipulation for lumbar intervertebral disk herniation. Journal of Manipulative and Physiological Therapeutics 16(2): 96–103
Chrisman OD, Mittnacht A, Snook GA 1964 A study of the results following rotatory manipulation in the lumbar intervertebral disc syndrome. Journal of Bone and Joint Surgery 46A: 517–524
Christian GF, Stanton GJ, Sissons D et al 1988 Immunoreactive ACTH, beta-endorphin and cortisol levels in plasma following spinal manipulative therapy. Spine 13: 1411–1417
Coplans CW 1978 The conservative treatment of low back pain. In: Helfet AJ, Gruebel Lee DM (eds) Disorders of the lumbar spine. Lippincott, Philadelphia, pp 145–183
Cox JM 1980 Low back pain, 3rd edn. Self-published, Fort Wayne, IN
Cox JM, Hazen LJ, Mungovan M 1993 Distraction manipulation reduction of an L5–S1 disk herniation. Journal of Manipulative and Physiological Therapeutics 16(5): 342
Coxhead CE, Inskip H, Meade TW, North WRS, Troug JDG 1981 Multicentre trial of physiotherapy in the management of sciatic symptoms. Lancet 1: 1065–1068
Coyer AB, Curwen IHM 1955 Low back pain treated by manipulation: a controlled series. British Medical Journal March 19: 705–707
Cramer GD, Tuck NR Jr, Knudsen JT, Fonda SD, Schliesser JS, Fournier JT, Patel P 2000 Effects of side-posture positioning and side-posture adjusting on the lumbar zygapophyseal joints as evaluated by magnetic resonance imaging: a before and after study with randomization. Journal of Manipulative Physiological Therapeutics 23(6): 380–394
Cyriax J 1971 Textbook of orthopaedic medicine, diagnosis of soft tissue lesions, vol 1, 6th edn. Baillière Tindall, London
Dettori JR, Bullock SH, Sutlive TG, Franklin RJ, Patience T 1995 The effects of spinal flexion and extension exercises and their associated postures in patients with acute low back pain. Spine 20(21): 2303–2312
Diebert P, England R 1972 Electromyographic studies. Part 1: consideration in the evaluation of osteopathic therapy. Journal of the American Osteopathic Association 72: 162–169
Doran DML, Newell DJ 1975 Manipulation in treatment of low back pain: a multicentre study. British Madical Journal 2: 161–164
Edwards BC 1969 Low back pain resulting from lumbar spine conditions. A comparison of treatment results. Australian Journal of Physiotherapy 15: 104–110
Elkins EC, Herrick JF, Grindlay JH, Mann FC, DeForrest RE 1953 Effect of various procedures on the flow of lymph. Archives of Physical Medicine 34: 31
Elnaggar IM, Nordin M, Sheikhzadeh A, Parnianpour M, Kahanovitz N 1991 Effects of spinal flexion and extension exercises on low-back pain and spinal mobility in chronic mechanical low-back pain patients. Spine 16(8): 967–972
Evans DP, Burke MS, Lloyd KN, Roberts EE, Roberts GM 1978 Lumbar spinal manipulation on trial. Part 1: clinical assessment. Rheumatology and Rehabilitation 17: 46–53
Faas A 1996 Exercises: which ones are worth trying, for which patients, and when? Spine 21(24): 2874–2878
Fahrni WH 1976 Backache and primal posture. Musqueam, Vancouver
Farrell JP, Twomey LT 1982 Acute low back pain. Comparison of two conservative treatment approaches. Medical Journal of Australia 1: 160–164
Ferrell BA, Josephson KR, Pollan AM, Loy S, Ferrell BR 1997 A randomized trial of walking versus physical methods for chronic pain management. Aging (Milano) 9(1–2): 99–105
Fisk JW 1979 A controlled trial of manipulation in a selected group of patients with low back pain favouring one side. New Zealand Medical Journal 645: 288–291
Gibson T, Grahame R, Harkness J et al 1985 Controlled comparison of short wave diathermy treatment with osteopathic treatment in non-specific low back pain. Lancet 1: 1258–1260
Giles LGF 1986 Lumbosacral and cervical zygapophyseal joint inclusions. Manual Medicine 2: 89–92
Giles LG, Muller R 1999 Chronic spinal pain syndromes: a clinical pilot trial comparing acupuncture, a nonsteroidal anti-inflammatory drug, and spinal manipulation. Journal of Manipulative and Physiological Therapeutics 22(6): 376–381
Giles LGF, Taylor JR 1982 Intra-articular synovial protrusions in the lower lumbar apophyseal joints. Bulletin of the Hospital for Joint Diseases Orthopaedic Institute 42: 248–254
Giles LGF, Taylor JR 1984 The effect of postural scoliosis on lumbar apophyseal joints. Scandinavian Journal of Rheumatology 13: 209–220
Giles LGF, Taylor JR 1985 Osteoarthritis in human cadaveric lumbo-sacral zygapophyseal joints. Journal of Manipulative and Physiological Therapeutics 8: 239–243
Glover JR, Morris JG, Khosla T 1974 Back pain: a randomized clinical trial of rotational manipulation of the trunk. British Journal of Industrial Medicine 31: 59–64
Glover JR, Morris JG, Khosla T 1977 A randomized clinical trial of rotational manipulation of the trunk. In: Buerger AA, Tobis JS (eds) Approaches to the validation of manipulation therapy. Thomas, Springfield, IL, pp 271–283
Godfrey CM, Morgan PP, Schatzker J 1984 A randomized trial of manipulation for low back pain in a medical setting. Spine 9: 301–304
Goodridge JP 1981 Muscle energy technique: definition, explanation, methods of procedure. Journal of the American Osteopathic Association 81: 249
Greco MA 1953 Chiropractic technique illustrated. Jarl, New York
Greenland S, Reisbord L, Haldeman S, Buerger AA 1979 Controlled clinical trials of manipulation: a review and proposal. Journal of Occupational Medicine 22: 670–676
Grice AA 1974 Muscle tonus changes following manipulation. Journal of the Canadian Chiropractic Association 19(4): 29–31
Grice AA, Tschumi PC 1985 Pre- and post-manipulation lateral bending radiographic study and relation to muscle function of

the low back. Annals of the Swiss Chiropractic Association 8: 149–165
Gross AR, Aker PD, Quartly C 1996 Manual therapy in the treatment of neck pain. Rheumatic Disease Clinics of North America 22(3): 579–598
Haldeman S 1978 The clinical basis for discussion of mechanisms of manipulative therapy. In: Korr IM (ed) Neurobiologic mechanisms in manipulative therapy. Plenum Press, New York, pp 53–75
Haldeman S 1980 Modern developments in the principles and practice of chiropractic. Appleton-Century-Crofts, New York
Haldeman S 1992 Principles and practice of chiropractic. Appleton-Century-Crofts, New York
Hansen FR, Bendix T, Skov P et al 1993 Intensive, dynamic back-muscle exercises, conventional physiotherapy, or placebo-control treatment of low-back pain. A randomized, observer-blind trial. Spine 18(1): 98–108
Hession EF, Donald GD 1993 Treatment of multiple lumbar disk herniations in an adolescent athlete utilizing flexion distraction and rotational manipulation. Journal of Manipulative and Physiological Therapeutics 16(3): 185–192
Hoehler FK, Tobis JS, Buerger AA 1981 Spinal manipulation for low back pain. Journal of the American Medical Association 245: 1835–1838
Hofkosh JM 1985 Classical massage. In: Basmajian JV (ed) Manipulation, traction and massage, 3rd edn. Williams & Wilkins, Baltimore
Holm S, Nachemson A 1982 Variations in the nutrition of canine intervertebral disc induced by motion. Orthopaedic Transactions 6: 48
Howe DH, Newcombe RG, Wade MT 1983 Manipulation of the cervical spine—a pilot study. Journal of the Royal College of General Practitioners 33: 574–579
Hoyt WH, Schafter F, Bard DA et al 1979 Osteopathic manipulation in the treatment of muscle contraction headache. Journal of the American Osteopathic Association 78: 325–332
Hsieh CY, Phillips RB, Adams AH, Pope MH 1992 Functional outcomes of low back pain: comparison of four treatment groups in a randomized controlled trial. Journal of Manipulative Physiological Therapeutics 15(1): 4–9
Hurwitz EL, Aker PD, Adams AH, Meeker WC, Shekelle PG 1996 Manipulation and mobilization of the cervical spine. A systematic review of the literature. Spine 21(15): 1746–1759
Hyman J, Liebenson C 1996 Spinal stabilization exercise program. In: Liebenson C (ed) Rehabilitation of the spine: a practitioner's manual. Williams & Wilkins, Baltimore, pp 293–318
Jackson CP, Brown MD 1983 Is there a role for exercise in the treatment of patients with low back pain? Clinical Orthopaedics and Related Research 179: 39–45
Jayson MIV 1986 A limited role for manipulation. British Medical Journal 293: 1454–1455
Jirout J 1972a The effect of mobilization of the segmental blockade on the sagittal component of the reaction on lateral flexion of the cervical spine. Neuroradiology 3: 210–215
Jirout J 1972b Changes in the sagittal component of the reaction of the cervical spine to lateroflexion after manipulation of blockade. Cesckoslovenska Neurologie a Neurochirurgie 35: 175–180
Johannsen F, Remvig L, Kryger P et al 1995 Exercises for chronic low back pain: a clinical trial. Journal of Orthopaedic and Sports Physical Therapy 22(2): 52–59
Jordan A, Bendix T, Nielsen H, Hansen FR, Host D, Winkel A 1998 Intensive training, physiotherapy, or manipulation for patients with chronic neck pain. A prospective, single-blinded, randomized clinical trial. Spine 23(3): 311–318
Kane R, Olsen D, Leymaster C 1974 Manipulating the patient: a comparison of the effectiveness of physician and chiropractor care. Lancet 1: 1333
Keller TS, Colloca CJ 2000 Mechanical force spinal manipulation increases trunk muscle strength assessed by electromyography: a comparative clinical trial. Journal of Manipulative and Physiological Therapeutics 23(9): 585–595
Kimberly PE 1979 Outline of osteopathic manipulative procedures. Kirksville College of Osteopathic Medicine, Kirksville
Koes BW, Bouter LM, Van Mameren H et al 1992a A blinded randomized clinical trial of manual therapy and physiotherapy for chronic back and neck complaints: physical outcome measures. Journal of Manipulative and Physiological Therapeutics 15(1): 16–23
Koes BW, Bouter LM, Van Mameren H et al 1992b The effectiveness of manual therapy, physiotherapy, and treatment by the general practitioner for nonspecific back and neck complaints. A randomized clinical trial. Spine 17(1): 28–35
Koes BW, Bouter LM, Van Mameren H et al 1993 A randomized clinical trial of manual therapy and physiotherapy for persistent back and neck complaints: subgroup analysis and relationship between outcome measures. Journal of Manipulative and Physiological Therapeutics 16(4): 211–219
Koes BW, Bouter LM, Van der Heijden GJ 1995 Methodological quality of randomized clinical trials on treatment efficacy in low back pain. Spine 20(2): 228–235
Koes BW, Assendelft WJ, Van der Heijden GJ, Bouter LM 1996 Spinal manipulation for low back pain. An updated systematic review of randomized clinical trials. Spine 21(24): 2860–2871
Leboeuf-Yde C, Hennius B, Rudber E, Leufvenmark P, Thunman M 1997 Chiropractic in Sweden: a short description of patients and treatment. Journal of Manipulative and Physiological Therapeutics 20(8): 507–510
Lehman GJ, McGill SM 1999 The influence of a chiropractic manipulation on lumbar kinematics and electromyography during simple and complex tasks: a case study. Journal of Manipulative and Physiological Therapeutics 22(9): 576–581
Lehman GJ, McGill SM 2001 Spinal manipulation causes variable spine kinematic and trunk muscle electromyographic responses. Clinical Biomechanics 16(4): 293–299
Lewith GT, Turner GMT 1982 Retrospective analysis of the management of acute low back pain. Practitioner 226: 1614–1618
Logan HB 1950 Textbook of Logan basic methods. LBM, St Louis
Maitland GD 1973 Vertebral manipulation, 3rd edn. Butterworth, London
Malmivera A, Hakkinen U, Aro T et al 1995 The treatment of acute low back pain—bed rest, exercises, or ordinary activity? New England Journal of Medicine 332(6): 351–355
Manniche C 1995 Assessment and exercise in low back pain. With special reference to the management of pain and disability following first time lumbar disc surgery. Danish Medical Bulletin 42(4): 301–313
Manniche C 1996 Clinical benefit of intensive dynamic exercises for low back. Scandinavian Journal of Medicine and Science in Sports 6(2): 82–87
Manniche C, Lundberg E, Christensen I, Bentzen L, Hesselsoe G 1991 Intensive dynamic back exercises for chronic low back pain: a clinical trial. Pain 47(1): 53–63
Manniche C, Skall HF, Braendholt L et al 1993 Clinical trial of postoperative dynamic back exercises after first lumbar discectomy. Spine 18(1): 92–97
Matthews JA, Yates DAH 1969 Reduction of lumbar disc prolapse by manipulation. British Medical Journal 20: 696–699
Matthews JA, Mills SB, Jenkins VM et al 1987 Back pain and sciatica: controlled trials of manipulation, traction, sclerosal and epidural injections. British Journal of Rheumatology 26: 416–423
McKenzie R 1985 The lumbar spine: mechanical diagnosis and therapy. Spinal Publications, Wellington, New Zealand

Meade TW, Dyher S, Browne W, Townsend J, Frank AO 1990 Low back pain of mechanical origin: randomized comparison of chiropractic and hospital outpatient treatment. British Medical Journal 300: 1431–1437
Meade TW, Dyer S, Browne W, Frank AO 1995 Randomized comparison of chiropractic and hospital outpatient management for low back pain: results from extended follow up. British Medical Journal 311(7001): 349–351
Mennell J McM 1960 Back pain—diagnosis and treatment using manipulative therapy. Little, Brown, Boston
Mooney V 1979 Surgery and post surgical management of the patient with low back pain. Physical Therapy 59: 1000–1006
Nelson BW, O'Reilly E, Miller M, Hogan M, Wegner JA, Kelly C 1995 The clinical effects of intensive, specific exercise on chronic low back pain: a controlled study of 895 consecutive patients with 1-year follow up. Orthopedics 18(10): 971–981
Nilsson N 1995 A randomized controlled trial of the effect of spinal manipulation in the treatment of cervicogenic headache. Journal of Manipulative and Physiological Therapeutics 18(7): 435–440
Nilsson N, Christensen HW, Hartvigsen J 1997 The effect of spinal manipulation in the treatment of cervicogenic headache. Journal of Manipulative and Physiological Therapeutics 20(5): 326–330
Nwuga VCB 1982 Relative therapeutic efficacy of vertebral manipulation and conventional treatment in back pain management. American Journal of Physical Medicine and Rehabilitation 61: 273–278
Nyberg R 1985 The role of physical therapists in spinal manipulation. In: Basmajian JV (ed) Manipulation, traction and massage, 3rd edn. Williams & Wilkins, Baltimore
Nyiendo J, Haldeman S 1987 A prospective study of 2000 patients attending a chiropractic college teaching unit. Medical Care 25: 516–527
Nyiendo J, Haas M, Goodwin P 2000 Patient characteristics, practice activities, and one-month outcomes for chronic, recurrent low-back pain treated by chiropractors and family medicine physicians: a practice-based feasibility study. Journal of Manipulative and Physiological Therapeutics 23(4): 239–245
Ongley MJ, Klein RG, Droman TA, Eck BC, Hubert LJ 1987 A new approach to the treatment of low back pain. Lancet 2: 143–146
O'Sullivan PB, Twomey L, Allison GTJ 1998 Altered abdominal muscle recruitment in patients with chronic back pain following a specific exercise intervention. Journal of Orthopaedic and Sports Physical Therapy 27(2): 114–124
Ottenbacher K, DiFabio RP 1985 Efficiency of spinal manipulation/mobilization therapy. A meta-analysis. Spine 10: 833–837
Parker GB, Tupling H, Pryor DS 1978 A controlled trial of cervical manipulation for migraine. Australian and New Zealand Journal of Medicine 8: 589–593
Polkinghorn BS 1998 Treatment of cervical disc protrusions via instrumental chiropractic adjustment. Journal of Manipulative and Physiological Therapeutics 21(2): 114–121
Polkinghorn BS, Colloca CJ 1998 Treatment of symptomatic lumbar disc herniation using activator methods chiropractic technique. Journal of Manipulative and Physiological Therapeutics 21(3): 187–196
Pope MH, Phillips RB, Haugh LD, Hsieh CY, MacDonald L, Haldeman S 1994 A prospective randomized three-week trial of spinal manipulation, transcutaneous muscle stimulation, massage and corset in the treatment of subacute low back pain. Spine 19(22): 2571–2577
Rasmussen GG 1979 Manipulation in low back pain: a randomized clinical trial. Manuelle Medizin 1: 8–10
Robison R 1992 The new back school prescription: stabilization training. Part I. Occupational Medicine 7(1): 17–31
Saal JA 1992 The new back school prescription: stabilization training. Part II. Occupational Medicine 7(1): 33–42
Sanders GE, Reinert O, Tepe R, Maloney P 1990 Chiropractic adjustive manipulation on subjects with acute low back pain: visual analog pain scores and plasma beta-endorphin levels. Journal of Manipulative and Physiological Therapeutics 13: 391–395
Shambaugh P 1987 Changes in electrical activity in muscles resulting from chiropractic adjustment: a pilot study. Journal of Manipulative and Physiological Therapeutics 10: 300–303
Shekelle PG, Adams AH, Chassin MR, Hurwitz EC, Brook RH 1992 Spinal manipulation for back pain. Annals of Internal Medicine 117: 590–598
Sims-Williams H, Jayson MIDC, Young SMS, Baddeley H, Collins E 1978 Controlled trial of mobilization and manipulation for patients with low back pain in general practice. British Medical Journal 2: 1338–1340
Sims-Williams H, Jayson MIC, Young SMS, Baddeley H, Collins E 1979 Controlled trial of mobilization and manipulation for patients with low back pain: hospital patients. British Medical Journal 2: 1318–1320
Skull CW 1945 Massage—physiologic basis. Archives of Physical Medicine 261: 159
Sloop PR, Smith DS, Boldenberg SRN, Dore C 1982 Manipulation for chronic neck pain. A double-blind controlled study. Spine 7: 532–535
Starling EH 1894 The influence of mechanical factors on lymph production. Journal of Physiology 16: 224
States AZ 1968 Spinal and pelvic technics. Atlas of chiropractic technic, 2nd edn. National College of Chiropractic, Lombard, IL
Stern PJ, Cote P, Cassidy JDJ 1995 A series of consecutive cases of low back pain with radiating leg pain treated by chiropractors. Journal of Manipulative and Physiological Therapeutics 18(6): 335–342
Stig LC, Nilsson O, Leboeuf-Yde C 2001 Recovery pattern of patients treated with chiropractic spinal manipulative therapy for long-lasting or recurrent low back pain. Journal of Manipulative and Physiological Therapeutics 24(4): 288–291
Terrett ACJ, Vernon H 1984 Manipulation and pain tolerance. A controlled study of the effects of spinal manipulation on paraspinal cutaneous pain tolerance levels. American Journal of Physical Medicine 63: 217–225
Thompson JC 1973 Thompson technique. Thompson, Davenport
Timm KE 1994 A randomized-control study of active and passive treatments for chronic low back pain following L5 laminectomy. Journal of Orthopaedic and Sports Physical Therapy 20(6): 276–286
Travell J 1976 Myofascial trigger points: clinical view. Advances in Pain Research and Therapy 1: 919–926
Triano JJ, McGregor M, Hondras MA, Brennan PC 1995 Manipulative therapy versus education programs in chronic low back pain. Spine 20(8): 948–955
Underwood MR, Morgan J 1998 The use of a back class teaching extension exercises in the treatment of acute low back pain in primary care. Family Practice 15(1): 9–15
Van Tulder MW, Koes BW, Bouter LM 1997 Conservative treatment of acute and chronic nonspecific low back pain. A systematic review of randomized controlled trials of the most common interventions. Spine 22(18): 2128–2156
Vear HJ 1972 A study into the complaints of patients seeking chiropractic care. Journal of the Canadian Chiropractic Association 16: 9–13
Vernon HT 1995 The effectiveness of chiropractic manipulation in the treatment of headache: an exploration in the literature. Journal of Manipulative and Physiological Therapeutics 18(9): 611–617
Vernon HT, Dhami MSI, Annett R 1985 Abstract, Canadian

Foundation for Spinal Research. Symposium of low back pain, Vancouver BC, March 15–16
Waagen GN, Haldeman S, Cook G, Lopez D, DeBoer KF 1986 Short term trial of chiropractic adjustments for the relief of chronic low back pain. Manual Medicine 2: 63–67
Waagen GN, DeBoer K, Hansen J, McGhee D, Haldeman S 1990 A prospective comparative trial of general practice medical care, chiropractic manipulative therapy and sham manipulation in the management of patients with chronic or repetitive low back pain. Abstract, International Society for the Study of the Lumbar Spine, Boston
Wakim KG 1980 Physiologic effects of massage. In: Rogoff JB (ed) Manipulation, massage and traction, 2nd edn. Williams & Wilkins, Baltimore
Wakim KG, Martin GM, Terrier JC, Elkins EC, Krusen EH 1949 The effects of massage on the circulation in normal and paralyzed extremities. Archives of Physical Medicine 30: 135
Wakim KG, Martin GM, Krusen EH 1955 Influence of centripetal rhythmic compression on localized edema of an extremity. Archives of Physical Medicine 36: 98
Waterworth RF, Hunter IA 1985 An open study of diflunisal, conservative and manipulative therapy in the management of acute mechanical low back pain. New Zealand Medical Journal 98: 327–328
Williams PC 1974 Low back and neck pain: causes and conservative treatment. Thomas, Springfield, IL
Wood ED 1974 Beard's massage principles and techniques. Saunders, Philadelphia
Zhao P, Feng TY 1997 Protruded lumbar intervertebral nucleus pulposus in a 12-year-old girl who recovered after nonsurgical treatment: a follow-up case report. Journal of Manipulative and Physiological Therapeutics 20(8): 551–556
Zhu Y, Starr A, Haldeman S, Seffinger MA, Su SH 1993 Paraspinal muscle evoked cerebral potentials in patients with unilateral low back pain. Spine 18(8): 1096–1102

Chapter 33

The placebo response

Patrick D Wall

Introduction

The placebo response is at the heart of understanding pain. It is inevitably a complete paradox to classic theories of pain mechanisms that consider pain to be a reliable sensation signalling injury. The placebo is, by definition, inactive and yet produces analgesia (Beecher 1959, 1968). How can that be?

Examples of the placebo response

Medicine

Analgesics

Thousands of placebo trials have been carried out on analgesics since they are legally obligatory. The correct manner of such trials is discussed in Chap. 26. In a critical repeat analysis of five of their own trials, McQuay et al (1995) describe the problems of variability in such trials. Individual patient placebo scores varied from 0 to 100% of the maximum possible pain relief. The proportion who obtained more than 50% of the maximum possible pain relief with placebo varied from 7 to 37% across the trials while, with the active drugs, the variation was from 5 to 63%. Although trials are formally double blind, it is difficult or impossible to blind the physician's expectation (Gracely et al 1985) and this expectation affects the patient.

A special example of analgesia Harden et al (1996) carried out a double-blind, randomized trial of injected ketorolac or meperidine or saline for acute headache crises. All three treatments produced a very significant reduction of pain ($P = 0.0001$) but there was no significant difference between the three treatments. The reason for the surprise at these results is that both active drugs had previously been shown superior to a placebo in a number of trials. The difference in this paper was that the patients had presented themselves with an acute headache crisis to a busy urban emergency department and were therefore in severe need with a very high expectation of powerfully effective therapy. Their pain dropped from a severe level of 3.5 on the pain index to a mild 1.5 for all three treatments. This example emphasizes the general problem that trials are necessarily carried out on a selected restricted sample and that the situation differs particularly in the patient's expectation.

Narcotics

From the time of Lasagna et al (1954), there have been many comparisons of narcotic analgesia with placebo effects. The subtlety of the phenomenon of the placebo reaction and the skill needed to design an experiment are shown by Benedetti et al (1998). They examined 33 patients after the famously painful operation of thoracotomy and lobectomy for lung cancer. After the operation, the patients were given 0.1 mg buprenorphine boluses at 30-min intervals until the pain was adequately reduced, which required up to six injections. The next day when their pain had returned to a high level, each was given a saline injection and the pain dropped an average of 2.5 points over 1 h.

However, this paper included two considerable advances on previous papers. All patients had given informed consent. An additional 24 patients who had received the same operation and adequate pain relief from postoperative buprenorphine were given no treatment when their pain had reached the same level as the group who received a placebo injection. The pain level of this no-treatment group rose an average of 0.5 points during the 1-h observation period. Therefore, the placebo group had a marked drop of pain while the no-treatment group experienced a pain increase. The second advance of this paper is that the authors examined the sensitivity of the individual patients to the narcotic and correlated this with their placebo response. Those patients whose pain was substantially reduced by small doses of buprenorphine were those who gave the largest placebo responses. Similarly, those patients relatively insensitive to small doses of buprenorphine gave small placebo responses. In another way of measuring the same effect, it was shown that the number of buprenorphine doses needed to establish adequate analgesia related to the strength of a single placebo response so that the strongest placebo reactors had required fewer doses of buprenorphine.

Placebo responses in conditions other than pain

There are many examples of placebo responses in pathological conditions such as asthma, diabetes, emesis, multiple sclerosis, ulcers, and parkinsonism. Similarly, mental states such as anxiety, depression, and insomnia may respond. These are extensively reviewed in White et al (1985) and Turner et al (1980). *Nocebo* ('I will harm') responses occur when unwanted effects are reported after the administration of an inactive therapy. These even happen in trials of analgesics where the subject has been warned of possible side effects such as nausea, dizziness, and headache. In 109 double-blind drug trials, 19% of healthy volunteers reported adverse effects after the placebo. There is a certain humour in these reports when one reads that coffee drinkers drinking decaffeinated coffee in a double-blind crossover study develop a tremor after both drinks, and in a test for drunkenness, 27–29% of the subjects were intoxicated by flavoured water in a crossover study with flavoured ethanol (0.8 ml/kg body weight) (O'Boyle et al 1994). These reports are important because the responses have exactly the same general structure as analgesic placebo responses and yet can hardly all depend on a single mechanism such as the release of endorphins.

Classes of explanation

Affective

Gracely et al (1978) originally proposed that the placebo effect works only on the unpleasantness of pain while leaving the intensity dimension unaffected. However, their experiments represent a special case that does not apply across the board, especially in clinical cases. Evans (1974), in another version of this approach, proposes that the placebo operates by decreasing anxiety. However, the results show that there is a weak and variable interaction with various types of anxiety, and it is not clear that anxiety reduction is not a component of the placebo effect rather than the cause of it. Montgomery and Kirsch (1996) review and discard emotional theories to explain placebos and favour cognitive-expectation mechanisms.

Cognitive

By far the commonest proposal is that the placebo effect depends on the expectation of the subject. There is nothing subtle about this. Placebo reactors can be identified before the trial by simply asking the subject what they expect to be the outcome of the therapy. Those who doubt that a therapy will be effective do not respond to the placebo while those with high expectations do. The very extensive literature on this is reviewed by Bootzin (1985). Lasagna et al (1954) investigated many aspects of postoperative patients who responded to placebos and to analgesic drugs and conclude: 'A positive placebo response indicated a psychological set predisposing to anticipation of pain relief'. They add: 'It is important to appreciate that this same anticipation of pain relief also predisposes to better response, to morphine and other pharmacologically active drugs'. In a trial of two drugs versus placebos on 100 patients, Nash and Zimring (1969) tested specifically for the role of expectation. The two drugs had no effect that would differentiate them from the placebo but there was a strong correlation between the measured expectation and the placebo effect. Expectation is given a number of related names—belief, faith, confidence, enthusiasm, response bias, meaning, credibility, transference, anticipation, etc.—in 30 of the papers in the bibliography of Turner et al (1980).

Expectation is a learned state and therefore young children do not respond to placebos as adults do since they have had neither the time nor the experience to learn. Similarly in adults, the learning of expected effects will depend on culture, background, experience, and personality. A desire to believe, please, and obey the doctor will increase the effect while hostility decreases it. Obviously, part of the expectation of the patient will depend on the expectation, enthusiasm, and charisma of the therapist, and therefore there are many reports on this doctor–patient interaction. Expectation in a laboratory experiment may be more limited than in a clinical setting, which may explain why rates and intensities of placebo effects tend to be less in the laboratory than in the clinic (Beecher 1959).

Conditioning

There are many reports of drug anticipatory responses in animals (Herrnstein 1965, Siegel 1985). These come in two forms. In the first, the animal has been given one or more trials on an active drug and is then subject to a saline injection and proceeds to mimic the behavioural or physiological response observed after the active drug. In the second type, the animal mimics the counteractions which it mobilizes to neutralize the effect of the active compound. For example, if animals have experienced a series of injections of insulin which lower the blood sugar, a saline injection in the same setting as the insulin injection results in a rise of blood sugar, which would be one of the animal's reactions to counteract the insulin-induced decrease (Siegel 1975). In cultures not raised on *Winnie the Pooh, Wind in the Willows*, and *Watership Down*, it is customary to deny animals the luxury of cognitive processing and to ascribe such phenomena to classic Pavlovian conditioning.

This led to the proposal that the human placebo response had the characteristics of a conditioned response (Reiss 1980, Wickramasekera 1980). The idea is that active powerful drugs produce a powerful objective physiological response in the same manner that food produces salivation—the unconditioned stimuli and responses. However, giving the drug is inevitably inadvertently associated with a pattern of other stimuli such as a hypodermic injection by a man in a white coat. It is proposed that these are the equivalent of unconditioned stimuli coupled with the conditioned stimulus. It is then proposed that if these incidentally coupled stimuli are given alone, they will provoke the same response as the original drug, just as in the dog, coupling a bell with food eventually leads to the ability of the bell by itself to provoke salivation. The similarity goes beyond the proposed production of a conditioned response. If a placebo is given repeatedly in some but not all trials, the effect declines. This is a characteristic of Pavlovian responses where simple repeated ringing of the bells leads to a steady decline of the salivation unless the conditioning is reinforced by occasional coupling of the bell with food.

The question of a decreased effectiveness of placebos on repeated application has an obviously important practical aspect if placebos were to be used in a constructive fashion. They have rarely been tested in this way. Montgomery and Kirsch (1997) show an increasing effectiveness of repeated placebo applications in an experimental situation. Since most patients expect medication to have a long-term decreasing effect and since the placebo response is locked to patient expectation, this by itself could lead to diminishing placebo responses.

All such comparisons between widely differing processes lead to argument about similarities and differences, identities and analogies (Wall and Safran 1986). However, the idea led to a series of clever experiments by Voudouris et al (1989, 1990). The first stage of this work was a repeat of a type of trial that had been reported many times before. Volunteer subjects were given rising electric shocks and the current was established in full view of the subject. The experiments determined the level at which the shock became painful and the level at which it become intolerable. Then a bland cream was rubbed on the area, the subjects were assured that it was a powerful anaesthetic, and the shock trial was run a second time. A small fraction of the subjects demonstrated a placebo response by reporting pain and intolerable pain at a higher shock level than they had on the first trial. This part of the experiment is of no general interest but it established the placebo response rate in these particular circumstances. They then started again with a new group of subjects and determined their threshold and tolerance shock levels. The cream was applied and now came the clever and novel part of the experiment; the strength of the electric shocks was secretly reduced unknown to the subject and observer. When the trial was now run, the subject observed that much higher numbers on the shock machine were achieved before pain was felt and before the pain reached the tolerance limit. These subjects believed that they had tested on themselves the truth of the remarkable anaesthetic properties of the cream. Next, after one such apparent demonstration of the efficacy of the cream, a trial was run in the original conditions; i.e., the strength of current was returned to its original level. The cream was put on and the shock level raised. On this trial large numbers of the subjects became placebo reactors. The only difference in these newly produced placebo responders was that they had 'experienced' in some fashion the apparently 'true' anaesthetic properties of the cream. Clearly, this result can have important practical implications. Whether the change in the subjects was cognitive or conditioned must remain an issue for debate and further experiment. Brewer (1974) concludes that 'There is no convincing evidence for operant or classical conditioning in adult humans' that is free of cognitive awareness of the situation. It may be that the passionately maintained differences between cognitive and conditioned responses may collapse on each other.

The question of whether the so-called conditioned placebo response contains a cognitive component has been approached in a very clever way by Montgomery and Kirsch 1997 (but see also Staats et al 1998 and Kirsch and Montgomery 1998). They repeated the Voudouris et al (1990) experiment with the same results but added a crucial group, who were verbally informed that the applied cream was not anaesthetic; this group failed to produce placebo responses. The importance of this strange but subtle experiment is that the subjects had experienced precisely the same shocks as the group who did become placebo responders. There are those, such as Price and Fields (1997), and unlike Brewer (1974), who believe that conditioning involves subconscious non-cognitive mechanisms. In the Kirsch and Montgomery experiments, the groups who failed to produce a placebo response had received all the same stimuli during the training trials except that they had been verbally informed that the cream was inert. Therefore they conclude that the placebo response was not simply learned by the pairing of stimuli with response but needed a verbally induced change of expectation.

A new proposal: the placebo is not a stimulus but an appropriate response

It is fatuous to regard a placebo as a stimulus in the ordinary sense of that word. By definition, if a placebo is administered in complete secrecy so that the patient is unaware that anything has been done, there is no reaction. An example would be the covert injection by way of a long line from a hidden source of saline of which the patient has no knowledge and to which the patient does not react. If the placebo is not a stimulus in this sense, what is it? In the introduction to the third edition of the *Textbook of Pain*, I proposed that sensation was appropriate to the overall situation. In the introduction to the fourth edition, I extended that idea to propose that sensation is not simply a report of a stimulus but an awareness of possible appropriate action. It is proposed that the sensation of pain is an awareness of a series of need states. The phrase 'need state' is used in contemporary psychology to replace the old word 'drive'. It is used particularly for reactions such as hunger and thirst which, like pain, show such a poor correlation with any objective stimulus. The onset of pain is associated with active avoidance in an attempt to abolish the stimulus. After the avoidance phase, a complex series of events start up to optimize the prevention of further damage. They include muscle contractions to splint the painful area and to guard the area. There follows the phase optimal for recovery, including rest and immobility and, in the case of humans, the seeking of aid and therapy. Therapy for an animal may be limited to licking the painful area but, for us, our personal experience and culture have added an elaborate array of potential actions. It is proposed that pain at this stage is a need state in need of appropriate therapy. Need states such as hunger, thirst, itching, and nausea are terminated by consummatory action. The need state of pain is hopefully terminated by taking the appropriate action, i.e., by seeking and accepting an apparently appropriate therapy. The sensation of the need state disappears once consummation is complete. This places the placebo in the category of appropriate response rather than as an appropriate stimulus.

References

Beecher HK 1959 Measurement of subjective responses. Oxford University Press, New York

Beecher HK 1968 Placebo effects: a quantitative study of suggestibility. In: Beecher HK (ed) Non-specific factors in drug therapy. Thomas, Springfield, IL, pp 27–39

Benedetti F, Amanzio M, Baldi S, Casadio C, Cavallo A 1998 The specific effects of prior opioid exposure on placebo analgesia and placebo respiratory depression. Pain 75: 313–319

Bootzin RR 1985 The role of expectancy in behaviour change. In: White LP, Tursky B, Schwarz GE (eds) Placebo: theory, research and mechanisms. Guilford Press, New York

Brewer WF 1974 There is no convincing evidence for operant or classical conditioning in adult humans. In: Weiner WB, Palermo

DS (eds) Cognition and the symbolic processes. Wiley, New York, pp 1–42
Evans FJ 1974 The placebo response in pain reduction. In: Bonica JJ (ed) Advances in neurology, vol 4. Raven Press, New York, pp 289–296
Gracely RH, McGrath P, Dubner R 1978 Validity and sensitivity of ratio scales. Manipulation of affect by diazepam. Pain 5: 19–29
Gracely RH, Dubner R, Deeter WR, Wolskee PJ 1985 Clinicians' expectations influence placebo analgesia. Lancet 1: 8419–8423
Harden RN, Gracely RH, Carter T, Warner G 1996 Placebo effect in acute pain management. Headache 36: 1–6
Herrnstein RJ 1965 Placebo effect in the rat. Science 138: 677–678
Kirsch I, Montgomery GH 1998 Reply to Staats et al. Pain 76: 269–270
Lasagna L, Mosteller F, Von Felsinger JM, Beecher HK 1954 A study of the placebo response. American Journal of Medicine 16: 770–779
McQuay H, Carroll D, Moore A 1995 Variation in the placebo effect in randomised controlled trials of analgesics: is all as blind as it seems. Pain 63: 1–5
Montgomery GH, Kirsch I 1996 Mechanisms of placebo pain reduction. Psychological Science 7: 174–176
Montgomery GH, Kirsch I 1997 Classical conditioning and the placebo effect. Pain 72: 107–113
Nash MM, Zimring FM 1969 Prediction of reaction of placebo. Journal of Abnormal Psychology 74: 569–573
O'Boyle DJ, Binns AS, Summer JJ 1994 On the efficacy of alcohol placebos in including feelings of intoxication. Psychopharmacology 115: 229–236
Price DD, Fields HL 1997 The contribution of desire and expectation to placebo analgesia. In: Harrington A (ed) The placebo effect. An interdisciplinary exploration. Harvard University Press, Cambridge, pp. 117–137
Reiss S 1980 Pavlovian conditioning and human fear. An expectancy model. Behaviour Therapy 11: 380–396
Siegel S 1975 Conditioning insulin effects. Journal of Comparative and Physiological Psychology 89: 189–199
Siegel S 1985 Drug anticipatory responses in animals. In: White LP, Tursky B, Schwarz GE (eds) Placebo: theory, research and mechanisms. Guilford Press, New York
Staats PS, Hekmat H, Staats AW 1998 Comment on Montgomery & Kirsch. Pain 76: 268–269
Turner JL, Gallimore R, Fox-Henning C 1980 An annotated bibliography of placebo research. Journal Supplement Abstract Service of the American Psychological Association 10(2): 22
Voudouris NJ, Peck CL, Coleman G 1989 Conditioned response models of placebo phenomena. Pain 38: 109–116
Voudouris NJ, Peck CL, Coleman G 1990 The role of conditioning and verbal expectancy in the placebo response. Pain 43: 121–128
Wall PD, Safran JW 1986 Artefactual intelligence. In: Rose S, Appignanesi L (eds) Science and beyond. Blackwell, Oxford
White L, Tursky B, Schwarz GE (eds) 1985 Placebo: theory, research and mechanisms. Guilford Press, New York
Wickramasekera I 1980 A conditioned response model of the placebo effect. Biofeedback and Self-Regulation 5: 5–18

Chapter 34

Relaxation and biofeedback

Vivienne X Gallegos

Introduction

Both relaxation and biofeedback are used to treat various types of pain. Relaxation is an integrated physiological response characterized by generalized decreases in the sympathetic nervous system and metabolic activity (Benson 1975). Relaxation is a characteristic part of most psychological interventions for pain (Turner and Chapman 1982a).

Biofeedback is the presentation to an individual of a sensory signal (usually visual or auditory) that changes in proportion to a biological process. The biological measures 'fed back' have included the electromyogram (EMG) of various muscles in different parts of the body, skin temperature, skin resistance, pulse volume, and waveforms of the electroencephalogram (EEG). Feedback has been presented under varying conditions of amplification and electronic modification. Subjects have received differing concurrent instruction, including forms of counselling and psychotherapy, have or have not utilized relaxation training and home practice, and have had the biofeedback sessions conducted in a deliberately neutral or encouraging manner. In addition, the activity level (passive versus active) or position of the body (sitting versus standing, etc.) has varied. Thus the term 'biofeedback' has come to refer to a constellation of procedures, having as their only common element the use of biofeedback itself, employing various physiological and self-report measures to assess the outcome of the intervention.

This chapter examines relaxation and biofeedback effects for the most frequently treated pain syndromes. Issues in aetiology, measurement, theory, and research are also considered.

Current status of relaxation and biofeedback

Relaxation and biofeedback as treatments for pain have been studied extensively and have been examined in many review articles (e.g., Blanchard and Ahles 1990).

Biofeedback has been used to treat a wide variety of pain syndromes. By far the most frequent application has been EMG feedback for muscle-contraction headaches. Next in frequency has been the use of vascular feedback (skin temperature or other measures of vascular activity) for migraine. It has also been applied less frequently to other pain problems such as back pain, paediatric pain, temporomandibular joint pain, Raynaud's disease, torticollis, neck problems, gynaecological problems, arthritis, phantom-limb pain, reflex sympathetic dystrophy, and other miscellaneous conditions.

In addition, research subjects of all types have varied substantially in their pain-problem histories and pretreatment pain episodes. Variability in pain syndromes, types of subject, and the measures recorded should be kept in mind when considering treatment outcome. Despite the preponderance of noncontrolled studies, enough systematic data have accumulated to permit some firm conclusions about treatment efficacy.

Scalp-muscle-contraction headache

This pain syndrome is the most widely studied for its responsiveness to relaxation and biofeedback. The *Classification of Chronic Pain* published by the International Association for the Study of Pain (IASP; Merskey and Bogduk 1994) defines scalp-muscle-contraction headache as 'virtually continuous dull aching head pain, usually symmetrical and frequently global. This headache is frequently, but not in all cases, associated with muscle 'tension'. The term *tension* is, nevertheless, retained; tension may also be taken to indicate stress, strain, anxiety, and emotional tension. There is a frequent association between these factors and also depressive states and this headache. In the later stages, exacerbations with a tinge of pounding headache and with nausea (and, less typically, vomiting) may occasionally occur, although less typically and with less intensity than in common migraine' (Merskey and Bogduk 1994).

The literatures on biofeedback and relaxation treatments for scalp-muscle-contraction headache are intertwined to an extent that they are best considered together. The studies reviewed here support relaxation training as the treatment of choice in muscle-contraction headache. As noted below, most of the controlled studies used this technique.

Thirteen controlled studies of scalp-muscle-contraction headache compared biofeedback or relaxation training in any of their forms to a no-treatment control group involving symptom monitoring, waiting list, or placebo. Eleven of those studies showed reduction in headache pain after treatment but not in the control condition (Lacroix et al 1986; Larsson et al 1987, 1990; Wisniewski et al 1988; Blanchard et al 1990a, 1991a; Melis et al 1991; Schoenen et al 1991b, c; Wallbaum et al 1991; Rokicki et al 1997). Two of these studies used relaxation training within the context of another therapeutic modality, hypnosis (Melis et al 1991), or chamber-restricted environment (Wallbaum et al 1991). In the other two controlled studies, relaxation taught in school failed to result in a decrease of students' headache activity in comparison to either a wait-list control (Fichtel and Larsson 2001) or a placebo group (Passchier et al 1990).

Nine group outcome studies with no control group found improvement (as reductions in headache activity or medication intake) after a variety of treatment conditions, including relaxation training (Arena et al 1988, Juprelle and Schoenen 1990), GSR biofeedback (Collet et al 1986), EMG biofeedback (Grazzi et al 1988, Juprelle and Schoenen 1990, Schoenen et al 1991a, Grazzi and Bussone 1993), cognitive therapy using relaxation instructions (Holroyd et al 1991), or both relaxation training and cognitive therapy (Attanasio et al 1987). One study found that EMG biofeedback was more effective than relaxation alone or relaxation plus temperature biofeedback (Cott et al 1992).

The long-term maintenance of benefits obtained after relaxation and biofeedback training was demonstrated in three follow-up studies of up to five years after initial treatment (Blanchard et al 1987a, b; Smith 1987).

In a meta-analysis carried out in 1980, Blanchard et al determined that 'the apparent effectiveness of EMG biofeedback for muscle-contraction headache varies moderately across the headache measures used. With some exceptions, headache frequency tends to decrease slightly more than duration or intensity'. These authors found that relaxation training or biofeedback reduced reported muscle-contraction-headache pain by about 60%. Other early reviews reached a similar figure, or occasionally slightly less, of about 50%. This improvement was almost always maintained during the following months. In contrast, the control comparison subjects, who received uninstructed self-relaxation, placebo medication, or no treatment for their muscle-contraction headaches consistently did not improve as much.

In considering the results for control group subjects *in the same studies* analysed by Blanchard et al (1980), other early reviewers found variable effects. Taking an average of subjects, measures, and studies, reported pain tends to increase by about 8–10% in the control groups and is occasionally reported to increase much more (Haynes et al 1975, Jessup et al 1979). However, the use of a false signal as a control procedure for EMG biofeedback leads more often to a decrease in headache symptoms of about 15%.

A later meta-analysis by Malone et al (1988)

reviewed 109 studies, of which 48 were used to calculate effect sizes. This sample of studies was called the effect-size sample while the remaining 61 studies were labelled the percentage-improved group. In the effect-size sample, 'All treatments were reported as extremely successful when compared with the estimated outcome effects of no-treatment control groups'. When type of outcome measure was examined, the outcome findings varied considerably, except number of symptoms, EMG recordings, and mood. When these variables were taken into account, improvement was observed consistently. In contrast to Blanchard et al (1980), pill placebo was found to be more effective than biofeedback or relaxation training. Autogenic training was found to be superior to pill placebo, confirming the finding of Blanchard et al (1980).

In the percentage-improved sample Malone et al (1988) concluded that 'only relaxation training is truly effective, biofeedback training is minimally effective and the other treatments are actually less effective than no treatment at all'. The criterion for considering improvement was a 25% or greater reduction in the outcome measures (activity level, duration, EMG or temperature recordings, frequency, etc.). The percentage of improvement reported was 84% for biofeedback, 95% for relaxation, 70% for pill placebo, 72% for treatment package, and 77% for no treatment. For a critique of Malone et al's meta-analysis see Holroyd and Penzien (1989).

Blanchard and Ahles (1990), in a review of the studies of tension headache, conclude that frontal EMG biofeedback alone or with adjunctive relaxation training is more effective than placebo and at least as effective as other active psychological treatments and drug treatments.

Both relaxation training and biofeedback are effective in reducing tension headache, but relaxation is simpler to administer and is more cost-effective. The equivalent benefits of relaxation training have been repeatedly noted by researchers and reviewers, such as Turner and Chapman (1982a). Viewed even more broadly, if EMG biofeedback is effective not as a specific muscle-training technique, but as a way of training relaxation, then the key question becomes the relative effectiveness of biofeedback and relaxation training for generating relaxation. Relaxation-training studies are subject to the same sources of variability as noted earlier for EMG biofeedback, leading to some conflicting findings.

What happens during treatment to cause improvement? One of the most incisive studies of this question was carried out by Andrasik and Holroyd (1980). They compared EMG biofeedback training for decreasing, increasing, or stabilizing frontalis muscle tension with a no-treatment group. The three treatment groups showed equivalent substantial improvement in tension headaches at a 3-month follow-up. All three treatments were equally superior to the no-treatment group. Andrasik and Holroyd (1980) concluded: 'These results suggest that the learned reduction of EMG activity may play only a minor role in outcomes obtained with biofeedback'.

Neither treatment duration nor the source of subjects have been important variables in determining treatment outcome. With regard to treatment, a minimum of 3 h of EMG biofeedback training is usually adequate, although most clinicians use about 6–8 h.

Schoenen et al in a series of studies (Schoenen et al 1991a, b, c; Juprelle and Schoenen 1990) found that EMG levels are not related to headache severity and concluded that EMG activity of the pericranial muscles is not the cause of headaches, but rather one of the changes associated with headaches. Their data supported the hypothesis that 'diffuse disruption of central pain-modulating systems, possibly due to a modified limbic input to the brain stem, is pivotal in the pathophysiology of muscle contraction headache' (Schoenen et al 1991c).

Migraine

The Subcommittee on Taxonomy of the IASP (Merskey and Bogduk 1994) has defined classic migraine as: 'Throbbing head pain in attacks, often with a prodromal state and usually preceded by an aura which frequently contains visual phenomena. The pain is typically unilateral but may be bilateral. Nausea, vomiting, photophobia and phonophobia often accompany the pain'.

Migraine headache has been treated with finger-temperature biofeedback. Sargent et al (1973) suggested that hand-warming biofeedback could alleviate migraine by reducing sympathetic arousal. Overall outcome effectiveness of finger-warming feedback for migraine, when objectively evaluated, has been somewhat weaker than that for EMG biofeedback applied to muscle-contraction headaches. A typical figure for migraine-symptom reduction during controlled studies of finger-warming biofeedback is about 30–35%, although occasionally no improvement has been reported. Virtually the same improvement is found in no-treatment groups, in which subjects simply keep records of their migraines, and in what should be counter-therapeutic groups, in which the subjects attempt to decrease their finger temperature (Kewman and Roberts 1980).

In their review article, Blanchard et al (1980) concluded that thermal biofeedback alone leads to a 52% improvement in migraine headache index (intensity × duration); thermal feedback with autogenic training, a 65% improvement; relaxation training, 53%; and medication placebo, 17%. Other exhaustive reviews (Chapman 1986, Litt 1986, Blanchard and Ahles 1990) all draw similar conclusions about treatment outcome when relaxation or biofeedback is used for migraine:

1. Thermal biofeedback and relaxation training are equally effective.
2. Frontalis EMG biofeedback and thermal biofeedback are equally effective in the treatment of migraine (Chapman 1986).
3. Improvement that occurs during relaxation or biofeedback continues at follow-up periods of at least up to 1 year.
4. Changes in headache parameters are not reliably associated with physiological changes postulated to mediate migraine.
5. To account best for the complex and seemingly contradictory findings in *clinical* practice, an interactional model that considers 'biochemical, specific vascular, general autonomic, cognitive/affective/behavioural, dyadic and social' processes is apt to be most useful (Litt 1986).

From 1986 to 2001, 21 studies involving populations of migraineurs who had been treated with biofeedback or relaxation training or both were published. Seven were controlled studies (Ellersten et al 1987; Gallegos and Espinoza 1989; Blanchard et al 1990b, c; Gauthier and Carrier 1991; Ilacqua 1994; McGrady et al 1994) and the rest were group outcome studies. The studies show that biofeedback in combination with relaxation or alone is more effective in the treatment of migraine headache than placebo treatment or no treatment (with the exception of Ilacqua 1994). However, none of the controlled studies clarified whether temperature biofeedback was a better treatment per se than other more cost-effective treatments.

Holroyd and Penzien (1990) in a meta-analytic review of 60 studies reported that relaxation/biofeedback training and propranolol medication are equally effective in the prophylactic treatment of migraine. Both treatments greatly reduced headache activity in patients with migraine and differed significantly from patients in non-treatment or placebo conditions. If propranolol and psychological treatment are equally effective, it would seem that many patients would prefer propranolol than a lengthy and more demanding treatment such as biofeedback or relaxation training. Nevertheless, it should be noted that individuals may have medication side effects (Wilkinson 1988), particularly with long-term ingestion of the drug, and that relaxation has beneficial effects for the individual's health beyond the reduction in migraine (e.g., in helping cope with stress).

Mixed headache

In contrast to the extensive literature on muscle-contraction headache and migraine headache, studies involving patients with combined headache (migraine and muscle contraction) or cluster headache are rather scarce. In some clinics, patients with muscle-contraction headache, migraine, or both are treated with a combined package of treatments, apparently with good results (Schwartz 1987). However, research studies of patients with combined headache and cluster headache are needed.

In a study involving biofeedback with or without home practice (Blanchard et al 1991b), patients with biofeedback treatment improved more than a monitoring group. However, there were no significant differences between the two feedback groups and migraineurs responded better (64%) than patients with mixed headaches (28%).

Evidence of the effectiveness of a combined treatment of relaxation training and biofeedback was reported by Smith (1987) with 318 mixed headache (muscle contraction, migraine, or mixed) patients contacted by telephone. All patients had received earlier EMG and thermal biofeedback, relaxation training, psychotherapy, and physical therapy. She found that patients who had had some previous biofeedback treatment reported reduction in headache frequency and associated symptoms. The reduction was maintained in the majority of the patients for 25 months or more.

Back pain

Twelve studies on biofeedback and relaxation for back pain were published between 1986 and 2001. The studies examined varied syndromes, and most subjects had recurring or nearly continuous medium to severe pain for at least 6 months. Pain histories in excess of 10 years have been typical in both clinical and research volunteer populations.

Degenerative, dysfunctional, structural, inflammatory, traumatic, postsurgical, and unknown aetiologies are evident. The most frequently studied conditions are fibrositis or diffuse myofascial pain syndrome, rheumatoid arthritis, chronic mechanical low back pain, and muscle-tension pain of psychological origin.

Between 20 and 85% of back pain patients do not have differentially diagnostic physical findings. The wide range in physical findings depends on what consideration one gives to degenerative changes that do not reliably produce pain (White and Gordon 1982). Consequently, outcome findings for relaxation and biofeedback treatments of back pain have varied widely.

Relaxation training has produced some evidence of being an effective treatment for low back pain. It also appears to be an effective component of multidimensional treatment packages (e.g., Middaugh et al 1991). It produced positive results in four of six relaxation studies (Stuckey et al 1986, Petrie and Azariah 1990, Spinhoven and Linssen 1991, Nicholas et al 1992).

The rationale for relaxation training is straightforward: sustained muscle contraction has been considered both a cause and an effect of chronic back pain, sustaining a cycle of pain–spasm–pain (Dolce and Raczynski 1985). Hence reduction of muscle contraction should be beneficial. However, muscle-tension levels in back pain patients have been found to be lower than, equal to, or higher than those in pain-free populations under various diagnostic, postural, and movement conditions (Dolce and Raczynski 1985). It is also important to consider reports pointing to the fact that relaxation training may not be effective for all patients (e.g., Degner and Barkwell 1991).

The problem of back pain is probably too complex and variable between patients to permit a simple, single-modality solution. Nonetheless, relaxation techniques are non-invasive, inexpensive, portable procedures that enjoy easy patient acceptance. They deserve further systematic study.

In general, when EMG has been used alone or in combination with other treatments, the results have been positive in terms of gains in muscular strength and physical mobility or reports in pain intensity (e.g., Hasenbring et al 1999). However, mixed results have also been reported (Dolce and Raczynski 1985).

The main aetiological issues relevant to relaxation and biofeedback training for back pain are the lack of reliable covariation between reported pain and EMG readings (Bush et al 1985) and evidence that for some painful back conditions training for increased rather than decreased EMG may be indicated. Diagnosis, patient gender, and EMG technique, including interactions of posture (Kravitz et al 1981), movement, and site of EMG electrode placement, as well as location and depth of placement of electrodes (Wolf et al 1989), are also proving to be significant factors affecting muscular activity in normal and painful backs. Although these findings are important and point to a new direction in biofeedback monitoring and treatment of low back pain, the small number of studies does not warrant definitive conclusions. Consequently, the relationship between EMG measures and back pain remains an open question.

Paediatric pain

Schechter (1985) notes that paediatric pain is a significant and psychophysiologically complex problem, involving the interaction of a neurophysiological response with age, cognitive set, personality, ethnic background, and emotional state.

Since caution has been advised regarding long-term drug therapy with children (Duckro and Cantwell-Simmons 1989), behavioural treatment seems to be a promising alternative and several researchers have studied the use of relaxation and biofeedback techniques for pain in children. The children's response to biofeedback and relaxation treatments is consistent with that of adults, but children have shown greater improvement in headache activity than adults with EMG biofeedback and temperature feedback (Sarafino and Goehring 2000). Duckro and Cantwell-Simmons (1989) reviewed 12 studies that in general supported the assumption that relaxation training with or without biofeedback is an effective treatment in the management of chronic headache in children and adolescents. Other studies in the literature point to the effectiveness of relaxation treatment (Engel et al 1992) and EMG biofeedback with mental imagery (Labbe and Ward 1990).

Other pain syndromes

Research on biofeedback treatment of a variety of pain syndromes other than functional headache shows outcomes similar to the headache research. Uncontrolled studies greatly outnumber systematic studies. Controlled research suggests that, as with headache, generalized relaxation is as effective as biofeedback and may mediate improvement in a number of syndromes.

Biofeedback treatments have been reported for the following syndromes: temporomandibular joint pain, Raynaud's disease, spasmodic torticollis, neck injury, menstrual stress, writer's cramp, duodenal ulcer, pyelonephritis, rheumatoid arthritis, phantom-limb pain, anginal pain, and posttraumatic headache. They have also been applied during childbirth.

In the case of temporomandibular joint pain, anecdotal case reports and group studies (Jessup et al 1979) suggest that masseter or temporalis muscle EMG biofeedback alone or in conjuction with cognitive–behavioural treatment is beneficial for temporomandibular joint pain and bruxism. Flor and Birbaumer (1993) randomly assigned 78 patients, including 21 suffering from temporomandibular pain, to one of three treatment groups: EMG biofeedback, cognitive therapy, or traditional medical treatment. They found improvement in all patients, with the biofeedback group showing more positive change than the others. Likewise, only the biofeedback group showed treatment gains at follow-up in a number of outcome measures, including pain severity and interference.

Three reviews of the literature on the treatment of Raynaud's disease reported contradictory findings. Sappington et al (1979) found that the most systematic studies showed that hand-warming biofeedback was no more effective than relaxation training. Rose and Carlson (1987) also reported inconsistent findings among major treatment studies. Several methodological and cost-effectiveness issues that make it difficult to generalize across studies, settings, and subject groups are raised. In contrast, Freedman (1985) reported in a review article that temperature biofeedback is an effective treatment for idiopathic Raynaud's disease. He points to the importance of differentiating patients with Raynaud's disease, which refers to the primary form of the disorder, and 'Raynaud's phenomenon', which may be present with other tissue disorders such as scleroderma and rheumatoid arthritis. Treatment with thermal biofeedback when scleroderma is present has not been as effective. The authors suggested that different aetiologies may be involved.

Freedman (1991) reported replications of controlled investigations that demonstrated that temperature biofeedback was effective in the treatment of patients suffering Raynaud's disease. Findings at the Freedman laboratory supported the hypothesis that feedback-induced vasodilatation and vasoconstriction are mediated by different physiological mechanisms, namely, vasodilatation through a β-adrenergic mechanism and vasoconstriction through the sympathetic nervous pathway. This may explain the inconsistencies between heart rate, skin conductance, and other parameters during temperature biofeedback in many studies reported so far.

Spasmodic torticollis is a painful twisting of the head to one side due to abnormal activity of the sternocleidomastoid muscles. Nine cases reported by Cleeland (1973) suggest that EMG biofeedback is effective for at least 90% of cases during treatment, including cases with long histories. Benefit continues for up to 3 years for about two-thirds of cases (Cleeland 1973). Not all cases show marked improvement and, even with biofeedback, sternocleidomastoid muscle tension may not decline to that of comparable controls (Martin 1981).

Menstrual stress (dysmenorrhoea) improved with individual or group relaxation training or a combination of relaxation training and vaginal-temperature feedback (Heczey 1978), and in a multiple-baseline study (Vargas et al 1987), 12 women suffering from dysmenorrhoea reported less pain after relaxation training.

Arthritic pain has been treated with frontalis muscle EMG biofeedback or relaxation training (e.g., Bradley et al 1987) with positive results, but negative inconclusive results have also been obtained (Noda 1979).

Phantom-limb pain was virtually eliminated in 10 of 16 cases and reduced to the point of no longer needing treatment in an additional four in a single-group study using relaxation training, EMG biofeedback, and provision of information (Sherman et al 1979). These findings are particularly encouraging because 14 of the cases had suffered chronic pain for an average duration of 12 years.

Pain associated with reflex sympathetic dystrophy (RSD) has been treated with thermal biofeedback, relaxation training, psychotherapy, and hypnotherapy, reducing subjective pain levels (Grunert et al 1990).

Other types of pain syndrome have been treated with biofeedback or relaxation or both and have improved to various degrees. Ham and Packard (1996) reported improvement of posttraumatic headache with biofeedback. Olson (1988) reported improvement in a sample of 563 psychiatric patients suffering from different pain syndromes after treatment with biofeedback and relaxation training, and a recent NIH Technology Assessment Panel on Integration of Behavioral and Relaxation Approaches into the Treatment of Chronic Pain and Insomnia (1996) concluded that there is strong evidence for the use of relaxation in reducing chronic pain in a variety of medical conditions (although Carroll and Seers 1998 argue that evidence for relaxation training reducing chronic pain is still insufficient). Relaxation has been reported to be effective in the relief of postoperative pain (e.g., Good et al 2001), although Seers and Carroll (1998) recommend caution when using relaxation for acute pain. Relaxation and imagery training reduced cancer treatment-related pain (Syrjala et al 1995, Wallace 1997).

In summary, the studies of biofeedback treatment of a variety of pain syndromes other than functional headache suggest that further inquiry is merited. However, as with biofeedback treatment of headache, relaxation training and other cognitive–behavioural interventions may prove to be at least as effective.

Treatment process considerations

Pain taxonomy

The *Classification of Chronic Pain* (Merskey and Bogduk 1994), by creating a coherent pain taxonomy, could significantly aid clarification of the processes operating in biofeedback and relaxation treatment for pain. However, pain taxonomy continues to be a particularly pressing problem in routine clinical practice, particularly in regard to headache patients (Schoenen and Maertens de Noordhout 1994). Furthermore, although generally accepted, the belief that tension of the frontalis muscle reliably causes muscle-contraction headache is not entirely supportable (Bakal 1975) and numerous exceptions to the general opinion have been documented. Whereas biofeedback and relaxation research are apt to aid further clarification of pain syndromes and subtypes (Carrobles et al 1981), subtypes of headache for which biofeedback and relaxation are specifically effective may yet be identified.

Pain–physiology desynchrony

Reduction in frontalis EMG is not necessary for improvement in muscle-contraction headaches. Evidence supporting this surprising conclusion comes from studies of the frontalis EMG–pain relationship. Muscle tension tends to be higher during muscle-contraction headaches, but many case-by-case exceptions have been observed (e.g., Haynes et al 1975). Frontalis EMG does not reliably covary with self-reported headache pain, even when a headache is occurring during EMG monitoring in the laboratory (Epstein et al 1978, Gray et al 1980).

Nuechterlein and Holroyd (1980) reviewed some of the complexities behind frontalis EMG–pain desynchrony, and emphasized the need for very discrete diagnosis (i.e., pain taxonomy) to clarify the considerable diversity within the tension headache population in the extent to which EMG alteration can be expected to change headache activity. Also noteworthy is the fact that Andrasik and Holroyd (1980) closely monitored biofeedback training that increased frontalis EMG to ensure that it would not exacerbate headache symptoms.

Although opinion is not unanimous (Basmajian 1976), reductions in frontalis EMG during biofeedback do not generalize to other, even adjacent muscles (Thompson et al 1981). Frontalis EMG level may not be reliably related to subjective reports of relaxation (Shedivy and Kleinman 1977). However, a generalized reduction in autonomic and cortical arousal, involving changes in heart rate, skin resistance, and EEG activity, has been found during extensive frontalis EMG training (Hoffman 1979). Whether the EMG biofeedback caused the generalized decrease in arousal could not be determined by Hoffman's study. However, the pattern is congruent with the state of low arousal that Benson (1975) termed the 'relaxation response'. Conceivably, EMG biofeedback treatment, like relaxation training, does lead to a generalized reduction in arousal that is nonetheless not synchronous across muscle systems, nor with self-report of experienced relaxation.

Flor and Turk (1989) carried out an exhaustive research review of the relationship between specific symptoms and psychophysiological responses in chronic-pain patients. Detailed evaluation of 60 studies against 12 theoretical and methodological criteria showed that 'baseline levels, regardless of type of physiological measure, are not generally elevated in chronic-pain patients. The presence of symptom-specific, stress-related psychophysiological responses is more commonly observed and the evidence on return to baseline is at this time inconclusive.' These findings should direct reseachers towards a more precise evaluation of biofeedback and relaxation training as methods for reducing stress-related responses.

Psychosocial processes

Other processes that are probably not necessary for improvement during biofeedback include socioeconomic status (Acosta and Yamamoto 1978), hypnotizability (Frischolz and Tryon 1980), and home practice during biofeedback training (Haynes et al 1975). Continued practice after training may be related to continued benefit (Reinking and Hutchings 1976).

A number of processes have been proposed as mediators for improvement during biofeedback and relaxation treatment, including personality × treatment interactions, anxiety reduction, enhanced sense of self-control, cognitive changes, behavioural changes, therapist contact, instructions to relax, somatic manoeuvres, and subtle changes in biological processes.

Two features of the list of possible mediators should be noted. First, the length and variety of the list suggest that no conclusive mediator has yet been found. As Turner and Chapman (1982b) note, this may reflect 'the difficulty of carrying out outcome evaluation research in the chronic-pain area. The problems are extremely complex, and many treatment packages involve a collage of interventions rather than single therapy.'

Second, a common theme of many of the mediators is increased perceived control over bodily processes and social life. Increased self-efficacy (Bandura 1977) may prove to be a potent common element explaining the similar effectiveness of diverse biofeedback, relaxation, and cognitive and behavioural pain treatments.

Personality variables may also be involved in mediating improvement in biofeedback treatments of pain (Jessup et al 1979). Qualls and Sheehan (1981) argued that different relaxation procedures, including feedback, interact with certain trait dimensions in different populations to produce reliably different effects. The dimensions put forward include trait anxiety, locus of control, capacity for absorption in mental imagery, and type of clinical disorder. The construct of a 'disease-prone personality' which involves 'depression, anger/hostility and anxiety' may also prove to be a relevant process variable in biofeedback and relaxation treatments of pain (Friedman and Booth-Kewley 1987).

Conclusions

Three main conclusions follow from the past four decades of biofeedback and relaxation research:

1. Biofeedback and relaxation training have been established as useful treatment interventions for a variety of pain conditions. They have been incorporated as components of standard treatment protocols in pain clinics throughout the world. In addition, biofeedback specifically can be helpful in some refractory cases. Now, however, research must focus on more specific relationships of environmental stimuli, specific physical reactivities, and clarity of aetiology.

2. Biofeedback started with strong roots in psychophysiology and evolved dynamically into clinical practice, but interest in research seems to have waned in the past decade, at least as reflected in the decreased number of empirical articles on biofeedback and relaxation in the treatment of pain. Further research is needed on basic physiological processes, as exemplified by the work of Flor and Turk (1989) on the psychophysiology of chronic pain and Freedman's (1991) research on biofeedback to elucidate the different physiological mechanisms of finger warming and cooling.

3. Regrettably, the research underscores the limited utility of poorly designed research. Aetiologies and syndromes have been confounded. Research hypotheses have been too simple, and the measurement strategies too crude. The addition of further confounding treatments to already equivocal findings has added to the confusion. Biofeedback and relaxation research in the treatment of pain is still lacking precision and sophistication.

References

Acosta FX, Yamamoto J 1978 Application of electromyographic biofeedback to the relaxation training of schizophrenic, neurotic, and tension headache patients. Journal of Consulting and Clinical Psychology 46: 383–384

Andrasik F, Holroyd KA 1980 A test of specific and nonspecific effects in the biofeedback treatment of tension headache. Journal of Consulting and Clinical Psychology 48: 575–586

Arena JG, Hightower NE, Chong GC 1988 Relaxation therapy for tension headache in the elderly: a prospective study. Psychology and Aging 3: 96–98

Attanasio V, Andrasik F, Blanchard EB 1987 Cognitive therapy and relaxation training in muscle contraction headache: efficacy and cost-effectiveness. Headache 27: 254–260

Bakal DA 1975 Headache: a biophysical perspective. Psychological Bulletin 82: 369–382

Bandura A 1977 Self efficacy: toward a unifying theory of behavioral change. Psychological Review 84: 191–215

Basmajian JV 1976 Facts vs. myths in EMG biofeedback. Biofeedback and Self-Regulation 1: 369–372

Benson H 1975 The relaxation response. Morrow, New York

Blanchard EB, Ahles TA 1990 Biofeedback therapy. In: Bonica JJ, Loeser JD, Chapman CR, Fordyce WE (eds) The management of pain, 2nd edn. Lea & Febiger, Philadelphia, pp 1722–1732

Blanchard E, Andrasik F, Ahles T, Teders S, O'Keefe D 1980 Migraine and tension headache: a meta-analytic review. Behavior Therapy 11: 613–631

Blanchard EB, Andrasik F, Guarnieri P, Neff DF, Rodichok D 1987a Two-, three-, and four-year follow-up on the self-regulatory treatment of chronic headache. Journal of Consulting and Clinical Psychology 55: 257–259

Blanchard EB, Appelbaum KA, Guarnieri P, Morrill B, Dentinger MP 1987b Five year prospective follow-up on the treatment of

chronic headache with biofeedback and/or relaxation. Headache 27: 580–583
Blanchard EB, Appelbaum KA, Radnitz CL et al 1990a Placebo-controlled evaluation of abbreviated progressive muscle relaxation and of relaxation combined with cognitive therapy in the treatment of tension headache. Journal of Consulting and Clinical Psychology 58: 210–215
Blanchard EB, Appelbaum KA, Radnitz CL et al 1990b A controlled evaluation of thermal biofeedback and thermal biofeedback combined with cognitive therapy in the treatment of vascular headache. Journal of Consulting and Clinical Psychology 58: 216–224
Blanchard EB, Appelbaum KA, Nicholson NL et al 1990c A controlled evaluation of the addition of cognitive therapy to a home-based biofeedback and relaxation treatment of vascular headache. Headache 30: 371–376
Blanchard EB, Nicholson NL, Taylor AE, Steffek BD, Radnitz CL, Appelbaum KA 1991a The role of regular home practice in the relaxation treatment of tension headache. Journal of Consulting and Clinical Psychology 59: 467–470
Blanchard EB, Nicholson NL, Radnitz CL, Steffek BD, Appelbaum KA, Dentinger MP 1991b The role of home practice in thermal biofeedback. Journal of Consulting and Clinical Psychology 59: 507–512
Bradley LA, Young LD, Anderson KO et al 1987 Effects of psychological therapy on pain behavior of rheumatoid arthritis patients. Arthritis and Rheumatism 30: 1105–1114
Bush C, Ditto B, Feuerstein M 1985 A controlled evaluation of paraspinal EMG biofeedback in the treatment of chronic low back pain. Health Psychology 4: 307–321
Carrobles JA, Cardona A, Santacreu J 1981 Shaping and generalization procedures in the EMG–biofeedback treatment of tension headaches. British Journal of Clinical Psychology 20: 49–56
Carroll D, Seers K 1998 Relaxation for the relief of chronic pain: a systematic review. Journal of Advanced Nursing 27: 476–487
Chapman SL 1986 A review and clinical perspective on the use of EMG and thermal biofeedback for chronic headaches. Pain 27: 1–43
Cleeland CS 1973 Behavior techniques in the modification of spasmodic torticollis. Neurology 23: 1241–1247
Collet L, Cottraux J, Juenet C 1986 GSR feedback and Schultz relaxation in tension headaches: a comparative study. Pain 25: 205–213
Cott A, Parkinson W, Fabich M, Bedard M, Marlin R 1992 Long-term efficacy of combined relaxation: biofeedback treatments for chronic headache. Pain 51: 49–56
Degner L, Barkwell D 1991 Nonanalgesic approaches to pain control. Cancer Nursing 14: 105–111
Dolce J, Raczynski J 1985 Neuromuscular activity and electromyography in painful backs: psychological and biomechanical models in assessment and treatment. Psychological Bulletin 97: 502–520
Duckro PN, Cantwell-Simmons E 1989 A review of studies evaluating biofeedback and relaxation training in the management of pediatric headache. Headache 29: 428–433
Ellersten B, Nordy H, Hammerorg D, Sigurdur Thorlacious 1987 Psychophysiologic response patterns in migraine before and after temperature feedback. Cephalalgia 7: 109–124
Engel JM, Rapoff MA, Pressman AR 1992 Long-term follow-up of relaxation training for pediatric headache disorders. Headache 32: 152–156
Epstein LH, Abel GG, Collins F, Parker L, Cinciripini PM 1978 The relationship between frontalis muscle activity and self-reports of headache pain. Behaviour Research and Therapy 16: 153–160
Fichtel A, Larsson B 2001 Does relaxation treatment have differential effects on migraine and tension-type headache in adolescents? Headache 41: 290–296
Flor H, Birbaumer N 1993 Comparison of the efficacy of electromyographic biofeedback, cognitive-behavioral therapy, and conservative medical interventions in the treatment of chronic musculoskeletal pain. Journal of Consulting and Clinical Psychology 61: 653–658
Flor H, Turk DC 1989 Psychophysiology of chronic pain: do chronic pain patients exhibit symptom-specific psychophysiological responses? Psychological Bulletin 105: 215–259
Freedman RR 1985 Behavioral treatment of Raynaud's disease and phenomenon. Advances in Microcirculation 12: 138–156
Freedman RR 1991 Physiological mechanisms of temperature biofeedback. Biofeedback and Self-Regulation 16: 95–114
Friedman H, Booth-Kewley S 1987 The 'disease-prone personality': a meta-analytic view of the construct. American Psychologist 42: 539–555
Frischolz EJ, Tryon WW 1980 Hypnotizability in relation to the ability to learn thermal biofeedback. American Journal of Clinical Hypnosis 23: 53–56
Gallegos X, Espinoza E 1989 Retroalimentacion biologica termal versus entrenamiento autogenico en el tratamiento de la migrana. Revista Mexicana de Psicologia 6: 55–63
Gauthier JG, Carrier S 1991 Long-term effects of biofeedback on migraine headache: A prospective follow-up study. Headache 31: 605–612
Good M, Stanton-Hicks M, Grass JA et al 2001 Relaxation and music to reduce postsurgical pain. Journal of Advanced Nursing 33: 208–215
Gray L, Lyle RC, McGuire RJ, Peck DF 1980 Electrode placement, EMG feedback, and relaxation for tension headaches. Behaviour Research and Therapy 18: 19–23
Grazzi L, Bussone G 1993 Effect of biofeedback treatment on sympathetic function in common migraine and tension-type headache. Cephalalgia 13: 197–200
Grazzi L, Frediani F, Zappacosta B, Boiardi A, Bussone G 1988 Psychological assessment in tension headache before and after biofeedback treatment. Headache 28: 337–338
Grunert BK, Devine CA, Sanger JR, Matloub HS, Green D 1990 Thermal self-regulation for pain control in reflex sympathetic dystrophy syndrome. Journal of Hand Surgery 15: 615–618
Ham LP, Packard RC 1996 A retrospective, follow-up study of biofeedback-assisted relaxation therapy in patients with posttraumatic headache. Biofeedback and Self-Regulation 21: 93–104
Hasenbring M, Ulrich HW, Hartmann M, Soyka D 1999 The efficacy of a risk factor-based cognitive behavioral intervention and electromyographyic biofeedback in patients with acute sciatic pain. An attempt to prevent chronicity. Spine 24: 2525–2535
Haynes SN, Griffin P, Mooney D, Parise M 1975 Electromyographic biofeedback and relaxation instructions for the treatment of muscle contraction headaches. Behavior Therapy 6: 672–678
Heczey MD 1978 Effects of biofeedback and autogenic training on menstrual experiences, relationships among anxiety, locus of control, and dysmenorrhea. Dissertation Abstracts International 38(B): 5571
Hoffman E 1979 Autonomic, EEG and clinical changes in neurotic patients during EMG biofeedback training. Research Communications in Psychology, Psychiatry and Behavior 4: 209–240
Holroyd KA, Penzien DB 1989 Meta-analysis minus the analysis: a prescription for confusion. Pain 39: 359–361
Holroyd KA, Penzien DB 1990 Pharmacological versus non-pharmacological prophylaxis of recurrent migraine headache: a meta-analytic review of clinical trials. Pain 42: 1–13
Holroyd KA, Nash JM, Pingel JD, Cordingley GE, Gerome A 1991 A comparison of pharmacological (amitriptyline HCL) and

nonpharmacological (cognitive-behavioral) therapies for chronic tension headaches. Journal of Consulting and Clinical Psychology 59: 387–393
Ilacqua GE 1994 Migraine headaches: coping efficacy of guided imagery training. Headache 34: 99–102
Jessup BA, Neufeld RWJ, Merskey H 1979 Biofeedback therapy for headache and other pain: an evaluative review. Pain 7: 225–270
Juprelle M, Schoenen J 1990 Relaxation avec biofeedback musculaire dans les cephalées de type tension: analyse multifactorielle d'un groupe de 31 patients. Revue Medicale de Liège 45: 630–637
Kewman DG, Roberts AH 1980 Skin temperature biofeedback and migraine headaches, a double blind study. Biofeedback and Self-Regulation 5: 327–345
Kravitz EA, Moore ME, Glaros A 1981 Paralumbar muscle activity in chronic low back pain. Archives of Physical Medicine and Rehabilitation 62: 172–176
Labbe EE, Ward CH 1990 Electromyographic biofeedback with mental imagery and home practice in the treatment of children with muscle-contraction headache. Journal of Developmental and Behavioral Pediatrics 11: 65–68
Lacroix JM, Clarke MA, Bock JC, Doxey NCS 1986 Physiological changes after biofeedback and relaxation training for multiple-pain tension-headache patients. Perceptual and Motor Skills 63: 139–153
Larsson B, Daleflod B, Hakansson L, Melin L 1987 Therapist-assisted versus self-help relaxation treatment of chronic headaches in adolescents: a school-based intervention. Journal of Child Psychology and Psychiatry and Allied Disciplines 28: 127–136
Larsson B, Melin L, Doberl A 1990 Recurrent tension headache in adolescents treated with self-help relaxation training and a muscle relaxant drug. Headache 30: 665–671
Litt M 1986 Mediating factors in non-medical treatment for migraine headache: toward an interactional model. Journal of Psychosomatic Research 30: 505–519
Malone MD, Strube MJ, Scogin FR 1988 Meta-analysis of non-medical treatments for chronic pain. Pain 34: 231–244
Martin PR 1981 Spasmodic torticollis: investigation and treatment using EMG feedback training. Behavior Therapy 12: 247–262
McGrady A, Wauquier A, McNeil A, Gerard G 1994 Effect of biofeedback-assisted relaxation on migraine headache and changes in cerebral blood flow velocity in the middle cerebral artery. Headache 34: 424–428
Melis PML, Rooimans W, Spierings ELH, Hoogduin CAL 1991 Treatment of chronic tension-type headache with hypnotherapy: a single-blind time controlled study. Headache 31: 686–689
Merskey H, Bogduk N (eds) 1994 Classification of chronic pain: descriptions of chronic pain syndromes and definitions of pain terms, 2nd edn. IASP Press, Seattle
Middaugh SJ, Woods SE, Kee WG, Harden RN, Peters JR 1991 Biofeedback-assisted relaxation training for the aging chronic pain patient. Biofeedback and Self-Regulation 16: 361–377
Nicholas MK, Wilson PH, Goyen J 1992 Comparison of cognitive–behavioral group treatment and an alternative non-psychological treatment for chronic low back pain. Pain 48: 339–347
NIH Technology Assessment Panel on Integration of Behavioral and Relaxation Approaches into the Treatment of Chronic Pain and Insomnia 1996 Integration of behavioral and relaxation approaches into the treatment of chronic pain and insomnia. Journal of the American Medical Association 276: 313–318
Noda HH 1979 An exploratory study of the effects of EMG and temperature biofeedback on rheumatoid arthritis. Dissertation Abstracts International 39(B): 3532–3533
Nuechterlein K, Holroyd J 1980 Biofeedback in the treatment of tension headache. Archives of General Psychiatry 37: 866–873
Olson P 1988 A long-term, single-group follow-up study of biofeedback therapy with chronic medical and psychiatric patients. Biofeedback and Self-Regulation 13: 331–346
Passchier J, Van den Bree MBM, Emmen HH, Osterhaus SOL, Orlebeke JF, Verhage F 1990 Relaxation training in school classes does not reduce headache complaints. Headache 30: 660–664
Petrie K, Azariah R 1990 Health promoting variables as predictors of response of a brief pain management program. Clinical Journal of Pain 6: 43–46
Qualls PJ, Sheehan PW 1981 Electromyograph biofeedback as a relaxation technique: a critical appraisal and reassessment. Psychological Bulletin 90: 21–42
Reinking R, Hutchings D 1976 Follow-up extension of 'Tension headaches—what method is most effective?' Proceedings of the Biofeedback Research Society Seventh Annual Meeting. Colorado Springs, p 60
Rokicki LA, Holroyd KA, France CR et al 1997 Change mechanisms associated with combined relaxation/EMG biofeedback training for chronic tension headache. Applied Psychophysiology and Biofeedback 22: 21–41
Rose GD, Carlson JG 1987 The behavioral treatment of Raynaud's disease: a review. Biofeedback and Self-Regulation 12: 257–273
Sappington J, Fiorito E, Brehony K 1979 Biofeedback as therapy in Raynaud's disease. Biofeedback and Self-Regulation 4: 155–169
Sarafino EP, Goehring P 2000 Age comparisons in acquiring biofeedback control and success in reducing headache pain. Annals of Behavioral Medicine 22: 10–16
Sargent J, Walters E, Green E 1973 Psychosomatic self-regulation of migraine headache. Seminars in Psychiatry 5: 415–428
Schechter N 1985 Pain and pain control in children. Current Problems in Pediatrics 15: 1–67
Schoenen J, Maertens de Noordhout A 1994 Headache. In: Wall PD, Melzack R (eds) Textbook of pain, 3rd edn. Churchill Livingstone, Edinburgh, p 517
Schoenen J, Gerard P, De Pasqua V, Sianard-Gainko J 1991a Multiple clinical and paraclinical analyses of chronic tension-type headache associated or unassociated with disorder of pericranial muscles. Cephalalgia 11: 135–139
Schoenen J, Gerard P, De Pasqua V, Juprelle M 1991b EMG activity in pericranial muscles during postural variation and mental activity in healthy volunteers and patients with chronic tension type headache. Headache 31: 321–324
Schoenen J, Bottin D, Hardy F, Gerard P 1991c Cephalic and extracephalic pressure pain thresholds in chronic tension-type headache. Pain 47: 145–149
Schwartz M 1987 Biofeedback and stress management in the treatment of headache. Journal of Craniomandibular Disorders 1: 41–45
Seers K, Carroll D 1998 Relaxation techniques for acute pain management: a systematic review. Journal of Advanced Nursing 27: 466–475
Shedivy DI, Kleinman KM 1977 Lack of correlation between frontalis EMG and either neck EMG or verbal ratings of tension. Psychophysiology 14: 182–186
Sherman RA, Gail N, Gormly J 1979 Treatment of phantom limb pain with muscular relaxation training to disrupt the pain-anxiety-tension cycle. Pain 6: 47–55
Smith WB 1987 Biofeedback and relaxation training: the effect on headache and associated symptoms. Headache 27: 511–514
Spinhoven P, Linssen ACG 1991 Behavioral treatment of chronic low back pain. I Relation of coping strategy use to outcome. Pain 45: 29–34
Stuckey SJ, Jacobs A, Goldfarb J 1986 EMG biofeedback training, relaxation training, and placebo for the relief of chronic back pain. Perceptual and Motor Skills 63: 1023–1036
Syrjala KL, Donaldson GW, Davis MW, Kippes ME, Carr JE 1995 Relaxation and imagery and cognitive-behavioral training

reduce pain during cancer treatment: a controlled clinical trial. Pain 63: 189–198
Thompson JK, Haber JD, Tearman BH 1981 Generalization of frontalis electromyographic feedback to adjacent muscle groups: a critical review. Psychosomatic Medicine 43: 19–24
Turner JA, Chapman CR 1982a Psychological interventions for chronic pain: a critical review. I. Relaxation training and biofeedback. Pain 12: 1–21
Turner JA, Chapman CR 1982b Psychological interventions for chronic pain: a critical review. II. Operant conditioning, hypnosis, and cognitive-behavioral therapy. Pain 12: 23–46
Vargas JJ, Ibanez J, Colotla VA 1987 Efecto de la relajacion en el reporte del dolor por dismenorrea. Revista Mexicana de Psicologia 4: 36–40
Wallace KG 1997 Analysis of recent literature concerning relaxation and imagery interventions for cancer pain. Cancer Nursing 20: 79–87
Wallbaum ABC, Pzewnicki R, Steele H, Svedfeld P 1991 Progressive muscle relaxation and restructured environmental stimulation therapy for chronic tension headache: a pilot study. International Journal of Psychosomatics 38: 33–39
White A, Gordon S 1982 Synopsis: workshop on idiopathic low-back pain. Spine 7: 141–149
Wilkinson M 1988 Treatment of migraine. Headache 28: 659–661
Wisniewski JJ, Genshaft JL, Mulick JA, Coury DL, Hammer D 1988 Relaxation therapy and compliance in the treatment of adolescent headache. Headache 28: 612–617
Wolf SL, Wolf LB, Segal RL 1989 The relationship of extraneous movements to lumbar paraspinal muscle activity: implications for EMG biofeedback training applications to low back pain patients. Biofeedback and Self-Regulation 14: 63–73

Chapter 35

Hypnotic analgesia

Ann Gamsa

Introduction

Attempts to define hypnosis bring to mind St. Augustine's remark on the subject of time: 'If no one asks me I know what it is. If I wish to explain it to him who asks me, I do not know' (1966, p. 343). From a clinical standpoint, hypnosis, however defined, has a long-standing history of relieving pain (Barber 1996, Patterson et al 1997). Less clear, however, are the mechanisms by which hypnosis produces its effects, and whether it is, as traditionally believed, a distinct state of consciousness, or as some propose, no more than a normal waking state in which social influence combines with a set of cognitive-behavioural skills to heighten suggestibility. These are the questions driving current research and debate.

Despite contentious views about whether hypnosis is a special state of consciousness, most agree on the following essential components: narrowed focus of attention, reduced awareness of external stimuli, absorption in hypnotic suggestions, increased responsiveness to hypnotic suggestions, and usually, though not always, deep relaxation (Barber 1996, Alden and Heap 1998, Peebles-Kleiger 2000). For relief of pain, hypnotic suggestions and imagery are used to divert attention from the usual experience of pain and to increase comfort.

Theoretical debate

According to proponents of state theory, hypnosis is a special state of consciousness, distinct from the normal waking state, characterized by heightened responsiveness to suggestions. Once the hypnotic state is induced, responses to suggestions, for example, relief of pain are experienced as non-voluntary and passive or 'automatic' (Eastwood et al 1998). In this view, some individuals ('high hypnotizables') are more able than others to enter into a deep hypnotic state, or 'trance', and are more responsive to suggestions.

Since the 1960s, cognitive-behavioural psychologists have argued that hypnotic phenomena are more simply explained by social and cognitive influences normally expected to increase suggestibility in motivated subjects, without need to invoke a special altered state (Spanos and Chaves 1989, Spanos et al 1994, Alden and Heap 1998). They hold that short non-hypnotic instructions to enhance expectations, motivation, relaxation, and the use of imaginative skills are sufficient to heighten responsiveness to suggestions for analgesia without use of a hypnotic induction, as such (Spanos et al 1994). In this view, the subject or patient is an active participant who enters an implicit contract to respond to desirable suggestions, such as reduction of pain. It has even been suggested that the appearance of an altered state is no more than the result of social compliance on the part of subjects (Spanos et al 1994). Montgomery and colleagues (2000) argue against this position on grounds that studies of hypnosis often show reduced need for pain medication during painful procedures (Wakeman and Kaplan 1978, Lang et al 1996), a result unlikely to be highly influenced by social 'role' or demand characteristics.

The debate has spawned a considerable body of theory-driven research. In fact, it has been possible to interpret and reinterpret studies in favour of either point of view (Dixon and Laurence 1992, Spanos et al 1994, Chaves 1997b). For example, in support of the state view, several experimental studies have shown that highly hypnotizable subjects report greater analgesia in response to suggestions in the hypnotized than in the non-hypnotized state (Stacher et al 1975, Hilgard et al 1978, Malone et al 1989). According to Spanos et al (1994) such findings reflect social compliance rather than a true reduction of pain.

Laurence (1997) contends that research unencumbered by theoretical bias would do more to advance our understanding of hypnosis. In fact, there may be no debate to win, only different aspects of the same phenomena to explore, reminiscent of the blind men arguing about the description of an elephant as each touches a different body-part. For example, sociocognitive theorists tend to discuss hypnosis in terms of the set of behavioural instructions given to subjects or patients, while proponents of state theory focus more on the subjective experience of the person receiving suggestions. With regard to hypnotic analgesia, the picture is complicated by the fact that both the experience of hypnosis and the experience of pain are subjective events, dependent on the subject's report. Barber (1996) suggests that interpretations of findings are largely a function of one's view of psychology, and possibly, whether one has had a hypnotic experience.

Neurophysiological research

Recent research in neurophysiology shows central nervous system changes in subjects undergoing hypnoanalgesia (Holroyd 1996, Hofbauer et al 2001).

As early as 1966, Duensing proposed multiple sites such as spinal cord, midbrain, and frontal lobes for pain-blocking action during hypnoanalgesia. Hawkins and LePage (1988) concurred that frontal lobes may inhibit upwards transmission of pain signals at the level of the brain stem, and Kissen (1986) suggested the inhibitory septal-hippocampus circuit accounted for increased EEG theta wave activity typically observed in altered states of consciousness. Gruzelier and Warren (1993) proposed that inhibitory functions of the frontal lobe and limbic systems may contribute to observed peripheral nervous system changes associated with hypnosis and pain modulation.

According to Holroyd (1996), neural inhibition likely contributes to hypnotic analgesia since inhibitory neurons continually down-regulate excitatory neurons in the brain and spinal cord to prevent overload of sensory stimulation. Recent studies of hypnotized subjects have shown changes in both excitatory and inhibitory patterns in the brain (Holroyd 1992, Crawford and Gruzelier 1992, Crawford 1994).

Studies by Arendt-Nielsen et al (1990) and Spiegel et al (1989) showed that amplitudes of EEG event-related potentials (ERPs) were reduced in hypnotic analgesia subjects given electric shock, indicating less awareness of pain. As well, suggestions to not feel an electric shock were followed by reductions in skin reflexes on the arm (Hernandez-Peon et al 1960), in muscle response in the ankle (Kiernan et al 1995), and in nerve response in the jaw (Sharav and Tal 1989), suggesting inhibition was occurring at the spinal cord level as well.

Research using positron emission tomography and somatosensory event-related potentials indicates that hypnotic analgesia decreases pain sensation by inhibiting thalamic-somatosensory cortex pathways and decreases subjective pain unpleasantness by inhibiting thalamic-frontal cortex-anterior cingulate pathways (Crawford et al 1998).

Taken together, results of neurophysiologic research on hypnotic analgesia offer strong evidence for the influence of active inhibitory control of incoming stimuli at various levels of the central nervous system, and possibly also at peripheral levels (Holroyd 1996, Peebles-Kleiger 2000).

Hilgard's well-known dissociation model proposes that in the hypnotic state there can be a dissociation of sensory and affective components of pain, possibly at the medial thalamus level, such that a nociceptive stimulus may be registered as pain by the body, but the information does not register in (is dissociated from) higher brain centres (Hilgard 1984, Hilgard and Hilgard 1994).

In Chapman's constructivist model, awareness is produced by a massive complex of parallel brain processes (Chapman and Nakamura 1998). Building on Melzack's (1996) neuromatrix model of pain, Chapman and Nakamura contend that central processing associated with hypnotic analgesia involves much greater complexity than could be accounted for by simple linear information processing in somatosensory pathways. A process called 'priming feedback', which alters the formation of schemata in a non-volitional manner during hypnosis, is proposed, thus producing the experience of effortlessness in response to analgesic suggestions.

Rainville and colleagues (1999) conducted an experimental study to examine neural mechanisms underlying the effects of hypnotic suggestions to alter pain during hand immersion in painfully hot water. Positron emission tomography was used to measure regional cerebral blood flow (rCBF), and electroencephalography (EEG) to measure brain electrical activity. The authors concluded that the observed occipital increases in rCBF and delta EEG activity reflect an alteration of consciousness. Corroborating evidence came from subjects' spontaneous reports of an altered state of consciousness, including feelings of deep relaxation, automatic responding, and a suspension of usual time orientation.

Hypnotizability

Early in the scientific study of hypnosis, scales were constructed to predict hypnotic suggestibility. Commonly used tests are the Hypnotic Induction Profile (Spiegel 1974), Harvard Group Scale of Hypnotic Susceptibility (Shor and Orne 1962), and the Stanford Hypnotic Susceptibility scale (Weitzenhoffer and Hilgard 1959). In these tests, subjects first undergo a hypnotic induction and are then rated on their responses to a series of behavioural suggestions. Hypnotizability is assessed by the number of suggestions subjects follow, with the assumption that responses are involuntary.

The predictive value of these scales in studies of hypnotic analgesia has been mixed. Subjects classified as high hypnotizables have shown greater pain relief than low hypnotizables in studies of conditions such as headache (Andreychuk and Skriver 1975, Cedercreutz et al 1976, Friedman and Taub 1985), labour pain (Harmon et al 1990), treatment-induced temporomandibular joint pain (Stam et al 1984), and burn pain (Schafer 1975). However, other studies failed to show a correlation between hypnotizability and responsiveness to suggested analgesia in conditions such as headache (Nolan et al 1989, Spanos et al 1994), obstetrical pain (Rock et al 1969, Samko and Schoenfeld 1975, Venn 1987), and dental pain (Gillett and Coe 1984).

Results are also variable in research on paediatric populations. For example, Hilgard and LeBaron (1982) found that following hypnotic induction, children previously identified as high hypnotizables showed less reported and observed procedural pain during bone marrow aspiration (BMA) than low hypnotizables, while no such relationship was found during BMA in a study by Wall and Womack (1989).

Spanos and colleagues (1994) argue that hypnotizability test results influence subjects' responses to suggestion by creating expectations about their ability to reduce pain in hypnotic situations. In research designed to investigate this question, subjects who scored low on the scales but did not know that results were expected to predict ability to reduce pain following suggestion, or who were led to expect they would do well in responding to suggestions for analgesia despite test results, reported pain reductions similar to highly hypnotizable subjects (Spanos and Voorneveld 1987, Spanos et al 1988, Andrews and Hall 1990). As well, several studies found no relationship between hypnotizability and pain relief when hypnotizability was measured after hypnotic intervention (Spanos et al 1993, Lang et al 1996). Furthermore, there is evidence that ability to control pain can improve with training in hypnoanalgesia (Lewis 1992, Crasilneck 1995), indicating that susceptibility to hypnotic suggestions may not be a stable trait.

Clinical conditions

This section describes the use of hypnotic analgesia in painful clinical conditions, without further commentary on theoretical viewpoint or critique of published reports. The term hypnosis is used as authors under discussion use it, and generally refers to a process involving focused attention, imagery, and suggestions for comfort, with or without a formal hypnotic induction.

Burn pain

Patients with burn injuries suffer not only from the severe pain of burn, but also from the excruciating pain of debridement and frequent dressing changes.

They must often undergo multiple painful procedures daily, sometimes for many months (Patterson 1996). While opioid medications are essential during these treatments, the adjunctive use of hypnosis can offer added benefit.

Controlled studies have shown that hypnotic analgesia can reduce pain as well as medication needs in hospitalized burn patients. For example, Wakeman and Kaplan (1978) found that burn patients in their hypnosis treatment group requested significantly less analgesic medication than those receiving only attention from a psychologist. In a study by Patterson and colleagues (1989), a group of 8 patients with burn injuries and high baseline levels of pain showed significant decreases in pain ratings after hypnotic treatment, while 14 historical control patients with high pain scores did not.

Several studies by Patterson and his colleagues have shown that patients with high initial pain scores benefit more from hypnotic analgesia, particularly during intensely painful procedures, such as wound cleaning and physical therapy (Patterson et al 1997). In one study, burn patients were randomly assigned to one of three groups: hypnotic treatment together with medication, pain medication only, and attention-control visits from a psychologist. Patients receiving both hypnotic and chemical anaesthesia showed greater reductions in their VAS pain scores than either of the two other groups. As well, the effect was consistent with nurses' ratings of patients' pain. The patients in this study all had high baseline levels of pain (Patterson et al 1992). These differences were not observed in a similar study looking at outcome independent of pain levels at baseline (Everett et al 1993). In a subsequent study, Patterson and Ptacek (1997) showed that pain ratings decreased significantly in the hypnotic analgesia group and not in the control group when baseline pain measures were high, but the distinction disappeared when baseline pain ratings were ignored, suggesting that initial pain level may be an important predictor of the usefulness of hypnotic analgesia in burn pain.

For an excellent discussion with examples of the use of hypnosis for burn care in the emergency room, the intensive care unit, and during acute care procedures, see Patterson (1996).

Cancer pain

Not all cancer patients suffer pain from their disease, although most have pain related to treatments or procedures. Pain from cancer occurs in about 30 to 40% of all cancer patients and from 60 to 90% of patients with advanced disease (Portenoy 1989, Cleeland et al 1994, Grond et al 1994).

There are different sources of pain associated with cancer, including for example, post-surgical pain, chemotherapy-caused pain, bone marrow aspirations, radiation burns, nociception from tumour invasion, gastrointestinal distress, and neuropathic pain from nerve root invasion (Syrjala and Roth-Roemer 1996).

In a study of patients with hyperthermia-induced cancer pain, Reeves and colleagues (1983) showed that those receiving a hypnotic intervention had significantly greater reduction in pain than those in the control group. Syrjala and colleagues (1987) found hypnotherapy to be more effective than cognitive-behavioural treatment in reducing oral pain secondary to chemotherapy and radiation.

A substantial body of literature on children with cancer-related pain shows that hypnosis or hypnosis-like methods can reduce pain and augment benefits of medication, especially during procedures (Zeltzer and LeBaron 1982, Katz et al 1987, Kuttner et al 1988, Wall and Womack 1989, Syrjala and Roth-Roemer 1996). Liossi and Hatira (1999) found that both hypnosis and cognitive-behavioural skills training alleviated pain and distress of paediatric patients undergoing bone marrow aspirations, but hypnosis was more effective in decreasing anxiety and behavioural signs of distress.

Pain in dentistry

One of the first uses of hypnosis, reported as far back as the early 1800s, was attenuation of pain during tooth extractions (Patel et al 2000). Currently, hypnosis in dentistry is used as much to allay anxiety as it is to manage procedural pain (Mulligan 1996, Patel et al 2000). This application is particularly important as 8–16% of the population stay away from the dentist because of fear (Gerschman 1988).

Hypnosis in dentistry is typically used as an adjunct to local anaesthetics, although in some patients with allergies to chemical anaesthesia it has been used alone (Morse and Wilcko 1979, Kleinhauz and Eli 1993). In one study, Barber (1977) reported the successful use of his rapid induction analgesia method in 99% of subjects undergoing a dental procedure without chemical anaesthesia.

Hypnosis has also been effective in modifying maladaptive oral habits, such as tongue thrust, bruxism, and clenching (Hartland 1989, Chaves 1997a), and improving tolerance for orthodontic or prosthodontic appliances (Patel et al 2000). Patel and colleagues (2000) discuss use of hypnosis in patients with chronic facial pain syndromes. For example, Gerschman and colleagues (1978) found that 68% of patients with various complaints, including temporomandibular joint dysfunction and atypical facial pain, showed significant improvement with the use of hypnosis.

Headache

Barber (1996) reports several well-documented cases of effective use of hypnosis with problems of migraine, vascular headache, muscle tension headache, cluster headache, and posttraumatic headache. Spanos and colleagues (1994) also cite evidence for relief of various types of head pain with hypnotic suggestion, but overall find no difference between hypnoanalgesia and other psychological interventions.

Friedman and Taub (1984) showed equal reductions in frequency and intensity of migraine headaches with thermal biofeedback, relaxation alone, hypnotic relaxation plus thermal imagery, and hypnotic relaxation alone, compared with no treatment. In a study comparing autogenic training and training in self-hypnosis, Spinhoven and colleagues (1992) found significant improvements in chronic tension headache and associated distress in both groups, but no differences between the groups. Melis et al (1991) showed that patients with chronic tension headache receiving a hypnosis treatment reported significantly greater reductions in frequency and intensity of headache than those in a waiting-list control group, but they made no comparisons with non-hypnotic intervention.

Hypnosis and similar techniques have also been shown to improve head pain in children and adolescents, and in some cases to reduce medication requirements (Holden et al 1999, Gysin 1999). Hypnosis may be particularly useful when chronic head pain fails to respond to medication, but often treatment will need to target emotional problems as well as pain.

Postoperative and interventional pain

In a literature review, Blankfield (1991) found consistent support for the use of hypnotic treatments in the postsurgical care of patients. According to Peebles-Kleiger (2000), hypnotic suggestions preceding surgery can decrease patients' postoperative ratings of pain and requirements for analgesic medication. Defechereux et al (2000) report that patients sedated by means of hypnoanaesthesia preceding thyroid surgery had less postoperative pain than those under general anaesthesia. In a study of patients receiving an intravenous drug for anxiety and pain during interventional radiologic procedures, the self-hypnosis group had fewer procedural interruptions, received seven times fewer drug units, and self-administered less analgesic medication than the control group. Interestingly, a hypnotizability measure administered after patients had recovered showed no correlation between degree of hypnotizability and outcome (Lang et al 1996).

Paediatric pain

A substantial body of literature has shown that hypnotic interventions can alleviate pain and anxiety in children. For example, Lambert (1996) found that paediatric surgical patients who received hypnosis with guided imagery had significantly lower postoperative pain ratings and shorter hospital stays than those in the control group. As well, Iserson (1999) provides evidence for the usefulness of hypnosis in children during examinations and procedures in the emergency room.

Research with pediatric patients undergoing bone marrow aspiration lumbar punctures shows greater decreases in pain and distress with hypnotic treatments combining deep breathing and guided imagery than with non-imaginal distraction (Zeltzer and LeBaron 1982, Katz et al 1987, Kuttner et al 1988, Wall and Womack 1989). For a comprehensive review of the literature on the use of hypnosis for paediatric cancer patients, see Steggles and colleagues' annotated bibliography (1997).

Anbar (2001) showed that self-hypnosis was effective in resolving functional abdominal pain in four out of five paediatric patients, and was also useful in treating pain and other symptoms of chronic dyspnoea in paediatric patients with normal lung function at rest, who had not responded to medical treatments.

Barber (1996) emphasizes the need to consider the child's stage of development when determining the method of hypnosis to be used. For example, younger children are routinely engaged in imaginative play, rendering a hypnotic induction, as such, unnecessary. This changes progressively between the ages of 9 and 12 as children's critical reasoning ability becomes stronger. As well, a child's coping style must be taken into account when planning psychological interventions for pain attenuation. The problem is complicated by the need to also consider parents' coping style to achieve best outcome.

Gastrointestinal disorders

There is some indication that hypnosis can relieve symptoms of chronic intestinal distress, including pain. In a study by Whorwell and colleagues (1984), 30 patients suffering from severe irritable bowel syndrome were randomly assigned to either a psychotherapy group or treatment with hypnosis. The hypnosis group received suggestions for control of smooth muscle, gut motility, and improved bowel function. At 12 weeks, the hypnosis group had significantly decreased distension and pain as well as increased well-being by comparison with the psychotherapy group. The results were sustained at 18 months (1987), and were replicated in a later study using both individual and group hypnotherapy (Harvey et al 1989). As well, Prior and colleagues (1990) showed that hypnotic suggestions significantly decreased rectal sensitivity in patients with irritable bowel syndrome.

Obstetrics

Numerous studies have found reductions in reported pain during labour in women who received hypnoanalgesia (Davidson 1962, Rock et al 1969, Davidson et al 1985, Harmon et al 1990). The study by Harmon and colleagues of 60 nulliparous women showed shorter stage-one labour and less medication use in the hypnosis group than in the comparison group, which used only relaxation and breathing techniques. Jenkins and Pritchard (1993) showed that participants in their hypnosis treatment groups used significantly less analgesic medication than those in control groups matched for age and first- or second-time delivery. By contrast, Freeman and colleagues (1986) found that although women with first pregnancies in a self-hypnosis group reported greater satisfaction with the experience of childbirth, they were in labour for a longer time and showed no difference in pain ratings by comparison with those in the control group who received standard care. The women in this study were not randomized into groups, but had been offered a choice between standard care and self-hypnosis, including suggestions for creating sensations of warmth and relaxation as well as glove anaesthesia transferred to the abdomen.

While there is good evidence to support the use of hypnotic analgesia for pain during labour in some women, the myth that hypnosis alone should be sufficient to control pain has created unnecessary suffering. As with other clinical situations, hypnotic analgesia is only one option amongst several for reducing pain. It should not be used instead of chemical anaesthesia where that is indicated.

Chronic pain

To date, there has been a paucity of research on hypnotic analgesia in chronic pain conditions, but a few studies have shown benefits. Haanen et al (1991) reported that patients diagnosed with fibromyalgia responded to hypnotic suggestions and instructions for relaxation with greater improvements in sleep, muscle pain, fatigue, and well-being than those who received relaxation training and massage. As well, patients in the hypnosis group reduced their intake of paracetamol by 80% as opposed to 35% for the comparison group. Studies of other conditions treated effectively with hypnotic analgesia include chronic pain secondary to peripheral irritation (Spiegel and Albert 1983) and pain associated with reflex sympathetic dystrophy (Gainer 1992). Eimer (2000) describes how clinical applications of hypnosis can facilitate treatment in goal-oriented pain management programmes.

There is pressing need for more research into the use of hypnosis for the growing problem of chronic pain, a condition that often fails to respond sufficiently to medications or interventional anaesthesia therapies.

Application of hypnotic analgesia

A variety of established hypnotherapy techniques can be used to treat pain. As important as knowledge of technique is the therapist's sensitivity and ability to adapt to the needs, coping styles, and defense patterns of the patient. For example, some patients respond more to an authoritarian approach, while others do better with a permissive and collaborative approach.

An essential first step in the use of hypnosis for pain management is assessment of the patient's experience of pain, coping style, capacity for imagery, and assumptions about hypnosis. Barber (1996) suggests that hypnosis be tried for relief of pain only if patients feel comfortable with its use and are sufficiently motivated to continue to practise on their own. To allay anxiety and gain the necessary trust, patients' fears and concerns about hypnosis must be respectfully addressed. Frequently expressed concerns include fears of: (a) behaving strangely or shamefully as sometimes witnessed in stage hypnosis, (b) giving up control or being 'taken over' by an authority figure, (c) being unable to come out of trance, and (d) entering an unknown state of consciousness. It helps patients to know they will be using skills they already possess, such as imagination and absorption, and that they will not engage in behaviours against their will. Examples of absorption familiar to patients, such as watching a movie, can be useful. If further assurance is required, they can be told to raise their hand or say 'stop' if they feel in any way uncomfortable.

The following basic steps are common across hypnotic techniques: (a) the patient's interest and cooperation are obtained, (b) the range of attention is narrowed, (c) attention is directed inwards, and usually, (d) a deeply relaxed state is induced. Once these steps are complete, the hypnotherapist offers suggestions to increase comfort and creates imagery to reduce pain. For example, if the patient visualizes the pain as a solid harsh red colour, it can gradually be lightened to pale pink, or a burning pain in the hand can be relieved by imagining a handful of cool water scooped up from the river. In the method of 'glove anaesthesia', the therapist provides suggestions to create numbness in a pain-free hand, and may pinch the skin on the back of the hand to demonstrate absence of sensation. The numb-ness can then be transferred by placing the 'anaesthetized' hand to the painful part of the body. Imagery can be used to change the quality of the pain into a more bearable sensation (e.g., from burning to warmth or tingling) or to transfer the pain to a different part of the body where it can be better tolerated. Post-hypnotic suggestions, including reinforcing the patient's competence to use the procedure at home, can also be offered. The hypnotic session is ended by gradually returning the patient's attention to the immediate surroundings while suggesting feelings of comfort and alertness upon coming out of hypnosis.

The 'authoritarian' approach uses directives, instructing patients how to feel and what to do, for example, 'I want you to listen to my voice and as you listen your body will gradually relax.' The 'permissive' approach uses softer language, gives patients options for how they might feel or what they may experience, and acknowledges the therapist's uncertainty about the patient's images and subjective experience. For example, the therapist might say, 'As you listen to my voice, you may notice a feeling of calm come over you, and maybe you'll imagine yourself in a calm comfortable place, perhaps a quiet meadow, or maybe by the sea, looking at waves. Whatever you see as your calm safe place is fine.'

Modulation of voice, phrasing, and rhythm are important. Typically the voice is soft, low, and monotonous, with frequent repetitions and pauses between words (without regard to grammar) to make room for the patient's imaginative process and response to suggestions. Positive suggestions, such as you will feel calm and comfortable are more advisable than negative ones such as 'you won't feel pain anymore.' Use of metaphor engages the patient's imaginative process, enhancing suggested imagery to relieve pain.

Case example

Mr. B. had severe dysaesthesia and burning pain (diagnosed as complex regional pain syndrome, type II) in the left shoulder and arm, as a result of a work injury. He had not been helped by a variety of medications including anticonvulsants, opioids, tricyclic antidepressants, and NSAIDS. Nor did he benefit from intensive physiotherapy, TENS, or stellate blocks. Celexa had recently offered some benefit for anxiety and depression. Preceding the injury, he had been a healthy, athletic, well-functioning individual. He presented as sad, quiet, and helpless, but talked about an inner rage associated with his attempt to fight unrelenting pain, which he described as a 'solid wall, thick, black, and impenetrable'. We conducted one session of hypnotherapy enlisting Mr. B.'s own imagery. The following is an excerpt from the session.

> And now, as you feel the comfort… and calm…maybe in the distance you see the thick black wall …far away…just look at it from the distance... slowly…as the wall comes closer, you may feel that with each exhalation of breath, you blow out in the direction of the wall...As you blow softly towards the wall, softly but firmly, the colour of the wall may start to gradually fade from a dark to a lighter shade of black. Gradually, as you continue to blow in the direction of the wall, the black may become tinged with grey, then all grey, then a lighter…and lighter…and lighter shade of grey until it gradually becomes a diffuse, vanishing, barely visible grey. And now, with each breath out you may see the pale gray turn into the shape of a light grey cloud, and maybe that cloud will turn white or maybe it will stay

slightly grey, I don't know, but gradually you might begin blowing gently at the cloud, watching it float, and disperse, until there are only a few wisps left. Those few wisps may stay, or they may go, I don't know…but they don't need to bother you. They're just up there way off in the distance. You can continue to look up into the sky if you want to, and feel calm and peaceful…enjoy the peace and calm and comfort… calm… calm... calm….

Posthypnotic suggestion: And as you enjoy the ease you feel, you can know that later, if you need to, when you want to…maybe it will be later today or maybe it will be tomorrow or the day after, I really can't know…when you need to, you can use your breath to gradually disperse any discomfort you may feel... blowing gently to lighten, loosen and disperse…and to feel a sense of comfort and calm. You will only need to become aware of your easy breathing, in….and…out…and know you can use your breath to blow away any uneasy feeling and restore your comfort and calm.

Upon opening his eyes Mr. B. was calm and showed no signs of pain. He expressed surprise at how easy it had been to use his breath to blow away the wall of pain. In his appointment two weeks later, he said the 'wall of pain' had returned a few times, but he was able to 'blow it away', even while walking down a crowded street. There had been no unmanageable episodes of pain, and he was generally coping better. The benefit was sustained at follow-up three weeks later. In a telephone follow-up at six months he reported that the pain was not gone, but he was managing to control it well most of the time using the same hypnotic imagery. He was no longer depressed and was now working in a library. Credit for some of the improvement in mood and better coping may also be due to an increased dose of Celexa.

This successful example demonstrates that in some patients hypnotic analgesia may be effective where other treatments have failed. However, hypnosis is not 'magic'; it is only one more tool in the armamentarium against pain. In general, it should be used as an adjunct to medication, not instead of it, although in some people it may be useful on its own.

Caution must be used in selection of patients for hypnoanalgesic treatment since those with psychiatric disturbance or psychological instability could become further destabilized. Otherwise, in the hands of a well-trained and sensitive clinician, hypnosis has the benefit of being without side effects. For the interested clinician, accredited training programmes are available in many countries (see Peebles-Kleiger 2000). The reader is also referred to the *Handbook of Clinical Hypnosis* (Rhue et al 1993), and the excellent guide by Barber (1996), *Hypnosis and Suggestion in the Treatment of Pain.*

Conclusion

A recent meta-analysis (Montgomery et al 2000) of published studies on hypnotically induced analgesia showed that: (1) 75% of the population obtain substantial pain relief from hypnosis, (2) hypnosis is at least as effective as other psychological interventions for pain, and (3) individuals classified as medium and high hypnotizables profit more from hypnotic analgesia than those who score low on suggestibility scales. From these results the authors conclude that hypnoanalgesia is an effective treatment for pain and fits the criteria of a 'well-established treatment' (Chambless and Hollon 1998).

Clinicians and researchers have yet to reach a consensus on how hypnosis works (Pinnell and Covino 2000) and how to define it. While theoretical debate persists and laboratory studies continue to search for explanatory mechanisms, the use of clinical hypnosis for pain continues pretty much as it has done historically, with a few refinements and variations in technique. Despite persisting uncertainties, a large body of convincing research shows that hypnosis can help to relieve pain, reduce medication use, and shorten hospital stays (Lang et al 1996, Lambert 1996, Montgomery et al 2000).

References

Alden P, Heap M 1998 Hypnotic pain control: some theoretical and practical issues. International Journal of Clinical and Experimental Hypnosis 46: 62–76

Anbar RD 2001 Self-hypnosis for management of chronic dyspnea in pediatric patients. Pediatrics 107: E21

Andrews VH, Hall HR 1990 The effects of relaxation/imagery training on recurrent aphthous stomatitis: a preliminary study. Psychosomatic Medicine 52: 526–535

Andreychuk T, Skriver C 1975 Hypnosis and biofeedback in the treatment of migraine headache. International Journal of Clinical and Experimental Hypnosis 23: 172–183

Arendt-Nielsen L, Zachariae R, Bjerring P 1990 Quantitative evaluation of hypnotically suggested hyperaesthesia and analgesia by painful laser stimulation. Pain 42: 243–251

Barber J 1977 Rapid induction analgesia: a clinical report. American Journal of Clinical Hypnosis 19: 138–145

Barber J 1996 Hypnosis and suggestion in the treatment of pain. Norton, New York

Blankfield RP 1991 Suggestion, relaxation, and hypnosis as adjuncts in the care of surgery patients: a review of the literature. American Journal of Clinical Hypnosis 33: 172–186
British Society of Medical and Dental Hypnosis 2001 A brief history of hypnosis in medicine. Available at http://www.bsmdh.org/history.htm
Bryan WJA 2001 A history of hypnosis. Available at http://www.infinityinst.com/articles/nartic.html
Cedercreutz C, Lahteenmaki R, Tulikoura J 1976 Hypnotic treatment of headache and vertigo in skull injured patients. International Journal of Clinical and Experimental Hypnosis 24: 195–201
Chambless DL, Hollon SD 1998 Defining empirically supported therapies. Journal of Consulting and Clinical Psychology 66: 7–18
Chapman CR, Nakamura Y 1998 Hypnotic analgesia: a constructivist framework. International Journal of Clinical and Experimental Hypnosis 46: 6–27
Chaves JF 1997a Hypnosis in dentistry. Hypnosis International Monographs
Chaves JF 1997b The state of the 'state' debate in hypnosis: a view from the cognitive-behavioral perspective. International Journal of Clinical and Experimental Hypnosis 45: 251–265
Chaves JF, Barber TX 1976 Hypnotic procedures and surgery: a critical analysis with applications to 'acupuncture analgesia'. American Journal of Clinical Hypnosis 18: 217–236
Crasilneck HB 1995 The use of the Crasilneck Bombardment Technique in problems of intractable organic pain. American Journal of Clinical Hypnosis 37: 255–266
Crawford HJ 1994 Brain systems involved in attention and disattention (hypnotic analgesia) to pain. In: Pribram KH (ed) Origins: brain and self organization. Lawrence Erlbaum, Hillsdale, NJ, pp 661–679
Crawford HJ, Gruzelier JH 1992 A midstream view of the neuropsychophysiology of hypnosis: recent research and future directions. In: Fromm E, Nash MR (eds) Contemporary hypnosis research. Guilford, New York, pp 227–266
Crawford HJ, Knebel T, Kaplan L, Vendemia JM, Xie M, Jamison S, Pribram KH 1998 Hypnotic analgesia: 1. Somatosensory event-related potential changes to noxious stimuli and 2. Transfer learning to reduce chronic low back pain. International Journal of Clinical and Experimental Hypnosis 46: 92–132
Davidson GP, Garbett ND, Tozer SG 1985 An investigation into audiotaped self-hypnosis training in pregnancy and labor. In: Waxman D, Misra PC, Gibson M, Basker MA (eds) Modern trends in hypnosis. Plenum, New York, pp 223–233
Davidson JA 1962 An assessment of the value of hypnosis in pregnancy and labour. British Medical Journal 2: 951–953
Defechereux T, Degauque C, Fumal I, Faymonville ME, Joris J, Hamoir E, Meurisse M 2000 [Hypnosedation, a new method of anesthesia for cervical endocrine surgery. Prospective randomized study]. Annales de Chirurgie 125: 539–546
Dixon M, Laurence J-R 1992 Two hundred years of hypnosis research: questions resolved? questions unanswered? In: Fromm E, Nash MR (eds) Contemporary hypnosis research. Gilford, New York, pp 34–66
Duensing F 1966 Level of consciousness in hypnosis and the experience of pain from a neurophysiological (point of) view. Psychotherapy and Psychosomatics 14: 365–378
Eastwood JD, Gaskovski P, Bowers KS 1998 The folly of effort: ironic effects in the mental control of pain. International Journal of Clinical and Experimental Hypnosis 46: 77–91
Eimer BN 2000 Clinical applications of hypnosis for brief and efficient pain management psychotherapy. American Journal of Clinical Hypnosis 43: 17–40
Everett JJ, Patterson DR, Burns GL, Montgomery B, Heimbach D 1993 Adjunctive interventions for burn pain control: comparison of hypnosis and ativan: the 1993 Clinical Research Award. Journal of Burn Care and Rehabilitation 14: 676–683
Freeman RM, Macaulay AJ, Eve L, Chamberlain GV, Bhat AV 1986 Randomised trial of self hypnosis for analgesia in labour. British Medical Journal (Clinical Research Ed.) 292: 657–658
Friedman H, Taub HA 1984 Brief psychological training procedures in migraine treatment. American Journal of Clinical Hypnosis 26: 187–200
Friedman H, Taub HA 1985 Extended follow-up study of the effects of brief psychological procedures in migraine therapy. American Journal of Clinical Hypnosis 28: 27–33
Gainer MJ 1992 Hypnotherapy for reflex sympathetic dystrophy. American Journal of Clinical Hypnosis 34: 227–232
Gerschman JA 1988 Dental fears and phobias. Australian Family Physician 17: 261–263, 266
Gerschman J, Burrows G, Reade P 1978 Hypnotherapy in the treatment of oro-facial pain. Australian Dental Journal 23: 492–496
Gillett PL, Coe WC 1984 The effects of rapid induction analgesia (RIA), hypnotic susceptibility and the severity of discomfort on reducing dental pain. American Journal of Clinical Hypnosis 27: 81–90
Gruzelier J, Warren K 1993 Neuropsychological evidence of reductions on left frontal tests with hypnosis. Psychological Medicine 23: 93–101
Gysin T 1999 [Clinical hypnotherapy/self-hypnosis for unspecified, chronic and episodic headache without migraine and other defined headaches in children and adolescents]. Forsch Komplementarmedizin 6 (Suppl 1): 44–46
Haanen HC, Hoenderdos HT, van Romunde LK, Hop WC, Mallee C, Terwiel JP, Hekster GB 1991 Controlled trial of hypnotherapy in the treatment of refractory fibromyalgia. Journal of Rheumatology 18: 72–75
Harmon TM, Hynan MT, Tyre TE 1990 Improved obstetric outcomes using hypnotic analgesia and skill mastery combined with childbirth education. Journal of Consulting and Clinical Psychology 58: 525–530
Hartland J 1989 Medical and dental hypnosis and its clinical applications, 3rd edn. Baillière, Tindall & Cossell, London
Harvey RF, Hinton RA, Gunary RM, Barry RE 1989 Individual and group hypnotherapy in treatment of refractory irritable bowel syndrome. Lancet 1: 424–425
Hawkins R, LePage K 1988 Hypnotic analgesia and reflex inhibition. Australian Journal of Clinical and Experimental Hypnosis 16: 133–139
Hernandez-Peon R, Dittborn J, Borlone M, Davidovich A 1960 Changes of spinal excitability during hypnotically induced anesthesia and hyperesthesia. American Journal of Clinical Hypnosis 3: 64
Hilgard ER 1984 The hidden observer and multiple personality. International Journal of Clinical and Experimental Hypnosis 32: 248–253
Hilgard ER, Hilgard JR 1994 Hypnosis in the relief of pain. Brunner/Mazel, New York
Hilgard ER, LeBaron S 1982 Relief of anxiety and pain in children and adolescents with cancer: quantitative measures and clinical observations. International Journal of Clinical and Experimental Hypnosis 30: 417–442
Hilgard ER, Hilgard JR, Macdonald H, Morgan AH, Johnson LS 1978 Covert pain in hypnotic analgesia: its reality as tested by the real–simulator design. Journal of Abnormal Psychology 87: 655–663
Hofbauer RK, Rainville P, Duncan GH, Bushnell MC 2001 Cortical representation of the sensory dimension of pain. Journal of Neurophysiology 86: 402–411
Holden EW, Deichmann MM, Levy JD 1999 Empirically supported treatments in pediatric psychology: recurrent pediatric

headache. Journal of Pediatric Psychology 24: 91–109
Holroyd J 1992 Hypnosis as a methodology in psychological research. In: Fromm E, Nash MR (eds) Contemporary hypnosis research. Guilford, New York, pp 201–226
Holroyd J 1996 Hypnosis treatment of clinical pain: understanding why hypnosis is useful. International Journal of Clinical and Experimental Hypnosis 44: 33–51
Iserson KV 1999 Hypnosis for pediatric fracture reduction. Journal of Emergency Medicine 17: 53–56
Jenkins MW, Pritchard MH 1993 Hypnosis: practical applications and theoretical considerations in normal labour. British Journal of Obstetrics and Gynaecology 100: 221–226
Katz ER, Kellerman J, Ellenberg L 1987 Hypnosis in the reduction of acute pain and distress in children with cancer. Journal of Pediatric Psychology 12: 379–394
Kiernan BD, Dane JR, Phillips LH, Price DD 1995 Hypnotic analgesia reduces R-III nociceptive reflex: further evidence concerning the multifactorial nature of hypnotic analgesia. Pain 60: 39–47
Kissen B 1986 Conscious and unconscious programs in the brain: psychobiology of human behaviour. Plenum, New York
Kleinhauz M, Eli I 1993 When pharmacologic anesthesia is precluded: the value of hypnosis as a sole anesthetic agent in dentistry. Special Care in Dentistry 13: 15–18
Kuttner L, Bowman M, Teasdale M 1988 Psychological treatment of distress, pain, and anxiety for young children with cancer. Journal of Developmental and Behavioral Pediatrics 9: 374–381
Lambert SA 1996 The effects of hypnosis/guided imagery on the postoperative course of children. Journal of Developmental and Behavioral Pediatrics 17: 307–310
Lang EV, Joyce JS, Spiegel D, Hamilton D, Lee KK 1996 Self-hypnotic relaxation during interventional radiological procedures: effects on pain perception and intravenous drug use. International Journal of Clinical and Experimental Hypnosis 44: 106–119
Laurence JR 1997 Hypnotic theorizing: spring cleaning is long overdue. International Journal of Clinical and Experimental Hypnosis 45: 280–290
Lewis DO 1992 Hypnoanalgesia for chronic pain: the response to multiple inductions at one session and to separate single inductions. Journal of the Royal Society of Medicine 85: 620–624
Liossi C, Hatira P 1999 Clinical hypnosis versus cognitive behavioral training for pain management with pediatric cancer patients undergoing bone marrow aspirations. International Journal of Clinical and Experimental Hypnosis 47: 104–116
Malone MD, Kurtz RM, Strube MJ 1989 The effects of hypnotic suggestion on pain report. American Journal of Clinical Hypnosis 31: 221–230
Melis PM, Rooimans W, Spierings EL, Hoogduin CA 1991 Treatment of chronic tension-type headache with hypnotherapy: a single-blind time controlled study. Headache 31: 686–689
Melzack R 1996 Gate control theory: on the evolution of pain concepts. Pain Forum 5: 128–138
Montgomery GH, DuHamel KN, Redd WH 2000 A meta-analysis of hypnotically induced analgesia: how effective is hypnosis? International Journal of Clinical and Experimental Hypnosis 48: 138–153
Morse DR, Wilcko JM 1979 Nonsurgical endodontic therapy for a vital tooth with meditation-hypnosis as the sole anesthetic: a case report. American Journal of Clinical Hypnosis 21: 258–262
Mulligan R 1996 Dental pain. In: Barber J (ed) Hypnosis and suggestion in the treatment of pain. Norton, New York, pp 185–208
Nolan R, Spanos NP, Hayward A, Scott H 1989 Hypnotic and nonhypnotic imagery based strategies in the treatment of tension and mixed tension/migraine headache. In:
Patel B, Potter C, Mellor AC 2000 The use of hypnosis in dentistry: a review. Dental Update 27: 198–202
Patterson DR 1996 Burn pain. In: Barber J (ed) Hypnosis and suggestion in the treatment of pain. Norton, New York, pp 267–302
Patterson DR, Ptacek JT 1997 Baseline pain as a moderator of hypnotic analgesia for burn injury treatment. Journal of Consulting and Clinical Psychology 65: 60–67
Patterson DR, Questad KA, de Lateur BJ 1989 Hypnotherapy as an adjunct to narcotic analgesia for the treatment of pain for burn debridement. American Journal of Clinical Hypnosis 31: 156–163
Patterson DR, Everett JJ, Burns GL, Marvin JA 1992 Hypnosis for the treatment of burn pain. Journal of Consulting and Clinical Psychology 60: 713–717
Patterson DR, Adcock RJ, Bombardier CH 1997 Factors predicting hypnotic analgesia in clinical burn pain. International Journal of Clinical and Experimental Hypnosis 45: 377–395
Peebles-Kleiger MJ 2000 The use of hypnosis in emergency medicine. Emergency Medicine Clinics of North America 18: 327–328
Pinnell CM, Covino NA 2000 Empirical findings on the use of hypnosis in medicine: a critical review. International Journal of Clinical and Experimental Hypnosis 48: 170–194
Prior A, Colgan SM, Whorwell PJ 1990 Changes in rectal sensitivity after hypnotherapy in patients with irritable bowel syndrome. Gut 31: 896–898
Rainville P, Hofbauer RK, Paus T, Duncan GH, Bushnell MC, Price DD 1999 Cerebral mechanisms of hypnotic induction and suggestion. Journal of Cognitive Neuroscience 11: 110–125
Reeves JL, Redd WH, Storm FK, Minagawa RY 1983 Hypnosis in the control of pain during hyperthermia treatment of cancer. In: Bonica JJ, Lindblom U, Iggo A (eds) Advances in pain research and therapy, vol 4. Raven Press, New York, pp 857–861
Rhue JW, Lynn SJ, Kirsch I (eds) 1993 Handbook of clinical hypnosis. American Psychological Association, Washington, DC
Rock NL, Shipley TE, Campbell C 1969 Hypnosis with untrained, nonvolunteer patients in labor. International Journal of Clinical and Experimental Hypnosis 17: 25–36
Samko MR, Schoenfeld LS 1975 Hypnotic susceptibility and the Lamaze childbirth experience. American Journal of Obstetrics and Gynecology 121: 631–636
Schafer DW 1975 Hypnosis use on a burn unit. International Journal of Clinical and Experimental Hypnosis 23: 1–14
Sharav Y, Tal M 1989 Masseter inhibitory periods and sensations evoked by electrical tooth-pulp stimulation in subjects under hypnotic anesthesia. Brain Research 479: 247–254
Shor RE, Orne MT 1962 The Harvard group scale of hypnotic susceptibility. Consulting Psychologists Press, Palo Alto, CA
Spanos NP, Chaves JF 1989 Hypnosis, analgesia and surgery: in defence of the social psychological position. British Journal of Experimental and Clinical Hypnosis 6: 131–140
Spanos NP, Voorneveld PW 1987 The mediating effects of expectation on hypnotic and nonhypnotic pain reduction. Imagination, Cognition and Personality 6: 321–337
Spanos NP, MacDonald DK, Gwynn MI 1988 Instructional set and the relative efficacy of hypnotic and waking analgesia. Canadian Journal of Behavioural Science 26: 64–72
Spanos NP, Burnley MC, Cross PA 1993 Response expectancies and interpretations as determinants of hypnotic responding. Journal of Personality and Social Psychology 65: 1237–1242
Spanos NP, Carmanico SJ, Ellis JA 1994 Hypnotic analgesia. In: Wall PD, Melzack R (eds) Textbook of pain, 3rd edn. Churchill Livingstone, Edinburgh, pp 1349–1366
Spiegel D, Albert LH 1983 Naloxone fails to reverse hypnotic alleviation of chronic pain. Psychopharmacology (Berlin) 81: 140–143

Spiegel D, Bierre P, Rootenberg J 1989 Hypnotic alteration of somatosensory perception. American Journal of Psychiatry 146: 749–754
Spiegel H 1974 Manual for hypnotic induction profile. Soni Medica, New York
Spinhoven P, Linssen AC, Van Dyck R, Zitman FG 1992 Autogenic training and self-hypnosis in the control of tension headache. General Hospital Psychiatry 14: 408–415
St-Augustine 1966 Confessions. Transl. by: V. Bourke. Catholic University of America Press, Washington, DC
Stacher G, Schuster P, Bauer P, Lahoda R, Schulze D 1975 Effects of suggestion of relaxation or analgesia on pain threshold and pain tolerance in the waking and in the hypnotic state. Journal of Psychosomatic Research 19: 259–265
Stam HJ, McGrath PA, Brooke RI 1984 The effects of a cognitive-behavioral treatment program on temporo-mandibular pain and dysfunction syndrome. Psychosomatic Medicine 46: 534–545
Steggles S, Damore-Petingola S, Maxwell J, Lightfoot N 1997 Hypnosis for children and adolescents with cancer: an annotated bibliography, 1985–1995. Journal of Pediatric Oncology Nursing 14: 27–32
Syrjala KL, Roth-Roemer S 1996 Cancer pain. In: Barber J (ed) Hypnosis and suggestion in the treatment of pain. Norton, New York, pp 121–157
Syrjala KL, Cummings C, Donaldson G, Chapman CR 1987 Hypnosis for oral pain following chemotherapy and irradiation. Paper presented at the 5th World Conference on Pain, Hamburg, West Germany
Venn J 1987 Hypnosis and Lamaze method—an exploratory study: a brief communication. International Journal of Clinical and Experimental Hypnosis 35: 79–82
Wakeman RJ, Kaplan JZ 1978 An experimental study of hypnosis in painful burns. American Journal of Clinical Hypnosis 21: 3–12
Wall VJ, Womack W 1989 Hypnotic versus active cognitive strategies for alleviation of procedural distress in pediatric oncology patients. American Journal of Clinical Hypnosis 31: 181–191
Weitzenhoffer AM, Hilgard ER 1959 Stanford hypnotic susceptibility scale. Consulting Psychologists Press, Palo Alto, CA
Whorwell PJ, Prior A, Faragher EB 1984 Controlled trial of hypnotherapy in the treatment of severe refractory irritable-bowel syndrome. Lancet 2: 1232–1234
Whorwell PJ, Prior A, Colgan SM 1987 Hypnotherapy in severe irritable bowel syndrome: further experience. Gut 28: 423–425
Zeltzer L, LeBaron S 1982 Hypnosis and nonhypnotic techniques for reduction of pain and anxiety during painful procedures in children and adolescents with cancer. Journal of Pediatrics 101: 1032–1035

Chapter 36

A cognitive-behavioural approach to pain management

Dennis C Turk and Akiko Okifuji

Introduction

The cognitive-behavioural (C-B) perspective on pain management evolved from research on a number of mental health problems (e.g., anxiety, depression and phobias). Following the initial empirical research on C-B techniques in the early 1970s, there have been a large number of research and clinical applications. The common denominators across different C-B approaches include:

1. interest in the nature and modification of a patient's thoughts, feelings, and beliefs, as well as behaviours; and
2. some commitment to behaviour therapy procedures in promoting change (such as graded practice, homework assignments, relaxation, relapse prevention training, and social skills training) (Turk et al 1983).

In general, the C-B therapist is concerned with using environmental manipulations, as are behaviour (operant conditioning) therapists, but for the C-B therapist such manipulations represent informational feedback trials that provide an opportunity for the patient to question, reappraise, and acquire self-control over maladaptive thoughts, feelings, behaviours, and physiological responses. Both the C-B perspective and the gate control model of pain (Melzack and Wall 1965) emphasize the important contribution of psychological variables such as the perception of control, the meaning of pain to the patient, and dysphoric affect (Turk and Flor 1999).

Overview of the cognitive-behavioural perspective

It is important to differentiate the C-B perspective from C-B treatments. The cognitive-behavioural perspective is based on five central assumptions (Table 36.1) and can be superimposed upon any treatment approach used with chronic pain patients. In many cases the perspective is as important as the content of the therapeutic modalities employed, somatic as well as psychological (Turk 1997).

The application of the C-B perspective to the treatment of chronic pain involves a complex clinical interaction and makes use of a wide range of tactics and techniques. Despite the specific techniques used, all C-B treatment approaches are characterized by being present focused, active, time limited, and structured. Therapists are not simply conveyers of information acting on passive patients but serve as educators, coaches, and trainers. They work in concert with the patient (and sometimes

Table 36.1 Assumptions of the cognitive-behavioural perspective

- Individuals are active processors of information and not passive reactors.
- Thoughts (e.g., appraisals, expectancies, beliefs) can elicit and influence mood, affect physiological processes, have social consequences, and can also serve as an impetus for behaviour; conversely, mood, physiology, environmental factors, and behaviour can influence the nature and content of thought processes.
- Behaviour is reciprocally determined by *both* the individual and environmental factors.
- Individuals can learn more adaptive ways of thinking, feeling, and behaving.
- Individuals should be active collaborative agents in changing their maladaptive thoughts, feelings, and behaviours.

family members) to achieve mutually agreed upon goals.

A growing body of research has demonstrated the important roles that cognitive factors (appraisals, beliefs, expectancies) play in exacerbating pain and suffering, contributing to disability, and influencing response to treatment (Turk and Rudy 1992). Thus, C-B interventions are designed to help patients identify maladaptive patterns and acquire, develop, and practise more adaptive ways of responding. Patients are encouraged to become aware of and to monitor the impact that negative pain-engendering thoughts and feelings play in the maintenance of maladaptive overt and covert behaviours. Additionally, patients are taught to recognize the connections linking cognitions, affective, behavioural, and physiological responses together with their joint consequences. Finally, patients are encouraged to undertake 'personal experiments' and to test the effects of their appraisals, expectations, and beliefs by means of selected homework assignments. The C-B therapist is concerned not only with the role that patients' thoughts play in contributing to their disorders but, equally important, with the nature and adequacy of the patients' behavioural repertoire, since this affects resultant intrapersonal and interpersonal situations.

In this chapter we will focus only on the psychological components of the C-B treatment; however, it is important to acknowledge that the psychological treatment modalities described need to be considered within a broader rehabilitation model that includes physical and vocational components and involvement of significant others. The

Table 36.2 Phases in cognitive-behavioural treatment

1. Initial assessment
2. Collaborative reconceptualization of the patient's view of pain
3. Skills acquisition and skills consolidation, including cognitive and behavioural rehearsal
4. Generalization, maintenance, and relapse prevention
5. Booster sessions and follow-up

C-B perspective should be considered not merely as a set of methods designed to address the psychological components of pain and disability, but as an organizing strategy for more comprehensive rehabilitation (Turk 1997). For example, patients' difficulties arising during physical therapy may be associated not only with physical limitations but also with the fear engendered by anticipation of increased pain or concern about injury. Therefore, from a C-B perspective, physical therapists need to address not only the patient's performance of physical therapy exercises and the accompanying attention to body mechanics, but also the patient's expectancies and fears as they will affect the amount of effort, perseverance in the face of difficulties, and adherence with the treatment plan (Meichenbaum and Turk 1987). These cognitive and affective processes, including self-management concerns, may be impediments to rehabilitation and thus need to be considered and addressed, along with traditional instructions regarding the proper performance of exercise. The attention paid to the individual's thoughts and expectancies by a psychologist should be adopted by all members of the interdisciplinary treatment team.

The C-B treatment consists of five overlapping phases listed in Table 36.2. Although the five treatment phases are listed separately, it is important to appreciate that they overlap. The distinction between phases is designed to highlight the different components of the multidimensional treatment. Moreover, although the treatment, as presented, follows a logical sequence, it should be implemented in a flexible, individually tailored fashion. Patients proceed at varying paces and the therapist must be sensitive to these individual differences. In short, treatment should not be viewed as totally scripted. Therapists must realize that flexibility and clinical skills must be brought to bear throughout the treatment programme.

The C-B treatment is not designed to eliminate patients' pain per se, although the intensity and frequency of their pain may be reduced as a result of

Table 36.3 Primary objectives of cognitive-behavioural treatment programmes

- To combat demoralization by assisting patients to change their view of their pain and suffering from overwhelming to manageable.
- To teach patients that there are coping techniques and skills that can be used to help them to adapt and respond to pain and the resultant problems.
- To assist patients to reconceptualize their view of themselves from being passive, reactive, and helpless to being active, resourceful, and competent.
- To help patients learn the associations between thoughts, feelings, and their behaviour, and subsequently to identify and alter automatic, maladaptive patterns.
- To teach patients specific coping skills and, moreover, when and how to utilize these more adaptive responses.
- To bolster self-confidence and to encourage patients to attribute successful outcomes to their own efforts.
- To help patients anticipate problems proactively and generate solutions, thereby facilitating maintenance and generalization.

increased activity, physical reconditioning achieved during physical therapy, and the acquisition of various cognitive and behavioural coping skills. Table 36.3 outlines the primary objectives of C-B treatment. The treatment programme can readily supplement other forms of somatic, pharmacological, and psychological treatment.

The over-riding message of the C-B approach is that people are not helpless in dealing with their pain and need not view pain as an all-encompassing determinant of their lives. Rather, a variety of resources are available for confronting pain, and pain should come to be viewed by patients in a more differentiated manner. The treatment encourages patients to maintain a problem-solving orientation and to develop a sense of resourcefulness, instead of the feelings of helplessness and withdrawal that revolve around bed, physicians, and pharmacists.

Phase 1: assessment

The assessment and reconceptualization phases are highly interdependent. The assessment phase serves several distinct functions as outlined in Table 36.4 (see Turk and Okifuji 2002 for a detailed review of assessment methods). During the assessment phase, psychosocial and behavioural factors that probably have an impact on disability are evaluated. Attention is given to identification of any factors that might impede rehabilitation. All this information is integrated with biomedical information used in treatment planning. There should be a close relationship between the data acquired during the assessment phase and the nature, focus, and goals of the therapeutic regimen.

Table 36.4 Functions of assessment

- To establish the extent of physical impairment.
- To identify levels and areas of psychological distress.
- To establish, collaboratively, behavioural goals covering such areas as activity level, use of the health care system, patterns of medication use, and response of significant others.
- To provide baseline measures against which the progress and success of treatment can be compared.
- To provide detailed information about the patient's perceptions of his or her medical condition, previous treatments, and expectations about current treatment.
- To detail the patient's occupational history and goals vis-à-vis work.
- To examine the important role of significant others in the maintenance and exacerbation of maladaptive behaviours and to determine how they can be positive resources in the change process.
- To begin the reconceptualization process by assisting patients and significant others to become aware of the situational variability of the pain and the psychological, behavioural, and social factors that influence the nature and degree of pain.

Phase 2: Reconceptualization

A central feature of C-B treatment is facilitation of a new conceptualization of pain, thereby permitting the patient's symptoms to be viewed as circumscribed and addressable problems rather than pain as a vague, undifferentiated, overwhelming experience. The reconceptualization process prepares the patient for future therapeutic interventions in a way designed to anticipate and minimize patient resistance and treatment non-adherence (see Meichenbaum and Turk 1987 and Turk and Rudy 1991 for discussions of methods available to increase treatment adherence).

First contact with the patient

As part of this initial contact, pain questionnaires designed to elicit information regarding patients' thoughts and feelings about their capacity to exert control over pain and many other aspects of their lives, the impact of pain, and responses by significant others are administered (see Turk and Melzack 2001, Turk et al 2002). In addition, by means of a structured interview, questions designed to help patients view their severest pain episodes as having a definite beginning, middle, and ending; to see pain episodes as variable but not life-threatening; to interpret them as responses that can be controlled; and to view them as responsive to the passage of time, situational factors, and life circumstances are asked. As part of this assessment, the therapist encourages the patient's spouse or significant other to identify the impact of the patient's pain on them and the effect of their behaviour on the patient, as well as providing the family members with an understanding of the self-management approach to rehabilitation.

The therapist introduces the concept of 'pain behaviours' and 'operant pain' (Fordyce 1976, 2001) and discusses the important role that significant others may play in unwittingly, inadvertently, and perhaps unknowingly reinforcing and maintaining the patient's overt expression of pain and suffering. Such behaviours as grimacing, lying down, avoiding certain activities and moaning, are offered as examples of 'pain behaviours'. The patient's significant other is encouraged to recall examples of the patient's specific pain behaviours and how the significant other responded to such behaviours. The spouse or significant other is also asked to complete a diary of the patient's pain behaviours and their own responses. This homework assignment serves to highlight the role pain has come to have in their lives and the importance of significant others in the treatment. The questions put to the spouse or significant other include: 'How do you know when your spouse is experiencing severe pain?', 'What do you do in response?', and 'What impact does it have?'

The patient may be asked to complete a self-report diary for 1–2 weeks. They are asked to record episodes each day when they view their pain as moderate to severe and also when they are feeling particularly upset or distressed. They are also asked to record the circumstances surrounding the episode, who was present, what they thought, how they felt, what they did, and whether what they did had any effect on the level of their pain. Diaries are designed so that the therapist will use them to assist patients to identify the links among thoughts, feelings, behaviours, pain intensity, and distress. This process illustrates how assessment and treatment are intermixed; an important aspect of the learning process.

Finally, the assessment should also focus on the patient's strengths and resources (e.g., coping abilities, competencies, social supports). These can be incorporated into subsequent treatment phases and contribute to the cognitive restructuring process described below.

Preliminary formulation of treatment goals

At this point the patient, spouse, and therapist *collaborate* in establishing treatment goals that will return the patient to optimal functioning in light of any physical restriction and that are consistent with the patient's wishes. From the C-B perspective, collaboration is essential because it helps patients to feel that they are responsible for what occurs in treatment and for the outcomes. It is often helpful to use the information obtained from the structured interview, such as 'How would your life be different if your pain could be relieved?', to generate specific goals. The goals must be specific and measurable. For example, a patient's goal 'to feel better' is inadequate. The patient needs to specify what they will be doing that will indicate such improvement. We have found it useful to establish short-term, intermediate, and long-term goals in order that reinforcement by goal achievement can occur early in treatment, thus enhancing patients' self-confidence.

Towards the end of the reconceptualization phase it is appropriate to provide a brief description of what will occur in subsequent sessions such as education and practice of specific cognitive and behavioural coping skills. It is important that patients and significant others understand the kinds of demands and expectancies of the programme and the likely impact their efforts will have on all phases of their lives. Clarification of the treatment demands at the earliest phases of the programme helps to circumvent problems that often arise later during therapy.

Graded exercise and activities

Many chronic pain patients have developed a sedentary lifestyle that can exacerbate pain by reducing endurance, strength, and flexibility. Thus, the therapist, in collaboration with a physiotherapist and the patient's physician, should develop a graded exercise and activity programme appropriate to the patient's physical status, age, and sex. Patients should maintain activity-level charts of achievable, incremental goals from which progress can be gauged by the patient, as well as by the therapist and other family and treatment team members. Initial goals are set at a level that the patient should have little trouble achieving to assure success, with the requirements increasing at a gradual rate.

Medication reduction

Another important issue to discuss with the patient is the use of analgesic medication. There is sufficient evidence to indicate that many patients are overmedicated and often are dependent on analgesics. Moreover, reduction in pain can coincide with medication reduction (Flor et al 1992). It is advantageous to help patients reduce and eventually eliminate all unnecessary medication. Since reduction of some drugs is known to be accompanied by serious side effects, consultation with the physician is imperative.

Since self-control and responsibility are major factors in this approach, the therapist encourages the patient to systematically reduce their medication, helps the patient design procedures by which this can be accomplished, and shares responsibility for medication control with the patient. The patient is required to record the quantity and time of medication intake. The importance of medication reduction is stressed and the patient's medication records are carefully monitored. If the patient does not follow the guidelines in reducing the dosage, then this becomes a focus of discussion. The attempt to control medication intake is looked upon as a personal responsibility and the reasons for failure are considered in depth.

Translation process

At this time the translation or reconceptualization process begins in a more formal manner. A simplified conceptualization of pain based on the gate control model of Melzack and Wall (1965) is presented and contrasted with the sensory-physiological model held by many patients. The interaction of thoughts, mood state, and sensory aspects of a situation is presented in a clear, understandable fashion using the patient's self-monitored experiences as illustrations (Turk et al 1983). For example, the impact of anxiety is briefly considered and related to the exacerbation of pain. Data from patient diaries are extremely useful to make this point more concrete. Patients can review recent stressful episodes and examine the course their pain followed at that time.

To facilitate this reappraisal process, the therapist introduces the notion that the patient's experience of pain can be viewed as consisting of several manageable phases, rather than one overwhelmingly undifferentiated assault. In this way the patient comes to view their pain as composed of several components that go through different phases that are, in part, influenced by their reactions. The patient is not the 'helpless victim' of pain nor need they be a passive pawn. The therapist and patient have collected data to support this more differentiated view of pain, thus providing the basis for the intervention programme that will follow.

Examples are offered to show how pain can be subdivided into several steps, each of which is manageable by the patient. For example, when the patient rates his or her pain as 0 or 1 on an 11-point scale (i.e., no pain or fairly low-level intensity), this is an opportunity for the patient to engage in productive coping activities. This period of low-intensity pain can function as a time when the patient can plan how to deal with more intense levels of pain by means of employing cognitive and behavioural coping strategies that the patient will learn by the end of the treatment programme. Similarly, the patient can develop coping skills to employ at the higher levels of pain intensity. The patient is encouraged to view pain as creating problems to be anticipated and solved. A useful analogy is the way athletic teams develop game plans. Preplanning lowers the risk of the patient becoming overwhelmed at times of more severe pain, while implicitly fostering an expectation that episodes of the most severe pain will fade. Patients are also encouraged to self-reinforce their efforts throughout by taking credit for their coping efforts.

Negative thoughts, pain-engendering appraisals, and attributions are reviewed in treatment so that the patient will not be surprised when and if they do arise. Rather, the patient is encouraged to use the negatively valenced cognitions and feelings as reminders or as cues to initiate more adaptive coping strategies. The pain diaries described earlier can provide information that becomes the focus of discussion. For example, patients who recorded thoughts that they felt 'incompetent' and 'helpless' in controlling their pain during a specific episode should be encouraged to become aware of when they engage in such thinking and to appreciate how such thoughts may exacerbate their pain and become a self-fulfilling prophecy. Alternative thoughts, such as a realistic appraisal of the situation and of their coping resources, are encouraged and patients reinforced for using one or more of the coping strategies covered during the skills training. The patient is encouraged to divide the situation into stages as described earlier and to acknowledge that the most severe pain is usually relatively transitory. Such 'cognitive restructuring' is incorporated throughout the treatment regimen. The therapist also incorporates examples of when the patient has been resourceful in their life and considers how these skills can be applied in the pain situation.

Phase 3: skills acquisition and skills consolidation

The skills acquisition and skills consolidation phase begins once the basic initial goals of the treatment programme have been agreed upon. During this third phase the therapist provides practice in the use of a variety of cognitive and behavioural coping skills geared toward the alteration of the patient's response to environmental contributors to pain, to bolstering coping skills (e.g., attention diversion, relaxation skills for dealing with specific symptoms), to changing maladaptive interpretations, and to changing factors that might contribute to stress (e.g., maladaptive communication patterns).

In addition to helping the patient develop specific coping skills, this phase is also designed to help patients use skills they already possess and to enhance the patient's belief in their ability to exercise control, further enhancing a sense of self-efficacy. The point to be underscored is that the C-B approach does not deal exclusively with the pain symptoms per se, but with those self-statements and environmental factors that may instigate or maintain less than optimal functioning and subsequent pain exacerbations. Alterations in lifestyle, problem solving, communication skills training, relaxation skills, and homework assignments are woven into the fabric of the treatment.

As was the case with exercise, skills training follows a graded sequence. Firstly, the therapist discusses the rationale for using a specific method. This is followed by assessing whether the skills are in the patients' repertoires, teaching the patients the necessary skills, and having them practise in the therapeutic setting. As patients develop proficiency, they are encouraged to use the skills in their homes, first in the least difficult circumstance and then building up to more stressful or difficult situations (when their pain is greater or when they are engaged in an interpersonal conflict).

Problem solving

A useful way to think about pain is as a set of sequential problems, rather than simply as the presence of pain being a single overwhelming problem. The C-B therapists suggest that chronic pain presents the sufferer with an array of small and large problems—familial, occupational, social, recreational, and financial, as well as physical. The therapist assists patients in identifying their problems in these areas and presents a process for dealing with these problems, namely generating a set of alternatives, weighing the relative advantages and disadvantages of each of these alternatives, trying different solutions, evaluating the outcomes, and recycling the process as needed.

There are several critical features of problem-solving skills training. The important first step in problem solving is to have patients 'operationalize' their problems in behaviourally prescriptive language (e.g., when X occurs in situation Y, I feel Z). The second step is to help patients identify what particular situations are associated with pain. The use of self-monitoring in patient diaries can help to identify such problematic situations. Patients need to think of the difficulties that they encounter as 'problems to be solved'. Next, they must try out the alternative to achieve the desired outcome. Patients need to learn that there is usually not a single solution to solving problems and they need to weigh alternatives. In this way, lack of success with any one attempt will not be taken as a complete failure, but rather such setbacks and lapses are viewed as learning trials and occasions to consider alternatives. Patients should be given the homework task of formally identifying problems, generating alternative solutions, rating the solutions for likely effectiveness, trying them out, and then reporting on the outcome.

Relaxation and controlled breathing

Relaxation and controlled breathing exercises are especially useful in the skills acquisition phase because they can be readily learned by almost all patients and they have a good deal of face validity. Instruction in the use of relaxation and controlled breathing is designed not only to teach an incompatible response, but also as a way of helping the patients develop a behavioural coping skill that they can use in any situation in which adaptive coping is required. The practice of relaxation and controlled breathing strengthens the patients' belief that they can exert control during periods of stress and pain and that they are not helpless. Patients are encouraged to employ the relaxation skills in situations where they perceive themselves becoming tense, anxious, or experiencing pain.

Relaxation is not achieved by only one method. There are many relaxation techniques in the literature. There is no evidence that one relaxation approach is any more effective than any other. What is most important is to explain these findings to patients and help them determine what relaxation technique, or set of techniques, is most effective for them. Thus, in a collaborative mode, the therapist will assist patients to learn coping strategies that they find acceptable. If the coping effort proves ineffective, this is not to be viewed as a failure of relaxation nor a reflection of the patient's incompetence, but rather an opportunity to seek another alternative. As in the case of problem solving described above, it is suggested that there may not be any one best coping alternative, but rather different ones for different people or for the same individual in different situations.

Attentional training

The role of attention is a major factor in perceptual activity and therefore of primary concern in examining and changing behaviour. The act of attending has been described as having both selective and amplifying functions. Several types of strategies are considered and the patient is encouraged to choose those that are most likely to evolve into personally relevant resources. Patients are also assisted in generating strategies and techniques that they believe might be useful. Again, attempts to actively involve patients in their own treatment are made.

The therapist notes that people can focus their attention on only one thing at a time and that people control, to some extent, what they attend to, although at times this may require active effort. Examples, metaphors, and analogies are used to make this point concrete (coming from the patient's experience whenever possible). For example, the therapist uses the analogy of the simultaneous availability of all channels on a TV 'but only one channel can be fully attended to at any one time. Attention is like a TV channel tuner: we can control what we attend to, what we avoid, and the channel to which we tune'. With instruction and practice, the patient can gain similar control over his or her attention. This discussion prepares the way for presentation of different cognitive coping strategies.

Both non-imagery and imagery-based strategies can be employed. Although imagery-based strategies (refocusing attention on pleasant pain-incompatible scenes and so forth) have received much attention, the results have not consistently demonstrated that any imagery strategies are uniformly effective for all patients (Fernandez and Turk 1989). The important component seems to be the patient's imaginative ability, involvement, and degree of absorption in using specific images. Guided imagery training is given to patients in order to enhance their abilities to employ all sensory modalities (e.g., imagine such scenes as a lemon being cut on a plate, a tennis match, or a pleasant scene that incorporates all five senses). The specifics of the images seem less important than the details of sensory modalities incorporated and the patient's involvement in these images (see Turk 1997 for detailed illustrations).

The therapist asks the patient to imagine circumstances along a continuum of pain and encourages the patient to see themselves employing the various images to cope with the pain more effectively. The purpose of the imagery and relaxation rehearsal is to foster a sense of 'learned resourcefulness' as compared to 'learned helplessness' that characterizes many pain patients.

Some patients will have difficulty learning relaxation or making use of imagery techniques. In such circumstances, it is often helpful to have patients use audiotapes or posters to help them focus their attention and to guide them with relaxation or imagery.

Phase 4: rehearsal and application training

After learning different skills, patients are asked to use them in imaginary situations in the therapist's office or the clinical setting. For example, after learning different relaxation methods, patients can be asked to imagine themselves in various stressful situations and to see themselves employing the relaxation and coping skills in those situations. For example, patients imagine the last time their pain intensity was rated between '6' and '10' on the pain intensity rating card and to see themselves using the relaxation and other coping techniques at those times. The intent is to have the patients learn that relaxation can be employed as a general coping skill in various situations of stress and discomfort and to prepare themselves for aversive sensations as they arise.

With success, the therapist can follow up with specific homework assignments that will consolidate the skills in the patient's natural environment. For example, patients are asked to practise relaxation techniques at home at least twice a day for 15 min with one of the practice sessions occurring prior to the times of the most intense pain, if such times have been identified on the pain intensity rating cards. Patients are also asked to anticipate potential problems that might arise in performing the homework assignment (e.g., they forget, they fall asleep) and to generate ways in which these obstacles might be addressed should they occur. In this way, attempts are made to anticipate potential difficulties before they arise and to convey the message to patients that they are capable of generating alternative solutions to problems.

Phase 5: generalization and maintenance

Generalization and maintenance are fostered throughout treatment by provision of guided exercise, imaginary and behavioural rehearsal, and homework assignments, each of which is designed to increase the patient's sense of self-efficacy. Following the skills acquisition and rehearsal phases, patients are encouraged to 'try out' the various skills that have been covered during the treatment in a broad range of situations and to identify any difficulties that arise. During these sessions, the patient is encouraged to consider potentially problematic situations and assisted in generating plans or scripts as to how they could handle these difficulties, should they arise. Plans are formulated for what the patient might do if they begin to lapse. The therapist attempts to anticipate problems and generate solutions, in a sense to 'inoculate' the patient against difficulties that may occur. Finally, the patient is encouraged to evaluate progress, review homework assignments, and, most importantly, to attribute progress and success to their own efforts.

It is not enough to have patients change—they must learn to 'take credit' for such changes that they have been able to bring about. The therapist asks the patient a series of questions to consolidate such self-attributions. For example: 'It worked? What did you do? How did you handle the situation this time differently from how you handled it last time? When else did you do this? How did that make you feel?'

Phase 6: treatment follow-up

At 1 month following termination, the patient is asked to return to review progress and the maintenance of skills. At 3 and 6 months and 1 year, follow-up appointments are made to consider any difficulties that have arisen. Patients are also encouraged to call for appointments between specific follow-up dates if they are having difficulty with any aspect of the training. Checking in with the therapist is not viewed as a sign of failure, but rather as an opportunity to re-evaluate coping options. It should be obvious that C-B therapy consists of more than implementing a set of skills. Rather, it is a way of helping patients change their views of themselves and their plight. The techniques are used to help bring about the change from passivity to active control. The intangibles of treatment, such as the patient–therapist relationship of collaboration and how information is communicated, are at least as important as any specific skills presented and taught.

Effectiveness of the cognitive-behavioural approach

C-B approaches have been evaluated in a number of clinical pain studies. The results tend to support the effectiveness of C-B therapy in reducing pain and improving funcitonal activities (Morley et al 1999)

The C-B approach offers promise for use with a variety of chronic pain syndromes across all developmental levels. The American Psychological Association Task Force on Treatment Efficacy designated cognitive-behavioural therapy for chronic pain as one of 20 applications of psychological treatments for which there was significant empirical support.

Taken as an aggregate, the available evidence suggests that the C-B approach has a good deal of potential as a treatment modality by itself and in conjunction with other treatment approaches. The cognitive-behavioural perspective is a reasonable way for health care providers to think about and deal with their patients regardless of the therapeutic modalities utilized.

References

Fernandez E, Turk DC 1989 The utility of cognitive coping strategies for altering pain perception: a meta-analysis. Pain 38: 123–135

Flor H, Fydrich T, Turk DC 1992 Efficacy of multidisciplinary pain treatment centers: a meta-analytic review. Pain 49: 221–230

Fordyce WE 1976 Behavioural methods for chronic pain and illness. Mosby, St Louis

Fordyce WE 2001 Contingency management. In: Loeser JD, Butler SD, Chapman CR, Turk DC (eds) Bonica's management of pain, 3rd edn. Lippincott Williams & Wilkins, Philadelphia

Meichenbaum D, Turk DC 1987 Faciliating treatment adherence: a practitioner's guidebook. Plenum Press, New York

Melzack R, Wall PD 1965 Pain mechanisms: a new theory. Science 150: 971–979

Morley S, Eccleston C, Williams A deC 1999 Systematic review and meta-analysis of randomized controlled trials of cognitive behaviour therapy and behavior therapy for chronic pain in adults, excluding headache. Pain 80: 1–13

Turk DC 1997 Psychological aspects of pain. In: Bakule P (ed) Expert pain management Springhouse, Springhouse, PA

Turk DC, Flor H 1999 Chronic pain: a biobehavioral perspective. In: Gatchel RJ, Turk DC (eds) Psychosocial factors in pain. Guilford Press, New York

Turk DC, Melzack R (eds) 2001 Handbook of pain assessment, 2nd edn. Guilford Press, New York
Turk DC, Okifuji A 2002 Clinical assessment of the person with chronic pain. In: Jensen TS, Wilson PR, Rice ASC (eds) Textbook of clinical pain management: chronic pain. Arnold, London
Turk DC, Rudy TE 1991 Neglected factors in chronic pain treatment outcome studies—relapse, noncompliance, and adherence enhancement. Pain 44: 24–43
Turk DC, Rudy TE 1992 Cognitive factors and persistent pain: a glimpse into Pandora's box. Cognitive Therapy and Research 16: 99–122
Turk DC, Meichenbaum D, Genest M 1983 Pain and behavioural medicine: a cognitive-behavioral perspective Guilford Press, New York
Turk DC, Monarch ES, Williams AD 2002 Psychological evaluation of patients diagnosed with fibromyalgia syndrome: comprehensive approach. Rheumatic Disease Clinics of North America 28: 219–233

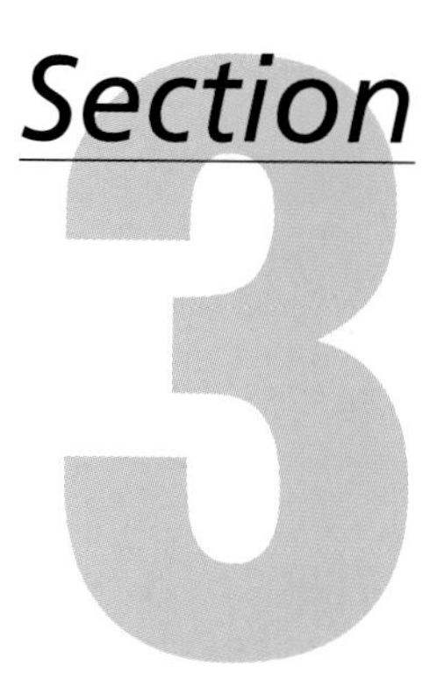

Special problems of assessment and management

Chapter 37

Pain in children

Charles B Berde and Bruce Masek

Introduction

Nociceptive functions develop during fetal life and show considerable maturity even in preterm neonates. Infants and children can receive treatment for acute and chronic pain with efficacy and safety comparable to adults. Pain assessment and measurement in infants and pre-verbal children is more difficult because of the inability to use self report, and requires judicious use of behavioural and physiologic measures. Fear and anxiety are prominent in hospitalized children. An essential aspect of paediatric pain management and supportive care lies in making medical encounters less terrifying. Cognitive-behavioural treatments can be used for children undergoing medical procedures or in treatment of a range of acute and chronic pain problems. Analgesic pharmacology differs in neonates because of certain pharmacokinetic and pharmacodynamic factors. Many age-related pharmacologic differences become less important after the first year of life.

In this chapter, we will review:

(1) the developmental neurobiology of pain sensation and perception,
(2) methods of pain assessment and measurement at different ages,
(3) analgesic pharmacology in children,
(4) specific pain syndromes in children,
(5) psychological factors in the child's responses to pain, illness, and the hospital environment, and
(6) nonpharmacologic methods of pain management.

Developmental neurobiology of pain

Pain is a powerful force in learning and neurologic development. Behaviour is shaped to a considerable degree by stimuli that evoke pain as well as pleasure. It would thus be expected that the afferent pathways for pain sensation and perception would develop early: there is considerable adaptive significance in avoiding things that hurt. A number of research groups over the past 20 years have characterized the ontogeny of pain pathways in the peripheral and central nervous system.

An important series of studies by Fitzgerald and her coworkers described neurobehavioural, neuroanatomic, and neurophysiologic aspects of the development of nociceptive systems in infant rats, with some correlative studies in infant humans (Andrews and Fitzgerald 1997). Sensory nerves project to peripheral targets during mid-gestation in rats and in humans.

The flexion withdrawal reflex is well developed in neonatal rats and humans (Fitzgerald et al 1988). Neonates respond to milder mechanical or thermal stimuli than older subjects. Human newborns receiving repeated heel sticks for blood sampling develop secondary hyperalgesia indicative of spinal plasticity.

Noxious stimuli evoke stronger responses in peripheral and spinal neurons in infant animals than in those in older organisms, and these responses are more 'spread out' spatially and temporally. Myelination of afferent pathways to the thalamus is well developed by 30 weeks. Thalamo-cortical projections begin synapse formation with cortical neurons by 20–24 weeks, and myelination of thalamo-cortical fibres is well developed by roughly 37 weeks.

Some reviewers have suggested, based on these studies, that the neonate may feel pain more intensely than older subjects. This interpretation should be made with caution, since neurophysiological and molecular studies do not clarify the nature of pain, viewed as suffering, in neonatal humans or animals. We know comparatively little about the supraspinal aspects of nociception in neonates, and even less about the affective dimension of their pain experiences.

Rather than addressing the nature of suffering in the neonate, one can more readily examine whether there are adverse short- or long-term consequences of noxious events in neonates, and whether these consequences can be ameliorated by analgesics or other pain-reducing interventions.

Short-term consequences of pain in the neonate

Noxious events, including needle procedures or surgery, evoke behavioural and physiologic signs of stress and distress in newborns. Surgery in inadequately anaesthetized newborns evokes a dramatic hormonal and metabolic stress response that can be associated with haemodynamic fluctuations, catabolism, and postsurgical complications (Anand et al 1987). Opioids (Robinson and Gregory 1981) and regional anaesthesia can be used safely and effectively in neonates. Both may blunt hormonal-metabolic and autonomic stress responses. In some cases, blunting of stress responses may improve outcomes (Anand and Hickey 1992). With proper expertise, neonates can be safely anaesthetized for any type of surgery (Berry and Gregory 1987, Berde 1998). There is no need to perform surgery in neonates without adequate general and/or regional anaesthesia.

Newborn circumcision is commonly performed without anaesthesia. Circumcision performed in this manner produces autonomic changes, including increases in heart rate and blood pressure, and hypoxaemia. Several methods have been studied to reduce the pain of circumcision, including dorsal penile nerve block (Stang et al 1988), ring block, and topical anaesthesia with a eutectic mixture of lidocaine (lignocaine) and prilocaine known as EMLA (Benini et al 1993, Taddio et al 1997). EMLA provides partial suppression of behavioural and physiologic signs of stress with circumcision; it appears more effective than placebo but less effective than ring block (Lander et al 1997). Non-pharmacologic measures, including oral ingestion of sucrose (Blass and Hoffmeyer 1991), also diminish distress with circumcision. The combination of pharmacologic and non-pharmacologic approaches may be optimal for this procedure.

Newborns in intensive care units commonly receive opioids and benzodiazepines, both for invasive procedures and for tolerating mechanical ventilation via endotracheal tubes. There is wide variation in analgesic and sedative use in this setting (Johnston et al 1997, Kahn et al 1998). A multicentre trial of ventilated neonates (Anand et al 1999) found evidence for improved neurologic outcomes in a group who received morphine infusions, compared with those receiving midazolam or placebo.

Potential long-term consequences of pain in the neonate

In a previous era, a common excuse for witholding analgesia from newborns was infants would not remember pain, and that there would be no long-term adverse sequelae of unrelieved pain in infancy. Some recent studies have attempted to address this issue. Responses to intramuscular injections for immunization were studied in 4- to 6-month-old boys who had participated as neonates in a randomized blinded comparison of EMLA to placebo for circumcision (Taddio et al 1997). In addition, there was a group of boys who were uncircumcised. Uncircumcised infants cried less and had lower pain ratings by blinded observers. For some measures, but not others, the EMLA group had statistically lower pain ratings than the placebo group. The authors could not explain away these group differences on the basis of baseline temperament or demographic variables. These findings are suggestive, but should be interpreted cautiously in view of a potential for confounding factors.

A study of heelstick procedures in preterm infants of varying previous histories (Johnston and Stevens 1996) found that neonates who had previously undergone the largest number of invasive procedures had the least behavioural responses to the heelstick procedure. This lack of responsiveness has been ascribed to interrupted neurologic development with critical illness, but may also reflect a degree of 'learned helplessness'.

Studies of children who had previously undergone newborn intensive care have found either fewer parental ratings of pain behaviours or a higher prevalence of somatized complaints in comparison to controls (Grunau et al 1994). These results are intriguing, although a range of alternative interpretations are possible, related to both a wide range of neurologic impairments in the survivors of newborn intensive care and effects of early trauma and illness on subsequent parent–child interactions.

Overall, the long-term consequences of untreated pain in infancy remain difficult to quantify, but merit further study. Since safe and effective treatments are available for many forms of pain, in our view the burden of proof lies with those who would withhold treatment, not with those who would treat pain aggressively with analgesics.

Pain assessment

In adults, self-report is most commonly relied upon for pain measurement and assessment. Visual analogue scales have a number of convenient and favourable properties. Children ages 8 and above can generally apply standard VAS scales successfully. Several self-report scales have been developed for children ages 3–8. These have been primarily in 3 groups: (1) scales that use pictures or drawings of faces, (2) scales that use graded colour intensity, generally red, and (3) scales that use numbers of objects, e.g., poker chips.

Faces scales have been quite popular, and these scales differ in several respects, including number of faces presented, the way the faces are drawn or photographed (Beyer et al 1992), and how the faces are ordered on the page (Wong and Baker 1988, Bieri et al 1990). In general, severe pain is depicted as a crying face, with eyes closed, brow furrowed, and nasolabial folds contracted. A recent study found that the pain ratings differ according to whether the 'no pain' end of the scale shows a neutral face or a happy face (Chambers and Craig 1998). Some children seem to be confused regarding ranking of happiness or well-being as opposed to absence of pain. Colour analogue scales (more pain corresponds to more intensely red colour) appear acceptable to most children ages 4 and older (Grossi et al 1983, McGrath et al 1996), and show convergent validity to VAS scales in older children.

Behavioural scales have been developed predominantly in two settings: in the assessment of toddlers and pre-school children undergoing brief painful procedures or surgery (Katz et al 1980, McGrath et al 1985) and in the assessment of neonates undergoing procedures or intensive care. Behavioural measures in neonates have examined facial expression, a range of gross motor behaviours, and analysis of cry acoustic properties. Facial expressions appear useful and valid as indicators of pain in neonates; they appear more robust and sensitive than measures of crying (Grunau et al 1990, Hadjistavropoulos et al 1994). Multidimensional measures that adjust for developmental stage such as the PIPP appear to be very appropriate for studies of preterm infants of different post-conceptional and postnatal ages (Johnston et al 1993; Stevens et al 1995, 1996).

Several behavioural scales in toddlers and older children have been labelled as 'distress' scales, because they record behaviours that may reflect combinations of pain, fear, or anxiety, but cannot distinguish among these states. Behavioural scales may overrate fear instead of pain in the setting of acute medical procedures, and may under-rate persistent pain, such as pain following surgery (Beyer et al 1990) or pain due to cancer. Many children with persistent pain due to cancer, surgery, burns, or sickle cell disease may lie still in bed, close their eyes, and inhibit their movements, not because they are comfortable or narcotized, but because it hurts too much to move; withdrawal from the surroundings is an adaptive response to unrelieved pain. Other behavioural measures developed for children with cancer incorporate assessment of social involvement and inhibition of movement (Gauvain-Piquard et al 1987). There is a need for additional validation and for modifications of these measures to make them more convenient and generalizable to other populations and clinical situations. Behavioural pain measures for children with developmental disabilities have been developed (Breau et al 2001).

Physiologic measures have seemed attractive because of their presumed objectivity. Pain evokes increases in heart rate, blood pressure, and respiratory rate, but these signs can be influenced by several physiologic conditions unrelated to pain.

Several investigators have examined variability in heart rate using a variety of mathematical algorithms in frequency domain or transfer function analyses to reflect sympathetic and parasympathetic contributions to the overall variability. Variability in heart rate has been widely used as an index of physiologic integrity and stress in fetal monitoring. Indices of 'vagal tone' have been used to measure stress and distress in neonates undergoing painful procedures (Porter et al 1988, Porter and Porges 1991), but some of these parameters may also be sensitive to factors unrelated to pain (Litvack et al 1995; Oberlander et al 1995, 1996). Variability in physiologic parameters, including heart rate, blood pressure, and end-tidal carbon dioxide, may be more useful than absolute trends in these physiologic parameters in painful situations (McIntosh et al 1994). Issues of sensitivity and specificity remain, since critical illness and other processes can also affect beat-to-beat variability of heart rate and blood pressure.

Stress hormones, including cortisol and epinephrine, and metabolites, such as glucose, are increased by surgical trauma, and analgesics and anaesthetics suppress these increased plasma concentrations, but there is little evidence for the specificity of any of these biochemical markers as a pain measure per se.

Overall, there is little immediate prospect for a unidimensional physiologic measure that is convenient and specific for pain in neonates.

Table 37.1 Factors that influence drug action in neonates

Factor	Clinical implications
Immature ventilatory reflexes	Greater potential for hypoventilation from opioids
Larger percent body mass as water, less as fat	Altered volumes of distribution
Immature hepatic enzyme systems	Diminished hepatic conjugation of drugs, accumulation of opioids and local anaesthetics with delayed toxicity during infusions
Diminished glomerular filtration and renal tubular secretion	Diminished renal excretion of opioid metabolites, with potential for delayed sedation and respiratory depression
Decreased plasma concentrations of albumen and α-1 acid glycoprotein	Decreased protein binding of drugs; greater first-pass local anaesthetic toxicity
Smaller size per se	With local anaesthetic blockade, the effective dose to block nerves scales weakly with body weight, while systemic toxicity scales directly with body weight, so that the therapeutic index for local anaesthetics is narrower in smaller subjects.

Developmental pharmacology

A number of pharmacokinetic and pharmacodynamic factors modify responses to analgesic medication in the newborn and young infant, as summarized in Table 37.1.

Analgesic pharmacology

Acetaminophen (paracetamol) is useful for treatment of mild pain and fever control. Acetaminophen replaced aspirin as the most commonly used routine analgesic and antipyretic in children in the 1970s, when it became apparent that aspirin could in rare circumstances cause Reye's hepatic encephalopathy, especially during viral illnesses. Acetaminophen overall appears very safe in children if dosing guidelines are followed. Children may receive single doses of 15–20 mg/kg, or repeated dosing of 10–15 mg/kg every 4 h. Toxicity appears related in part to cumulative dosing. Conservative daily dose limits based on available pharmacokinetic data are 90 mg/kg/day in children, 75 mg/kg/day in infants, 60 mg/kg/day in term neonates, and 45 mg/kg/day in preterm neonates from 32 weeks onwards (Lin et al 1997). Rectal absorption is slow, with peak concentrations over 70 min after administration. Single rectal doses of 35–40 mg/kg achieve therapeutic plasma concentrations, with slow clearance (Birmingham et al 1997). Therefore, following a first dose of 35 mg/kg, subsequent doses should extend the interval to 6–8 h, and should use smaller doses as limited by the daily maximum guidelines above.

Nonsteroidal anti-inflammatory drugs (NSAIDs) are useful for many forms of pain, including postoperative pain, arthritis, and other inflammatory conditions, and pain in sickle cell disease. A large number of NSAIDs have been examined for perioperative use in children, including indomethacin (Maunuksela et al 1988), ibuprofen, diclofenac, and ketorolac (Rusy et al 1995). They are effective via oral, intravenous, rectal, and intramuscular routes. There is no reason to use intramuscular injection for most children, as it is painful. The intravenous route is convenient for administration during or immediately after surgery, although evidence indicates no unique efficacy of this route compared with oral or rectal administration. NSAIDs reduce the requirement for opioids in many paediatric postoperative studies, and in some of these studies, this results in a reduction of opioid-related side effects (Vetter and Heiner 1994). There is little evidence for differences between NSAIDs in analgesic effectiveness, and many studies do not compare them at a range of doses that would permit proper comparison of analgesia and side effects (Tramer et al 1998).

When compared with aspirin in children with rheumatoid arthritis, ibuprofen appeared equally effective and better tolerated (Giannini et al 1990). Short-term use of ibuprofen in children in paediatric office practice has a very low risk of gastric irritation or bleeding (Lesko and Mitchell 1995). Overall, the safety of NSAIDs in children seems quite good, although rare cases of gastrointestinal bleeding and nephropathy have been reported. NSAIDs should be used with caution in types of surgery where bleeding is of major concern. Some studies of children undergoing tonsillectomy suggest an increased incidence of postoperative bleeding (Judkins et al 1996). The safety and efficacy of NSAIDs used as analgesics in newborns has not been established. NSAIDs are used in prematures primarily to facilitate closure of the ductus arteriosus.

Few data are available at present regarding the cyclo-oxygenase 2 (COX2) specific inhibitors in children. Available data in adults suggests that their lack of impairment of haemostasis may be especially useful for paediatric postoperative use and for children with cancer pain.

Table 37.2 Dosing of non-opioid analgesics in children

Drug	Recommended dosing
Acetaminophen	10–15 mg/kg orally every 4 h 20–30 mg/kg rectally every 6 h Daily maximum Children 90 mg/kg Infants 75 mg/kg Term neonates 60 mg/kg Preterm 45 mg/kg Neonates (≥32 weeks postconceptional age)
Aspirin	10–15 mg/kg orally every 4 h Daily maximum 90–120 mg/kg (children)
Ibuprofen	8–10 mg/kg every 6 h
Naproxen	6–8 mg/kg every 8–12 h

Opioids can be used for infants and children of all ages with proper understanding of age-related changes in pharmacokinetics (Olkkola et al 1995) and pharmacodynamics. A number of opioids have received pharmacokinetic study in infants and children, including morphine (Olkkola et al 1988), fentanyl (Gauntlett et al 1988), and sufentanil (Greeley et al 1987). The general pattern emerges that clearances, normalized by body weight, are diminished in the first months of life, and reach mature values over the first 3–9 months of age. Neonates and young infants are thus susceptible to drug accumulation and delayed sedation and respiratory depression if infusions are extrapolated based on recommended dosing in older children. The time course of maturation may depend in part on medical condition. For example, infants undergoing noncardiac surgery tend to show mature morphine clearances by 1–3 months of age, while infants undergoing cardiac surgery show reduced clearances through the first 6–9 months of life (Lynn et al 1998). Recommended opioid dosing is shown in Table 37.3.

Ventilatory reflexes to hypoxia and hypercarbia are immature in human newborns, and mature over the first months of life (Cohen et al 1997). Healthy infants ages 3 months and older in several postoperative studies show analgesic and respiratory depressant effects similar to those among adults at comparable plasma opioid concentrations. Systemic and epidural opioid infusions have shown generally good analgesia and safety, although opioids via either route produce a fairly high frequency of side effects, including itching, nausea, ileus, and urinary retention (Haberkern et al 1996).

Overall, opioid infusions in younger infants are useful and generally safe, but their dosing and titration are nontrivial, and they require expertise and vigilance. Since pain assessment in infants is imprecise, titration to clinical effect is more difficult. There is neither consensus or conclusive evidence to say which forms of electronic monitoring are most useful for detecting hypoxaemia or hypoventilation. Impedance apnoea monitoring is widely available with telemetry alarms that can ring in a hallway or at the nurses' station on a hospital ward. There are case reports of significant hypoxaemia in infants receiving opioids despite normal respiratory rates (Karl et al 1996). For this reason, some clinicians have advocated continuous oximetry as a method of monitoring. Oximetry is useful for detection of hypoxaemia, but has practical limitations related to motion artefacts. More importantly, remote telemetry of oximeters is not widely available. Oximeter alarms may thus go

Table 37.3 Opioid analgesic initial dosage guidelines

Drug	Equianalgesic doses		Usual starting IV or SC doses and intervals		Parenteral/ oral dose ratio	Usual starting oral doses and intervals	
	Parenteral	Oral	Child < 50 kg	Child > 50 kg		Child < 50 kg	Child >50 kg
Codeine	N/R	200 mg	N/R	N/R	1:2	0.5–1 mg/kg every 3–4 h	30–60 mg every 3–4 h
Morphine	10 mg	10–15 mg	Bolus: 0.1 mg/kg every 2–4 h Infusion: 0.03 mg/kg/h	Bolus: 5–8 mg every 2–4 h Infusion: 1.5 mg/h	1:3	Immediate release: 0.3 mg/kg every 3–4 h Sustained release: 20–35 kg: 10–15 mg every 8–12 h 35–50 kg: 15–30 mg every 8–12 h	Immediate release: 15–20 mg every 3–4 h Sustained release: 30–45 mg every 8–12 h
Oxycodone	N/A	10–15 mg	N/A	N/A	N/A	0.1–0.2 mg/kg every 3–4 h	5–10 mg every 3–4 h
Methadone	10 mg	15 mg	0.1 mg/kg every 4–8 h	1:2	1:2	0.2 mg/kg every 4–8 h	10 mg every 4–8 h
	Methadone requires additional vigilance, because it can accumulate and produce delayed sedation. If sedation occurs, doses should be withheld until sedation resolves. Thereafter, doses should be substantially reduced and/or the dosing interval should be extended to 8–12 h.						
Fentanyl	100 μg (0.1 mg)	N/A	Bolus: 0.5–1 μg/kg every 1–2 h Infusion: 0.5–1.5 μg/kg/h	Bolus: 25–50 μg every 1–2 h Infusion: 25–75 μg/h	N/A	N/A	N/A
Hydromorphone	1.5–2 mg	6–8 mg	Bolus: 0.02 mg every 2–4 h Infusion: 0.006 mg/kg/h	Bolus: 1 mg every 2–4 h Infusion: 0.3 mg/hr	1:4	0.04–0.08 mg/kg every 3–4 h	4 mg every 3–4 h
Meperidine (pethidine)	75 mg	300 mg	Bolus: 0.8–1 mg/kg every 2–3 h	Bolus: 50–75 mg every 2–3 h	1:4	2–3 mg/kg every 3–4 h	100–150 mg every 3–4 h
	Meperidine should generally be avoided if other opioids are available, especially with chronic use, because its metabolite can cause seizures.						

Doses refer to patients > 6 months of age. In infants < 6 months, initial doses/kg should begin at roughly 25% of the doses/kg recommended here. All doses are approximate and should be adjusted according to clinical circumstances.

undetected in a hospital room and provide a false sense of security. Convenient, low-cost, motion-insensitive oximetry with telemetry to a central site on a ward would be extremely useful. Electronic surveillance is not a substitute for clinical assessment and understanding of factors that modify opioid requirements and risk.

Patient-controlled analgesia has been used for children for the past 14 years with excellent safety, good efficacy, and excellent patient acceptance. Compared with bolus administration, PCA provides better pain scores, better patient acceptance, and no increase in opioid use or opioid side effects (Berde et al 1991). Compared with continuous opioid infusions, PCA provides either equivalent or better pain scores, but with a reduction of opioid use and opioid side effects (Mackie et al 1991). PCA is generally well used by children ages 6 and above. Optimal choice of dosing parameters has been studied. Short lockout intervals (e.g., 5–7 min) are safe, and allow more rapid 'catch-up' in the setting of unrelieved pain. Basal infusions should be individualized according to medical risk factors, as well as psychological factors (Wermeling et al 1992). They may increase patient satisfaction (Doyle et al 1993), but may result in more episodic night-time oxygen desaturation (McNeely and Trentadue 1997).

For infants and children who are unable to self-administer opioids, nurse-controlled analgesia appears effective, safe, and convenient (Monitto et al 2000). There is greater controversy surrounding parent-controlled analgesia. With PCA administered by the patient, the inherent safety lies in the fact that when the patient gets narcotized, they fall asleep, stop dosing, and the plasma concentration falls, thereby reducing the risk of hypoventilation during sleep. There is generally a very good experience with home dosing of PCA pumps by parents for infants and children in palliative care. What is more problematic is having parents push the button for opioid-naïve children, particularly in a postoperative setting. The arguments in favour of parental dosing are that parents are the child's primary caregivers, and they are in an ideal position to assess their needs. The counter argument is that without specific training and monitoring, on rare occasions, their well-meaning efforts may lead to overdose. We are aware of several cases around the world in which this has occurred, with disastrous consequences. Until this has received further study, it would be prudent to recommend that, if parent-controlled PCA is to be used in non-palliative situations, there should be a formal programme of parent education, and an increased level of patient observation.

Local anaesthetics

Local anaesthetics are used increasingly for regional anaesthesia in children, as well as for topical analgesia and infiltration. Maximum doses for single injection are recommended in Table 37.4.

Excessive doses of local anaesthetics cause convulsions, arrhythmias, and cardiac depression that can be very difficult to treat. Studies using a rat model found that infant animals have a narrower therapeutic index for local anaesthetics than adult animals on the basis of scaling factors, since the effective dose to block nerves scales comparatively weakly with body size, while toxic doses scale more directly with body size (Kohane et al 1998).

Topical local anaesthetics are widely used for needle procedures and for superficial procedures, including suture of lacerations or removal of skin lesions. For intact skin, the most widely used preparation is a eutectic mixture of lidocaine (lignocaine) and prilocaine known as EMLA (Maunuksela and Korpela 1986). EMLA has proved to be extremely safe in infants and children of all ages. It requires about 1 h for adequate cutaneous analgesia. Longer application will enhance depth and quality of analgesia, and after roughly 2 h it will produce cutaneous vasodilatation, which may facilitate venipuncture or venous cannulation. Although high systemic concentrations of prilocaine can produce methaemoglobinaemia, this has not been a significant clinical problem in widespread use, even with repeated or prolonged dosing in younger infants. Tetracaine gel (amethocaine) is an alternative preparation with excellent safety and efficacy, slightly more rapid onset, and early vasodilatation; it is available in Canada and Europe, but not the United States (Lawson et al 1995).

For application to cut skin, especially for suture of lacerations, combinations of local anaesthetics with vasoconstrictors are widely used. The combination of tetracaine (amethocaine) with epinephrine (adrenalin) and cocaine is known as TAC. Several studies have shown that these preparations are effective when used in emergency departments for repair of lacerations (Bonadio 1989). TAC should be avoided in the vicinity of end-arteries, since ischaemic complications have occurred. Larger doses applied to mucosal surfaces have produced

Table 37.4 Conservative dosing guidelines for local anaesthetics (mg/kg for single injection; mg/kg/h for infusions)

Drug	Single injection 0–6 months – epi	+ epi	> 1 year – epi	+ epi	Prolonged infusion 0–6 months	> 1 year
Lidocaine (lignocaine)	4	5	5	7	0.8	1.6
Bupivacaine	1.8	2	2	2.5	0.2	0.4
Chloroprocaine	20	30	20	30	30	30
Ropivacaine	2	2.5	3	3.5	0.3	0.6

convulsions and deaths due to rapid absorption of the tetracaine (amethocaine) and cocaine. More recent studies have found equivalent effectiveness using preparations with the cocaine omitted, and combinations of tetracaine (amethocaine) and phenylephrine appear useful in this setting (Smith et al 1997).

Regional anaesthesia in infants and children can be performed by specific modifications of techniques used in adults. The reader is referred to Dalens' excellent textbook for an illustrated summary. A variety of peripheral nerve blocks can provide analgesia after surgery with an excellent safety and side effect profile (Dalens et al 1989a, b; Giaufre et al 1996). Regional anaesthesia is generally performed in children asleep, as a method of providing postoperative analgesia.

For major thoracic, abdominal, pelvic, and lower extremity operations, epidural analgesia can provide outstanding analgesia and, when optimally managed, may facilitate recovery of high-risk patients. (Meignier et al 1983, McNeely 1991). Single-shot caudal blockade with local anaesthetics is generally safe and effective for many minor lower-body procedures, although there is a need to provide longer duration than is afforded by bupivacaine alone. α_2-Adrenergics, such as clonidine, prolong local anaesthetic action, and have received promising study in children (Mikawa et al 1996, Constant et al 1998). Combinations of opioids and local anaesthetics have excellent efficacy, and are particularly effective when the catheter tip can be placed in the dermatomes involved in the surgery, either by direct placement or by cephalad advancement from the caudal route (Bosenberg et al 1988). Placement and cephalad advancement can be further confirmed by two recent novel techniques based either on electrical nerve stimulation or on ECG patterns (Tsui et al 1999).

Other analgesics

There have been comparatively few clinical trials of other drug classes for pain in children. Although clinicians widely prescribe tricyclic antidepressants, anticonvulsants, and a range of other medications for several chronic pain conditions in children, most dosing is based on anecdote or extrapolation from adult experience. There are clinical trials of trazodone (Battistella et al 1993) and calcium channel blockers (Sorge and Marano 1985) in childhood migraine that show efficacy. Sumatriptan, which is quite effective in interupting adult migraine attacks, had equivocal results in one paediatric trial (Hamalainen et al 1997), and more positive results in subsequent trials (Ueberall and Wenzel 1999). Propranolol appears minimally effective in migraine prophylaxis in children (Olness et al 1987). There is a need for more controlled trials of a range of analgesics in children, especially in the setting of chronic or recurrent pain.

Management of specific types of pain in children

Postoperative pain

Amelioration of postoperative pain is best accomplished by coordinated efforts among parents, paediatricians, surgeons, anaesthesiologists, nurses, pharmacists, psychologists, child-life specialists, and others involved in perioperative care. Proper preoperative preparation can reduce anxiety and fear, which can amplify pain. Children should receive explanations that are appropriate to their developmental stage. Preoperative education programmes are now available at many paediatric centres, and these may be helpful in this process. Techniques of anaesthetic induction should strive to be atraumatic. Parental presence for mask induction may reduce distress for many children. EMLA or other topical anaesthetics may reduce the distress of intravenous induction. Oral premedication can also reduce anxiety for many children.

Kehlet and others have championed the concept of multimodal analgesia for adults undergoing surgery (Kehlet 1998). It is likely that this concept applies for children as well. Combinations of opioids, local anaesthetics, and NSAIDs may be ideal in many settings.

Acute pain services can be useful for advocacy and for ensuring that pain management is a priority. In many paediatric centres, these have been developed and appear to provide extremely useful services. Standardized protocols are useful to ensure consistency in management, to ensure that side effects are treated promptly, and to minimize dosing errors. Decimal point errors are common in paediatric hospitals, and protocolized dosing facilitates cross-checking for erroneous orders. If children are to be cared for in general hospitals, it is ideal to have paediatric specialists be involved in creation of specific pain management protocols for children. A number of models for pain treatment can be used, and the choice of participants and specialists may depend on local expertise and availability.

Trauma and burns

In many respects, children sustaining major trauma and burns should be managed according to the principles set out for postoperative pain. Historically, these forms of pain have been often undertreated in children (Perry and Heidrich 1982). Often, the duration of pain may be quite prolonged (Szyfelbein et al 1985). Particularly with major burns, marked opioid dose escalation is often required. As pain subsides, dosing may require gradual tapering to prevent withdrawal.

Cancer and palliative care

Cancer pain and palliative care in children are discussed in detail in Chap. 44. Many of the principles outlined in adult palliative care apply to children (Miser et al 1983, Stevens et al 1994, Collins et al 1995). Pharmacologic management by the WHO analgesic ladder is effective for most children with pain due to widespread cancer (Kasai et al 1995). Some of the differences in the approach to palliative care for children involves consideration of the child's emotional and cognitive development and the family's roles in support and palliative care (Goldman 1996).

Brief diagnostic and therapeutic procedures

Needle procedures are a significant source of distress for children. Healthy infants and children receive subcutaneous and intramuscular injections for immunizations. Children with acute and chronic illness may in addition receive more frequent procedures, including venipuncture, intravenous cannulation, lumbar puncture, and bone marrow aspiration. Approaches to these procedures must be individualized according to the child's age, cognitive development, coping style, and health status. Appropriate explanation and support can be helpful.

Cognitive-behavioural techniques, including guided imagery, hypnosis, and relaxation, can diminish the distress of these procedures for many children (Zeltzer and LeBaron 1982, McGrath and deVeber 1986, Zeltzer et al 1989, Kuttner 1989, Jay et al 1995). These techniques are used very widely, and can be taught to most children ages 5–7 and above. Some experts use them for children ages 3–5 as well (McGrath and deVeber 1986).

For children receiving oncology procedures, gastrointestinal endoscopy, or radiologic procedures, many do well with 'conscious sedation', often using sedative-anxiolytics, especially benzodiazepines (Sievers et al 1991), combined with either opioid analgesics or low-dose ketamine (Marx et al 1997). For higher risk or highly uncooperative children, or for more extensive procedures, general anaesthesia may be a more effective alternative. There is considerable controversy regarding the appropriate personnel (i.e., anaesthetist versus non-anaesthetist), choice of agents, depth of sedation required, relative risks, benefits, efficacy, costs, and comparative safety of conscious sedation versus brief general anaesthesia (Maxwell and Yaster 1996).

Sickle cell anaemia

Sickle haemoglobinopathies are genetic disorders occurring predominantly in people of African and Middle Eastern descent. Abnormal haemoglobin molecules polymerize under certain conditions, including hypoxaemia, acidosis, hypothermia, and erythrocycte cell water loss. Haemoglobin polymerization leads to abnormal erythrocyte shape (sickling) and reduced deformability and impaired rheology of small vessels, leading to vaso-occlusion and ischaemic pain. Pain in sickle cell disease is extremely variable in its frequency and severity (Platt et al 1991). The majority of patients manage their persistent and episodic pains as outpatients, using oral hydration, NSAIDs, and episodic oral opioids. A subgroup of patients has more severe episodes of vaso-occlusive pain that require hospitalization. Opioids should be given as needed to provide comfort (Benjamin 1989). Opioid titration may require some additional care, since hypoxaemia and hypercarbia further exacerbate sickling of erythrocytes. Recent studies emphasize home management (Shapiro et al 1995), oral opioid dosing, avoidance of a 'crisis' model, and teaching of cognitive-behavioural (Thomas et al 1984, Dinges et al 1997) and coping (Gil et al 1997) techniques.

HIV/AIDS

HIV disease in children is now most commonly acquired by congenital infection. The natural history of HIV in infants has improved greatly in developed countries in recent years with multidrug treatment regimens. Children with HIV receive a large number of painful diagnostic and therapeutic procedures (Hirschfeld et al 1996). Infants with encephalopathy and severe developmental delay sometimes present with persistent irritability and screaming. Many of these infants respond to opioids; in other cases, anticonvulsants may be helpful, even when clinical seizures are not evident.

Neuropathic pains

Neuropathic pains in children can be a source of considerable distress and suffering (Ollson and Berde 1993). In our clinic, the most common causes are postsurgical/posttraumatic localized peripheral nerve injuries, complex regional pain syndrome type 1 (CRPS1)/reflex sympathetic dystrophy (RSD), pains associated with metabolic neuropathies, pain after spinal cord injury, and neuropathic cancer pain. Phantom pain following amputation is not rare, and may be persistent and severe (Krane et al 1991). We commonly extrapolate approaches used in adults, including liberal prescribing of tricyclic antidepressants and anticonvulsants.

CRPS1/RSD in children and adolescents has a marked female predominance (roughly 6:1), a marked lower extremity predominance (roughly 6:1), and an apparently high association with competitive sports (Pillemer and Micheli 1988), gynastics, and dance (Wilder et al 1992). The reasons for this association are unclear. Some clinicians regard this as a psychogenic condition (Sherry and Weisman 1988), although evidence of causation, as opposed to association, is weak. Approaches to treatment of CRPS1/RSD have been extremely varied, ranging from rehabilitative (Bernstein et al 1978) to more interventionist. In our view, physical therapy and biobehavioural approaches should be emphasized (Lee et al 2002, in press), and sympathetic blockade should be used sparingly and not in isolation.

Chronic 'benign' pains of childhood

Chronic and recurrent pains in children have a different epidemiology from those in adults. Back pain and neck pain are less common in children. Trigeminal neuralgia is extraordinarily rare in children, and herpes zoster is much less likely to produce a postherpetic neuralgia.

Children commonly experience recurrent pains of the head, chest, abdomen, and limbs. These conditions typically involve painful episodes alternating with pain-free times in a child who is otherwise healthy. These conditions are very common, and population-based surveys suggest that between 4 and 10% of children experience these symptoms with some regularity (Apley and Naish 1958, Oster 1972, Oster and Nielson 1972, Coleman 1984, Bille 1997). Both migraine and tension-type headaches increase in prevalence during the school age years and into adolescence. A number of chronic and recurrent pain conditions in children show a female gender predominance, particularly among adolescents.

Most children presenting with these complaints will be determined to be medically well. The primary paediatrician or general practitioner should develop a screening approach that emphasizes a sensitive medical history and physical examination that detects the small subset of patients who need further evaluation (Levine and Rappaport 1984). It is wise to de-emphasize unfocused laboratory testing, which is generally of low yield in these conditions. Lifestyle interventions may be helpful, and questions regarding family and school circumstances, diet, sleep, sports, and a range of activities should be included. In some situations, modifications of diet, school stressors, and exercise may have considerable benefit. For example, a subgroup of children with recurrent abdominal pain may improve by treatment of constipation or by treating lactose intolerance with oral lactase enzyme replacement or avoidance of milk products (Barr et al 1979).

Physical therapeutic approaches are extremely helpful for many chronic painful conditions in children. Physical therapists should be integral participants in multidisciplinary chronic pain programmes for children. Aerobic conditioning and strength training may have both specific, localized benefits, e.g., for an adolescent with myofascial pain, and more generalized beneficial effects on mood, sleep, and general well-being.

Psychological factors in pain in children

As with adults, in children the experience of pain is modulated by biologic variation, past pain experiences, meaning of the pain, context, fear, anxiety, depression, and a range of other factors. In children, there is the additional aspect of the impact of development on the cognitive and emotional aspects of pain responses.

A number of the recurrent benign pains of childhood have been commonly regarded as 'psychogenic'. The evidence that most children with these symptoms are psychiatrically ill is generally weak (McGrath and Unruh 1987, Walker et al 1993); many children and adolescents with these symptoms in fact are well-adjusted and cope well. Barr, Oberlander, Rappaport, and others have argued against dichotomizing these conditions as purely 'psychogenic' or purely 'organic' (Oberlander and Rappaport 1993).

School absenteeism and disability

In adults, chronic pain is a major social, economic, and political problem both because it produces suffering and because low back pain in particular is an enormous cause of disability. A medical model alone cannot explain the natural history and patterns of disability.

School absenteeism and school avoidance are common among patients referred to paediatric pain clinics. It is helpful to regard school avoidance in many (but not all) cases as a disability syndrome with analogies to work absenteeism in adults with chronic pain. Just as the workmen's compensation system in adults sometimes reinforces disability, home tutoring programmes for some children with chronic pain may facilitate a sick role away from the mainstream of life in a school setting. Multidisciplinary paediatric pain management should address the process of return to school (Bursch et al 1998).

Biobehavioural treatment

Evidence supports the efficacy of biobehavioural interventions for several paediatric disorders, including migraine (Mehegan et al 1987), recurrent abdominal pain (Scharff 1997), juvenile rheumatoid arthritis (Varni 1992), neuropathic pain (Bursch et al 1998), and pain associated with sickle cell disease (Gil et al 1993). Biobehavioural treatment techniques can be grouped into four categories: biofeedback, including electromyographic (EMG) and thermal; relaxation therapies, including hypnosis; operant (or contingency) pain behaviour management; and a more general category of cognitive-behavioural techniques employing self-monitoring, coping strategies, and environmental modification.

References

Abbott FV, Guy ER 1995 Effects of morphine, pentobarbital and amphetamine on formalin-induced behaviors in infant rats: sedation versus specific suppression of pain. Pain 62: 303–312

Anand KJ, Hickey PR 1992 Halothane-morphine compared with high-dose sufentanil for anesthesia and postoperative analgesia in neonatal cardiac surgery—see comments. New England Journal of Medicine 326: 1–9

Anand KJS, Sippell WG, Aynsley-Green A 1987 A randomised trial of fentanyl anaesthesia in preterm neonates undergoing surgery: effects on the stress response, Lancet 1: 62–66

Anand KJ, Barton BA et al 1999 Analgesia and sedation in preterm neonates who require ventilatory support: results from the NOPAIN trial. Neonatal outcome and prolonged analgesia in neonates. Archives of Pediatric and Adolescent Medicine 153(4): 331–338

Andrews K, Fitzgerald M 1997 Biological barriers to paediatric pain management. Clinical Journal of Pain 13(2): 138–143

Apley J, Naish N 1958 Recurrent abdominal pains: A field survey of 1,000 school children, Archives of Disease in Childhood 33: 165

Barr RG, Watkins JB, Levine MD 1979 Recurrent abdominal pain (RAP) of childhood due to lactose intolerance: a prospective study. New England Journal of Medicine 300: 1449–1452

Battistella P, Ruffilli R, Cernetti R, Pettenazzo A, Baldin L, Bertoli S, Zacchello F 1993 A placebo-controlled crossover trial using trazodone in pediatric migraine. Headache 33: 36–39

Benini F, Johnston CC, Faucher D, Aranda JV 1993 Topical anesthesia during circumcision in newborn infants. Journal of the American Medical Association 270: 850–853

Benjamin LJ 1989 Pain in sickle cell disease. In: Current therapy of pain. BC Decker, Toronto, pp 90–104

Berde CB 1998 Anesthesia and analgesia. In: Cloherty JP, Stark AR (eds) Manual of neonatal care. Lippincott-Raven, Philadelphia, pp 667–675

Berde CB, Lehn BM, Yee JD, Sethna NF, Russo D 1991 Patient-controlled analgesia in children and adolescents: a randomized, prospective comparison with intramuscular administration of morphine for postoperative analgesia. Journal of Pediatrics 118: 460–466

Bernstein BH, Singsen BH, Kent JT, Kornreich H, King K, Hicks R, Hanson V 1978 Reflex neurovascular dystrophy in childhood. Journal of Pediatrics 93: 211–215

Berry FA, Gregory GA 1987 Do premature infants require anesthesia for surgery? Anesthesiology 67: 291–293

Beyer JE, McGrath PJ, Berde CB 1990 Discordance between self-report and behavioral pain measures in children aged 3–7 years after surgery. Journal of Pain and Symptom Management 5: 350–356

Beyer JE, Denyes MJ, Villarruel AM 1992 The creation, validation, and continuing development of the Oucher: a measure of pain intensity in children. Journal of Pediatric Nursing 7: 335–346

Bieri D, Reeve RA, Champion GD, Addicoat L, Ziegler JB 1990 The Faces Pain Scale for the self-assessment of the severity of pain experienced by children: development, initial validation, and preliminary investigation for ratio scale properties. Pain 41: 139–150

Bille B 1997 A 40-year follow-up of school children with migraine. Cephalalgia 17(4): 488–491

Birmingham P, Tobin M, Henthorn T, Fisher D, Berkelhamer M, Smith F, Fanta K, Cote C 1997 Twenty-four-hour pharmacokinetics of rectal acetaminophen in children: an old drug with new recommendations. Anesthesiology 87(2): 244–252

Blass EM, Hoffmeyer LB 1991 Sucrose as an analgesic for newborn infants. Pediatrics 87: 215–218

Bonadio W 1989 TAC: a review. Pediatric Emergency Care 128

Bosenberg A, Bland B, Schulte-Steinberg O et al 1988 Thoracic epidural anesthesia via the caudal route in infants. Anesthesiology 69: 265–269

Breau LM, Camfield C et al 2001 Measuring pain accurately in children with cognitive impairments: refinement of a caregiver scale. Journal of Pediatrics 138(5): 721–727

Bursch B, Walco GA, Zeltzer L 1998 Clinical assessment and management of chronic pain and pain-associated disability syndrome. Journal of Developmental and Behavioral Pediatrics 19: 45–53

Chambers CT, Craig KD 1998 An intrusive impact of anchors in children's faces pain scales. Pain 78(1): 27–37

Coggeshall R, Jennings E, Fitzgerald M 1996 Evidence that large myelinated primary afferent fibers make synaptic contacts in lamina II of neonatal rats. Brain Research 92(1): 81–90

Cohen G, Malcolm G et al 1997 Ventilatory response of the newborn infant to mild hypoxia. Pediatric Pulmonology 24(3): 163–172

Coleman WL 1984 Recurrent chest pain in children. Pediatric Clinics of North America 31: 1007

Collins J, Grier H, Kinney H, Berde C 1995 Control of severe pain in children with terminal malignancy. Journal of Pediatrics 126: 653–657

Constant I, Gall O, Gouyet L, Chauvin M, Murat I 1998 Addition of clonidine or fentanyl to local anaesthetics prolongs the duration of surgical analgesia after single shot caudal block in children. British Journal of Anaesthesia 80: 294–298

Dalens B, Vanneuville G, Dechelotte P 1989a Penile block via the subpubic space in 100 children. Anesthesia and Analgesia 69: 41–45

Dalens B, Vanneuville G, Tanguy A 1989b Comparison of the fascia iliaca compartment block with the 3-in-1 block in children. Anesthesia and Analgesia 69: 705–713

Dinges D, Whitehouse W, Orne E, Bloom P, Carlin M, Bauer N, Gillen K, Shapiro B, Ohene-Frempong K, Dampier C, Orne M 1997 Self-hypnosis training as an adjunctive treatment in the management of pain associated with sickle cell disease. International Journal of Clinical and Experimental Hypnosis 45: 417–432

Doyle E, Harper I, Morton N 1993 Patient-controlled analgesia with low dose background infusions after lower abdominal surgery in children. British Journal of Anaesthesia 71: 818–822

Fitzgerald M, Shaw A, MacIntosh N 1988 Postnatal development of the cutaneous flexor reflex: comparative study of preterm infants and newborn rat pups. Developmental Medicine and Child Neurology 30: 520–526

Gauntlett IS, Fisher DM, Hertzka RE, Kuhls E, Spellman MJ, Rudolph C 1988 Pharmacokinetics of fentanyl in neonatal humans and lambs: effects of age. Anesthesiology 69: 683–687

Gauvain-Piquard A, Rodary C, Rezvani A, Lemerle J 1987 Pain in children aged 2–6 years: a new observational rating scale elaborated in a pediatric oncology unit—preliminary report. Pain 31: 177–188

Giannini E, Brewer E, Miller M et al 1990 Ibuprofen suspension in the treatment of juvenile rheumatoid arthritis. Journal of Pediatrics 117: 645–652

Giaufre E, Dalens B, Gombart A 1996 Epidemiology and morbidity of regional anesthesia in children: a one-year prospective survey of the French-Language Society of Pediatric Anesthesiologists. Anesthesia and Analgesia 83: 904–912

Gil K, Thomson R, Keith B, Tota-Faucette M, Noll S, Kinney T 1993 Sickle cell disease pain in children and adolescents: change in pain frequency and coping strategies over time. Journal of Pediatric Psychology 18: 621–637

Gil K, Wilson J, Edens J 1997 The stability of pain coping strategies in young children, adolescents, and adults with sickle cell disease over an 18-month period. Clinical Journal of Pain 13: 110–115

Goldman A 1996 Home care of the dying child. Journal of Palliative Care 12: 16–19

Greeley WJ, de Bruijn NP, David DP 1987 Sufentanil pharmacokinetics in pediatric cardiovascular patients. Anesthesia and Analgesia 66: 1067–1072

Grossi E, Borghi C, Cerchiari EL et al 1983 Analogue chromatic continuous scale: a new method for pain assessment. Clinical and Experimental Rheumatology 1: 337–340

Grunau RV, Johnston CC, Craig KD 1990 Neonatal facial and cry responses to invasive and non-invasive procedures. Pain 42: 295–305

Grunau RV, Whitfield MF, Petrie JH, Fryer EL 1994 Early pain experience, child and family factors, as precursors of somatization: a prospective study of extremely premature and full-term children. Pain 56: 353–359

Haberkern CM, Lynn AM, Geiduschek JM, Nespeca MK, Jacobson LE, Bratton SL, Pomietto M 1996 Epidural and intravenous bolus morphine for postoperative analgesia in infants. Canadian Journal of Anaesthesia 43: 1203–1210

Hadjistavropoulos HD, Craig KD, Grunau RV, Johnston CC 1994 Judging pain in newborns: facial and cry determinants. Journal of Pediatric Psychology 19: 485–491

Hamalainen M, Hoppu K, Santavuori P 1997 Sumatriptan for migraine attacks in children: a randomized placebo-controlled study. Do children with migraine respond to oral sumatriptan differently from adults? Neurology 48(4): 1100–1103

Hirschfeld S, Moss H, Dragisic K, Smith W, Pizzo PA 1996 Pain in pediatric human immunodeficiency virus infection: incidence and characteristics in a single-institution pilot study. Pediatrics 98: 449–452

Jay S, Elliott CH, Fitzgibbons I, Woody P, Siegel S 1995 A comparative study of cognitive behavior therapy versus general anesthesia for painful medical procedures in children. Pain 62: 3–9

Jennings E, Fitzgerald M 1996 C-fos can be induced in the neonatal rat spinal cord by both noxious and innocuous peripheral stimulation. Pain 68(2–3): 301–306

Johnston CC, Stevens BJ 1996 Experience in a neonatal intensive care unit affects pain response. Pediatrics 98: 925–930

Johnston CC, Stevens B, Craig KD, Grunau RV 1993 Developmental changes in pain expression in premature, full-term, two- and four-month-old infants. Pain 52: 201–208

Johnston CC, Collinge JM, Henderson SJ, Anand KJ 1997 A cross-sectional survey of pain and pharmacological analgesia in Canadian neonatal intensive care units. Clinical Journal of Pain 13: 308–312

Judkins JH, Dray TG, Hubbell RN 1996 Intraoperative ketorolac and post-tonsillectomy bleeding. Archives of Otolaryngology—Head and Neck Surgery 122: 937–940

Kahn DJ, Richardson DK, Gray JE, Bednarek F, Rubin LP, Shah B, Frantz ID, III, Pursley DM 1998 Variation among neonatal intensive care units in narcotic administration. Archives of Pediatrics and Adolescent Medicine 152: 844–851

Kanagasundaram S, Cooper M, Lane L 1997 Nurse-controlled analgesia using a patient-controlled analgesia device: an alternative strategy in the management of severe cancer pain in children. Journal of Paediatrics and Child Health 33(4): 352–355

Karl HW, Tyler DC, Krane EJ 1996 Respiratory depression after low-dose caudal morphine. Canadian Journal of Anaesthesia 43: 1065–1067

Kasai H, Sasaki K, Tsujinaga H, Hoshino T 1995 Pain management in advanced pediatric cancer patients—a proposal of the two-step analgesic ladder. Masui—Japanese Journal of Anesthesiology 44: 885–889

Katz ER, Kellerman J, Siegel SE 1980 Behavioral distress in children with cancer undergoing medical procedures: developmental considerations. Journal of Consulting and Clinical Psychology 48: 356–365

Kehlet H 1998 Balanced analgesia: a prerequisite for optimal recovery. British Journal of Surgery 85: 3–4

Kohane D, Sankar W, Shubina M, Hu D, Rifai N, Berde C 1998 Sciatic nerve blockade in infant, adolescent and adult rats: a comparison of ropivacaine with bupivacaine. Anesthesiology 89: 1199–1208

Krane EJ, Heller LB, Pomietto ML 1991 Incidence of phantom sensation and pain in pediatric amputees. Anesthesiology 75: A691

Kuttner L 1989 Management of young children's acute pain and anxiety during invasive medical procedures. Pediatrician 16: 39–44

Lander J, Brady-Fryer B, Metcalfe J, Nazarali S, Muttitt S 1997 Comparison of ring block, dorsal penile nerve block, and topical anesthesia for neonatal circumcision: a randomized controlled trial. Journal of the American Medical Association 278: 2157–2162

Lawson RA, Smart NG, Gudgeon AC, Morton NS 1995 Evaluation of an amethocaine gel preparation for percutaneous analgesia before venous cannulation in children. British Journal of Anaesthesia 75: 282–285
Lesko S, Mitchell A 1995 An assessment of the safety of pediatric ibuprofen. A practitioner-based randomized clinical trial. Journal of the American Medical Association 273(12): 929–933
Levine M, Rappaport LA 1984 Recurrent abdominal pain in school children: the loneliness of the long distance physician. Pediatric Clinics of North America 31: 969–991
Lin YC, Sussman HH, Benitz WE 1994 Plasma concentrations after rectal administration of acetaminophen in preterm neonates. Paediatric Anaesthesia 7: 457–459
Litvack DA, Oberlander TF, Carney LH, Saul JP 1995 Time and frequency domain methods for heart rate variability analysis: a methodological comparison. Psychophysiology 32: 492–504
Lynn A, Nespeca MK, Bratton SL, Strauss SG, Shen DD 1998 Clearance of morphine in postoperative infants during intravenous infusion: the influence of age and surgery. Anesthesia and Analgesia 86: 958–963
Mackie AM, Coda BC, Hill HF 1991 Adolescents use patient-controlled analgesia effectively for relief from prolonged oropharyngeal mucositis pain. Pain 46: 265–269
Marx CM, Stein J, Tyler MK, Nieder ML, Shurin SB, Blumer JL 1997 Ketamine-midazolam versus meperidine-midazolam for painful procedures in pediatric oncology patients. Journal of Clinical Oncology 15: 94–102
Maunuksela E, Korpela R 1986 Double-blind evaluation of a lignocaine-prilocaine cream (EMLA) in children. Effect on the pain associated with venous cannulation. British Journal of Anaesthesia 58: 1242–1245
Maunuksela EL, Olkkola KT, Korpela R 1988 Does prophylactic intravenous infusion of indomethacin improve the management of postoperative pain in children? Canadian Journal of Anaesthesia 35: 123–127
Maxwell LG, Yaster M 1996 The myth of conscious sedation. Archives of Pediatrics and Adolescent Medicine 150: 665–667
McGrath P, deVeber L 1986 The management of acute pain evoked by medical procedures in children with cancer. Journal of Pain and Symptom Management 1: 145–150
McGrath PJ, Unruh AM 1987 Psychogenic pain; in pain in children and adolescents. Elsevier Science, Amsterdam
McGrath PJ, Johnson G, Goodman JT, Schillinger J, Dunn J 1985 The CHEOPS: a behavioral scale to measure postoperative pain in children. In: Chapman J, Fields HL, Dubner R, Cervero F (eds) Advances in pain research and therapy, vol 9. Raven Press, New York, pp 395–402
McGrath P, Seifert C, Speechley K, Booth J, Stitt L, Gibson M 1996 A new analogue scale for assessing children's pain: an initial validation study. Pain 64: 435–443
McIntosh N, van Veen L, Brameyer H 1994 Alleviation of the pain of heel prick in preterm infants. Archives of Disease in Childhood Fetal and Neonatal Edition 70: F177–181
McNeely JK, Trentadue NC 1997 Comparison of patient-controlled analgesia with and without nighttime morphine infusion following lower extremity surgery in children. Journal of Pain and Symptom Management 13: 268–273
McNeely JM 1991 Comparison of epidural opioids and intravenous opioids in the postoperative management of pediatric antireflux surgery. Anesthesiology 75: A689
Mehegan J, Masek BJ, Harrison W et al 1987 A multi-component behavioral treatment for pediatric migraine. Clinical Journal of Pain 2: 191–196
Meignier M, Souron R, Leneel J 1983 Postoperative dorsal epidural analgesia in the child with respiratory disabilities. Anesthesiology 59(5): 473–475
Mikawa K, Nishina K, Maekawa N, Obara H 1996 Oral clonidine premedication reduces postoperative pain in children. Anesthesia and Analgesia 82: 225–230
Miser AW, Davis DM, Hughes CS, Mulne AF, Miser JS 1983 Continuous subcutaneous infusion of morphine in children with cancer. American Journal of Diseases of Childhood 137: 383–385
Monitto CL, Greenberg RS et al 2000 The safety and efficacy of parent-/nurse-controlled analgesia in patients less than six years of age. Anesthesia and Analgesia 91(3): 573–579
Oberlander TF, Rappaport LA 1993 Recurrent abdominal pain during childhood. Pediatrics in Review 14: 313–319
Oberlander TF, Berde CB, Lam KH, Rappaport LA, Saul JP 1995 Infants tolerate spinal anesthesia with minimal overall autonomic changes: analysis of heart rate variability in former premature infants undergoing hernia repair. Anesthesia and Analgesia 80: 20–27
Oberlander TF, Berde CB, Saul JP 1996 Halothane and cardiac autonomic control in infants: assessment with quantitative respiratory sinus arrhythmia. Pediatric Research 40: 710–717
Olkkola KT, Maunuksela EL, Korpela R, Rosenberg PH 1988 Kinetics and dynamics of postoperative intravenous morphine in children. Clinical Pharmacology and Therapeutics 44: 128–136
Olkkola K, Hamunen K, Maunuksela E 1995 Clinical pharmacokinetics and pharmacodynamics of opioid analgesics in infants and children. Clinical Pharmacokinetics 28: 385–404
Ollson G, Berde CB 1993 Neuropathic pain in children and adolescents. In: Schechter NL, Berde CB, Yaster M (eds) Pain in infants, children and adolescents. Williams & Wilkins, Baltimore, pp 473–489
Olness K, MacDonald J, Uden D 1987 Comparison of self-hypnosis and propranolol in the treatment of juvenile classic migraine. Pediatrics 79: 593–597
Oster J 1972 Recurrent abdominal pain, headache and limb pain in children and adolescents. Pediatrics 50: 429–436
Oster J, Nielson A 1972 Growing pains: a clinical investigation of a school population, Acta Paediatrica Scandinavica 61: 321
Perry S, Heidrich G 1982 Management of pain during debridement: a survey of USA burns units. Pain 13: 267–280
Pillemer FG, Micheli LJ 1988 Psychological considerations in youth sports. Clinics in Sports Medicine 7: 679–689
Platt OS, Thorington BD, Brambilla DJ, Milner PF, Rosse WF, Vichinsky E, Kinney TR 1991 Pain in sickle cell disease. Rates and risk factors. New England Journal of Medicine 325: 11–16
Porter F, Porges S 1991 Vagal tone: an index of stress and pain in high risk newborn infants. Journal of Pain Symptom Management 6: 206
Porter FL, Porges SW, Marshall RE 1988 Newborn pain cries and vagal tone: parallel changes in response to circumcision. Child Development 59: 495–505
Robinson S, Gregory G 1981 Fentanyl air oxygen anesthesia for patent ductus arteriosus in pre-term infants. Anesthesia and Analgesia 60: 331–334
Rusy LM, Houck CS, Sullivan LJ, Ohlms LA, Jones DT, McGill TJ, Berde CB 1995 A double-blind evaluation of ketorolac tromethamine versus acetaminophen in pediatric tonsillectomy: analgesia and bleeding. Anesthesia and Analgesia 80: 226–229
Scharff L 1997 Recurrent abdominal pain in children: a review of psychological factors and treatment. Clinical Psychology Review 17: 145–166
Shapiro B, Dinges D, Orne E et al 1995 Home management of sickle cell-related pain in children and adolescents: natural history and impact on school attendance. Pain 61: 139–144
Sherry DD, Weisman R 1988 Psychologic aspects of childhood reflex neurovascular dystrophy. Pediatrics 81: 572–578
Sievers TD, Yee JD, Foley ME, Blanding PJ, Berde CB 1991

Midazolam for conscious sedation during pediatric oncology procedures: safety and recovery parameters. Pediatrics 88: 1172–1179
Smith G, Strausbaugh S, Harbeck-Weber C, Cohen D, Shields B, Powers J 1997 New non-cocaine-containing topical anesthetics compared with tetracaine-adrenaline-cocaine during repair of lacerations. Pediatrics 100: 825–830
Sorge F, Marano E 1985 Flunarizine v. placebo in childhood migraine. A double-blind study. Cephalalgia 5 (Suppl 2): 145–148
Stang HJ, Gunnar MR, Snellman L, Condon LM, Kestenbaum R 1988 Local anesthesia for neonatal circumcision. Effects on distress and cortisol response. Journal of the American Medical Association 259: 1507–1511
Stevens BJ, Johnston CC, Grunau RV 1995 Issues of assessment of pain and discomfort in neonates. Journal of Obstetric, Gynecologic, and Neonatal Nursing 24: 849–855
Stevens B, Johnston C, Petryshen P, Taddio A 1996 Premature Infant Pain Profile: development and initial validation. Clinical Journal of Pain 12: 13–22
Stevens M, Dalla Pozza L, Cavalletto B, Cooper M, Kilham H 1994 Pain and symptom control in paediatric palliative care. Cancer Surveys 21: 211–231
Szyfelbein SK, Osgood PF, Carr DB 1985 The assessment of pain and plasma B-endorphin immunoactivity in burned children. Pain 22: 173–182
Taddio A, Katz J, Ilersich A, Koren G 1995 Effect of neonatal circumcision on pain response during subsequent routine vaccination. Lancet 349: 599–603
Taddio A, Stevens B, Craig K, Rastogi P, Ben-David S, Shennan A, Mulligan P, Koren G 1997 Efficacy and safety of lidocaine-prilocaine cream for pain during circumcision. New England Journal of Medicine 336: 1197–1201
Thomas JE, Koshy M, Patterson L, Dorn L, Thomas K 1984 Management of pain in sickle cell disease using biofeedback therapy: a preliminary study. Biofeedback and Self Regulation 9: 413–420
Tramer MR, Williams JE et al 1998 Comparing analgesic efficacy of non-steroidal anti-inflammatory drugs given by different routes in acute and chronic pain: a qualitative systematic review. Acta Anaesthesiologica Scandinavica 42(1): 71–79
Tsui BC, Seal R et al 1999 Thoracic epidural analgesia via the caudal approach using nerve stimulation in an infant with CATCH22. Canadian Journal of Anaesthesia 46(12): 1138–1142
Uberall MA, Wenzel D 1999 Intranasal sumatriptan for the acute treatment of migraine in children. Neurology 52(7): 1507–1510
Varni JW 1992 Evaluation and management of pain in children with juvenile rheumatoid arthritis. Journal of Rheumatology 19: 32–35
Vetter T, Heiner E 1994 Intravenous ketorolac as an adjuvant to pediatric patient-controlled analgesia with morphine. Journal of Clinical Anesthesia 6: 110–113
Walker LS, Garber J, Greene JW 1993 Psychosocial correlates of recurrent childhood pain: a comparison of pediatric patients with recurrent abdominal pain, organic illness, and psychiatric disorders. Journal of Abnormal Psychology 102: 248–258
Way W, Costley E, Way E 1965 Respiratory sensitivity of the newborn infant to meperidine and morphine. Clinical Pharmacology and Therapeutics 6: 454–461
Wermeling DP, Greene SA, Boucher BA, Lehman ME, Briggs GG, Bezarro ER, Foster TS 1992 Patient controlled analgesia: the relation of psychological factors to pain and analgesic use in adolescents with postoperative pain. Clinical Journal of Pain 8: 215–221
Wilder RT, Berde CB, Wolohan M, Vieyra MA, Masek BJ, Micheli LJ 1992 Reflex sympathetic dystrophy in children. Clinical characteristics and follow-up of seventy patients. Journal of Bone and Joint Surgery 74A: 910–919
Wong DL, Baker CM 1988 Pain in children: comparison of assessment scales. Pediatric Nursing 14: 9–17
Zeltzer L, LeBaron S 1982 Hypnotic and nonhypnotic techniques for reduction of pain and anxiety during painful procedures in children and adolescents with cancer. Journal of Pediatrics 101: 1032–1035
Zeltzer L, Jay S, Fisher D 1989 The management of pain associated with pediatric procedures. Pediatric Clinics of North America 36: 941–964

Chapter 38

Pain in the elderly

Lucia Gagliese and Ronald Melzack

Introduction

As the population ages, health care workers are increasingly called upon to provide effective pain assessment and management to elderly patients. Fortunately, information regarding age-related patterns of pain, disability, and psychological distress has become more readily available over the past decade. This chapter presents an overview of this rapidly growing area of research.

Pain assessment

Measures of pain intensity

Appropriate pain assessment is the first step to effective pain management. However, most pain scales were designed for use with younger adults, and may have different psychometric properties when used with elderly people.

The most frequently assessed component of pain is intensity, and the most commonly used measures of pain intensity are visual analogue scales (VAS), verbal descriptor scales (VDS), and numerical rating scales (NRS) (see Jensen and Karoly 2001 for a review). Although preliminary, the available data support the use of VDSs and NRSs, but suggest that caution is necessary when using VASs with elderly patients (see review by Gagliese 2001). Increasing age has been associated with a higher frequency of incomplete or unscorable responses on the VAS but not on the VDS, the behavioural rating scale (BRS), or the NRS (Kremer et al 1981, Jensen et al 1986, Gagliese and Melzack 1997a). Another potential difficulty with the VAS is a lack of agreement with other measures, including the VDS and BRS, in estimates of pain intensity (Herr and Mobily 1993, Gagliese and Melzack 1997a). This pattern was not found in young and middle-aged chronic pain patients (Gagliese and Melzack 1997a). Furthermore, the elderly report that the VAS is more difficult to complete and is a poorer description of pain than scales made up of verbal descriptors (Herr and Mobily 1993, Benesh et al 1997). These data raise important problems for the use of the VAS with the elderly.

The McGill Pain Questionnaire

The McGill Pain Questionnaire (MPQ) measures the sensory, affective, evaluative, and miscellaneous components of pain (Melzack 1975). There is much evidence for its validity, reliability, and discriminative abilities when used with younger adults (Melzack and Katz 2001). Recent evidence suggests that the psychometric properties of the MPQ are not age related. Specifically, the latent structure, internal consistency, and pattern of subscale correlations of the MPQ are very similar in young and elderly chronic pain patients who have been matched for pain diagnosis, location, and duration, and for gender (Gagliese et al 1998). Similarly, in a sample of adults with chronic arthritis pain, there were no age differences in error rates on the short form of the MPQ (SF-MPQ) (Gagliese and Melzack 1997a). Although the elderly endorsed fewer words than younger subjects, the same adjectives were chosen most frequently to describe arthritis pain regardless of age (Gagliese and Melzack 1997a). Although further studies are needed, these results suggest that the MPQ is appropriate for use with older patients. It appears to measure the same constructs in the same way across the adult lifespan.

It is evident that the assessment of pain in elderly people should include a verbal descriptor or numeric scale measure of pain intensity and the MPQ in either its original or short form (Gagliese 2001). Furthermore, pain maps—that is, outlines of the human body—have been validated for the elderly and provide useful information about the location and spatial distribution of pain (Escalante et al 1995). As with younger patients, assessment of the elderly person with chronic pain must include more than measures of pain. A comprehensive assessment should include, but is certainly not limited to, measures of physical disability, interference of pain in the performance of daily activities, and psychological distress. Self-report and objective measures of many of these constructs have been developed and are in frequent use in both the research and clinical setting (Turk and Melzack 2001). However, few of these measures have been validated for elderly pain patients (Gagliese 2001).

Clinical pain

Epidemiological studies

Age-related patterns of pain prevalence vary across studies and may depend on the type of pain symptom assessed. While the majority of studies report that the prevalence of pain complaints (Andersson et al 1993), tension headache (Schwartz et al 1998), migraine (Cook et al 1989), and low back pain (de Zwart et al 1997) peaks in middle age and decreases thereafter, there are also reports of an age-related increase in the prevalence of persistent (Crook et al 1984) and recurrent (Brattberg et al 1997) pain, musculoskeletal pain (de Zwart et al 1997), and fibromyalgia (Wolfe et al 1995). Finally, there are also reports of an age-related decrease in the prevalence of pain problems for all sites other than the joints (Sternbach 1986).

Several reasons for these inconsistent results have been proposed, including increased mortality among the elderly with chronic pain, age differences in the willingness to report painful symptoms, and variability in the definitions of chronic and acute pain (Bressler et al 1999, Helme and Gibson 1999). Another possibility is that the inconsistent results reflect actual differences in the prevalence of various painful symptoms as a function of age. There is no a priori reason to expect all types of pain to change in a comparable way with age given that different pathophysiological mechanisms may be involved. Documenting these pain-specific patterns is fundamental to identifying the mechanisms underlying the age differences.

Regardless of age-related patterns, these studies indicate that a considerable proportion of elderly people experience pain. Approximately 2–27% report migraine or tension headache (Lipton et al 1993), 14–49% report low back pain (Sternbach 1986, Valkenburg 1988), and 24–71% report joint pain (Sternbach 1986, Valkenburg 1988). Pain may be even more common among the institutionalized elderly with 71–83% of patients reporting at least one current pain problem (Roy and Thomas 1986, Ferrell et al 1990).

The characteristics and impact of these pain complaints have not been clarified. Most elderly people report mild to moderate, intermittent pain (Lavsky-Shulan et al 1985, Roy and Thomas 1986, Ferrell et al 1990, Cook and Thomas 1994). Although the pain may interfere with activities (Ferrell et al 1990), the extent of activity restriction due to pain in the elderly may be as great as that reported by middle-aged people (Brattberg et al 1989). Surprisingly, activity levels and use of health care services among elderly people with and without chronic pain do not differ (Roy and Thomas 1987, Cook and Thomas 1994).

Acute pain

The most striking and consistently reported age differences are in the experience of acute pain related to specific, brief injuries or infections. In general, the elderly present with few of the symptoms typically associated with acute clinical syndromes, including pain. Pathological conditions painful to young adults may, in the elderly, produce only behavioural changes such as confusion, restlessness, aggression, anorexia, and fatigue (Butler and Gastel 1980). When pain is reported, it may be referred from the site of origin in an atypical manner. These features may contribute to delayed seeking of treatment and misdiagnosis in the elderly (Albano et al 1975, Mehta et al 2001). For example, the incidence and prevalence of asymptomatic and atypical myocardial infarction increases dramatically with age (Sigurdsson et al 1995, Mehta et al 2001). Although uncommon in younger patients, up to 30% of elderly survivors of myocardial infarction did not report any acute symptoms, while another 30% had an atypical presentation (see review by Ambepitiya et al 1993). Similar age differences have been documented in the presentation of duodenal ulcer (Scapa et al 1989), acute intra-abdominal infection (Cooper et al 1994), appendicitis (Albano et al 1975), and pancreatitis (Gullo et al 1994). Decreased intensity of acute pain associated with duodenal ulcers and myocardial infarction with age has also been reported (Scapa et al 1992). Mechanisms for the differences in acute pain with age are poorly understood.

Postoperative pain

After surgical procedures, the elderly are at greater risk than younger patients for unrelieved pain (Melzack et al 1987), prolonged analgesic use (Gagliese et al 2000), and impaired long-term recovery (White et al 1997, Beltrami 1998). Proper assessment and management of acute postoperative pain is a priority for both research and clinical practice because postoperative confusion (Lynch et al 1998), suppression of the immune and respiratory systems (Cousins 1994), and high rates of mortality (Ergina et al 1993) have been associated with inadequate pain control. Unfortunately, we have only a rudimentary understanding of how postoperative pain differs in young and elderly people. Several studies have suggested that elderly patients report lower pain intensity than younger patients (Bellville et al 1971, Oberle et al 1990), while others have not found age differences (Giuffre et al 1991, Duggleby and Lander 1994).

Postoperative pain management continues to be inadequate in the elderly, even though many of the standard treatment strategies, especially the use of opioids and NSAIDs, are effective (Pasero and McCaffery 1996). The elderly are more vulnerable to the adverse effects of these drugs, and it has been recommended that initial doses be reduced to 25–50% of those given to younger patients (Pasero and McCaffery 1996). Age-related increases in the analgesic efficacy of opioids have been consistently reported (Kaiko 1980, Moore et al 1990). Elderly patients obtain greater analgesia than younger patients in response to a fixed dose of opioids (Bellville et al 1971, Kaiko 1980). As well, they self-administer less opioid than young patients but obtain comparable pain relief using patient-controlled analgesia (PCA) (Burns et al 1989, Giuffre et al 1991, Macintyre and Jarvis 1995, Gagliese et al 2000). In this modality, patients press a button when they require pain relief to obtain a fixed dose of an analgesic through an intravenous or epidural line (Lehmann 1991). PCA is associated with good pain control and high satisfaction among younger patients (Egan and Ready 1994, Perry et al 1994, Miaskowski et al 1999), and there is growing evidence that PCA also may provide adequate analgesia in elderly patients (Egbert et al 1990, Macintyre and Jarvis 1995, Badaoui et al 1996, Gagliese et al 2000), with fewer adverse effects than intramuscular injection of opioids (Egbert et al 1990).

Increased analgesic efficacy of opioids with age may be related to slower or altered metabolism of these drugs (Owen et al 1983, Baillie et al 1989, Laizure et al 1993). Although it has been suggested that the elderly self-administer less opioid using PCA than younger patients due to decreased ability to use the PCA equipment and increased fears of addiction and adverse events (Hofland 1992, Pasero and McCaffery 1996), a recent study found that the effective use of PCA by older patients was not hindered by beliefs about postoperative pain and opioid analgesia (Gagliese et al 2000). In fact, younger and older patients had similar concerns about PCA equipment failure, opioid-related adverse effects, and opioid addiction. Most importantly, the older patients were able to use the PCA apparatus to attain levels of pain relief comparable to those of younger patients (Gagliese et al 2000).

Chronic pain

Age differences in the experience of chronic pain remain controversial. Despite occasional reports that pain intensity decreases (Parker et al 1988, Turk et al 1995) or increases (Puder 1988, Wilkieson et al 1993) with age, most studies have not found age differences in pain intensity (Harkins 1988, Middaugh et al 1988, Sorkin et al 1990, Benbow et al 1995, Harkins et al 1995). However, advancing age may be associated with lower MPQ scores (Lichtenberg et al 1984, Corran et al 1997, but see Lichtenberg et al 1986). Interestingly, studies that employ multiple measures of pain in the same sample have found no age differences in the intensity of pain, but that the elderly obtain lower MPQ scores than younger groups (Gagliese and

Melzack 1997a, Gagliese and Melzack 2001). Unfortunately, the large cross-study variability in age range, pain tools, sample size, and study design limit conclusions.

Taken together, however, the results suggest that age differences in chronic pain are less likely to be evident on measures of intensity than on the McGill Pain Questionnaire. There are several possible explanations for this: one may be that there are age-related changes in the quality but not the intensity of chronic pain; another is that age differences in pain language could lead to the lower MPQ scores independent of actual changes in pain. This explanation is not likely given that the most frequently chosen adjectives are the same across age groups (Gagliese and Melzack 1997a, Gagliese and Melzack 2001). This pattern of word selection suggests that, while there may be changes in the quality of pain with age, the elderly also adopt a more parsimonious response style than younger subjects. They may be endorsing only the most salient qualities of the experience. This possibility has yet to be tested.

The cognitive dimension of chronic pain

Cognitive factors, including beliefs about pain and the use of various coping strategies, have consistently been associated with levels of pain intensity, disability, and emotional distress (Weisenberg 1999). It has been proposed that the elderly believe that pain is a normal part of ageing and to be tolerated rather than treated (Hofland 1992). In addition, the elderly may be more reluctant than younger people to acknowledge the contribution of psychological factors to pain (Blazer and Houpt 1979). However, many elderly people do not agree with statements reflecting beliefs that pain is a normal part of ageing (Brockopp et al 1996). In fact, Gagliese and Melzack (1997c) found no age differences in pain beliefs in both pain-free adults and in those with arthritis pain. The elderly were not more likely than the younger groups to believe that pain was normal at their age, nor were they more likely to associate pain with the normal ageing process than with organic factors such as tissue damage. Furthermore, they did not deny the importance of psychological factors in pain experience.

Age differences in other aspects of the cognitive dimension of pain have been reported. Health locus of control may be more external with advancing age. Specifically, the elderly are more likely than younger patients to relinquish control of their health to powerful others (Melding 1997) and to prefer less information and behavioural control over their health care (Gagliese et al 2000). Although external locus of control has been associated with increased depression, pain, and impairment (Crisson and Keefe 1988), these age differences are very subtle, and their implications for treatment have not been fully explored.

Similarly, subtle differences in the use of coping strategies have been reported. The elderly are more likely than younger patients to employ externally mediated passive coping strategies such as praying and hoping (Keefe and Williams 1990, Sorkin et al 1990). These differences, however, are not large, and their clinical significance is not clear. Overall, the pattern of coping strategies seems more similar than dissimilar across age groups (Sorkin et al 1990). A lack of significant age differences in perceived effectiveness of coping strategies and in perceived ability to control pain has been consistently reported (Harkins 1988, Keefe and Williams 1990, Gagliese and Melzack 1997c). This pattern of results implies that the elderly with chronic pain may be more amenable to psychological pain management strategies than has previously been assumed.

The affective dimension of chronic pain

Pain and anxiety The affective consequences of chronic pain are most often conceptualized in terms of depression and/or anxiety. Age differences in anxiety have received far less empirical attention than depression. There is evidence that anxiety levels do not differ in younger and older patients (Middaugh et al 1988). Furthermore, anxious elderly individuals report more pain complaints and pain of greater intensity than those with lower levels of anxiety (Parmelee et al 1991). This relationship may be independent of concurrent depressive symptomatology (Parmelee et al 1991). These data suggest that, in elderly chronic pain patients, anxiety may be a significant problem that requires assessment and treatment.

Pain and depression Similar to younger individuals (Fishbain et al 1997), there is significant comorbidity of pain and depression in the elderly. In fact, the prevalence and intensity of depression among chronic pain patients is similar across age groups (Sorkin et al 1990, Turk et al 1995, Gagliese and Melzack 1997b). Interestingly, Turk et al (1995) reported that the relationship between pain intensity and depression may differ in young and elderly chronic pain patients. Although the relationship between these variables is mediated by perceived life control and the extent to which pain interferes with functioning in both age groups, it is only in elderly patients that the direct relationship between depression and pain intensity may be significant. As such, in elderly, but not younger, patients changes in pain intensity may directly influence levels of depression and vice versa, independent of other factors. Consistent with this possibility, depressed elderly people report more intense pain and more pain complaints than do non-depressed elderly (Parmelee et al 1991, Casten et al 1995). In addition, elderly people with chronic pain obtain higher scores on depression scales than those who are pain free (Williamson and Schulz 1992, Black et al 1998, but see Ferrell et al 1990).

Clinical differentiation of these states among the elderly may be difficult (Herr and Mobily 1991) especially since many of the most common symptoms of depression, such as sleep and appetite disturbance, may be part of normal ageing (Parmelee 1997). In addition, the elderly are more likely to have atypical presentation of both pain (see above) and depression (Gallo and Rabins 1999). Importantly, the suspicion of depression does not reduce the necessity of a comprehensive pain assessment including an evaluation of psychological well-being.

Although there are several well-validated instruments for the assessment of depression in the elderly (Brink et al 1982), high levels of comorbidity and atypical presentation may present significant problems for these measures. Many of the items assess the vegetative or somatic symptoms of depression that may also be associated with age-related increases in comorbidity, including pain, independent of depression. This would inflate the scores obtained on these scales by the elderly, especially those with chronic pain (Irwin et al 1999, Papassotiropoulos and Heun 1999). Clinicians and researchers are advised to use only scales validated for younger and older people with chronic pain (Gagliese 2001).

Chronic pain and impairment

Both chronic pain (Brattberg et al 1989) and increasing age (Forbes et al 1991) are associated with impairment in functional abilities and the performance of activities of daily living (ADL). Elderly people with chronic pain report more disability and ADL impairment than pain-free elderly people (March et al 1998, Scudds and Robertson 2000). However, several studies have not found this relationship (Roy and Thomas 1987, Ross and Crook 1998, Werner et al 1998).

There has been insufficient empirical attention to age differences in the relationship between pain, disability, and adaptation. Older and younger chronic pain patients report similar levels of interference of pain in their relationships and performance of activities (Brattberg et al 1989, Sorkin et al 1990, Corran et al 1997). However, pain-related impairment may be more emotionally distressing for younger than older people (Williamson and Schulz 1995). The limited data suggest that the relationship between these variables changes with age and that the overall adaptation made to chronic pain may be influenced by slightly different factors in younger and older people (Turk et al 1995, Corran et al 1997).

Pain and dementia

Pain in the cognitively impaired elderly has recently begun to receive empirical attention. The relationship of dementia-related neurodegeneration to pain prevalence, incidence, intensity, and impairment remains to be elucidated. Differential diagnosis between pain and dementia is often necessary in the elderly patient. Pain complaints may be the first signs of dementia (Kisely et al 1992), or may be used to explain or hide mild cognitive impairment (Harkins 1984). Also, acute pathologies, which often are associated with pain in younger patients, may manifest only as confusion in the elderly (see above). Experimental pain threshold does not differ between the cognitively impaired and intact elderly (Cornu 1975, Jonsson et al 1977). In the clinical setting, the prevalence and intensity of painful conditions (Marzinski 1991, Parmelee et al 1993, Scherder et al 1999) and administration of analgesic medications (Scherder and Bouma 2000) decrease as dementia progresses. However, these results must be interpreted with great caution because a reliable and valid assessment protocol has yet to be developed. Among the cognitively impaired elderly who are capable of verbal report, memory and language impairments may confound reports of pain independent of actual changes in the experience of pain (Farrell et al 1996).

Consistent with this, several problems have been identified regarding self-report of pain among people with mild to moderate cognitive impairment. Not surprisingly, many patients are unable to complete self-report measures (Ferrell et al 1995, Miller et al 1996, Hadjistavropoulos et al 1997, Feldt et al 1998). Among those who can, the validity and reliability of the responses remain to be established (Ferrell et al 1995, Feldt et al 1998, Weiner et al 1999). These studies have not provided evidence that the cognitively impaired patients understood the demands of the task. Specifically, it is not clear that the protocols assessed each patient's understanding of the concept of pain or of the method used to quantify intensity. The challenge of developing a reliable, quantitative pain assessment instrument for use with this population remains.

An alternative to self-report may be to rely on the observation of pain behaviours or facial expressions. This may be especially important as dementia progresses and self-report becomes impossible. At this point, valuable information may be obtained from significant others (Werner et al 1998) or through direct observation of behaviour (Weiner et al 1996), especially abrupt changes in behaviour or disruption in usual functioning (Marzinski 1991). Several pain behaviour checklists have been developed for this group (Hurley et al 1992, Feldt et al 1998), although the full-range of their psychometric properties remains to be established (Gagliese 2001). Interestingly, pain behaviours may be more frequent among cognitively impaired than intact patients (Feldt et al 1998). As yet, it is not clear which behaviours are most important for the assessment of pain nor how the behaviours change with the progression of dementia.

Facial expressions may provide reliable indicators of painful states among nonverbal populations (Craig et al 2001). However, there is little information regarding the facial expression of pain among the demented elderly. In three small studies, an increase in the number of facial movements during exposure to noxious stimuli was found, but the responses were highly variable. Specific facial movements associated with pain could not be identified, and complex facial expressions were not seen (Asplund et al 1991, Porter et al 1996, Hadjistavropoulos et al 1997). Interestingly, in response to venipuncture, the cognitively impaired demonstrated blunted physiological responses (heart rate) but increased facial expressiveness during the actual stick (Porter et al 1996). The authors speculate that this may be related to the impaired elderly subjects' inability to prepare for the aversive event leading to greater 'surprise' and expression during the event than is experienced by cognitively intact elderly. On the other hand, the apparent dissociation between physiological and facial responses may be related to generalized emotional disinhibition rather than pain perception per se among the cognitively impaired elderly (Porter et al 1996).

Management of pain in the elderly

Many elderly people do not receive adequate pain treatment. Approximately 47–80% of community-dwelling (Roy and Thomas 1987, Woo et al 1994) and 16–27% of institutionalized elderly do not receive any treatment for their pain (Roy and Thomas 1986, Lichtenberg and McGrogan 1987). Although inadequate pain management is not limited to the elderly, several unique factors may contribute to the poor treatment of pain in this group. These include, but are not limited to, increased risks of pharmacotherapy, misconceptions regarding the efficacy of non-pharmacological pain management strategies, and a reluctance to offer multidisciplinary treatments to the elderly.

Pharmacological therapy

Pharmacotherapy, including the use of opioids, is safe for the elderly when used with appropriate medical supervision (Popp and Portenoy 1996). Nonetheless, it is well documented that the elderly are more likely than younger patients to develop adverse reactions to most classes of analgesic drugs at much lower dosages (Popp and Portenoy 1996). This may be due to age-associated changes in the metabolism and clearance rates of drugs which lead to altered pharmacokinetics and pharmacodynamics (Popp and Portenoy 1996). The AGS (American Geriatrics Society) Panel on Chronic Pain in Older Persons (1998) has developed detailed clinical practice guidelines, which are applicable to all classes of analgesic medication. Because pharmacotherapy requires special attention in this group, it is important to recognize that there are alternative, potentially safer, modalities of therapy available for chronic pain management. These include both physical and psychological treatments.

Psychological treatment

The efficacy of psychological interventions for the management of chronic pain has been well established for younger patients (Gatchel and Turk 1996). Comparable data from elderly samples are limited yet promising (Gagliese and Melzack 1997b). The elderly have been shown to benefit from cognitive-behavioural therapy (Puder 1988), relaxation and biofeedback training (Nicholson and Blanchard 1993), and behaviour therapy (Miller and LeLieuvre 1982). In some of these studies, the elderly made treatment gains comparable to those of younger patients (Middaugh et al 1988, Puder 1988), although modifications to the interventions may be required to maximize compliance and treatment benefits (Arena et al 1988, 1991). These modifications have not been tested with younger patients and may prove to be of equal benefit across the adult lifespan (Gagliese and Melzack 1997b).

Physical therapies

Elderly patients benefit from physical interventions such as transcutaneous electrical nerve stimulation (Thorsteinsson 1987), massage (Eisenberg et al 1993), and the application of heat and cold (Eisenberg et al 1993). In addition to these more passive strategies, there is considerable evidence that elderly chronic pain patients, especially those with musculoskeletal pain, may derive substantial benefit from regular exercise (Ferrell et al 1997). An additional advantage to these treatment modalities is that they involve little risk of adverse events when carried out under appropriate medical supervision (AGS Panel on Chronic Pain in Older Persons 1998).

Multidisciplinary treatment

Although multidisciplinary treatment is recognized as the gold standard for younger patients (Flor et al 1992), data concerning the elderly are scant and often contradictory. It has been suggested that the elderly may not have access to such treatment (Harkins and Price 1992, Kee et al 1998). However, the age distribution of patients referred to pain clinics is consistent with both the age-related patterns in the prevalence of many common pain disorders and the proportion of elderly in the general population (Benbow et al 1995, Gagliese and Melzack 1997b). Therefore, it is not clear that the elderly are underrepresented in these clinics. Importantly, studies have not found age-related differences in treatment expectations (Harkins and Price 1992), acceptance, compliance, or dropout rates (Sorkin et al 1990).

Although there have been reports that increasing age is a predictor of poor outcome following multidisciplinary pain management (Graff-Radford and Naliboff 1988), there is also evidence that the elderly may derive substantial benefit, comparable to that seen with younger patients (Middaugh et al 1988, Cutler et al 1994). Multidisciplinary treatment should be considered for all geriatric patients with significant pain complaints.

Acknowledgements

This work was supported by a University of Toronto, Faculty of Medicine Dean's Grant to LG.

References

AGS Panel on Chronic Pain in Older Persons 1998 The management of chronic pain in older persons. Journal of the American Geriatrics Society 46: 635–651

Albano WA, Zielinski CM, Organ CH 1975 Is appendicitis in the aged really different? Geriatrics 30: 81–88

Ambepitiya GB, Iyengar EN, Roberts ME 1993 Review: silent exertional myocardial ischaemia and perception of angina in elderly people. Age and Ageing 22: 302–307

Andersson HI, Ejilertsson G, Leden I, Rosenberg C 1993 Chronic pain in a geographically defined population: studies of differences in age, gender, social class and pain localization. Clinical Journal of Pain 9: 174–182

Arena JG, Hightower NE, Chong GC 1988 Relaxation therapy for tension headache in the elderly: a prospective study. Psychology and Aging 3: 96–98

Arena JG, Hannah SL, Bruno GM, Meador KJ 1991 Electromyographic biofeedback training for tension headache in the elderly: a prospective study. Biofeedback and Self-Regulation 16: 379–390

Asplund K, Norberg A, Adolfsson R, Waxman HM 1991 Facial expressions in severely demented patients: a stimulus-response study of four patients with dementia of the Alzheimer type. International Journal of Geriatric Psychiatry 6: 599–606

Badaoui R, Riboulot M, Ernst C, Ossart M 1996 L'analgésie postopératoire autocontrolée par le patient agé. Cahiers d'Anesthésiologie 44: 519–522

Baillie SP, Bateman DN, Coates PE, Woodhouse KW 1989 Age and the pharmacokinetics of morphine. Age and Ageing 18: 258–262

Bellville JW, Forrest WH, Miller E, Brown BW 1971 Influence of age on pain relief from analgesics. Journal of the American Medical Association 217: 1835–1841

Beltrami V 1998 Age related risk and prevention of postoperative complications. Clinica Terapeutica 149: 435–438

Benbow SJ, Cossins L, Bowsher D 1995 A comparison of young and elderly patients attending a regional pain centre. Pain Clinic 8: 323–332

Benesh LR, Szigeti E, Ferraro FR, Gullicks JN 1997 Tools for assessing chronic pain in rural elderly women. Home Healthcare Nurse 15: 207–211

Black SA, Goodwin JS, Markides KS 1998 The association between chronic diseases and depressive symptomatology in older Mexican Americans. Journal of Gerontology: Medical Sciences 53A: M188–M194

Blazer DG, Houpt JL 1979 Perception of poor health in the healthy older adult. Journal of the American Geriatrics Society 27: 330–334

Brattberg G, Thorslund M, Wikman A 1989 The prevalence of pain in a general population. The results of a postal survey in a county of Sweden. Pain 37: 215–222

Brattberg G, Parker MG, Thorslund M 1997 A longitudinal study of pain: reported pain from middle age to old age. Clinical Journal of Pain 13: 144–149

Bressler HB, Keyes WJ, Rochon PA, Badley E 1999 The prevalence of low back pain in the elderly. A systematic review of the literature. Spine 24: 1813–1819

Brink TL, Yesavage JA, Lum O, Heersema PH, Adey M, Rose TL 1982 Screening tests for geriatric depression. Clinical Gerontologist 1: 37–43

Brockopp D, Warden S, Colclough G, Brockopp G 1996 Elderly people's knowledge of and attitudes to pain management. British Journal of Nursing 5: 556–562

Burns JW, Hodsman NBA, McLintock TTC, Gillies GWA, Kenny GNC, McArdle CS 1989 The influence of patient characteristics on the requirements for postoperative analgesia. Anaesthesia 44: 2–6

Butler RN, Gastel B 1980 Care of the aged: Perspectives on pain and discomfort, In: Ng LK, Bonica J (eds) Pain, discomfort and humanitarian care. Elsevier, New York, pp 297–311

Casten RJ, Parmelee PA, Kleban MH, Lawton MP, Katz IR 1995 The relationships among anxiety, depression, and pain in a geriatric institutionalized sample. Pain 61: 271–276

Cook AJ, Thomas MR 1994 Pain and the use of health services among the elderly. Journal of Aging and Health 6: 155–172

Cook NR, Evans DA, Funkenstein HH, Scherr PA, Ostfeld AM, Taylor JA, Hennekens CH 1989 Correlates of headache in a population-based cohort of elderly. Archives of Neurology 46: 1338–1344

Cooper GS, Shlaes DM, Salata RA 1994 Intraabdominal infection: differences in presentation and outcome between younger patients and the elderly. Clinical Infectious Diseases 19: 146–148

Cornu FR 1975 Disturbances of the perception of pain among persons with degenerative dementia. Journal de Psychologie Normale et Pathologique 72: 461–464

Corran TM, Farrell MJ, Helme RD, Gibson SJ 1997 The classification of patients with chronic pain: age as a contributing factor. Clinical Journal of Pain 13: 207–214

Cousins M 1994 Acute and postoperative pain. In: Wall PD, Melzack R (eds) Textbook of pain. Churchill Livingstone, Edinburgh, pp 284–305

Craig KD, Prkachin KM, Grunau RE 2001 The facial expression of pain. In: Turk DC, Melzack R (eds) Handbook of pain assessment. Guilford Press, New York, pp 153–169

Crisson JE, Keefe FJ 1988 The relationship of locus of control to pain coping strategies and psychological distress in chronic pain patients. Pain 35: 147–154

Crook J, Rideout E, Browne G 1984 The prevalence of pain complaints in a general population. Pain 18: 299–314

Cutler RB, Fishbain DA, Rosomoff RS, Rosomoff HL 1994 Outcomes in treatment of pain in geriatric and younger age groups. Archives of Physical Medicine and Rehabilitation 75: 457–464

de Zwart BCH, Broersen JPJ, Frings-Dresen MHW, van Dijk FJH 1997 Musculoskeletal complaints in the Netherlands in relation to age, gender and physically demanding work. International Archives of Occupational and Environmental Health 70: 352–360

Duggleby W, Lander J 1994 Cognitive status and postoperative pain: older adults. Journal of Pain and Symptom Management 9: 19–27

Egan KJ, Ready LB 1994 Patient satisfaction with intravenous PCA or epidural morphine. Canadian Journal of Anaesthesia 41: 6–11

Egbert AM, Parks LH, Short LM, Burnett ML 1990 Randomized trial of postoperative patient-controlled analgesia vs intramuscular narcotics in frail elderly men. Archives of Internal Medicine 150: 1897–1903

Eisenberg DM, Kessler RC, Foster C 1993 Unconventional medicine in the United States: prevalence, costs and patterns of use. New England Journal of Medicine 328: 246–252

Ergina PL, Gold SL, Meakins JL 1993 Perioperative care of the elderly patient. World Journal of Surgery 17: 192–198

Escalante A, Lichtenstein MJ, White K, Rios N, Hazuda HP 1995 A method for scoring the pain map of the McGill Pain Questionnaire for use in epidemiologic studies. Aging (Milano) 7: 358–366

Farrell MJ, Katz B, Helme RD 1996 The impact of dementia on the pain experience. Pain 67: 7–15

Feldt KS, Ryden MB, Miles S 1998 Treatment of pain in cognitively impaired compared with cognitively intact older patients with hip-fracture. Journal of the American Geriatrics Society 46: 1079–1085

Ferrell BA, Ferrell BR, Osterweil D 1990 Pain in the nursing home. Journal of the American Geriatrics Society 38: 409–414

Ferrell BA, Ferrell BR, Rivera L 1995 Pain in cognitively impaired nursing home residents. Journal of Pain and Symptom Management 10: 591–598

Ferrell BA, Josephson KR, Pollan AM, Loy S, Ferrell BR 1997 A randomized trial of walking versus physical methods for chronic pain management. Aging: Clinical and Experimental Research 9: 99–105

Fishbain DA, Cutler RB, Rosomoff HL, Rosomoff RS 1997 Chronic pain-associated depression: Antecedent or consequence of chronic pain? A review. Clinical Journal of Pain 13: 116–137

Flor H, Fydrich T, Turk DC 1992 Efficacy of multidisciplinary pain treatment centers: a meta-analytic review. Pain 49: 221–230

Forbes WF, Hatward LM, Agwani N 1991 Factors associated with the prevalence of various self-reported impairments among older people residing in the community. Canadian Journal of Public Health 82: 240–244

Gagliese L 2001 Assessment of pain in the elderly. In: Turk DC, Melzack R (eds) Handbook of pain assessment. Guilford Press, New York, pp 119–133

Gagliese L, Melzack R 1997a Age differences in the quality of chronic pain: A preliminary study. Pain Research and Management 2: 157–162

Gagliese L, Melzack R 1997b Chronic pain in elderly people. Pain 70: 3–14

Gagliese L, Melzack R 1997c Lack of evidence for age differences in pain beliefs. Pain Research and Management 2: 19–28

Gagliese L, Melzack R 2001 The Canadian chronic pain centre patient: age differences and similarities in pain and psychosocial characteristics. Submitted for publication

Gagliese L, Stratford JG, Hickey D, Gamsa A, Melzack R 1998 The psychometric properties of the McGill Pain Questionnaire in young and elderly chronic pain patients. Pain Research and Management 3: 58

Gagliese L, Jackson M, Ritvo P, Wowk A, Katz J 2000 Age is not an impediment to effective use of patient controlled analgesia by surgical patients. Anesthesiology 93: 601–610

Gallo JJ, Rabins PV 1999 Depression without sadness: alternative presentations of depression in late life. American Family Physician 60: 820–826

Gatchel RJ, Turk DC 1996 Psychological approaches to pain management. Guilford Press, New York

Giuffre M, Asci J, Arnstein P, Wilkinson C 1991 Postoperative joint replacement pain: description and opioid requirements. Journal of Post Anesthesia Nursing 6: 239–245

Graff-Radford SB, Naliboff BD 1988 Age predicts treatment outcome in postherpetic neuralgia. Clinical Journal of Pain 4: 1–4

Gullo L, Sipahi HM, Pezzilli R, 1994 Pancreatitis in the elderly. Journal of Clinical Gastroenterology 19: 64–68

Hadjistavropoulos T, Craig KD, Martin N, Hadjistavropoulos H, McMurtry B 1997 Toward a research outcome measure of pain in frail elderly in chronic care. Pain Clinic 10: 71–79

Harkins SW 1984 Pain and the elderly. In: Benedetti C (Ed) Advances in pain research and therapy, vol 7. Raven Press, New York, pp 103–121

Harkins SW 1988 Pain in the elderly. In: Dubner R, Gebhart FG, Bond MR (eds) Proceedings of the 5th world congress on pain. Elsevier, Amsterdam, pp 355–357

Harkins SW, Price DD 1992 Assessment of pain in the elderly. In: Turk DC, Melzack R (eds) Handbook of pain assessment. Guilford Press, New York, pp 315–331

Harkins SW, Lagua BT, Price DD, Small RE 1995 Geriatric pain. In: Roy R (ed) Chronic pain in old age. University of Toronto, Toronto, pp 127–159

Helme RD, Gibson SJ 1999 Pain in older people. In: Crombie IK, Croft PR, Linton SJ, LeResche L,Von Korff M (eds) Epidemiology of pain. IASP Press, Seattle, pp 103–112

Herr KA, Mobily PR 1991 Complexities of pain assessment in the elderly: clinical considerations. Journal of Gerontological Nursing 17: 12–19

Herr KA, Mobily PR 1993 Comparison of selected pain assessment tools for use with the elderly. Applied Nursing Research 6: 39–46

Hofland SL 1992 Elder beliefs: blocks to pain management. Journal of Gerontological Nursing 18: 19–24

Hurley AC, Volicer BJ, Hanrahan PA, Houde S, Volicer L 1992 Assessment of discomfort in advanced Alzheimer patients. Research in Nursing and Health 15: 369–377

Irwin M, Artin KH, Oxman MN 1999 Screening for depression in the older adult: criterion validity of the 10-item Center for Epidemiological Studies Depression Scale (CES-D). Archives of Internal Medicine 159: 1701–1704

Jensen MP, Karoly P 2001 Self-report scales and procedures for assessing pain in adults. In: Turk DC, Melzack R (Eds) Handbook of pain assessment. Guilford Press, New York, pp 15–34

Jensen MP, Karoly P, Braver S 1986 The measurement of clinical pain intensity: a comparison of six methods. Pain 27: 117–126

Jonsson CO, Malhammar G, Waldton S 1977 Reflex elicitation thresholds in senile dementia. Acta Psychiatrica Scandinavica 55: 81–96

Kaiko RF 1980 Age and morphine analgesia in cancer patients with post-operative pain. Clinical Pharmacology and Therapeutics 28: 823–826

Kee WG, Middaugh SJ, Redpath S, Hargadon R 1998 Age as a factor in admission to chronic pain rehabilitation. Clinical Journal of Pain 14: 121–128

Keefe FJ, Williams DA 1990 A comparison of coping strategies in chronic pain patients in different age groups. Journal of Gerontology: Psychological Sciences 45: P161–165

Kisely S, Tweddle D, Pugh EW 1992 Dementia presenting with sore eyes. British Journal of Psychiatry 161: 120–121

Kremer E, Atkinson JH, Ignelzi RJ 1981 Measurement of pain: patient preference does not confound pain measurement. Pain 10: 241–249

Laizure SC, Miller JH, Stevens RC, Donahue DJ, Laster RE, Brown D 1993 The disposition and cerebrospinal fluid penetration of morphine and its two major glucuronidated metabolites in adults undergoing lumbar myelogram. Pharmacotherapy 13: 471–475

Lavsky-Shulan M, Wallace RB, Kohout FJ, Lemke JH, Morris MC, Smith IM 1985 Prevalence and functional correlates of low back pain in the elderly: the Iowa 65+ rural health study. Journal of the American Geriatrics Society 33: 23–28

Lehmann KA 1991 Patient-controlled intravenous analgesia for postoperative pain relief. In: Max M, Portenoy R, Laska E (eds) Advances in pain research and therapy. Raven Press, New York, pp 481–505

Lichtenberg PA, McGrogan AJ 1987 Chronic pain in elderly psychiatric inpatients. Clinical Biofeedback and Health 10: 3–7

Lichtenberg PA, Skehan MW, Swensen CH 1984 The role of personality, recent life stress and arthritic severity in predicting pain. Journal of Psychosomatic Research 28: 231–236

Lichtenberg PA, Swensen CH, Skehan MW 1986 Further investigation of the role of personality, lifestyle and arthritic severity in predicting pain. Journal of Psychosomatic Research 30: 327–337

Lipton RB, Pfeffer D, Newman LC, Solomon S 1993 Headaches in the elderly. Journal of Pain and Symptom Management 8: 87–97

Lynch EP, Lazor MA, Gellis JE, Orav J, Goldman L, Marcantonio ER 1998 The impact of postoperative pain on the development of postoperative delirium. Anesthesia and Analgesia 86: 781–785

Macintyre PE, Jarvis DA 1995 Age is the best predictor of postoperative morphine requirements. Pain 64: 357–364

March LM, Brnabic AJM, Skinner JC, Schwarz JM, Finnegan T, Druce J, Brooks PM 1998 Musculoskeletal disability among elderly people in the community. Medical Journal of Australia 168: 439–442

Marzinski LR 1991 The tragedy of dementia: clinically assessing pain in the confused, nonverbal elderly. Journal of Gerontological Nursing 17: 25–28

Mehta RH, Rathore SS, Radford MJ, Wang Y, Krumholz HM 2001 Acute myocardial infarction in the elderly: differences by age. Journal of the American College of Cardiology 38: 736–741

Melding PS 1997 Coping with pain in old age. In: Mostofsky DI, Lomranz J (eds) Handbook of pain and aging. Plenum Press, New York, pp 167–184

Melzack R 1975 The McGill Pain Questionnaire: major properties and scoring methods. Pain 1: 277–299

Melzack R, Katz J 2001 The McGill Pain Questionnaire: appraisal and current status. In: Turk DC, Melzack R (eds) Handbook of pain assessment. Guilford Press, New York, pp 35–52

Melzack R, Abbott FV, Zackon W, Mulder DS, Davis MWL 1987 Pain on a surgical ward: a survey of the duration and intensity of pain and the effectiveness of medication. Pain 29: 67–72

Miaskowski C, Crews J, Ready LB, Paul SM, Ginsberg B 1999 Anesthesia-based pain services improve the quality of postoperative pain management. Pain 80: 23–29

Middaugh SJ, Levin RB, Kee WG, Barchiesi FD, Roberts JM 1988 Chronic pain: its treatment in geriatric and younger patients. Archives of Physical Medicine and Rehabilitation 69: 1021–1025

Miller C, LeLieuvre RB 1982 A method to reduce chronic pain in elderly nursing home residents. Gerontologist 22: 314–317

Miller J, Neelon V, Dalton J, Ng'andu N, Bailey D, Jr., Layman E, Hosfeld A 1996 The assessment of discomfort in elderly confused patients: a preliminary study. Journal of Neuroscience Nursing 28: 175–182

Moore AK, Vilderman S, Lubenskyi W, McCans J, Fox GS 1990 Differences in epidural morphine requirements between elderly and young patients after abdominal surgery. Anesthesia and Analgesia 70: 316–320

Nicholson NL, Blanchard EB 1993 A controlled evaluation of behavioral treatment of chronic headache in the elderly. Behavior Therapy 24: 395–408

Oberle K, Paul P, Wry J, Grace M 1990 Pain, anxiety and analgesics: a comparative study of elderly and younger surgical patients. Canadian Journal of Aging 9: 13–22

Owen JA, Sitar DS, Berger L, Brownell L, Duke PC, Mitenko PA 1983 Age-related morphine kinetics. Clinical Pharmacology and Therapeutics 34: 364–368

Papassotiropoulos A, Heun R 1999 Screening for depression in the elderly: a study on misclassification by screening instruments and improvement of scale performance. Progress in Neuro-Psychopharmacology and Biological Psychiatry 23: 431–446

Parker J, Frank R, Beck N, Finan M, Walker S, Hewett JE, Broster C, Smarr K, Smith E, Kay D 1988 Pain in rheumatoid arthritis: relationship to demographic, medical, and psychological factors. Journal of Rheumatology 15: 433–437

Parmelee PA 1997 Pain and psychological function in late life. In: Lomranz J, Mostofsky DI (eds) Handbook of pain and aging. Plenum Press, New York, pp 207–226

Parmelee PA, Katz IR, Lawton MP 1991 The relation of pain to depression among institutionalized aged. Journal of Gerontology, Psychological Sciences 46: p15–p21

Parmelee PA, Smith B, Katz IR 1993 Pain complaints and cognitive status among elderly institution residents. Journal of the American Geriatrics Society 41: 517–522

Pasero CL, McCaffery M 1996 Managing postoperative pain in the elderly. American Journal of Nursing 96: 38–45

Perry F, Parker RK, White PF, Clifford PA 1994 Role of psychological factors in postoperative pain control and recovery with patient-controlled analgesia. Clinical Journal of Pain 10: 57–63

Popp B, Portenoy RK 1996 Management of chronic pain in the elderly: Pharmacology of opioids and other analgesic drugs. In: Ferrell BR, Ferrell BA (eds) Pain in the elderly. IASP Press, Seattle, pp 21–34

Porter FL, Malhorta KM, Wolf CM, Morris JC, Miller JP, Smith MC 1996 Dementia and the response to pain in the elderly. Pain 68: 413–421
Puder RS 1988 Age analysis of cognitive-behavioral group therapy for chronic pain outpatients. Psychology and Aging 3: 204–207
Ross MM, Crook J 1998 Elderly recipients of home nursing services: Pain, disability and functional competence. Journal of Advanced Nursing 27: 1117–1126
Roy R, Thomas M 1986 A survey of chronic pain in an elderly population. Canadian Family Physician 32: 513–516
Roy R, Thomas MR 1987 Elderly persons with and without pain: a comparative study. Clinical Journal of Pain 3: 102–106
Scapa E, Horowitz M, Waron M, Eshchar J 1989 Duodenal ulcer in the elderly. Journal of Clinical Gastroenterology 11: 502–506
Scapa E, Horowitz M, Avtalion J, Waron M, Eshchar J 1992 Appreciation of pain in the elderly. Israel Journal of Medical Science 28: 94–96
Scherder EJ, Bouma A 2000 Acute versus chronic pain experience in Alzheimer's disease. A new questionnaire. Dementia and Geriatric Cognitive Disorders 11: 11–16
Scherder EJ, Bouma A, Borkent M, Rahman O 1999 Alzheimer patients report less pain intensity and pain affect than non-demented elderly. Psychiatry 62: 265–272
Schwartz BS, Stewart WF, Simon D, Lipton RB 1998 Epidemiology of tension-type headache. Journal of the American Medical Association 279: 381–383
Scudds RJ, Robertson JM 2000 Pain factors associated with physical disability in a sample of community-dwelling senior citizens. Journals of Gerontology. Series A, Biological Sciences and Medical Sciences 55: M393–M399
Sigurdsson E, Thorgeirsson G, Sigvaldason H, Sigfusson N 1995 Unrecognized myocardial infarction: epidemiology, clinical characteristics, and the prognostic role of angina pectoris. Annals of Internal Medicine 122: 96–102
Sorkin BA, Rudy TE, Hanlon RB, Turk DC, Stieg RL 1990 Chronic pain in old and young patients: differences appear less important than similarities. Journal of Gerontology: Psychological Sciences 45: P64–68
Sternbach RA 1986 Survey of pain in the United States: the Nuprin pain report. Clinical Journal of Pain 2: 49–53
Thorsteinsson G 1987 Chronic pain: use of TENS in the elderly. Gerontology 42: 75–82
Turk DC, Melzack R 2001 Handbook of pain assessment. Guilford Press, New York
Turk DC, Okifuji A 1999 A cognitive-behavioral approach to pain management. In: Wall PD, Melzack R (eds) Textbook of pain. Churchill Livingstone, Edinburgh, pp 1431–1444
Turk DC, Okifuji A, Scharff L 1995 Chronic pain and depression: role of perceived impact and perceived control in different age cohorts. Pain 61: 93–101
Valkenburg HA 1988 Epidemiological considerations of the geriatric population. Gerontology 34 (Suppl. 1): 2–10
Weiner D, Peiper C, McConnell E, Martinez S, Keefe FJ 1996 Pain measurement in elders with chronic low back pain: traditional and alternative approaches. Pain 67: 461–467
Weiner D, Peterson B, Keefe F 1999 Chronic pain-associated behaviors in the nursing home: resident versus caregiver perceptions. Pain 80: 577–588
Weisenberg M 1999 Cognitive aspects of pain. In: Wall PD, Melzack R (eds) Textbook of pain. Churchill Livingstone, Edinburgh, pp 345–358
Werner P, Cohen-Mansfield J, Watson V, Pasis S 1998 Pain in participants of adult day care centers: assessment by different raters. Journal of Pain and Symptom Management 15: 8–17
White CL, LeFort SM, Amsel R, Jeans ME 1997 Predictors of the development of chronic pain. Research in Nursing and Health 20: 309–318
Wilkieson CA, Madhok R, Hunter JA, Capell HA 1993 Toleration, side-effects and efficacy of sulphasalazine in rheumatoid arthritis patients of different ages. Quarterly Journal of Medicine 86: 501–505
Williamson GM, Schulz R 1992 Pain, activity restriction and symptoms of depression among community-residing elderly adults. Journal of Gerontology 47: P367–372
Williamson GM, Schulz R 1995 Activity restriction mediates the association between pain and depressed affect: A study of younger and older adult cancer patients. Psychology and Aging 10: 369–378
Wolfe F, Ross K, Anderson J, Russell IJ, Hebert L 1995 The prevalence and characteristics of fibromyalgia in the general population. Arthritis and Rheumatism 38: 19–28
Woo J, Ho SC, Lau J, Leung PC 1994 Musculoskeletal complaints and associated consequences in elderly Chinese aged 70 and over. Journal of Rheumatology 21: 1927–1931

Chapter 39

Sex and gender differences in pain

Anita Holdcroft and Karen J Berkley

Introduction

In the past decade, increasing societal respect for sex and gender differences has widely influenced basic and clinical research, from molecular-genetic to sociocultural, as well as public policy on health, resulting in an expanding literature (Wisemann and Pardue 2001). In this context, gender is defined as the sex with which an individual identifies. Evidence for sex and gender differences in pain has developed significantly leading to reviews by Fillingim and Maixner (1995), Jensvold et al (1996), Unruh (1996), Berkley (1997a), Ciccone and Holdcroft (1998), Riley et al (1998), and Fillingim (2000). Significant advances have occurred in our understanding of pain modulation from fetus to old age, with concomitant development of new therapeutic strategies for individuals of either sex in pain. This chapter summarizes the evidence for sex differences in pain, the mechanisms that might underlie them, the clinical relevance of this information, and future directions.

What are the differences?

Evidence for sex differences in human pain derives from four main areas of research: community epidemiology, disease prevalence, psychophysics, and reproductive variations.

Epidemiology and sex prevalence in disease

Community epidemiological studies consistently reveal (Unruh 1996, Berkley 1997a) that women compared to men report more severe pain intensity, more frequent pain, pain in more areas of the body, and pain of longer duration.

In addition there are many painful diseases that have female > male prevalence (Table 39.1, Berkley and Holdcroft 1999), e.g., those sited in the head and neck, those of musculoskeletal origin, those in the visceral/internal organs, and those of auto-immune aetiology. Some authors have attributed this apparent female vulnerability to an increased willingness for women to report pain and seek health care. While that may be a factor, it is only one of many. Thus, much of the female prevalence can be accounted for by parturition or gynaecological problems. In addition, overall prevalence patterns in both sexes for many types of pain (such as those of temporomandibular joint disorder, fibromyalgia, migraine, chest, abdomen, and joints) change across the lifespan (Von Korff et al 1988, LeResche

Table 39.1 Sex prevalence of some common painful syndromes and potential contributing causes[a]

Female prevalence	Male prevalence
Head and neck	
Migraine headache with aura	Migraine without aura
Chronic tension headache	Cluster headache
Postdural puncture headache	Post-traumatic headache
Cervicogenic headache	Paratrigeminal syndrome[b]
Tic douloureux	
Temporomandibular disorder	
Occipital neuralgia	
Atypical odontalgia	
Burning tongue	
Carotidynia	
Temporal arteritis	
Chronic paroxysmal hemicrania	
Limbs	
Carpal tunnel syndrome	Thromboangiitis obliterans[c]
Raynaud's disease	Haemophilic arthropathy*
Chilblains	Brachial plexus neuropathy
Reflex sympathetic dystrophy	
Chronic venous insufficiency	
Piriformis syndrome	
Peroneal muscular atrophy[d]*	
Internal organs	
Oesophagitis	Pancoast tumour[e,†]
Gallbladder disease[†]	Pancreatic disease
Irritable bowel syndrome	Duodenal ulcer
Interstitial cystitis	
Proctalgia fugax	
Chronic constipation	
General	
Fibromyalgia syndrome	Postherpetic neuralgia
Multiple sclerosis[‡]	
Rheumatoid arthritis[‡]	
Acute intermittent porphyria*	
Lupus erythematosis[‡]	

[a]Sex prevalences were taken mainly from Merskey and Bogduk (1994) and cross-checked using Medline and other search sources.
[b]Raeder's syndrome.
[c]Buerger's disease.
[d]Charcot–Marie–Tooth disease.
[e]Bronchogenic carcinoma.
Potential contributory causes: *sex-linked inheritance; [†]lifestyle; [‡]autoimmune.

et al 1997, LeResche and Von Korff 1998). Thus, the sex prevalence of some painful disorders can diminish or reverse with age. Further complicating the issue is that in some disorders, such as irritable bowel syndrome, acute appendicitis, migraine headaches, rheumatoid arthritis, and coronary heart disease, the clinical signs differ between the sexes (Berkley 1997a, b; Weyand et al 1998). And finally, in the context of major disease or illness, sex differences in pain reports disappear (Turk and Okifuji 1998). Thus, while overall women are more vulnerable than men to acute, intermittent, and chronic pain, the pertinent individual circumstances vary and there are many exceptions (Unruh 1996).

Psychophysical studies

A meta-analysis of experimental psychophysical studies of healthy individuals on sex differences in the attribution of somatic stimulation as painful showed that women have lower pain thresholds, higher ratings, and less tolerance than men (Riley et al 1998). Thus, even in safe experimental settings where the subject experiences brief pain, females generally report more pain than men. Is this pain sensitivity a response bias or 'somatosensory amplification' or a greater awareness of potential harm, or are other factors operative (Berkley 1997b)?

The direction of the sex differences are affected by *stimulus* type and presentation. Thus, pressure and electrical stimuli produce larger sex differences than thermal or ischaemic stimuli (Riley et al 1998), but when thermal stimuli are delivered repeatedly the difference increases (Fillingim et al 1998). Sex differences are also affected by the *testing paradigm* (e.g., thresholds vs tolerance; Riley et al 1998), the *stimulus location* (males show greater sensitivity than females when the stimuli are applied to areas near the genitalia; Giamberardino et al 1997), *situational variables* (e.g., sex and attractiveness of the experimenter, or whether the setting is a clinic or science laboratory), and *psychological variables*, such as anxiety, or efficacy and control beliefs. Physiological factors are also important: *blood pressure* is inversely related to pain sensitivity, even for normotensive subjects (Fillingim and Maixner 1996); the presence of *stress* induces analgesia, the effects being different in the two sexes (Sternberg and Liebeskind 1995); *nutrition* (sugar and fat intake) and the presence of certain *disease* conditions can significantly increase or decrease pain sensitivity (Berkley 1997a).

Reproductive biology/gynaecology/urology

New data from humans and animals are emerging that clinical and experimental pain can vary with reproductive status, especially at puberty, during the reproductive cycle, pregnancy, postpartum, menopause, and andropause, and in situations where exogenous sex hormones are administered (Murray and Holdcroft 1989; Fillingim and Maixner 1995; Marcus 1995; Unruh 1996; Berkley 1997a, b; Jones 1997; Fillingim et al 1998; LeResche and Von Korff 1998). Interestingly the reported effects vary but overall the important conclusion is that there is more variability in women's pains than in men.

How might these differences occur?

The varied and sometimes contradictory findings of the many studies of sex differences in both experimentally induced and endogenous pain, together with fluctuations associated with reproductive and hormonal status, necessitate a consideration of potential mechanisms derived from diverse fields of research on animals and humans.

Genetics

Genetic differences in pain-related traits have been increasingly studied (Mogil et al 1996, 2000). These differences can manifest themselves in several ways:

(1) *Sex-linked genetic diseases* associated with pain syndromes, e.g., haemophilia, porphyria, and the X-linked recessive type of peroneal muscular atrophy (Charcot–Marie–Tooth, Merskey and Bogduk 1994).

(2) *Metabolizing enzyme systems* such as sex-related genetic variations in the cytochrome P450 enzyme family (Jensvold et al 1996, Ciccone and Holdcroft 1998).

(3) Differences in both *nociception and responses to manipulations of exogenous and endogenous analgesics* in rodents. Using quantitative trait locus (QTL) mapping techniques, Mogil et al (1997a) localized a male-specific QTL on chromosome 4 that appears to account for variability between two strains of mice in δ-opioid associated nociception as assessed by the hot-plate assay method. This same group also localized, on chromosome 8, a female-specific QTL that accounts for variability in stress-induced analgesia (SIA; Mogil et al 1997b). They concluded that it may be part of the basis for a female-specific SIA mechanism in rats that is ontogenetically organized, is non-opioid, varies with reproductive status, and is oestrogen-dependent.

(4) Oestrogen regulation of *gene expression*, recently discovered in rats for neurofilament proteins, nerve growth factor, and substance P (Sohrabji et al 1994, Scoville et al 1997, Villablanca and Hanley 1997).

Physiology

Women relative to men have a higher percentage body fat, smaller muscle mass, lower blood pressure, amd fluctuations associated with reproductive conditions in gastrointestinal time, urinary creatinine clearance, metabolism, and thermoregulation. These differences in body composition have implications not only for sex prevalence differences in pain sites (e.g., musculoskeletal), but also for drug pharmacodynamics and pharmacokinetics (Jensvold et al 1996, Ciccone and Holdcroft 1998). Furthermore, pain estimates are inversely proportional to resting blood pressure, a situation that, due to higher blood pressure in males, may be one of the contributors to male hypoalgesia relative to silent ischaemia (Fillingim and Maixner 1995).

Anatomy

Differences in pelvic organ structures and arrangements create large sex differences in pain (see Chap. 12). In addition, as argued by Berkley (1997a), sex differences in the reproductive tract create in females a greater vulnerability to both local and remote central sensitization. This situation could partly explain the greater vulnerability in women for multiple referred pains, particularly in muscles and the clinical signs of diseases, e.g., coronary heart disease (Douglas and Ginsberg 1996, described later).

Stress/psychoneuroimmunology

There are enormous sex differences in responses to and the effects of stress in every realm of biology, including the hypothalamic–pituitary axis, which, while most well known for the integration of sexual and reproductive functions, is differentially affected by stress in males and females (Aloisi et al 1996; Aloisi 1997, 2000); exercise-induced cardiovascular, respiratory, and pain responses, studied mainly in the context of angina, that differ in males and females (Forslund et al 1998); mechanisms of stress-induced analgesia that exhibit sex differences in opioid/non-opioid involvement (Sternberg et al 1995, Sternberg and Liebeskind 1995); and stressful major life events accompanied by changes in sex steroid hormones (puberty, pregnancy, parturition, menopause, andropause; Jones 1997).

Sex steroid hormones

The influence of gonadal hormones has been described as having 'organizing' or 'activating' effects. Organizing effects occur during embryonic development to set up sex differences in the adult that are either independent of or activated by contemporary hormonal conditions. For hormone-dependent situations, three aspects are relevant: cellular genomic and non-genomic activity, sex hormone concentrations and their dynamics, and changes across the lifespan from embryo to senescence.

Sex steroid cellular organizing and activating effects modify the functions of virtually every organ, e.g., metabolism (drug action discussed later); the immune system (painful autoimmune diseases are up to nine times more common in women; Fox 1995); trauma-induced inflammation (modulated by sex hormones, e.g., Ashcroft et al 1997, Roof et al 1997); the hypothalamic–pituitary axis (with interactions between stress, pain, and cardiovascular variables; Fillingim and Maixner 1995, Forslund et al 1998, Aloisi 2000); and neuroactive agents (discussed later).

As summarized in Table 39.2, it is known that some clinical pains are influenced by changes in sex hormones, but the mechanisms have not been studied intensively. Part of the problem is that until recently most studies have not analysed these factors. Another reason is the difficulty of measuring hormones (Stern and McClintock 1996). As more information accumulates, hormone manipulation may become a positive adjuvant for the treatment of hormone-related painful conditions.

Table 39.2 Clinical examples of alterations in pain associated with alterations in the hormone milieu

Progesterone ↑	Migraine resolves during pregnancy Pains reduced midluteal (menstrual cycle) Experimental animal nociception is reduced during lactation
Oestrogen ↓	Joint pains increase after the menopause
Testosterone ↓	Angina frequency increases in older men
Testosterone ↑	Cluster headaches in men at puberty
Progesterone, oestrogen, and testosterone ↓	Decreased abdominal pain, migraine, tension headaches
Progesterone, oestrogen, and testosterone ↑	Increased temporomandibular joint pain

Central nervous system function and neuroactive agents

Although many would agree that there are sex differences in the brain and spinal cord, the evidence for and functional significance of sex differences in the *size* of these differences is debatable (e.g., Bishop and Wahlsten 1997). The organizing and activating effects of sex steroid hormones on CNS pain mechanisms (Jensvold et al 1996, Majewska 1996) is at present largely unknown, mainly because the relevance and importance of these influences is only now being appreciated by pain researchers (Ruda 1998). It is likely that the relationship will prove to be wide ranging and complex.

Brain imaging studies

The results of SPECT, PET, or fMRI activation studies are consistent in two ways. Firstly, they show surprising activations of widespread regions of the brain, including many not traditionally associated with pain. Secondly, they show large intersubject variations. Thus, there are multiple CNS 'targets' within which sex steroid hormones, together with sociocultural and lifespan factors (see later), can act in individuals to effect a myriad of sex differences in pain (Derbyshire 1997).

Two recent studies support this conclusion. The first (Berman et al 2000) used PET to compare brain activation patterns produced by distension of the distal intestine in men and women suffering from irritable bowel syndrome (IBS) with normal subjects. There were no sex differences in the normal activation pattern, but in IBS the left prefrontal cortex became more active, and the perigenual anterior cingulate cortex less active. Among the IBS patients, activation was observed in the right premotor cortex and left anterior insula only in the men. The second study (Becerra et al 1998) used fMRI to compare brain activation patterns induced by noxious thermal stimulation in men and women in two stages of their menstrual cycle (midfollicular stage—low progesterone/oestradiol, high testosterone, and midluteal stage—high progesterone/oestradiol, low testosterone). Their results showed similar patterns of activation of multiple regions in men and women in their midfollicular stage, but significant reduction of activity in the anterior cingulate, insula, and frontal lobes in women during their midluteal phase, despite identical pain ratings in the two phases. These data suggest that if we are to understand sex differences and other individual variations in pain mechanisms, it is imperative to adopt some form of an 'ensemble' (or 'distributed') conceptualization of neural mechanisms for pain in which the brain networks that create pain in an individual can vary between individuals and with experience within an individual (Melzack 1989, Berkley and Hubscher 1995).

One of the interesting outcomes of imaging studies of pain is the activation of regions of areas normally thought of as 'motor', which fits with the view that pain is a context-dependent experience created by the nervous system as a means to motivate the individual to plan her/his own care (Wall 1994). As discussed above, some of these regions, for example, cerebellum, striatum, and inferior olive, show potent sex differences in sex steroidal influences on their somatosensory functions.

Activating effects of sex steroid hormones

Sex steroids exert sex-specific effects on neurones throughout the CNS in regions associated not only with reproductive but also 'non-reproductive' functions (McEwen and Alves 1999). The pain-related consequences of such effects are only just beginning to be appreciated (Berkley et al 2002). The effects are exerted directly or via modification of the action of other neuroactive agents such as preproenkephalin, enkephalins, dopamine, serotonin, galanin, *N*-methyl-D-aspartate (NMDA), γ-aminobutyric acid (GABA), glutamate, cholecystokinin, bombesin, substance P, neurokinin A, nitric oxide, cytokines, and growth factors, located in 'non-reproductive' areas (such as the neocortex, hippocampus, basal forebrain, striatum, central grey, cerebellum, inferior olive, dorsal column and trigeminal nuclei, and spinal cord) where there are one or more of the following: quantitative sex differences in their distribution; quantititive variations in immunoreactivity, receptors, or function with reproductive status; colocalization with sex steroid hormones or their receptors; and modulation by hormones of their gene expression (for detailed discussion and references see Berkley and Holcroft 1999).

Sympathetic nervous system

The organization of the sympathetic nervous system and neuromodulatory action of its adrenergic and other chemicals (e.g., nitric oxide and purinergic agents) may increase female vulnerability to neuropathic and 'sympathetically mediated' pain conditions (Coyle et al 1995, Newton and Hamill 1996, Berkley 1997a).

Central sensitization

The now-popular concept of central sensitization is an important component of putative neural mechanisms underlying hyperalgesia and persistent pain, and involves changes in gene expression related to NMDA, cytokines, growth factors, excitatory amino acids (e.g., glutamate), and peptides such as substance P and CGRP. As discussed above, all of these agents are potently affected by sex steroids and some show sex differences, suggesting that reproductive and/or hormonal status at the time of trauma may be important for the subsequent development of chronic pains.

CNS opioid sensitivity

There appear to be organizationally determined sex differences in CNS sensitivity to opioids. Studies show that female compared with male rats have opioid, oestrogen-dependent SIA (see above). Human studies of acute dental pain indicate that κ opioids may produce greater analgesia in females than males (Gear et al 1996), an observation that likely relates to the finding that analgesia during pregnancy in rats involves a κ-opioid mechanism (Dawson-Basoa and Gintzler 1996). These data may prove to be one of the contributory components for females seemingly having a wider range of mechanisms than men for alleviating pain.

Lifespan events, lifestyle, and sociocultural roles

Individual differences in pain are clearly influenced by major life events (e.g., associated with reproductive status and ageing), by personal characteristics (termed 'lifestyle'), and by sociocultural roles. Despite their psychological importance, these factors have been only loosely integrated into our conceptualizations of pain mechanisms and individualized treatment strategies. However, this situation is changing as society moves away from disease models. One emerging direction is to explore how the changing characteristics of each stage of development accumulate their potential influences on sex differences.

Fetus, childhood, puberty

Major sex differences in future bodily structure, physiology, and brain function (including some aspects of nociceptive sensitivity and stress modulation) are organized during fetal life, gradually manifesting themselves during childhood. These factors, together with family lifestyle and schooling, all influenced by sociocultural sex roles, operate uniquely on each child, gradually producing overall sex-specific patterns of reported pain sensitivity and other behaviours. During puberty and adolescence, dramatic alterations in hormonal status (Jones 1997) exert their activating effects to produce lifelong sex-specific traits. It is at this time that some pain-relevant, sex-different lifestyle patterns begin to be established, all influenced by the cultural milieu, such as tendency towards risk-taking behaviours (smoking, dangerous activities, violent behaviours), occupational goals, social roles, and attitudes towards injury and disease in both oneself and others. Sex differences in some painful disorders also emerge at this time (e.g., cluster headaches in males, dysmenorrhoea in females).

Fertile adulthood

It is during the long period of fertile adulthood that an individual's occupation, social roles, and lifestyle, while slowly changing, become entrenched. Although societal attitudes are evolving in many cultures, most women still predominate as caregivers and organizers with wide-ranging obligations and duties spanning family and workplace realms, while men still predominate in aggressive and focused, physically demanding occupational and leisure activities with a relatively narrower range than women of social obligations and duties. Such differences have enormous implications for sex differences as follows: vulnerability to different types of injury (work- or sport-related for men; assault/rape for women); greater female duty, obligations, and willingness to seek health care; higher female sensitivity towards the recognition of conditions as being 'painful' (i.e., those that demand tending) both in others and in themselves; greater female freedom to access health care; and, finally, sex-specific attitudes of health care givers towards the significance of pain in their patients.

Lifestyle differences present as injury-induced conditions, such as brachial plexus neuropathy, more commonly in men (e.g., motor bike crashes), and pelvic pains, more commonly in women (physical assault; see Chap. 10). Smoking- and alcohol-associated disorders are more common in men, e.g., thromboangiitis obliterans (Buerger's disease), which, interestingly, is increasing in women because more are smoking. Gallbladder disorders are more common in women, but sex differences in lifestyle are only part of a complex multifactorial aetiology that can be traced to a combination of nutritional, metabolic pathways, and hormone effects.

Sex differences in lifestyle explain in large part female vulnerability to pain, with its companion strategy of marshalling multiple approaches to deal with it. The repetitive pain cycles of dysmenorrhoea, pregnancy, and parturition exaggerate lifestyle differences. Severe dysmenorrhoea suffered by a substantial proportion of women induces a constant and generalized muscle hyperalgesia (Giamberardino et al 1997). During pregnancy and premenstrually, fluid retention can increase tissue pressure around nerves, thereby precipitating or exacerbating painful neuropathies such as carpal tunnel syndrome and lateral femoral cutaneous nerve pain (Zager et al 1998). The trauma associated with parturition clearly generates its own extremely severe pain (Melzack 1993), and can increase the severity of postpartum pain after subsequent deliveries (Murray and Holdcroft 1989) as well as sensitivity to noxious stimulation in a manner similar to that in men resulting from comparable experiences, such as severe injury sustained during war or sport, a phenomenon that appears to be associated with long-term changes in gene expression induced by injury in animals.

Menopause, andropause, and senescence

Following the fertile years, there is at first, for women, a 5- to 10-year period of menopausal alterations in hormone patterns terminating in their sharp decline, while in men more complex changes in hormone metabolism occur over a longer period between the ages of about 48 and 70 (Vermeulen 2000). Accompanying these alterations are changes in general metabolism, physiology, and structure. Lifestyle changes also occur relatively rapidly during this period, as children leave home and both occupational duties and leisure activities are altered. An increasing disease burden arises for both sexes, with alterations of drug metabolism that while most dramatic for women also occur in men, and with modified attitudes towards and access of health care. While the net result is a decrease in many sex differences in pain, especially as chronic disease burden becomes significant in both sexes (Turk and Okifuju 1998), sex differences in strategic therapeutic approaches by individuals persist.

What are the clinical implications?

Clearly, diagnostic and treatment strategies are best carried out by focusing on the individual, regardless of sex. However, as more information accumulates and is classified, sex differences in reported pain experience and pain mechanisms will have increasingly potent and useful implications for both diagnosis and treatment as well as for health economics.

Diagnosis

It is during the first steps of the diagnostic process (symptoms, signs, and drug usage) that knowledge about sex differences will lead clinicians to improve their differential diagnoses and treatment decisions. Details to be obtained include signs and symptoms that are distant as well as focused on the presenting illness; the timing characteristics of those symptoms (by memory and diary); family history of painful disease and how it was dealt with; history of major life events; detailed characteristics of the individual's lifestyle (including such things as risk-taking behaviours, smoking, occupational goals, leisure activities, attitudes towards health care); and reproductive status.

For women such details will include knowledge of parosity, menstrual history, or menopausal status (possibly with hormone levels) and for both sexes usage of supplemental hormones. Other relevant details for both sexes include a history of abuse or other trauma, and assessment of tenderness or pain symptoms throughout the body, including 'minor' complaints the patient discounts or fails to report.

To examine how this strategy could improve diagnosis, let us consider coronary heart disease as an example. When a patient presents with chest pain, it is often difficult to assess whether coronary artery disease is present, and whether further invasive and expensive testing is necessary. Douglas and Ginsberg (1996) have developed a clear set of sex differential features.

The likelihood of coronary heart disease in women is higher than men if: (1) pain distribution is altered, e.g., chest pain is present at rest, or on exercise other symptoms such as neck and shoulder pain are present apart from typical angina; (2) diabetes or other associated medical conditions are present, and (3) in the elderly hypertension is present. Thus, when a patient presents with 'atypical' chest pain, it might not in the past have been considered relevant to ask about other pains. However, by including as diagnostic a detailed history of pain complaints and their distribution, as well as, particularly for the postmenopausal woman, observing that she is diabetic and hypertensive, could be lifesaving.

Therapy

There are three broad categories of pain therapies—drugs, somatic manipulations, and situational adjustments. Often now only one is selected by a clinician (primarily drugs), but strategies are slowly changing towards suitable combinations chosen in partnership with the patient. Each category is considered with a view to developing strategies for pain relief that include considerations of the patient's sex and reproductive condition. Pain therapies targeted to incorporate management supportive of individual variations have implications for health economics as follows: diagnostic strategies lead to more effective treatments; awareness of simpler forms of somatic and situational therapies for men could reduce costs; recognition of sex differences in pharmacokinetics and pharmacodynamics in the early stages of drug trials could improve safety and effectiveness in the general population; and estimates of quality assurance could be improved if the results were stratified by sex- and hormone-related factors.

Drugs

Potential sources of sex differences in drug action Body composition and sex hormone-related differences between women and men can modify drug pharmacokinetics and pharmacodynamics (Jensvold et al 1996, Ciccone and Holdcroft 1998). Potential sources of sex differences in *pharmacokinetics* include drug absorption, protein binding, volume of distribution, renal excretion, total drug clearance, and metabolism (Gleiter and Gundert-Remy 1996).

Regarding absorption, women are affected by changes in gastric function during the menstrual cycle, leading to decreased absorption during the periovulatory stage (mid-cycle) of some drugs such as aspirin (and alcohol). Intestinal transit times are longer for women in the late luteal phase, as well as during pregnancy and hormone supplementation. Regarding protein binding, levels of α_1-acid glycoprotein are slightly lower in women than in men and change with birth control medication and pregnancy, so that free lidocaine (lignocaine) is increased if used in nerve blocks.

Body compositional differences would seem relevant to the volume of distribution, but they appear not to be, even if the drug is highly lipophilic. They do, however, alter renal excretion. Creatinine clearance is higher in men than in women, because of a larger muscle mass and glomerular filtration being proportional to body weight. When total drug clearance is considered, measurements do not differentiate between the various excretory processes. Age is an important factor in this process and clear sex differences have been demonstrated for the short-acting opioid drug alfentanil (Lemmens et al 1990). Thus, in females and males of similar weight, total median alfentanil clearance was highest in women less than 50 years of age, decreasing thereafter to rates similar to men at older ages.

The sex-specific effects in hepatic metabolism of drugs are, firstly, that some components of the CYP2 enzyme family display genetic polymorphism, and some of the CYP3 family (that metabolize drugs such as lidocaine (lignocaine) and midazolam) are regulated by androgens. Secondly, exogenous sex steroid hormones can have facilitatory or inhibitory activity on drug-metabolizing enzyme systems; e.g., the half-life of prednisolone used as an adjunct in pain medication increases when birth control medication is prescribed. Thirdly, there are quantitative and qualitative differences in enzyme activity; e.g., the metabolic fate of mephobarbital, a chiral anticonvulsant, is sex specific, with its clearance greater and elimination half-life shorter in young men than in women or older men (Hooper and Qing 1990). Thus as chiral drugs are introduced to reduce the side effects of racemic mixtures or to enhance potency, some may be metabolized in a sex-specific manner.

In the developing area of human sex differences in pharmacodynamics, the analgesic effectivess of partial κ opioids such as nalbuphine, buprenophine, and pentazocine for postoperative pain relief, compared with morphine, was significantly better in young females than in males (Gear et al 1996). Because, as described above, sex hormones have been shown in animals to affect the function of many neuroactive agents associated with pain, it is likely that new drugs with similar mechanisms will also exhibit sex differences in their pharmacodynamics.

Adverse drug events At least two aspects of drug usage lead to sex differences in adverse effects. Firstly, the prevalence of such effects is twice as much for women than men (Haddi et al 1990), probably not a result of differences in body composition (e.g., weight), but of drug sensitivity and interactions through increased use by women of all medications including supplemental hormones (25% of childbearing women, Jensvold et al 1996). Secondly, new evidence is emerging for sex differences in side effects of drugs. For example, morphine reduces the slope of the ventilatory response to carbon dioxide more in young adult women than in men (Dahan et al 1998).

Implications for drugs currently in use for pain

- The efficacy of some classes of drugs (such as opioids) could be improved by selecting different specific agonists for women and men or by titrating dosage in women to account for variations with age (e.g., alfentanil). Adjustments of dosage by sex, reproductive status, and supplemental hormone use may improve efficacy for analgesics and their adjuvants.
- While a cyclical history of pain may or may not be diagnostic of any particular pain condition, its impact could be used to better advantage, e.g., increasing the drug dose just before pain is expected to increase and reducing it when pain decreases. Such strategies could also be coordinated with other therapies, such as exercise titrated to cyclical conditions. For example, in women with rheumatoid arthritis who exhibit exacerbations of their pain and mobility perimenstrually, doses of their non-steroidal anti-inflammatory drugs (NSAIDs) might be increased perimenstrually and activities requiring dexterity scheduled during other menstrual stages (Wetherby 1995).
- Because of drug interactions, it is important to collect information *routinely* about the patient's supplemental sex hormone usage (as well as other medications) and to adjust drug choice and dose appropriately. Safety could be further improved for some drugs by using dosing schedules related to body weight.
- Adjuvant hormones or similar agents are likely to prove useful as important components of pain prevention and management.
- The speed with which new clinically applicable information is being published on sex and hormonal influences on the efficacy and safety of all drugs (including those used for pain management) warrants continuous attention by clinicians.

Future drug development and clinical trials Sex differences and hormone interactions in the specificity of pharmacological action and half-life or clearance are likely for some new drugs, particularly chiral forms. If such factors were considered initially at the outset of drug development, needless potential adverse drug effects may be avoided or differences in effectiveness discovered. This same logic applies to phase-one (toxicity) trials, which in the United States, but not Europe, are now being carried out routinely in both sexes. During all clinical trials, much is to be gained from analyses stratified by sex, age, menstrual stage, menopause, andropause, and supplemental hormone use.

Somatic (physical) interventions

Little is known about sex differences in the effectiveness of some of the simpler forms of somatic therapies. Nevertheless, women are generally more willing to use effective forms such as relaxation, heat or cold application, massage, and vibration, suggesting that men might benefit if encouraged and educated. Interestingly, psychophysical studies in healthy women show that their sensitivity to some forms of somatic stimuli (pressure, thermal) can change with menstrual status (see above), which could affect efficacy when heat, cold, vibration, or massage is used for pain alleviation by women. Regarding exercise and physical therapy, sports medicine studies report greater risks of injury in women than men (Jones et al 1993), and more problems for women perimenstrually. In addition, the differences in exercise-induced cardiovascular responses in males and females may affect pain either by way of the relationship between blood pressure and pain discussed above or by other mechanisms (Fillingim and Maixner 1996, Forslund et al 1998). For surgical interventions, emerging evidence suggests that hormonal or menstrual status may in some cases affect surgical outcome through changes in vascular growth factors (Hrushesky 1996). Therapists who select surgical interventions in pain management should be aware that in a prospective study of 4173 patients (45% female) women had more 'minor' postoperative pains of sore throat, headache, and backache than men (Myles et al 1997). This difference may relate to drugs used during anaesthesia (such as succinylcholine, known to produce more muscle pain in women than men), or to the choice of postoperative analgesics, or to reporting bias. A review of postoperative drug usage has shown that the dose of morphine accessed by men through patient-controlled analgesia devices is significantly higher than that used by women (Miakowski et al 2000). The reasons for this result are speculative and include sex differences in the side effect profile of morphine and coping strategies.

Situational manipulations

When pain is chronic, situational changes in the patient's environment and social interactions may not eliminate the pain, but there is much evidence that they reduce it by changing expectations, enhancing productive activity, and improving quality of life. Several studies of relevance here indicate not only that women are more likely than men to use many of these therapies, but also that they may derive benefit, particularly from cognitive ones. Part of the basis for this difference may lie in women's greater verbal abilities (reviewed in Harasty et al 1997), their lifestyles, and their occupations, but whatever the cause(s), it is important to consider that males more than females need education and encouragement to consider situational adjustments, including not only changes in their personal environment (music, diet, meditation, etc.), but also in their use of various interactive services. In addition, the clinician should recognize that her/his attitudes are also major factors. These attitudes, warranting continual reassessment, include the clinician's general beliefs about the differences between women and men in the validity of their pain reports or responses to treatment, and about the value of various situational manipulations (Unruh 1996, Berkley 1997a).

Deliberate combinations of therapies

The treatment plan that best serves these objectives is a design incorporating a flexible combination of drugs, somatic therapies, and situational manipulations. The different approach by men and women to seek and combine therapies should be rationalized so that the wide array of strategies is selected on individual and research evidence (diagnosis, age, sex, etc) rather than at random.

References

Aloisi AM 1997 Sex differences in pain-induced effects on the septo-hippocampal system. Brain Research Reviews 25: 397–406

Aloisi AM 2000 Sensory effects of gonadal hormones. In: Fillingim R (ed) Sex, gender and pain. Progress in pain research and management, vol 17. IASP Press, Seattle pp 7–24

Aloisi AM, Albonetti ME, Carli G 1996 Formalin-induced changes in adrenocorticotropic hormone and corticosterone plasma levels and hippocampal choline acetyltransferase activity in male and female rats. Neuroscience 74: 1019–1024

Ashcroft GS, Dodsworth J, van Boxtel E et al 1997 Estrogen accelerates cutaneous wound healing associated with an increase in TGF-beta 1 levels. Nature Medicine 3: 1209–1215

Becerra L, Comite A, Breiter H, Gonzalez RG, Borsook D 1998 Differential CNS activation following a noxious thermal stimulus in men and women: an fMRI study. Society for Neuroscience Abstracts 24 (1998) 1136

Berkley KJ 1997a Sex differences in pain. Behavioral and Brain Sciences 20: 371–380

Berkley KJ 1997b Female vulnerability to pain and the strength to deal with it. Behavioral and Brain Sciences 20: 473–479

Berkley KJ, Holdcroft A 1999 Sex and gender differences in pain. In: Melzack R, Wall PD (eds) Textbook of pain, 4th edn. Churchill Livingstone, Edinburgh, pp 951–965

Berkley KJ, Hubscher CH 1995 Are there separate central nervous pathways for touch and pain? Nature Medicine 1: 766–773

Berkley KJ, Hoffman G, Murray AZ, Holdcroft A 2002 Pain sex/gender differences. In: Pfaaf D, Arnold A, Etgen A, Fahrbach S, Rubin R (eds) Hormones, brain and behavior. Academic Press, London

Berman S, Munakata J, Naliboff BD et al 2000 Gender differences in regional brain response to visceral pressure in IBS patients. European Journal of Pain 4: 157–172

Bishop KM, Wahlsten D 1997 Sex differences in the human corpus callosum: myth or reality? Neuroscience and Biobehavioral Reviews 21: 581–601

Ciccone G, Holdcroft A 1998 Drugs and sex differences: a review of drugs relating to anaesthesia. British Journal of Anaesthesia 82: 255–265
Coyle DE, Sehlhorst CS, Mascari C 1995 Female rats are more susceptible to the development of neuropathic pain using the partial sciatic nerve ligation (PSNL) model. Neuroscience Letters 186: 135–138
Dahan A, Sarton E, Teppema L, Olievier C 1998 Sex-related differences in the influence of morphine on ventilatory control in humans. Anesthesiology 88: 903–913
Dawson-Basoa ME, Gintzler AR 1996 Estrogen and progesterone activate spinal kappa-opiate receptor analgesic mechanisms. Pain 64: 608–615
Derbyshire SWG 1997 Sources of variation in assessing male and female responses to pain. New Ideas in Psychology 15: 83–95
Douglas PS, Ginsberg GS 1996 The evaluation of chest pain in women. New England Journal of Medicine 334: 1311–1315
Fillingim RB (ed) 2000 Sex, gender, and pain. Progress in pain research and management, vol 17. IASP Press, Seattle
Fillingim RB, Maixner W 1995 Gender differences in the responses to noxious stimuli. Pain Forum 4: 209–221
Fillingim RB, Maixner W 1996 The influence of resting blood pressure and gender on pain responses. Psychosomatic Medicine 58: 326–332
Fillingim RB, Maixner W, Kincaid S, Silva S 1998 Sex differences in temporal summation but not sensory-discriminative processing of thermal pain. Pain 75: 121–127
Forslund L, Hjemdahl P, Held C, Bjorkander I, Eriksson SV, Rehnqvist N 1998 Ischaemia during exercise and ambulatory monitoring in patients with stable angina pectoris and healthy controls. Gender differences and relationships to catecholamines. European Heart Journal 19: 578–587
Fox HS 1995 Sex steroids and the immune system. In: Bock GR, Goode JA (eds) Non-reproductive actions of sex steroids. Wiley, Chichester, pp 203–217
Gear RW, Miaskowski C, Gordon NC, Paul SM, Heller PH, Levine JD 1996 Kappa-opioids produce significantly greater analgesia in women than in men. Nature Medicine 2: 1248–1250
Giamberardino MA, Berkley KJ, Iezzi S, de Bigontina P, Vecchiet L 1997 Pain threshold variations in somatic wall tissues as a function of menstrual cycle, segmental site and tissue depth in non-dysmenorrheic women, dysmenorrheic women and men. Pain 71: 187–197
Gleiter CH, Gundert-Remy U 1996 Gender differences in pharmacokinetics. European Journal of Drug Metabolism and Pharmacokinetics 21: 123–128
Haddi E, Sharpin D, Tafforeau M 1990 Atopy and systemic reactions to drugs. Allergy 45: 1–4
Harasty J, Double KL, Halliday GM, Kril JJ, McRitchie DA 1997 Language-associated cortical regions are proportionally larger in the female brain. Archives of Neurology 54: 171–176
Hooper WD, Qing MS 1990 The influence of age and gender on the stereoselective metabolism and pharmacokinetics of mephobarbital in humans. Clinical Pharmacology and Therapeutics 48: 633–640
Hrushesky WJM 1996 Breast cancer, timing of surgery, and the menstrual cycle: call for prospective trial. Journal of Women's Health 5: 555–566
Jensvold MF, Halbreich U, Hamilton JA (eds) 1996 Psychopharmacology and women. Sex gender and hormones. American Psychiatric Press, Washington, DC
Jones BH, Bovee MW, Harris JM III, Cowan DN 1993 Intrinsic risk factors for exercise-related injuries among male and female army trainees. American Journal of Sports Medicine 21: 705–710
Jones RE 1997 Human reproductive biology, 2nd edn. Academic Press, San Diego
Lemmens HJM, Burm AGL, Hennis PJ, Gladines MPPR, Bovill JG 1990 Influence of age on the pharmacokinetics of alfentanil: gender dependence. Clinical Pharmacokinetics 19: 416–422
LeResche L, Von Korff M 1998 Epidemiology of chronic pain. In: Block AR, Kremer EF, Fernandez E (eds) Handbook of pain syndromes: biopsychosocial perspectives. Lawrence Erlbaum, Mahwah, NJ, pp 3–22
LeResche L, Saunders K, Von Korff MR, Barlow W, Dworkin SF 1997 Use of exogenous hormones and risk of temporomandibular disorder pain. Pain 69: 153–160
Majewska MD 1996 Sex differences in brain morphology and pharmacodynamics. In: Jensvold MF, Halbreich U, Hamilton JA (eds) Psychopharmacology and women. Sex gender and hormones. American Psychiatric Press, Washington, DC, pp 73–83
Marcus DA 1995 Interrelationships of neurochemicals, estrogen, and recurring headache. Pain 62: 129–141
McEwen BS, Alves SE 1999 Estrogen actions in the central nervous system. Endocrine Review 20: 279–307
Melzack R 1989 Phantom limbs, the self and the brain (the D.O. Hebb memorial lecture). Canadian Psychology 30: 1–16
Melzack R 1993 Labor pain as a model of acute pain. Pain 53: 117–120
Merskey H, Bogduk N (eds) 1994 Classification of chronic pain: descriptions of chronic pain syndromes and definitions of pain terms, 2nd edn. IASP Press, Seattle
Miakowski C, Gear RW, Levine JD 2000 Sex-related differences in analgesic responses. In: Fillingim R (ed) Sex, gender and pain. Progress in pain research and management, vol 17. IASP Press, Seattle, pp 218–219
Mogil JS, Sternberg WF, Marek P, Sadowski B, Belknap JK, Liebeskind JC 1996 The genetics of pain and pain inhibition. Proceedings of the National Academy of Sciences of the USA 93: 3048–3055
Mogil JS, Richards SP, O'Toole LA et al 1997a Identification of a sex-specific quantitative trait locus mediating nonopioid stress-induced analgesia in female mice. Journal of Neuroscience 17: 7995–8002
Mogil JS, Richards SP, O'Toole LA, Helms ML, Mitchell SR, Belknap JK 1997b Genetic sensitivity to hot-plate nociception in DBA/2J and C57BL/6J inbred mouse strains: possible sex-specific mediation by delta2-opioid receptors. Pain 70: 267–277
Mogil JS, Yu L, Basbaum AI 2000 Pain genes?: natural variation and transgenic mutants. Annual Review of Neuroscience 23: 777–811
Murray A, Holdcroft A 1989 Incidence and intensity of postpartum lower abdominal pain. British Medical Journal 298: 1619
Myles PS, Hunt JO, Moloney JT 1997 Postoperative 'minor' complications: comparison between men and women. Anaesthesia 52: 300–306
Newton BW, Hammill RW 1996 Sexual differentiation of the autonomic nervous system. In: Unsicker K (ed) Autonomic–endocrine interactions. Harwood Academic, Amsterdam, pp 425–463
Riley III JL, Robinson ME, Wise EA, Myers CD, Fillingim RB 1998 Sex differences in the perception of noxious experimental stimuli: a meta-analysis. Pain 74: 181–187
Roof RL, Hoffman SW, Stein DG 1997 Progesterone protects against lipid peroxidation following traumatic brain injury in rats. Molecular and Chemical Neuropathology 31: 1–11
Ruda MA 1998 Gender and pain: a focus on how pain impacts women differently than men. Conference sponsored by National Institutes of Health Pain Research Consortium, Bethesda
Scoville SA, Bufton SM, Liuzzi FJ 1997 Estrogen regulated neurofilament gene expression in adult female rat dorsal root ganglion neurons. Experimental Neurology 146: 596–599

Sohrabji F, Miranda RC, Toran-Allerand DC 1994 Estrogen differentially regulates estrogen and nerve growth factor receptor mRNAs in adult sensory neurons. Journal of Neuroscience 14: 459–471

Stern KN, McClintock MM 1996 Individual variation in biological rhythms: accurate measurement of preovulatory LH surge and menstrual cycle phase. In: Jensvold MF, Halbreich U, Hamilton JA (eds) Psychopharmacology and women. Sex gender and hormones. American Psychiatric Press, Washington, DC, pp 393–413

Sternberg WF, Liebeskind JC 1995 The analgesic response to stress: genetic and gender considerations. European Journal of Anaesthesiology 10: 14–17

Sternberg WF, Mogil JS, Kest B et al 1995 Neonatal testosterone exposure influences neurochemistry of non-opioid swim stress-induced analgesia in adulthood. Pain 63: 321–326

Turk DC, Okifuji A 1999 Does sex make a difference in the prescription of treatments and the adaptation to chronic pain by cancer and non-cancer patients? Pain 92: 139–48

Unruh AM 1996 Gender variations in clinical pain experience. Pain 65: 123–167

Vermeulen A 2000 Andropause. Maturitas 34: 5–15

Villablanca AC, Hanley MR 1997 17beta-estradiol stimulates substance P receptor gene expression. Molecular and Cellular Endocrinology 135: 109–117

Von Korff M, Dworkin SF, Le Resche L, Kruger A 1988 An epidemiologic comparison of pain complaints. Pain 32: 173–183

Wall PD 1994 Introduction to the edition after this one. In: Wall PD, Melzack R (eds) Textbook of pain, 3rd edn. Churchill Livingstone, Edinburgh, pp 1–7

Wetherby MMC 1995 Fluctuations of pain and the menstrual cycle in rheumatoid arthritis. Thesis, Florida State University

Weyand CM, Schmidt D, Wagner U, Goronzy JJ 1998 The influence of sex on the phenotype of rheumatoid arthritis. Arthritis and Rheumatism 41: 817–822

Wisemann T, Pardue M-L (eds) 2001 Exploring the biological contributions to human health. Does sex matter? National Academy Press, Washington, DC

Zager EL, Pfeifer SM, Brown MJ, Torosian MH, Hackney DB 1998 Catamenial mononeuropathy and radiculopathy: a treatable neuropathic disorder. Journal of Neurosurgery 88: 827–830

Chapter 40

Peripheral neuropathic pain: an approach to management

Howard L Fields

Introduction

Pain is characteristic of some peripheral neuropathic diseases (e.g., diabetic and alcohol-deficiency neuropathies and herpes zoster). There are two broad classes of patients with painful peripheral nerve disease: focal and multifocal (e.g., traumatic, ischaemic, inflammatory) or generalized (e.g., toxic/metabolic, hereditary, or inflammatory). Although our knowledge of the mechanisms of peripheral neuropathic pain has grown, treatment remains largely empirical. This chapter outlines a systematic approach to management.

Diagnosis

Peripheral neuropathic pain has several distinct clinical characteristics. First, there is almost always an area of abnormal sensation and the patient's maximum pain is topographically coextensive with an area of sensory deficit. The sensory deficit is usually to noxious and thermal stimuli, indicating damage to small-diameter afferent fibres. Second, there is often a hyperpathic state characterized by allodynia, summation, and radiation of pain. Allodynia is present when gentle mechanical stimuli evoke pain. Summation is the progressive worsening of pain evoked by slow repetitive stimulation with mildly noxious stimuli. Third, neuropathic pain commonly has a burning and/or shooting quality with numbness, tingling, crawling, or electrical sensations (dysaesthesiae). When these features are present, the diagnosis of neuropathic pain is likely.

Mechanisms that may contribute to neuropathic pain (See Chaps. 16–21)

Peripheral mechanisms

Sensitization and ectopic impulse generation in primary afferent nociceptors

Injured peripheral nerves develop spontaneous activity and exquisite mechanical sensitivity (Wall and Gutnick 1974, Scadding 1981, Kajander and Bennett 1992). Primary afferent axons need not be transected to become hyperactive. Intact primary afferent nociceptors in a partially damaged nerve become spontaneously active (Bennett 1993, Ali et al 1999). Furthermore, ectopic impulses may be generated at sites other than the damaged and regenerating distal axon terminals. For example, when a peripheral nerve is damaged, a region near the dorsal root ganglion (which is distant from the site of injury) becomes capable of generating 'spontaneous' impulses (Devor and Rappaport 1990, Kajander et al 1992).

There is evidence that hyperactive nociceptors contribute to pain in patients with postherpetic neuralgia (PHN). In some PHN patients pain relief can be produced by cooling the skin, applying local anaesthetics or cyclo-oxygenase inhibitors topically (De Benedittis and Lorenzetti 1996, Rowbotham et al 1996), or inactivating C nociceptors by repeated application of capsaicin (Watson et al 1993). These observations indicate that sensitized C fibres can generate an ongoing discharge that contributes to neuropathic pain.

Sympathetically maintained pain

Causalgia is the classic example of a sympathetically maintained pain associated with nerve injury. It is characterized by autonomic changes, severe allodynia, and a distal burning sensation exacerbated by cold and strong emotions (Mitchell 1865). Early in the course of the disease, most patients obtain virtually complete relief with sympathetic blocks. Damaged primary afferents including nociceptors acquire adrenergic sensitivity (Devor and Janig 1981, Scadding 1981, Janig et al 1996). For example, electrical stimulation of the sympathetic trunk can activate C nociceptors that have regenerated following nerve injury (Habler et al 1987). Furthermore, after partial nerve injury, electrical stimulation of the sympathetic trunk (Sato and Perl 1991) and local application of adrenergic agonists can activate or sensitize intact unmyelinated nociceptors (Ali et al 1999). Sympatholytic procedures can alleviate rodent pain behaviours that develop after partial nerve injury (Shir and Seltzer 1991).

These animal studies are supported by human research demonstrating that adrenaline (epinephrine) applied directly to a neuroma produces severe burning pain (Chabal et al 1992). Furthermore, intraoperative stimulation of the sympathetic chain increases spontaneous pain in patients with causalgia (Walker and Nulsen 1948). In post-traumatic neuralgias, intracutaneous application of noradrenaline (norepinephrine) into a symptomatic area rekindles spontaneous pain and mechanical hyperalgesia after they are relieved by sympathetic blockade (Torebjork et al 1995). Thus, damage to a peripheral nerve induces a novel state of sensitivity to sympathetic activity and noradrenaline (norepinephrine) in primary afferent nociceptors.

Inflammation of the nerve trunk

Because the connective tissue sheath surrounding a peripheral nerve is innervated by nociceptive primary afferents (*nervi nervorum*) (Hromada 1963, Bahns et al 1986, Bove and Light 1995), peripheral nerve can be a source of pain in conditions with an inflammatory component. Consistent with this idea, certain diseases are associated with localized pain and tenderness along the trunk of the nerve, rather than pain referred to its innervation territory. The acute pain of a herniated inflamed disc, or that seen with brachial neuritis or acute inflammatory demyelinating neuropathy (Guillain–Barré syndrome), probably represents pain mediated by nociceptive *nervi nervorum* (Asbury and Fields 1984).

In experimental animals, activation of macrophages and a proliferation of endoneurial blood vessels have been demonstrated in injured peripheral nerve (Sommer and Myers 1996). The cytokine tumour necrosis factor alpha (TNFα) produced by activated macrophages is a potential cause of pain (Sommer et al 1998, Wagner et al 1998) by inducing ectopic activity in primary afferent nociceptors (Sorkin et al 1997). Consistent with this view, the TNFα inhibitor thalidomide is reported to reduce pain in inflammatory lepromatous neuropathy (Partida-Sanchez et al 1998).

Central mechanisms

Central sensitization

Prolonged or repeated activation of nociceptive C fibres produces central sensitization so that innocuous stimuli produce pain (allodynia) and noxious stimuli produce more intense pain (hyperalgesia). Central sensitization occurs in any situation with prolonged or intense C-fibre input. In neuropathic pains like postherpetic neuralgia, where there is evidence of ongoing C-fibre activity, central sensitization seems to play a significant role in maintaining pain and allodynia (Koltzenburg et al 1992, Petersen et al 2000). Glutamate acting at the *N*-methyl-D-aspartate (NMDA) receptor contributes to central sensitization, and thus NMDA antagonists are potential therapeutic targets in some patients with neuropathic pain (Dougherty et al 1994, Dickenson 1997).

Deafferentation hyperactivity

Following dorsal rhizotomy or peripheral nerve damage, many dorsal horn cells begin to fire spontaneously at high frequencies (Lombard and Larabi 1983, Laird and Bennett 1993). Such a mechanism may underlie the pain that occurs following extensive denervating injuries. For example, pain is a characteristic sequela of the deafferentation produced by brachial plexus avulsion (Wynn-Parry 1980), and this pain seems to respond to surgical procedures that destroy nociceptive dorsal horn neurons (Nashold and Ostdahl 1979).

Reorganization of the central connections of primary afferents

In models of peripheral nerve injury, loss of the central terminals of unmyelinated primary afferents to dorsal horn neurons leads to sprouting of large-diameter primary afferents. These afferents, which respond maximally to gentle mechanical stimulation, sprout to directly innervate the deafferented nociceptive dorsal horn neurons (Shortland and Woolf 1993). Although it is difficult to prove that this is a mechanism of pain in any clinical situation, some patients with postherpetic neuralgia have exquisite allodynia in a region of skin that shows a profound nociceptive deficit (Baron and Saguer 1993).

Loss of large-fibre afferent inhibition

Because selective blockade of large-diameter myelinated sensory axons increases pain, Melzack and Wall (1965) proposed that these axons normally inhibit pain-transmitting spinal-cord neurons and that the pain of nerve injury is due to selective damage to these large axons. This hypothesis predicts that selective activation of large-diameter, non-nociceptive myelinated primary afferents, for example by electrical stimulation of a peripheral nerve, would decrease pain. In fact, there are cases of dramatic pain relief produced by transcutaneous electrical nerve stimulation (TENS) in patients with painful traumatic mononeuropathies (Meyer and Fields 1972). Furthermore, there are reports that dorsal column stimulation, which would selectively activate the central branches of large-diameter primary afferents, is effective for some patients with neuropathic pain (Broggi et al 1994, Kumar et al 1996). Thus it seems likely that release of dorsal horn pain transmission cells from inhibition by myelinated axons contributes to the pain that occurs in some cases of peripheral nerve injury.

The treatment of neuropathic pain

Except for trigeminal neuralgia, which responds reliably and specifically to anticonvulsant medications, the treatment of neuropathic pain is largely empirical and often unsatisfactory. Fortunately, data from clinical trials have led to improvements in the medical management of neuropathic pain (Kingery 1997).

Pharmacological approaches

Antidepressants

Tricyclic antidepressants (TCAs) are currently the best documented therapy for neuropathic pain (Onghena and Van Houdenhove 1992, McQuay et al 1996, Kingery 1997). These compounds are inhibitors of the reuptake of monoaminergic transmitters. They are believed to potentiate the effects of biogenic amines in CNS pain-modulating pathways. On the other hand, the effectiveness of TCAs in neuropathic pain may depend on their broad range of pharmacological actions. In addition to blocking serotonin and noradrenaline (norepinephrine) reuptake, these drugs block voltage-dependent sodium channels (Jett et al 1997) and α-adrenergic receptors. All three of these actions could contribute to their analgesic effect.

Of the TCAs, amitriptyline is currently the best established for the treatment of chronic pain. Amitriptyline produces pain relief in diabetic neuropathy and postherpetic neuralgia (McQuay et al 1996, Sindrup and Jensen 1999). The mean dose required for pain reduction (75–150 mg/day) is usually smaller than the doses necessary to achieve antidepressant effects. Improvement of sleep, mood, and anxiety are an added benefit of antidepressant therapy. Amitriptyline and other TCAs have significant side effects (Richelson 1990). They can produce orthostatic hypotension, due largely to an α-adrenergic blocking action. Because of its histamine receptor blockade, amitriptyline is also a potent sedating drug, which can be a desirable action if patients are having difficulty sleeping. Other significant problems include urinary retention, memory loss, and cardiac conduction abnormalities (largely due to the muscarinic anticholinergic actions of the drug). Patients, especially the elderly, who are to be treated with this drug should be started at a very low dose, even as low as 10 mg, and built up slowly by about 25 mg every fourth day until optimal pain relief is achieved.

Desipramine and nortriptyline, both of which have predominant noradrenaline (norepinephrine) reuptake blocking action, appear to be almost as effective as amitriptyline in postherpetic neuralgia and painful diabetic neuropathy. Patients respond to desipramine and nortriptyline at doses comparable to those of amitriptyline but with fewer anticholinergic side effects and significantly less sedation.

All patients undergoing treatment with any TCA should have a cardiogram at the onset of treatment. Cardiac conduction defects are a contraindication to their use. Plasma drug levels and repeated cardiograms should be taken if the dose is pushed above 100 mg/24 h, especially in elderly or cognitively impaired patients.

There are very few studies of antidepressants other than TCAs for pain management. Serotonin selective reuptake inhibitors (SSRIs) are currently the most commonly used drugs for the treatment of depression. SSRIs may have some efficacy for neuropathic pain but are significantly less effective than TCAs (Max et al 1992, McQuay et al 1996, Sindrup and Jensen 1999). Furthermore, there is evidence that noradrenaline (norepinephrine) reuptake blockade is more effective in producing analgesia than pure serotonin reuptake blockade (Atkinson et al 1999). On the other hand, SSRIs have virtually none of the serious side effects common with desipramine or amitriptyline. They are non-sedating, and devoid of the adrenergic-, histaminergic-, and muscarinic-antagonist-induced side effects. Thus, even if SSRIs are less effective for neuropathic pain per se, they are effective antidepressants and some patients report an improvement in pain as their depression clears. Thus, when using antidepressants, especially in patients with clinically significant depression, the drug dose should be pushed until limiting side effects ensue or the maximum recommended plasma concentration is achieved.

There are some newer antidepressants that are neither TCAs nor SSRIs. Venlafaxine is an example of such a drug. It blocks both serotonin and noradrenaline (norepinephrine) reuptake (Lang et al 1996). There are some early positive reports on the usefulness of this drug (Sumpton and Moulin 2001). However, above a daily dose of 300 mg it has a tendency to elevate blood pressure and to cause headaches.

Anticonvulsants and antiarrhythmics

In contrast to the antidepressants, anticonvulsants such as phenytoin and carbamazepine are helpful for a more restricted group of neuropathic pain patients. Carbamazepine is very effective in trigeminal neuralgia (McQuay et al 1995, Fields 1996). However, carbamazepine is less helpful in other types of neuropathic pain. These anticonvulsants are more likely to be helpful if a patient reports pain with a sharp shooting or electric shock-like component.

Gabapentin is an interesting drug that was originally developed and marketed for seizure control. Its mechanism of action is unknown; however, recent placebo-controlled trials show that it is effective in diabetic neuropathy (Backonja et al 1998) and postherpetic neuralgia (Rowbotham et al 1998). Its relatively benign side-effect profile compared to TCAs has encouraged many physicians to use it as a first-line drug for nerve injury pain.

The antiarrhythmic drugs lidocaine (lignocaine), mexiletine, and tocainide block voltage-dependent sodium channels. Caution should be exercised when administering these compounds. Contraindications include electrocardiac abnormalities, reduced left ventricular function, and coronary heart disease. Lidocaine (lignocaine) by intravenous infusion produces significant relief for patients with postherpetic neuralgia (Rowbotham et al 1991), diabetic neuropathy (Kastrup et al 1987), and a variety of other neuropathic pain syndromes (Glazer and Portenoy 1991). Mexiletine has been shown to be effective for pain in diabetic neuropathy (Dejgard et al 1988) and other peripheral neuropathic conditions (Chabal et al 1992, Wallace et al 2000). A positive response to intravenous lidocaine (lignocaine) significantly predicts longer-term relief with oral mexiletine (Galer et al 1996).

Drugs that affect gamma-aminobutyric acid receptors

Several drugs that enhance or mimic the effects of the inhibitory transmitter gamma-aminobutyric acid (GABA) are clinically available (Dickenson et al 1997). Baclofen is an agonist of the GABA-B receptors and in the spinal cord acts presynaptically to prevent the release of excitatory neurotransmitters. Baclofen in useful in trigeminal neuralgia (Fields 1996). Some GABA receptor modulating agents may have a place in the treatment of painful muscle spasms, particularly when these are associated with spasticity. In some cases of neuropathic pain clonazepam has been shown to be effective (Bartusch et al 1996).

Opioid analgesics

Opioids are clearly effective in postoperative, inflammatory, and cancer pain. However, the use of narcotic analgesics for patients with chronic neuropathic pain is highly controversial, even among experts in the field of pain management. Acute infusions of morphine or fentanyl give significant relief to patients with postherpetic neuralgia (Rowbotham et al 1991) and a mixed group of neuropathic pain patients respectively (Dellemijn and Vanneste 1997). Furthermore, sustained efficacy has been demonstrated for oral oxycodone (Watson and Babul 1998) and tramadol (Harati et al 2000) in postherpetic neuralgia and painful diabetic neuropathy respectively.

Our (anecdotal) experience and that of others (Portenoy et al 1990) is that many patients with pain due to central and peripheral nerve injury can be successfully and safely treated with stable doses of narcotic analgesics. However, the use of opioids requires caution in patients with a history of chemical dependence or pulmonary disease. We recommend using long-acting opioid analgesics (transdermal fentanyl, levorphanol, or a sustained-release morphine preparation) when alternative approaches to treatment have failed.

N-methyl-D-aspartate-receptor antagonists

Clinically available substances with *N*-methyl-D-aspartate (NMDA) receptor blocking properties include ketamine, dextromethorphan, memantine, and amantadine. Typical side effects include sedation, nausea, disagreeable psychological disturbances, and even frank hallucinations.

Studies of small cohorts have generally confirmed the analgesic effects of ketamine in patients suffering from post-herpetic neuralgia (Eide et al 1994, 1995) and other kinds of neuropathic pain (Eide et al 1995, Max et al 1995, Mercadante et al 1995, Felsby et al 1996, Nikolajsen et al 1996). Dextromethorphan was effective in painful diabetic neuralgia (Nelson et al 1997) but was without beneficial effect in postherpetic neuralgia or in a mixed population of patients with neuropathic pain (McQuay et al 1994, Nelson et al 1997). Amantadine relieved surgical neuropathic pain in cancer patients (Pud et al 1998).

Topical medications

Several topical agents have been used for neuropathic pain, particularly when patients have cutaneous hypersensitivity. Capsaicin is an agonist of the vanilloid receptor, VR1, which is present on the sensitive peripheral terminal of primary nociceptive afferents (Lynn 1990, Caterina et al 1997). On initial application it has an excitatory action and produces burning pain and hyperalgesia, but with repeated or prolonged application it inactivates the receptive terminals of nociceptors (Bjerring et al 1990). Therefore, this approach may help patients whose pain is maintained by anatomically intact, sensitized primary nociceptors.

Capsaicin extracts are commercially available in a 0.025 and a 0.075% preparation (Rains and Bryson 1995). Both preparations have been reported to reduce the pain of postherpetic neuralgia (Bernstein et al 1989, Watson et al 1993) and postmastectomy pain (Watson et al 1992). The 0.075% preparation has also been advocated for pain in diabetic neuropathy (Group 1991). However, these capsaicin preparations often produce intolerable burning so that many patients discontinue their use. There is anecdotal evidence that application of relatively high concentrations (greater than 5%) of capsaicin can produce prolonged pain relief in some patients with neuropathic pain (Robbins et al 1998). This produces burning so severe that spinal anaesthesia is required for the patients to tolerate the procedure.

A second promising topical medication for neuropathic pain is local anaesthetics. The rationale is similar to that discussed above in the section on anticonvulsants and antiarrhymics. Efficacy for a 5% patch preparation has been established (Rowbotham et al 1995, 1996). Topical application of aspirin in either a chloroform or ethyl ether suspension has been reported to produce profound pain relief for some patients with postherpetic neuralgia (King 1988, De Benedittis and Lorenzetti 1996).

In summary, the medical management of neuropathic pain consists of four main classes of oral medication (serotonin/noradrenaline (norepinephrine) reuptake blockers, anticonvulsants, antiarrhythmics, opioids) and several categories of topical medications for patients with cutaneous hyperalgesia (cyclooxygenase inhibitors, capsaicin in either 0.025 or 0.075% preparations, and local anaesthetics).

Non-pharmacological approaches

Transcutaneous electrical nerve stimulation

The advantages of peripheral nerve stimulation techniques are the lack of side effects and complications and the fact that the treatment can be easily repeated (see Chap. 30). Furthermore, efficacy can be determined rapidly. Therefore, a trial should be performed when feasible (Meyer and Fields 1972, Kumar and Marshall 1997, Finsen et al 1998). Invasive techniques, i.e., epidural spinal cord stimulation (SCS) and deep brain stimulation, may be effective in special cases of neuropathic pain (Broggi et al 1994, Tasker and Vilela Filho 1995, Kumar et al 1996). Complications include dislocation of the electrodes, infection of the system, and occasionally bleeding.

Neurosurgical destructive techniques (see Chap. 29)

Techniques such as neurectomy, rhizotomy, dorsal root entry zone lesions (DREZ), cordotomy and thalamotomy may provide short-term pain relief. Because destructive techniques increase the amount of deafferentation, sometimes even more severe pain will result from the procedure. Outside of trigeminal neuralgia there are no surgical approaches with established efficacy in neuropathic pain (Fields 1996).

A systematic approach to patients with neuropathic pain

The ideal in medicine is to treat the cause of the disease rather than the symptom. Since neuropathic pain is often multifactorial and its causes are usually uncertain, a treatment algorithm is required (Fig. 40.1). Entrapment neuropathies can be treated by neurolysis, transposition, or decompression (Dawson et al 1983). If scar-induced mechanical traction is a factor, this approach is particularly worthwhile. Transcutaneous electrical stimulation of nerves (TENS) is a viable option for some patients with focal nerve injury, particularly if the nerve trunk can be stimulated proximal to the site of injury. The majority of patients, however, require medical management. When cutaneous hyperalgesia and/or allodynia are present, topical agents are a good starting point, with either local anaesthetic, cyclo-oxygenase inhibitor, or capsaicin.

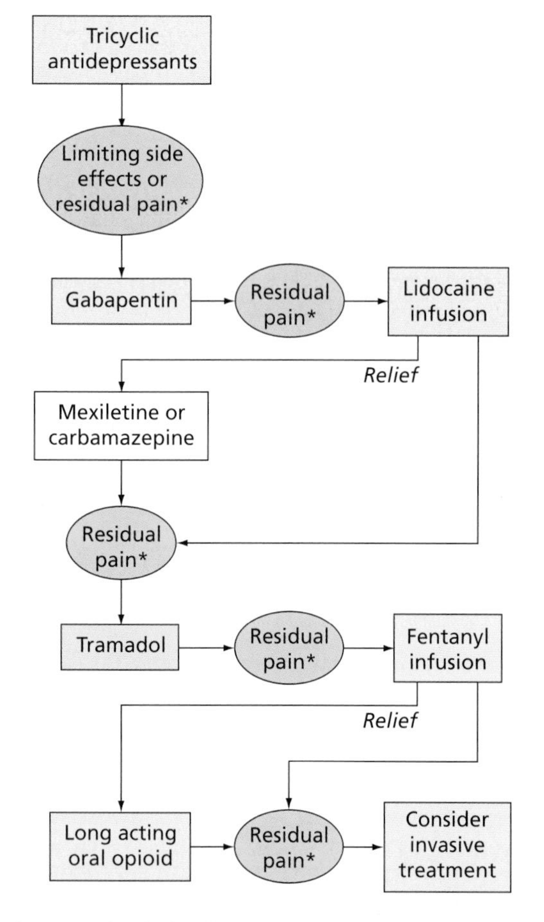

Fig. 40.1 Algorhythm for systematic management of neuropathic pain. See text for explanation.

In patients with focal neuropathies, a sympathetic block can be a useful procedure (Dellemijn et al 1994, Baron and Maier 1996). We use a local anaesthetic block of the sympathetic chain early if there is evidence of a sympathetically maintained component to the patient's problem (see Chap 18). Such evidence includes unilateral distal extremity pain, swelling, and vasomotor and sudomotor asymmetries. Patients with sympathetically maintained pain may obtain relief from a series of sympathetic blocks combined with vigorous physical therapy, provided this is done early in the course of the disease. In general, if sympathetic blocks are going to be helpful, they will provide sustained or at least increasing durations of post-block relief. If local anaesthetic blocks achieve sympatholysis as indicated by skin temperature change or a Horner's syndrome but no relief beyond 6 h, this approach is not promising. Furthermore, we have seldom found that surgical sympathectomy is helpful. There are two serious interpretive problems with sympathetic blocks (Dellemijn et al 1994). The first is systemic absorption of lidocaine (lignocaine), because even low plasma concentrations can relieve neuropathic pain independent of a sympathetic component to the problem. The second is the production of a somatic block by diffusion of local anaesthetic to the nearby nerve plexus.

If there is no strong evidence of sympathetically maintained pain or sympatholytic interventions do not provide significant relief, we proceed to systemic medication. General treatment principles are the individualization of therapy and the titration of a given drug depending on effect on the one hand and side effects on the other. Non-response should not be accepted unless a sufficient dose has been given and until a sufficient period of time has passed to judge the drug's benefit. A rigorous systematic sequential approach is useful, if progression of the disease and pain profile are stationary.

Once the decision is made to pursue systematic medical management, we currently use the algorithm illustrated in Fig. 40.1. Because of the extensive literature supporting their use, we usually begin with TCAs; however, in some patients we begin therapy with gabapentin, especially in elderly patients or those with evidence of cardiac conduction block. With TCAs patients must be warned about side effects such as drowsiness, dry mouth, and orthostasis and then therapy should be initiated with an appropriately low dose (e.g., 10–25 mg). It is equally important to increase the dose gradually to optimize pain relief. In some patients it is necessary to raise the dose into the antidepressant range (over 200 mg/day). It is essential to check plasma levels of antidepressant medications before concluding that they are of no value. If side effects prevent raising the dose into the antidepressant range, switch to another TCA (desipramine and nortriptyline are less sedating and less anticholinergic than amitriptyline or doxepin), to gabapentin, or to a non-tricyclic antidepressant with noradrenergic reuptake blocking action such as venlafaxine, maprotiline, or mirtazapine.

If patients obtain inadequate relief from antidepressants and plasma levels are at the top of the recommended therapeutic range, or if they do not tolerate the side effects, then begin a trial of gabapentin. This drug can be pushed to relatively high doses (e.g., over 3200 mg/day). If the patient still has significant pain consider using an oral antiarrhythmic or other anticonvulsant drugs. Begin with a lidocaine (lignocaine) infusion. If the patient does get a good response with the lidocaine (lignocaine) infusion, then begin treatment with either mexiletine, or an anticonvulsant such as carbamazepine.

If the patient does not obtain relief with a lidocaine (lignocaine) infusion our experience is that the pain is much less likely to respond to drugs of this class (Galer et al 1996). At this point, therapy is often commenced with tramadol. If this drug is ineffective we give the patient a fentanyl infusion to determine the opioid sensitivity of his pain. With a good response to fentanyl we initiate opioid therapy. At the present time, levorphanol, sustained-release morphine, or oxycodone are our first-line drugs. These medications are used on a scheduled rather than on-demand basis. Because of the problem of tolerance and physical dependence, it is our impression that the longer-acting drugs (levorphanol, methadone, and the sustained-release opioid preparations) are more effective because they avoid the exacerbation of pain by a mini-abstinence state during the falling phase of the plasma concentration of the opioid. The majority of our patients require a combination of therapies for optimal results.

Although this algorithm casts a broad net across potential pain mechanisms and is gratifying for those patients who obtain significant relief, many still have significant pain after all currently available options have been exhausted. As newer drugs are brought into use and other pain mechanisms are targeted, it is our belief that more patients can be helped.

References

Ali Z, Ringkamp M, Hartke T et al 1999 Uninjured C-fiber nociceptors develop spontaneous activity and alpha-adrenergic sensitivity following L6 spinal nerve ligation in monkey. Journal of Neurophysiology 81: 455–466

Asbury AK, Fields HL 1984 Pain due to peripheral nerve damage: an hypothesis. Neurology 34: 1587–1590

Atkinson J, Slater M, Wahlgren D et al 1999 Effects of noradrenergic and serotonergic antidepressants on chronic low back pain intensity. Pain 83: 137

Backonja M, Beydoun A, Edwards K et al 1998 Gabapentin for the symptomatic treatment of painful neuropathy in patients with diabetes mellitus: a randomized controlled trial. Journal of the American Medical Association 280: 1831–1836

Bahns E, Ernsberger U, Janig W, Nelke A 1986 Discharge properties of mechanosensitive afferents supplying the retroperitoneal space. Pflugers Archiv. European Journal of Physiology 407: 519–525

Baron R, Maier C 1996 Reflex sympathetic dystrophy: skin blood flow, sympathetic vasoconstrictor reflexes and pain before and after surgical sympathectomy. Pain 67: 317–326

Baron R, Saguer M 1993 Postherpetic neuralgia. Are C-nociceptors involved in signalling and maintenance of tactile allodynia? Brain 116: 1477–1496

Bartusch S, Sanders B, D'alessio J, Jernigan J 1996 Clonazepam for the treatment of lancinating phantom limb pain. Clinical Journal of Pain 12: 59–62

Bennett G 1993 An animal model of neuropathic pain: a review. Muscle and Nerve 16: 1040–1048

Bernstein JE, Korman NJ, Bickers DR, Dahl MV, Millikan LE 1989 Topical capsaicin treatment of chronic postherpetic neuralgia. Journal of the American Academy of Dermatology 21: 265–270

Bjerring P, Arendt-Nielsen L, Soderberg U 1990 Argon laser induced cutaneous sensory and pain thresholds in postherpetic neuralgia. Quantitative modulation by topical capsaicin. Acta Dermato-Venereologica 70: 121–125

Bove GM, Light AR 1995 Unmyelinated nociceptors of rat paraspinal tissues. Journal of Neurophysiology 73: 1752–1762

Broggi G, Servello D, Dones I, Carbone G 1994 Italian multicentric study on pain treatment with epidural spinal cord stimulation. Stereotactic and Functional Neurosurgery 62: 273–278

Caterina MJ, Schumacher MA, Tominaga M, Rosen TA, Levine JD, Julius D 1997 The capsaicin receptor: a heat-activated ion channel in the pain pathway. Nature 389: 816–824

Chabal C, Jacobson L, Mariano A, Chaney E, Britell CW 1992 The use of oral mexiletine for the treatment of pain after peripheral nerve injury. Anesthesiology 76: 513–517

Dawson D, Hallet M, Millender L 1983 Entrapment neuropathies. Little, Brown, Boston

De Benedittis G, Lorenzetti A 1996 Topical aspirin/diethyl ether mixture versus indomethacin and diclofenac/diethyl ether mixtures for acute herpetic neuralgia and postherpetic neuralgia: a double-blind crossover placebo-controlled study. Pain 65: 45–51

Dejgard A, Petersen P, Kastrup J 1988 Mexiletine for treatment of chronic painful diabetic neuropathy. Lancet I: 9

Dellemijn P, Vanneste J 1997 Randomised double-blind active-placebo-controlled crossover trial of intravenous fentanyl in neuropathic pain. Lancet 349: 753–758

Dellemijn PL, Fields HL, Allen RR, Mckay WR, Rowbotham MC 1994 The interpretation of pain relief and sensory changes following sympathetic blockade. Brain 117: 1475–1487

Devor M, Janig W 1981 Activation of myelinated afferents ending in a neuroma by stimulation of the sympathetic supply in the rat. Neuroscience Letters 24: 43–47

Devor M, Rappaport ZH 1990 Pain and pathophysiology of damaged nerves. In: Fields Hl (ed) Pain syndromes in neurology. Butterworth, London, pp 47–84

Dickenson AH 1997 NMDA receptor antagonists: interactions with opioids. Acta Anaesthesiologica Scandinavica 41: 112–115

Dickenson AH, Chapman V, Green GM 1997 The pharmacology of excitatory and inhibitory amino acid-mediated events in the transmission and modulation of pain in the spinal cord. General Pharmacology 28: 633–638

Dougherty PM, Palecek J, Paleckova V, Willis WD 1994 Neurokinin 1 and 2 antagonists attenuate the responses and NK1 antagonists prevent the sensitization of primate spinothalamic tract neurons after intradermal capsaicin. Journal of Neurophysiology 72: 1464–1475

Eide PK, Jorum E, Stubhaug A, Bremnes J, Breivik H 1994 Relief of post-herpetic neuralgia with the N-methyl-D-aspartic acid receptor antagonist ketamine: a double-blind, cross-over comparison with morphine and placebo. Pain 58: 347–354

Eide P, Stubhaug A, Stenehjem A 1995 Central dysesthesia pain after traumatic spinal cord injury is dependent on N-methyl-D-aspartate receptor activation. Neurosurgery 37: 1080–1087

Felsby S, Nielsen J, Arendt-Nielsen L, Jensen T 1996 NMDA receptor blockade in chronic neuropathic pain: a comparison of ketamine and magnesium chloride. Pain 64: 283–291

Fields H 1996 Treatment of trigeminal neuralgia. New England Journal of Medicine 334: 1125

Finsen V, Persen L, Lovlien M 1998 Transcutaneous electrical nerve stimulation after major amputation. Journal of Bone and Joint Surgery 70B: 109

Galer B, Harle J, Rowbotham M 1996 Response to intravenous lidocaine infusion predicts subsequent response to oral mexiletine: a prospective study. Journal of Pain and Symptom Management 12: 161–167

Glazer S, Portenoy R 1991 Systemic local anesthetics in pain control. Journal of Pain and Symptom Management 6: 30–39

Group TCS 1991 Treatment of painful diabetic neuropathy with topical capsaicin. A multicenter, double-blind, vehicle-controlled study. Archives of Internal Medicine 151: 2225

Habler H, Janig W, Koltzenberg M 1987 Activation of unmyelinated afferents in chronically lesioned nerves by adrenaline and excitation of sympathetic efferents in the cat. Neuroscience Letter 82: 35

Harati Y, Gooch C, Swenson M et al 2000 Maintenence of the long-term effectiveness of tramadol in treatment of the pain of diabetic neuropathy. Journal of Diabetes and its Complications 14: 65–70

Hromada J 1963 On the nerve supply to the connective tissue of some peripheral nervous system components. Acta Anatomica 55: 343

Janig W, Levine JD, Michaelis M 1996 Interactions of sympathetic and primary afferent neurons following nerve injury and tissue trauma. Progress in Brain Research 113: 161–184

Jett MF, McGuirk J, Waligora D, Hunter JC 1997 The effects of mexiletine, desipramine and fluoxetine in rat models involving central sensitization. Pain 69: 161–169

Kajander KC, Bennett GJ 1992 Onset of a painful peripheral neuropathy in rat: a partial and differential deafferentation and spontaneous discharge in a beta and a delta primary afferent neurons. Journal of Neurophysiology 68: 734–744

Kajander KC, Wakisaka S, Bennett GJ 1992 Spontaneous discharge originates in the dorsal root ganglion at the onset of a painful peripheral neuropathy in the rat. Neuroscience Letter 138: 225–228

Kastrup J, Petersen P, Dejgard A, Angelo HR, Hilsted J 1987 Intravenous lidocaine infusion—a new treatment of chronic painful diabetic neuropathy? Pain 28: 69–75

King RB 1988 Concerning the management of pain associated with herpes zoster and of postherpetic neuralgia. Pain 33: 73–78

Kingery WS 1997 A critical review of controlled clinical trials for peripheral neuropathic pain and complex regional pain syndromes. Pain 73: 123

Koltzenburg M, Lundberg LE, Torebjork HE 1992 Dynamic and static components of mechanical hyperalgesia in human hairy skin. Pain 51: 207–219

Kumar D, Marshall H 1997 Diabetic peripheral neuropathy: amelioration of pain with transcutaneous electrostimulation. Diabetes Care 20: 1702–1705

Kumar K, Toth C, Nath RK 1996 Spinal cord stimulation for chronic pain in peripheral neuropathy. Surgical Nuerology 46: 363

Laird JM, Bennett GJ 1993 An electrophysiological study of dorsal horn neurons in the spinal cord of rats with an experimental peripheral neuropathy. Journal of Neurophysiology 69: 2072–2085

Lang E, Hord A, Denson D 1996 Venlafaxine hydrochloride (effexor) relieves thermal hyperalgesia in rats with an experimental mononeuropathy. Pain 68: 151

Lombard MC, Larabi Y 1983 Electrophysiological study of cervical dorsal horn cells in partially deafferented rats. In: Bonica JJ (ed) Advances in pain research and therapy. Raven Press, New York, pp 147–154

Lynn B 1990 Capsaicin: actions on nociceptive C-fibres and therapeutic potential. Pain 41: 61–69

Max M, Lynch S, Muir J, Shoaf S, Smoller B, Dubner R 1992 Effects of desipramine, amitriptyline, and fluoxetine on pain in diabetic neuropathy. New England Journal of Medicine 326: 1250

Max M, Byas-Smith M, Gracely R, Bennett G 1995 Intravenous infusion of the NMDA antagonist, ketamine, in chronic posttraumatic pain with allodynia: a double-blind comparison to alfentanil and placebo. Clinical Neuropharmacology 18: 360–368

McQuay HJ, Carroll D, Jadad AR et al 1994 Dextromethorphan for the treatment of neuropathic pain: a double-blind randomised controlled crossover trial with integral n-of-1 design. Pain 59: 127–133

McQuay H, Carroll D, Jadad A, Wiffen P, Moore A 1995 Anticonvulsant drugs for management of pain: a systematic review. British Medical Journal 311: 1047

McQuay HJ, Tramer M, Nye BA, Carroll D, Wiffen PJ, Moore RA 1996 A systematic review of antidepressants in neuropathic pain. Pain 68: 217–227

Melzack R, Wall PD 1965 Pain mechanisms: a new theory. Science 150: 971–979

Mercadante S, Lodi F, Sapio M, Calligara M, Serretta R 1995 Long-term ketamine subcutaneous continuous infusion in neuropathic cancer pain. Journal of Pain and Symptom Management 10: 564–568

Meyer RA, Fields HL 1972 Causalgia treated by selective large fibre stimulation of peripheral nerve. Brain 95: 163–168

Mitchell SW 1865 Injuries of nerves and their consequences. Dover, New York

Nashold BS, Jr, Ostdahl RH 1979 Dorsal root entry zone lesions for pain relief. Journal of Neurosurgery 51: 59–69

Nelson K, Park K, Robinovitz E 1997 High-dose oral dextromethorphan versus plecebo in painful diabetic neuropathy and postherpetic neuralgia. Neurology 48: 1212

Nikolajsen L, Hansen C, Nielsen J, Keller J, Arendt-Nielsen L, Jensen T 1996 The effect of ketamine on phantom pain: a central neuropathic disorder maintained by peripheral input. Pain 67: 69–77

Onghena P, Van Houdenhove B 1992 Antidepressant-induced analgesia in chronic non-malignant pain: a meta-analysis of 39 placebo-controlled studies. Pain 49: 205

Partida-Sanchez S, Favila-Castillo L, Pedraza-Sanchez S et al 1998 IgG antibody subclasses, tumor necrosis factor and IFN-gamma levels in patients with type II lepra reaction on thalidomide treatment. International Archives of Allergy and Applied Immunology 116: 60–66

Petersen K, Fields H, Brennum J, Sandroni P, Rowbotham M 2000 Capsaicin evoked pain and allodynia in post-herpetic neuralgia. Pain 88: 125–133

Portenoy R, Foley K, Inturrisi C 1990 The nature of opioid responsiveness and its implications for neuropathic pain: new hypotheses derived from studies of opioid infusions. Pain 43: 273–286

Pud D, Eisenberg E, Spitzer A, Adler R, Fried G, Yarnitsky D 1998 The NMDA receptor antagonist amantadine reduces surgical nueropathic pani in cancer patients: a double blind, randomized, placebo controlled trial. Pain 75: 349–354

Rains C, Bryson HM 1995 Topical capsaicin. A review of its pharmacological properties and therapeutic potential in post-herpetic neuralgia, diabetic neuropathy and osteoarthritis. Drugs and Aging 7: 317–328

Richelson E 1990 Antidepressants and brain neurochemistry. Mayo Clinic Proceedings 65: 1227–1236

Robbins W, Staats P, Levine J 1998 Treatment of intractable pain with topical large-dose capsaicin: preliminary report. Anesthesia and Analgesia 86: 579

Rowbotham MC, Reisner-Keller LA, Fields HL 1991 Both intravenous lidocaine and morphine reduce the pain of postherpetic neuralgia. Neurology 41: 1024–1028

Rowbotham MC, Davies PS, Fields HL 1995 Topical lidocaine gel relieves postherpetic neuralgia. Annals of Neurology 37: 246–253

Rowbotham MC, Davies PS, Verkempinck C, Galer BS 1996 Lidocaine patch: double-blind controlled study of a new treatment method for post-herpetic neuralgia. Pain 65: 39–44

Rowbotham M, Harden N, Stacey B, Bernstein P, Magnus-Miller L 1998 Gabapentin for the treatment of postherpetic neuralgia: a randomized controlled trial. Journal of the American Medical Association 280: 1837–1842

Sato J, Perl ER 1991 Adrenergic excitation of cutaneous pain receptors induced by peripheral nerve injury. Science 251: 1608–1610

Scadding JW 1981 Development of ongoing activity, mechanosensitivity, and adrenaline sensitivity in severed peripheral nerve axons. Experimental Neurology 73: 345–364

Shir Y, Seltzer Z 1991 Effects of sympathectomy in a model of causalgiform pain produced by partial sciatic nerve injury in rats. Pain 45: 309

Shortland P, Woolf CJ 1993 Chronic peripheral nerve section results in a rearrangement of the central axonal arborizations of axotomized A beta primary afferent neurons in the rat spinal cord. Journal of Comparative Neurology 330: 65–82

Sindrup S, Jensen T 1999 Efficacy of pharmacological treatments of neuropathic pain: an update and effect related to mechanism of drug action. Pain 83: 389–400

Sommer C, Myers RR 1996 Vascular pathology in CCI neuropathy: a quantitative temporal study. Experimental Neurology 141: 113–119

Sommer C, Marziniak M, Myers RR 1998 The effect of thalidomide treatment on vascular pathology and hyperalgesia caused by chronic constriction injury. Pain 74: 83–91

Sorkin L, Xiao W, Wagner R, Myers R 1997 Tumour necrosis factor-A induces ectopic activity in nociceptive primary afferent fibers. Neuroscience 81: 255–262

Sumpton J, Moulin D 2001 Treatment of neuropathic pain with venlafaxine. Annals of Pharmacotherapy 35: 557–559

Tasker R, Vilela Filho O 1995 Deep brain stimulation for neuropathic pain. Stereotactic and Functional Neurosurgery 65: 122–124

Torebjork E, Wahren L, Wallin G, Hallin R, Koltzenburg M 1995 Noradrenaline-evoked pain in neuralgia. Pain 63: 11–20

Wagner R, Janjigian M, Myers RR 1998 Anti-inflammatory interleukin-10 therapy in CCI neuropathy decreases thermal hyperalgesia, macrophage recruitment, and endoneurial TNF-alpha expression. Pain 74: 35–42

Walker AE, Nulsen F 1948 Electrical stimulation of the upper thoracic portion of the sympathetic chain in man. Archives of Neurology and Psychiatry 59: 559–560

Wall PD, Gutnick M 1974 Ongoing activity in peripheral nerves: the physiology and pharmacology of impulses originating from a neuroma. Experimental Neurology 43: 580–593

Wallace M, Magnuson S, Ridgeway B 2000 Efficacy of oral mexiletine for neuropathic pain with allodynia: a double-blind, placebo-controlled, crossover study. Regional Anesthesia and Pain Medicine 25: 459–467

Watson C, Babul N 1998 Efficacy of oxycodone in neuropathic pain: a randomized trial in postherpetic neuralgia. Neurology 50: 1837–1841

Watson CP, Chipman M, Reed K, Evans RJ, Birkett N 1992 Amitriptyline versus maprotiline in postherpetic neuralgia: a randomized, double-blind, crossover trial. Pain 48: 29–36

Watson C, Tyler K, Bickers D 1993 A randomized vehicle-controlled trial of topical capsaicin in the treatment of postherpetic neuralgia. Clinical Therapy 15: 510

Wynn-Parry CB 1980 Pain in avulsion lesions of the brachial plexus. Pain 9: 41–53

Chapter 41

Pain of burns

Manon Choinière

Introduction

Providing optimal analgesia to burn patients presents a major challenge. Burn pain is difficult to control because of its multiple components and changing pattern over time. It also involves repeated traumas or manipulations of the injured painful sites. The sometimes-excruciating pain, along with extreme intra- and inter-individual variability in severity, complicates the task of providing analgesia to burn patients.

Clinical characteristics

Components of burn pain

Burn pain involves several components that cause severe pain (Ashburn 1995, Latarjet and Choinière 1995, Kowalske and Tanelian 1997, Pal et al 1997, Henry and Foster 2000, Meyer et al 2002). The *background pain* is felt at the wound sites and surrounding areas. This pain is relatively constant and can be exacerbated (*breakthrough pain*) by movements such as changing position, turning in bed, walking, or even breathing. Donor sites—areas of normal skin that have been harvested for skin grafts—also elicit pain since nerve terminals are exposed to stimulation.

The second component of burn pain—*procedural pain*—is related to the multiple therapeutic procedures carried out during the course of treatment. These procedures, which occur daily or even several times a day, include dressing changes, wound cleansing, and physiotherapy sessions. Other sources of pain related to treatment include the enforced immobilization of limbs in splints or garments, and multiple surgical interventions (e.g., skin grafting, reconstructive surgery).

Finally, the third component of burn pain is related to the tissue regeneration and the healing process. When skin grafting is required, the necrotic tissue—i.e., the eschar—is excised until viable tissue is reached, thereby damaging intact nerves. When these nerves regenerate along with those destroyed at the time of the injury, pain is commonly experienced along with intense tingling or itching sensations. In such a setting, the pain may resemble *neuropathic pain* rather than acute pain due to thermal injury (Atchison et al 1991, Latarjet and Choinière 1995, Silbert et al 1998, Coderre and Choinière 2000). The healing process may last for months to years, and pain or paresthesic sensations may persist afterwards (Ward et al 1989, Choinière et al 1991, Malenfant et al 1996, Dauber et al 2002).

Malenfant et al (1996) found that more than 70% of the 236 burn patients interviewed one year or more after their accident reported paraesthesic sensations (e.g., itching, tingling, cold sensations, etc) and 36% complained of pain at the burn injury site. These problems may persist for many years, be present every week, and interfere with daily living activities. Weather-related variations in sensations (Ward et al 1989, Malenfant et al 1996) suggest that the prevalence of chronic postburn neuralgia may vary in different climates.

Pain intensity and sources of variation

The depth, size, and location of the burns determine the severity of the injury, which, in turn, influences pain intensity and clinical outcome. More severe burns usually require longer hospitalizations, and multiple manipulations and surgical interventions, which add to the patient's pain. In contrast, minor burns of less than 10–15% of the body surface which do not require skin grafting, can be managed on an outpatient basis although they can be as painful or more painful initially than deeper burns that require hospitalization (Baxter and Wackerie 1988, Demling 1990).

The relationship between burn severity and pain intensity is complex and often inconsistent, even within the same patient throughout the treatment course. Some studies (Perry et al 1981, Everett et al 1994, Byers et al 2001) have failed to find any significant correlation between pain intensity and burn severity. Others (Choinière et al 1989, Atchison et al 1991, Ptacek et al 2000) have shown that patients with larger burn injuries tend to report more pain at rest and/or during procedures. Clinically, it is generally recognized that superficial second-degree burns (which constitute the largest number of burns treated on an outpatient basis) are the most painful initially. As the inflammatory response progresses, the pain increases at the wound site (primary hyperalgesia) and spreads to surrounding areas (secondary hyperalgesia). First-degree burns cause less pain since they damage only the superficial layer of the epidermis, and nerve terminals are not exposed as in superficial second-degree burns. In deep partial-thickness burns (deep second degree), which usually require skin grafting for healing, nerve terminals can be damaged or destroyed such that some of the areas may show little or no response initially when a sharp stimulus is applied. The same is true for full-thickness or third-degree burns in which the dermis is entirely destroyed along with the rich network of nerve terminals. Yet, a patient may complain of pain in these areas since deep burns are most often intermixed with and/or surrounded by more superficial burns in which nerve terminals are intact and exposed (Latarjet and Choinière 1995, Silbert et al 1998, Meyer et al 2002).

Burn pain is described by many patients as the worst they had ever experienced. However, it would be erroneous to believe that burn patients suffer atrocious pain continuously. Furthermore, the most severe pain does not appear to be related to the injury itself but to intermittent trauma caused by the various therapeutic procedures. Burn adults and children report that the greatest pain is usually related to therapeutic procedures and can reach excruciating levels (Perry et al 1981, Choinière et al 1989, Atchison et al 1991, Weinberg et al 2000, Byers et al 2001).

Another factor that makes burn pain difficult to treat is its variability. Pain intensity varies considerably from one burn patient to another, especially during therapeutic procedures (Choinière et al 1989, Atchison et al 1991, Everett et al 1994, Jonsson et al 1998, Ptacek et al 2000). Variations in the procedures may explain some of the variation in pain scores. Patient's age, sex, ethnicity, education, occupation, or socioeconomic status are not significant predictors of pain intensity in adults or children. The interrelationship between pain, anxiety and depression is complex in burn adults and children. Several studies indicate that more anxious and/or depressed patients tend to report more pain while others failed to find any significant relationship between these factors (Choinière et al 1989, Geisser et al 1995, Ulmer et al 1997, Weinberg et al 2000, Ptacek et al 2000, Byers et al 2001).

Time course of the pain

Burn pain usually begins a few minutes after the injury. However, some victims may experience a pain-free period, which persists from several minutes to hours (Choinière et al 1989). Wall (1979) has proposed that pain may be inhibited for a period after an injury to permit other behavioural and physiological responses that have greater biological priorities for adaptation and survival. This may explain why burn victims often perform astonishing actions such as rescuing others, walking miles to find help, with apparently little or no pain. Individual differences in pain onset may also be related to a state of stress or psychological shock. Finally, pain may be diminished because nerve endings have been destroyed.

After hospitalization, pain persists on a daily basis and, unlike postsurgical pain, does not decline with time because new sources of pain are introduced during treatment (Ashburn 1995, Latarjet and Choinière 1995, Kowalske and Tanelian 1997, Meyer et al 2002). For example, the patients may feel less pain at the injury site as healing progresses or when skin grafts are applied, but they now have to endure other pains such as the pain associated with nerve regeneration or the pain at the donor site.

Choinière et al (1989) found wide fluctuations in pain intensity ratings from day to day, confirmed by Jonsson et al (1998) and Ptacek et al (2000). These findings have important clinical implications in terms of the patients' analgesic requirements. Due to the fear of addiction or a misconception about burn pain, the medical staff may be inclined to decrease the patient's medication as times goes on.

The intensity of the pain experienced during therapeutic procedures may also increase rather than decrease over time. Rapid escalation of the patients' analgesic needs, especially during repetitive dressing changes, can be an important problem for the clinician (Wermeling et al 1986, Osgood and Szyfelbein 1989, Williams et al 1998). This problem may result from insufficient analgesics.

Towards the end of hospitalization, the pain usually decreases. However, some patients develop postburn neuralgia at the site of injury, which can persist for variable periods of time ranging from weeks to several years (Ward et al 1989, Choinière et al 1991, Malenfant et al 1996, Dauber et al 2002).

Pain-generating mechanisms

Silbert et al (1998) and Coderre and Choinière (2000) have recently reviewed the neural and chemical mechanisms involved in burn injuries. Several authors including Pederson and Kelhet (1998) studied the persistent hyperalgesia in the injured site (primary hyperalgesia) and surrounding areas (secondary hyperalgesia), and found that they involve peripheral nociceptive and inflammatory mechanisms as well as changes in the central nervous system that facilitate afferent signals and cause spontaneous pain.

Furthermore, any manipulation of the burn sites (e.g., movement, dressing changes, debridement) can also trigger these neural and chemical mechanisms. Recurrent inputs from damaged and redamaged tissue contribute to short- and long-term changes in central nervous system (CNS) activity and subsequent pain sensitivity.

Deficiencies in the reinnervation of the scarred tissue and abnormalities of neural excitability of damaged or regenerated nerve endings and fibres may give rise to abnormal inputs and produce persisting neuralgic sensations. Moreover, the healing process may lead to the formation of contractures and hypertrophic scars in injured areas and donor sites that have been harvested more than once. It is therefore not surprising that burn patients may develop chronic sensory problems (pain, paraesthesia) at the site of their injuries.

Pain management

Local treatment

Covering open wounds with dressings reduces burn-wound pain. However, these dressings must be changed frequently, causing considerable discomfort to the patient. Early excision of the wounds and skin grafting alleviate the pain and obviates the need for long, painful, and debilitating sessions of bedside debridement. Temporary coverage with cadaver skin represents another option. Application of synthetic wound dressings or skin substitutes can reduce or even eliminate the pain at the wound site or skin donor site. As these dressings also remain in place for several days, fewer dressing changes are required.

Pharmacological treatment

Deficiencies and problems in analgesic therapy for burn patients

Several studies in the 1980s documented inadequacies in burn pain management and advocated more aggressive analgesic interventions (Perry and Heidrich 1982, Choinière et al 1989, Atchison et al 1991, Van der Does 1989). What is the situation today? Recent literature suggests that it has changed little. The administration of opioids is standard care for burn pain in many facilities (Ashburn 1995, Latarjet and Choinière 1995, Sheridan et al 1997, Kowalske and Taenelian 1997, Meyer et al 2002), but others avoid opioids because of concerns about potential adverse effects (Foertsch et al 1995). Some burn units continue to give patients less than 50% of the prescribed dose (Ulmer 1997), and others give low doses that are barely in the range required to control much less intense types of pain (e.g., Geisser et al 1995, Meyer et al 1997, Patterson et al 1997, Rae et al 2000). Finally, insufficient doses are often prescribed to elderly patients (Honari et al 1997) and to the vast population (about 95% of all burn injuries) treated on an outpatient basis (Friedland et al 1997, Smith et al 1997).

Various factors influence prescribing habits, and one of these is the fear that patients will develop addiction and tolerance to opioids. Interestingly, not one case of iatrogenic addiction has been documented in a nationwide survey of 93 burn centres, which had treated more than 10 000 patients (Perry and Heidrich 1982). With regard to the development of opioid tolerance, it can be treated effectively by increasing the dose (Foley 1991). Awareness of this phenomenon should alert the clinician to make upward adjustments in dosage of opioids. However, the complexity of the problem of opioid tolerance must be kept in mind. Several studies in cancer pain patients and more recently in patients suffering chronic, non-malignant pain show that even after years of treatment with strong opioids, patients do not necessarily require dose escalation or experience decreased pain relief. When increases in opioid dosing are required, they appear to be most often related to disease progression (Cherny and Portenoy 1999, Dertwinkel et al 1999). However, distressing paradoxical effects of opioids have also been described recently (Daeninck and Bruera 1999). Hyperalgesia and allodynia were reported in patients with cancer who receive very large doses of opioids for prolonged periods of time, generally in association with psychoactive medication—a situation often encountered in severely burned patients. This phenomenon of 'paradoxical pain' is of clinical relevance since clinicians may misinterpret it by not recognizing it as a neurotoxic adverse effect, and respond by further increasing the opioid dose in an attempt to control the pain.

Anecdotal reports and clinical experience (e.g., Wermeling et al 1986, Osgood and Szyfelbein 1989, Williams et al 1998) suggest that dose escalation may occur in burn patients when opioids are administered over an extended period of time. Sharply increasing doses of opioids may be required to maintain pain relief at rest or during dressing changes. As mentioned earlier, this problem may result from insufficient analgesia, especially at times of frequent dressing changes. Increased doses of opioids may also be needed because true tolerance occurs or because more pain is felt as a result of the healing process (e.g., of third-degree burns). Burn patients may continue to experience intense pain despite escalating opioid dosage because over time their pain changes to involve different mechanisms. Deep burn injuries can damage or destroy nerve terminals, causing neuropathic pain that responds less well to opioids (Bennett 1999). It is clear that further research is needed to study the effects of long-term opioid therapy in burn patients.

The fear that drug metabolism is altered in burn patients may make medical staff reluctant to use high doses of opioids. Although this concern may be justified during the immediate postinjury phase (see below), it is not warranted during the later phases of treatment of burn patients, as suggested by several reports on the pharmacokinetics of morphine, meperidine, sufentanyl, and methadone (see reviews by Martyn 1990, Meyer et al 2002). Burn patients are known to be hypermetabolic and resistant to many drugs used in anaesthetic practice. They are also known to require high doses of opioids to achieve adequate pain relief. Whether this is due to pharmacokinetic or pharmacodynamic alterations in the drug has not been completely established (Martyn 1990, MacLennan et al 1998).

The place of prevention in burn pain management

The need for aggressive analgesic intervention and the adverse effects of pain are increasingly recognized (Ashburn 1995, Latarjet and Choinière 1995, Kowalske and Tanelian 1997, Ulmer 1998, Henry and Foster 2000, Meyer et al 2002). Severe, persistent pain can be devastating; it can affect sleep and appetite, and may thus impede recovery from injury, and in a weakened individual like a burn patient, it may make the difference between life and death (Melzack 1990).

Current research suggests that early, vigorous analgesic intervention is crucial to prevent the adverse consequences of uncontrolled pain. For example, the burn patient who has learned to associate dressing changes with agonizing pain will be extremely difficult to treat, even with massive doses of opioids (Watkins et al 1992). Prompt, aggressive analgesia is critical to prevent the establishment of a pain–anxiety–pain cycle and to minimize other adverse psychological effects of pain commonly encountered in burn patients (Patterson et al 1993, Baur et al 1998, Yu and Dimsdale 1999, Martin-Herz et al 2000, Thurber et al 2000, Thomas et al 2002).

Equally important are the adverse physiological, chemical, and neural consequences of pain: the nervous system's 'memory' of pain (Carr 1998). Recent evidence on postburn hyperalgesia, central hyperexcitability, and opioid sensitivity (Silbert et al 1998, Coderre and Choinière 2000), provides evidence that burn patients would certainly benefit from an analgesic approach that involves strategies aimed at preventing or reducing the neural 'memory' of pain (preemptive analgesia) and includes the use of more than one treatment modality (multimodal analgesia) (Carr 1998, Kehlet et al 1999). Introduced to improve analgesic efficacy and reduce drug side effects in postoperative patients, the concept of 'pre-emptive/multimodal' analgesia implies a combination of two or more drugs with different mechanisms of action (e.g., local anaesthetics, non-steroidal anti-inflammatory agents (NSAIDS), opioids) applied before, during, and after surgery at different targets (at the periphery or centrally) along with non-pharmacological techniques to reduce stress and anxiety.

The 'pre-emptive/multimodal' analgesic approach is not fully applicable to burn patients. The risk of infection precludes spinal analgesia in most burn patients (Latarjet and Choinière 1995). Topical application of local anaesthetics on burns is often of limited usefulness due to their systemic toxicity (Pal et al 1997). However, some studies (Brofeldt et al 1989, Owen and Dye 1990, Jellish et al 1999) show interesting results with topically applied lidocaine (lignocaine) in small burn areas or in skin donor sites. All feasible strategies to reduce peripheral and/or central sensitization resulting from manipulation of painful burn sites should be applied, particularly at times of dressing changes.

Basic considerations in analgesic pharmacotherapy for burn patients

Pharmacotherapy is the mainstay for pain management in burn patients. The unique characteristics of burn pain call for specific strategies to maximize pharmacological treatment efficacy. Several key principles have been outlined in recent review articles (Ashburn 1995, Latarjet and Choinière 1995, Kowalske and Tanelian 1997, Pal et al 1997, Ulmer 1998, Henry and Foster 2000, Meyer et al 2002):

1. Evaluate and treat separately the two main components of burn pain—i.e., the background pain and the procedural pain.
2. Administer analgesics regularly (not 'as needed' or PRN) as long as the pain is present most of the day.
3. Individualize medication dosage, set flexible doses, and make frequent dose adjustments to account for wide variations in patients' analgesic requirements and the changing condition of their wounds.
4. Measure pain and treatment efficacy at regular intervals, and chart the information in the patient's file to provide a documented rationale for adjusting the medication for background and procedural pains.
5. Carefully monitor opioid side effects and use strategies to prevent or treat them rather than undermedicating the patient.
6. Always consider using non-opioid analgesics along with strong opioids because the different actions of these drugs enhance analgesia and reduce side effects.
7. Monitor anxiety and mood; use anxiolytic and/or antidepressant medication along with psychological interventions to complement, not replace, analgesics.

The place of opioids in burn pain management (see Chap. 24)

Strong opioids are the cornerstone of pain management in burn patients. What must be changed, however, is the way these drugs are used. One of the foremost causes of inadequate pain relief in burn patients is undermedication. Strong opioids are effective when administered according to basic principles such as those outlined above. One of the biggest problems when administering opioids to burns patients is how to provide sufficient medication during painful therapeutic procedures (e.g., dressing changes) without leaving the patient oversedated afterwards. However, strong opioids can be used very effectively in burn patients, and their dosage (as well as side effects) reduced by coadministering agents that block nociceptive or inflammatory afferent input, glutamate release, and/or activation of *N*-methyl-D-aspartate (NMDA) receptors (Silbert et al 1998, Choinière 2001).

With regard to opioid choice, morphine is probably the most widely used agent in burn patients: it is effective for moderate to severe pain, and it is not expensive compared to other opioid agonists (e.g., hydromorphone, fentanyl). Meperidine is of limited usefulness because repeated doses result in the accumulation of normeperidine, an active metabolite of meperidine that produces neurotoxic reactions. Methadone, a long-acting opioid, is well suited to provide a sustained level of analgesia. In contrast, synthetic opioid agonists, with a more rapid onset of action and a shorter duration of effect (e.g., fentanyl, alfentanyl, remifentanil), have gained a lot of popularity for alleviating pain at times of therapeutic procedures. Partial opioid agonists (e.g., buprenorphine, nalbuphine) can also be employed but it should be pointed out that they may precipitate withdrawal symptoms in patients who have previously received pure agonists (e.g., morphine). Finally, mild opioids (e.g., codeine) alone or in combination with acetaminophen (e.g., paracetamol) can provide sufficient analgesia when the pain is less intense.

Opioids are preferentially administered in burn patients by using the intravenous (I.V.) or oral route. Intramuscular (I.M.) administration is avoided, not only on account of poor absorption, but because the pain associated with the injections makes this route impractical for prolonged pain. The I.V. route has the advantage of rapid effect and ease of titration, and repeated injections into the I.V. line does not cause any pain. As soon as the I.V. route is no longer required, the oral route should be employed.

Pharmacotherapy for pain at rest

In the immediate postinjury phase, analgesic needs may be reduced or even absent in some burn patients who experience variable pain-free periods. However, most patients require prompt and effective pain medication. During the emergency or resuscitative phase of treament (1–2 days after injury), small but frequent bolus doses along with a continuous infusion of I.V. opioids are recommended. Other routes of administration should be avoided during this phase because burn injuries covering greater than 10% of the total body surface may decrease blood flow to organs and tissues, and thereby delay drug absorption and lead to respiratory depression, especially if high dosages have been administered to overcome poor absorption (Martyn 1990). The role of anxiety and fear must be carefully assessed at this stage since the patient's agitation may be interpreted as a pain response. Reassurance and information may help considerably in managing agitation while anxiolytic medication may contribute to reducing the analgesic needs. However, anxiolytic medications must be used with great care because of their possible potentiation of the respiratory depressive effects of opioids, especially in patients in shock.

Once the initial resuscitation phase is over, sufficient analgesia should be given for the pain felt at rest. The primary goal is to provide adequate baseline analgesia. This can be achieved with a continuous I.V. infusion of opioids with rescue boluses (Kealey 1995, Latarjet and Choinière 1995, Sheridan et al 2001, Meyer et al 2002). Another useful technique for alleviating pain at rest is patient-controlled analgesia (PCA). PCA has been shown to be safe and effective in burn adults and children (Wermeling et al 1986, Kinsella et al 1988, Gaukrogere et al 1991, Choinière et al 1992). However, the PCA method may not suffice for the intense pain levels felt during therapeutic procedures. Less-than-optimal analgesia with PCA can also be observed at rest simply because patients do not adequately medicate themselves, preferring to experience pain rather than drug side effects (Lehmann 1995). Another problem with PCA is that it requires the patient to be both awake and responsive in order to maintain adequate drug delivery. Thus, changes in dosing regimens at night must be planned to prevent the patient awaking in pain. This can be done by adding a continuous I.V. infusion of morphine at night. As pointed out by Lehmann (1995) and Meyer et al (2002), PCA is not different from any other analgesic regimen; it must be highly individualized and frequently adjusted to be most effective. In patients who can take medication by mouth, oral opioids with a long duration of action (e.g., slow-release morphine, methadone) are useful in providing stable analgesia when the patient is at rest.

The finding of opioid receptors on peripheral nerve terminals in inflammatory states such as thermal injuries (Stein 1995) suggests that the peripheral administration of morphine may decrease burn pain. Recent reports suggest promising results with this simple mode of treatment for painful skin ulcers in various medical conditions (Krajnik et al 1999, Twillman et al 1999) and for small burns (Long et al 2001). The efficacy and safety of peripheral opioid administration in burn patients merit evaluation as this mode of treatment constitutes an interesting therapeutic avenue to explore, especially as part of a multimodal regimen.

Combination of opioids and non-opioid analgesics should always be considered for controlling the pain at rest. For example, acetaminophen or NSAIDs in combination with opioids (Meyer et al 1997, 2002; Pal et al 1997; Ulmer 1998; Choinière 2001) could be used as a basic treatment for background pain. Traditional analgesic regimens usually neglect or completely ignore the inflammatory component of burn pain, but it is extremely important, especially during early treatment. Traditional NSAIDs are not recommended in burn patients who require extensive excision and grafting procedures because their antiplatelet effects may increase blood loss. However, this class of drugs might help burn patients who require minimal skin grafts to reduce pain at donor sites (Ulmer 1998, Choinière 2001). The same might be true for those burn patients with superficial injuries who are treated on an outpatient basis. Also interesting is the new generation of NSAIDs, the cycloxygenase-2 (COX2) inhibitors (e.g., rofecoxib, celecoxib) that have been shown to provide efficient analgesia with few side effects, including minimal inhibition of platelet function (Hawkey 1999). These drugs may constitute a major advance in the treatment of burn pain and merit further investigation.

NMDA-receptor antagonists may offer specific advantages for treating postburn hyperalgesia and lessening opioid dose escalation (Silbert et al 1998, Wiesenfield-Hallin 1998, Williams et al 1998). Several reports on the use of methadone in burn adults and children have substantiated the advantages of this long-acting agent for providing stable analgesia for background pain (Concilus et al 1989, Shir et al 1998, Williams et al 1998). Ketamine at low doses—i.e., at analgesic doses rather than anaesthetic doses—may be used in combination with an opioid such as morphine to control the pain at rest (Cederholm et al 1990). The usefulness of a PCA regimen that combines morphine and ketamine (Schmid et al 1999) also merits evaluation as it could represent an interesting therapeutic avenue for burn patients.

Two recent case reports (Lyons et al 1996, Kariya et al 1998) suggest that clonidine, an α_2-adrenoceptor agonist, could be a useful sedative-analgesic adjunctive medication in burn pain management. Clonidine could not only reduce opioid requirements but also drug side effects as it does not cause pruritus or respiratory depression (Pal et al 1997).

As mentioned earlier, when persistent burn pain cannot be adequately controlled despite increasing the dose of opioids, other diagnoses such as the presence of a neuropathic pain component should be considered. Drugs that are effective for this type of pain, such as tricyclic antidepressants, anticonvulsants, and/or membrane-stabilizing drugs, may be indicated for controlling burn pain (Latarjet and Choinière 1995, Pal et al 1997, Meyer et al 2002). Results reported by Jonsson et al (1991) suggest that continous infusion of low doses of lidocaine (lignocaine), which is known to alleviate neuropathic pain in other settings, may be a valuable additional option for pain control in burn patients.

When the background pain is mild and less persistent, weak opioids (e.g., codeine), non-opioids (e.g., acetaminophen), or combined preparations of analgesics (e.g., codeine plus acetaminophen) may be sufficient to make the patient comfortable. Finally, treatment for painful or paraesthesic sensations in healed wounds may involve experimenting with a variety of medications employed for neuropathic pain including methadone (Altier et al 2001).

Since fear and anxiety are almost universal responses to burn injury, anxiolytics (e.g., benzodiazepines) may be useful supplements to the analgesic medication given to the resting patient. Many patients are anxious when they are in pain but are calm once the pain is relieved. If the anxiety persists, for reasons other than anticipation of painful treatments, anxiolytics may be used. These drugs and/or hypnotics can also be given at bedtime to favour optimal sleep. Antidepressant drugs may also be necessary in burn patients hospitalized for prolonged periods of time and who develop problems of depression. Antidepressant drugs are helpful not only in elevating mood but they may also relieve pain and improve sleep and appetite (Watkins et al 1992, Pal et al 1997, Meyer et al 2002).

Pharmacotherapy for pain due to therapeutic procedures

As mentioned earlier, the most intense pain in burn patients results from therapeutic procedures such as dressing changes, wound debridement, and physiotherapy sessions. Strong opioids such as morphine or fentanyl are typically required to bring the pain under control for dressing changes both in adults and children (Ashburn 1995, Latarjet and Choinière 1995, Kowalske and Tanelian 1997, Henry and Foster 2000, Meyer et al 2002). Because these procedures are usually performed at the bedside, the biggest challenge for the clinician is to provide proper analgesia without interfering with the patient's awareness during and after the procedure. Compared to morphine, opioids such as fentanyl or alfentanyl have major advantages in that they act rapidly, have short duration, and avoid oversedation following the procedures. Intravenous morphine, which is less costly, is preferable for more lengthy procedures for which short-acting opioids have no real advantages. When therapeutic procedures are less painful, premedication with oral morphine or milder opioids may be sufficient. Flexible doses of drugs coupled with frequent evaluation of the resulting analgesia are necessary. The need to administer oral preparation drugs far enough in advance to be maximally effective must also be taken into account.

Analgesia for procedural pain in burn children deserves special comments. Several studies have demonstrated that burn children are much less likely than adults to receive adequate analgesia for dressing changes despite the fact that a burn is not less painful in a child than in an adult (Osgood and Szyfelbein 1989, Latarjet and Choinière 1995, Henry and Foster 2000, Meyer et al 2002). In fact, the same therapeutic modalities adjusted for age and size should be used for burn children. However, it is often not the case. Several authors (Osgood and Szyfelbein 1989, Atchison et al 1991) have pointed out the inadequacy of oral preparations such as Percocet (oxycodone + acetaminothen) for controlling severe pain during dressing changes. Oral preparations of short-acting morphine or hydromorphone are more likely to be effective and can easily be administered in the form of an elixir or tablet. Increasingly popular is the transmucosal fentanyl citrate in the form of lollipops that provide a new user-friendly form of treating pain in burn children (Henry and Foster 2000, Meyer et al 2002). In a recent double-blind study, Sharar et al (1998) compared fentanyl lollipops and oral hydromorphone for wound care analgesia in hospitalized burn children. They concluded that the fentanyl lollipops are safe and effective but they found only minor benefits in terms of analgesia and anxiolysis over oral hydromorphone pretreatment. However, sample size was small in this study and further studies involving larger samples of patients are needed to assess the benefits of fentanyl lollipops.

Depending upon the patient's anxiety level, opioids can be administered alone or in combination with a benzodiazepine before the therapeutic procedure. Since undermedication for pain can escalate anxiety, early optimal control of pain is crucial to minimize anxiety for future procedures and to prevent the continual use of benzodiazepines for controlling anticipatory anxiety. As pointed out by Watkins et al (1992), once the patient has learned to associate burn treatment with agonizing pain, even massive increases in opioids will fail to provide adequate pain relief. In such a case, the addition of a benzodiazepine (e.g., lorazepam, midazolam) can be most beneficial (Ashburn 1995, Pal et al 1997, Patterson et al 1997).

In some cases, procedures such as extensive dressing changes and wound debridements can produce pain so severe that the conscious patient simply cannot tolerate it. Conscious sedation may then be required while deep sedation or general anaesthesia may be the only choices (Dimick et al 1993, Latarjet and Choinière 1995, MacLennan 1998, Ebach et al 1999). Considering the various adverse side effects of anaesthetic agents, there is an obvious reluctance to repeatedly expose burn patients to general anaesthesia. Furthermore, the repeated administration of some anaesthetic agents requires the withholding of food prior to each intervention and for some time afterwards, thereby interrupting the intensive nutritional support so important for the recovery of burn patients.

Self-administration of inhalational agents such as nitrous oxide with oxygen has been shown to provide successful analgesia for dressing changes in burn adults and children. However, there is some controversy in the burn literature with respect to the side effects and potential toxicity of nitrous oxide (with particular concern about bone marrow suppression) with repeated exposure over prolonged periods of time (Pal et al 1997, MacLennan et al 1998, Meyer et al 2002).

Ketamine has been one of the most extensively used anaesthetics for burn patients. Several studies (see reviews by Kowalske and Tanelian 1997 and Meyer et al 2002) indicate that subanaesthetic doses of ketamine provide very effective analgesia for burn dressings and wound debridement. Ketamine often causes dysphoria with unpleasant hallucinations but these reactions can be minimized with benzodiazepine premedication. As mentioned earlier, ketamine also has NMDA-receptor antagonist activity. Therefore, if ketamine is used with an opioid such as morphine or fentanyl for relieving pain at times of therapeutic procedures, this regimen could not only have opioid-sparing actions but also reduce opioid-related side effects, including the hyperalgesia sometimes seen with high opioid dose (Schmid et al 1999).

Propofol is another agent that has gained popularity for providing sedation during prolonged painful procedures in burn patients. It is a sedative-hypnotic agent with a very rapid onset of action but no analgesic activity. Its dosage can be accurately titrated for sedation or total anaesthesia; recovery after its use is rapid, and emergence after a single bolus or short infusion is free of the 'hangover' associated with the use of most other I.V. anaesthetic drugs. However, benefits of deep sedation with propofol is not without risks (e.g., hypotension) (Bryson et al 1995, Meyer et al 2002).

Other treatment methods

To be severely burned is a devastating experience, not only from a physical but also from a psychological point of view. The injury itself is frightening and, during hospitalization, the patient must face helplessness, pain, dependency, and the possibility of disfigurement, deformity, and death. Many burn patients experience various forms of psychological distress during their hospitalization. These reactions can take the form of a normal process of psychological adaptation to the injury (e.g., sadness, depression, sleep disturbance, anger, frustration, fear, anxiety, dread) or frank psychiatric disorders (e.g. delirium, adjustment disorders, major depression, posttraumatic stress disorder). Comprehensive reviews of these reactions are provided by Watkins et al (1988), Patterson et al (1993), and Thomas et al (2002).

That psychological disturbances can influence or be influenced by pain in burn patients is well documented in the literature. Therefore, psychological interventions can also be helpful in the treatment of burn pain, and several techniques have been used with varying degrees of success in burn adults and children (see reviews by Patterson et al 1993, Patterson 1995, Martin-Hertz et al 2000, Meyer et al 2002). These approaches, which have been used alone or in combination, include hypnosis, relaxation training (breathing exercises, progressive muscle relaxation), biofeedback, behaviour modification (respondant and operant techniques), desensitization, stress inoculation training, cognitive-behavioural strategies (guided imagery, distraction techniques, coping skills training), and group or individual psychotherapy. Unfortunately, many of the published reports are anecdotal. Others studies suffer from methodological deficiencies. Nevertheless, several well-designed studies suggest that burn patients can be helped to control their pain and anxiety through hypnosis, cognitive-behavioural, and stress reduction techniques. All of these techniques can help the patient to relax and maintain a sense of control (Patterson 1995, Martin-Hertz et al 2000, Thurber et al 2000, Meyer et al 2002).

Considering the severity of burn pain, it is very unlikely, however, that psychological techniques alone can provide complete pain relief. Furthermore, hospitalized burn patients are often too stressed, fatigued, disoriented, or sick to engage in psychological interventions that require time and discipline. This does not mean, however, that psychological techniques cannot serve as useful adjuncts to opioids in burn pain control. Coupled with adequate and effective medication, psychological interventions can be helpful in optimizing pain relief in selected categories of patients. Additional well-designed studies are needed to document which types of burn patients are most likely to benefit from one type of intervention or another and at what stages of burn care these techniques could be most beneficial. More research must also be conducted to determine the practicality and cost-effectiveness of some of these techniques (e.g., hypnosis) compared to a combination of drug regimens (e.g., use of opioids plus benzodiazepines).

Conclusion

Burn pain management is most likely to be maximally effective if individualized preemptive–multimodal strategies are employed. Studies on combination of drug regimens and their side effects are required in this population. As important if not more important is the need to evaluate the short- and long-term effect of early aggressive analgesic treatment. Whether effective burn pain control has any effect beyond immediate reduction of suffering is an extremely important question. If positive, such studies could help to convince clinicians of the importance of providing adequate analgesia for burn and non burn patients. Whether effective burn pain relief will improve immune function and wound healing, hasten recovery, and decrease psychological complications are other important issues to investigate. But to avoid useless suffering remains the ultimate goal both from the patient's and clinician's point of view.

References

Altier N, Dion D, Boulanger A, Choinière M 2001 Successful use of methadone in the treatment of chronic neuropathic pain arising from burn injuries: a case-study. Burns 27: 771–775

Ashburn MA 1995 Burn pain: the management of procedure-related pain. Journal of Burn Care and Rehabilitation 16: 365–371

Atchison NE, Osgood PF, Carr DB, Szylfelbein SK 1991 Pain during burn dressing change in children: relationship to burn area, depth and analgesic regimens. Pain 47: 41–45

Baur KM, Hardy PE, Van Dorsten B 1998 Postraumatic stress disorder in burn populations: a critical review of the literature. Journal of Burn Care and Rehabilitation 19: 230–240

Baxter CR, Wackerie JF 1988 Emergency treatment of burn injury. Annals of Emergency Medicine 17: 1305–1315

Bennett GJ 1999 Opioids and painful peripheral neuropathy. In: Kalso E, McQuay HJ, Wiesenfeld-Hallin Z (eds) Opioid sensitivity of chronic noncancer pain, progress in pain research and management, vol 14. IASP Press, Seattle, pp 319–326

Brofeldt BT, Cornwell P, Doherty D, Batra K, Gunther RA 1989 Topical lidocaine in the treatment of partial-thickness burns. Journal of Burn Care and Rehabilitation 10: 63–68

Bryson HM, Fulton BR, Faulds D 1995 Propofol: an update on its use in anesthesia and conscious sedation. Drugs 50: 513–559

Byers JF, Bridges S, Kijek J, LaBorde P 2001 Burn patient's pain and anxiety experiences. Journal of Burn Care and Rehabilitation 22: 144–149

Carr DB 1998 Preempting the memory of pain. Journal of the American Medical Association, 278: 114–115

Cederholm I, Bengtsson M, Bjorkman S, Choonara I, Rane A 1990 Long-term high dose morphine, ketamine, and midazolam infusion in a child with burns. British Journal of Clinical Pharmacology 30: 901–905

Cherny NI, Portenoy RK 1999 Practical issues in the management of cancer pain. In: Wall PD, Melzack R (eds) Textbook of pain, 4th edn. Churchill Livingstone, Edinburgh, pp 1479–1491

Choinière M 2001 Burn pain: a unique challenge – Pain Clinical Updates – IASP Press, Seattle, Vol IX, p 1–4

Choinière M, Melzack R, Rondeau J, Girard N, Paquin MJ 1989 The pain of burns: characteristics and correlates. Journal of Trauma 29: 1531–1539

Choinière M, Melzack R, Papillon J 1991 Pain and paraesthesia in patients with healed burns: an exploratory study. Journal of Pain and Symptom Management 6: 437–444

Choinière M, Grenier R, Paquette C 1992 Patient-controlled analgesia: a double-blind study in burned patients. Anaesthesia 47: 467–472

Coderre TJ, Choinière M 2000 Neuronal plasticity associated with burn injury and its relevance for perception and management of pain in burn patients. Pain Research and Management 5: 205–213

Concilus R, Denson DD, Knarr D, Warden G, Raj P 1989 Continuous intravenous infusion of methadone for control of burn pain. Journal of Burn Care and Rehabilitation 10: 406–409

Daeninck PJ, Bruera E 1999 Opioid use in cancer pain. Is a more liberal approach enchancing toxicity? Acta Anaesthesiologica Scandinavia 43: 924–938

Dauber A, Osgood PF, Breslau AJ et al 2002 Chronic persistent pain after severe burns: a survery of 358 burn survivors. Pain Medicine 3: 6–17
Demling RH 1990 Pathophysiological changes after cutaneous burns and approach to initial resuscitation. In: Martyn JAJ (ed) Acute management of the burned patient. Saunders, Philadelphia, pp 12–24
Dertwinkel R, Zenz M, Strumpf M, Donner B 1999 Clinical status of opioid tolerance in long-term therapy of chronic non-cancer pain. In: Kalso E, McQuay HJ, Wiesenfeld-Hallin Z (eds) Opioid sensitivity of chronic noncancer pain, progress in pain research and management, vol 14. IASP Press, Seattle, pp 129–141
Dimick P, Helvig E, Heimbach D et al 1993 Anesthesia assisted procedures in a burn care intensive unit procedure room: benefits and complications. Journal of Burn Care and Rehabilitation 14: 446–449
Ebach DR, Foglia RP, Jones MB et al 1999 Experience with procedural sedation in a pediatric burn center. Journal of Pediatric Surgery 34: 955–958
Everett JJ, Patterson DR, Marvin JA et al 1994 Pain assessment from patients with burns and their nurses. Journal of Burn Care and Rehabilitation 15: 194–198
Foertsch CE, O'Hara M, Kealey GP, Foster LD, Schumacher EA 1995 A quasi-experimental, dual-center study of morphine efficacy in patients with burns. Journal of Burn Care and Rehabilitation 16: 118–126
Foley KM 1991 Clinical tolerance to opioids. In: Basbaum AI, Besson JM (eds) Towards a new pharmacology of pain. Wiley, Chichester, pp 181–203
Freund PR, Marvin JA 1990 Postburn pain. In: Bonica JJ (ed) The management of pain, 2nd edn. Lea & Febiger, Philadelphia, pp 481–489
Friedland LR, Pancioli AM, Duncan KM 1997 Pediatric emergency department analgesic practice. Pediatric Emergency Care 13: 103–106
Galizia JP, Cantineau D, Selosse A, Crepy A, Scherpereel PH 1987 Essai comparatif du propofol et de la kétamine au cours de l'anesthésie pour bain des grands brûlés. Annales Françaises d'Anesthésie et de Réanimation 6: 320–323
Gallagher G, Rae CP, Kenny GNC, Kinsella J 2000 The use of a target-controlled infusion of alfentanil to provide analgesia for burn dressing changes. Anaesthesia 55: 1159–1163
Gaukroger PB, Chapman MJ, Davey RB 1991 Pain control in paediatric burns—the use of patient-controlled analgesia. Burns 17: 396–399
Geisser ME, Bingham HG, Robinson ME 1995 Pain and anxiety during burn dressing changes: concordance between patients' and nurses' ratings and relation to medication administration and patient variables. Journal of Burn Care and Rehabilitation 16: 165–171
Hawkey CJ 1999 COX-2 inhibitors. Lancet 353: 307–314
Henry DB, Foster RL 2000 Burn pain management in children. Pediatric Clinics of North America 47: 681–698
Honari S, Patterson DR, Gibbons J et al 1997 Comparison of pain control medication in three age groups of elderly patients. Journal of Burn Care and Rehabilitation 18: 500–504
Jellish WS, Gamelli RL, Furry PA, McGill VL, Fluder EM 1999 Effect of topical local anesthetic application to skin harvest sites for pain management in burn patients undergoing skin-grafting procedures. Annals of Surgery 229: 115–120
Jonsson A, Cassuto J, Hanson B 1991 Inhibition of burn pain by intravenous lignocaine infusion. Lancet 338: 151–152
Jonsson CE, Holmsten A, Dahlström L, Jonsson K 1998 Background pain in burn patients: routine measurement and recording of pain intensity in a burn unit. Burns 24: 448–454
Kariya N, Shindoh M, Nishi S, Yukioka H, Asada A 1998 Oral clonidine for sedation and analgesia in burn patient. Journal of Clinical Anesthesia 10: 514–517
Kealey GP 1995 Pharmacologic management of background pain in burn victims. Journal of Burn Care and Rehabilitation 19: 358–362
Kehlet H, Werner M, Perkins F 1999 Balanced analgesia: what is it and what are its advantages in postoperative pain? Drugs 58: 793–797
Kinsella J, Glavin R, Reid WH 1988 Patient-controlled analgesia for burned patients: a preliminary report. Burns 14: 500–503
Kowalske K, Tanelian D 1997 Burn pain—evaluation and management. Anesthesiology Clinics of North America 15: 269–283
Krajnik M, Zylicz Z, Finlay I, Luczak J, van Sorge AA 1999 Potential uses of topical opioids in palliative care—report of 6 cases. Pain 80: 121–125
Latarjet J, Choinière M 1995 Pain in burn patients. Burns 21: 344–348
Lehmann KA 1995 New developments in patient-controlled postoperative analgesia. Annals of Medicine 27: 271–282
Long TD, Cathers TA, Twillman R et al 2001 Morphine-infused silver sulfadiazine (MISS) cream for burn analgesia: a pilot study. Journal of Burn Care and Rehabilitation 22: 118–123
Lyons B, Casey W, Doherty P, McHugh M, Moore KP 1996 Pain relief with low-dose intravenous clonidine in a child with severe burns. Intensive Care Medicine 22: 249–251
MacLennan N, Heimbach D, Cullen B 1998 Anesthesia for major thermal injury. Anesthesiology 89: 749–770
Malenfant A, Forget R, Amsel R et al 1996 Prevalence and characteristics of chronic and sensory problems in burn patients. Pain 67: 493–500
Martin-Herz SP, Thurber CA, Patterson DR 2000 Psychological principles of burn wound pain in children. Part II: treatment applications. Journal of Burn Care and Rehabilitation 21: 451–478
Martyn JAJ 1990 Clinical pharmacology and therapeutics in burns. In: Martyn JAJ (ed) Acute management of the burned patient. Saunders, Philadelphia, pp 180–200
Marvin JA, Muller MJ, Blakeney PE, Meyer WJ 1996 Pain response and pain control. In: Herdon DN (ed) Total burn care. Saunders, London, pp 529–543
Melzack R 1990 The tragedy of needless suffering. Scientific American 262: 27–33
Meyer WJ, Nichols RJ, Cortiella J, Villarreal C, Marvin JA 1997 Acetaminophen in the management of background pain in children post-burn. Journal of Pain and Symptom Management 13: 50–55
Meyer WJ, Marvin JA, Patterson DR, Thomas C, Blakeney P 2002 Management of pain and other discomforts in burned patients. In: Herdon DN (ed) Total burn care, 2nd edn. Saunders, London, pp 747–765
Osgood PF, Szyfelbein SK 1989 Management of burn pain in children. Pediatric Clinics of North America 36: 1001–1013
Osgood PF, Szyfelbein SK 1990 Management of pain. In: Martyn JAJ (ed) Acute management of the burned patient. Saunders, Philadelphia, pp 201–216
Owen TD, Dye D 1990 The value of topical lignocaine gel in pain relief on skin graft donor sites. British Journal of Plastic Surgery 43: 480–482
Pal SK, Cortiella J, Herndon D 1997 Adjunctive methods of pain control in burns. Burns 23: 404–412
Patterson DR 1995 Non-opioid-based approaches to burn pain. Journal Burn Care and Rehabilitation 16: 372–376
Patterson DR, Everett JJ, Bombardier CH et al 1993 Psychological effects of severe burn injuries. Psychological Bulletin 133: 362–378
Patterson DR, Ptacek JT, Carrougher GJ, Sharar SR 1997 Lorazepam as an adjunct to opioid analgesic in the treatment of burn pain. Pain 72: 367–374

Pederson JL, Kelhlet H 1998 Hyperalgesia in a human model of acute inflammatory pain: a methodological study. Pain 74: 139–151
Perry S, Heidrich G 1982 Management of pain during debridement: a survey. Pain 13: 267–280
Perry S, Heidrich G, Ramos E 1981 Assessment of pain by burned patients. Journal of Burn Care and Rehabilitation 2: 322–326
Ptacek JT, Patterson DR, Doctor J 2000 Describing and predicting the nature of procedural pain after thermal injuries: implications for research. Journal of Burn Care and Rehabilitation 21: 318–326
Rae CP, Gallagher G, Watson S, Kinsella J 2000 An audit of pain perception compared with medical and nursing staff estimation of pain during burn dressing changes. European Journal of Anaesthesiology 17: 43–45
Schmid RL, Sandler AN, Katz J 1999 Use and efficacy of low-dose ketamine in the management of acute postoperative pain: a review of current techniques and outcomes. Pain 82: 111–125
Sharar SR, Bratton SL, Garrougher GJ et al 1998 A comparison of oral transmucosal fentanyl citrate and oral hydromorphone for inpatient pediatric burn wound care analgesia. Journal of Burn Care and Rehabilitation 19: 516–521
Sheridan RL, Hinson M, Nackel A et al 1997 Development of a pediatric burn pain and anxiety management program. Journal of Burn Care and Rehabilitation 18: 455–459
Sheridan R, Stoddard F, Querzoli E 2001 Management of background pain and anxiety in critically burned children requiring protracted mechanical ventilation. Journal of Burn Care and Rehabilitation 22: 150–153
Shir Y, Shenkman Z, Shavelson V, Davidson EM, Rosen G 1998 Oral methadone for the treatment of severe pain in hospitalized children: a report of five cases. Clinical Journal of Pain 14: 350–353
Silbert BS, Osgood PR, Carr DB 1998 Burn pain In: Yaksh TL, Lynch C, Zapol WM et al (eds) Anesthesia biologic foundations. Lippincott–Raven, Philadelphia, pp 759–773
Smith S, Duncan M, Mobley J, Kagan R 1997 Emergency room management of minor burn injuries: a quality management evaluation. Journal Burn Care and Rehabilitation 18: 76–80
Stein C 1995 The control of pain in peripheral tissue by opioid. New England Journal of Medicine 332: 1685–1690
Thomas CR, Meyer WJ, Blakeney PE 2002 Psychiatric disorders associated with burn injury. In: Herdon DN (ed) Total burn care, 2nd edn. Saunders, London, pp 766–773
Thurber CA, Martin-Herz SP, Patterson DR 2000 Psychological principles of burn wound pain in children. Journal of Burn Care and Rehabilitation 21: 376–387
Twillman RR, Long TD, Cathers TA, Mueller DW 1999 Treatment of painful skin ulcers with topical opioids. Journal of Pain and Symptom Management 17: 288–292
Ulmer JF 1997 An exploratory study of pain, coping, and depressed mood following burn injury. Journal of Pain and Symptom Management 13: 148–157
Ulmer JF 1998 Burn pain management: a guideline-based approach. Journal of Burn Care and Rehabilitation 19: 151–159
Van der Does AJ 1989 Patients' and nurses' ratings of pain and anxiety during burn wound care. Pain 39: 95–101
Wall PD 1979 On the relationship of injury to pain. Pain 6: 253–264
Ward RS, Jeffrey PT, Saffle R, Schnebly A, Hayes-Lundy C, Reddy R 1989 Sensory loss over grafted areas in patients with burns. Journal of Burn Care and Rehabilitation 10: 536–538
Ward RS, Tuckett R 1991 Quantitative threshold change in cutaneous sensation of patients with burns. Journal of Burn Care and Rehabilitation 12: 560–575
Watkins PN, Cook EL, May R, Ehleben CM 1988 Psychological stages in adaptation following burn injury: a method for facilitating psychological recovery of burn victims. Journal of Burn Care and Rehabilitation 9: 376–384
Watkins PN, Cook EL, May R, Still JM 1992 The role of the psychiatrist in the team treatment of the adult patient with burns. Journal of Burn Care and Rehabilitation 13: 19–27
Weinberg K, Birdsall C, Vail D et al 2000 Pain an anxiety with burn dressing changes: patient self-report. Journal of Burn Care and Rehabilitation 21: 157–161
Wermeling DP, Record KE, Foster TS 1986 Patient-controlled high dose morphine therapy in a patient with electrical burns. Clinical Pharmacy 5: 832–835
Wiesenfeld-Hallin Z 1998 Combined opioid-NMDA antagonist therapies. What advantages do they offer for the control of pain syndromes? Drugs 55: 1–4
Williams PI, Sarginson RE, Ratcliffe JM 1998 Use of methadone in the morphine-tolerant burned paediatric patient. British Journal of Anaesthesia 80: 92–95
Yu BH, Dimsdale JE 1999 Postraumatic stress disorder in patients with burn injuries. Journal of Burn Care and Rehabilitation 20: 426–433

Chapter 42

Cancer pain syndromes

Nathan I Cherny

Introduction

Surveys indicate a pain prevalence of 28% among patients with newly diagnosed cancer (Vuorinen 1993), 50–70% among patients receiving active anticancer therapy (Portenoy et al 1992, 1994), and 64–80% among patients with far advanced disease (Donnelly and Walsh 1995, Caraceni and Portenoy 1999). Unrelieved pain interferes with physical functioning and social interaction, and is strongly associated with heightened psychological distress (Ferrell and Dean 1995). The high prevalence of acute and chronic pain among cancer patients and the profound psychological and physical burdens engendered by this symptom oblige all treating clinicians to be skilled in pain management (Emanuel 1996). Relief of pain in cancer patients is an ethical imperative, and it is incumbent upon clinicians to maximize the knowledge, skill, and diligence needed to attend to this task.

The undertreatment of cancer pain, which continues to be common (Cherny and Catane 1995, Stjernsward et al 1996), has many causes, among the most important of which is inadequate assessment (Grossman et al 1991, Von Roenn et al 1993).

Cancer pain syndromes—problems of classification

A woman with breast cancer who presents with shoulder pain may have any one of a number of pain syndromes including postoperative frozen shoulder, drug-associated proximal myalgias, metastases in the bony structures of the shoulder, or a benign pathology unrelated to the cancer. To arrive at an appropriate therapeutic plan the treating clinician must be aware of the range of possible causes of the pain, their distinguishing clinical features, and efficient diagnostic strategies to isolate the specific cause as quickly and easily as possible. Lack of awareness of the range of diagnostic possibilities may result in undertreatment.

Since the seminal work of John Bonica (1953a), various attempts have been made to develop a taxonomy for cancer pain (Foley 1987b, Cherny and Portenoy 1999). The description of cancer pain syndromes has facilitated a wider understanding of the causes of pain among cancer patients and enhanced the possibility of specific treatment approaches based upon better understanding of the underlying pathological process.

Cancer pain syndromes are defined by the association of particular pain characteristics and physical signs with specific consequences of the underlying disease or its treatment. Syndromes are associated with distinct aetiologies and pathophysiologies, and have important prognostic and therapeutic implications. Pain syndromes associated with cancer can be either acute or chronic. Whereas acute pains experienced by cancer patients are usually related to diagnostic and therapeutic interventions, chronic pains are most commonly caused by direct tumour infiltration. Adverse consequences of cancer therapy, including surgery, chemotherapy, and radiation therapy, account for 15–25% of chronic cancer pain problems, and a small proportion of the chronic pains experienced by cancer patients are caused by pathology unrelated to either the cancer or the cancer therapy.

Acute pain syndromes

Cancer-related acute pain syndromes are most commonly due to diagnostic or therapeutic interventions (Stull et al 1996) (Table 42.1) and they generally pose little diagnostic difficulty. Although some tumour-related pains have an acute onset (such as pain from a pathological fracture), most of these will persist unless effective treatment for the underlying lesion is provided. A comprehensive pain assessment in such patients is usually valuable, potentially yielding important information about the extent of disease or concurrent issues relevant to therapy.

Table 42.1 Cancer-related acute pain syndromes

Acute pain associated with diagnostic and therapeutic interventions
Acute pain associated with diagnostic interventions
Lumbar puncture headache
Transthoracic needle biopsy
Arterial or venous blood sampling
Bone marrow biopsy
Lumbar puncture
Colonoscopy
Myelography
Percutaneous biopsy
Thoracocentesis
Acute postoperative pain
Acute pain caused by other therapeutic interventions
Pleurodesis
Tumour embolization
Suprapubic catheterization
Intercostal catheter
Nephrostomy insertion
Cryosurgery associated pain and cramping
Acute pain associated with analgesic techniques
Local anaesthetic infiltration pain
Opioid injection pain
Opioid headache
Spinal opioid hyperalgesia syndrome
Epidural injection pain
Acute pain associated with anticancer therapies
Acute pain associated with chemotherapy infusion techniques
Intravenous infusion pain
Venous spasm
Chemical phlebitis
Vesicant extravasation
Anthracycline associated flare reaction
Hepatic artery infusion pain
Intraperitoneal chemotherapy abdominal pain
Acute pain associated with chemotherapy toxicity
Mucositis
Corticosteroid-induced perineal discomfort
Taxol-induced arthralgias
Steroid pseudorheumatism
Painful peripheral neuropathy
Headache
Intrathecal methotrexate meningitic syndrome
L-Asparaginase associated dural sinuses thrombosis
trans-Retinoic acid headache
Diffuse bone pain
trans-Retinoic acid
Colony-stimulating factors
5-Fluorouracil-induced anginal chest pain
Palmar–plantar erythrodysaesthesia syndrome
Postchemotherapy gynaecomastia
Chemotherapy-induced acute digital ischaemia
Acute pain associated with hormonal therapy
Leutenizing hormone releasing factor tumour flare in prostate cancer
Hormone-induced pain flare in breast cancer
Acute pain associated with immunotherapy
Interferon-induced acute pain

Acute pain associated with diagnostic and therapeutic interventions

Acute pain associated with diagnostic interventions

Lumbar puncture headache Lumbar puncture (LP) headache is the best characterized acute pain syndrome associated with a diagnostic intervention. This syndrome is characterized by the delayed development of a positional headache, which is precipitated or markedly exacerbated by upright posture. The pain is believed to be related to reduction in cerebrospinal fluid volume, due to ongoing leakage through the defect in the dural sheath, and compensatory expansion of the pain-sensitive intracerebral veins (Morewood 1993, Bakshi et al 1999). The incidence of headache is related to the caliber of the LP needle (0–2% with 27- to 29-gauge, 0.5–7% with 25- to 26-gauge, 5–8% with 22-gauge, 10–15% with 20-gauge, and 20–30%

Table 42.1 Cancer-related acute pain syndromes (*cont'd*)

Acute pain associated with growth factors
Colony-stimulating factor-induced musculoskeletal pains
Erythropoietin injection pain
Acute pain associated with radiotherapy
Incident pains associated with positioning
Oropharyngeal mucositis
Acute radiation enteritis and proctocolitis
Early onset brachial plexopathy
Subacute radiation myelopathy
Strontium-89 induced pain flare
Acute pain associated with infection
Acute herpetic neuralgia
Acute pain associated with vascular events
Acute thrombosis pain
Lower-extremity deep venous thrombosis
Upper-extremity deep venous thrombosis
Superior vena cava obstruction

with 18-gauge needles) (Bonica 1953b, McConaha et al 1996, Lambert et al 1997). Using a regular bevelled needle, the overall incidence can be reduced by the use of a small gauge needle and by longitudinal insertion of the needle bevel, which presumably induces less trauma to the longitudinal elastic fibres in the dura (Kempen and Mocek 1997). Use of a non-traumatic, conical tipped needle with a lateral opening spreads the dural fibres, and is associated with a substantially lesser risk of post-lumbar-puncture headaches than regular cannulae (Prager et al 1996, Corbey et al 1997, Lambert et al 1997, Vallejo et al 2000). The evidence that recumbency after LP reduces the incidence of this syndrome is controversial (Gonzalez 2000).

LP headache, which usually develops hours to several days after the procedure, is typically described as a dull occipital discomfort that may radiate to the frontal region or to the shoulders. Pain is commonly associated with nausea and dizziness. When severe, the pain may be associated with diaphoresis and vomitting (Lybecker et al 1995, Vilming and Kloster 1998a). The duration of the headache is usually 1–7 days (Lybecker et al 1995, Vilming and Kloster 1998b), and routine management relies on rest, hydration, and analgesics (Evans 1998). Persistent headache may necessitate application of an epidural blood patch (Evans 1998). Although a recent controlled study suggested that prophylactic administration of a blood patch may reduce this complication (Martin et al 1994), the incidence and severity of the syndrome do not warrant this treatment. Severe headache has also been reported to respond to treatment with intravenous or oral caffeine (Morewood 1993).

Transthoracic needle biopsy Transthoracic fine-needle aspiration of intrathoracic mass is generally a non-noxious procedure. Severe pain has, however been associated with this procedure when the underlying diagnosis was a neurogenic tumour (Jones et al 1993).

Transrectal prostatic biopsy Transrectal ultrasound-guided prostate biopsy is an essential procedure in the diagnosis and management of prostate cancer. In a prospective study 16% of the patients reported pain of moderate or greater severity (PAS PI ≥ 5) and 19% would not agree to undergo the procedure again without anaesthesia (Irani et al 1997). Transrectal ultrasound-guided prostatic nerve blockade is effective in relieving discomfort associated with this procedure (Nash et al 1996).

Mammography pain Breast compression associated with mammography can cause moderate and rarely severe pain (Leaney and Martin 1992, Aro et al 1996). Unless patients are adequately counselled and treated, occasional patients will refuse repeat mammograms because of pain (Leaney and Martin 1992).

Acute pain associated with therapeutic interventions

Postoperative pain Acute postoperative pain is universal unless adequately treated. Unfortunately, undertreatment is endemic despite the availability of adequate analgesic and anaesthetic techniques (Marks and Sachar 1973, Edwards 1990, Agency for Health Care Policy and Research: Acute Pain Management Panel 1992). Guidelines for management have been reviewed (Ready 1991, Agency for Health Care Policy and Research: Acute Pain Management Panel 1992). Postoperative pain that exceeds the normal duration or severity should prompt a careful evaluation for the possibility of infection or other complications.

Cryosurgery-associated pain and cramping Cryosurgery of the cervix in the treatment of intraepithelial neoplasm commonly produces an acute cramping pain syndrome. The severity of the pain is related to the duration of the freeze period, and it is not diminished by the administration of prophylactic NSAIDs (Harper 1994).

Other interventions Invasive interventions other than surgery are commonly used in cancer therapy and may also result in predictable acute pain syndromes. Examples include the pains associated with tumour embolization techniques (Chen et al 1997) and chemical pleurodesis (Prevost et al 1998).

Acute pain associated with analgesic techniques

Local anaesthetic infiltration pain Intradermal and subcutaneous infiltration of lidocaine (lignocaine) produces a transient burning sensation before the onset of analgesia. This can be modified with the use of buffered solutions (Palmon et al 1998). Other manoeuvres including warming of the solution (Martin et al 1996) or slowing rate of injection (Scarfone et al 1998) do not diminish injection pain.

Opioid injection pain Intramuscular (IM) and subcutaneous (SC) injections are painful. When repetitive dosing is required, the IM route of administration is not recommended (Agency for Health Care Policy and Research: Acute Pain Management Panel 1992, Agency for Health Care Policy and Research 1994). The pain associated with subcutaneous injection is influenced by the volume injected and the chemical characteristics of the injectant.

Opioid headache Rarely, patients develop a reproducible generalized headache after opioid administration. Although its cause is not known, speculation suggests that it may be caused by opioid-induced histamine release.

Spinal opioid hyperalgesia syndrome Intrathecal and epidural injection of high opioid doses is occasionally complicated by pain (typically perineal, buttock, or leg), hyperalgesia, and associated manifestations including segmental myoclonus, piloerection, and priapism. This is an uncommon phenomenon that remits after discontinuation of the infusion (Glavina and Robertshaw 1988, De Conno et al 1991, Cartwright et al 1993).

Epidural injection pain Back, pelvic, or leg pain may be precipitated by epidural injection or infusion. The incidence of this problem has been estimated at approximately 20% (De Castro et al 1991). It is speculated that it may be caused by the compression of an adjacent nerve root by the injected fluid (De Castro et al 1991).

Acute pain associated with anticancer therapies

Acute pain associated with chemotherapy infusion techniques

Intravenous infusion pain Pain at the site of cytotoxic infusion is a common problem. Four pain syndromes related to intravenous infusion of chemotherapeutic agents are recognized: venous spasm, chemical phlebitis, vesicant extravasation, and anthracycline-associated flare. Venous spasm causes pain not associated with inflammation or phlebitis, and which may be modified by application of a warm compress or reduction of the rate of infusion. Chemical phlebitis can be caused by cytotoxic medications including amasarcine, decarbazine, and carmustine (Hundrieser 1988, Mrozek-Orlowski et al 1991), vinorelbine (Rittenberg et al 1995), as well as the infusion of potassium chloride and hyperosmolar solutions (Pucino et al 1988). The pain and linear erythema associated with chemical phlebitis must be distinguished from the more serious complication of a vesicant cytotoxic extravasation (Table 42.2) (Bertelli 1995, Boyle and Engelking 1995). Vesicant extravasation may produce intense pain followed by desquamation and ulceration (Bertelli 1995, Boyle and Engelking 1995). Finally, a brief venous flare reaction is often associated with intravenous administration of the anthracycline, doxorubicin. The flare is typically associated with local urticaria and occasional patients report pain or stinging (Vogelzang 1979, Curran et al 1990).

Table 42.2 Commonly used tissue vesicant cytotoxic drugs

Amasarcine
BCNU
cis-Platinum
Decarbazine
Daunorubicin
Doxorubicin
Etoposide
Mitomycin-C
Mitoxantrone (mitozantrone)
Streptozotocin
Teniposide
Vinblastine
Vincristine
Vindesine

Hepatic artery infusion pain Cytotoxic infusions into the hepatic artery (for patients with hepatic metastases) are often associated with the development of a diffuse abdominal pain (Kemeny 1991). Continuous infusions can lead to persistent pain. In some patients, the pain is due to the development of gastric ulceration or erosions (Shike et al 1986), or cholangitis (Batts 1998). If the latter complications do not occur, the pain usually resolves with discontinuation of the infusion. A dose relationship is suggested by the observation that some patients will comfortably tolerate reinitiating of the infusion at a lower dose (Kemeny 1992)

Intraperitoneal chemotherapy pain Abdominal pain is a common complication of intraperitoneal chemotherapy (IPC). A transient mild abdominal pain, associated with sensations of fullness or bloating, is reported by approximately 25% of patients (Almadrones and Yerys 1990). A further 25% of patients report moderate or severe pain, necessitating opioid analgesia or discontinuation of therapy (Almadrones and Yerys 1990). Moderate or severe pain is usually caused by chemical serositis or infection (Markman 1986). Drug selection may be a factor in the incidence of chemical serositis; it is a common complication of intraperitoneal of the anthracycline agents mitoxantrone (mitozantrone) and doxorubicin and with taxol, but it is relatively infrequent with 5-fluorouracil or *cis*-platinum. Abdominal pain associated with fever and leukocytosis in blood and peritoneal fluid is suggestive of infectious peritonitis (Kaplan et al 1985).

Intravesical chemo or immunotherapy Intravesical bacillus Calmette-Guerin (BCG) therapy for transitional cell carcinoma of the urinary bladder usually causes a transient bladder irritability syndrome characterized by frequency and/or micturition pain (Uekado et al 1994). Rarely, treatment may trigger a painful polyarthritis (Kudo et al 1991). Similarly, intravesical doxorubicin often causes a painful chemical cystitis (Matsumura et al 1992).

Acute pain associated with chemotherapy toxicity

Mucositis Severe mucositis is an almost invariable consequence of the myeloablative chemotherapy and radiotherapy that precedes bone marrow transplantation, but it is less common with standard intensity therapy (Rider 1990, Verdi 1993, Dose 1995). Damaged mucosal surfaces may become superinfected with microorganisms, such as candida albicans and herpes simplex. The latter complication is most likely in neutropenic patients, who are also predisposed to systemic sepsis arising from local invasion by aerobic and anaerobic oral flora.

Corticosteroid-induced perineal discomfort A transient burning sensation in the perineum is described by some patients following rapid infusion of large doses (20–100 mg) of dexamethasone (Bell 1988). Patients need to be warned that such symptoms may occur. Clinical experience suggests that this syndrome is prevented by slow infusion.

Steroid pseudorheumatism The withdrawal of corticosteroids may produce a pain syndrome that manifests as diffuse myalgias, arthralgias, and tenderness of muscles and joints. These symptoms occur with rapid or slow withdrawal and may occur in patients taking these drugs for long or short periods of time. Treatment consists of reinstituting the steroids at a higher dose and withdrawing them more slowly (Rotstein and Good 1957).

Painful peripheral neuropathy Chemotherapy-induced painful peripheral neuropathy, which is usually associated with vinca alkaloids, *cis*-platinum, and paclitaxel can have an acute course. The vinca alkaloids (particularly vincristine) are also associated with other, presumably neuropathic acute pain syndromes, including pain in the jaw, legs, arms, or abdomen that may last from hours to days (Sandler et al 1969, Rosenthal and Kaufman 1974, McCarthy and Skillings 1992). Vincristine-induced orofacial pain in the distribution of the trigeminal and glossopharyngeal nerves occurs in approximately 50% of patients at the onset of vincristine treatment (McCarthy and Skillings 1992). The pain, which is severe in about half of those affected, generally begins 2–3 days after vincristine administration and lasts for 1–3 days. It is usually self-limiting and if recurrence occurs, it is usually mild (McCarthy and Skillings 1992). The neuropathy associated with paclitaxel neuropathy is dose related and is generally subacute in onset with a tendency to resolution after the completion of therapy (Postma et al 1995).

Headache Intrathecal methotrexate in the treatment of leukaemia or leptomeningeal metastases produces an acute meningitic syndrome in 5–50% of patients (Weiss et al 1974). Headache is the prominent symptom and may be associated with vomiting, nuchal rigidity, fever, irritability, and lethargy. Symptoms usually begin hours after intrathecal treatment and persist for several days.

Cerebrospinal fluid (CSF) examination reveals a pleocytosis that may mimic bacterial meningitis. Patients at increased risk for the development of this syndrome include those who have received multiple intrathecal injections and those patients undergoing treatment for proven leptomeningeal metastases (Weiss et al 1974). The syndrome tends not to recur with subsequent injections.

Systemic administration of L-asparaginase for the treatment of acute lymphoblastic leukaemia produces thrombosis of cerebral veins or dural sinuses in 1–2% of patients (Priest et al 1982). This complication typically occurs after a few weeks of therapy, but its onset may be delayed until after the completion of treatment. Headache is the most common initial symptom, and seizures, hemiparesis, delirium, vomiting, or cranial nerve palsies may also occur. The diagnosis may be established by angiography or by gradient echo sequences on MRI scan (Schick et al 1989).

trans-Retinoic acid therapy, which may be used in the treatment of acute promyelocytic leukaemia (APML), can cause a transient severe headache (Visani et al 1996). The mechanism may be related to pseudotumour cerebri induced by hypervitaminosis A.

Diffuse bone pain *trans*-Retinoic acid therapy in patients with APML often produces a syndrome of diffuse bone pain (Castaigne et al 1990, Ohno et al 1993). The pain is generalized, of variable intensity, and closely associated with a transient neutrophilia. The latter observation suggests that the pain may be due to marrow expansion, a phenomenon that may underlie a similar pain syndrome that occurs following the administration of colony-stimulating factors (Hollingshead and Goa 1991).

Taxol-induced arthralgia and myalgia Administration of paclitaxel generates a syndrome of diffuse arthralgias and myalgia in 10–20% of patients (Rowinsky et al 1993, Muggia et al 1995). Diffuse joint and muscle pains generally appear 1–4 days after drug administration and persist for 3–7 days.

5-Fluorouracil-induced anginal chest pain Patients receiving continuous infusions of 5-fluorouracil (5-FU) may develop ischaemic chest pain (Freeman and Costanza 1988). Continuous ambulatory electrocardiographic (ECG) monitoring of patients undergoing 5-FU infusion demonstrated a near threefold increase in ischaemic episodes over pre-treatment recordings (Rezkalla et al 1989); these ECG changes were more common among patients with known coronary artery disease. It is widely speculated that coronary vasospasm may be the underlying mechanism (Freeman and Costanza 1988, Rezkalla et al 1989, Eskilsson and Albertsson 1990).

Palmar–plantar erythrodysaesthesia syndrome Protracted infusion of 5-fluorouracil can be complicated by the development of a tingling or burning sensation in the palms and soles followed by the development of an erythematous rash. The rash is characterized by a painful, sharply demarcated, intense erythema of the palms and/or soles followed by bulla formation, desquamation, and healing. Continuous low-dose 5-FU infusion (200–300 $mg/m^2/day$) will produce this palmar–plantar erythrodysaesthesia syndrome in 40–90% of patients (Lokich and Moore 1984, Leo et al 1994). It occurs rarely with patients undergoing 96- to 120-h infusions (Bellmunt et al 1988). The pathogenesis is unknown. The eruption is self-limiting in nature and it does not usually require discontinuation of therapy. Symptomatic measures are often required (Bellmunt et al 1988), and treatment with pyridoxine has been reported to induce resolution of the lesions (Fabian et al 1990). Palmar–plantar erythrodysaesthesia caused by capecitabine, an orally administered 5-FU prodrug, may warrant discontinuation of therapy if severe (Dooley and Goa 1999). A similar syndrome has recently been reported with liposomal doxorubicin, which is thought to be relatively sequestered in skin (Alberts and Garcia 1997). As with 5-FU, this is also a dose-related adverse effect related to repeated dosing. Uncommonly, palmar–plantar erythrodysaesthesia has been observed with paclitaxel (Vukelja et al 1993).

Postchemotherapy gynaecomastia Painful gynaecomastia can occur as a delayed complication of chemotherapy. Testis cancer is the most common underlying disorder (Aki et al 1996), but it has been reported after therapy for other cancers as well (Glass and Berenberg 1979, Trump et al 1982). Gynaecomastia typically develops after a latency of 2–9 months and resolves spontaneously within a few months. Persistent gynaecomastia is occasionally observed (Trump et al 1982). Cytotoxic-induced disturbance of androgen secretion is the probable cause of this syndrome (Aki et al 1996). In the patient with testicular cancer, this syndrome must be differentiated from tumour-related gynaecomastia, which may be associated with early recurrence (see below) (Saeter et al 1987, Trump and Anderson 1983).

Chemotherapy-induced acute digital ischaemia Raynaud's phenomenon or transient ischaemia of the toes is a common complication of bleomycin, vinblastine, and cisplatin (PVB) treatment for testicular cancer (Aass et al 1990). Rarely, irreversible digital ischaemia leading to gangrene has been reported after bleomycin (Elomaa et al 1984).

Chemotherapy induced tumour pain Pain at the site of tumour is reported to occur in some patients (7%) after treatment with vinorelbine. Typically, pain begins within a few minutes of the vinorelbine infusion, is moderate to severe in intensity, and requires analgesic therapy. Premedication with ketorolac may prevent recurrence in some cases (Colleoni et al 1995, Kornek et al 1996, De Marco et al 1999).

Acute pain associated with hormonal therapy

Leutenizing hormone releasing factor (LHRF) tumour flare in prostate cancer Initiation of LHRF hormonal therapy for prostate cancer produces a transient symptom flare in 5–25% of patients (Chrisp and Goa 1991, Chrisp and Sorkin 1991). The flare is presumably caused by an initial stimulation of leutenizing hormone release before suppression is achieved. The syndrome typically presents as an exacerbation of bone pain or urinary retention; spinal cord compression and sudden death have been reported (Thompson et al 1990). Symptom flare is usually observed within the first week of therapy, and lasts 1–3 weeks in the absence of androgen antagonist therapy. Coadministration of an androgen antagonist during the initiation of LHRF agonist therapy can prevent this phenomenon (Labrie et al 1987). Among patients with prostate cancer that is refractory to first-line hormonal therapy, transient tumour flares have been observed with androstenedione (Shearer et al 1990, Davies et al 1992) and medroxyprogesterone (Fossa and Urnes 1986).

Hormone-induced pain flare in breast cancer Any hormonal therapy for metastatic breast cancer can be complicated by a sudden onset of diffuse musculoskeletal pain commencing within hours to weeks of the initiation of therapy (Plotkin et al 1978). Other manifestations of this syndrome include erythema around cutaneous metastases, changes in liver function studies, and hypercalcaemia. Although the underlying mechanism is not understood, this does not appear to be caused by tumour stimulation, and it is speculated that it may reflect normal tissue response (Reddel and Sutherland 1984).

Acute pain associated with immunotherapy

Interferon (IFN)-induced acute pain Virtually all patients treated with IFN experience an acute syndrome consisting of fever, chills, myalgias, arthralgias, and headache (Quesada et al 1986). The syndrome usually begins shortly after initial dosing and frequently improves with continued administration of the drug (Quesada et al 1986). The severity of symptoms is related to type of IFN, route of administration, schedule, and dose. Doses of 1–9 million units of α-interferon are usually well tolerated, but doses greater than or equal to 18 million units usually produce moderate to severe toxicity (Quesada et al 1986). Acetaminophen pretreatment is often useful in ameliorating these symptoms.

Acute pain associated with bisphosphonates

Bisphosphonate-induced bone pain Bisphosphonates are widely used in the care of patients with bony metastases, especially among patients with breast cancer and myeloma (Hillner et al 2000). Infusion of bisphosphonates is sometimes associated with the development of multifocal bone pain and/or myalgia. Typically, pain occurs within 24 h of infusion and may last up to 3 days. Pain intensity is variable and may be severe. The condition is self-limiting but may require analgesic therapy (Coukell and Markham 1998).

Acute pain associated with growth factors

Colony-stimulating factors (CSFs) are haematopoietic growth hormones that stimulate the production, maturation, and function of white blood cells. Granulocyte-macrophage CSF (GM-CSF) and granulocyte CSF (G-CSF) and interleukin-3 commonly produce mild to moderate bone pain and constitutional symptoms such as fever, headache, and myalgias during the period of administration (Veldhuis et al 1995, Vial and Descotes 1995). Subcutaneous administration of r-HuEPO alpha is associated with pain at the injection site in about 40% of cases (Frenken et al 1991). Subcutaneous injection of r-HuEPO alpha is more painful than r-HuEPO beta (Morris et al 1994). Alpha erythropoietin injection pain can be reduced by dilution of the vehicle with benzyl alcohol saline, reduction of the volume of the vehicle to 1.0 to 0.1 ml (Frenken et al 1994) or addition of lidocaine (lignocaine) (Alon et al 1994).

Acute pain associated with radiotherapy

Incident pains can be precipitated by transport and positioning of the patient for radiotherapy. Other pains can be caused by acute radiation toxicity, which is most commonly associated with inflammation and ulceration of skin or mucous membranes within the radiation port. The syndrome produced is dependent upon the involved field: head and neck irradiation can cause a stomatitis or pharyngitis (Rider 1990), treatment of the chest and oesophagus can cause an oesophagitis (Vanagunas et al 1990), and pelvic therapy can cause a proctitis, cystitis-urethritis, vaginal ulceration, or radiation dermatitis.

Oropharyngeal mucositis Radiotherapy-induced mucositis is invariable with doses above 1000 cGy, and ulceration is common at doses above 4000 cGy. Although the severity of the associated pain is variable, it is often severe enough to interfere with oral alimentation. Painful mucositis can persist for several weeks after the completion of the treatment (Rider 1990, Epstein and Stewart 1993).

Acute radiation enteritis and proctocolitis Acute radiation enteritis occurs in as many as 50% of patients receiving abdominal or pelvic radiotherapy. Involvement of the small intestine can present with cramping abdominal pain associated with nausea and diarrhoea (Yeoh and Horowitz 1988). Pelvic radiotherapy can cause a painful proctocolitis, with tenesmoid pain associated with diarrhoea, mucous discharge, and bleeding (Babb 1996). These complications typically resolve shortly after completion of therapy, but may have a slow resolution over 2–6 months (Yeoh and Horowitz 1988, Nussbaum et al 1993, Babb 1996). Acute enteritis is associated with an increased risk of late onset radiation enteritis (see below).

Early onset brachial plexopathy A transient brachial plexopathy has been described in breast cancer patients immediately following radiotherapy to the chest wall and adjacent nodal areas. In retrospective studies, the incidence of this phenomenon has been variably estimated as 1.4–20% (Salner et al 1981, Pierce et al 1992); clinical experience suggests that lower estimates are more accurate. The median latency to the development of symptoms was 4.5 months (3–14 months) in one survey (Salner et al 1981). Paraesthesias are the most common presenting symptom, and pain and weakness occur less frequently. The syndrome is self-limiting and does not predispose to the subsequent development of delayed onset, progressive plexopathy.

Subacute radiation myelopathy Subacute radiation myelopathy is an uncommon phenomenon that may occur following radiotherapy of extraspinal tumours (Ang and Stephens 1994, Schultheiss 1994). It is most frequently observed involving the cervical cord after radiation treatment of head and neck cancers and Hodgkin's disease. In the latter case, patients develop painful, shock-like pains in the neck that are precipitated by neck flexion (Lhermitte's sign); these pains may radiate down the spine and into one or more extremities. The syndrome usually begins weeks to months after the completion of radiotherapy, and typically resolves over a period of 3–6 months (Ang and Stephens 1994).

Radiopharmaceutical-induced pain flare Strontium-89, Rhenium-186 hydroxyethylidene diphosphonate, and Samarium-153 are systemically administered beta-emitting calcium analogues taken up by bone in areas of osteoblastic activity and which may help relieve pain caused by blastic bony metastases (McEwan 1997). A 'flare' response, characterized by transient worsening of pain 1–2 days after administration, occurs in 15–20% of patients (Robinson et al 1995). This flare usually resolves after 3–5 days and most affected patients subsequently develop a good analgesic response (Robinson et al 1995).

Acute pain associated with infection

Acute herpetic neuralgia

A significantly increased incidence of acute herpetic neuralgia occurs among cancer patients, especially those with haematological or lymphoproliferative malignancies and those receiving immunosuppressive therapies (Portenoy et al 1986, Rusthoven et al 1988). Pain or itch usually precedes the development of the rash by several days and may occasionally occur without the development of skin eruption (Portenoy et al 1986, Galer and Portenoy 1991). The pain, which may be continuous or lancinating, usually resolves within 2 months (Galer and Portenoy 1991). Pain persisting beyond this interval is referred to as postherpetic neuralgia (see below). Patients with active tumour are more likely to have a disseminated infection (Rusthoven et al 1988). In those predisposed by chemotherapy, the infection usually develops less than 1 month after the completion of treatment. The dermatomal location of the infection is often associated with the site of the malignancy (Rusthoven et al 1988). Patients with primary tumours of gynaecologic and genitourinary origin have a predilection to lumbar and sacral involvement, and those with breast or lung carcinomas tend to present with thoracic involvement; patients with haematologic tumours appear to be predisposed to cervical lesions. The infection also occurs twice as frequently in previously irradiated dermatomes as non-radiated areas.

Acute pain associated with vascular events

Acute thrombosis pain

Thrombosis is the most frequent complication and the second cause of death in patients with overt malignant disease (Donati 1994). Thrombotic episodes may precede the diagnosis of cancer by months or years and represent a potential marker for occult malignancy (Agnelli 1997). Postoperative deep vein thrombosis is more frequent in patients operated for malignant diseases than for other disorders, and both chemotherapy and hormone therapy are associated with an increased thrombotic risk (Agnelli 1997).

Possible prothrombic factors in cancer include the capacity of tumour cells and their products to interact with platelets, clotting and fibrinolytic systems, endothelial cells, and tumour-associated macrophages. Cytokine release, acute phase reaction, and neovascularization may contribute to in vivo clotting activation (Donati 1994, Agnelli 1997). Patients with pelvic tumours (Clarke-Pearson and Olt 1989), pancreatic cancer (Heinmoller et al 1995), gastric cancer, advanced breast cancer (Levine et al 1994), and brain tumours (Sawaya and Ligon 1994) are at greatest risk.

Lower-extremity deep venous thrombosis Pain and swelling are the commonest presenting features of lower-extremity deep vein thrombosis (Criado and Burnham 1997). The pain is variable in severity and it is often mild. It is commonly described as a dull cramp, or diffuse heaviness. The pain most commonly affects the calf but may involve the sole of the foot, the heel, the thigh, the groin or pelvis. Pain usually increases on standing and walking. On examination, suggestive features include swelling, warmth, dilatation of superficial veins, tenderness along venous tracts, and pain induced by stretching (Criado and Burnham 1997).

Rarely patients may develop tissue ischaemia or frank gangrene, even without arterial or capillary occlusion; this syndrome is called phlegmasia cerulea dolens. It is most commonly seen in patients with underlying neoplasm (Hirschmann 1987, Lorimer et al 1994) and is characterized by severe pain, extensive oedema, and cyanosis of the legs. Gangrene can occur unless the venous obstruction is relieved. When possible, optimal therapy is anticoagulation and thrombectomy (Perkins et al 1996). The mortality rate for ischaemic venous thrombosis is about 40%, the cause of death usually being the underlying disease or pulmonary emboli (Hirschmann 1987).

Upper-extremity deep venous thrombosis Only 2% of all cases of deep venous thrombosis involve the upper extremity, and the incidence of pulmonary embolism related to thrombosis in this location is approximately 12% (Nemmers et al 1990). The three major clinical features of upper-extremity venous thrombosis are oedema, dilated collateral circulation, and pain (Burihan et al 1993). Approximately two-thirds of patients have arm pain. Among patients with cancer the most common causes are central venous catheterization and extrinsic compression by tumour (Burihan et al 1993). Although thrombosis secondary to intrinsic damage usually responds well to anticoagulation alone and rarely causes persistent symptoms, when extrinsic obstruction is the cause, persistent arm swelling and pain are commonplace (Donayre et al 1986).

Superior vena cava obstruction Superior vena cava (SVC) obstruction is most commonly caused by extrinsic compression by enlarged mediastinal lymph nodes (Escalante 1993). In contemporary series lung cancer and lymphomas are the most commonly associated conditions. Increasingly, thrombosis of the superior vena cava is caused by intravascular devices (Morales et al 1997), particularly with left-sided ports and when the catheter tip lies in the upper part of the vena (Puel et al 1993). Patient usually present with facial swelling and dilated neck and chest wall veins. Chest pain, headache, and mastalgia are less common presentations.

Acute mesenteric vein thrombosis Acute mesenteric vein thrombosis is most commonly associated with hypercoaguability states. Rarely it has been associated with extrinsic venous compression by malignant lymphdenopathy (Traill and Nolan 1997), extension of venous thrombosis (Vigo et al 1980), or as a result of iatrogenic hypercoaguable state (Sahdev et al 1985).

Chronic pain syndromes

Most chronic cancer-related pains are caused directly by the tumour (Table 42.3). Data from the largest prospective survey of cancer pain syndromes

Table 42.3 Cancer-related chronic pain syndromes

Tumour-related pain syndromes

- Bone pain
  - Multifocal or generalized bone pain
    - Multiple bony metastases
    - Marrow expansion
  - Vertebral syndromes
    - Atlantoaxial destruction and odontoid fractures
    - C7–T1 syndrome
    - T12–L1 syndrome
    - Sacral syndrome
  - Back pain and epidural compression
  - Pain syndromes of the bony pelvis and hip
    - Hip joint syndrome
  - Acrometastases

- Arthritides
  - Hypertrophic pulmonary osteoarthropathy
  - Other polyarthritides

- Muscle pain
  - Muscle cramps
  - Skeletal muscle tumours

- Headache and facial pain
  - Intracerebral tumour
  - Leptomeningeal metastases
  - Base of skull metastases
    - Orbital syndrome
    - Parasellar syndrome
    - Middle cranial fossa syndrome
    - Jugular foramen syndrome
    - Occipital condyle syndrome
    - Clivus syndrome
    - Sphenoid sinus syndrome
  - Painful cranial neuralgias
    - Glossopharyngeal neuralgia
    - Trigeminal neuralgia

- Tumour involvement of the peripheral nervous system
  - Tumour-related radiculopathy
    - Postherpetic neuralgia
  - Cervical plexopathy
  - Brachial plexopathy
    - Malignant brachial plexopathy
    - Idiopathic brachial plexopathy associated with Hodgkin's disease
  - Malignant lumbosacral plexopathy
  - Tumour-related mononeuropathy
  - Paraneoplastic painful peripheral neuropathy
    - Subacute sensory neuropathy
    - Sensorimotor peripheral neuropathy

- Pain syndromes of the viscera and miscellaneous tumour-related syndromes
  - Hepatic distension syndrome
  - Midline retroperitoneal syndrome
  - Chronic intestinal obstruction
  - Peritoneal carcinomatosis
  - Malignant perineal pain
    - Malignant pelvic floor myalgia
  - Adrenal pain syndrome
  - Ureteric obstruction
  - Ovarian cancer pain
  - Lung cancer pain

Table 42.3 Cancer-related chronic pain syndromes (*cont'd*)

- Paraneoplastic nociceptive pain syndromes
  - Tumour-related gynaecomastia
  - Paraneoplastic pemphigus

Chronic pain syndromes associated with cancer therapy

- Postchemotherapy pain syndromes
  - Chronic painful peripheral neuropathy
  - Avascular necrosis of femoral or humeral head
  - Plexopathy associated with intraarterial infusion
  - Raynaud's phenomenon

- Chronic pain associated with hormonal therapy
  - Gynaecomastia with hormonal therapy for prostate cancer

- Chronic postsurgical pain syndromes
  - Postmastectomy pain syndrome
  - Postradical neck dissection pain
  - Post-thoracotomy pain
  - Postoperatve frozen shoulder
  - Phantom pain syndromes
    - Phantom limb pain
    - Phantom breast pain
    - Phantom anus pain
    - Phantom bladder pain
  - Stump pain
  - Postsurgical pelvic floor myalgia

- Chronic postradiation pain syndromes
  - Plexopathies
    - Radiation-induced brachial and lumbosacral plexopathies
    - Radiation-induced peripheral nerve tumour
  - Chronic radiation myelopathy
  - Chronic radiation enteritis and proctitis
  - Burning perineum syndrome
  - Osteoradionecrosis

revealed that almost one-quarter of the patients experienced two or more pains. Over 90% of the patients had one or more tumour-related pains and 21% had one or more pains caused by cancer therapies. Somatic pains (71%) were more common than neuropathic (39%) or visceral pains (34%) (Caraceni and Portenoy 1999). Bone pain and compression of neural structures are the two most common causes (Banning et al 1991, Daut and Cleeland 1982, Foley 1987a, Grond et al 1996, Twycross et al 1996).

Bone pain

Bone metastases are the most common cause of chronic pain in cancer patients (Banning et al 1991, Daut and Cleeland 1982, Foley 1987a, Grond et al 1996, Twycross et al 1996). Cancers of the lung, breast, and prostate most often metastasize to bone, but any tumour type may be complicated by painful bony lesions. Although bone pain is usually associated with direct tumour invasion of bony structures, more than 25% of patients with bony metastases are pain-free (Wagner 1984), and patients with multiple bony metastases typically report pain in only a few sites. The factors that convert a painless lesion to a painful one are unknown. Bone metastases could potentially cause pain by any of multiple mechanisms, including endosteal or periosteal nociceptor activation (by mechanical distortion or release of chemical mediators) or tumour growth into adjacent soft tissues and nerves (Mercadante 1997). Recent studies have demonstrated that tumour osteolysis may be mediated by a cascade involving the secretion of tumour-produced parathyroid hormone-related protein (PTHrP), which stimulates osteoclastic bone resorption, thus releasing transforming growth factor beta (TGF-β), which is abundant in bone matrix. The released TGF-β further promotes osteolysis by stimulating PTHrP production by tumour cells (Guise 2000).

Bone pain due to metastatic tumour needs to be differentiated from less common causes. Non-neoplastic causes in this population include osteoporotic fractures (including those associated with multiple myeloma), focal osteonecrosis, which may be idiopathic or related to chemotherapy, corticosteroids (Socie et al 1997) or radiotherapy (see below) and osteomalacia (Shane et al 1997).

Multifocal or generalized bone pain

Bone pain may be focal, multifocal, or generalized. Multifocal bone pains are most commonly experienced by patients with multiple bony metastases. A generalized pain syndrome is also rarely produced by replacement of bone marrow (Jonsson et al 1990, Wong et al 1993). This bone marrow replacement syndrome has been observed in haematogenous malignancies (Golembe et al 1979, Lembersky et al 1988) and, less commonly, solid tumours (Wong et al 1993). This syndrome can occur in the absence of abnormalities on bone scintigraphy or radiography, increasing the difficulty of diagnosis. Rarely, a paraneoplastic osteomalacia can mimic multiple metastases (Shane et al 1997).

Vertebral syndromes

The vertebrae are the most common sites of bony metastases. More than two-thirds of vertebral metastases are located in the thoracic spine; lumbosacral and cervical metastases account for approximately 20 and 10%, respectively (Gilbert et al 1978, Sorensen et al 1990). Multiple-level involvement is common, occurring in greater than 85% of patients (Constans et al 1983). The early recognition of pain syndromes due to tumour invasion of vertebral bodies is essential, since pain usually precedes compression of adjacent neural structures and prompt treatment of the lesion may prevent the subsequent development of neurologic deficits. Several factors often confound accurate diagnosis, referral of pain is common, and the associated symptoms and signs can mimic a variety of other disorders, both malignant (e.g., paraspinal masses) and non-malignant.

Atlantoaxial destruction and odontoid fracture Nuchal or occipital pain is the typical presentation of destruction of the atlas or fracture of the odontoid process. Pain often radiates over the posterior aspect of the skull to the vertex and is exacerbated by movement of the neck, particularly flexion (Phillips and Levine 1989). Pathologic fracture may result in secondary subluxation with compression of the spinal cord at the cervico-medullary junction. This complication is usually insidious and may begin with symptoms or signs in one or more extremity. Typically, there is early involvement of the upper extremities and the occasional appearance of so-called 'pseudo-levels' suggestive of more caudal spinal lesions; these deficits can slowly progress to involve sensory, motor, and autonomic functions (Sundaresan et al 1981). MRI is probably the best method for imaging this region of the spine (Bosley et al 1985), but clinical experience suggests that CT is also sensitive. Plain radiography, tomography, and bone scintigraphy should be viewed as ancillary procedures.

C7–T1 syndrome Invasion of the C7 or T1 vertebra can result in pain referred to the interscapular region. These lesions may be missed if radiographic evaluation is mistakenly targeted to the painful area caudal to the site of damage. Additionally, visualization of the appropriate region on routine radiographs may be inadequate due to obscuration by overlying bone and mediastinal shadows. Patients with interscapular pain should therefore undergo radiography of both the cervical and the thoracic spine. Bone scintigraphy may assist in targeting additional diagnostic imaging procedures, such as CT or MRI. The latter procedures can be useful in assessing the possibility that pain is referred from an extraspinal site, such as the paraspinal gutter.

T12–L1 syndrome A T12 or L1 vertebral lesion can refer pain to the ipsilateral iliac crest or the sacroiliac joint. Imaging procedures directed at pelvic bones can miss the source of the pain.

Sacral syndrome Severe focal pain radiating to buttocks, perineum, or posterior thighs may accompany destruction of the sacrum (Hall and Fleming 1970, Feldenzer et al 1989, Porter et al 1994). The pain is often exacerbated by sitting or lying and is relieved by standing or walking. The neoplasm can spread laterally to involve muscles that rotate the hip (e.g., the pyriformis muscle). This may produce severe incident pain induced by motion of the hip, or a malignant 'pyriformis syndrome', characterized by buttock or posterior leg pain exacerbated by internal rotation of the hip. Local extension of the tumour mass may also involve the sacral plexus.

Imaging investigations of bone pain

The two most important imaging modalities for the evaluation of bone pain are plain radiography and nuclear bone scan. In general, CT and MRI scans are reserved for situations when the diagnosis cannot be discerned from clinical information and these baseline tests or when there are specific diagnostic issues to be resolved that require special techniques. Imaging investigations of bone pain are discussed in Cherny and Portenoy (1999).

Back pain and epidural compression (EC)

Epidural compression of the spinal cord or cauda equina is the second most common neurologic complication of cancer, occurring in up to 10% of patients (Posner 1987). In the community setting, EC is often the first recognized manifestation of malignancy (Stark et al 1982); at a cancer hospital it is the presenting syndrome in only 8% of cases (Posner 1987). Most EC is caused by posterior extension of vertebral body metastasis to the epidural space. Occasionally, EC is caused by tumour extension from the posterior arch of the vertebra or infiltration of a paravertebral tumour through the intervertebral foramen.

Untreated, EC leads inevitably to neurological damage. Effective treatment can potentially prevent these complications. The most important determinate of the efficacy of treatment is the degree of neurological impairment at the time therapy is initiated. Seventy-five percent of patients who begin treatment while ambulatory remain so; the efficacy of treatment declines to 30–50% for those who begin treatment while markedly paretic, and is 10–20% for those who are plegic (Gilbert et al 1978, Barcena et al 1984, Portenoy et al 1989, Ruff and Lanska 1989, Rosenthal et al 1992, Maranzano and Latini 1995, Huddart et al 1997, Milross et al 1997, Razak and Sappani 1998, Cowap et al 2000). Despite this, delays in diagnosis are commonplace (Husband 1998).

Back pain is the initial symptom in almost all patients with EC (Posner 1987), and in 10% it is the only symptom at the time of diagnosis (Greenberg et al 1980) Since pain usually precedes neurologic signs by a prolonged period, it should be viewed as a potential indicator of EC, which can lead to treatment at a time that a favourable response is most likely. Back pain, however, is a non-specific symptom that can result from bony or paraspinal metastases without epidural encroachment, from retroperitoneal or leptomeningeal tumour, epidural lipomatosis due to steroid administration (Stranjalis et al 1992), or from a large variety of other benign conditions. Since it is infeasible to pursue an extensive evaluation in every cancer patient who develops back pain, the complaint should impel an evaluation that determines the likelihood of EC and thereby selects patients appropriate for definitive imaging of the epidural space. The selection process is based on symptoms and signs and the results of simple imaging techniques.

Clinical features of epidural extension Some pain characteristics are particularly suggestive of epidural extension (Helweg-Larsen and Sorensen 1994). Rapid progression of back pain in a crescendo pattern is an ominous occurrence (Rosenthal et al 1992). Radicular pain, which can be constant or lancinating, has similar implications (Helweg-Larsen and Sorensen 1994). It is usually unilateral in the cervical and lumbosacral regions and bilateral in the thorax, where it is often experienced as a tight, belt-like band across the chest or abdomen (Helweg-Larsen and Sorensen 1994). The likelihood of EC is also greater when back or radicular pain is exacerbated by recumbency, cough, sneeze, or strain (Ruff and Lanska 1989). Other types of referred pain are also suggestive, including Lhermitte's sign (Ventafridda et al 1991) and central pain from spinal cord compression, which usually is perceived some distance below the site of the compression and is typically a poorly localized, non-dermatomal dysaesthesia (Posner 1987).

Weakness, sensory loss, autonomic dysfunction, and reflex abnormalities usually occur after a period of progressive pain (Helweg-Larsen and Sorensen 1994). Weakness may begin segmentally if related to nerve root damage or in a multisegmental or pyramidal distribution if the cauda equina or spinal cord, respectively, is injured. The rate of progression of weakness is variable; in the absence of treatment, following the onset of weakness one-third of patients will develop paralysis within 7 days (Barron et al 1959). Patients whose weakness progresses slowly have a better prognosis for neurologic recovery with treatment than those who progress rapidly (Helweg-Larsen et al 1990, Helweg-Larsen 1996). Without effective treatment, sensory abnormalities, which may also begin segmentally, may ultimately evolve to a sensory level, with complete loss of all sensory modalities below site of injury. The upper level of sensory findings may correspond to the location of the epidural tumour or be below it by many segments (Helweg-Larsen and Sorensen 1994). Ataxia without pain is the initial presentation of epidural compression in 1% of patients; this finding is presumably due to early involvement of the spinocerebellar tracts (Gilbert et al 1978). Bladder and bowel dysfunction occur late, except in patients with a conus medullaris lesion who may present with acute urinary retention and constipation without preceding motor or sensory symptoms (Helweg-Larsen and Sorensen 1994).

Other features that may be evident on examination of patients with EC include scoliosis, asymmetrical wasting of paravertebral musculature, and a gibbus (palpable step in the spinous processes). Spinal tenderness to percussion, which may be severe, often accompanies the pain.

Imaging modalities Definitive imaging of the epidural space confirms the existence of EC (and thereby indicates the necessity and urgency of treatment), defines the appropriate radiation portals, and determines the extent of epidural encroachment (which influences prognosis and may alter the therapeutic approach) (Portenoy et al 1987). The options for definitive imaging include MRI, myelography, and CT-myelography or spiral CT without myelographic contrast, and are discussed in Cherny and Portenoy (1999).

Algorithm for the investigation of cancer patients with back pain Given the prevalence and the potential for dire consequences of EC, and the recognition that back pain is a marker of early (and therefore treatable) EC, algorithms to guide the evaluation of back pain in the cancer patient have been developed. The objective of these algorithms is to select a subgroup of patients who should undergo definitive imaging of the epidural space from amongst the large number of patients who develop back pain (Portenoy et al 1987). Effective treatment of EC before irreversible neurological compromise occurs is the overriding goal of these approaches.

One such algorithm defines both the urgency and course of the evaluation (Fig. 42.1). Patients with emerging symptoms and signs indicative of spinal cord or cauda equina dysfunction are designated Group 1. The evaluation (and if appropriate, treatment) of these patients should proceed on an emergency basis. In most cases, these patients should receive an intravenous dose of corticosteroid before epidural imaging is performed.

Patients with symptoms and signs of radiculopathy or stable or mild signs of spinal cord or cauda equina dysfunction are designated Group 2. These patients are also usually treated presumptively with a corticosteroid and are scheduled for definitive imaging of the epidural space as soon as possible. Group 3 patients have back pain and no symptoms or signs suggesting EC. These patients should be evaluated in routine fashion starting with plain spine radiographs. The presence at the appropriate level of any abnormality consistent with neoplasm indicates a high probability (60%) of EC (Rodichok et al 1986, Hill et al 1993). This likelihood varies, however, with the type of radiological abnormality; for example, one study noted that EC occurred in 87% of patients with greater than 50% vertebral body collapse, 31% with pedicle erosion, and only 7% with tumour limited to the body of the vertebra without collapse (Graus et al 1986). Definitive imaging of the epidural space is thus strongly indicated in patients who have > 50% vertebral body collapse, and is generally recommended for patients with pedicle erosion. Some patients with neoplasm limited to the vertebral body can be followed expectantly; imaging should be performed if pain progresses or changes (e.g., become radicular), or if radiographic evidence of progression is obtained.

Among patients with vertebral collapse it is often difficult to distinguish malignant from non-malignant pathology. Vertebral metastases are suggested by destruction of the anterolateral or posterior cortical bone of the vertebral body, the cancellous bone or vertebral pedicle, a focal paraspinal soft-tissue mass, and an epidural mass. Non-malignant causes are suggested by cortical fractures of the vertebral body without cortical bone destruction, retropulsion of a fragment of the posterior cortex of the vertebral body into the spinal canal, fracture lines within the cancellous bone of the vertebral body, an intravertebral vacuum phenomenon, and a thin diffuse paraspinal soft-tissue mass (Laredo et al 1995). For further details see Cherny and Portenoy (1999).

Pain syndromes of the bony pelvis and hip

The pelvis and hip are common sites of metastatic involvement. Lesions may involve any of the three

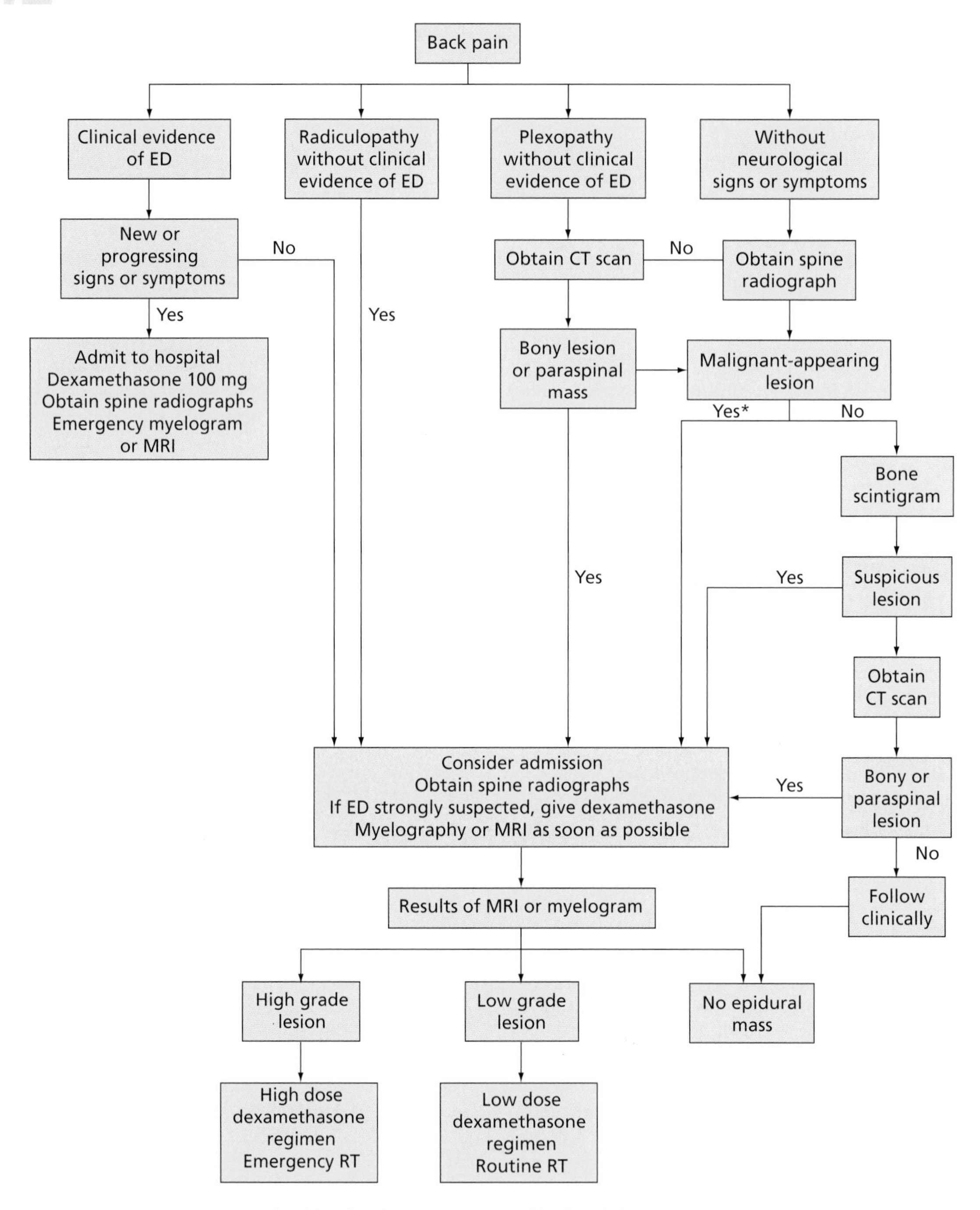

Fig. 42.1 Algorithm for the management of back pain in the cancer patient.

anatomic regions of the pelvis (ischiopubic, iliosacral, or periacetabular), the hip joint itself, or the proximal femur (Sim 1992). The weight-bearing function of these structures, essential for normal ambulation, contributes to the propensity of disease at these sites to cause incident pain with ambulation.

Hip joint syndrome Tumour involvement of the acetabulum or head of femur typically produces localized hip pain that is aggravated by weight bearing and movement of the hip. The pain may radiate to the knee or medial thigh, and occasionally, pain is limited to these structures

(Graham 1976, Sim 1992). Medial extension of an acetabular tumour can involve the lumbosacral plexus as it traverses the pelvic sidewall.

Acrometastases

Acrometastases, metastases in the hands and feet, are rare and often misdiagnosed or overlooked (Healey et al 1986). In the feet, the larger bones containing the higher amounts of red marrow, such as the os calcis, are usually involved (Freedman and Henderson 1995). Symptoms may be vague and can mimic other conditions, such as osteomyelitis, gouty rheumatoid arthritis, Reiter's syndrome, Paget's disease, osteochondral lesions, and ligamentous sprains.

Arthritides

Hypertrophic pulmonary osteoarthropathy

Hypertrophic pulmonary osteoarthropathy (HPOA) is a paraneoplastic syndrome that incorporates clubbing of the fingers, periostitis of long bones, and occasionally a rheumatoid-like polyarthritis (Martinez-Lavin 1997). Periosteitis and arthritis can produce pain, tenderness, and swelling in the knees, wrists, and ankles. The onset of symptoms is usually subacute, and it may proceed the discovery of the underlying neoplasm by several months. It is most commonly associated with non-small cell lung cancer. Less commonly it is associated with benign mesothelioma (Briselli et al 1981), pulmonary metastases from other sites (Davies et al 1991), smooth muscle tumours of the oesophagus (Kaymakcalan et al 1980), breast cancer (Shapiro 1987), and metastatic nasopharyngeal cancer (Daly 1995). Effective antitumour therapy is sometimes associated with symptom regression (Hung et al 2000). HPOA is diagnosed on the basis of physical findings, radiological appearance, and radionuclide bone scan (Greenfield et al 1967, Sharma 1995, Martinez-Lavin 1997).

Other polyarthritides

Rarely, rheumatoid arthritis, systemic lupus erythematosus, and an asymmetrical polyarthritis may occur as paraneoplastic phenomena that resolve with effective treatment of the underlying disease (Pines et al 1984, Rogues et al 1993). A syndrome of palmar–plantar fasciitis and polyarthritis, characterized by palmar and digital with polyarticular painful capsular contractions, has been associated with ovarian (Shiel et al 1985) and breast (Saxman and Seitz 1997) cancers.

Muscle pain

Muscle cramps

Persistent muscle cramps in cancer patients are usually caused by an identifiable neural, muscular, or biochemical abnormality (Siegal 1991). In one series of 50 patients, 22 had peripheral neuropathy, 17 had root or plexus pathology (including 6 with leptomeningeal metastases), 2 had polymyositis, and 1 had hypomagnesaemia. In this series, muscle cramps were the presenting symptom of recognizable and previously unsuspected neurologic dysfunction in 64% (27 of 42) of the identified causes (Steiner and Siegal 1989).

Skeletal muscle tumours

Soft-tissue sarcomas arising from fat, fibrous tissue, or skeletal muscle are the most common tumours involving the skeletal muscles. Skeletal muscle is one of the most unusual sites of metastasis from any malignancy (Sridhar et al 1987, Araki et al 1994). Lesions are usually painless but they may present with persistent ache.

Headache and facial pain

Headache in the cancer patient results from traction, inflammation, or infiltration of pain-sensitive structures in the head or neck. Early evaluation with appropriate imaging techniques may identify the lesion and allow prompt treatment, which may reduce pain and prevent the development of neurological deficits (Vecht et al 1992).

Intracerebral tumour

Among 183 patients with new onset chronic headache, as an isolated symptom, investigation revealed underlying tumour in 15 cases (Vazquez-Barquero et al 1994). The prevalence of headache in patients with brain metastases or primary brain tumours is 60–90% (Forsyth and Posner 1993, Suwanwela et al 1994). The headache is presumably produced by traction on pain-sensitive vascular and dural tissues. Patients with multiple metastases and those with posterior fossa metastases are more likely to report this symptom (Forsyth and Posner 1993). The pain may be focal, overlying the site of the lesion, or generalized. Headache has lateralizing value, especially in patients with supratentorial lesions (Suwanwela et al 1994). Posterior fossa lesions often cause a bifrontal headache. The quality of the headache is usually throbbing or steady, and the intensity is usually mild to moderate (Suwanwela et al 1994).

Among children, clinical features predictive of underlying tumour include sleep-related headache, headache in the absence of a family history of migraine, vomiting, absence of visual symptoms, headache of less than 6 months duration, confusion, and abnormal neurologic examination findings (Medina et al 1997).

The headache is often worse in the morning and is exacerbated by stooping, sudden head movement, or valsalva manoeuvres (cough, sneeze, or strain) (Suwanwela et al 1994). In patients with increased intracranial pressure, these manoeuvres can also precipitate transient elevations in intracranial pressure called 'plateau waves'. These plateau waves, which may also be spontaneous, can be associated with short periods of severe headache, nausea, vomiting, photophobia, lethargy, and transient neurological deficits (Matsuda et al 1979, Hayashi et al 1991). Occasionally these plateau waves produce life-threatening herniation syndromes (Matsuda et al 1979, Hayashi et al 1991).

Leptomeningeal metastases

Leptomeningeal metastases, which are characterized by diffuse or multifocal involvement of the subarachnoid space by metastatic tumour occur in 1–8% in patients with systemic cancer (Grossman and Krabak 1999). Non-Hodgkin's lymphoma and acute lymphocytic leukemia both demonstrate predilection for meningeal metastases (Grossman and Krabak 1999); the incidence is lower for solid tumours alone. Of solid tumours, adenocarcinomas of the breast and small cell lung cancer predominate (Jayson and Howell 1996).

Leptomeningeal metastases present with focal or multifocal neurological symptoms or signs that may involve any level of the neuraxis (Wasserstrom et al 1982, Grossman and Krabak 1999, van Oostenbrugge and Twijnstra 1999). More than one-third of patients present with evidence of cranial nerve damage, including double vision, hearing loss, facial numbness, and decreased vision (Wasserstrom et al 1982, van Oostenbrugge and Twijnstra 1999); this is particularly true among patients with underlying haematologic malignancy (van Oostenbrugge and Twijnstra 1999). Less common features include seizures, papilloedema, hemiparesis, ataxic gait, and confusion (Balm and Hammack 1996). Generalized headache and radicular pain in the low back and buttocks are the most common pains associated with leptomeningeal metastases (Wasserstrom et al 1982, Kaplan et al 1990, van Oostenbrugge and Twijnstra 1999). The headache is variable and may be associated with changes in mental status (e.g., lethargy, confusion, or loss of memory), nausea, vomiting, tinnitus, or nuchal rigidity. Pains that resemble cluster headache (DeAngelis and Payne 1987) or glossopharyngeal neuralgia with syncope (Sozzi et al 1987) have also been reported.

The diagnosis of leptomeningeal metastases is confirmed through analysis of the CSF, which may reveal elevated pressure, elevated protein, depressed glucose, and/or lymphocytic pleocytosis. Ninety percent of patients ultimately show positive cytology, but multiple evaluations may be required (see Cherny and Portenoy 1999).

Base of skull metastases

Base of skull metastases are associated with well-described clinical syndromes (Greenberg et al 1981), which are named according to the site of metastatic involvement: orbital, parasellar, middle fossa, jugular foramen, occipital condyle, clivus, and sphenoid sinus. Cancers of the breast, lung, and prostate are most commonly associated with this complication (Greenberg et al 1981, Hawley et al 1999), but any tumour type that metastasizes to bone may be responsible. When base of skull metastases are suspected, axial imaging with CT (including bone window settings) is the usual initial procedure (Greenberg et al 1981). MRI is more sensitive for assessing soft-tissue extension, and CSF analysis may be needed to exclude leptomeningeal metastases.

Orbital syndrome Orbital metastases usually present with progressive pain in the retro-orbital and supraorbital area of the affected eye. Blurred vision and diplopia may be associated complaints. Signs may include proptosis, chemosis of the involved eye, external ophthalmoparesis, ipsilateral papilloedema, and decreased sensation in the ophthalmic division of the trigeminal nerve. Imaging with MRI or CT scan can delineate the extent of bony damage and orbital infiltration.

Parasellar syndrome The parasellar syndrome typically presents as unilateral supraorbital and frontal headache, which may be associated with diplopia (Bitoh et al 1985). There may be ophthalmoparesis or papilloedema, and formal visual field testing may demonstrate hemianopsia or quadrantinopsia.

Middle cranial fossa syndrome The middle cranial fossa syndrome presents with facial numbness, paraesthesias, or pain, which is usually referred to the cheek or jaw (in the distribution of second or third divisions of the trigeminal nerve) (Lossos and Siegal 1992). The pain is typically described as a dull continual ache, but may also be paroxysmal or lancinating. On examination, patients may have hypaesthesia in the trigeminal nerve distribution and signs of weakness in the ipsilateral muscles of mastication. Occasional patients have other neurological signs, such as abducens palsy (Greenberg et al 1981, Bullitt et al 1986).

Jugular foramen syndrome The jugular foramen syndrome usually presents with hoarseness or dysphagia. Pain is usually referred to the ipsilateral ear or mastoid region and may occasionally present as glossopharyngeal neuralgia, with or without syncope (Greenberg et al 1981). Pain may also be referred to the ipsilateral neck or shoulder. Neurologic signs include ipsilateral Horner's syndrome, and paresis of the palate, vocal cord, sternocleidomastoid, or trapezius. Ipsilateral paresis of the tongue may also occur if the tumour extends to the region of the hypoglossal canal.

Occipital condyle syndrome The occipital condyle syndrome presents with unilateral occipital pain that is worsened with neck flexion (Loevner and Yousem 1997, Moris et al 1998). The patient may complain of neck stiffness. Pain intensity is variable, but can be severe. Examination may reveal a head tilt, limited movement of the neck, and tenderness to palpation over the occipitonuchal junction. Neurological findings may include ipsilateral hypoglossal nerve paralysis and sternocleidomastoid weakness.

Clivus syndrome The clivus syndrome is characterized by vertex headache, which is often exacerbated by neck flexion. Lower cranial nerve (VI–XII) dysfunction follows and may become bilateral.

Sphenoid sinus syndrome A sphenoid sinus metastasis often presents with bifrontal and/or retro-orbital pain, which may radiate to the temporal regions (Lawson and Reino 1997). There may be associated features of nasal congestion and diplopia. Physical examination is often unremarkable, although unilateral or bilateral sixth nerve paresis can be present.

Painful cranial neuralgias

As noted, specific cranial neuralgias can occur from metastases in the base of skull or leptomeninges. They are most commonly observed in patients with prostate and lung cancer (Gupta et al 1990). Invasion of the soft tissues of the head or neck or involvement of sinuses can also eventuate in such lesions. Each of these syndromes has a characteristic presentation. Early diagnosis may allow effective treatment of the underlying lesion before progressive neurologic injury occurs.

Glossopharyngeal neuralgia Glossopharyngeal neuralgia has been reported in patients with leptomeningeal metastases (Sozzi et al 1987), the jugular foramen syndrome (Greenberg et al 1981), or head and neck malignancies (Dykman et al 1981, Giorgi and Broggi 1984, Metheetrairut and Brown 1993). This syndrome presents as severe pain in the throat or neck, which may radiate to the ear or mastoid region. Pain may be induced by swallowing. In some patients, pain is associated with sudden orthostasis and syncope.

Trigeminal neuralgia Trigeminal pains may be continual, paroxysmal, or lancinating. Pain that mimics classical trigeminal neuralgia can be induced by tumours in the middle or posterior fossa (Bullitt et al 1986, Cheng et al 1993, Barker et al 1996, Hirota et al 1998) or leptomeningeal metastases (DeAngelis and Payne 1987). Continual pain in a trigeminal distribution may be an early sign of acoustic neuroma (Payten 1972). All cancer patients who develop trigeminal neuralgia should be evaluated for the existence of an underlying neoplasm.

Ear and eye pain syndromes

Otalgia Otalgia is the sensation of pain in the ear, while referred otalgia is pain felt in the ear but originating from a non-otologic source. The rich sensory innervation of the ear derives from four cranial nerves and two cervical nerves that also supply other areas in the head, neck, thorax, and abdomen. Pain referred to the ear may originate in areas far removed from the ear itself. Otalgia is reported among patients with carcinoma of the oropharynx or hypopharynx (Aird et al 1983, Talmi et al 1997), acoustic neuroma (Morrison and Sterkers 1996), and metastases to the temporal bone or infratemporal fossa (Hill and Kohut 1976, Shapshay et al 1976).

Eye pain Blurring of vision and eye pain are the two most common symptoms of choridal metastases (Hayreh et al 1982, Servodidio and Abramson 1992, Swanson 1993). More commonly chronic eye pain is related to metastases to the bony orbit, intraorbital structures such as the rectus muscles (Weiss et al 1984, Friedman et al 1990), or optic nerve (Laitt et al 1996).

Uncommon causes of headache and facial pain

Headache and facial pain in cancer patients may have many other causes. Unilateral facial pain can be the initial symptom of an ipsilateral lung tumour (Bongers et al 1992, Schoenen et al 1992, Capobianco 1995, Shakespeare and Stevens 1996). Presumably, this referred pain is mediated by vagal afferents. Facial squamous cell carcinoma of the skin may present with facial pain due to extensive perineural invasion (Schroeder et al 1998). Patients with Hodgkin's disease may have transient episodes of neurological dysfunction that has been likened to migraine (Dulli et al 1987). Headache may occur with cerebral infarction or haemorrhage, which may be due to non-bacterial thrombotic endocarditis or disseminated intravascular coagulation. Headache is also the usual presentation of sagittal sinus occlusion, which may be due to tumour infiltration, hypercoaguable state, or treatment with L-asparaginase therapy (Sigsbee et al 1979). Headache due to pseudotumour cerebri has also been reported to be the presentation of superior vena caval obstruction in a patient with lung cancer (Portenoy et al 1983). Tumours of the sinonasal tract may present with deep facial or nasal pain (Marshall and Mahanna 1997).

Neuropathic pains involving the peripheral nervous system

Neuropathic pains involving the peripheral nervous system are common. The syndromes include painful radiculopathy, plexopathy, mononeuropathy, or peripheral neuropathy.

Painful radiculopathy

Radiculopathy or polyradiculopathy may be caused by any process that compresses, distorts, or inflames nerve roots. Painful radiculopathy is an important presentation of epidural tumour and leptomeningeal metastases (see above).

Postherpetic neuralgia Postherpetic neuralgia is defined solely by the persistence of pain in the region of a zoster infection. Although some authors apply this term if pain continues beyond lesion healing, most require a period of weeks to months before this label is used; a criterion of pain persisting beyond 2 months after lesion healing is recommended (Portenoy et al 1986). One study suggests that postherpetic neuralgia is two to three times more frequent in the cancer population than the general population (Rusthoven et al 1988). In patients with postherpetic neuralgia and cancer, changes in the intensity or pattern of pain, or the development of new neurologic deficits, may indicate the possibility of local neoplasm and should be investigated.

Cervical plexopathy

The ventral rami of the upper four cervical spinal nerves join to form the cervical plexus between the deep anterior and lateral muscles of the neck. Cutaneous branches emerge from the posterior border of the sternocleidomastoid. In the cancer population, plexus injury is frequently due to tumour infiltration or treatment (including surgery or radiotherapy) to neoplasms in this region (Jaeckle 1991). Tumour invasion or compression of the cervical plexus can be caused by direct extension of a primary head and neck malignancy or neoplastic (metastatic or lymphomatous) involvement of the cervical lymph nodes (Jaeckle 1991). Pain may be experienced in the preauricular (greater auricular nerve) or postauricular (lesser and greater occipital nerves) regions, or the anterior neck (transverse cutaneous and supraclavicular nerves). Pain may refer to the lateral aspect of the face or head, or to the ipsilateral shoulder. The overlap in the pain referral patterns from the face and neck may relate to the close anatomic relationship between the central connections of cervical afferents and the afferents carried in cranial nerves V, VII, IX, and X in the upper cervical spinal cord. The pain may be aching, burning, or lancinating, and is often exacerbated by neck movement or swallowing. Associated features can include ipsilateral Horner's syndrome or hemidiaphragmatic paralysis. The diagnosis must be distinguished from epidural compression of the cervical spinal cord and leptomeningeal metastases. MRI or CT imaging of the neck and cervical spine is usually required to evaluate the etiology of the pain.

Brachial plexopathy

The two most common causes of brachial plexopathy in cancer patients are tumour infiltration and radiation injury. Less common causes of painful brachial plexopathy include trauma during surgery or anaesthesia, radiation-induced second neoplasms, acute brachial plexus ischaemia, and paraneoplastic brachial neuritis.

Malignant brachial plexopathy Plexus infiltration by tumour is the most prevalent cause of brachial plexopathy. Malignant brachial plexopathy is most common in patients with lymphoma, lung cancer, or breast cancer. The invading tumour usually arises from adjacent axillary, cervical, and supraclavicular lymph nodes (lymphoma and breast cancer) or from the lung (superior sulcus tumours or so-called Pancoast tumours) (Kori et al 1981, Kori 1995). Pain is nearly universal, occurring in 85% of patients, and often precedes neurologic signs or symptoms by months (Kori 1995). Lower plexus involvement (C7, C8, T1 distribution) is typical, and is reflected in the pain distribution, which usually involves the elbow, medial forearm, and fourth and fifth fingers. Pain may sometimes localize to the posterior arm or elbow. Severe aching is usually reported, but patients may also experience constant or lancinating dysaesthesias along the ulnar aspect of the forearm or hand.

Tumour infiltration of the upper plexus (C5–C6 distribution) is less common. This lesion is characterized by pain in the shoulder girdle, lateral arm, and hand. Seventy-five percent of patients presenting with upper plexopathy subsequently develop a panplexopathy, and 25% of patients present with panplexopathy (Kori et al 1981).

Cross-sectional imaging is essential in all patients with symptoms or signs compatible with plexopathy. In one study, CT scanning had 80–90% sensitivity in detecting tumour infiltration (Cascino et al 1983); others have demonstrated improved diagnostic yield with a multiplanar imaging technique (Fishman et al 1991). Although there are no comparative data on the sensitivity and specificity of CT and MRI in this setting, MRI does have the theoretical advantage of reliably assessing the integrity of the adjacent epidural space (Thyagarajan et al 1995).

Electrodiagnostic studies may be helpful in patients with suspected plexopathy, particularly when neurological examination and imaging studies are normal (Synek 1986). Although not specific for tumour, abnormalities on electromyography (EMG) or somatosensory-evoked potentials may establish the diagnosis of plexopathy, and thereby confirm the need for additional evaluation.

Patients with malignant brachial plexopathy are at high risk for epidural extension of the tumour (Portenoy et al 1989, Jaeckle 1991). Epidural disease can occur as the neoplasm grows medially and invades vertebrae or tracks along nerve roots through the intervertebral foramina. In the latter case, there may be no evidence of bony erosion on imaging studies. The development of Horner's syndrome, evidence of panplexopathy, or finding of paraspinal tumour or vertebral damage on CT or MRI are highly associated with epidural extension and should lead to definitive imaging of the epidural tumour (Portenoy et al 1989, Jaeckle 1991).

Radiation-induced brachial plexopathy Two distinct syndromes of radiation-induced brachial plexopathy have been described: (1) early onset transient plexopathy (see above) and (2) delayed onset progressive plexopathy. The latter can occur 6 months to 20 years after a course of radiotherapy that included the plexus in the radiation portal. In contrast to tumour infiltration, pain is a relatively uncommon presenting symptom (18%), and when present, is usually less severe (Kori et al 1981). Weakness and sensory changes predominate in the distribution of the upper plexus (C5, C6 distribution) (Mondrup et al 1990, Olsen et al 1990, Vecht 1990). Radiation changes in the skin and lymphoedema are commonly associated. The CT scan usually demonstrates diffuse infiltration that cannot be distinguished from tumour infiltration. There is no specific advantage to MRI scanning. In particular, increased T2 signal in or near the brachial plexus is commonly seen in both radiation plexopathy and tumour infiltration (Thyagarajan et al 1995). Electromyography may demonstrate myokymia (Lederman and Wilbourn 1984, Mondrup et al 1990, Esteban and Traba 1993). Although a careful history, combined with neurologic findings and the results of CT scanning and electrodiagnostic studies, can strongly suggest the diagnosis of radiation-induced injury, repeated assessments over time may be needed to confirm the diagnosis. Rare patients require surgical exploration of the plexus to exclude neoplasm and establish the aetiology. When due to radiation, plexopathy is usually progressive (Killer and Hess 1990, Jaeckle 1991), although some patients plateau for a variable period of time.

Uncommon causes of brachial plexopathy Malignant peripheral nerve tumour or a second primary tumour in a previously irradiated site can account for pain recurring late in the patient's course (Richardson et al 1979, Gorson et al 1995). Pain has been reported to occur as a result of brachial plexus entrapment in a lymphoedematous shoulder (Vecht 1990), and as a consequence of acute ischaemia many years after axillary radiotherapy (Gerard et al 1989). An idiopathic brachial plexopathy has also been described in patients with Hodgkin's disease (Lachance et al 1991).

Lumbosacral plexopathy

The lumbar plexus, which lies in the paravertebral psoas muscle, is formed primarily by the ventral rami of L1–4. The sacral plexus forms in the sacroiliac notch from the ventral rami of S1–3 and the lumbosacral trunk (L4–5), which courses caudally over the sacral ala to join the plexus (Chad and

Bradley 1987). Lumbosacral plexopathy may be associated with pain in the lower abdomen, inguinal region, buttock, or leg (Jaeckle et al 1985). In the cancer population, lumbosacral plexopathy is usually caused by neoplastic infiltration or compression. Radiation-induced plexopathy also occurs, and occasional patients develop the lesion as a result of surgical trauma, infarction, cytotoxic damage, infection in the pelvis or psoas muscle, abdominal aneurysm, or idiopathic lumbosacral neuritis. Polyradiculopathy from leptomeningeal metastases or epidural metastases can mimic lumbosacral plexopathy.

Malignant lumbosacral plexopathy The primary tumours most frequently associated with malignant lumbosacral plexopathy include colorectal, cervical, breast, sarcoma, and lymphoma (Jaeckle et al 1985, Jaeckle 1991). Most tumours involve the plexus by direct extension from intrapelvic neoplasm; metastases account for only one-fourth of the cases. In one study, two-thirds of patients developed plexopathy within 3 years of their primary diagnosis and one-third presented within one year (Jaeckle et al 1985). Pain is, typically, the first symptom, it is experienced by almost all patients at some point, and it is the only symptom in almost 20% of patients. The quality is aching, pressure-like, or stabbing; dysaesthesias are relatively uncommon. Most patients develop numbness, paraesthesias, or weakness weeks to months after the pain begins. Common signs include leg weakness that involves multiple myotomes, sensory loss that crosses dermatomes, reflex asymmetry, focal tenderness, leg oedema, and positive direct or reverse straight leg-raising signs.

An upper plexopathy occurs in almost one-third of patients with lumbosacral plexopathy (Jaeckle et al 1985). This lesion is usually due to direct extension from a low abdominal tumour, most frequently colorectal. Pain may be experienced in the back, lower abdomen, flank or iliac crest, or the anterolateral thigh. Examination may reveal sensory, motor, and reflex changes in a L1–4 distribution. A subgroup of these patients presents with a syndrome characterized by pain and paraesthesias limited to the lower abdomen or inguinal region, variable sensory loss, and no motor findings. CT scan may show tumour adjacent to the L1 vertebra (the L1 syndrome) (Jaeckle et al 1985) or along the pelvic sidewall, where it presumably damages the ilioinguinal, iliohypogastric, or genitofemoral nerves. Another subgroup has neoplastic involvement of the psoas muscle and presents with a syndrome characterized by upper lumbosacral plexopathy, painful flexion of the ipsilateral hip, and positive psoas muscle stretch test; this has been termed the malignant psoas syndrome (Stevens and Gonet 1990). Similarly, pain in the distribution of the femoral nerve has been observed in the setting of recurrent retroperitoneal sarcoma (Zografos and Karakousis 1994), and tumour in the iliac crest can compress the lateral cutaneous nerve of the thigh, producing a pain that mimics meralgia parasthetica (Tharion and Bhattacharji 1997).

A lower plexopathy occurs in just over 50% of patients with malignant lumbosacral plexopathy (Jaeckle et al 1985). This lesion is usually due to direct extension from a pelvic tumour, most frequently rectal cancer, gynaecological tumours, or pelvic sarcoma. Pain may be localized in the buttocks and perineum, or referred to the posterolateral thigh and leg. Associated symptoms and signs conform to an L4–S1 distribution. Examination may reveal weakness or sensory changes in the L5 and S1 dermatomes and a depressed ankle jerk. Other findings include leg oedema, bladder or bowel dysfunction, sacral or sciatic notch tenderness, and a positive straight leg-raising test. A pelvic mass may be palpable. Other, relatively rare plexopathies are described in Cherny and Portenoy (1999).

Painful mononeuropathy

Tumour-related mononeuropathy Tumour-related mononeuropathy usually results from compression or infiltration of a nerve from tumour arising in an adjacent bony structure. The most common example of this phenomenon is intercostal nerve injury in a patient with rib metastases. Constant burning pain and other dysaesthesias in the area of sensory loss are the typical clinical presentation. Other examples include the cranial neuralgias previously described, sciatica associated with tumour invasion of the sciatic notch, and common peroneal nerve palsy associated with primary bone tumours of the proximal fibula and lateral cutaneous nerve of the thigh neuralgia associated with iliac crest tumours.

Other causes of mononeuropathy Cancer patients also develop mononeuropathies from many other causes. Postsurgical syndromes are well described (see below) and radiation injury of a peripheral nerve occurs occasionally. Rarely, cancer patients develop nerve entrapment syndromes (such as carpal tunnel syndrome) related to oedema or direct compression by tumour (Desta et al 1994).

Painful peripheral neuropathies

Painful peripheral neuropathies have multiple causes, including nutritional deficiencies, other metabolic derangements (e.g., diabetes and renal dysfunction), neurotoxic effects of chemotherapy, and, rarely, paraneoplastic syndromes.

Toxic peripheral neuropathy Chemotherapy-induced peripheral neuropathy is a common problem typically manifested by painful paraesthesias in the hands and/or feet, and signs consistent with an axonopathy, including 'stocking-glove' sensory loss, weakness, hyporeflexia, and autonomic dysfunction (McDonald 1991). The pain is usually characterized by continuous burning or lancinating pains, either of which may be increased by contact. The drugs most commonly associated with a peripheral neuropathy are the vinca alkaloids (especially vincristine) (Rosenthal and Kaufman 1974, Forman 1990), *cis*-platinum (Mollman et al 1988, Siegal and Haim 1990), and oxaliplatin (Culy et al 2000). Procarbazine, carboplatinum, misonidazole, and hexamethylmelamine have also been implicated as causes for this syndrome (Weiss et al 1974a, b). Data from several studies indicates that the risk of neuropathy associated with *cis*-platinum can be diminished by the coadministration of the radioprotective agent amifostine at the time of treatment (Spencer and Goa 1995).

Paraneoplastic painful peripheral neuropathy Paraneoplastic painful peripheral neuropathy can be related to injury to the dorsal root ganglion (also known as subacute sensory neuronopathy or ganglionopathy) or injury to peripheral nerves (Grisold and Drlicek 1999). These syndromes may be the initial manifestation of an underlying malignancy. Except for the neuropathy associated with myeloma (Kissel and Mendell 1996, Rotta and Bradley 1997) their course is usually independent of the primary tumour (Dalmau and Posner 1997, Grisold and Drlicek 1999)].

Subacute sensory neuronopathy is characterized by pain (usually dysaesthetic), paraesthesias, sensory loss in the extremities, and severe sensory ataxia (Brady 1996). Although it is usually associated with small cell carcinoma of the lung (van Oosterhout et al 1996), other tumour types, including breast cancer (Peterson et al 1994), Hodgkin's disease (Plante-Bordeneuve et al 1994), and varied solid tumours, are rarely associated. Both constant and lancinating dysaesthesias occur and typically predate other symptoms. Neuropathic symptoms (pain, paraesthesia, sensory loss) were asymmetric at onset, with a predilection for the upper limbs. Indeed, in one instance a painful bilateral ulnar neuropathy is described (Sharief et al 1999). The pain usually develops before the tumour is evident and its course is typically independent. Coexisting autonomic, cerebellar, or cerebral abnormalities are common (Brady 1996). The syndrome, which results from an inflammatory process involving the dorsal root ganglia, may be part of a more diffuse autoimmune disorder that can affect the limbic region, brainstem, and spinal cord (Brady 1996, Dalmau and Posner 1997, Toepfer et al 1999). An antineuronal IgG antibody ('anti-Hu'), which recognizes a low-molecular-weight protein present in most small cell lung carcinomas, has been associated with the condition (Dalmau and Posner 1997).

A sensorimotor peripheral neuropathy, which may be painful, has been observed in association with diverse neoplasms, particularly Hodgkin's disease and paraproteinaemias (Brady 1996, Dalmau and Posner 1997). The peripheral neuropathies associated with multiple myeloma, Waldenstrom's macroglobulinaemia, small-fibre amyloid neuropathy, and osteosclerotic myeloma, are thought to be due to antibodies that cross-react with constituents of peripheral nerves (Kissel and Mendell 1996). Clinically evident peripheral neuropathy occurs in approximately 15% of patients with multiple myeloma, and electrophysiologic evidence of this lesion can be found in 40% (Kissel and Mendell 1996). The pathophysiology of the neuropathy is unknown.

Pain syndromes of the viscera and miscellaneous tumour-related syndromes

Pain may be caused by pathology involving the luminal organs of the gastrointestinal or genitourinary tracts, the parenchymal organs, the peritoneum, or the retroperitoneal soft tissues. Obstruction of hollow viscus, including intestine, biliary tract, and ureter, produces visceral nociceptive syndromes that are well described in the surgical literature (Silen 1983). Pain arising from retroperitoneal and pelvic lesions may involve mixed nociceptive and neuropathic mechanisms if both somatic structures and nerves are involved.

Hepatic distension syndrome

Pain-sensitive structures in the region of the liver include the liver capsule, blood vessels, and biliary tract (Coombs 1990). Nociceptive afferents that innervate these structures travel via the celiac plexus, the phrenic nerve, and the lower right intercostal nerves. Extensive intrahepatic metastases, or gross hepatomegaly associated with cholestasis, may produce discomfort in the right subcostal region, and less commonly in the right mid-back or flank

(Coombs 1990, Mulholland et al 1990, De Conno and Polastri 1996). Referred pain may be experienced in the right neck or shoulder, or in the region of the right scapula (Mulholland et al 1990). The pain, usually described as a dull aching, may be exacerbated by movement, pressure in the abdomen, and deep inspiration. Pain is commonly accompanied by symptoms of anorexia and nausea. Physical examination may reveal a hard irregular subcostal mass that descends with respiration and is dull to percussion. Other features of hepatic failure may be present. Imaging of the hepatic parenchyma by either ultrasound or CT will usually identify the presence of space occupying lesions or cholestasis.

Occasional patients who experience chronic pain due to hepatic distension develop an acute intercurrent subcostal pain that may be exacerbated by respiration. Physical examination may demonstrate a palpable or audible rub. These findings suggest the development of an overlying peritonitis, which can develop in response to some acute event, such as a haemorrhage into a metastasis.

Midline retroperitoneal syndrome

Retroperitoneal pathology involving the upper abdomen may produce pain by injury to deep somatic structures of the posterior abdominal wall, distortion of pain-sensitive connective tissue and vascular and ductal structures, local inflammation, and direct infiltration of the celiac plexus. The most common causes are pancreatic cancer (Kelsen et al 1995, 1997; Grahm and Andren-Sandberg 1997) and retroperitoneal lymphadenopathy (Krane and Perrone 1981, Neer et al 1981, Sponseller 1996), particularly coeliac lymphadenopathy (Schonenberg et al 1991). The reasons for the high frequency of perineural invasion and the presence of pain in pancreatic cancer may be related to locoregional secretion and activation of growth factor (NGF) and its high-affinity receptor TrkA. These factors are involved in stimulating epithelial cancer cell growth and perineural invasion (Zhu et al 1999). In some instances of pancreatic cancer, obstruction of the main pancreatic duct with subsequent ductal hypertension generates pain that can be relieved by stenting of the pancreatic duct (Tham et al 2000). The pain is experienced in the epigastrium, in the low thoracic region of the back, or in both locations. It is often diffuse and poorly localized. It is usually dull and boring in character, exacerbated with recumbency, and improved by sitting. The lesion can usually be demonstrated by CT, MRI, or ultrasound scanning of the upper abdomen. If tumour is identified in the paravertebral space, or vertebral body destruction is identified, consideration should be given to careful evaluation of the epidural space (Portenoy et al 1989).

Chronic intestinal obstruction

Abdominal pain is an almost invariable manifestation of chronic intestinal obstruction, which may occur in patients with abdominal or pelvic cancers (Baines 1994, Ripamonti 1994). The factors that contribute to this pain include smooth muscle contractions, mesenteric tension, and mural ischaemia. Obstructive symptoms may be due primarily to the tumour, or more likely, to a combination of mechanical obstruction and other processes, such as autonomic neuropathy and ileus from metabolic derangements or drugs. Both continuous and colicky pains, which may be referred to the dermatomes represented by the spinal segments supplying the affected viscera, occur. Vomiting, anorexia, and constipation are important associated symptoms.

Peritoneal carcinomatosis

Peritoneal carcinomatosis occurs most often by transcoelomic spread of abdominal or pelvic tumour; excepting breast cancer, haematogenous spread of an extra-abdominal neoplasm in this pattern is rare. Carcinomatosis can cause peritoneal inflammation, mesenteric tethering, malignant adhesions, and ascites, all of which can cause pain. Pain and abdominal distension are the most common presenting symptoms. Mesenteric tethering and tension appears to cause a diffuse abdominal or low back pain. Tense malignant ascites can produce diffuse abdominal discomfort and a distinct stretching pain in the anterior abdominal wall. Adhesions can also cause obstruction of hollow viscus, with intermittent colicky pain (Averbach and Sugarbaker 1995). CT scanning may demonstrate evidence of ascites, omental infiltration, and peritoneal nodules (Archer et al 1996).

Malignant perineal pain

Tumours of the colon or rectum, female reproductive tract, and distal genitourinary system are most commonly responsible for perineal pain (Stillman 1990, Boas et al 1993, Hagen 1993, Miaskowski 1996, Rigor 2000). Severe perineal pain following antineoplastic therapy may precede evidence of detectable disease and should be viewed as a potential harbinger of progressive or recurrent cancer (Stillman 1990, Boas et al 1993, Rigor 2000). There is evidence to suggest that this phenomenon is caused by microscopic perineural invasion by recurrent disease (Seefeld and Bargen 1943). The pain, which is typically described as constant and aching, is often aggravated by sitting or standing, and may be associated with tenesmus or bladder spasms (Stillman 1990).

Tumour invasion of the musculature of the deep pelvis can also result in a syndrome that appears similar to the so-called 'tension myalgia of the pelvic floor' (Sinaki et al 1977). The pain is typically described as a constant ache or heaviness that exacerbates with upright posture. When due to tumour, the pain may be concurrent with other types of perineal pain. Digital examination of the pelvic floor may reveal local tenderness or palpable tumour.

Adrenal pain syndrome

Large adrenal metastases, common in lung cancer, may produce unilateral flank pain and, less commonly, abdominal pain. Pain is of variable severity, and it can be severe (Berger et al 1995).

Ureteric obstruction

Ureteric obstruction is most frequently caused by tumour compression or infiltration within the true pelvis (Kontturi and Kauppila 1982, Harrington et al 1995). Less commonly, obstruction can be more proximal, associated with retroperitoneal lymphadenopathy, an isolated retroperitoneal metastasis, mural metastases, or intraluminal metastases. Cancers of the cervix, ovary, prostate, and rectum are most commonly associated with this complication. Non-malignant causes, including retroperitoneal fibrosis resulting from radiotherapy or graft versus host disease, occur rarely (Sklaroff et al 1978, Muram et al 1981, Goodman and Dalton 1982).

Pain may or may not accompany ureteric obstruction. When present, it is typically a dull chronic discomfort in the flank, with radiation into the inguinal region or genitalia. If pain does not occur, ureteric obstruction may be discovered when hydronephrosis is discerned on abdominal imaging procedures or renal failure develops. Ureteric obstruction can be complicated by pyelonephritis or pyonephrosis, which often present with features of sepsis, loin pain, and dysuria. Diagnosis of ureteric obstruction can usually be confirmed by the demonstration of hydronephrosis on renal sonography. The level of obstruction can be identified by pyelography, and CT scanning techniques will usually demonstrate the cause (Greenfield and Resnick 1989).

Ovarian cancer pain

Moderate to severe chronic abdominopelvic pain is the most common symptom of ovarian cancer; it is reported by almost two-thirds of patients in the 2 weeks prior to the onset or recurrence of the disease (Portenoy et al 1994). In patients who have been previously treated it is an important symptom of potential recurrence (Portenoy et al 1994).

Lung cancer pain

Even in the absence of involvement of the chest wall or parietal pleura, lung tumours can produce a visceral pain syndrome. In a large case series of lung cancer patients pain was unilateral in 80% of the cases and bilateral in 20%. Among patients with hilar tumours the pain was reported to the sternum or the scapula. Upper and lower lobe tumours referred to the shoulder and to the lower chest respectively (Marino et al 1986, Marangoni et al 1993). As previously mentioned, early lung cancers can generate ipsilateral facial pain (Des Prez and Freemon 1983, Schoenen et al 1992, Capobianco 1995, Shakespeare and Stevens 1996). It is postulated that this pain syndrome is generated via vagal afferent neurones.

Other uncommon visceral pain syndromes

Sudden onset severe abdominal or loin pain may be caused by non-traumatic rupture of a visceral tumour. This has been most frequently reported with hepatocellular cancer (Miyamoto et al 1991). Kidney rupture due to a renal metastasis from an adenocarcinoma of the colon (Wolff et al 1994) and metastasis-induced perforated appendicitis (Ende et al 1995) have been reported. Torsion of pedunculated visceral tumours can produce a cramping abdominal pain (Abbott 1990, Reese and Blocker 1994, Andreasen and Poulsen 1997).

Paraneoplastic nociceptive pain syndromes

Tumour-related gynaecomastia Tumours that secrete chorionic gonadotrophin (HCG), including malignant and benign tumours of the testis (Tseng et al 1985, Haas et al 1989, Mellor and McCutchan 1989, Cantwell et al 1991) and rarely cancers from other sites (Wurzel et al 1987, Forst et al 1995), may be associated with chronic breast tenderness or gynaecomastia. Approximately 10% of patients with testis cancer have gynaecomastia or breast tenderness at presentation, and the likelihood of gynaecomastia is greater with increasing HCG level (Tseng et al 1985). Breast pain can be the first presentation of an occult tumour (Haas et al 1989, Mellor and McCutchan 1989, Cantwell et al 1991).

Paraneoplastic pemphigus Paraneoplastic pemphigus is a rare mucocutaneous disorder associated with non-Hodgkin's lymphoma: chronic lymphocytic leukaemia. The condition is characterized by widespread shallow ulcers with haemorrhagic crusting of the lips, conjunctival bullae, and, uncommonly, pulmonary lesions. Characteristically, histopathology reveals intra-epithelial and subepithelial clefting, and immunoprecipitation studies reveal autoantibodies directed against desmoplakins and desmogleins (Camisa et al 1992, Allen and Camisa 2000).

Chronic pain syndromes associated with cancer therapy

Most treatment-related pains are caused by tissue-damaging procedures. These pains are acute, predictable, and self-limited. Chronic treatment-related pain syndromes are associated with either a persistent nociceptive complication of an invasive treatment (such as a postsurgical abscess) or, more commonly, neural injury. In some cases, these syndromes occur long after the therapy is completed, resulting in a difficult differential diagnosis between recurrent disease and a complication of therapy.

Postchemotherapy pain syndromes

Chronic painful peripheral neuropathy Although most patients who develop painful peripheral neuropathy due to cytotoxic therapy gradually improve, some develop a persistent pain. In particular, peripheral neuropathy associated with *cis*-platinum may continue to progress months after discontinuation of therapy and may persist for months to years (Rosenfeld and Broder 1984, LoMonaco et al 1992). This is less common with vincristine or paclitaxol (Hilkens et al 1996). The characteristics of this pain syndrome were described previously.

Avascular (aseptic) necrosis of femoral or humeral head Avascular necrosis of the femoral or humeral head may occur either spontaneously or as a complication of intermittent or continuous corticosteroid therapy (Ratcliffe et al 1995, Thornton et al 1997). Osteonecrosis may be unilateral or bilateral. Involvement of the femoral head is most common and typically causes pain in the hip, thigh, or knee. Involvement of the humeral head usually presents as pain in the shoulder, upper arm, or elbow. Pain is exacerbated by movement and relieved by rest. There may be local tenderness over the joint, but this is not universal. Pain usually precedes radiological changes by weeks to months; bone scintigraphy and MRI are sensitive and complementary diagnostic procedures. Early treatment consists of analgesics, decrease or discontinuation of steroids, and sometimes surgery. With progressive bone destruction, joint replacement may be necessary.

Plexopathy Lumbosacral or brachial plexopathy may follow *cis*-platinum infusion into the iliac artery (Castellanos et al 1987) or axillary artery (Kahn et al 1989), respectively. Affected patients develop pain, weakness, and paraesthesias within 48 h of the infusion. The mechanism for this syndrome is thought to be due to small vessel damage and infarction of the plexus or nerve. The prognosis for neurologic recovery is not known.

Raynaud's phenomenon Among patients with germ cell tumours treated with cisplatin, vinblastine, and bleomycin, persistent Raynaud's phenomenon is observed in 20–30% (Aass et al 1990, Gerl 1994). This effect has also been observed in patients with carcinoma of the head and neck treated with a combination of cisplatin, vincristine, and bleomycin (Kukla et al 1982). Pathophysiological studies have demonstrated that a hyper-reactivity in the central sympathetic nervous system results in a reduced function of the smooth muscle cells in the terminal arterioles (Hansen et al 1990).

Chronic pain associated with hormonal therapy

Gynaecomastia with hormonal therapy for prostate cancer Chronic gynaecomastia and breast tenderness are common complications of anti-androgen therapies for prostate cancer. The incidence of this syndrome varies among drugs; it is frequently associated with diethylstilbestrol (Srinivasan et al 1972) and bicalutamide (Soloway et al 1996), is less common with flutamide (Brogden and Chrisp 1991) and cyproterone (Goldenberg and Bruchovsky 1991), and is uncommon among patients receiving LHRF agonist therapy (Chrisp and Goa 1991, Chrisp and Sorkin 1991). Gynaecomastia in the elderly must be distinguished from primary breast cancer or a secondary cancer in the breast (Olsson et al 1984, Ramamurthy and Cooper 1991).

Chronic postsurgical pain syndromes

Surgical incision at virtually any location may result in chronic pain. Although persistent pain is occasionally encountered after nephrectomy, sternotomy, craniotomy, inguinal dissection, and other procedures, these pain syndromes are not well described in the cancer population. In contrast, several syndromes are now clearly recognized as sequelae of specific surgical procedures. The predominant underlying pain mechanism in these syndromes is neuropathic, resulting from injury to peripheral nerves or plexus.

Breast surgery pain syndromes Chronic pain of variable severity is a common sequel of surgery for breast cancer. In two large surveys pain, paraesthesias and strange sensations were reported by 30–50% the patients (Tasmuth et al 1995, 1996; Carpenter et al 1998; Smith et al 1999). The most common sites of pain were the breast scar region and the ipsilateral arm. Pain was more common among women who underwent breast conserving treatments than those who underwent mastectomy. The highest incidence of pain was reported by patients who had had both radio- and chemotherapy (Tasmuth et al 1995). Data from a retrospective survey of 408 mastectomy patients revealed that this phenomenon was more common among younger patients and that the pain severity attenuated over time (Smith et al 1999).

Although chronic pain has been reported to occur after almost any surgical procedure on the breast (from lumpectomy to radical mastectomy), it is most common after procedures involving axillary dissection (Vecht et al 1989, Vecht 1990, Hladiuk et al 1992, Maunsell et al 1993). Pain may begin immediately or as late as many months following surgery. The natural history of this condition appears to be variable, and both subacute and chronic courses are possible (International Association for the Study of Pain: Subcommittee on Taxonomy 1986). The onset of pain later than 18 months following surgery is unusual, and a careful evaluation to exclude recurrent chest wall disease is recommended in this setting.

Postmastectomy pain is characterized as a constricting and burning discomfort localized to the medial arm, axilla, and anterior chest wall (Wood 1978, Granek et al 1983, Vecht et al 1989, Paredes et al 1990, van Dam et al 1993); on examination, there is often an area of sensory loss within the region of the pain (van Dam et al 1993). The aetiology is believed to be related to damage to the intercostobrachial nerve, a cutaneous sensory branch of T1,2,3 (Vecht et al 1989, van Dam et al 1993). There is marked anatomic variation in the size and distribution of the intercostobrachial nerve, and this may account for some of the variability in the distribution of pain observed in patients with this condition (Assa 1974).

In some cases of pain after breast surgery a trigger point can be palpated in the axilla or chest wall. The patient may restrict movement of the arm leading to frozen shoulder as a secondary complication.

Postradical neck dissection pain Longstanding locoregional pain after radical neck dissection is uncommon (Talmi et al 2000). Several types of postradical neck dissection pain are recognized. A persistent neuropathic pain can develop weeks to months after surgical injury to the cervical plexus. Tightness, along with burning or lancinating dysaesthesias in the area of the sensory loss, are the characteristic symptoms. More commonly, chronic pain can result from musculoskeletal imbalance in the shoulder girdle following surgical removal of neck muscles (Talmi et al 2000). Similar to the droopy shoulder syndrome (Swift and Nichols 1984), this syndrome can be complicated by development of a thoracic outlet syndrome or suprascapular nerve entrapment, with selective weakness and wasting of the supraspinatus and infraspinatus muscles (Brown et al 1988). Data from a a large survey demonstrated that neck dissections sparing CN XI, and not dissecting level V of the neck when CN XI is spared, are associated with less shoulder and neck pain (Terrell et al 2000).

Escalating pain in patients who have undergone radical neck dissection may signify recurrent tumour or soft-tissue infection. These lesions may be difficult to diagnose in tissues damaged by radiation and surgery. Repeated CT or MRI scanning may be needed to exclude tumour recurrence. Empiric treatment with antibiotics should be considered (Bruera and MacDonald 1986, Coyle and Portenoy 1991).

Post-thoracotomy pain There have been two major studies of post-thoracotomy pain (Kanner et al 1982, Keller et al 1994). In the first (Kanner et al 1982), three groups were identified: The largest (63%) had prolonged postoperative pain that abated within 2 months after surgery. Recurrent pain, following resolution of the postoperative pain, was usually due to neoplasm. A second group (16%) experienced pain that persisted following the thoracotomy, then increased in intensity during the follow-up period. Local recurrence of disease and infection were the most common causes of the increasing pain. A final group had a prolonged period of stable or decreasing pain that gradually resolved over a maximum 8-month period. This pain was not associated with tumour recurrence. Overall, the development of late or increasing post-thoracotomy pain was due to recurrent or persistent tumour in greater than 95% of patients. This finding was corroborated in the more recent study, which evaluated the records of 238 consecutive patients who underwent thoracotomy and identified recurrent pain in 20 patients, all of whom were found to have tumour regrowth (Keller et al 1994).

Patients with recurrent or increasing post-thoracotomy pain should be carefully evaluated, preferably with a chest CT scan or MRI. Chest radiographs are insufficient to evaluate recurrent chest disease. In some patients, post-thoracotomy pain appears to be caused by a taut muscular band within the scapular region. In such cases, pain may be amenable to trigger point injection of local anaesthetic (Hamada et al 2000).

Postoperative frozen shoulder Patients with post-thoracotomy or postmastectomy pain are at risk for the development of a frozen shoulder (Maunsell et al 1993). This lesion may become an independent focus of pain, particularly if complicated by reflex sympathetic dystrophy. Adequate postoperative analgesia and active mobilization of the joint soon after surgery are necessary to prevent these problems.

Phantom pain syndromes Phantom limb pain is perceived to arise from an amputated limb, as if the limb were still contiguous with the body. Phantom pain is experienced by 60 to 80% of patients following limb amputation but is only severe in about 5 to 10% of cases (Ehde et al 2000, Nikolajsen and Jensen 2000). Phantom pain is more prevalent after tumour-related than traumatic amputations, and postoperative chemotherapy is an additional risk factor (Smith and Thompson 1995). Some patients have spontaneous partial remission of the pain. The recurrence of pain after such a remission, or the late onset of pain in a previously painless phantom limb, suggests the appearance of a more proximal lesion, including recurrent neoplasm (Chang et al 1997). A phantom anus pain syndrome occurs in approximately 15% of patients who undergo abdominoperineal resection of the rectum (Ovesen et al 1991, Boas et al 1993). Phantom anus pain may develop either in the early postoperative period or after a latency of months to years. Late onset pain is almost always associated with tumour recurrence (Ovesen et al 1991, Boas et al 1993). Phantom pain after removal of a breast or bladder is described in Cherny and Portenoy (1999).

Stump pain Stump pain occurs at the site of the surgical scar several months to years following amputation (Davis 1993). It is usually the result of neuroma development at a site of nerve transection. This pain is characterized by burning or lancinating dysaesthesias, which are often exacerbated by movement or pressure and blocked by an injection of a local anaesthetic.

Postsurgical pelvic floor myalgia Surgical trauma to the pelvic floor can cause a residual pelvic floor myalgia, which, like the neoplastic syndrome described previously, mimics so-called tension myalgia (Sinaki et al 1977). The risk of disease recurrence associated with this condition is not known, and its natural history has not been defined. In patients who have undergone anorectal resection, this condition must be differentiated from the phantom anus syndrome (see above).

Chronic postradiation pain syndromes

Chronic pain complicating radiation therapy tends to occur late in the course of a patient's illness. These syndromes must always be differentiated from recurrent tumour.

Radiation-induced brachial and lumbosacral plexopathies Radiation-induced brachial and lumbosacral plexopathies were described previously (see above).

Chronic radiation myelopathy Chronic radiation myelopathy is a late complication of spinal cord irradiation. The latency is highly variable but is most commonly 12–14 months. The most common presentation is a partial transverse myelopathy at the cervicothoracic level, sometimes in a Brown–Sequard pattern (Schultheiss and Stephens 1992). Sensory symptoms, including pain, typically precede the development of progressive motor and autonomic dysfunction (Schultheiss and Stephens 1992). The pain is characterized as a burning dysaesthesia localized to the area of spinal cord damage or below.

Chronic radiation enteritis and proctitis Chronic enteritis and proctocolitis occur as a delayed complication in 2–10% of patients who undergo abdominal or pelvic radiation therapy (Yeoh and Horowitz 1987, Nussbaum et al 1993). The rectum and rectosigmoid are more commonly involved than the small bowel, a pattern that may relate to the retroperitoneal fixation of the former structures. The latency is variable (3 months–30 years) (Yeoh and Horowitz 1987, Nussbaum et al 1993). Chronic radiation injury to the rectum can present as proctitis (with bloody diarrhoea, tenesmus, and cramping pain), obstruction due to stricture formation, or fistulae to the bladder or vagina. Small bowel radiation damage typically causes colicky abdominal pain, which can be associated with chronic nausea or malabsorption. Barium studies may demonstrate a narrow tubular bowel segment resembling Crohn's disease or ischaemic colitis. Endoscopy and biopsy may be necessary to distinguish suspicious lesions from recurrent cancer.

Radiation cystitis Radiation therapy used in the treatment of tumours of the pelvic organs (prostate, bladder, colon/rectum, uterus, ovary, and vagina/vulva) may produce a chronic radiation cystitis (Pillay et al 1984, Joly et al 1998, Perez et al 1999). The late sequelae of radiation injury to the bladder can range from minor temporary irritative voiding symptoms and asymptomatic hematuria to more severe complications such as gross haematuria, contracted non-functional bladder, persistent incontinence, and fistula formation. The clinical presentation can include frequency, urgency, dysuria, haematuria, incontinence, hydronephrosis, pneumaturia, and fecaluria.

Lymphoedema pain One-third of patients with lymphoedema as a complication of breast cancer or its treatment experience pain and tightness in the arm (Newman et al 1996). Some patients develop nerve entrapment syndromes of the carpal tunnel syndrome or brachial plexus (Ganel et al 1979, Vecht 1990). Severe or increasing pain in a lymphoedematous arm is strongly suggestive of tumour invasion of the brachial plexus (Kori et al 1981, Kori 1995).

Burning perineum syndrome Persistent perineal discomfort is an uncommon delayed complication of pelvic radiotherapy. After a latency of 6–18 months, burning pain can develop in the perianal region; the pain may extend anteriorly to involve the vagina or scrotum (Minsky and Cohen 1988). In patients who have had abdominoperineal resection, phantom anus pain and recurrent tumour are major differential diagnoses.

Osteoradionecrosis Osteoradionecrosis is another late complication of radiotherapy. Bone necrosis, which occurs as a result of endarteritis obliterans, may produce focal pain. Overlying tissue breakdown can occur spontaneously or as a result of trauma, such as dental extraction or denture trauma (Epstein et al 1987, 1997). Delayed development of a painful ulcer must be differentiated from tumour recurrence.

Breakthrough pain

Transitory exacerbations of severe pain over a baseline of moderate pain or less may be described as 'breakthrough pain' (Portenoy and Hagen 1990). Breakthrough pains are common in both acute or chronic pain states. These exacerbations may be precipitated by volitional actions of the patient (so-called incident pains), such as movement, micturition, cough, or defecation, or by non-volitional events, such as bowel distension. Spontaneous fluctuations in pain intensity can also occur without an identifiable precipitant.

Breakthrough pains must be distinguished from exacerbations of pain associated with failure of analgesia. 'End-of-dose failure (of analgesia)' is commonly observed as therapeutic levels of analgesic fall. This phenomenon is observed most commonly when the interval between scheduled doses exceeds the known duration of action of short half-life analgesics. Since there is substantial interindividual differences in drug metabolism and excretion, some analgesics that may typically have a 4-h duration of action may be effective for only 2–3 h in some individuals. Similarly, variability in the duration of analgesic effect is observed with long-acting formulations such as oral morphine or transdermal fentanyl. End-of-dose failure is addressed through either dose or schedule modification.

In a survey by Portenoy and Hagen (1990) of 63 cancer patients with pain requiring opioid analgesics, 41 (64%) reported breakthrough pain. Patients had a median of 4 episodes per day, the duration of which ranged seconds to hours (median/range: 30 min/1–240 min). Pain characteristics were extremely varied. Twenty-two (43%) of the pains were paroxysmal in onset; the remainder were more gradual and 21 (41%) were both paroxysmal and brief (lancinating pain). Fifteen (29%) of the pains were related to end-of-dose failure from a fixed dose of opioid on a regular schedule. Twenty-eight (55%) of the pains were precipitated; of these, 22 were caused by an action of the patient (incident pain), and 6 were associated with a non-volitional precipitant, such as flatulence. The pathophysiology of the pain was believed to be somatic in 17 (33%), visceral in 10 (20%), neuropathic in 14 (27%), and mixed in 10 (20%). Pain was related to the tumour in 42 (82%), the effects of therapy in 7 (14%), and neither in 2 (4%). Diverse interventions were employed to manage these pains, with variable efficacy. In a study of 194 cancer patients with pain, Jacobsen et al (1994) reported that 61% reported one or more episodes of breakthrough pain. These episodes were typically paroxysmal (56%), predictable (63%), and precipitated by patient action (67%). They had a mean duration of 20 min (range 5 s–1.5 h) and occurred an average of 10 times/day (range 1–80). In a survey of 22 hospice patients by Fine and Busch (1998), 86% reported breakthrough pain, with an average of 2.9 episodes per 24-h period and a mean pain intensity of 7 on a 10-point scale. These episodes lasted an average of

52 min (range 1–240). The range of time to relief of breakthrough pains was 5–60 min, with a mean of 30 min.

Syndromes of breakthrough pain

Pain exacerbations represent a heterogeneous phenomenon. The clinical approach to these problems is influenced by the specific underlying mechanism. It is useful, therefore, to define the specific breakthrough pain syndrome: (1) somatic movement-related pain (volitional and non-volitional), (2) somatic non-movement-related pain, and (3) neuropathic movement-related pain.

Conclusion

Adequate assessment is a necessary precondition for effective pain management. In the cancer population, assessment must recognize the dynamic relationship between the symptom, the illness, and larger concerns related to quality of life. Syndrome identification and inferences about pain pathophysiology are useful elements that may simplify this complex undertaking.

References

Aass N, Kaasa S, Lund E, Kaalhus O, Heier MS, Fossa SD 1990 Long-term somatic side-effects and morbidity in testicular cancer patients. British Journal of Cancer 61: 151–155

Abbott J 1990 Pelvic pain: lessons from anatomy and physiology. Journal of Emergency Medicine 8: 441–447

Agency for Health Care Policy and Research 1994 Management of cancer pain: adults. Cancer Pain Guideline Panel. Agency for Health Care Policy and Research. American Family Physician 49: 1853–1868

Agency for Health Care Policy and Research: Acute Pain Management Panel 1992 Acute pain management: operative or medical procedures and trauma. US Department of Health and Human Services, Washington, DC

Agnelli G 1997 Venous thromboembolism and cancer: a two-way clinical association. Thrombosis and Haemostasis 78: 117–120

Aird DW, Bihari J, Smith C 1983 Clinical problems in the continuing care of head and neck cancer patients. Ear Nose and Throat Journal 62: 230–243

Aki FT, Tekin MI, Ozen H 1996 Gynecomastia as a complication of chemotherapy for testicular germ cell tumors. Urology 48: 944–946

Alberts DS, Garcia DJ 1997 Safety aspects of pegylated liposomal doxorubicin in patients with cancer. Drugs 54 (Suppl 4): 30–35

Allen CM, Camisa C 2000 Paraneoplastic pemphigus: a review of the literature. Oral Diseases 6: 208–214

Almadrones L, Yerys C 1990 Problems associated with the administration of intraperitoneal therapy using the Port-A-Cath system. Oncological Nursing Forum 17: 75–80

Alon US, Allen S, Rameriz Z, Warady BA, Kaplan RA, Harris DJ 1994 Lidocaine for the alleviation of pain associated with subcutaneous erythropoietin injection. Journal of the American Society of Nephrology 5: 1161–1162

Andreasen DA, Poulsen J 1997 [Intra-abdominal torsion of the testis with seminoma (see comments)]. Ugeskrift fur Laeger 159: 2103–2104

Ang KK, Stephens LC 1994 Prevention and management of radiation myelopathy. Oncology (Huntingt) 8: 71–76; discussion 78, 81–82

Araki K, Kobayashi M, Ogata T, Takuma K 1994 Colorectal carcinoma metastatic to skeletal muscle. Hepatogastroenterology 41: 405–408

Archer AG, Sugarbaker PH, Jelinek JS 1996 Radiology of peritoneal carcinomatosis. Cancer Treatment Research 82: 263–288

Aro AR, Absetz YP, Eerola T, Pamilo M, Lonnqvist J 1996 Pain and discomfort during mammography. European Journal of Cancer 32A: 1674–1679

Assa J 1974 The intercostobrachial nerve in radical mastectomy. Journal of Surgical Oncology 6: 123–126

Averbach AM, Sugarbaker PH 1995 Recurrent intraabdominal cancer with intestinal obstruction. International Surgery 80: 141–146

Babb RR 1996 Radiation proctitis: a review. American Journal of Gastroenterology 91: 1309–1311

Baines MJ 1994 Intestinal obstruction. Cancer Survey 21: 147–156

Bakshi R, Mechtler LL, Kamran S, Gosy E, Bates VE, Kinkel PR, Kinkel WR 1999 MRI findings in lumbar puncture headache syndrome: abnormal dural-meningeal and dural venous sinus enhancement. Clinical Imaging 23: 73–76

Balm M, Hammack J 1996 Leptomeningeal carcinomatosis. Presenting features and prognostic factors [see comments]. Archives of Neurology 53: 626–632

Banning A, Sjogren P, Henriksen H 1991 Pain causes in 200 patients referred to a multidisciplinary cancer pain clinic. Pain 45: 45–48

Barcena A, Lobato RD, Rivas JJ, Cordobes F, de Castro S, Cabrera A, Lamas E 1984 Spinal metastatic disease: analysis of factors determining functional prognosis and the choice of treatment. Neurosurgery 15: 820–827

Barker FG II, Jannetta PJ, Babu RP, Pomonis S, Bissonette DJ, Jho HD 1996 Long-term outcome after operation for trigeminal neuralgia in patients with posterior fossa tumors. Journal of Neurosurgery 84: 818–825

Barron KD, Hirano A, Araki S et al 1959 Experience with metastatic neoplasms involving the spinal cord. Neurology 9: 91–100

Batts KP 1998 Ischemic cholangitis. Mayo Clinic Proceedings 73: 380–385

Bell A 1988 Preventing perineal burning from i.v. dexamethasone. Oncological Nursing Forum 15: 199

Bellmunt J, Navarro M, Hidalgo R, Sole LA 1988 Palmar-plantar erythrodysesthesia syndrome associated with short-term continuous infusion (5 days) of 5-fluorouracil. Tumori 74: 329–331

Berger MS, Cooley ME, Abrahm JL 1995 A pain syndrome associated with large adrenal metastases in patients with lung cancer. Journal of Pain and Symptom Management 10: 161–166

Berna L, Torres G, Carrio I, Estorch M, Germa JR, Alonso C 1994 Antigranulocyte antibody bone marrow scans in cancer patients with metastatic bone superscan appearance. Clinical Nuclear Medicine 19: 121–128

Bertelli G 1995 Prevention and management of extravasation of cytotoxic drugs. Drug Safety 12: 245–255

Bitoh S, Hasegawa H, Ohtsuki H, Obashi J, Kobayashi Y 1985 Parasellar metastases: four autopsied cases. Surgical Neurological 23: 41–48

Boas RA, Schug SA, Acland RH 1993 Perineal pain after rectal amputation: a 5-year follow-up. Pain 52: 67–70

Bongers KM, Willigers HM, Koehler PJ 1992 Referred facial pain from lung carcinoma. Neurology 42: 1841–1842

Bonica JJ 1953a The management of pain. Lea & Febiger, Philadelphia

Bonica JJ 1953b Headache and other visceral disorders of the head and neck. In: The management of pain, 1st edn. Lea & Febiger, Philadelphia, pp 1263–1309
Bosley TM, Cohen DA, Schatz NJ, Zimmerman RA, Bilaniuk LT, Savino PJ, Sergott RS 1985 Comparison of metrizamide computed tomography and magnetic resonance imaging in the evaluation of lesions at the cervicomedullary junction. Neurology 35: 485–492
Boyle DM, Engelking C 1995 Vesicant extravasation: myths and realities. Oncological Nursing Forum 22: 57–67
Brady AM 1996 Management of painful paraneoplastic syndromes. Hematology/Oncology Clinics of North America 10: 801–809
Briselli M, Mark EJ, Dickersin GR 1981 Solitary fibrous tumors of the pleura: eight new cases and review of 360 cases in the literature. Cancer 47: 2678–2689
Brogden RN, Chrisp P 1991 Flutamide. A review of its pharmacodynamic and pharmacokinetic properties, and therapeutic use in advanced prostatic cancer. Drugs and Aging 1: 104–115
Brown H, Burns S, Kaiser CW 1988 The spinal accessory nerve plexus, the trapezius muscle, and shoulder stabilization after radical neck cancer surgery. Annals of Surgery 208: 654–661
Bruera E, MacDonald N 1986 Intractable pain in patients with advanced head and neck tumors: a possible role of local infection. Cancer Treatment Report 70: 691–692
Bullitt E, Tew JM, Boyd J 1986 Intracranial tumors in patients with facial pain. Journal of Neurosurgery 64: 865–871
Burihan E, de Figueiredo LF, Francisco Junior J, Miranda Junior F 1993 Upper-extremity deep venous thrombosis: analysis of 52 cases, Cardiovascular Surgery 1: 19–22
Camisa C, Helm TN, Liu YC, Valenzuela R, Allen C, Bona S, Larrimer N, Korman NJ 1992 Paraneoplastic pemphigus: a report of three cases including one long-term survivor. Journal of the American Academy of Dermatology 27: 547–553
Cantwell BM, Richardson PG, Campbell SJ 1991 Gynaecomastia and extragonadal symptoms leading to diagnosis delay of germ cell tumours in young men [see comments]. Postgraduate Medical Journal 67: 675–677
Capobianco DJ 1995 Facial pain as a symptom of nonmetastatic lung cancer. Headache 35: 581–585
Caraceni A, Portenoy RK 1999 An international survey of cancer pain characteristics and syndromes. IASP Task Force on Cancer Pain. International Association for the Study of Pain. Pain 82: 263–274
Carpenter JS, Andrykowski MA, Sloan P, Cunningham L, Cordova MJ, Studts JL, McGrath PC, Sloan D, Kenady DE 1998 Postmastectomy/postlumpectomy pain in breast cancer survivors. Journal of Clinical Epidemiology 51: 1285–1292
Cartwright PD, Hesse C, Jackson AO 1993 Myoclonic spasms following intrathecal diamorphine. Journal of Pain and Symptom Management 8: 492–495
Cascino TL, Kori S, Krol G, Foley KM 1983 CT of the brachial plexus in patients with cancer. Neurology 33: 1553–1557
Castaigne S, Chomienne C, Daniel MT, Ballerini P, Berger R, Fenaux P, Degos L 1990 All-trans retinoic acid as a differentiation therapy for acute promyelocytic leukemia. I. Clinical results [see comments]. Blood 76: 1704–1709
Castellanos AM, Glass JP, Yung WK 1987 Regional nerve injury after intra-arterial chemotherapy. Neurology 37: 834–837
Chad DA, Bradley WG 1987 Lumbosacral plexopathy. Seminars in Neurology 7: 97–107
Chang VT, Tunkel RS, Pattillo BA, Lachmann EA 1997 Increased phantom limb pain as an initial symptom of spinal-neoplasia. Journal of Pain and Symptom Management 13: 362–364 [Erratum 1997 Journal of Pain and Symptom Management 14(3): 135]
Chen C, Chen PJ, Yang PM, Huang GT, Lai MY, Tsang YM, Chen DS 1997 Clinical and microbiological features of liver abscess after transarterial embolization for hepatocellular carcinoma. American Journal of Gastroenterology 92: 2257–2259
Cheng TM, Cascino TL, Onofrio BM 1993 Comprehensive study of diagnosis and treatment of trigeminal neuralgia secondary to tumors. Neurology 43: 2298–2302
Cherny NI, Catane R 1995 Professional negligence in the management of cancer pain. A case for urgent reforms [editorial; comment]. Cancer 76: 2181–2185
Cherny NI, Portenoy RK 1999 Cancer pain: principles of assessment and syndromes. In: Wall PD, Melzack R (eds) Textbook of pain, 4th edn. Churchill Livingstone, Edinburgh, pp 1017–1064
Chrisp P, Goa KL 1991 Goserelin. A review of its pharmacodynamic and pharmacokinetic properties, and clinical use in sex hormone-related conditions. Drugs 41: 254–288
Chrisp P, Sorkin EM 1991 Leuprorelin. A review of its pharmacology and therapeutic use in prostatic disorders. Drugs and Aging 1: 487–509
Clarke-Pearson DL, Olt G 1989 Thromboembolism in patients with Gyn tumors: risk factors, natural history, and prophylaxis. Oncology (Huntingt) 3: 39–45; discussion 45, 48
Colleoni M, Gaion F, Vicario G, Nelli P, Pancheri F, Sgarbossa G, Manente P 1995 Pain at tumor site after vinorelbine injection: description of an unexpected side effect. Tumori 81: 194–196
Constans JP, de Divitiis E, Donzelli R, Spaziante R, Meder JF, Haye C 1983 Spinal metastases with neurological manifestations. Review of 600 cases. Journal of Neurosurgery 59: 111–118
Coombs DW 1990 Pain due to liver capsular distention. In: Ferrer-Brechner T (ed) Common problems in pain management. Year Book Medical Publishers, Chicago, pp 247–253
Corbey MP, Bach AB, Lech K, Frorup AM 1997 Grading of severity of postdural puncture headache after 27-gauge Quincke and Whitacre needles. Acta Anaesthesiologica Scandinavica 41: 779–784
Coukell AJ, Markham A 1998 Pamidronate. A review of its use in the management of osteolytic bone metastases, tumour-induced hypercalcaemia and Paget's disease of bone. Drugs and Aging 12: 149–168
Cowap J, Hardy JR, A'Hern R 2000 Outcome of malignant spinal cord compression at a cancer center: implications for palliative care services. Journal of Pain and Symptom Management 19: 257–264
Coyle N, Portenoy RK 1991 Infection as a cause of rapidly increasing pain in cancer patients. Journal of Pain and Symptom Management 6: 266–269
Criado E, Burnham CB 1997 Predictive value of clinical criteria for the diagnosis of deep vein thrombosis. Surgery 122: 578–583
Culy CR, Clemett D, Wiseman LR 2000 Oxaliplatin. A review of its pharmacological properties and clinical efficacy in metastatic colorectal cancer and its potential in other malignancies [In Process Citation]. Drugs 60 895–924
Curran CF, Luce JK, Page JA 1990 Doxorubicin-associated flare reactions. Oncological Nursing Forum 17: 387–389
Dalmau JO, Posner JB 1997 Paraneoplastic syndromes affecting the nervous system. Seminars in Oncology 24: 318–328
Daly BD 1995 Thoracic metastases from nasopharyngeal carcinoma presenting as hypertrophic pulmonary osteoarthropathy: scintigraphic and CT findings. Clinical Radiology 50: 545–547
Daut RL, Cleeland CS 1982 The prevalence and severity of pain in cancer. Cancer 50: 1913–1918
Davies JH, Dowsett M, Jacobs S, Coombes RC, Hedley A, Shearer RJ 1992 Aromatase inhibition: 4-hydroxyandrostenedione (4-OHA, CGP 32349) in advanced prostatic cancer. British Journal of Cancer 66: 139–142
Davies RA, Darby M, Richards MA 1991 Hypertrophic pulmonary osteoarthropathy in pulmonary metastatic disease. A case

report and review of the literature. Clinical Radiology 43: 268–271 [The above report is in Macintosh/PC/UNIX text/html format.]
Davis RW 1993 Phantom sensation, phantom pain, and stump pain. Archives of Physical Medicine and Rehabilitation 74: 79–91
DeAngelis LM, Payne R 1987 Lymphomatous meningitis presenting as atypical cluster headache. Pain 30: 211–216
De Castro MD, Meynadier MD, Zenz MD 1991 Regional opioid analgesia, vol 20. Kluwer Academic, Dordrecht
De Conno F, Polastri D 1996 [Clinical features and symptomatic treatment of liver metastasis in the terminally ill patient]. Annals Italiani Chirurgia 67: 819–826
De Conno F, Caraceni A, Martini C, Spoldi E, Salvetti M, Ventafridda V 1991 Hyperalgesia and myoclonus with intrathecal infusion of high-dose morphine. Pain 47: 337–339
De Marco S, Fabi A, Ceribelli A, Carlini P, Pollera CF, Cognetti F 1999 Does pain at tumor site during vinorelbine infusion affect treatment of recurrent head and neck cancer patients? [letter] Annals of Oncology 10: 865–866
Des Prez RD, Freemon FR 1983 Facial pain associated with lung cancer: a case report. Headache 23: 43–44
Desta K, O'Shaughnessy M, Milling MA 1994 Non-Hodgkin's lymphoma presenting as median nerve compression in the arm. Journal of Hand Surgery [Br] 19 289–291
Donati MB 1994 Cancer and thrombosis. Haemostasis 24: 128–131
Donayre CE, White GH, Mehringer SM, Wilson SE 1986 Pathogenesis determines late morbidity of axillosubclavian vein thrombosis. American Journal of Surgery 152: 179–184
Donnelly S, Walsh D 1995 The symptoms of advanced cancer. Seminars in Oncology 22: 67–72
Dooley M, Goa KL 1999 Capecitabine. Drugs 58: 69–76; discussion 77–78
Dose AM 1995 The symptom experience of mucositis, stomatitis, and xerostomia. Seminars in Oncological Nursing 11: 248–255
Dulli DA, Levine RL, Chun RW, Dinndorf P 1987 Migrainous neurologic dysfunction in Hodgkin's disease [letter]. Archives of Neurology 44: 689
Dykman TR, Montgomery EB Jr, Gerstenberger PD, Zeiger HE, Clutter WE, Cryer PE 1981 Glossopharyngeal neuralgia with syncope secondary to tumor. Treatment and pathophysiology. American Journal of Medicine 71: 165–170
Edwards WT 1990 Optimizing opioid treatment of postoperative pain. Journal of Pain and Symptom Management 5: S24–S36
Ehde DM, Czerniecki JM, Smith DG, Campbell KM, Edwards WT, Jensen MP, Robinson LR 2000 Chronic phantom sensations, phantom pain, residual limb pain, and other regional pain after lower limb amputation. Archives of Physical Medicine and Rehabilitation 81: 1039–1044
Elomaa I, Pajunen M, Virkkunen P 1984 Raynaud's phenomenon progressing to gangrene after vincristine and bleomycin therapy. Acta Medica Scandinavica 216: 323–326
Emanuel EJ 1996 Pain and symptom control. Patient rights and physician responsibilities. Hematology/Oncology Clinics of North America 10: 41–56
Ende DA, Robinson G, Moulton J 1995 Metastasis-induced perforated appendicitis: an acute abdomen of rare aetiology. Australian and New Zealand Journal of Surgery 65: 62–63
Epstein J, van der Meij E, McKenzie M, Wong F, Lepawsky M, Stevenson-Moore P 1997 Postradiation osteonecrosis of the mandible: a long-term follow-up study. Oral Surgery, Oral Medicine, Oral Pathology, Oral Radiology, and Endodontics 83: 657–662
Epstein JB, Rea G, Wong FL, Spinelli J, Stevenson-Moore P 1987 Osteonecrosis: study of the relationship of dental extractions in patients receiving radiotherapy. Head and Neck Surgery 10: 48–54
Epstein JB, Stewart KH 1993 Radiation therapy and pain in patients with head and neck cancer. European Journal of Cancer B: Oral Oncology 29B: 191–199
Escalante CP 1993 Causes and management of superior vena cava syndrome. Oncology (Huntingt) 7: 61–68; discussion 71–72, 75–77
Eskilsson J, Albertsson M 1990 Failure of preventing 5-fluorouracil cardiotoxicity by prophylactic treatment with verapamil. Acta Oncologica 29: 1001–1003
Esteban A, Traba A 1993 Fasciculation-myokymic activity and prolonged nerve conduction block. A physiopathological relationship in radiation-induced brachial plexopathy. Electroencephalography and Clinical Neurophysiology 89: 382–391
Evans RW 1998 Complications of lumbar puncture. Neurologic Clinics 16: 83–105
Fabian CJ, Molina R, Slavik M, Dahlberg S, Giri S, Stephens R 1990 Pyridoxine therapy for palmar-plantar erythrodysesthesia associated with continuous 5-fluorouracil infusion. Investigational New Drugs 8: 57–63
Feldenzer JA, McGauley JL, McGillicuddy JE 1989 Sacral and presacral tumors: problems in diagnosis and management. Neurosurgery 25: 884–891
Ferrell BR, Dean G 1995 The meaning of cancer pain. Seminars in Oncological Nursing 11: 17–22
Fine PG, Busch MA 1998 Characterization of breakthrough pain by hospice patients and their caregivers. Journal of Pain and Symptom Management 16: 179–183
Fishman EK, Campbell JN, Kuhlman JE, Kawashima A, Ney DR, Friedman NB 1991 Multiplanar CT evaluation of brachial plexopathy in breast cancer. Journal of Computer Assisted Tomography 15: 790–795
Foley KM 1987a Pain syndromes in patients with cancer. Medical Clinics of North America 71: 169–184
Foley KM 1987b Cancer pain syndromes. Journal of Pain and Symptom Management 2: 513–517
Forman A 1990 Peripheral neuropathy in cancer patients: clinical types, etiology, and presentation. Part 2. Oncology (Huntingt) 4: 85–89
Forst T, Beyer J, Cordes U, Pfutzner A, Kustner E, Moll R, Bockisch A, Lehnert H 1995 Gynaecomastia in a patient with a hCG producing giant cell carcinoma of the lung. Case report. Experimental and Clinical Endocrinology and Diabetes 103: 28–32
Forsyth PA, Posner JB 1993 Headaches in patients with brain tumors: a study of 111 patients. Neurology 43: 1678–1683
Fossa SD, Urnes T 1986 Flare reaction during the initial treatment period with medroxyprogesterone acetate in patients with hormone-resistant prostatic cancer. European Urology 12: 257–259
Freedman DM, Henderson RC 1995 Metastatic breast carcinoma to the os calcis presenting as heel pain. Southern Medical Journal 88: 232–234
Freeman NJ, Costanza ME 1988 5-Fluorouracil-associated cardiotoxicity. Cancer 61: 36–45
Frenken LA, van Lier HJ, Gerlag PG, den Hartog M, Koene RA 1991 Assessment of pain after subcutaneous injection of erythropoietin in patients receiving haemodialysis. British Medical Journal 303: 288
Frenken LA, van Lier HJ, Koene RA 1994 Analysis of the efficacy of measures to reduce pain after subcutaneous administration of epoetin alfa [see comments]. Nephrology, Dialysis, Transplantation 9: 1295–1298
Friedman J, Karesh J, Rodrigues M, Sun CC 1990 Thyroid carcinoma metastatic to the medial rectus muscle. Ophthalamic Plastic and Reconstructive Surgery 6: 122–125

Galer BS, Portenoy RK 1991 Acute herpetic and postherpetic neuralgia: clinical features and management. Mt Sinai Journal of Medicine 58: 257–266
Ganel A, Engel J, Sela M, Brooks M 1979 Nerve entrapments associated with postmastectomy lymphedema. Cancer 44: 2254–2259
Gerard JM, Franck N, Moussa Z, Hildebrand J 1989 Acute ischemic brachial plexus neuropathy following radiation therapy. Neurology 39: 450–451
Gerl A 1994 Vascular toxicity associated with chemotherapy for testicular cancer. Anticancer Drugs 5: 607–614
Gilbert RW, Kim JH, Posner JB 1978 Epidural spinal cord compression from metastatic tumor: diagnosis and treatment. Annals of Neurology 3: 40–51
Giorgi C, Broggi G 1984 Surgical treatment of glossopharyngeal neuralgia and pain from cancer of the nasopharynx. A 20-year experience. Journal of Neurosurgery 61: 952–955
Glass AR, Berenberg J 1979 Gynecomastia after chemotherapy for lymphoma. Archives of Internal Medicine 139: 1048–1049
Glavina MJ, Robertshaw R 1988 Myoclonic spasms following intrathecal morphine. Anaesthesia 43: 389–390
Goldenberg SL, Bruchovsky N 1991 Use of cyproterone acetate in prostate cancer. Urologic Clinics of North America 18: 111–122
Golembe B, Ramsay NK, McKenna R, Nesbit ME, Krivit W 1979 Localized bone marrow relapse in acute lymphoblastic leukemia. Medical and Pediatric Oncology 6: 229–234
Gonzalez DP 2000 Lumbar puncture headache exacerbated by recumbent position [editorial]. Mil Med 165: vi, 690
Goodman M, Dalton JR 1982 Ureteral strictures following radiotherapy: incidence, etiology and treatment guidelines. Journal of Urology 128: 21–24
Gorson KC, Musaphir S, Lathi ES, Wolfe G 1995 Radiation-induced malignant fibrous histiocytoma of the brachial plexus. Journal of Neurooncology 26: 73–77
Graham DF 1976 Hip pain as a presenting symptom of acetabular metastasis. British Journal of Surgery 63: 147–148
Grahm AL, Andren-Sandberg A 1997 Prospective evaluation of pain in exocrine pancreatic cancer. Digestion 58: 542–549
Granek I, Ashikari R, Foley KM 1983 Postmastectomy pain syndrome: clinical and anatomic correlates. Proceedings American Society of Clinical Oncology 3: Abstract 122
Graus F, Krol G, Foley K 1986 Early diagnosis of spinal epidural metastasis: correlation with clinical and radiological findings. Proceedings American Society of Clinical Oncology 5: Abstract 1047
Greenberg HS, Kim JH, Posner JB 1980 Epidural spinal cord compression from metastatic tumor: results with a new treatment protocol. Annals of Neurology 8: 361–366
Greenberg HS, Deck MD, Vikram B, Chu FC, Posner JB 1981 Metastasis to the base of the skull: clinical findings in 43 patients. Neurology 31: 530–537
Greenfield A, Resnick MI 1989 Genitourinary emergencies. Seminars in Oncology 16: 516–520
Greenfield GB, Schorsch HA, Shkolnik A 1967 The various roentgen appearances of pulmonary hypertrophic osteoarthropathy. American Journal of Roentgenology Radium Therapy and Nuclear Medicine 101: 927–931
Grisold W, Drlicek M 1999 Paraneoplastic neuropathy. Current Opinions in Neurology 12: 617–625
Grond S, Zech D, Diefenbach C, Radbruch L, Lehmann KA 1996 Assessment of cancer pain: a prospective evaluation in 2266 cancer patients referred to a pain service. Pain 64: 107–114
Grossman SA, Krabak ML 1999 Leptomeningeal carcinomatosis. Cancer Treatment Reviews 25: 103–119
Grossman SA, Sheidler VR, Swedeen K, Mucenski J, Piantadosi S 1991 Correlation of patient and caregiver ratings of cancer pain. Journal of Pain and Symptom Management 6: 53–57
Guise TA 2000 Molecular mechanisms of osteolytic bone metastases. Cancer 88: 2892–2898
Gupta SR, Zdonczyk DE, Rubino FA 1990 Cranial neuropathy in systemic malignancy in a VA population [see comments]. Neurology 40: 997–999
Haas GP, Pittaluga S, Gomella L, Travis WD, Sherins RJ, Doppman JL, Linehan WM, Robertson C 1989 Clinically occult Leydig cell tumor presenting with gynecomastia. Journal of Urology 142: 1325–1327
Hagen NA 1993 Sharp, shooting neuropathic pain in the rectum or genitals: pudendal neuralgia. Journal of Pain and Symptom Management 8: 496–501
Hall JH, Fleming JF 1970 The 'lumbar disc syndrome' produced by sacral metastases. Canadian Journal of Surgery 13: 149–156
Hamada H, Moriwaki K, Shiroyama K, Tanaka H, Kawamoto M, Yuge O 2000 Myofascial pain in patients with postthoracotomy pain syndrome. Regional Anesthesia and Pain Medicine 25: 302–305
Hanna SL, Fletcher BD, Fairclough DL, Jenkins JHD, Le AH 1991 Magnetic resonance imaging of disseminated bone marrow disease in patients treated for malignancy. Skeletal Radiology 20: 79–84
Hansen SW, Olsen N, Rossing N, Rorth M 1990 Vascular toxicity and the mechanism underlying Raynaud's phenomenon in patients treated with cisplatin, vinblastine and bleomycin [see comments]. Annals of Oncology 1: 289–292
Harper DM 1994 Pain and cramping associated with cryosurgery. Journal of Family Practice 39: 551–557
Harrington KJ, Pandha HS, Kelly SA, Lambert HE, Jackson JE, Waxman J 1995 Palliation of obstructive nephropathy due to malignancy. British Journal of Urology 76: 101–107
Hawley RJ, Patel A, Lastinger L 1999 Cranial nerve compression from breast cancer metastasis [letter; comment]. Surgical Neurology 52: 431–432
Hayashi M, Handa Y, Kobayashi H, Kawano H, Ishii H, Horose S 1991 Plateau-wave phenomenon (I). Correlation between the appearance of the plateau waves and CSF circulation in patients with intracranial hypertension. Brain 114(pt 6): 2681–2691
Hayreh SS, Blodi FC, Silbermann NN, Summers TB, Potter PH 1982 Unilateral optic nerve head and choroidal metastases from a bronchial carcinoma. Ophthalmologica 185: 232–241
Healey JH, Turnbull AD, Miedema B, Lane JM 1986 Acrometastases. A study of twenty-nine patients with osseous involvement of the hands and feet. Journal of Bone and Joint Surgery [Am] 68: 743–746
Heinmoller E, Schropp T, Kisker O, Simon B, Seitz R, Weinel RJ 1995 Tumor cell-induced platelet aggregation in vitro by human pancreatic cancer cell lines. Scandinavian Journal of Gastroenterology 30: 1008–1016
Helweg-Larsen S 1996 Clinical outcome in metastatic spinal cord compression. A prospective study of 153 patients. Acta Neurologica Scandinavica 94: 269–275
Helweg-Larsen S, Sorensen PS 1994 Symptoms and signs in metastatic spinal cord compression: a study of progression from first symptom until diagnosis in 153 patients. European Journal of Cancer 30A: 396–398
Helweg-Larsen S, Rasmusson B, Sorensen PS 1990 Recovery of gait after radiotherapy in paralytic patients with metastatic epidural spinal cord compression. Neurology 40: 1234–1236
Hilkens PH, Verweij J, Stoter G, Vecht CJ, van Putten WL, van den Bent MJ 1996 Peripheral neurotoxicity induced by docetaxel [see comments]. Neurology 46: 104–108
Hill BA, Kohut RI 1976 Metastatic adenocarcinoma of the temporal bone. Archives of Otolaryngology 102: 568–571
Hill ME, Richards MA, Gregory WM, Smith P, Rubens RD 1993 Spinal cord compression in breast cancer: a review of 70 cases. British Journal of Cancer 68: 969–973

Hillner BE, Ingle JN, Berenson JR, Janjan NA, Albain KS, Lipton A, Yee G, Biermann JS, Chlebowski RT, Pfister DG 2000 American Society of Clinical Oncology guideline on the role of bisphosphonates in breast cancer. American Society of Clinical Oncology Bisphosphonates Expert Panel. Journal of Clinical Oncology 18: 1378–1391
Hirota N, Fujimoto T, Takahashi M, Fukushima Y 1998 Isolated trigeminal nerve metastases from breast cancer: an unusual cause of trigeminal mononeuropathy [in process citation]. Surgical Neurology 49: 558–561
Hirschmann JV 1987 Ischemic forms of acute venous thrombosis. Archives of Dermatology 123: 933–936
Hladiuk M, Huchcroft S, Temple W, Schnurr BE 1992 Arm function after axillary dissection for breast cancer: a pilot study to provide parameter estimates. Journal of Surgical Oncology 50: 47–52
Hollingshead LM, Goa KL 1991 Recombinant granulocyte colony-stimulating factor (rG-CSF). A review of its pharmacological properties and prospective role in neutropenic conditions. Drugs 42: 300–330
Huddart RA, Rajan B, Law M, Meyer L, Dearnaley DP 1997 Spinal cord compression in prostate cancer: treatment outcome and prognostic factors. Radiotherapy and Oncology 44: 229–236
Hundrieser J 1988 A non-invasive approach to minimizing vessel pain with DTIC or BCNU. Oncological Nursing Forum 15: 199
Hung GU, Kao CH, Lin WY, Wang SJ 2000 Rapid resolution of hypertrophic pulmonary osteoarthropathy after resection of a lung mass caused by xanthogranulomatous inflammation [in process citation]. Clinical Nuclear Medicine 25: 1029–1030
Husband DJ 1998 Malignant spinal cord compression: prospective study of delays in referral and treatment. British Medical Journal 317: 18–21
International Association for the Study of Pain: Subcommittee on Taxonomy 1986 Classification of chronic pain. Pain 3 (suppl): 135–138
Irani J, Fournier F, Bon D, Gremmo E, Dore B, Aubert J 1997 Patient tolerance of transrectal ultrasound-guided biopsy of the prostate. British Journal of Urology 79: 608–610
Jacobsen P, Kriegstein O, Portenoy R 1994 Breakthrough pain: prevalence and characteristics (meeting abstract). Proceedings Annual Meeting American Society of Clinical Oncology 13: abstract 1643
Jaeckle KA 1991 Nerve plexus metastases. Neurologic Clinics 9: 857–866
Jaeckle KA, Young DF, Foley KM, 1985 The natural history of lumbosacral plexopathy in cancer. Neurology 35: 8–15
Jayson GC, Howell A 1996 Carcinomatous meningitis in solid tumours. Annals of Oncology 7: 773–786
Joly F, Brune D, Couette JE, Lesaunier F, Heron JF, Peny J, Henry-Amar M 1998 Health-related quality of life and sequelae in patients treated with brachytherapy and external beam irradiation for localized prostate cancer. Annals of Oncology 9: 751–757
Jones HM, Conces DJ Jr, Tarver RD 1993 Painful transthoracic needle biopsy: a sign of neurogenic tumor. Journal of Thoracic Imaging 8: 230–232
Jonsson OG, Sartain P, Ducore JM, Buchanan GR 1990 Bone pain as an initial symptom of childhood acute lymphoblastic leukemia: association with nearly normal hematologic indexes. Journal of Pediatrics 117: 233–237
Kahn CE Jr, Messersmith RN, Samuels BL 1989 Brachial plexopathy as a complication of intraarterial cisplatin chemotherapy. Cardiovascular and Interventional Radiology 12: 47–49
Kanner R, Martini N, Foley KM 1982 Nature and incidence of postthoracotomy pain. Proceedings American Society of Clinical Oncology 1: Abstract 590
Kaplan JG, DeSouza TG, Farkash A et al 1990 Leptomeningeal metastases: comparison of clinical features and laboratory data of solid tumors, lymphomas and leukemias. Journal of Neurooncology 9: 225–229
Kaplan RA, Markman M, Lucas WE, Pfeifle C, Howell SB 1985 Infectious peritonitis in patients receiving intraperitoneal chemotherapy. American Journal of Medicine 78: 49–53
Kaymakcalan H, Sequeria W, Barretta T, Ghosh BC, Steigmann F 1980 Hypertrophic osteoarthropathy with myogenic tumors of the esophagus. American Journal of Gastroenterology 74: 17–20
Keller SM, Carp NZ, Levy MN, Rosen SM 1994 Chronic post thoracotomy pain. Journal of Cardiovascular Surgery (Torino) 35: 161–164
Kelsen DP, Portenoy R, Thaler H, Tao Y, Brennan M 1997 Pain as a predictor of outcome in patients with operable pancreatic carcinoma. Surgery 122: 53–59
Kelsen DP, Portenoy RK, Thaler HT, Niedzwiecki D, Passik SD, Tao Y, Banks W, Brennan MF, Foley KM 1995 Pain and depression in patients with newly diagnosed pancreas cancer. Journal of Clinical Oncology 13: 748–755
Kemeny MM 1991 Continuous hepatic artery infusion (CHAI) as treatment of liver metastases. Are the complications worth it? Drug Safety 6: 159–165
Kemeny N 1992 Review of regional therapy of liver metastases in colorectal cancer. Seminars in Oncology 19: 155–162
Kempen PM, Mocek CK 1997 Bevel direction, dura geometry, and hole size in membrane puncture: laboratory report. Regional Anesthesia 22: 267–272
Killer HE, Hess K 1990 Natural history of radiation-induced brachial plexopathy compared with surgically treated patients. Journal of Neurology 237: 247–250
Kissel JT, Mendell JR 1996 Neuropathies associated with monoclonal gammopathies. Neuromuscular Disorders 6: 3–18
Kontturi M, Kauppila A 1982 Ureteric complications following treatment of gynaecological cancer. Annals Chirurgiae et Gynaecologiae 71: 232–238
Kori SH 1995 Diagnosis and management of brachial plexus lesions in cancer patients. Oncology (Huntingt) 9: 756–760; discussion 765
Kori SH, Foley KM, Posner JB 1981 Brachial plexus lesions in patients with cancer: 100 cases. Neurology 31: 45–50
Kornek GV, Kornfehl H, Hejna M, Raderer M, Zochbauer S, Scheithauer W 1996 Acute tumor pain in patients with head and neck cancer treated with vinorelbine [letter]. Journal of the National Cancer Institute 88: 1593
Krane RJ, Perrone TL 1981 A young man with testicular and abdominal pain. New England Journal of Medicine 305: 331–336
Kudo S, Tsushima N, Sawada Y, Saito F, Motomura F, Takashima T, Kogawa T, Suzuki T, Kurotaki H, Masumori J et al 1991 [Serious complications of intravesical bacillus Calmette-Guerin therapy in patients with bladder cancer]. Nippon Hinyokika Gakkai Zasshi 82: 1594–1602
Kukla LJ, McGuire WP, Lad T, Saltiel M 1982 Acute vascular episodes associated with therapy for carcinomas of the upper aerodigestive tract with bleomycin, vincristine, and cisplatin. Cancer Treatment Reports 66: 369–370
Labrie F, Dupont A, Belanger A, Lachance R 1987 Flutamide eliminates the risk of disease flare in prostatic cancer patients treated with a luteinizing hormone-releasing hormone agonist. Journal of Urology 138: 804–806
Lachance DH, O'Neill BP, Harper CM Jr, Banks PM, Cascino TL 1991 Paraneoplastic brachial plexopathy in a patient with Hodgkin's disease. Mayo Clinic Proceedings 66: 97–101
Laitt RD, Kumar B, Leatherbarrow B, Bonshek RE, Jackson A 1996 Cystic optic nerve meningioma presenting with acute proptosis. Eye 10: 744–746

Lambert DH, Hurley RJ, Hertwig L, Datta S 1997 Role of needle gauge and tip configuration in the production of lumbar puncture headache. Regional Anesthesia 22: 66–72

Laredo JD, Lakhdari K, Bellaiche L, Hamze B, Janklewicz P, Tubiana JM 1995 Acute vertebral collapse: CT findings in benign and malignant nontraumatic cases. Radiology 194: 41–48

Lawson W, Reino AJ 1997 Isolated sphenoid sinus disease: an analysis of 132 cases. Laryngoscope 107: 1590–1595

Leaney BJ, Martin M 1992 Breast pain associated with mammographic compression. Australasian Radiology 36: 120–123

Lederman RJ, Wilbourn AJ 1984 Brachial plexopathy: recurrent cancer or radiation? Neurology 34: 1331–1335

Lembersky BC, Ratain MJ, Golomb HM 1988 Skeletal complications in hairy cell leukemia: diagnosis and therapy. Journal of Clinical Oncology 6: 1280–1284

Leo S, Tatulli C, Taveri R, Campanella GA, Carrieri G, Colucci G 1994 Dermatological toxicity from chemotherapy containing 5-fluorouracil. Journal of Chemotherapy 6: 423–426

Levine M, Hirsh J, Gent M, Arnold A, Warr D, Falanga A, Samosh M, Bramwell V, Pritchard KI, Stewart D et al 1994 Double-blind randomised trial of a very-low-dose warfarin for prevention of thromboembolism in stage IV breast cancer [see comments]. Lancet 343: 886–889

Loevner LA, Yousem DM 1997 Overlooked metastatic lesions of the occipital condyle: a missed case treasure trove. Radiographics 17: 1111–1121

Lokich JJ, Moore C 1984 Chemotherapy-associated palmar-plantar erythrodysesthesia syndrome. Annals of Internal Medicine 101: 798–799

LoMonaco M, Milone M, Batocchi AP, Padua L, Restuccia D, Tonali P 1992 Cisplatin neuropathy: clinical course and neurophysiological findings. Journal of Neurology 239: 199–204

Lorimer JW, Semelhago LC, Barber GG 1994 Venous gangrene of the extremities [see comments]. Canadian Journal of Surgery 37 379–384

Lossos A, Siegal T 1992 Numb chin syndrome in cancer patients: etiology, response to treatment, and prognostic significance [see comments]. Neurology 42: 1181–1184

Lybecker H, Djernes M, Schmidt JF 1995 Postdural puncture headache (PDPH): onset, duration, severity, and associated symptoms. An analysis of 75 consecutive patients with PDPH. Acta Anaesthesiologica Scandinavica 39: 605–612

Marangoni C, Lacerenza M, Formaglio F, Smirne S, Marchettini P 1993 Sensory disorder of the chest as presenting symptom of lung cancer. Journal of Neurology, Neurosurgery and Psychiatry 56: 1033–1034

Maranzano E, Latini P 1995 Effectiveness of radiation therapy without surgery in metastatic spinal cord compression: final results from a prospective trial [see comments]. International Journal of Radiation Oncology–Biology–Physics 32: 959–967

Marino C, Zoppi M, Morelli F, Buoncristiano U, Pagni E 1986 Pain in early cancer of the lungs. Pain 27: 57–62

Markman M 1986 Cytotoxic intracavitary chemotherapy. American Journal of Medical Sciences 291: 175–179

Marks RM, Sachar EJ 1973 Undertreatment of medical inpatients with narcotic analgesics. Annals of Internal Medicine 78: 173–181

Marshall JA, Mahanna GK 1997 Cancer in the differential diagnosis of orofacial pain. Dental Clinics of North America 41: 355–365

Martin R, Jourdain S, Clairoux M, Tetrault JP 1994 Duration of decubitus position after epidural blood patch. Canadian Journal of Anaesthesia 41: 23–25

Martin S, Jones JS, Wynn BN 1996 Does warming local anesthetic reduce the pain of subcutaneous injection? American Journal of Emergency Medicine 14: 10–12

Martinez-Lavin M 1997 Hypertrophic osteoarthropathy. Current Opinions in Rheumatology 9: 83–86

Matsuda M, Yoneda S, Handa H, Gotoh H 1979 Cerebral hemodynamic changes during plateau waves in brain-tumor patients. Journal of Neurosurgery 50: 483–488

Matsumura Y, Akaza H, Isaka S, Kagawa S, Koiso K, Kotake T, Machida T, Niijima T, Obata K, Ohashi Y et al 1992 The 4th study of prophylactic intravesical chemotherapy with adriamycin in the treatment of superficial bladder cancer: the experience of the Japanese Urological Cancer Research Group for Adriamycin. Cancer Chemotherapy and Pharmacology 30 (Suppl): S10–S14

Maunsell E, Brisson J, Deschenes L 1993 Arm problems and psychological distress after surgery for breast cancer. Canadian Journal of Surgery 36: 315–320

McCarthy GM, Skillings JR 1992 Jaw and other orofacial pain in patients receiving vincristine for the treatment of cancer. Oral Surgery, Oral Medicine, Oral Pathology 74: 299–304

McConaha C, Bastiani AM, Kaye WH 1996 Significant reduction of post-lumbar puncture headaches by the use of a 29-gauge spinal needle. Biological Psychiatry 39: 1058–1060

McDonald DR 1991 Neurological complications of chemotherapy. Neurology Clinics 9: 955–967

McEwan AJ 1997 Unsealed source therapy of painful bone metastases: an update. Seminars in Nuclear Medicine 27: 165–182

Medina LS, Pinter JD, Zurakowski D, Davis RG, Kuban K, Barnes PD 1997 Children with headache: clinical predictors of surgical space-occupying lesions and the role of neuroimaging. Radiology 202: 819–824

Mellor SG, McCutchan JD 1989 Gynaecomastia and occult Leydig cell tumour of the testis. British Journal of Urology 63: 420–422

Mercadante S 1997 Malignant bone pain: pathophysiology and treatment. Pain 69: 1–18

Metheetrairut C, Brown DH 1993 Glossopharyngeal neuralgia and syncope secondary to neck malignancy. Journal of Otolaryngology 22: 18–20

Miaskowski C 1996 Special needs related to the pain and discomfort of patients with gynecologic cancer. Journal of Obstetrics, Gynecologic and Neonatal Nursing 25: 181–188

Milross CG, Davies MA, Fisher R, Mameghan J, Mameghan H 1997 The efficacy of treatment for malignant epidural spinal cord compression. Australasian Radiology 41: 137–142

Minsky BD, Cohen AM 1988 Minimizing the toxicity of pelvic radiation therapy in rectal cancer. Oncology (Huntingt) 2: 21–25, 28–29

Miyamoto M, Sudo T, Kuyama T 1991 Spontaneous rupture of hepatocellular carcinoma: a review of 172 Japanese cases. American Journal of Gastroenterology 86: 67–71

Mollman JE, Hogan WM, Glover DJ, McCluskey LF 1988 Unusual presentation of cis-platinum neuropathy. Neurology 38: 488–490

Mondrup K, Olsen NK, Pfeiffer P, Rose C 1990 Clinical and electrodiagnostic findings in breast cancer patients with radiation-induced brachial plexus neuropathy. Acta Neurologica Scandinavica 81: 153–158

Morales M, Llanos M, Dorta J 1997 Superior vena cava thrombosis secondary to Hickman catheter and complete resolution after fibrinolytic therapy. Support Care Cancer 5: 67–69

Morewood GH 1993 A rational approach to the cause, prevention and treatment of postdural puncture headache [see comments]. Canadian Medical Association Journal 149: 1087–1093

Moris G, Roig C, Misiego M, Alvarez A, Berciano J, Pascual J 1998 The distinctive headache of the occipital condyle syndrome: a report of four cases. Headache 38: 308–311

Morris KP, Hughes C, Hardy SP, Matthews JN, Coulthard MG 1994 Pain after subcutaneous injection of recombinant human erythropoietin: does Emla cream help? Nephrology, Dialysis, Transplantation 9: 1299–1301

Morrison GA, Sterkers JM 1996 Unusual presentations of acoustic tumours. Clinics in Otolaryngology 21: 80–83

Mrozek-Orlowski M, Christie J, Flamme C, Novak J 1991 Pain associated with peripheral infusion of carmustine. Oncologic Nursing Forum 18: 942

Muggia FM, Vafai D, Natale R, Israel V, Zaretsky S, McRae A, Rogers M, Jeffers S 1995 Paclitaxel 3-hour infusion given alone and combined with carboplatin: preliminary results of dose-escalation trials. Seminars in Oncology 22: 63–66

Mulholland MW, Debas H, Bonica JJ 1990 Diseases of the liver, biliary system and pancreas. In: Bonica JJ (ed) The management of pain, vol 2. Lea & Febiger, Philadelphia, pp 1214–1231

Muram D, Oxorn H, Curry RH, Drouin P, Walters JH 1981 Postradiation ureteral obstruction: a reappraisal. American Journal of Obstetrics and Gynecology 139: 289–293

Nash PA, Bruce JE, Indudhara R, Shinohara K 1996 Transrectal ultrasound guided prostatic nerve blockade eases systematic needle biopsy of the prostate. Journal of Urology 155: 607–609

Neer RM, Ferrucci JT, Wang CA, Brennan M, Buttrick WF, Vickery AL 1981 A 77-year-old man with epigastric pain, hypercalcemia, and a retroperitoneal mass. New England Journal of Medicine 305: 874–883

Nemmers DW, Thorpe PE, Knibbe MA, Beard DW 1990 Upper extremity venous thrombosis. Case report and literature review. Orthopedic Review 19: 164–172

Newman ML, Brennan M, Passik S 1996 Lymphedema complicated by pain and psychological distress: a case with complex treatment needs. Journal of Pain and Symptom Management 12: 376–379

Nikolajsen L, Jensen TS 2000 Phantom limb pain. Current Reviews of Pain 4: 166–170

Nussbaum ML, Campana TJ, Weese JL 1993 Radiation-induced intestinal injury. Clinics in Plastic Surgery 20: 573–580

Ohno R, Yoshida H, Fukutani H, Naoe T, Ohshima T, Kyo T, Endoh N, Fujimoto T, Kobayashi T, Hiraoka A et al 1993 Multi-institutional study of all-trans-retinoic acid as a differentiation therapy of refractory acute promyelocytic leukemia. Leukaemia Study Group of the Ministry of Health and Welfare. Leukemia 7: 1722–1727

Olsen NK, Pfeiffer P, Mondrup K, Rose C 1990 Radiation-induced brachial plexus neuropathy in breast cancer patients. Acta Oncologica 29: 885–890

Olsson H, Alm P, Kristoffersson U, Landin-Olsson M 1984 Hypophyseal tumor and gynecomastia preceding bilateral breast cancer development in a man. Cancer 53: 1974–1977

Ovesen P, Kroner K, Ornsholt J, Bach K 1991 Phantom-related phenomena after rectal amputation: prevalence and clinical characteristics. Pain 44: 289–291

Palmon SC, Lloyd AT, Kirsch JR 1998 The effect of needle gauge and lidocaine pH on pain during intradermal injection. Anesthesia and Analgesia 86: 379–381

Paredes JP, Puente JL, Potel J 1990 Variations in sensitivity after sectioning the intercostobrachial nerve. American Journal of Surgery 160: 525–528

Payten RJ 1972 Facial pain as the first symptom in acoustic neuroma. Journal of Laryngology and Otology 86: 523–534

Perez CA, Grigsby PW, Lockett MA, Chao KS, Williamson J 1999 Radiation therapy morbidity in carcinoma of the uterine cervix: dosimetric and clinical correlation. International Journal of Radiation Oncology–Biology–Physics 44: 855–866

Perkins JM, Magee TR, Galland RB 1996 Phlegmasia caerulea dolens and venous gangrene [see comments]. British Journal of Surgery 83: 19–23

Peterson K, Forsyth PA, Posner JB 1994 Paraneoplastic sensorimotor neuropathy associated with breast cancer. Journal of Neurooncology 21: 159–170

Phillips E, Levine AM 1989 Metastatic lesions of the upper cervical spine. Spine 14: 1071–1077

Pierce SM, Recht A, Lingos TI, Abner A, Vicini F, Silver B, Herzog A, Harris JR 1992 Long-term radiation complications following conservative surgery (CS) and radiation therapy (RT) in patients with early stage breast cancer [see comments]. International Journal of Radiation Oncology–Biology–Physics 23: 915–923

Pillay PK, Teh M, Chua EJ, Tan EC, Tung KH, Foo KT 1984 Haemorrhagic chronic radiation cystitis—following treatment of pelvic malignancies. Annals, Academy of Medicine, Singapore 13: 634–638

Pines A, Kaplinsky N, Olchovsky D, Frankl O 1984 Rheumatoid arthritis-like syndrome: a presenting symptom of malignancy. Report of 3 cases and review of the literature. European Journal of Rheumatology and Inflammation 7: 51–55

Plante-Bordeneuve V, Baudrimont M, Gorin NC, Gherardi RK 1994 Subacute sensory neuropathy associated with Hodgkin's disease. Journal of the Neurological Sciences 121: 155–158

Plotkin D, Lechner JJ, Jung WE, Rosen PJ 1978 Tamoxifen flare in advanced breast cancer. Journal of the American Medical Association 240: 2644–2646

Portenoy RK, Hagen NA 1990 Breakthrough pain: definition, prevalence and characteristics [see comments]. Pain 41: 273–281

Portenoy RK, Abissi CJ, Robbins JB 1983 Increased intracranial pressure with normal ventricular size due to superior vena cava obstruction [letter]. Archives of Neurology 40: 598

Portenoy RK, Duma C, Foley KM 1986 Acute herpetic and postherpetic neuralgia: clinical review and current management. Annals of Neurology 20: 651–664

Portenoy RK, Lipton RB, Foley KM 1987 Back pain in the cancer patient: an algorithm for evaluation and management. Neurology 37: 134–138

Portenoy RK, Galer BS, Salamon O et al 1989 Identification of epidural neoplasm. Radiography and bone scintigraphy in the symptomatic and asymptomatic spine. Cancer 64: 2207–2213

Portenoy RK, Miransky J, Thaler HT, Hornung J, Bianchi C, Cibas-Kong I, Feldhamer E, Lewis F, Matamoros I, Sugar MZ et al 1992 Pain in ambulatory patients with lung or colon cancer. Prevalence, characteristics, and effect. Cancer 70: 1616–1624

Portenoy RK, Kornblith AB, Wong G, Vlamis V, Lepore JM, Loseth DB, Hakes T, Foley KM, Hoskins WJ 1994 Pain in ovarian cancer patients. Prevalence, characteristics, and associated symptoms. Cancer 74: 907–915

Porter AD, Simpson AH, Davis AM, Griffin AM, Bell RS 1994 Diagnosis and management of sacral bone tumours [see comments]. Canadian Journal of Surgery 37: 473–478

Posner JB 1987 Back pain and epidural spinal cord compression. Medical Clinics of North America 71: 185–205

Postma TJ, Vermorken JB, Liefting AJ, Pinedo HM, Heimans JJ 1995 Paclitaxel-induced neuropathy. Annals of Oncology 6: 489–494

Prager JM, Roychowdhury S, Gorey MT, Lowe GM, Diamond CW, Ragin A 1996 Spinal headaches after myelograms: comparison of needle types. American Journal of Roentgenology 167: 1289–1292

Prevost A, Nazeyrollas P, Milosevic D, Fernandez-Valoni A 1998 Malignant pleural effusions treated with high dose intrapleural doxycycline: clinical efficacy and tolerance. Oncology Reports 5: 363–366

Price DD 2000 Psychological and neural mechanisms of the affective dimension of pain. Science 288: 1769–1772

Priest JR, Ramsay NK, Steinherz PG, Tubergen DG, Cairo MS, Sitarz AL, Bishop AJ, White L, Trigg ME, Levitt CJ, Cich JA, Coccia PF 1982 A syndrome of thrombosis and hemorrhage complicating L-asparaginase therapy for childhood acute lymphoblastic leukemia. Journal of Pediatrics 100: 984–989

Pucino F, Danielson BD, Carlson JD, Strommen GL, Walker PR, Beck CL, Thiege DJ, Gill DS 1988 Patient tolerance to intravenous potassium chloride with and without lidocaine. Drug Intelligence and Clinical Pharmacology 22: 676–679
Puel V, Caudry M, Le Metayer P, Baste JC, Midy D, Marsault C, Demeaux H, Maire JP 1993 Superior vena cava thrombosis related to catheter malposition in cancer chemotherapy given through implanted ports. Cancer 72: 2248–2252
Quesada JR, Talpaz M, Rios A, Kurzrock R, Gutterman JU 1986 Clinical toxicity of interferons in cancer patients: a review. Journal of Clinical Oncology 4: 234–243
Ramamurthy L, Cooper RA 1991 Metastatic carcinoma to the male breast. British Journal of Radiology 64: 277–278
Ratcliffe MA, Gilbert FJ, Dawson AA, Bennett B 1995 Diagnosis of avascular necrosis of the femoral head in patients treated for lymphoma. Hematological Oncology 13: 131–137
Razak M, Sappani K 1998 Neurological recovery following posterior decompression of spinal secondaries. Medical Journal of Malaysia 53: 6–11
Ready LB 1991 The treatment of post operative pain. In: Bond MR, Charlton JE, Woolf CJ (eds) Proceedings of the VIth world congress on pain, vol 4. Elsevier, Amsterdam, pp 53–58
Reddel RR, Sutherland RL 1984 Tamoxifen stimulation of human breast cancer cell proliferation in vitro: a possible model for tamoxifen tumour flare. European Journal of Cancer and Clinical Oncology 20: 1419–1424
Reese JA, Blocker SH 1994 Torsion of pedunculated hepatocellular carcinoma. Report of a case in a young woman presenting with abdominal pain. Missouri Medicine 91: 594–595
Rezkalla S, Kloner RA, Ensley J, al-Sarraf M, Revels S, Olivenstein A, Bhasin S, Kerpel-Fronious S, Turi ZG 1989 Continuous ambulatory ECG monitoring during fluorouracil therapy: a prospective study. Journal of Clinical Oncology 7: 509–514
Richardson RR, Siqueira EB, Oi S, Nunez C 1979 Neurogenic tumors of the brachial plexus: report of two cases. Neurosurgery 4: 66–70
Rider CA 1990 Oral mucositis. A complication of radiotherapy. New York State Dental Journal 56: 37–39
Rigor BM 2000 Pelvic cancer pain. Journal of Surgical Oncology 75: 280–300
Ripamonti C 1994 Management of bowel obstruction in advanced cancer. Current Opinions in Oncology 6: 351–357
Rittenberg CN, Gralla RJ, Rehmeyer TA 1995 Assessing and managing venous irritation associated with vinorelbine tartrate (Navelbine). Oncologic Nursing Forum 22: 707–710
Robinson RG, Preston DF, Schiefelbein M, Baxter KG 1995 Strontium 89 therapy for the palliation of pain due to osseous metastases. Journal of the American Medical Association 274: 420–424
Rodichok LD, Ruckdeschel JC, Harper GR et al 1986 Early detection and treatment of spinal epidural metastases: the role of myelography. Annals of Neurology 20: 696–702
Rogues AM, Vidal E, Boudinet F, Loustaud V, Arnaud M, Liozon F 1993 Breast cancer with systemic manifestations mimicking Still's disease. Journal of Rheumatology 20: 1786–1787
Rosenfeld CS, Broder LE 1984 Cisplatin-induced autonomic neuropathy. Cancer Treatment Reports 68: 659–660
Rosenthal MA, Rosen D, Raghavan D, Leicester J, Duval P, Besser M, Pearson, B 1992 Spinal cord compression in prostate cancer. A 10-year experience. British Journal of Urology 69: 530–533
Rosenthal S, Kaufman S 1974 Vincristine neurotoxicity. Annals of Internal Medicine 80: 733–737
Rotstein J, Good RA 1957 Steroid pseudorheumatism. Archives of Internal Medicine 99: 545–555
Rotta FT, Bradley WG 1997 Marked improvement of severe polyneuropathy associated with multifocal osteosclerotic myeloma following surgery, radiation, and chemotherapy. Muscle Nerve 20: 1035–1037
Rowinsky EK, Chaudhry V, Cornblath DR, Donehower RC 1993 Neurotoxicity of Taxol. Journal of National Cancer Institute Monographs (15): 107–115
Ruff RL, Lanska DJ 1989 Epidural metastases in prospectively evaluated veterans with cancer and back pain. Cancer 63: 2234–2241
Rusthoven JJ, Ahlgren P, Elhakim T, Pinfold P, Reid J, Stewart L, Feld R 1988 Varicella-zoster infection in adult cancer patients. A population study. Archives of Internal Medicine 148: 1561–1566
Saeter G, Fossa SD, Norman N 1987 Gynaecomastia following cytotoxic therapy for testicular cancer. British Journal of Urology 59: 348–352
Sahdev P, Wolff M, Widmann WD 1985 Mesenteric venous thrombosis associated with estrogen therapy for treatment of prostatic carcinoma. Journal of Urology 134: 563–564
Salner AL, Botnick LE, Herzog AG, Goldstein MA, Harris JR, Levene MB, Hellman S 1981 Reversible brachial plexopathy following primary radiation therapy for breast cancer. Cancer Treatment Reports 65: 797–802
Sandler SG, Tobin W, Henderson ES 1969 Vincristine-induced neuropathy. A clinical study of fifty leukemic patients. Neurology 19: 367–374
Sawaya RE, Ligon BL 1994 Thromboembolic complications associated with brain tumors. Journal of Neurooncology 22: 173–181
Saxman SB, Seitz D 1997 Breast cancer associated with palmar fasciitis and arthritis. Journal of Clinical Oncology 15: 3515–3516
Scarfone RJ, Jasani M, Gracely EJ 1998 Pain of local anesthetics: rate of administration and buffering. Annals of Emergency Medicine 31: 36–40
Schick RM, Jolesz F, Barnes PD, Macklis JD 1989 MR diagnosis of dural venous sinus thrombosis complicating L-asparaginase therapy. Computerized Medical Imaging and Graphics 13: 319–327
Schoenen J, Broux R, Moonen G 1992 Unilateral facial pain as the first symptom of lung cancer: are there diagnostic clues? Cephalalgia 12: 178–179
Schonenberg P, Bastid C, Guedes J, Sahel J 1991 [Percutaneous echography-guided alcohol block of the celiac plexus as treatment of painful syndromes of the upper abdomen: study of 21 cases]. Schweizerische Medizinische Wochenschrift 121: 528–531
Schroeder TL, Farlane DF, Goldberg LH 1998 Pain as an atypical presentation of squamous cell carcinoma [in process citation]. Dermatologic Surgery 24: 263–266
Schultheiss TE 1994 Spinal cord radiation tolerance [editorial]. International Journal of Radiation Oncology–Biology–Physics 30: 735–736
Schultheiss TE, Stephens LC 1992 Invited review: permanent radiation myelopathy. British Journal of Radiology 65: 737–753
Seefeld PH, Bargen JA 1943 The spread of carcinoma of the rectum: invasion of lymphatics, veins and nerves. Annals of Surgery 118: 76–90
Servodidio CA, Abramson DH 1992 Presenting signs and symptoms of choroidal melanoma: what do they mean? Annals of Ophthalmology 24: 190–194
Shakespeare TP, Stevens MJ 1996 Unilateral facial pain and lung cancer. Australasian Radiology 40: 45–46
Shane E, Parisien M, Henderson JE, Dempster DW, Feldman F, Hardy MA, Tohme JF, Karaplis AC, Clemens TL 1997 Tumor-induced osteomalacia: clinical and basic studies. Journal of Bone and Mineral Research 12: 1502–1511
Shapiro JS 1987 Breast cancer presenting as periostitis. Postgraduate Medicine 82: 139–140
Shapshay SM, Elber E, Strong MS 1976 Occult tumors of the infratemporal fossa: report of seven cases appearing as

preauricular facial pain. Archives of Otolaryngology 102: 535–538
Sharief MK, Robinson SF, Ingram DA, Geddes JF, Swash M 1999 Paraneoplastic painful ulnar neuropathy. Muscle Nerve 22: 952–955
Sharma OP 1995 Symptoms and signs in pulmonary medicine: old observations and new interpretations. Disease-a-Month 41: 577–638
Shearer RJ, Davies JH, Dowsett M, Malone PR, Hedley A, Cunningham D, Coombes RC 1990 Aromatase inhibition in advanced prostatic cancer: preliminary communication. British Journal of Cancer 62: 275–276
Shiel WC Jr, Prete PE, Jason M, Andrews BS 1985 Palmar fasciitis and arthritis with ovarian and non-ovarian carcinomas. New syndrome. American Journal of Medicine 79: 640–644
Shike M, Gillin JS, Kemeny N, Daly JM, Kurtz RC 1986 Severe gastroduodenal ulcerations complicating hepatic artery infusion chemotherapy for metastatic colon cancer. American Journal of Gastroenterology 81: 176–179
Siegal T 1991 Muscle cramps in the cancer patient: causes and treatment. Journal of Pain and Symptom Management 6: 84–91
Siegal T, Haim N 1990 Cisplatin-induced peripheral neuropathy. Frequent off-therapy deterioration, demyelinating syndromes, and muscle cramps. Cancer 66: 1117–1123
Sigsbee B, Deck MD, Posner JB 1979 Nonmetastatic superior sagittal sinus thrombosis complicating systemic cancer. Neurology 29: 139–146
Silen W 1983 Cope's early diagnosis of the acute abdomen. Oxford, New York
Sim FH 1992 Metastatic bone disease of the pelvis and femur. Instructional Course Lectures 41: 317–327
Sinaki M, Merritt JL, Stillwell GK 1977 Tension myalgia of the pelvic floor. Mayo Clinic Proceedings 52: 717–722
Sklaroff DM, Gnaneswaran P, Sklaroff RB 1978 Postirradiation ureteric stricture. Gynecologic Oncology 6: 538–545
Smith J, Thompson JM 1995 Phantom limb pain and chemotherapy in pediatric amputees. Mayo Clinic Proceedings 70: 357–364
Smith WC, Bourne D, Squair J, O'Phillips D, Alastair Chambers W 1999 A retrospective cohort study of post mastectomy pain syndrome. Pain 83: 91–95
Socie G, Cahn JY, Carmelo J, Vernant JP, Jouet JP, Ifrah N, Milpied N, Michallet M, Lioure B, Pico JL, Witz F, Molina L, Fischer A, Bardou VJ, Gluckman E, Reiffers J 1997 Avascular necrosis of bone after allogeneic bone marrow transplantation: analysis of risk factors for 4388 patients by the Societe Francaise de Greffe de Moelle (SFGM). British Journal of Haematology 97: 865–870
Soloway MS, Schellhammer PF, Smith JA, Chodak GW, Kennealey GT 1996 Bicalutamide in the treatment of advanced prostatic carcinoma: a phase II multicenter trial. Urology 47: 33–37; discussion 48–53
Sorensen S, Borgesen SE, Rohde K, Rasmusson B, Bach F, Boge-Rasmussen T, Stjernholm P, Larsen BH, Agerlin N, Gjerris F et al 1990 Metastatic epidural spinal cord compression. Results of treatment and survival. Cancer 65: 1502–1508
Sozzi G, Marotta P, Piatti L 1987 Vagoglossopharyngeal neuralgia with syncope in the course of carcinomatous meningitis. Italian Journal of Neurological Sciences 8: 271–275
Spencer CM, Goa KL 1995 Amifostine. A review of its pharmacodynamic and pharmacokinetic properties, and therapeutic potential as a radioprotector and cytotoxic chemoprotector. Drugs 50: 1001–1031
Sponseller PD 1996 Evaluating the child with back pain. American Family Physician 54: 1933–1941
Sridhar KS, Rao RK, Kunhardt B 1987 Skeletal muscle metastases from lung cancer. Cancer 59: 1530–1534
Srinivasan V, Miree J Jr, Lloyd FA 1972 Bilateral mastectomy and irradiation in the prevention of estrogen induced gynecomastia. Journal of Urology 107: 624–625
Stark RJ, Henson RA, Evans SJ 1982 Spinal metastases. A retrospective survey from a general hospital. Brain 105: 189–213
Steiner I, Siegal T 1989 Muscle cramps in cancer patients. Cancer 63: 574–577
Stevens MJ, Gonet YM 1990 Malignant psoas syndrome: recognition of an oncologic entity. Australasian Radiology 34: 150–154
Stillman M 1990 Perineal pain: Diagnosis and management, with particular attention to perineal pain of cancer. In: Foley KM, Bonica JJ, Ventafrida V (eds) Second international congress on cancer pain, vol 16. Raven Press, New York, pp 359–377
Stjernsward J, Colleau SM, Ventafridda V 1996 The World Health Organization Cancer Pain and Palliative Care Program. Past, present, and future. Journal of Pain and Symptom Management 12: 65–72
Stranjalis G, Jamjoom A, Torrens M 1992 Epidural lipomatosis in steroid-treated patients. Spine 17: 1268
Stull DM, Hollis LS, Gregory RE, Sheidler VR, Grossman SA 1996 Pain in a comprehensive cancer center: more frequently due to treatment than underlying tumor (meeting abstract). Proceedings Annual Meeting of the American Society of Clinical Oncologists 15: abstract 1717
Sundaresan N, Galicich JH, Lane JM, Greenberg HS 1981 Treatment of odontoid fractures in cancer patients. Journal of Neurosurgery 54: 187–192
Suwanwela N, Phanthumchinda K, Kaoropthum S 1994 Headache in brain tumor: a cross-sectional study. Headache 34: 435–438
Swanson MW 1993 Ocular metastatic disease. Optometry Clinics 3: 79–99
Swift TR, Nichols FT 1984 The droopy shoulder syndrome. Neurology 34: 212–215
Synek VM 1986 Validity of median nerve somatosensory evoked potentials in the diagnosis of supraclavicular brachial plexus lesions. Electroencephalography and Clinical Neurophysiology 65: 27–35
Talmi YP, Waller A, Bercovici M, Horowitz Z, Pfeffer MR, Adunski A, Kronenberg J 1997 Pain experienced by patients with terminal head and neck carcinoma. Cancer 80: 1117–1123
Talmi YP, Horowitz Z, Pfeffer MR, Stolik-Dollberg OC, Shoshani Y, Peleg M, Kronenberg J 2000 Pain in the neck after neck dissection. Otolaryngology Head and Neck Surgery 123: 302–306
Tasmuth T, von Smitten K, Hietanen P, Kataja M, Kalso E 1995 Pain and other symptoms after different treatment modalities of breast cancer. Annals of Oncology 6: 453–459
Tasmuth T, von Smitten K, Kalso E 1996 Pain and other symptoms during the first year after radical and conservative surgery for breast cancer. British Journal of Cancer 74: 2024–2031
Terrell JE, Welsh DE, Bradford CR, Chepeha DB, Esclamado RM, Hogikyan ND, Wolf GT 2000 Pain, quality of life, and spinal accessory nerve status after neck dissection [in process citation]. Laryngoscope 110: 620–626
Tham TC, Lichtenstein DR, Vandervoort J, Wong RC, Slivka A, Banks PA, Yim HB, Carr-Locke DL 2000 Pancreatic duct stents for 'obstructive type' pain in pancreatic malignancy. American Journal of Gastroenterology 95: 956–960
Tharion G, Bhattacharji S 1997 Malignant secondary deposit in the iliac crest masquerading as meralgia paresthetica. Archives of Physical Medicine and Rehabilitation 78: 1010–1011
Thompson IM, Zeidman EJ, Rodriguez FR 1990 Sudden death due to disease flare with luteinizing hormone-releasing hormone agonist therapy for carcinoma of the prostate [see comments]. Journal of Urology 144: 1479–1480
Thornton MJ, O'Sullivan G, Williams MP, Hughes PM 1997

Avascular necrosis of bone following an intensified chemotherapy regimen including high dose steroids. Clinical Radiology 52: 607–612
Thyagarajan D, Cascino T, Harms G 1995 Magnetic resonance imaging in brachial plexopathy of cancer. Neurology 45: 421–427
Toepfer M, Schroeder M, Unger JW, Lochmuller H, Pongratz D, Muller-Felber W 1999 Neuromyotonia, myocloni, sensory neuropathy and cerebellar symptoms in a patient with antibodies to neuronal nucleoproteins (anti-Hu-antibodies). Clinical Neurology and Neurosurgery 101: 207–209
Traill ZC, Nolan DJ 1997 Metastatic oesophageal carcinoma presenting as small intestinal ischaemia: imaging findings. European Radiology 7: 341–343
Trump DL, Anderson SA 1983 Painful gynecomastia following cytotoxic therapy for testis cancer: a potentially favorable prognostic sign? Journal of Clinical Oncology 1: 416–420
Trump DL, Pavy MD, Staal S 1982 Gynecomastia in men following antineoplastic therapy. Archives of Internal Medicine 142: 511–513
Tseng A Jr, Horning SJ, Freiha FS, Resser KJ, Hannigan JF Jr, Torti FM 1985 Gynecomastia in testicular cancer patients. Prognostic and therapeutic implications. Cancer 56: 2534–2538
Twycross R, Harcourt J, Bergl S 1996 A survey of pain in patients with advanced cancer. Journal of Pain and Symptom Management 12: 273–282
Uekado Y, Hirano A, Shinka T, Ohkawa T 1994 The effects of intravesical chemoimmunotherapy with epirubicin and bacillus Calmette-Guerin for prophylaxis of recurrence of superficial bladder cancer: a preliminary report. Cancer Chemotherapy and Pharmacology 35 (Suppl): S65–S68
Vallejo MC, Mandell GL, Sabo DP, Ramanathan S 2000 Postdural puncture headache: a randomized comparison of five spinal needles in obstetric patients. Anesthesia and Analgesia 91: 916–920
van Dam MS, Hennipman A, de Kruif JT, van der Tweel I, de Graaf PW 1993 [Complications following axillary dissection for breast carcinoma (see comments)]. Nederlands Tijdschrift voor Geneeskunde 137: 2395–2398
van Oostenbrugge RJ, Twijnstra A 1999 Presenting features and value of diagnostic procedures in leptomeningeal metastases. Neurology 53: 382–385
van Oosterhout AG, van de Pol M, ten Velde GP, Twijnstra A 1996 Neurologic disorders in 203 consecutive patients with small cell lung cancer. Results of a longitudinal study. Cancer 77: 1434–1441
Vanagunas A, Jacob P, Olinger E 1990 Radiation-induced esophageal injury: a spectrum from esophagitis to cancer. American Journal of Gastroenterology 85: 808–812
Vazquez-Barquero A, Ibanez FJ, Herrera S, Izquierdo JM, Berciano J, Pascual J 1994 Isolated headache as the presenting clinical manifestation of intracranial tumors: a prospective study [see comments]. Cephalalgia 14: 270–272
Vecht CJ 1990 Arm pain in the patient with breast cancer. Journal of Pain and Symptom Management 5: 109–117
Vecht CJ, Van de Brand HJ, Wajer OJ 1989 Post-axillary dissection pain in breast cancer due to a lesion of the intercostobrachial nerve. Pain 38: 171–176
Vecht CJ, Hoff AM, Kansen PJ, de Boer MF, Bosch DA 1992 Types and causes of pain in cancer of the head and neck. Cancer 70: 178–184
Veldhuis GJ, Willemse PH, van Gameren MM, Aalders JG, Mulder NH, Mull B, Biesma B, de Vries EG 1995 Recombinant human interleukin-3 to dose-intensify carboplatin and cyclophosphamide chemotherapy in epithelial ovarian cancer: a phase I trial. Journal of Clinical Oncology 13: 733–740
Ventafridda V, Caraceni A, Martini C, Sbanotto A, De Conno F 1991 On the significance of Lhermitte's sign in oncology. Journal of Neurooncology 10: 133–137
Verdi CJ 1993 Cancer therapy and oral mucositis. An appraisal of drug prophylaxis. Drug Safety 9: 185–195
Vial T, Descotes J 1995 Clinical toxicity of cytokines used as haemopoietic growth factors. Drug Safety 13: 371–406
Vigo M, De Faveri D, Biondetti PR Jr, Benedetti L 1980 CT demonstration of portal and superior mesenteric vein thrombosis in hepatocellular carcinoma. Journal of Computer Assisted Tomography 4: 627–629
Vilming ST, Kloster R 1998a Pain location and associated symptoms in post-lumbar puncture headache [see comments]. Cephalalgia 18: 697–703
Vilming ST, Kloster R 1998b The time course of post-lumbar puncture headache [see comments]. Cephalalgia 18: 97–100
Visani G, Bontempo G, Manfroi S, Pazzaglia A, D'Alessandro R, Tura S 1996 All-trans-retinoic acid and pseudotumor cerebri in a young adult with acute promyelocytic leukemia: a possible disease association [see comments]. Haematologica 81: 152–154
Vogelzang NJ 1979 'Adriamycin flare': a skin reaction resembling extravasation. Cancer Treatment Reports 63: 2067–2069
Von Roenn JH, Cleeland CS, Gonin R, Hatfield AK, Pandya KJ 1993 Physician attitudes and practice in cancer pain management. A survey from the Eastern Cooperative Oncology Group. Annals of Internal Medicine 119(2): 121–126
Vukelja SJ, Baker WJ, Burris HAD, Keeling JH, Von Hoff D 1993 Pyridoxine therapy for palmar-plantar erythrodysesthesia associated with taxotere [letter]. Journal of the National Cancer Institute 85: 1432–1433
Vuorinen E 1993 Pain as an early symptom in cancer. Clinical Journal of Pain 9: 272–278
Wagner G 1984 Frequency of pain in patients with cancer. Recent Results in Cancer Research 89: 64–71
Wasserstrom WR, Glass JP, Posner JB 1982 Diagnosis and treatment of leptomeningeal metastases from solid tumors: experience with 90 patients. Cancer 49: 759–772
Weiss HD, Walker MD, Wiernik PH 1974a Neurotoxicity of commonly used antineoplastic agents (first of two parts). New England Journal of Medicine 291: 75–81
Weiss HD, Walker MD, Wiernik PH 1974b Neurotoxicity of commonly used antineoplastic agents (second of two parts). New England Journal of Medicine 291: 127–133
Weiss R, Grisold W, Jellinger K, Muhlbauer J, Scheiner W, Vesely M 1984 Metastasis of solid tumors in extraocular muscles. Acta Neuropathologica (Berlin) 65: 168–171
Wolff JM, Boeckmann W, Jakse G 1994 Spontaneous kidney rupture due to a metastatic renal tumour. Case report. Scandinavian Journal of Urology and Nephrology 28: 415–417
Wong KF, Chan JK, Ma SK 1993 Solid tumour with initial presentation in the bone marrow—a clinicopathologic study of 25 adult cases. Hematological Oncology 11: 35–42
Wood KM 1978 Intercostobrachial nerve entrapment syndrome. Southern Medical Journal 71: 662–663
Wurzel RS, Yamase HT, Nieh PT 1987 Ectopic production of human chorionic gonadotropin by poorly differentiated transitional cell tumors of the urinary tract. Journal of Urology 137: 502–504
Yeoh E, Horowitz M 1988 Radiation enteritis. British Journal of Hospital Medicine 39: 498–504
Yeoh EK, Horowitz M 1987 Radiation enteritis. Surgery, Gynecology and Obstetrics 165: 373–379
Zhu Z, Friess H, di Mola FF, Zimmermann A, Graber HU, Korc M, Büchler MW 1999 Nerve growth factor expression correlates with perineural invasion and pain in human pancreatic cancer. Journal of Clinical Oncology 17: 2419–2428
Zografos GC, Karakousis CP 1994 Pain in the distribution of the femoral nerve: early evidence of recurrence of a retroperitoneal sarcoma. European Journal of Surgical Oncology 20: 692–693

Chapter 43

The management of cancer pain

Nathan I Cherny

Introduction

Optimal management of cancer pain requires familiarity with a wide range of therapeutic options including antineoplastic therapies, analgesic pharmacotherapy, and anaesthetic, neurosurgical, psychological, and rehabilitation techniques. Successful pain management is characterized by the implementation of the techniques with the most favourable therapeutic index for the prevailing circumstances along with provision for repeated evaluations so that a favourable balance between pain relief and adverse effects is maintained. Currently available techniques using specific analgesic approaches can provide adequate relief to a large majority of patients. Anaesthetic and neurosurgical techniques should be considered for the patient who has not obtained satisfactory pain relief. In all cases, these treatments must be skilfully integrated with the management of other symptoms.

Primary therapy

The assessment process may reveal a cause for the pain that is amenable to primary therapy (i.e., therapy that is directed at the aetiology of the pain). This therapy may improve comfort, function, or duration of survival. For example, pain generated by tumour infiltration may respond to antineoplastic treatment with surgery, radiotherapy, or chemotherapy, and pain caused by infections may be relieved with antibiotic therapy or drainage procedures. Specific analgesic treatments are usually required as an adjunct to the primary therapy.

Radiotherapy

The analgesic effectiveness of radiotherapy is documented by abundant data and a favourable clinical experience in the treatment of painful bone metastases (Janjan 1997), epidural neoplasm (Bates 1992), and headache due to cerebral metastases (Vermeulen 1998). In other settings, however, there is a lack of data, and the use of radiotherapy is largely anecdotal. For example, the results with perineal pain due to low sacral plexopathy appear to be encouraging (Dobrowsky and Schmid 1985), and hepatic radiotherapy (e.g., 2000–3000 cGy) can be well tolerated and effective for the pain of hepatic capsular distension in 50–90% of patients (Leibel et al 1987).

Chemotherapy

Despite a paucity of data concerning the specific analgesic benefits of chemotherapy, there is a strong clinical impression that tumour shrinkage is generally associated with relief of pain. Although there are some reports of analgesic value even in the absence of significant tumour shrinkage (Thatcher et al 1995, Rothenberg 1996), the likelihood of a favourable effect on pain is generally related to the likelihood of tumour response. In all situations, the decision to administer chemotherapy solely for the treatment of symptoms should be promptly reconsidered unless the patient demonstrates a clearly favourable balance between relief and adverse effects.

Surgery

Surgery may have a role in the relief of symptoms caused by specific problems, such as obstruction of a hollow viscus, unstable bony structures, and compression of neural tissues (Harris et al 1996). The potential benefits must be weighed against the risks of surgery, the anticipated length of hospitalization and convalescence, and the predicted duration of benefit (Boraas 1985). Clinical experience has generally been most favourable when surgery has been used to stabilize pathological fractures (Algan and Horowitz 1996), relieve bowel obstructions, or drain symptomatic ascites. Large volume (up to 5–10 L) paracentesis, for example, may provide prompt and prolonged relief from the pain and discomfort of tense ascites (Ross et al 1989), with a small risk of hypotension (Cruikshank and Buchsbaum 1973, Ross et al 1989) or hypoproteinaemia (Lifshitz and Buchsbaum 1976). Radical surgery to excise locally advanced disease in patients with no evidence of metastatic spread may be palliative, and potentially increase the survival of some patients (Estes et al 1993, Avradopoulos et al 1996).

Antibiotic therapy

Antibiotics may be analgesic when the source of the pain involves infection. Illustrative examples include cellulitis, chronic sinus infections, pelvic abscess, pyonephrosis, and osteitis pubis. In some cases, infection may be occult and confirmed only by the symptomatic relief provided by empiric treatment with these drugs (Coyle and Portenoy 1991).

Analgesic drug therapy

There is universal agreement that analgesic pharmacotherapy remains the mainstay of cancer pain management. Controversy, however, has arisen regarding the validity and application of the 'three-step analgesic ladder' of the World Health Organization, which advocated three basic steps of therapy according to the severity of the presenting pain problem (Fig. 43.1) (World Health Organization 1986). Despite data from a series of validation studies that demonstrated that this approach, combined with appropriate dosing guidelines, provides adequate relief to 70–90% of patients (Takeda 1985, Ventafridda et al 1987, Walker et al 1988, Goisis et al 1989, Schug et al 1990, Grond et al 1991), a review of these studies concluded that there was a lack of evidence for the long-term efficacy of this approach (Jadad and Browman 1995). Additionally, the recent production of low-dose formulations of pure opioid agonists traditionally used for severe pain and the introduction of other agents, such as tramadol, has blurred the distinction between Steps 2 and 3.

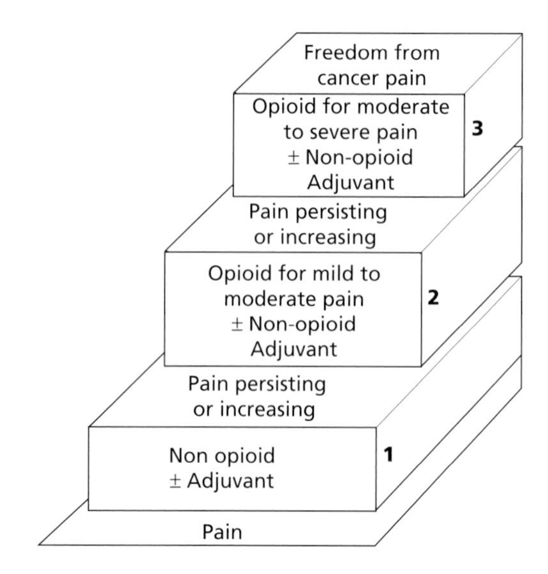

Fig. 43.1 WHO analgesic ladder (reprinted with permission).

Systemic analgesic pharmacotherapy

Non-opioid analgesics

The non-opioid analgesics (aspirin, acetaminophen, and the non-steroidal anti-inflammatory drugs (NSAIDs)) are useful alone for mild to moderate pain (Step 1 of the analgesic ladder) and provide additive analgesia when combined with opioid drugs in the treatment of more severe pain (Eisenberg et al 1994). They are useful in a broad range of pain syndromes of diverse mechanisms

Table 43.1 Commonly used non-opioid analgesics

Chemical class	Generic name
COX2 specific	Meloxicam Nemesulide Rofecoxib Celecoxib
Non-acidic	Acetaminophen
Acidic	
Salicylates	Aspirin Diflunisal Choline magnesium trisalicylate Salsalate
Proprionic acids	Ibuprofen Naproxen Fenoprofen Ketoprofen Flurbiprofen Suprofen
Acetic acids	Indometacin Tolmentin Sulindac Diclofenac Ketorolac
Oxicams	Piroxicam
Fenemates	Mefenamic acid Meclofenamic acid

but there are no data to support therapeutic superiority to alternative options in a particular setting other than inflammation (Eisenberg et al 1994). Unlike opioid analgesics, the non-opioid analgesics have a 'ceiling' effect for analgesia and produce neither tolerance nor physical dependence.

The non-opioid analgesics constitute a heterogeneous group of compounds that differ in chemical structure but share many pharmacological actions (Table 43.1). The NSAID drugs are competitive blockers of cyclooxygenase. It has recently been found that there are at least two isoforms of cylooxygenase with distinct roles in analgesia and toxicity (Vane et al 1998). Cyclooxygenase-1 is responsible for the synthesis of the protective prostaglandins that preserve the integrity of the stomach lining and maintain normal renal function in a compromised kidney and cyclooxygenase-2 is an inducible enzyme involved in inflammation, pain, and fever. Recently a range of relatively selective cyclooxygenase-2 inhibitors including meloxicam, nemesulide, rofecoxib, and celecoxib have been introduced and approved as analgesics. Early data indicate that these agents are equianalgesic with the non-selective inhibitors and that they are associated with less gastroduodenal morbidity (Brooks and Day 2000, Watson et al 2000). Other adverse effects, such as interference with antihypertensive agents and the potential to produce renal dysfunction in patients with compromised renal function, are similar to those of non-selective NSAIDs (Brooks and Day 2000, Perazella and Eras 2000, Eras and Perazella 2001).

Safely administering non-opioid analgesics requires familiarity with their potential adverse effects (Brooks and Day 1991, Bennett et al 1996, Laine 1996, Lehmann et al 1997). Aspirin and the other NSAIDs have a broad spectrum of potential toxicity; bleeding diathesis due to inhibition of platelet aggregation, gastroduodenopathy (including peptic ulcer disease), and renal impairment are the most common (Lehmann et al 1997). Less common adverse effects include confusion, precipitation of cardiac failure, and exacerbation of hypertension. Acetaminophen rarely produces gastrointestinal toxicity and there are no adverse effects on platelet function; hepatic toxicity is possible, however, and patients with chronic alcoholism and liver disease can develop severe hepatotoxicity at the usual therapeutic doses (Makin and Williams 1997).

Particular caution is required in the administration of these agents to patients at increased risk of adverse effects, including the elderly and those with blood clotting disorders, predilection to peptic ulceration, impaired renal function, and concurrent corticosteroid therapy. The risk of gastrointestinal bleeding can be influenced by drug selection and the use of peptic cytoprotective agents (Lanas and Hirschowitz 1999, Wolfe et al 1999). Of the NSAIDs, the relatively selective cyclooxygenase-2 inhibitors (nabumetone, nemsulide, and meloxicam) (Lancaster 1995, Masferrer et al 1996) or the non-acetylated salicylates (choline magnesium trisalicylate and salsalate) (Johnson and Miller 1994) are preferred in patients who have a predilection to peptic ulceration or bleeding; these drugs have less effect on platelet aggregation and no effect on bleeding time at the usual clinical doses. Data from randomized trials support the use of either omeprazole (Hawkey 1998), pantoprazole, misoprostol (Valentini et al 1995), or high-dose famotidine (80 mg/day) (Taha et al 1996) as the preferred agent for the prevention of NSAID-related peptic ulceration. In some countries a combined formulation of diclofenac and misoprostol is available as a convenient and cost-effective option (McKenna 1998, Plosker and Lamb 1999).

The optimal administration of non-opioid analgesics requires an understanding of their clinical pharmacology. There is no certain knowledge of the minimal effective analgesic dose, ceiling dose, or toxic dose for any individual patient with cancer pain. These doses may be higher or lower than the usual dose ranges recommended for the drug involved. Recommended doses are usually derived from studies performed in relatively healthy patients who have an inflammatory disease, a population clearly dissimilar from those with cancer pain, who often have coexistent organ failure and may be receiving multiple other drugs. Given that the effects of these drugs are (at least partially) dose-dependent, in the cancer population the minimal effective analgesic dose is unknown. These observations support an approach to the administration of NSAIDs that incorporates both low initial doses and dose titration. Through a process of gradual dose escalation, it may be possible to identify the ceiling dose and reduce the risk of significant toxicity.

Based on clinical experience, an upper limit for dose titration is usually set at 1.5–2 times the standard recommended dose of the drug in question. Since failure with one NSAID can be followed by success with another, sequential trials of several NSAIDs may be useful to identify a drug with a favourable balance between analgesia and side effects.

Opioid analgesics—basic pharmacology

A trial of systemic opioid therapy should be administered to all cancer patients with pain of moderate or greater severity regardless of the pain mechanism. Although somatic and visceral pain appear to be relatively more responsive to opioid analgesics than neuropathic pain, a neuropathic mechanism does not confer 'opioid resistance', and appropriate dose escalation will identify many patients with neuropathic pain who can achieve adequate relief (Portenoy et al 1990, Hanks and Forbes 1997).

Optimal use of opioid analgesics requires a sound understanding of the general principles of opioid pharmacology, the pharmacological characteristics of each of the commonly used drugs, and principles of administration, including drug selection, routes of administration, dosing and dose titration, and the prevention and management of adverse effects.

Important principles in opioid drug therapy

Classification Opioid compounds can be divided into agonist, agonist–antagonist, and antagonist classes based on their interactions with the various receptor subtypes (Table 43.2). In the management of cancer pain, the pure agonists are most commonly used. The mixed agonist–antagonist opioids and the partial agonist opioids play a minor role in the management of cancer pain because of the existence of a ceiling effect for analgesia, the potential for precipitation of withdrawal in patients physically dependent on opioid agonists, and in the case of mixed agonist–antagonists, the problem of dose-dependent psychotomimetic side effects that exceed those of pure agonist drugs (Hanks 1987).

Table 43.2 Classification of opioid analgesics

Agonists	Partial agonists	Agonists/ antagonists
Morphine	Buprenorphine	Pentazocine
Codeine	Dezocine	Butorphanol
Oxycodone		Nalbuphine
Heroin		
Oxymorphone		
Meperidine		
Levorphanol		
Hydromorphone		
Methadone		
Fentanyl		
Sufentanil		
Alfentanil		
Propoxyphene		

Dose–response relationship The pure agonist drugs do not have a ceiling dose; as the dose is raised analgesic effects increase in a semi-log–linear function, until either analgesia is achieved or the patient develops dose-limiting adverse effects such as nausea, vomiting, confusion, sedation, myoclonus, or respiratory depression.

The equianalgesic dose ratio Relative analgesic potency of opioids is commonly expressed in terms of the equianalgesic dose ratio. This is the ratio of the dose of two analgesics required to produce the same analgesic effect. By convention, the relative potency of each of the commonly used opioids is based upon a comparison to 10 mg of parenteral morphine (Houde et al 1966). Equianalgesic dose information (Table 43.3) provides guidelines for dose selection when the drug or route of administration is changed.

Several principles are critical in interpreting the data presented in equianalgesic dose tables. The

Table 43.3 Opioid agonist drugs

Drug	Dose (mg) equianalgesic to 10 mg I.M. morphine I.M.	P.O.	Half-life (h)	Duration of action (h)	Comments
Codeine	130	200	2–3	2–4	Usually combined with a non-opioid.
Oxycodone	7–10	15–20	2–3	2–4	
Propoxyphene	100	50	2–3	2–4	Usually combined with non-opioid. Norpropoxyphene toxicity may cause seizures.
Morphine	10	30	2–3	3–4	Multiple routes of administration and formulations available. M6G accumulation in renal failure.
Hydromorphone	2–3	7.5	2–3	2–4	Multiple routes of administration and formulations available.
Methadone	1–3	2–6	15–190	4–8	Plasma accumulation may lead to delayed toxicity. Dosing should be initiated on a PRN basis.
Pethidine	75	300	2–3	2–4	Low oral bioavailability. Norpethidine toxicity limits utility. Contraindicated in patients with renal failure and those receiving MAO inhibitors.
Oxymorphone	1	10 (P.R.)	2–3	3–4	No oral formulation available. Less histamine release.
Fentanyl transdermal system		Empirically transdermal fentanyl 100 μg/h = 2–4 mg/h intravenous morphine		48–72	Patches available to deliver 25, 50, 75, and 100 μg/h.

commonly quoted values do not reflect the substantial variability observed in both single-dose and multidose cross-over studies. Numerous variables may influence the appropriate dose for the individual patient, including pain severity, prior opioid exposure (and the degree of cross-tolerance this confers), age, route of administration, level of consciousness, and genetically determined metabolic or receptor heterogeneity. For most agents the equianalgesic dose relationship to morphine is linear; for methadone, however, the relationship appears to be curvilinear with the equianalgesic dose ratio falling as the dose of prior morphine increases: at low doses of morphine (30–300 mg oral morphine) the equianalgesic ratio for oral methadone to oral morphine is 1:4–1:6 and at high doses (> 300 mg oral morphine) 1:10–1:12 (Ripamonti et al 1998).

Selecting an appropriate opioid

The factors that influence opioid selection in chronic pain states include pain intensity, pharmacokinetic and formulatory considerations, previous adverse effects, and the presence of co-existing disease.

Traditionally, patients with moderate pain have been conventionally treated with a combination product containing acetaminophen or aspirin plus codeine, dihydrocodeine, hydrocodone, oxycodone, and propoxyphene. The doses of these combination products can be increased until the maximum dose of the non-opioid co-analgesic is attained (e.g., 4000 mg acetaminophen). Recent years have witnessed the proliferation of new opioid formulations that may improve the convenience of drug administration for patients with moderate pain. These include controlled release formulations of codeine, dihydrocodeine, oxycodone, morphine, and tramadol in dosages appropriate for moderate pain.

Patients who present with strong pain are usually treated with morphine, hydromorphone, oxycodone, oxymorphone, fentanyl, or methadone. Of these, the short half-life opioid agonists (morphine, hydromorphone, fentanyl, oxycodone, or oxymorphone) are generally favoured because they are easier to titrate than the long half-life drugs which require a longer period to approach steady-state plasma concentrations. Morphine is generally preferred since it has a short half-life and is easy to titrate in its immediate release form, and it is also available as a controlled release preparation that allows an 8- to 12-h dosing interval.

If the patient is currently using an opioid that is well tolerated, it is usually continued unless difficulties in dose titration occur or the required dose cannot be administered conveniently. A switch to an alternative opioid is considered if the patient develops dose-limiting toxicity which precludes adequate relief of pain without excessive side effects or if a specific formulation, not available with the current drug, either is needed or may substantially improve the convenience of opioid administration.

Some patients will require sequential trials of several different opioids before a drug that is effective and well tolerated is identified (Cherny et al 1995, de Stoutz et al 1995). This strategy has been variably labelled opioid-rotation, or opioid-switching. The existence of incomplete cross-tolerance to various opioid effects (analgesia and side effects) may explain the utility of these sequential trials. It is strongly recommended that clinicians be familiar with at least 3 opioid drugs used in the management of severe pain and have the ability to calculate appropriate starting doses using equianalgesic dosing data when switching between drugs.

Selecting the appropriate route of systemic opioid administration

Non-invasive routes Opioids should be administered by the least invasive and safest route capable of providing adequate analgesia. Usually, the oral route is preferred. Alternative routes are necessary for patients who have impaired swallowing or gastrointestinal dysfunction, those who require a very rapid onset of analgesia, and those who are unable to manage either the logistics or side effects associated with the oral route.

The development of transdermal fentanyl has provided a convenient and non-invasive alternative to oral administration. Transdermal patches capable of delivering 25, 50, 75, and 100 μg/h are available. The dosing interval for each patch is usually 72 h (Varvel et al 1989) but some patients require a 48-h schedule (Jeal and Benfield 1997). Recent data from controlled studies indicate that the transdermal administration of fentanyl is associated with a lesser incidence of constipation than oral morphine and is often preferred (Donner et al 1996, Ahmedzai and Brooks 1997, Payne et al 1998).

Other non-invasive routes are less commonly used. Rectal suppositories containing oxycodone, hydromorphone, oxymorphone, and morphine have been formulated, and controlled-release morphine tablets can also be administered per rectum (Maloney et al 1989, Kaiko et al 1992). The potency of opioids administered rectally is approximately equivalent to that achieved by the oral route (European Association for Palliative Care 1996).

The sublingual route has limited value due to the lack of formulations, poor absorption of most drugs, and the inability to deliver high doses or prevent swallowing of the dose. An oral transmucosal formulation of fentanyl, which incorporates the drug into a candy base, has recently been approved for use in the management of breakthrough pain (Simmonds 1997).

Invasive routes A parenteral route may be considered when the oral route is precluded or there is need for rapid onset of analgesia, or a more convenient regimen. Repeated parenteral bolus injections, which may be administered by the intravenous (I.V.), intramuscular (I.M.) or subcutaneous (S.C.) routes, provide the most rapid onset and shortest duration of action. Parenteral boluses are most commonly used to treat very severe pain, in which case doses can be repeated at an interval as brief as that determined by the time-to-peak effect, until adequate relief is achieved (Hagen et al 1997). Repeated bolus doses without frequent skin punctures can be accomplished through the use of an indwelling I.V. or S.C. infusion device such as a 25- to 27-gauge infusion device (a 'butterfly'), which can be left under the skin for up to a week (Coyle et al 1994).

Continuous parenteral infusions are useful for many patients who cannot be maintained on oral opioids. Long-term infusions may be administered I.V. or S.C. In practice, the major indication for continuous infusion occurs among patients who are unable to swallow or absorb opioids. Continuous infusion is also used in some patients whose high opioid requirement renders oral treatment impractical. Ambulatory patients can easily use continuous S.C. infusion. A range of pumps is available varying in complexity, cost, and ability to provide patient-controlled 'rescue doses' as an adjunct to a continuous basal infusion (Coyle et al 1994). Opioids suitable for continuous S.C. infusion must be soluble, well absorbed, and non-irritant. Extensive experience has been reported with heroin, hydromorphone, oxymorphone, morphine, and fentanyl. Methadone appears to be relatively irritating and is not recommended. To maintain the comfort of an infusion site, the S.C. infusion rate should not exceed 3–5 cc/h. Patients who require high doses may benefit from the use of concentrated solutions. A high-concentration hydromorphone (10 mg/cc) is available commercially and the organic salt of morphine, morphine tartrate, is available in some countries as an 80 mg/cc solution.

Changing routes of administration The switch between oral and parenteral routes should be guided by knowledge of relative potency (Table 47.3) to avoid subsequent over- or under-dosing. In calculating the equianalgesic dose, the potencies of the I.V., S.C., and I.M. routes are considered equivalent. In recognition of the imprecision in the accepted equianalgesic doses and the risk of toxicity from potential overdose, a modest reduction in the equianalgesic dose is prudent.

Scheduling of opioid administration

The schedule of opioid administration should be individualized to optimize the balance between patient comfort and convenience. 'Around the clock' dosing and 'as needed' dosing both have a place in clinical practice.

'Around the clock' dosing with 'rescue doses' 'Around the clock' dosing provides the chronic pain patient with continuous relief by preventing the pain from recurring. Controlled release preparations of opioids can lessen the inconvenience associated with the use of 'around the clock' administration of drugs with a short duration of action. Patients should also be provided with a so-called 'rescue dose', which is a supplemental dose offered on an 'as needed' basis to treat pain that breaks through the regular schedule (Cleary 1997).

The frequency with which the rescue dose can be offered depends on the route of administration and the time-to-peak effect for the particular drug. Oral rescue doses are usually offered up to every 1–2 h and parenteral doses can be offered as frequently as every 15–30 min. Clinical experience suggests that the initial size of the rescue dose should be equivalent to approximately 50–100% of the dose administered every 4 h for oral or parenteral bolus medications, or 50–100% of the hourly infusion rate for patients receiving continuous infusions. Alternatively, this may be calculated as 5–15% of the 24-h baseline dose. The magnitude of the rescue dose should be individualized and some patients with low baseline pain but severe exacerbations may require rescue doses that are substantially higher (Lyss 1997). The drug used for the rescue dose is usually identical to that administered on a scheduled basis.

This approach provides a method for safe and rational stepwise dose escalation, which is applicable to all routes of opioid administration. Patients requiring more than 4–6 rescue doses per day should generally undergo escalation of the baseline dose. The quantity of the rescue medication consumed can be used to guide the dose increment. Alternatively, each dose increment can be set at 33–50% of the pre-existing dose. In all cases, escalation of the baseline dose should be accompanied by a proportionate increase in the rescue dose, so that the size of the supplemental dose remains a constant percentage of the fixed dose.

'As-needed' (PRN) dosing Opioid administration on an 'as needed' basis, without an 'around the clock' dosing regimen, may provide additional safety during the initiation of opioid therapy, particularly when rapid dose escalation is needed or therapy with a long half-life opioid such as methadone or levorphanol is begun. 'As needed' dosing may also be appropriate for patients who have rapidly decreasing analgesic requirement or intermittent pains separated by pain-free intervals.

Patient-controlled analgesia (PCA) Patient-controlled analgesia (PCA) generally refers to a technique of parenteral drug administration in which the patient controls an infusion device that delivers a bolus of analgesic drug 'on demand' according to parameters set by the physician. Long-term PCA in cancer patients is most commonly accomplished via the subcutaneous route using an ambulatory infusion device (Ripamonti and Bruera 1997). In most cases, PCA is added to a basal infusion rate and acts essentially as a rescue dose (Ripamonti and Bruera 1997). Rare patients have benefited from PCA alone to manage episodic pains characterized by an onset so rapid that an oral dose could not provide sufficiently prompt relief.

Dose selection and titration

Selecting a starting dose A patient who is relatively non-tolerant, having had only some exposure to an opioid typically used on the second rung of the 'analgesic ladder' for moderate pain, should generally begin one of the opioids typically used for severe pain at a dose equivalent to 5–10 mg morphine I.M. every 4 h (European Association for Palliative Care 1996). If morphine is used, a P.O.:I.M. relative potency ratio of 2:1–3:1 is conventional (European Association for Palliative Care 1996).

Dose adjustment Inadequate relief should be addressed through gradual escalation of dose until adequate analgesia is reported or excessive side effects supervene. Because opioid response increases linearly with the log of the dose, a dose increment of less than 30–50% is not likely to significantly improve analgesia. The absolute dose is immaterial as long as administration is not compromised by excessive side effects, inconvenience, discomfort, or cost.

Rate of dose titration The rate of dose titration depends on the severity of the pain, the medical condition of the patient, and the goals of care. Patients who present with very severe pain are sometimes best managed by repeated parenteral administration of a dose every 15–30 min until pain is partially relieved. Patients with moderate pain may not require a loading dose of the opioid, but rather the initiation of a regular dose with provision for rescue doses and gradual dose titration. In this situation dose increments of 30–50% can be administered at intervals greater than that required to reach steady state following each change. The dose of morphine (tablets or elixir), hydromorphone, or oxycodone can be increased on a twice daily basis, and the dose of controlled release oral morphine or transdermal fentanyl can be increased every 24–48 h.

The problem of tolerance When the need for dose escalation arises, disease progression (Paice 1988, Schug et al 1992), increasing psychological distress, or changes in the pharmacokinetics of an analgesic drug are much more common than true analgesic tolerance. True analgesic tolerance, which could compromise the utility of treatment, can only be said to occur when a patient manifests the need for increasing opioid doses in the absence of other factors (e.g., progressive disease) that would be capable of explaining the increase in pain.

Management of opioid adverse effects

Successful opioid therapy requires that the benefits of analgesia clearly outweigh treatment-related adverse effects. This implies that a detailed understanding of adverse opioid effects and the strategies used to prevent and manage them are essential skills for all involved in cancer pain management. The adverse effects frequently observed in patients receiving oral morphine and other opioids are summarized in Table 43.4.

Among adverse effects there is substantial variability in their dose–response relationship. A dose–response relationship is most commonly evident with regards to the central nervous system adverse effects of sedation, cognitive impairment, hallucinations, myoclonus, and respiratory depression. Even among these, however, there is very substantial interindividual variability to many of these effects. Additionally, as tolerance develops to some effects, the spectrum of adverse effects varies with prolonged use. Commonly, patients who have had prolonged opioid exposure have a lesser tendency to develop sedation or respiratory depression, and the predominant central nervous system effects become the neuroexcitatory ones of delirium and myoclonus. Gastrointestinal adverse effects generally have a weaker dose–response relationship. Some, like nausea and vomiting, are common with the initiation with therapy but are subsequently unpredictable wth resolution among some patients and persistence among others. Constipation is virtually universal and it demonstrates a very weak dose relationship.

Factors predictive of opioid adverse effects

Drug related Overall, there is very little reproducible evidence suggesting that any one pure opioid agonist has a substantially better adverse effect profile than any other. Meperidine is not recommended in the management of chronic cancer pain because of concerns regarding its side effect profile. Recent data from controlled studies indicate that the transdermal administration of fentanyl is associated with a lesser incidence of constipation than oral morphine (Donner et al 1996, Ahmedzai and Brooks 1997, Payne et al 1998).

Table 43.4 Common opioid-induced adverse effects

Gastrointestinal	Nausea Vomiting Constipation
Autonomic	Xerostomia Urinary retention Postural hypotension
Central nervous system	Drowsiness Cognitive impairment Hallucinations Delirium Respiratory depression Myoclonus Seizure disorder Hyperalgesia
Cutaneous	Itch Sweating

Route related There is very limited evidence to suggest differences in adverse effects associated with specific routes of systemic administration. Compared to the oral morphine administration, small studies have demonstrated less nausea and vomiting with rectal (Babul et al 1998) and subcutaneous administration (McDonald et al 1991). Three studies comparing transdermal fentanyl to oral morphine demonstrated less constipation among the patients receiving transdermal fentanyl. It is not clear as to whether this is a route- or drug-related effect (Donner et al 1996, Ahmedzai and Brooks 1997, Payne et al 1998).

Patient related For reasons that are not well explained, there is striking interindividual variability in the sensitivity to adverse effects from morphine and other opioid drugs. Genetic variability in prelinical studies clearly affect the sensitivity to opioids, and it is reasonable to assume that the genetic background plays a similar important role clinically.

Some of this variability is related to comorbidity. Ageing is associated with altered pharmacokinetics particularly characterized by diminished clearance and volume of distribution. This has been well evaluated for morphine (Baillie et al 1989) and fentanyl (Bentley et al 1982, Holdsworth et al 1994). In a study of morphine use in the management of chronic cancer pain in the elderly, overall elderly patients required lower doses than their younger counterparts without exhibiting an enhanced risk for opioid-induced adverse effects (Rapin 1989). In patients with impaired renal function there is delayed clearance of an active metabolite of morphine, morphine-6-glucuronide (Osborne et al 1993). Anecdotally, high concentrations of M6G have been associated with toxicity (Osborne et al 1986, Hagen et al 1991, Sjogren et al 1993); however, in a prospective study of patients with opioid-induced delirium or myoclonus no relationship with renal function was observed (Tiseo et al 1995).

Other patient-related factors that may enhance the risk of adverse effects include the coadministration of drugs that may have cumulative toxicity or other concurrent comorbidity (Table 43.5).

Opioid initiation and dose escalation Some adverse effects appear transiently and spontaneously abate after the initiation of an opioid or after dose escalation. This phenomenon has been well demonstrated in a prospective study on the effect of morphine dose escalation on cognitive performance (Bruera et al 1989). This study demonstrated that cognitive impairment commonly improved after 7 days. This phenomenon, though often

Table 43.5 Comorbidity that may mimic opioid-induced adverse effects

Cause		Adverse effects
Central nervous system	Cerebral metastases	Drowsiness, cognitive impairment, nausea, vomiting
	Leptomeningeal metastases	Drowsiness, cognitive impairment, nausea, vomiting
	Cerebrovascular event	Drowsiness, cognitive impairment
	Extradural haemorrhage	Drowsiness, cognitive impairment
Metabolic	Dehydration	Drowsiness, cognitive impairment
	Hypercalcaemia	Drowsiness, cognitive impairment, nausea, vomiting
	Hyponatraemia	Drowsiness, cognitive impairment
	Renal failure	Drowsiness, cognitive impairment, nausea, vomiting, myoclonus
	Liver failure	Drowsiness, cognitive impairment, nausea, vomiting, myoclonus
	Hypoxaemia	Drowsiness, cognitive impairment
Sepsis/infection		Drowsiness, cognitive impairment, nausea, vomiting
Mechanical	Bowel obstruction	Nausea, vomiting
Iatrogenic	Tricyclics	Drowsiness, cognitive impairment, constipation
	Benzodiazepines	Drowsiness, cognitive impairment
	Antibiotics	Nausea and vomiting
	Vinca alkaloids	Constipation
	Flutamide	Constipation
	Steroids	Agitated delirium
	Non-steroidal anti-inflammatory drugs	Nausea, drowsiness
	Chemotherapy	Nausea, vomiting, drowsiness, cognitive impairment
	Radiotherapy	Nausea, vomiting, drowsiness

described, has not been formally studied in regards to other adverse effects.

Differential diagnosis

Adverse changes in patient well-being among patients taking opioids are not always caused by the opioid. Adverse effects must be differentiated from other causes of comorbidity that may develop in the treated patient and from drug interections. Common causes of comorbidity that may mimic opioid-induced adverse effects are presented in Table 43.5.

Indeed, the appearance of a new adverse change in patient well-being that occurs in the setting of stable opioid dosing is rarely caused by the opioid, and an alternate explanation should be vigorously sought. Since polypharmacy is common among patients with advanced cancer, it is essential to scrutinize medication records and patient report of medication administration to evauate for possible drug interactions or some other drug-related explanation for the reported symptoms.

Overview of the alternative approaches to treating opioid adverse effects

In general, four different approaches to the management of opioid adverse effects have been described:

1. Dose reduction of systemic opioid
2. Specific therapy to reduce the adverse effect
3. Opioid rotation
4. Change route of administration

Dose reduction of systemic opioid Reducing the dose of administered opioids usually results in a reduction in dose-related adverse effects. When patients have well-controlled pain, gradual reduction in the opioid dose will often result in the resolution of dose-related adverse effeects whilst preserving adequate pain relief (Fallon and O'Neill 1998).

When opioid doses cannot be reduced without the loss of pain control, reduction in dose must be accompanied by the addition of an accompanying synergist approach. Extensive experience has been reported with four accompanying approaches:

1. The addition of a non-opioid coanalgesic. The analgesia achieved from non-opioid coanalgesics from the non-steroidal anti-inflammatory class of agents is additive and often synergistic with that achieved by opioids. This is supported from a number of prospective studies (Sevarino et al 1992, Bjorkman et al 1993, Joishy and Walsh 1998, Minotti et al 1998) and from one retrospective drug utilization survey (Zech et al 1995).
2. The addition of an adjuvant analgesic that is appropriate to the pain syndrome and mechanism. Adjuvant analgesics (see below) may be combined with primary analgesics to improve the outcome for patients who cannot otherwise attain an acceptable balance between relief and side effects (Portenoy 1996). There is great interindividual variability in the response to all adjuvant analgesics and, for most, the likelihood of benefit is limited. Furthermore, many of the adjuvant analgesics have the potential to cause side effects that may be additive to the opioid-induced adverse effects already problematic. In evaluating the utility of an adjuvant agent in a particular patient setting, one must consider the likelihood of benefit, the risk of adverse effects, the ease of administration, and patient convenience.
3. The application of a therapy targetting the cause of the pain. Specific antitumour therapies, such as radiotherapy, chemotherapy, or surgery targetting the cause of cancer-related pain can provide substantial relief and thus lower the need for opioid analgesia. Radiotherapy is of established benefit in the treatment of painful bone metastases (Bates 1992, Hoskin 1995, Janjan 1997), epidural neoplasm (Bates 1992), and headache due to cerebral metastases (Coia 1992, Sneed et al 1996, Vermeulen 1998). In other settings there is a lack of well-established supportive data, and the use of radiotherapy is largely anecdotal. Despite a paucity of evidence concerning the specific analgesic benefits of chemotherapy (Queisser 1984, Rubens et al 1992), there is a strong clinical impression that tumour shrinkage is generally associated with relief of pain. Although there are some reports of analgesic value even in the absence of significant tumour shrinkage (Patt et al 1985, Thatcher et al 1995, Rothenberg 1996), the likelihood of a favourable effect on pain is generally related to the likelihood of tumour response. Surgery may have a role in the relief of symptoms caused by specific problems, such as obstruction of a hollow viscus (Jong et al 1995, Mainar et al 1996, Parker and Baines 1996, Barbalias et al 1997), unstable bony structures (Braun and Rohe 1984, Tarn and Lee 1994, Algan and Horowitz 1996), and compression of neural tissues (Sucher et al 1994, Gokaslan 1996, Harris et al 1996).
4. The application of a regional anaesthetic or neuroablative intervention (see below). The results of the WHO 'analgesic ladder' validation studies suggest that 10–30% of patients with cancer pain do not achieve a satisfactory balance

between relief and side effects using systemic pharmacotherapy alone without unacceptable drug toxicity (Takeda 1985, Ventafridda et al 1987, Walker et al 1988, Goisis et al 1989, Schug et al 1990, Grond et al 1991). Anaesthetic and neurosurgical techniques may reduce or eliminate the requirement for systemically administered opioids to achieve adequate analgesia. In general, regional analgesic techniques such as intraspinal opioid and local anaesthetic administration or intrapleural local anaesthetic administration are usually considered first because they can achieve this end without compromising neurological integrity. Neurodestructive procedures, however, are valuable in a small subset of patients, and some of these procedures, such as celiac plexus blockade in patients with pancreatic cancer, may have a favourable enough risk:benefit ratio that early treatment is warranted.

Symptomatic management of the adverse effect Symptomatic drugs used to prevent or control opioid adverse effects are commonly employed. Most of these approaches are based on cumulative anecdotal experience. With few exceptions, the literature describing these approaches is anecdotal or 'expert opinion'. Very few studies have prospectively evaluated efficacy, and no studies have evaluated the toxicity of these approaches over the long term. In general, this approach involves the addition of a new medication, adding to medication burden and with it the associated risks of adverse effects or drug interaction.

Opioid rotation Over the past 10 years numerous clinicians and cancer pain services have reported successful reduction in opioid side effects by switching to an alternative opioid (Galer et al 1992; Bruera et al 1995, 1996; Cherny et al 1995; de Stoutz et al 1995; Paix et al 1995; Thomas and Bruera 1995; Maddocks et al 1996; Vigano et al 1996; Fitzgibbon and Ready 1997; Hagen and Swanson 1997; Lawlor et al 1997; Makin and Ellershaw 1998; Ripamonti et al 1998; Ashby et al 1999). Improvements in cognitive impairment, sedation, hallucinations, nausea, vomiting, and myoclonus have been commonly reported. This approach requires familiarity with a range of opioid agonists and with the use of equianalgesic tables to convert doses when switching between opioids. While this approach has the practical advantage of minimizing polypharmacy, outcomes are variable and unpredictable. When switching between opioids, even with prudent use of equianalgesic tables, patients are at risk of under- or overdosing by virtue of individual sensitivities.

The biologic basis for the observed intraindividual variability in sensitivity to opioid analgesia and adverse effects is multifactorial. Preclinical studies show that opioids can act on different receptors or sub-type receptors (de Stoutz et al 1995, Pasternak and Standifer 1995, Zadina et al 1995, Rossi et al 1997), and individual receptor profiles may influence the analgesia as well as the side effects. The genetic makeup of the individual plays an important role in analgesia for some opioids (Brosen et al 1993, Sindrup et al 1993, Fromm et al 1995, Sindrup and Brosen 1995, Poulsen et al 1996, Kirkwood et al 1997, Heiskanen et al 1998), and similar phenomena may contribute to variability in adverse effect sensitivity.

Switching route of systemic administration Limited data indicates that some adverse side effects among patients receiving oral morphine can be relieved by switching the route of admission to the subcutaneous route. In one small study this phenomenon was reported for nausea and vomiting (McDonald et al 1991); in another there was less constipation, drowsiness, and nausea (Drexel et al 1989).

Initial management of the patient receiving opioids who presents with adverse effects

Among patients receiving opioid analgesic therapy there are two key steps in the initial management of adverse effects. Firstly, the clinician must distinguish between morphine adverse effects from comorbidity or drug interactions. This step requires careful evaluation of the patient for factors outlined in Table 43.5. If present, these factors should be redressed. Metabolic disorders, dehydration, or sepsis should be treated; non-essential drugs that may be producing an adverse interaction should be discontinued. Symptomatic measures may be required until effect is observed.

Secondly, if indeed it seems that there is a true adverse effect of an opioid, consideration should be given to reducing the opioid dose. If the patient has good pain control, reduce morphine dose by 25%.

Adverse drug interactions In patients with advanced cancer side effects due to drug combinations are common. The potential for additive side effects and serious toxicity from drug combinations must be recognized. The sedative effect of an opioid may add to that produced by numerous other centrally acting drugs, such as anxiolytics, neuroleptics, and antidepressants (Pies 1996). Likewise, drugs with anticholinergic effects probably worsen the constipatory effects of opioids. As noted previously, a severe adverse reaction, including excitation, hyperpyrexia, convulsions, and death, has been reported after the administration of meperidine to patients treated with a monoamine oxidase inhibitor (Browne and Linter 1987).

Gastrointestinal side effects The gastrointestinal adverse effects of opioids are common. In general they are characterized by having a weak dose–response relationship. *Constipation* is the most common adverse effect of chronic opioid therapy (Fallon and O'Neill 1997). The likelihood of opioid-induced constipation is so great that laxative medications should be prescribed prophylactically to most patients. Opioids may produce *nausea* and *vomiting* through both central and peripheral mechanisms. These drugs stimulate the medullary chemoreceptor trigger zone, increase vestibular sensitivity, and have effects on the gastrointestinal tract (including increased gastric antral tone, diminished motility, and delayed gastric emptying). With the initiation of opioid therapy, patients should be informed that nausea can occur and that it is usually transitory and controllable. Routine prophylactic administration of an antiemetic is not necessary, except in patients with a history of severe opioid-induced nausea and vomiting, but patients should have access to an antiemetic at the start of therapy if the need for one arises. Anecdotally, the use of prochlorperazine and metoclopromide has usually been sufficient.

Central nervous system side effects The CNS side effects of opioids are generally dose related. The specific pattern of CNS adverse effects is influenced by individual patient factors, duration of opioid exposure, and dose.

Sedation Initiation of opioid therapy or significant dose escalation commonly induces sedation that persists until tolerance to this effect develops, usually in days to weeks. It is useful to forewarn patients of this potential, and thereby reduce anxiety and encourage avoidance of activities, such as driving, that may be dangerous if sedation occurs (Vainio et al 1995). Some patients have a persistent problem with sedation, particularly if other confounding factors exist. These factors include the use of other sedating drugs or coexistent diseases such as dementia, metabolic encephalopathy, or brain metastases. Both dextroamphetamine and methylphenidate have been widely used in the treatment of opioid-induced sedation (Portenoy 1994). Treatment with methylphenidate or dextroamphetamine is typically begun with 2.5 to 5 mg in the morning, which is repeated at midday if necessary to maintain effects until evening. Doses are then increased gradually if needed. Few patients require more than 40 mg per day in divided doses. This approach is relatively contraindicated among patients with cardiac arrhythmias, agitated delirium, paranoid personality, and past amphetamine abuse.

Confusion and delirium Mild cognitive impairment is common following the initiation of opioid therapy or doses. Similar to sedation, however, pure opioid-induced encephalopathy appears to be transient in most patients, persisting from days to a week or two. Although persistent confusion attributable to opioids alone occurs, the aetiology of persistent delirium is usually related to the combined effect of the opioid and other contributing factors, including electrolyte disorders, neoplastic involvement of central nervous system, sepsis, vital organ failure, and hypoxaemia (Portenoy 1994). A stepwise approach to management (Table 43.6) often culminates in a trial of a neuroleptic drug. Haloperidol in low doses (0.5–1.0 mg P.O. or 0.25–0.5 mg I.V. or I.M.) is most commonly recommended because of its efficacy and low incidence of cardiovascular and anticholinergic effects.

Respiratory depression When sedation is used as a clinical indicator of CNS toxicity and appropriate steps are taken, respiratory depression is rare. When, however, it does occur it is always accompanied by other signs of central nervous system depression, including sedation and mental clouding. Respiratory compromise accompanied by

Table 43.6 Management of opioid-induced delirium

1) Discontinue non-essential centrally acting medications
2) If analgesia is satisfactory, reduce opioid dose by 25%
3) Exclude sepsis or metabolic derangement
4) Exclude CNS involvement by tumour
5) If delirium persists, consider:
   - trial of neuroleptic (e.g., haloperidol)
   - change to an alternative opioid drug
   - a change in opioid route to the intraspinal route (± local anaesthetic)
   - a trial of other anaesthetic or neurosurgical options

tachypnoea and anxiety is never a primary opioid event.

With repeated opioid administration, tolerance appears to develop rapidly to the respiratory depressant effects of the opioid drugs; consequently clinically important respiratory depression is a very rare event in the cancer patient whose opioid dose has been titrated against pain.

The ability to tolerate high doses of opioids is also related to the stimulus-related effect of pain on respiration in a manner that is balanced against the depressant opioid effect. Opioid-induced respiratory depression can occur, however, if pain is suddenly eliminated (such as may occur following neurolytic procedures) and the opioid dose is not reduced (Wells et al 1984).

When respiratory depression occurs in patients on chronic opioid therapy, administration of the specific opioid antagonist, naloxone, usually improves ventilation. This is true even if the primary cause of the respiratory event was not the opioid itself, but rather an intercurrent cardiac or pulmonary process. A response to naloxone, therefore, should not be taken as proof that the event was due to the opioid alone and an evaluation for these other processes should ensue.

Naloxone can precipitate a severe abstinence syndrome and should be administered only if strongly indicated. If the patient is bradypnoeic but readily arousable, and the peak plasma level of the last opioid dose has already been reached, the opioid should be withheld and the patient monitored until improved. If severe hypoventilation occurs (regardless of the associated factors that may be contributing to respiratory compromise), or the patient is bradypnoeic and unarousable, naloxone should be administered. To reduce the risk of severe withdrawal following a period of opioid administration, dilute naloxone (1:10) should be used in doses titrated to respiratory rate and level of consciousness. In the comatose patient, it may be prudent to place an endotracheal tube to prevent aspiration following administration of naloxone.

Multifocal myoclonus All opioid analgesics can produce myoclonus. Mild and infrequent myoclonus is common. In occasional patients, however, myoclonus can be distressing or contribute to breakthrough pain that occurs with involuntary movement. If the dose cannot be reduced due to persistent pain, consideration should be given either to switching to an alternative opioid (Cherny et al 1995) or to symptomatic treatment with a benzodiazepine (particularly clonazepam or midazolam), dantrolene, or an anticonvulsant (Portenoy 1994).

Other effects

Urinary retention Opioid analgesics increase smooth muscle tone and can occasionally cause bladder spasm or urinary retention (due to an increase in sphincter tone). This is an infrequent problem usually observed in elderly male patients. Tolerance can develop rapidly but catheterization may be necessary to manage transient problems.

Adjuvant analgesics

The term 'adjuvant analgesic' describes a drug that has a primary indication other than pain but is analgesic in some conditions. In the cancer population, these drugs may be combined with primary analgesics in any of the three steps of the 'analgesic ladder' to improve the outcome for patients who cannot otherwise attain an acceptable balance between relief and side effects. The potential utility of an adjuvant analgesic is usually suggested by the characteristics of the pain or by the existence of another symptom that may be amenable to a non-analgesic effect of the drug.

There is great interindividual variability in the response to all adjuvant analgesics. Although patient characteristics, such as advanced age or coexistent major organ failure, may increase the likelihood of some (usually adverse) responses, neither favourable effects nor specific side effects can be reliably predicted in the individual patient. Furthermore, there is remarkable intraindividual variability in the response to different drugs, including those within the same class. These observations suggest the potential utility of sequential trials of adjuvant analgesics. The process of sequential drug trials, like the use of low initial doses and dose titration, should be explained to the patient at the start of therapy to enhance compliance and reduce the distress that may occur if treatments fail.

In the management of cancer pain, adjuvant analgesics can be broadly classified based on conventional use. Four groups are distinguished:

1. Multipurpose adjuvant analgesics.
2. Adjuvant analgesics used for neuropathic pain.
3. Adjuvant analgesics used for bone pain.
4. Adjuvant analgesics used for visceral pain.

Multipurpose adjuvant medications

Corticosteroids Corticosteroids are among the most widely used adjuvant analgesics (Watanabe and Bruera 1994). They have been demonstrated to have analgesic effects, to significantly improve quality of life; and to have beneficial effects on appetite, nausea, mood, and malaise in the cancer population. Painful conditions that commonly respond to corticosteroids include raised intracranial pressure headache, acute spinal cord compression, superior vena cava syndrome, metastatic bone pain, neuropathic pain due to infiltration or compression by tumour, symptomatic lymphoedema, and hepatic capsular distension (Watanabe and Bruera 1994). The mechanism of analgesia produced by these drugs may involve antioedema effects, anti-inflammatory effects, and a direct influence on the electrical activity in damaged nerves (Devor et al 1985). The most commonly used drug is dexamethasone, a choice that gains theoretical support from the relatively low mineralocorticoid effect of this agent. Dexamethasone also has been conventionally used for raised intracranial pressure and spinal cord compression.

Patients with advanced cancer who experience pain and other symptoms may respond favourably to a relatively small dose of corticosteroid (e.g., dexamethasone 1–2 mg twice daily). In some settings, however, a high-dose regimen may be appropriate. For example, patients with spinal cord compression, an acute episode of very severe bone pain, or neuropathic pain that cannot be promptly reduced with opioids may respond dramatically to a short course of relatively high doses (e.g., dexamethasone 100 mg, followed initially by 96 mg per day in divided doses) (Sorensen et al 1994). This dose can be tapered over weeks, concurrent with initiation of other analgesic approaches, such as radiotherapy.

Although the effects produced by corticosteroids in patients with advanced cancer are often very gratifying, side effects are potentially serious and increase with prolonged usage (Twycross 1994). The most common adverse effects include oropharyngeal candidiasis, oedema or cushingoid habitus; dyspepsia, weight gain, neuropsychological changes and ecchymoses, hyperglycaemia, and myopathy. The risk of peptic ulcer is approximately doubled in patients chronically treated with corticosteroids, and coadministration of corticosteroid with aspirin or an NSAID further increases the risk of gastroduodenopathy and is not recommended (Ellershaw and Kelly 1994). Active peptic ulcer disease, systemic infection, and unstable diabetes are relative contraindications to the use of corticosteroids as adjuvant analgesics.

Topical local anaesthetics Topical local anaesthetics can be used in the management of painful cutaneous and mucosal lesions, and as a premedication prior to skin puncture. Eutectic mixture of 2.5% lidocaine (lignocaine) and 2.5% prilocaine (EMLA) is effective in reducing pain associated with venipuncture, lumbar puncture, and arterial puncture. It has also been used for painful ulcerating skin lesions. Viscous lidocaine (lignocaine) is frequently used in the management of oropharyngeal ulceration. Although the risk of aspiration appears to be very small, caution with eating is required after oropharyngeal anaesthesia.

Adjuvants used for neuropathic pain

Neuropathic pains are generally less responsive to opioid therapy than nociceptive pain, and in many cases the outcome of pharmacotherapy may be improved by the addition of an adjuvant analgesic.

Antidepressant drugs Antidepressant drugs are commonly used to manage continuous neuropathic pains and the evidence for analgesic efficacy is greatest for the tertiary amine tricyclic drugs, such as amitriptyline, doxepin, and imipramine (McQuay et al 1996). The secondary amine tricyclic antidepressants (such as desipramine, clomipramine, and nortryptyline) have fewer side effects and are preferred when concern about sedation, anticholinergic effects, or cardiovascular toxicity is high (McQuay et al 1996). The selective serotonin uptake inhibitor antidepressants are much less effective in the management of neuropathic pain and are generally not recommended for this purpose.

The starting dose of a tricyclic antidepressant should be low, e.g., amitriptyline 10 mg in the elderly and 25 mg in younger patients. Doses can be increased every few days, and the initial dosing increments are usually the same size as the starting dose. When doses have reached the usual effective range (e.g., amitriptyline 75–150 mg), it is prudent to observe effects for a week before continuing upward dose titration. It is reasonable to continue upward dose titration beyond the usual analgesic doses in patients who fail to achieve benefit and have no limiting side effects. Plasma drug concentration, if available, may provide useful information and should be followed during the course of therapy.

Anticonvulsant drugs Selected anticonvulsant drugs appear to be analgesic for the lancinating dysaesthesias that characterize diverse types of neuropathic pain (McQuay et al 1995). Although most practitioners prefer to begin with carbamazepine because of the very good response rate observed in trigeminal neuralgia (McQuay et al 1995), this drug must be used cautiously in cancer patients with thrombocytopenia, those at risk for marrow failure (e.g., following chemotherapy), and those whose blood counts must be monitored to determine disease status. If carbamazepine is used, a complete blood count should be obtained prior to the start of therapy, after 2 and 4 weeks, and then every 3–4 months thereafter. A leukocyte count below 4000 is usually considered to be a contraindication to treatment, and a decline to less than 3000, or an absolute neutrophil count of less than 1500 during therapy should prompt discontinuation of the drug. Other anticonvulsant drugs may also be useful, and published reports and clinical experience support trials with gabapentin, phenytoin, clonazepam, and valproate (McQuay et al 1995). When anticonvulsant drugs are used as adjuvant analgesics it is recommended that dosing follow the dosing guidelines customarily employed in the treatment of seizures.

Oral local anaesthetic drugs Occasionally, systemically administered local anaesthetic drugs may be useful in the management of neuropathic pains characterized by either continuous or lancinating dysaesthesias. It is reasonable to undertake a trial with an oral local anaesthetic in patients with continuous dysaesthesias who fail to respond adequately, or who cannot tolerate, the tricyclic antidepressants, and in patients with lancinating pains refractory to trials of anticonvulsant drugs and baclofen. Mexiletine is the safest of the oral local anaesthetics (CAST Investigators 1989, Ruskin 1989) and is preferred. Analgesic response to a trial of intravenous lidocaine (lignocaine; 5 mg/kg, over 45 min) may predict the likelihood of response to oral mexiletine (Galer et al 1996). Dosing with mexiletine should usually be started at 100–150 mg per day. If intolerable side effects do not occur, the dose can be increased by a similar amount every few days, until the usual maximum dose of 300 mg three times per day is reached.

Less compelling data support the use of clonidine, baclofen, calcitonin, and subcutaneously administered ketamine (Lipman 1996).

Adjuvant analgesics used for bone pain

The management of bone pain frequently requires the integration of opioid therapy with multiple ancillary approaches. Although a meta-analysis of NSAID therapy in cancer pain that reviewed data from 1615 patients in 21 trials found no specific efficacy in bone pain and analgesic effects equivalent only to 'weak' opioids (Eisenberg et al 1994), some patients appear to benefit greatly from the addition of such a drug. Corticosteroids are often advocated in difficult cases (Watanabe and Bruera 1994).

Bisphosphonates Bisphosphonates are analogues of inorganic pyrophosphate that inhibit osteoclast activity and reduce bone resorption in a variety of illnesses. Controlled and uncontrolled trials of intravenous pamidronate in patients with advanced cancer have demonstrated significant reduction of bone pain (Strang 1996). The analgesic effect of pamidronate appears to be dose and schedule dependent: a dose response is evident at doses between 15 and 30 mg/week and it has been noted that 30 mg every 2 weeks is less effective than 60 mg every 4 weeks (Strang 1996). Similar effects have been observed with orally administered clodronate (Ernst et al 1997).

Radiopharmaceuticals Radiolabelled agents absorbed into areas of high bone turnover have been evaluated as potential therapies for metastatic bone disease. It has the advantages of addressing all sites of involvement and relatively selective absorption, thus limiting radiation exposure to normal tissues. Excellent clinical responses with acceptable haematological toxicity have been observed with a range of radiopharmaceuticals. The best studied and most commonly used radionuclide is strontium-89. Large, prospectively randomized clinical trials have demonstrated its efficacy as a first-line therapy (Robinson et al 1995) or as an adjuvant to external-beam radiotherapy (Porter et al 1993). This approach is contraindicated with patients who have a platelet count less than 60 000 or a WCC < 2.4 and is not advised for patients with very poor performance status (Schmeler and Bastin 1996). Using another approach, bone-seeking radiopharmaceuticals that link a radioisotope with a bisphosphonate compound have been synthesized. Positive experience has been reported with samarium-153-ethylenediaminetetramethylene phosphonic acid, and rhenium-186-hydroxyethylidene diphosphonate.

Adjuvant analgesics for visceral pain

There are limited data that support the potential efficacy of a range of adjuvant agents for the management of bladder spasm, tenesmoid pain, and colicky intestinal pain. Oxybutynin chloride, a tertiary amine with anticholinergic and papaverine-like, direct muscular antispasmodic effects, is often helpful for bladder spasm pain (Paulson 1978) as is flavoxate (Baert 1974). Based on limited clinical experience and *in vitro* evidence that prostaglandins play a role in bladder smooth-muscle contraction, a trial of NSAIDs may be justified for patients with painful bladder spasms (Abrams and Fenely 1976). Limited data support a trial of intravesical capsaicin (Barbanti et al 1993, Lazzeri et al 1996).

There is no well-established pharmacotherapy for painful rectal spasms. A recent double-blinded study demonstrated that nebulized salbutamol can reduce the duration and severity of attacks (Eckardt et al 1996). There is anecdotal support for trials of diltiazem (Boquet et al 1986, Castell 1985), clonidine (Swain 1987), chlorpromazine (Patt et al 1994), and benzodiazepines (Hanks 1984).

Colicky pain due to inoperable bowel obstruction has been treated empirically with intravenous scopolamine (hyoscine) butylbromide (Baines 1997, De Conno et al 1991, Ventafridda et al 1990) and sublingual scopolamine (hyoscine) hydrobromide (Baines 1994). Limited data support the use of octreotide for this indication (Mercadante 1994b).

Other non-invasive analgesic techniques

Psychological therapies in cancer pain

Psychological approaches are an integral part of the care of the cancer patient with pain. All patients can benefit from psychological assessment and support, and some are good candidates for specific psychological interventions including those commonly used in the management of pain. Cognitive-behavioural interventions can help some patients decrease the perception of distress engendered by the pain through the development of new coping skills and the modification of thoughts, feelings, and behaviours (Spiegel and Moore 1997). Relaxation methods may be able to reduce muscular tension and emotional arousal, or enhance pain tolerance (Arathuzik 1994). Other approaches reduce anticipatory anxiety that may lead to avoidant behaviours, or lessen the distress associated with the pain (Turk and Feldman 1992). Successful implementation of these approaches in the cancer population requires a cognitively intact patient and a dedicated, well-trained physician (Fishman 1992).

Physiatric techniques

Physiatric techniques can be used to optimize the function of the patient with chronic cancer or enhance analgesia through application of modalities such as electrical stimulation, heat, or cryotherapy. The treatment of lymphoedema by use of wraps, pressure stockings, or pneumatic pump devices can both improve function and relieve pain and heaviness (Brennan et al 1996, Marcks 1997). The use of orthotic devices can immobilize and support painful or weakened structures, and assistive devices can be of great value to patients with pain precipitated by weight bearing or ambulation.

Transcutaneous electrical nerve stimulation

The mechanisms by which transcutaneous electrical stimulation reduces pain are not well defined; local neural blockade and activation of a central inhibitory system have been proposed as explanations. Clinical experience suggests that this modality can be a useful adjunct in the management of mild to moderate musculoskeletal or neuropathic pain (Sykes et al 1997).

Invasive analgesic techniques

Anaesthetic and neurosurgical techniques

The results of the WHO 'analgesic ladder' validation studies suggest that 10–30% of patients with cancer pain do not achieve a satisfactory balance between relief and side effects using systemic pharmacotherapy alone without unacceptable drug toxicity (World Health Organization 1996). Anaesthetic and neurosurgical techniques (Table 43.7) may reduce or eliminate the requirement for systemically administered opioids to achieve adequate analgesia.

Consideration of invasive approaches requires a word of caution. Interpretation of data regarding the use of alternative analgesic approaches and extrapolation to the presenting clinical problem requires care. The literature is characterized by the lack of uniformity in patient selection, inadequate reporting of previous analgesic therapies, inconsistencies in outcome evaluation, and paucity of long-term follow-up. Furthermore, reported outcomes in the literature may not predict the outcomes of a procedure performed on a medically ill patient by a physician who has more limited experience with the techniques involved.

When indicated, the use of invasive and neurodestructive procedures should be based on an evaluation of the likelihood and duration of analgesic benefit, the immediate and long-term risks, the likely duration of survival, the availability of local expertise, and the anticipated length of hospitalization.

For most pain syndromes there exists a range of techniques that may theoretically be applied.

Table 43.7 A guide to the selection of invasive analgesic techniques according to the site of pain

Site	Procedure
Face—unilateral	Gasserian gangliolysis Trigeminal neurolysis Intraventricular opioid
Pharyngeal	Glossopharyngeal neurolysis Intraventricular opioid
Arm/brachial plexus	Spinal opioid ± local anaesthetic Chemical rhizotomy Surgical rhizotomy
Chest wall	Spinal opioid ± local anaesthetic Intercostal neurolysis Paravertebral neurolysis Chemical rhizotomy Surgical rhizotomy
Abdominal somatic	Spinal opioid ± local anaesthetic Chemical rhizotomy Surgical rhizotomy Cordotomy (unilateral pain)
Upper abdomen: visceral	Celiac plexus neurolysis
Low abdomen: visceral	Hypogastric neurolysis Ganglion impar neurolysis
Perineum	Spinal opioid ± local anaesthetic Chemical rhizotomy Surgical rhizotomy Transsacral S4 neurolysis
Pelvis + lower limb	Spinal opioid ± local anaesthetic Chemical rhizotomy Surgical rhizotomy
Unilateral lower quadrant	Cordotomy
Multifocal or generalized pain	Pituitary ablation Cingulotomy

In choosing between a range of procedures the following principles are salient:

1. Ablative procedures are deferred as long as pain relief is obtainable by non-ablative modalities.
2. The procedure most likely to be effective should be selected. If there is a choice, however, the one with the fewest and least serious adverse effects is preferred.
3. In progressive stages of cancer, pain is likely to be multifocal, and a procedure aimed at a single locus of pain, even if completed flawlessly, is unlikely to yield complete relief of pain until death. A realistic and sound goal is a lasting decrease in pain to a level manageable by pharmacotherapy with minimal side effects.
4. Whenever possible, neurolysis should be preceded by the demonstration of effective analgesia with a local anaesthetic prognostic block.
5. Since there is a learning curve with all of the procedures, performance by a physician experienced in the specific intervention may improve the likelihood of a successful outcome.

In general, regional analgesic techniques such as intraspinal opioid and local anaesthetic administration or intrapleural local anaesthetic administration are usually considered first because they can achieve this end without compromising neurological integrity. Neurodestructive procedures, however, are valuable in a small subset of patients; and some of these procedures, such as coeliac plexus blockade in patients with pancreatic cancer, may have a favourable enough risk:benefit ratio that early treatment is warranted.

Regional analgesia

Epidural and intrathecal opioids

The delivery of low opioid doses near the sites of action in the spinal cord may decrease supraspinally mediated adverse effects. In the absence of randomized trials that compare the various intraspinal techniques with other analgesic approaches, the indications for the spinal route remain empirical but they are based on relative therapeutic index. One survey reported that only 16 of 1205 cancer patients with pain required intraspinal therapy (Hogan et al 1991). Compared to neuroablative therapies, spinal opioids have the advantage of preserving sensation, strength, and sympathetic function. Contraindications include bleeding diathesis, profound leukopenia, and sepsis. A temporary trial of spinal opioid therapy should be performed to assess the potential benefits of this approach before implantation of a permanent catheter.

Opioid selection for intraspinal delivery is influenced by several factors. Hydrophilic drugs, such as morphine and hydromorphone, have a prolonged half-life in cerebrospinal fluid and significant rostral redistribution (Brose et al 1991). Lipophilic opioids, such as fentanyl and sufentanil, have less rostral redistribution and may be preferable for segmental analgesia at the level of spinal infusion. The addition of a low concentration of a local anaesthetic, such as 0.125–0.25% bupivacaine, to an epidural (Du Pen and Williams 1992) or intrathecal opioid (Mercadante 1994a, Sjoberg et al 1994, Nitescu et al 1995) has been demonstrated to increase analgesic effect without increasing toxicity. Other agents have also been coadministered with intraspinal opioids, including clonidine (Eisenach et al 1995), octreotide (Penn et al 1992), ketamine (Yaksh 1996, Yang et al 1996), and calcitonin (Blanchard et al 1990), but additional studies are required to assess their potential utility.

There have been no trials comparing the intrathecal and epidural routes in cancer pain, and extensive experience has been reported with both approaches. Longitudinal studies of epidural or intrathecal opioid infusions for cancer pain suggest that the risks associated with these techniques are similar (Nitescu et al 1990, Hassenbusch et al 1995, Gestin et al 1997). The potential morbidity for these procedures indicates the need for a well-trained clinician and long-term monitoring.

Intraventricular opioids

A growing international experience suggests that the administration of low doses of an opioid (particularly morphine) into the cerebral ventricles can provide long-term analgesia in selected patients (Cramond and Stuart 1993, Karavelis et al 1996). This technique has been used for patients with upper body or head pain or severe diffuse pain and has been generally very well tolerated. Schedules have included both intermittent injection via an Ommaya reservoir (Cramond and Stuart 1993, Karavelis et al 1996) and continual infusion using an implanted pump (Dennis and DeWitty 1990).

Regional local anaesthetic

Several authors have described the use of intrapleural local anaesthetics in the management of chronic post-thoracotomy pain (Symreng et al 1989) and cancer-related pains involving the head, neck, chest, arms, and upper abdominal viscera (Dionne 1992, Lema et al 1992). Although a single bolus may provide a prolonged analgesia, continuous infusion of local anaesthetic has been recommended for patients with chronic pain due to advanced cancer (Myers et al 1993). For patients with localized upper limb pain, intermittent infusion of bupivicaine through an interscalene brachial plexus catheter may be of benefit (Cooper et al 1994).

Anaesthetic techniques for sympathetically maintained pain and visceral pain

Celiac plexus block

Neurolytic celiac plexus blockade can be considered in the management of pain caused by neoplastic infiltration of the upper abdominal viscera, including the pancreas, upper retroperitoneum, liver, gall bladder, and proximal small bowel (Eisenberg et al 1995, Caraceni and Portenoy 1996). In addition to an extensive anecdotal experience, this technique is supported by two controlled studies of the percutaneous approach (Mercadante 1993, Kawamata et al 1996) and a controlled trial of intraoperative neurolysis (Lillemoe et al 1993). Reported analgesic response rates in patients with pancreatic cancer are 50–90%, and the reported duration of effect is generally 1–12 months (Eisenberg et al 1995, Caraceni and Portenoy 1996). Given the generally favourable response to this approach and supportive data from two small studies (Mercadante 1993, Kawamata et al 1996), some clinicians recommend this intervention at an early stage; other experts differ and recommend coeliac plexus block only for patients who do not maintain an adequate balance between analgesia and side effects from an oral opioid (Caraceni and Portenoy 1996). Common transient complications include postural hypotension and diarrhoea. Rarely the procedure can produce a paraplegia due to an acute ischaemic myelopathy (probably caused by involvement of Adamkievicz's artery) (Wong and Brown 1995, Hayakawa et al 1997). Posterior spread of neurolytic solution can occasionally lead to involvement of lower thoracic and lumbar somatic nerves, which can potentially result in a neuropathic pain syndrome. Other uncommon complications include pneumothorax and retroperitoneal haematoma.

Sympathetic blocks for pelvic visceral pain

Limited anecdotal experience has been reported for two techniques. Phenol ablation of the superior hypogastric nerve plexus, which lies anterior to the sacral promontory, has been reported to relieve chronic cancer pain arising from the descending colon and rectum and the lower genitourinary structures in 40–80% of patients (Plancarte et al 1990, 1997). Similarly, neurolysis of the ganglion impar (ganglion of Walther, a solitary retroperitoneal structure at the sacrococcygeal junction that marks the termination of the paired paravertebral sympathetic chains) has been reported to relieve visceral sensations referred to the rectum, perineum, or vagina caused by locally advanced cancers of the pelvic visceral structures (Plancarte et al 1993, Wemm and Saberski 1995, Nebab and Florence 1997).

Sympathetic blockade of somatic structures

Sympathetically maintained pain syndromes may be relieved by interruption of sympathetic outflow to the affected region of the body. Lumbar sympathetic blockade should be considered for sympathetically maintained pain involving the legs, and stellate ganglion blockade may be useful for sympathetically maintained pain involving the face or arms (Lamacraft and Cousins 1997).

Neuroablative techniques for somatic and neuropathic pain

Rhizotomy

Segmental or multisegmental destruction of the dorsal sensory roots (rhizotomy), achieved by surgical section, chemical neurolysis, or radiofrequency lesion, can be an effective method of pain control for patients with otherwise refractory localized pain syndromes. These techniques are most commonly used in the management of chest wall pain due to tumour invasion of somatic and neural structures (Patt and Reddy 1994). Other indications include refractory upper limb, lower limb, pelvic, or perineal pain (Saris et al 1986). Chemical rhizotomy may be produced by the instillation of a neurolytic solution into either the epidural or intrathecal space (Patt and Reddy 1994). Chemical rhizotomies can be performed at any level up to the mid-cervical region, above which the spread of the neurolytic agent to the medullary centres carries unacceptable risk of cardiorespiratory collapse. To minimize the risk of excessive spread and lysis beyond the target segments, catheter tip position should be confirmed radiographically and phenol should be injected in small volumes (1–2 ml) (Salmon et al 1992).

Satisfactory analgesia is achieved in about 50% of patients (Patt and Reddy 1994), and the average duration of relief is 3–4 months but with a wide range of distribution. Adverse effects can be related to the injection technique (e.g., spinal headache, infection, and arachnoiditis) or to the destruction of non-nociceptive nerve fibres. Specific complications of the procedure depend on the site of neurolysis. For example, the complications of lumbosacral neurolysis include paresis (5–20%), sphincter dysfunction (5–60%), impairment of touch and proprioception, and dysaesthesias. Although neurological deficits are usually transient, the risk of increased disability through weakness, sphincter incompetence, and loss of positional sense suggests that these techniques should be reserved for patients with limited function and pre-existent urinary diversion. Patient counselling regarding the risks involved is essential.

Neurolysis of primary afferent nerves or their ganglia

Neurolysis of primary afferent nerves may also provide significant relief for selected patients with localized pain. The utility of these approaches is limited by the potential for concurrent motor or sphincteric dysfunction. Refractory unilateral facial or pharyngeal pain may be amenable to trigeminal neurolysis (gasserian gangliolysis) or glossopharyngeal neurolysis (Rizzi et al 1985, Ischia et al 1990). Unilateral pain involving the tongue or floor of mouth may be amenable to blockade of the sphenopalatine ganglion (Prasanna and Murthy 1993). Intercostal or paravertebral neurolysis are an alternative to rhizotomy for patients with chest wall pain. Unilateral shoulder pain may be amenable to suprascapular neurolysis (Meyer-Witting and Foster 1992). Arm pain that is more extensive may be effectively relieved by brachial plexus neurolysis, but this approach will result in weakness (Neill 1979). Anecdotally, refractory leg pain has been relieved without compromise of motor function by injection of 10 ml of 10% phenol injected into the psoas muscle sheath (Calava et al 1996). Severe somatic pain limited to the perineum may be treated by neurolysis of the S4 nerve root via the ipsilateral posterior sacral foramen, a procedure that carries a minimal risk of motor or sphincter dysfunction (Robertson 1983).

Regeneration of peripheral nerves is sometimes accompanied by the development of neuropathic pain; however, the threat of postablative dysaesthesia is of limited consequence when life expectancy is very limited or intractable pain already exceeds the limits of tolerance.

Cordotomy

During cordotomy, the anterolateral spinothalamic tract is ablated to produce contralateral loss of pain and temperature sensibility (Stuart and Cramond 1993, Sanders and Zuurmond 1995). The patient with severe unilateral pain arising in the torso or lower extremity is most likely to benefit from this procedure (Stuart and Cramond 1993, Sanders and Zuurmond 1995). Impressive results have also been observed in patients with chest wall pain (Sanders and Zuurmond 1995). The percutaneous technique is generally preferred (Stuart and Cramond 1993, Sanders and Zuurmond 1995); open cordotomy is usually reserved for patients who are unable to lie in the supine position or are not cooperative enough to undergo a percutaneous procedure.

Significant pain relief is achieved in more than 90% of patients during the period immediately following cordotomy (Stuart and Cramond 1993, Sanders and Zuurmond 1995). Fifty percent of surviving patients have recurrent pain after one year (Cowie and Hitchcock 1982). Repeat cordotomy can sometimes be effective. The neurological complications of cordotomy include paresis, ataxia, and bladder and 'mirror-image' pain (Sanders and Zuurmond 1995). The complications are usually transient, but are protracted and disabling in approximately 5% of cases (Sanders and Zuurmond 1995). Rarely, patients with a long duration of survival (> 12 months) develop a delayed-onset dysaesthetic pain (Cowie and Hitchcock 1982). The most serious potential complication is respiratory dysfunction, which may occur in the form of phrenic nerve paralysis or as sleep-induced (Chevrolet et al 1983, Polatty and Cooper 1986). Because of the latter concern, bilateral high cervical cordotomies or a unilateral cervical cordotomy ipsilateral to the site of the only functioning lung are not recommended.

Pituitary ablation

Pituitary ablation by chemical or surgical hypophysectomy has been reported to relieve diffuse and multifocal pain syndromes that have been refractory to opioid therapy and are unsuitable for any regional neuroablative procedure (Gonski and Sackelariou 1984, Levin and Ramirez 1984). Relief from pain due to both hormone-dependent and -independent tumours has been observed (Gonski and Sackelariou 1984, Levin and Ramirez 1984).

Cingulotomy

Anecdotal reports also support the efficacy of MRI-guided stereotactic cingulotomy in the management of diffuse pain syndromes that have been refractory to opioid therapy (Hassenbusch et al 1990, Wong et al 1997). Although this appears to be a safe procedure with minimal neurological or psychological morbidity, the duration of analgesia is often limited (Hassenbusch et al 1990, Wong et al 1997). The mode of action is unknown and the procedure is rarely considered.

Sedation as pain therapy

Through the vigilant application of analgesic care pain is often relieved adequately without compromising the sentience or function of the patient beyond that caused by the natural disease process itself. Occasionally, however, this cannot be achieved and pain is perceived to be 'refractory' (Cherny and Portenoy 1994). In deciding that a pain is refractory, the clinician must perceive that the further application of standard interventions is either (1) incapable of providing adequate relief, (2) associated with excessive and intolerable acute or chronic morbidity, or (3) unlikely to provide relief within a tolerable time frame. In this situation, sedation may be the only therapeutic option capable of providing adequate relief. This approach is described as 'sedation in the management of refractory symptoms at the end of life' (Cherny and Portenoy 1994).

The justification of sedation in this setting is that it is appropriate and proportionate. At the end of life, when the overwhelming goal of care is the preservation of patient comfort, the provision of adequate relief of symptoms must be pursued even in the setting of a narrow therapeutic index for the necessary palliative treatments (President's Commission for the Study of Ethical Problems in Medical and Biomedical and Behavioural Research 1983, American Medical Association 1996, Burt 1997). In this context, sedation is a medically indicated and proportionate therapeutic response to refractory symptoms, which cannot be otherwise relieved. Appeal to patients' rights also underwrites the moral legitimacy of sedation in the management of otherwise intolerable pain at the end of life. Patients have a right, recently affirmed by the Supreme Court, to palliative care in response to unrelieved suffering (Burt 1997).

Once a clinical consensus exists that pain is refractory, it is appropriate to present this option to the patient or their surrogate. When presented to a patient with refractory symptoms, the offer of sedation can demonstrate the clinician's commitment to the relief of suffering. This can enhance trust in the doctor–patient relationship and influence the patient's appraisal of their capacity to cope. Indeed, patients commonly decline sedation, acknowledging that pain will be incompletely relieved but secure in the knowledge that if the situation becomes intolerable to them, this option remains available. Other patients reaffirm comfort as the predominating consideration and request the initiation of sedation.

The published literature describing the use of sedation in the management of refractory pain at the end of life is anecdotal and refers to the use of opioids, neuroleptics, benzodiazepines, barbiturates, and propofol (Cherny and Portenoy 1994). In the absence of relative efficacy data, guidelines for drug selection are empirical. Irrespective of the agent or agents selected, administration initially requires dose titration to achieve adequate relief, followed subsequently by provision of ongoing therapy to ensure maintenance of effect.

Conclusion

The goal of analgesic therapy in the cancer population is to optimize analgesia with the minimum of side effects and inconvenience. Currently available techniques can provide adequate relief to a vast majority of patients. Most will require ongoing pain treatment, and analgesic requirements often change as the disease progresses. Patients with refractory pain, or unremitting suffering related to other losses or distressing symptoms, should have access to specialists in pain management or palliative medicine who can provide an approach capable of addressing these complex problems.

References

Abrams P, Fenely R 1976 The action of prostaglandins on smooth muscle of the human urinary tract in vitro. British Journal of Urology 47: 909–915

Ahmedzai S, Brooks D 1997 Transdermal fentanyl versus sustained-release oral morphine in cancer pain: preference, efficacy, and quality of life. The TTS-Fentanyl Comparative Trial Group Journal of Pain and Symptom Management 13: 254–261

Algan SM, Horowitz SM 1996 Surgical treatment of pathologic hip lesions in patients with metastatic disease. Clinical Orthopaedics 332: 223–231

American Medical Association 1996 Good care of the dying patient. Council on Scientific Affairs, American Medical Association. Journal of the American Medical Association 275: 474–478

Arathuzik D 1994 Effects of cognitive-behavioral strategies on pain in cancer patients. Cancer Nursing 17: 207–214

Ashby MA, Martin P, Jackson KA 1999 Opioid substitution to reduce adverse effects in cancer pain management. Medical Journal of Australia 170: 68–71

Avradopoulos KA, Vezeridis MP, Wanebo HJ 1996 Pelvic exenteration for recurrent rectal cancer. Advances in Surgery 29: 215–233

Babul N, Provencher L, Laberge F, Harsanyi Z, Moulin D 1998 Comparative efficacy and safety of controlled-release morphine suppositories and tablets in cancer pain. Journal of Clinical Pharmacology 38: 74–81

Baert L 1974 Controlled double-blind trail of flavoxate in painful conditions of the lower urinary tract. Current Medical Research and Opinion 2: 631–635

Baillie SP, Bateman DN, Coates PE, Woodhouse KW 1989 Age and the pharmacokinetics of morphine. Age and Ageing 18: 258–262

Baines MJ 1994 Management of intestinal obstruction in patients with advanced cancer. Annals, Academy of Medicine, Singapore 23: 178–182

Baines MJ 1997 ABC of palliative care. Nausea, vomiting, and intestinal obstruction. British Medical Journal 315: 1148–1150

Barbalias GA, Siablis D, Liatsikos EN, Karnabatidis D, Yarmenitis S, Bouropoulos K, Dimopoulos J 1997 Metal stents: a new treatment of malignant ureteral obstruction. Journal of Urology 158: 54–58

Barbanti G, Maggi CA, Beneforti P, Baroldi P, Turini D 1993 Relief of pain following intravesical capsaicin in patients with hypersensitive disorders of the lower urinary tract. British Journal of Urology 71: 686–691

Bates T 1992 A review of local radiotherapy in the treatment of bone metastases and cord compression. International Journal of Radiation Oncology–Biology–Physics 23: 217–221

Bennett WM, Henrich WL, Stoff JS 1996 The renal effects of nonsteroidal anti-inflammatory drugs: summary and recommendations. American Journal of Kidney Disease 28: S56–S62

Bentley JB, Borel JD, Nenad RE Jr, Gillespie TJ 1982 Age and fentanyl pharmacokinetics. Anesthesia and Analgesia 61: 968–971

Bjorkman R, Ullman A, Hedner J 1993 Morphine-sparing effect of diclofenac in cancer pain. European Journal of Clinical Pharmacology 44: 1–5

Blanchard J, Menk E, Ramamurthy S, Hoffman J 1990 Subarachnoid and epidural calcitonin in patients with pain due to metastatic cancer. Journal of Pain and Symptom Management 5: 42–45

Boquet J, Moore N, Lhuintre JP, Boismare F 1986 Diltiazem for proctalgia fugax [letter]. Lancet 1: 1493

Boraas MC 1985 Palliative surgery. Seminars in Oncology 12: 368–374

Braun A, Rohe K 1984 Orthopedic surgery for management of tumor pain. Recent Results in Cancer Research 89: 157–170

Brennan MJ, DePompolo RW, Garden FH 1996 Focused review: postmastectomy lymphedema. Archives of Physical Medicine and Rehabilitation 77: S74–S80

Brooks PM, Day RO 1991 Nonsteroidal antiinflammatory drugs—differences and similarities. New England Journal of Medicine 324: 1716–1725

Brooks PM, Day RO 2000 COX-2 inhibitors. Medical Journal of Australia 173: 433–436

Brose WG, Tanelian DL, Brodsky JB, Mark JB, Cousins MJ 1991 CSF and blood pharmacokinetics of hydromorphone and morphine following lumbar epidural administration. Pain 45: 11–15

Brosen K, Sindrup SH, Skjelbo E, Nielsen KK, Gram LF 1993 Role of genetic polymorphism in psychopharmacology—an update. Psychopharmacology Ser 10: 199–211

Browne B, Linter S 1987 Monoamine oxidase inhibitors and narcotic analgesics. A critical review of the implications for treatment. British Journal of Psychiatry 151: 210–212

Bruera E, Macmillan K, Hanson J, MacDonald RN 1989 The cognitive effects of the administration of narcotic analgesics in patients with cancer pain. Pain 39: 13–16

Bruera E, Franco JJ, Maltoni M, Watanabe S, Suarez-Almazor M 1995 Changing pattern of agitated impaired mental status in patients with advanced cancer: association with cognitive monitoring, hydration, and opioid rotation. Journal of Pain and Symptom Management 10: 287–291

Bruera E, Pereira J, Watanabe S, Belzile M, Kuehn N, Hanson J 1996 Opioid rotation in patients with cancer pain. A retrospective comparison of dose ratios between methadone, hydromorphone, and morphine. Cancer 78: 852–857

Burt RA 1997 The Supreme Court speaks—not assisted suicide but a constitutional right to palliative care. New England Journal of Medicine 337: 1234–1236

Calava JM, Patt RB, Reddy S, Varma DG, Chiang J 1996 Psoas sheath chemical neurolysis for management of intractable leg pain from metastatic liposarcoma. Clinical Journal of Pain 12: 69–75

Caraceni A, Portenoy RK 1996 Pain management in patients with pancreatic carcinoma. Cancer 78: 639–653

Cardiac Arrhythmia Suppression Trial (CAST) Investigators 1989 Preliminary report: effect of encainide and flecainide on mortality in a randomized trial of arrhythmia suppression after myocardial infarction. New England Journal of Medicine 321: 406–412

Castell DO 1985 Calcium-channel blocking agents for gastrointestinal disorders. American Journal of Cardiology 55: 210B–213B

Cherny NI, Portenoy RK 1994 Sedation in the management of refractory symptoms: guidelines for evaluation and treatment. Journal of Palliative Care 10: 31–38

Cherny NJ, Chang V, Frager G, Ingham JM, Tiseo PJ, Popp B, Portenoy RK, Foley KM 1995 Opioid pharmacotherapy in the management of cancer pain: a survey of strategies used by pain physicians for the selection of analgesic drugs and routes of administration. Cancer 76: 1283–1293

Chevrolet JC, Reverdin A, Suter PM, Tschopp JM, Junod AF 1983 Ventilatory dysfunction resulting from bilateral anterolateral high cervical cordotomy. Dual beneficial effect of aminophylline. Chest 84: 112–115

Cleary JF 1997 Pharmacokinetic and pharmacodynamic issues in the treatment of breakthrough pain. Seminars in Oncology 24 (Suppl 16): 13–19

Coia LR 1992 The role of radiation therapy in the treatment of brain metastases. International Journal of Radiation Oncology–Biology–Physics 23: 229–238

Cooper MG, Keneally JP, Kinchington D 1994 Continuous brachial plexus neural blockade in a child with intractable cancer pain. Journal of Pain and Symptom Management 9: 277–281

Cowie RA, Hitchcock ER 1982 The late results of antero-lateral cordotomy for pain relief. Acta Neurochirurgia (Wien) 1: 39–50

Coyle N, Portenoy RK 1991 Infection as a cause of rapidly increasing pain in cancer patients. Journal of Pain and Symptom Management 6: 266–269

Coyle N, Cherny NI, Portenoy RK 1994 Subcutaneous opioid infusions at home. Oncology (Huntingt) 8: 21–27; discussion 31–32, 37

Cramond T, Stuart G 1993 Intraventricular morphine for intractable pain of advanced cancer. Journal of Pain and Symptom Management 8: 465–473

Cruikshank DP, Buchsbaum HJ 1973 Effects of rapid paracentesis. Cardiovascular dynamics and body fluid composition. Journal of the American Medical Association 225: 1361–1362

De Conno F, Caraceni A, Zecca E, Spoldi E, Ventafridda V 1991 Continuous subcutaneous infusion of hyoscine butylbromide reduces secretions in patients with gastrointestinal obstruction. Journal of Pain and Symptom Management 6: 484–486

Dennis GC, DeWitty RL 1990 Long-term intraventricular infusion of morphine for intractable pain in cancer of the head and neck Neurosurgery 26: 404–407; discussion 407–408

de Stoutz ND, Bruera E, Suarez-Almazor M 1995 Opioid rotation for toxicity reduction in terminal cancer patients. Journal of Pain and Symptom Management 10: 378–384

Devor M, Govrin-Lippmann R, Raber P 1985 Corticosteroids suppress ectopic neural discharge originating in experimental neuromas. Pain 22: 127–137

Dionne C 1992 Tumour invasion of the brachial plexus: management of pain with intrapleural analgesia [letter]. Canadian Journal of Anaesthesia 39: 520–521

Dobrowsky W, Schmid AP 1985 Radiotherapy of presacral recurrence following radical surgery for rectal carcinoma. Diseases of Colon and Rectum 28: 917–919

Donner B, Zenz M, Tryba M, Strumpf M 1996 Direct conversion from oral morphine to transdermal fentanyl: a multicenter study in patients with cancer pain. Pain 64: 527–534

Drexel H, Dzien A, Spiegel RW, Lang AH, Breier C, Abbrederis K, Patsch JR, Braunsteiner H 1989 Treatment of severe cancer pain by low-dose continuous subcutaneous morphine. Pain 36: 169–176

Du Pen SL, Williams AR 1992 Management of patients receiving combined epidural morphine and bupivacaine for the treatment of cancer pain. Journal of Pain and Symptom Management 7: 125–127

Eckardt VF, Dodt O, Kanzler G, Bernhard G 1996 Treatment of proctalgia fugax with salbutamol inhalation. American Journal of Gastroenterology 91: 686–689

Eisenach JC, Du Pen S, Dubois M, Miguel R, Allin D 1995 Epidural clonidine analgesia for intractable cancer pain. The Epidural Clonidine Study Group. Pain 61: 391–399

Eisenberg E, Berkey CS, Carr DB, Mosteller F, Chalmers TC 1994 Efficacy and safety of nonsteroidal antiinflammatory drugs for cancer pain: a meta-analysis. Journal of Clinical Oncology 12: 2756–2765

Eisenberg E, Carr DB, Chalmers TC 1995 Neurolytic celiac plexus block for treatment of cancer pain: a meta-analysis. Anesthesia and Analgesia 80: 290–295 [Erratum 1995 Anesthesia and Analgesia 81: 213]

Ellershaw JE, Kelly MJ 1994 Corticosteroids and peptic ulceration. Palliative Medicine 8: 313–319

Eras J, Perazella MA 2001 NSAIDs and the kidney revisited: are selective cyclooxygenase-2 inhibitors safe? American Journal of the Medical Sciences 321: 181–190

Ernst DS, Brasher P, Hagen N, Paterson AH, MacDonald RN, Bruera E 1997 A randomized, controlled trial of intravenous clodronate in patients with metastatic bone disease and pain. Journal of Pain and Symptom Management 13: 319–326

Estes NC, Thomas JH, Jewell WR, Beggs D, Hardin CA 1993 Pelvic exenteration: a treatment for failed rectal cancer surgery. American Surgery 59: 420–422

European Association for Palliative Care 1996 Morphine in cancer pain: modes of administration. Expert Working Group of the European Association for Palliative Care. British Medical Journal 312: 823–826

Fallon M, O'Neill B 1997 ABC of palliative care. Constipation and diarrhoea. British Medical Journal 315: 1293–1296

Fallon MT, O'Neill B 1998 Substitution of another opioid for morphine. Opioid toxicity should be managed initially by decreasing the opioid dose [letter; comment]. British Medical Journal 317: 81

Fishman B 1992 The cognitive behavioral perspective on pain management in terminal illness. Hospital Journal 8: 73–88

Fitzgibbon DR, Ready LB 1997 Intravenous high-dose methadone administered by patient controlled analgesia and continuous infusion for the treatment of cancer pain refractory to high-dose morphine. Pain 73: 259–261

Fromm MF, Hofmann U, Griese EU, Mikus G 1995 Dihydrocodeine: a new opioid substrate for the polymorphic CYP2D6 in humans. Clinical Pharmacology and Therapeutics 58: 374–382

Galer BS, Coyle N, Pasternak GW, Portenoy RK 1992 Individual variability in the response to different opioids: report of five cases. Pain 49: 87–91

Galer BS, Harle J, Rowbotham MC 1996 Response to intravenous lidocaine infusion predicts subsequent response to oral mexiletine: a prospective study. Journal of Pain and Symptom Management 12: 161–167

Gestin Y, Vainio A, Pegurier AM 1997 Long-term intrathecal infusion of morphine in the home care of patients with advanced cancer. Acta Anaesthesiologica Scandinavica 41: 12–17

Goisis A, Gorini M, Ratti R, Luliri P 1989 Application of a WHO protocol on medical therapy for oncologic pain in an internal medicine hospital. Tumori 75: 470–472

Gokaslan ZL 1996 Spine surgery for cancer. Current Opinion in Oncology 8: 178–181

Gonski A, Sackelariou R 1984 Cryohypophysectomy for the relief of pain in malignant disease. Medical Journal of Australia 140: 140–142

Grond S, Zech D, Schug SA, Lynch J, Lehmann KA 1991 Validation of World Health Organization guidelines for cancer pain relief during the last days and hours of life. Journal of Pain and Symptom Management 6: 411–422

Hagen N, Swanson R 1997 Strychnine-like multifocal myoclonus and seizures in extremely high-dose opioid administration: treatment strategies [see comments]. Journal of Pain and Symptom Management 14: 51–58

Hagen NA, Foley KM, Cerbone DJ, Portenoy RK, Inturrisi CE 1991 Chronic nausea and morphine-6-glucuronide. Journal of Pain and Symptom Management 6: 125–128
Hagen NA, Elwood T, Ernst S 1997 Cancer pain emergencies: a protocol for management. Journal of Pain and Symptom Management 14: 45–50
Hanks GW 1984 Psychotropic drugs. Postgraduate Medical Journal 60: 881–885
Hanks GW 1987 The clinical usefulness of agonist–antagonistic opioid analgesics in chronic pain. Drug and Alcohol Dependence 20: 339–346
Hanks GW, Forbes K 1997 Opioid responsiveness. Acta Anaesthesiologica Scandinavica 41: 154–158
Harris JK, Sutcliffe JC, Robinson NE 1996 The role of emergency surgery in malignant spinal extradural compression: assessment of functional outcome. British Journal of Neurosurgery 10: 27–33
Hassenbusch SJ, Pillay PK, Barnett GH 1990 Radiofrequency cingulotomy for intractable cancer pain using stereotaxis guided by magnetic resonance imaging. Neurosurgery 27: 220–223
Hassenbusch SJ, Stanton-Hicks M, Covington EC, Walsh JG, Guthrey DS 1995 Long-term intraspinal infusions of opioids in the treatment of neuropathic pain. Journal of Pain and Symptom Management 10: 527–543
Hawkey CJ 1998 Progress in prophylaxis against nonsteroidal anti-inflammatory drug-associated ulcers and erosions. Omeprazole NSAID Steering Committee. American Journal of Medicine 104: 67S–74S; discussion 79S–80S
Hayakawa J, Kobayashi O, Murayama H 1997 Paraplegia after intraoperative celiac plexus block. Anesthesia and Analgesia 84: 447–448
Heiskanen T, Olkkola KT, Kalso E 1998 Effects of blocking CYP2D6 on the pharmacokinetics and pharmacodynamics of oxycodone. Clinical Pharmacology and Therapeutics 64: 603–611
Hogan Q, Haddox JD, Abram S, Weissman D, Taylor ML, Janjan N 1991 Epidural opiates and local anesthetics for the management of cancer pain. Pain 46: 271–279
Holdsworth MT, Forman WB, Killilea TA, Nystrom KM, Paul R, Brand SC, Reynolds R 1994 Transdermal fentanyl disposition in elderly subjects. Gerontology 40: 32–37
Hoskin PJ 1995 Radiotherapy for bone pain. Pain 63: 137–139
Houde RW, Wallenstein SL, Beaver WT 1966 Evaluation of analgesics in patients with cancer pain. In: Lasagna L (ed) International encyclopedia of pharmacology and therapeutics, vol 1. Pergamon Press, New York, pp 59–67
Ischia S, Luzzani A, Polati E 1990 Retrogasserian glycerol injection: a retrospective study of 112 patients. Clinical Journal of Pain 6: 291–296
Jadad AR, Browman GP 1995 The WHO analgesic ladder for cancer pain management. Stepping up the quality of its evaluation [see comments]. Journal of the American Medical Association 274: 1870–1873
Janjan NA 1997 Radiation for bone metastases: conventional techniques and the role of systemic radiopharmaceuticals. Cancer 80: 1628–1645
Jeal W, Benfield P 1997 Transdermal fentanyl. A review of its pharmacological properties and therapeutic efficacy in pain control. Drugs 53: 109–138
Johnson JR, Miller AJ 1994 The efficacy of choline magnesium trisalicylate (CMT) in the management of metastatic bone pain: a pilot study. Palliative Medicine 8: 129–135
Joishy SK, Walsh D 1998 The opioid-sparing effects of intravenous ketorolac as an adjuvant analgesic in cancer pain: application in bone metastases and the opioid bowel syndrome. Journal of Pain and Symptom Management 16: 334–339
Jong P, Sturgeon J, Jamieson CG 1995 Benefit of palliative surgery for bowel obstruction in advanced ovarian cancer. Canadian Journal of Surgery 38: 454–457
Kaiko RF, Fitzmartin RD, Thomas GB, Goldenheim PD 1992 The bioavailability of morphine in controlled-release 30-mg tablets per rectum compared with immediate-release 30-mg rectal suppositories and controlled-release 30-mg oral tablets. Pharmacotherapy 12: 107–113
Karavelis A, Foroglou G, Selviaridis P, Fountzilas G 1996 Intraventricular administration of morphine for control of intractable cancer pain in 90 patients. Neurosurgery 39: 57–61
Kawamata M, Ishitani K, Ishikawa K, Sasaki H, Ota K, Omote K, Namiki A 1996 Comparison between celiac plexus block and morphine treatment on quality of life in patients with pancreatic cancer pain. Pain 64: 597–602
Kirkwood LC, Nation RL, Somogyi AA 1997 Characterization of the human cytochrome P450 enzymes involved in the metabolism of dihydrocodeine. British Journal of Clinical Pharmacology 44: 549–555
Laine L 1996 Nonsteroidal anti-inflammatory drug gastropathy. Gastrointestinal and Endoscopy Clinics of North America 6: 489–504
Lamacraft G, Cousins MJ 1997 Neural blockade in chronic and cancer pain. International Anesthesiology Clinics 35: 131–153
Lanas A, Hirschowitz BI 1999 Toxicity of NSAIDs in the stomach and duodenum. European Journal of Gastroenterology and Hepatology 11: 375–381
Lancaster C 1995 Effective nonsteroidal anti-inflammatory drugs devoid of gastrointestinal side effects: do they really exist? Digestive Diseases 13 (Suppl 1): 40–47
Lawlor P, Turner K, Hanson J, Bruera E 1997 Dose ratio between morphine and hydromorphone in patients with cancer pain: a retrospective study. Pain 72: 79–85
Lazzeri M, Beneforti P, Benaim G, Maggi CA, Lecci A, Turini D 1996 Intravesical capsaicin for treatment of severe bladder pain: a randomized placebo controlled study. Journal of Urology 156: 947–952
Lehmann T, Day RO, Brooks PM 1997 Toxicity of antirheumatic drugs. Medical Journal of Australia 166: 378–383
Leibel SA, Pajak TF, Massullo V, Order SE, Komaki RU, Chang CH, Wasserman TH, Phillips TL, Lipshutz J, Durbin LM 1987 A comparison of misonidazole sensitized radiation therapy to radiation therapy alone for the palliation of hepatic metastases: results of a Radiation Therapy Oncology Group randomized prospective trial. International Journal of Radiation Oncology–Biology–Physics 13: 1057–1064
Lema MJ, Myers DP, De Leon-Casasola O, Penetrante R 1992 Pleural phenol therapy for the treatment of chronic esophageal cancer pain. Regional Anesthesia 17: 166–170
Levin AB, Ramirez LL 1984 Treatment of cancer pain with hypophysectomy: surgical and chemical. Advances in Pain Research and Therapy 7: 631–645
Lifshitz S, Buchsbaum HJ 1976 The effect of paracentesis on serum proteins. Gynecological Oncology 4: 347–353
Lillemoe KD, Cameron JL, Kaufman HS, Yeo CJ, Pitt HA, Sauter PK 1993 Chemical splanchnicectomy in patients with unresectable pancreatic cancer. A prospective randomized trial. Annals of Surgery 217: 447–455; discussion 456–457
Lipman AG 1996 Analgesic drugs for neuropathic and sympathetically maintained pain. Clinics in Geriatric Medicine 12: 501–515
Lyss AP 1997 Long-term use of oral transmucosal fentanyl citrate (OTFC) for breakthrough pain in cancer patients (meeting abstract). Proceedings Annual Meeting of the American Society of Clinical Oncologists
Maddocks I, Somogyi A, Abbott F, Hayball P, Parker D 1996 Attenuation of morphine-induced delirium in palliative care by

substitution with infusion of oxycodone. Journal of Pain and Symptom Management 12: 182–189
Mainar A, Tejero E, Maynar M, Ferral H, Castaneda-Zuniga W 1996 Colorectal obstruction: treatment with metallic stents. Radiology 198: 761–764
Makin AJ, Williams R 1997 Acetaminophen-induced hepatotoxicity: predisposing factors and treatments. Advances in Internal Medicine 42: 453–483
Makin MK, Ellershaw JE 1998 Substitution of another opioid for morphine. Methadone can be used to manage neuropathic pain related to cancer [letter; comment]. British Medical Journal 317: 81
Maloney CM, Kesner RK, Klein G, Bockenstette J 1989 The rectal administration of MS Contin: clinical implications of use in end stage cancer. American Journal of Hospital Care 6: 34–35
Marcks P 1997 Lymphedema. Pathogenesis, prevention, and treatment. Cancer Practice 5: 32–38
Masferrer JL, Isakson PC, Seibert K 1996 Cyclooxygenase-2 inhibitors: a new class of anti-inflammatory agents that spare the gastrointestinal tract. Gastroenterology Clinics of North America 25: 363–372
McDonald P, Graham P, Clayton M, Buhagiar A, Stuart-Harris R 1991 Regular subcutaneous bolus morphine via an indwelling cannula for pain from advanced cancer. Palliative Medicine 5: 323–329
McKenna F 1998 Diclofenac/misoprostol: the European clinical experience. Journal of Rheumatology 51 (Suppl): 21–30
McQuay H, Carroll D, Jadad AR, Wiffen P, Moore A 1995 Anticonvulsant drugs for management of pain: a systematic review. British Medical Journal 311: 1047–1052
McQuay HJ, Tramer M, Nye BA, Carroll D, Wiffen PJ, Moore RA 1996 A systematic review of antidepressants in neuropathic pain. Pain 68: 217–227
Mercadante S 1993 Celiac plexus block versus analgesics in pancreatic cancer pain. Pain 52: 187–192
Mercadante S 1994a Intrathecal morphine and bupivacaine in advanced cancer pain patients implanted at home. Journal of Pain and Symptom Management 9: 201–207
Mercadante S 1994b The role of octreotide in palliative care. Journal of Pain and Symptom Management 9: 406–411
Meyer-Witting M, Foster JM 1992 Suprascapular nerve block in the management of cancer pain. Anaesthesia 47: 626
Minotti V, De Angelis V, Righetti E, Celani MG, Rossetti R, Lupatelli M, Tonato M, Pisati R, Monza G, Fumi G, Del Favero A 1998 Double-blind evaluation of short-term analgesic efficacy of orally administered diclofenac, diclofenac plus codeine, and diclofenac plus imipramine in chronic cancer pain. Pain 74: 133–137
Myers DP, Lema MJ, de Leon-Casasola OA, Bacon DR 1993 Interpleural analgesia for the treatment of severe cancer pain in terminally ill patients. Journal of Pain and Symptom Management 8: 505–510
Nebab EG, Florence IM 1997 An alternative needle geometry for interruption of the ganglion impar [letter]. Anesthesiology 86: 1213–1214
Neill RS 1979 Ablation of the brachial plexus. Control of intractable pain, due to a pathological fracture of the humerus. Anaesthesia 34: 1024–1027
Nitescu P, Appelgren L, Linder LE, Sjoberg M, Hultman E, Curelaru I 1990 Epidural versus intrathecal morphine-bupivacaine: assessment of consecutive treatments in advanced cancer pain. Journal of Pain and Symptom Management 5: 18–26
Nitescu P, Sjoberg M, Appelgren L, Curelaru I 19995 Complications of intrathecal opioids and bupivacaine in the treatment of 'refractory' cancer pain. Clinical Journal of Pain 11: 45–62
Osborne RJ, Joel SP, Slevin ML 1986 Morphine intoxication in renal failure: the role of morphine-6-glucuronide. British Medical Journal (Clin Res Ed) 292: 1548–1549
Osborne R, Joel S, Grebenik K, Trew D, Slevin M 1993 The pharmacokinetics of morphine and morphine glucuronides in kidney failure [see comments]. Clinical Pharmacology and Therapeutics 54: 158–167
Paice JA 1988 The phenomenon of analgesic tolerance in cancer pain management. Oncology Nursing Forum 15: 455–460
Paix A, Coleman A, Lees J, Grigson J, Brooksbank M, Thorne D, Ashby M 1995 Subcutaneous fentanyl and sufentanil infusion substitution for morphine intolerance in cancer pain management. Pain 63: 263–269
Parker MC, Baines MJ 1996 Intestinal obstruction in patients with advanced malignant disease. British Journal of Surgery 83: 1–2
Pasternak GW, Standifer KM 1995 Mapping of opioid receptors using antisense oligodeoxynucleotides: correlating their molecular biology and pharmacology [see comments]. Trends in Pharmacologic Sciences 16: 344–350
Patt RB, Reddy S 1994 Spinal neurolysis for cancer pain: indications and recent results. Annals, Academy of Medicine, Singapore 23: 216–220
Patt RB, Proper G, Reddy S 1994 The neuroleptics as adjuvant analgesics. Journal of Pain and Symptom Management 9: 446–453
Patt YZ, Peters RE, Chuang VP, Wallace S, Claghorn L, Mavligit G 1985 Palliation of pelvic recurrence of colorectal cancer with intra-arterial 5-fluorouracil and mitomycin. Cancer 56: 2175–2180
Paulson DF 1978 Oxybutynin chloride in control of post-transurethral vesical pain and spasm. Urology 11: 237–238
Payne R, Mathias SD, Pasta DJ, Wanke LA, Williams R, Mahmoud R 1998 Quality of life and cancer pain: satisfaction and side effects with transdermal fentanyl versus oral morphine. Journal of Clinical Oncology 16: 1588–1593
Penn RD, Paice JA, Kroin JS 1992 Octreotide: a potent new non-opiate analgesic for intrathecal infusion [see comments]. Pain 49: 13–19
Perazella MA, Eras J 2000 Are selective COX-2 inhibitors nephrotoxic? American Journal of Kidney Disease 35: 937–940
Pies R 1996 Psychotropic medications and the oncology patient. Cancer Practice 4: 164–166
Plancarte R, Amescua C, Patt RB, Aldrete JA 1990 Superior hypogastric plexus block for pelvic cancer pain. Anesthesiology 73: 236–239
Plancarte R, Velazquez R, Patt RB 1993 Neurolytic block of the sympathetic axis. In: Patt RB (ed) Cancer pain. Lippincott, Philadelphia, pp 377–425
Plancarte R, de Leon-Casasola OA, El-Helaly M, Allende S, Lema MJ 1997 Neurolytic superior hypogastric plexus block for chronic pelvic pain associated with cancer. Regional Anesthesia 22: 562–568
Plosker GL, Lamb HM 1999 Diclofenac/misoprostol. Pharmacoeconomic implications of therapy. Pharmacoeconomics 16: 85–98
Polatty RC, Cooper KR 1986 Respiratory failure after percutaneous cordotomy. Southern Medical Journal 79: 897–899
Portenoy RK 1994 Management of common opioid side effects during long-term therapy of cancer pain. Annals, Academy of Medicine, Singapore 23: 160–170
Portenoy RK 1996 Adjuvant analgesic agents. Hematology/Oncology Clinics of North America 10: 103–119
Portenoy RK, Foley KM, Inturrisi CE 1990 The nature of opioid responsiveness and its implications for neuropathic pain: new hypotheses derived from studies of opioid infusions [see comments]. Pain 43: 273–286
Porter AT, McEwan AJ, Powe JE, Reid R, McGowan DG, Lukka H, Sathyanarayana JR, Yakemchuk VN, Thomas GM, Erlich LE et al 1993 Results of a randomized phase-III trial to evaluate the efficacy of strontium-89 adjuvant to local field external beam

irradiation in the management of endocrine resistant metastatic prostate cancer. International Journal of Radiation Oncology–Biology–Physics 25: 805–813
Poulsen L, Brosen K, Arendt-Nielsen L, Gram LF, Elbaek K, Sindrup SH 1996 Codeine and morphine in extensive and poor metabolizers of sparteine: pharmacokinetics, analgesic effect and side effects. European Journal of Clinical Pharmacology 51: 289–295
Prasanna A, Murthy PS 1993 Sphenopalatine ganglion block and pain of cancer [letter]. Journal of Pain and Symptom Management 8: 125
President's Commission for the Study of Ethical Problems in Medical and Biomedical and Behavioral Research 1983 Deciding to forgo life sustaining treatment: ethical and legal issues in treatment decisions. US Government Printing Office, Washington, DC
Queisser W 1984 Chemotherapy for the treatment of cancer pain. Recent Results in Cancer Research 89: 171–177
Rapin CH 1989 The treatment of pain in the elderly patient. The use of oral morphine in the treatment of pain. Journal of Palliative Care 5: 54–55
Raskin JB 1999 Gastrointestinal effects of nonsteroidal anti-inflammatory therapy. American Journal of Medicine 106: 3S–12S
Ripamonti C, Bruera E 1997 Current status of patient-controlled analgesia in cancer patients. Oncology (Huntingt) 11: 373–380, 383–384; discussion 384–386
Ripamonti C, Groff L, Brunelli C, Polastri D, Stavrakis A, De Conno F 1998 Switching from morphine to oral methadone in treating cancer pain: what is the equianalgesic dose ratio? [see comments] Journal of Clinical Oncology 16: 3216–3221
Rizzi R, Terrevoli A, Visentin M 1985 Long-term results of alcoholization and thermocoagulation of trigeminal nerve for cancer pain. The Pain Clinic I. In: Erdmann W, Oyama T, Pernak MJ (eds) Proceedings of the first international symposium. Vnu Science Press, Utrecht, The Netherlands
Robertson DH 1983 Transsacral neurolytic nerve block. An alternative approach to intractable perineal pain. British Journal of Anaesthesia 55: 873–875
Robinson RG, Preston DF, Schiefelbein M, Baxter KG 1995 Strontium 89 therapy for the palliation of pain due to osseous metastases. Journal of the American Medical Association 274: 420–424
Ross GJ, Kessler HB, Clair MR, Gatenby RA, Hartz WH, Ross LV 1989 Sonographically guided paracentesis for palliation of symptomatic malignant ascites. American Journal of Roentgenology 153: 1309–1311
Rossi GC, Leventhal L, Pan YX, Cole J, Su W, Bodnar RJ, Pasternak GW 1997 Antisense mapping of MOR-1 in rats: distinguishing between morphine and morphine-6beta-glucuronide antinociception. Journal of Pharmacology and Experimental Therapeutics 281: 109–114
Rothenberg ML 1996 New developments in chemotherapy for patients with advanced pancreatic cancer. Oncology (Huntingt) 10: 18–22
Rubens RD, Towlson KE, Ramirez AJ, Coltart S, Slevin ML, Terrell C, Timothy AR 1992 Appropriate chemotherapy for palliating advanced cancer. British Medical Journal 304: 35–40
Ruskin JN 1989 The cardiac arrhythmia suppression trial (CAST). New England Journal of Medicine 321: 386–388
Salmon JB, Finch PM, Lovegrove FT, Warwick A 1992 Mapping the spread of epidural phenol in cancer pain patients by radionuclide admixture and epidural scintigraphy. Clinical Journal of Pain 8: 18–22
Sanders M, Zuurmond W 1995 Safety of unilateral and bilateral percutaneous cervical cordotomy in 80 terminally ill cancer patients. Journal of Clinical Oncology 13: 1509–1512
Saris SC, Silver JM, Vieira JF, Nashold BS Jr 1986 Sacrococcygeal rhizotomy for perineal pain. Neurosurgery 19: 789–793
Schmeler K, Bastin K 1996 Strontium-89 for symptomatic metastatic prostate cancer to bone: recommendations for hospice patients. Hospital Journal 11: 1–10
Schug SA, Zech D, Dorr U 1990 Cancer pain management according to WHO analgesic guidelines. Journal of Pain and Symptom Management 5: 27–32
Schug SA, Zech D, Grond S, Jung H, Meuser T, Stobbe B 1992 A long-term survey of morphine in cancer pain patients. Journal of Pain and Symptom Management 7: 259–266
Sevarino FB, Sinatra RS, Paige D, Ning T, Brull SJ, Silverman DG 1992 The efficacy of intramuscular ketorolac in combination with intravenous PCA morphine for postoperative pain relief. Journal of Clinical Anesthesia 4: 285–288
Simmonds MA 1997 Oral transmucosal fentanyl citrate produces pain relief faster than medication typically used for breakthrough pain in cancer patients (Meeting abstract). Proceedings, Annual Meeting of the American Society of Clinical Oncologists 16: A180
Sindrup SH, Brosen K 1995 The pharmacogenetics of codeine hypoalgesia. Pharmacogenetics 5: 335–346
Sindrup SH, Poulsen L, Brosen K, Arendt-Nielsen L, Gram LF 1993 Are poor metabolisers of sparteine/debrisoquine less pain tolerant than extensive metabolisers? Pain 53: 335–339
Sjoberg M, Nitescu P, Appelgren L, Curelaru I 1994 Long-term intrathecal morphine and bupivacaine in patients with refractory cancer pain. Results from a morphine:bupivacaine dose regimen of 0.5:4.75 mg/ml. Anesthesiology 80: 284–297
Sjogren P, Dragsted L, Christensen CB 1993 Myoclonic spasms during treatment with high doses of intravenous morphine in renal failure. Acta Anaesthesiologica Scandinavica 37: 780–782
Sneed PK, Larson DA, Wara WM 1996 Radiotherapy for cerebral metastases. Neurosurgery Clinics of North America 7: 505–515
Sorensen S, Helweg-Larsen S, Mouridsen H, Hansen HH 1994 Effect of high-dose dexamethasone in carcinomatous metastatic spinal cord compression treated with radiotherapy: a randomised trial. European Journal of Cancer 30A: 22–27
Spiegel D, Moore R 1997 Imagery and hypnosis in the treatment of cancer patients. Oncology (Huntingt) 11: 1179–1189; discussion 1189–1195
Strang P 1996 Analgesic effect of bisphosphonates on bone pain in breast cancer patients: a review article. Acta Oncologica 5: 50–54
Stuart G, Cramond T 1993 Role of percutaneous cervical cordotomy for pain of malignant origin. Medical Journal of Australia 158: 667–670
Sucher E, Margulies JY, Floman Y, Robin GC 1994 Prognostic factors in anterior decompression for metastatic cord compression. An analysis of results. European Spine Journal 3: 70–75
Swain R 1987 Oral clonidine for proctalgia fugax. Gut 28: 1039–1040
Sykes J, Johnson R, Hanks GW 1997 ABC of palliative care. Difficult pain problems. British Medical Journal 315: 867–869
Symreng T, Gomez MN, Rossi N 1989 Intrapleural bupivacaine v saline after thoracotomy—effects on pain and lung function—a double-blind study [see comments]. Journal of Cardiothoracic Anesthesia 3: 144–149
Taha AS, Hudson N, Hawkey CJ, Swannell AJ, Trye PN, Cottrell J, Mann SG, Simon TJ, Sturrock RD, Russell RI 1996 Famotidine for the prevention of gastric and duodenal ulcers caused by nonsteroidal antiinflammatory drugs [see comments]. New England Journal of Medicine 334: 1435–1439
Takeda F 1985 Japanese field-testing of WHO guidelines. PRN Forum 4: 4–5
Tarn TS, Lee TS 1994 Surgical treatment of metastatic tumors of the long bones, Chung Hua I Hsueh Tsa Chih (Taipei) 54: 170–175
Thatcher N, Anderson H, Betticher DC, Ranson M 1995

Symptomatic benefit from gemcitabine and other chemotherapy in advanced non-small cell lung cancer: changes in performance status and tumour-related symptoms. Anticancer Drugs 6 (Suppl 6): 39–48

Thomas Z, Bruera E 1995 Use of methadone in a highly tolerant patient receiving parenteral hydromorphone. Journal of Pain and Symptom Management 10: 315–317

Tiseo PJ, Thaler HT, Lapin J, Inturrisi CE, Portenoy RK, Foley KM 1995 Morphine-6-glucuronide concentrations and opioid-related side effects: a survey in cancer patients. Pain 61: 47–54

Turk DC, Feldman CS 1992 Noninvasive approaches to pain control in terminal illness: the contribution of psychological variables. Hospital Journal 8: 1–23

Twycross R 1994 The risks and benefits of corticosteroids in advanced cancer. Drug Safety 11: 163–178

Vainio A, Ollila J, Matikainen E, Rosenberg P, Kalso E 1995 Driving ability in cancer patients receiving long-term morphine analgesia. Lancet 346: 667–670

Valentini M, Cannizzaro R, Poletti M, Bortolussi R, Fracasso A, Testa V, Sozzi M, Fornasarig M, Bortoluzzi F, Grazioli I 1995 Nonsteroidal antiinflammatory drugs for cancer pain: comparison between misoprostol and ranitidine in prevention of upper gastrointestinal damage. Journal of Clinical Oncology 13: 2637–2642

Vane JR, Bakhle YS, Botting RM 1998 Cyclooxygenases 1 and 2. Annual Review of Pharmacology and Toxicology 38: 97–120

Varvel JR, Shafer SL, Hwang SS, Coen PA, Stanski DR 1989 Absorption characteristics of transdermally administered fentanyl. Anesthesiology 70: 928–934

Ventafridda V, Tamburini M, Caraceni A, De Conno F, Naldi F 1987 A validation study of the WHO method for cancer pain relief. Cancer 59: 850–856

Ventafridda V, Ripamonti C, Caraceni A, Spoldi E, Messina L, De Conno F 1990 The management of inoperable gastrointestinal obstruction in terminal cancer patients. Tumori 76: 389–393

Vermeulen SS 1998 Whole brain radiotherapy in the treatment of metastatic brain tumors. Seminars in Surgical Oncology 14: 64–69

Vigano A, Fan D, Bruera E 1996 Individualized use of methadone and opioid rotation in the comprehensive management of cancer pain associated with poor prognostic indicators. Pain 67: 115–119

Walker VA, Hoskin PJ, Hanks GW, White ID 1988 Evaluation of WHO analgesic guidelines for cancer pain in a hospital-based palliative care unit. Journal of Pain and Symptom Management 3: 145–149

Watanabe S, Bruera E 1994 Corticosteroids as adjuvant analgesics. Journal of Pain and Symptom Management 9: 442–445

Watson DJ, Harper SE, Zhao PL, Quan H, Bolognese JA, Simon TJ 2000 Gastrointestinal tolerability of the selective cyclooxygenase-2 (COX-2) inhibitor rofecoxib compared with nonselective COX-1 and COX-2 inhibitors in osteoarthritis. Archives of Internal Medicine 160: 2998–3003

Wells CJ, Lipton S, Lahuerta J 1984 Respiratory depression after percutaneous cervical anterolateral cordotomy in patients on slow-release oral morphine [letter]. Lancet 1: 739

Wemm K Jr, Saberski L 1995 Modified approach to block the ganglion impar (ganglion of Walther) [letter]. Regional Anesthesia 20: 544–545

Wolfe MM, Lichtenstein DR, Singh G 1999 Gastrointestinal toxicity of nonsteroidal antiinflammatory drugs. New England Journal of Medicine 340: 1888–1899

Wong ET, Gunes S, Gaughan E, Patt RB, Ginsberg LE, Hassenbusch SJ, Payne R 1997 Palliation of intractable cancer pain by MRI-guided cingulotomy. Clinical Journal of Pain 13: 260–263

Wong GY, Brown DL 1995 Transient paraplegia following alcohol celiac plexus block. Regional Anesthesia 20: 352–355

World Health Organization 1986 Cancer pain relief. World Health Organization, Geneva

World Health Organization 1996 Cancer pain relief, 2nd edn. World Health Organization, Geneva

Yaksh TL 1996 Epidural ketamine: a useful, mechanistically novel adjuvant for epidural morphine? Regional Anesthesia 21: 508–513

Yang CY, Wong CS, Chang JY, Ho ST 1996 Intrathecal ketamine reduces morphine requirements in patients with terminal cancer pain. Canadian Journal of Anaesthesia 43: 379–383

Zadina JE, Kastin AJ, Harrison LM, Ge LJ, Chang SL 1995 Opiate receptor changes after chronic exposure to agonists and antagonists. Annals of the New York Academy of Science 757: 353–361

Zech DF, Grond S, Lynch J, Hertel D, Lehmann KA 1995 Validation of World Health Organization Guidelines for cancer pain relief: a 10-year prospective study. Pain 63: 65–76

Chapter 44

Cancer pain and palliative care in children

Charles B Berde and John J Collins

Introduction

In this chapter, we outline approaches to pain and symptom management, supportive care, and palliative care for children with life-threatening illnesses. Much of the literature on palliative care in adults and children concerns cancer, and we will focus in large measure on cancer in this chapter, but will also address a range of other life-threatening conditions, including neurodegenerative disorders, AIDS, and more rapidly progressive cases of cystic fibrosis. Each of the latter conditions differs from cancer in its natural history, clinical course, patterns of symptoms, and prognosis; these differences are important to individualized approaches to palliative care.

Curative, supportive, and palliative care should be regarded as a continuum. Aspects of a supportive care approach should be incorporated in the care of all children with life-threatening illnesses, even while curative or life-prolonging therapies continue. While pain is a prominent symptom in many cases, it should be emphasized that palliative care efforts must address the full spectrum of non-painful symptoms as well as the emotional and spiritual suffering of patients at the end of life. A survey of parents' impressions following the death of their child with cancer reinforces the need to improve efforts to address these broader issues (Wolfe et al 2000).

Cancer in children: epidemiology and prognosis

The treatment of childhood cancer has seen much more dramatic improvements in survival than most adult cancers. Over 60% of children diagnosed with malignancy in developed countries, who have access to state-of-the-art treatment, will have long-term disease-free survival. Acute lymphoblastic leukaemia, the most common childhood cancer, was uniformly fatal in the early 1950s; now disease-free long-term survival rates exceed 70%. Prognosis is less optimistic with some of the primary CNS neoplasms, although recent advances have improved survival.

Compared with adults, multimodal treatment with chemotherapy, radiation therapy, and surgery is performed more commonly with curative intent. Cancer therapy in children can be arduous, requiring a year or longer of repetitive cycles of chemotherapy, frequent diagnostic and therapeutic procedures, with associated medical complications, pain, nausea, and other symptoms.

Many children with widely advanced cancer participate in experimental protocols of chemotherapeutic agents and other novel treatment approaches. They and their families are often willing to undertake treatments with low a priori probability of cure.

The gains in survival in childhood cancer are not shared worldwide. Many developing countries lack the resources to provide the medications, blood products, radiation therapy, surgical expertise, and intensive medical support required to deliver curative therapy. It was with recognition of these economic realities that the WHO Cancer Unit emphasized straightforward, cost-effective, non-technologic methods of palliative care. Regulatory barriers continue to limit access to effective analgesics (Joranson and Gilson 1998).

Pain and distress at the time of initial diagnosis of cancer

At initial diagnosis, many children report tumour-related pain (Miser et al 1987a), commonly involving bone, viscera, soft tissues, and nerves. Bone pain may be due to periosteal stretch, as with bone sarcomas. Leukaemias and other malignancies that proliferate in the bone marrow can cause pain due to filling and compression of bone marrow spaces. Leukaemias, lymphomas, and neuroblastomas proliferate in abdominal viscera, especially in liver and spleen, and cause pain due to capsular stretch. Headache is common among children presenting with brain tumours, although others present first with neurologic deficits. The majority of children with spinal cord tumours have back or neck pain at diagnosis (Hahn and McLone 1984). Metastatic spinal cord compression is unusual at diagnosis and is more likely to occur later in the child's illness (Lewis et al 1986). Back pain, as a sign of spinal cord compression in children, usually occurs before abnormal neurological signs or symptoms (Lewis et al 1986).

Analgesics are often required for short periods of time following initial diagnosis. Initiation of cancer therapy brings relief of pain in the majority of cases, typically within 2 weeks. Resolution of bone marrow and visceral pain is particularly rapid for haematologic malignancies, and somewhat slower for children with solid tumours. Headache from brain tumours may improve with cortico-steroid therapy, or with relief of increased intra-cranial pressure, either from surgical resection or from shunting of cerebrospinal fluid.

Children and their families are 'shell-shocked' at the time of diagnosis, and experience fear, anxiety, anger, denial, and panic. Explanations should be simple, forthright, and calmly stated. Patients and parents may not process or remember instructions or descriptions.

Psychological support should be provided and individualized with consideration of the child's development and coping style, and the family's cultural and spiritual values. For many children and families, support by clergy provides great comfort. A range of interventions for emotional and spiritual support should be available. Many children express their fears and emotions through play, art, or music. Child life programmes have taken a lead in advocating for the emotional support of children and families facing illness (Brazelton and Thompson 1988, Anonymous 1993, Ruffin et al 1997) (Table 44.1).

Pain due to cancer treatment

As the treatment progresses, treatment-related rather than tumour-related causes of pain predominate (Miser et al 1987a, b). These include post-operative and procedure-related pain, mucositis, phantom limb pain, infection, and pain due to chemotherapy.

Table 44.1 Reasons to view palliative care as a continuum rather than an abrupt transition of care

1. Patients at all stages of care, not just end-of-life, benefit from psychosocial support and broad-based symptom management. Kindness should not be restricted only to the dying patient.
2. Issues of quality of life and goals of care should be raised at all stages of treatment, not just when treatments appear futile.
3. Prediction of longevity is a very inexact science.
4. Patients, parents, and health providers often differ among themselves in their views of chances of cure and futility.
5. A child who is terrorized and isolated during the initial phase of curative treatment will more likely feel fearful and isolated during late-stage care. In many cases, inadequate treatment of symptoms and inadequate support during treatment has led to adolescents refusing further treatment with a high likelihood of cure.
6. Conversely, if the child feels safe and cared-for during curative treatment, they may better face subsequent curative treatments, as well as coping better during end-of-life care.
7. An abrupt shift in the goals of care and therapeutic approach may make the patient and family feel abandoned. Physicians, nurses, psychologists, and child life specialists who have cared for the child during their long illness have formed a unique connection to the child that can continue in palliative care.

Painful diagnostic and therapeutic procedures

Needle procedures are a major source of distress for children with cancer (Zeltzer et al 1989). Common procedures include venipuncture, venous cannulation, lumbar puncture, bone marrow aspirate and biopsy, and removal of central venous lines. Radiation therapy is not painful per se, but often requires sedation or general anaesthesia to facilitate cooperation and immobility.

It is crucial to treat the pain and distress of the initial diagnostic procedures very effectively. Children need adequate preparation before needle procedures to minimize their fear and anxiety. This preparation includes involving the child's parents, to obtain an insight into their child's coping style, to explain to them the nature of the procedure, and to enlist their support. An age-appropriate explanation to the child should follow with consideration of a particular child's previous experience and coping style (Zeltzer et al 1989).

Effective initial treatment will set a pattern of trust and confidence for patients and families. Conversely, if a first bone marrow aspirate or lumbar puncture is a horrific experience, there will be a carry-over effect of persistent fear and distress over future procedures. A follow-up study of children in a clinical trial supports this belief. A randomized controlled trial compared a method of rapid opioid delivery, oral transmucosal fentanyl citrate (OTFC), versus placebo for the pain of lumbar puncture and bone marrow aspirate (Schechter et al 1995). (Regulatory agencies insisted on a placebo group, despite objections of some of the investigators.) Investigators were permitted to give OTFC unblinded to all patients for subsequent procedures. The group who had received the active agent for the first procedure showed less distress and pain for the group of subsequent procedures, implying a persistent carry-over effect of inadequately treated pain (Weisman et al 1998).

Management of painful and distressing procedures is best done by a combination of non-pharmacologic and pharmacologic approaches individualized to the particular child's developmental level, coping style, medical and psychological condition, and type of procedure (Berde 1995). Some aspects of the non-pharmacologic approach are common-sense, as outlined in Table 44.2.

In addition to these common-sense measures, there are a number of specific psychological techniques for managing pain and distress of procedures, including hypnosis, relaxation training, and guided imagery (Kuttner 1989, Steggles et al 1997). Other cognitive-behavioural interventions include preparatory information, positive coping statements, modelling, and/or behavioural rehearsal. There are many variations of these methods, and the optimal techniques depend on the experience of the practitioners and the developmental level and personal style of the child. Training programmes are provided by many organizations; the Society for Behavioral Pediatrics has taken a lead in this regard in North America.

Evidence supports the efficacy of psychological techniques for managing painful procedures in children with cancer (Jay et al 1987, 1995). In our opinion, these should be taught to children with cancer whenever possible. They have several advantages. They are exceedingly safe, and the child can develop a sense of mastery and confidence that can be generalized to new situations. Conversely, hypnosis should not be used as an excuse for withholding adequate analgesics for moderate to severe pain. Some children may be too traumatized to use these techniques, or may have developmental or cognitive limitations that prevent their use.

Cutaneous analgesia can be provided by several local anaesthetic formulations and delivery systems, including a eutectic mixture of the local anaesthetics lidocaine (lignocaine) and prilocaine (EMLA), tetracaine gel (amethocaine), and lidocaine iontophoresis. EMLA (Maunuksela and Korpela 1986, Halperin et al 1989) is available either as a

Table 44.2 Common-sense, but frequently forgotten, aspects of paediatric procedures

1. Minimize unnecessary procedures, especially repeated venipuncture.
2. Use age-appropriate explanations.
3. Involve the parents to support the child and be allies, not to assist or restrain the child.
4. In most cases, use a treatment room rather than the patient's room, so that their own room remains a 'safe' place.
5. Skilled and expeditious, but not rushed, performance shortens the period of distress. Get all supplies and equipment prepared beforehand, so that the procedure goes as quickly as possible.
6. Assign practitioners' pagers ('beepers') to other clinicians during the procedure whenever feasible, to minimize interruptions.
7. Where feasible, trainees should learn first by watching, by *in vitro* models, and in some cases by supervised performance of procedures on anaesthetized patients.

patch or as a cream, which is applied under an occlusive dressing. While the standard recommendation is to apply EMLA for 60 min, the depth and reliability of analgesia increases with longer application times, e.g., 90–120 min (Bjerring and Arendt-Nielsen 1993). EMLA has proven safe, with low plasma local anaesthetic concentrations, and a negligible risk of methaemoglobinaemia. Tetracaine gel (amethocaine, Ametop) appears similarly effective as EMLA, and may have more rapid onset (Doyle et al 1993). Tetracaine gel is commercially available in much of Europe and Canada, but not in the United States at present. Topical cooling using ice or fluorocarbon coolant sprays has been used with some success (Abbott and Fowler-Kerry 1995). Both skin cooling and EMLA may produce vasoconstriction, which may make venous cannulation more difficult. Iontophoresis employs electric current to accelerate drug penetration through skin. A formulation of lidocaine (lignocaine) is marketed as 'Numby-Stuff'. Iontophoresis can produce skin analgesia rapidly and with good depth of penetration (Zeltzer et al 1991).

Topical local anaesthetics are useful, and should be widely available, but they are not a panacea. For a child who has experienced repeated distressing procedures, they will likely remain anxious despite use of EMLA, because of their fear and lack of trust.

Local anesthetic infiltration can reduce pain from deeper needle procedures. Prior use of topical anaesthesia can reduce the discomfort of the infiltrating needle. Neutralizing the commercially supplied acidic local anaesthetic solutions immediately prior to use with sodium bicarbonate, in the following ratios, can also reduce the pain of infiltration: sodium bicarbonate (8.4% w/v) 1 part to either lidocaine (lignocaine; 1%) 9 parts or bupivacaine (0.25%) 25 parts, respectively (Peterfreund et al 1989).

'Conscious' sedation and general anaesthesia (Table 44.3)

For painful or extensive procedures, or for children who have limited ability to cope or cooperate, conscious sedation or general anaesthesia should both be readily available. Conscious sedation refers to administration of anxiolytics and analgesics to render the child sedated and comfortable, but able to respond to stimuli and able to maintain airway reflexes and ventilation. For both conscious sedation and general anaesthesia, safe practice necessitates administration by practitioners with expertise in airway management and with knowledge of the relevant pharmacology and medical issues. Protocols for monitoring and drug dosing can help reduce risk. Monitoring with oximetry is widely recommended.

Pure sedatives, such as pentobarbital, chloral hydrate, and midazolam are widely used for painless procedures such as radiation therapy that require immobility. Where procedures involve significant pain that cannot be relieved by local anaesthesia, such as a bone marrow aspirate, we generally prefer combining a sedative-anxiolytic, such as midazolam (Sievers et al 1991), with an analgesic, either an opioid or ketamine. The combination of midazolam with either fentanyl or low-dose ketamine is generally safe and effective (Marx et al 1997, Parker et al 1997). The intravenous route is useful because of rapid onset, complete bioavailability, and the ability to titrate incremental doses to effect.

Ketamine has received widespread use because it produces analgesia, dissociation, and stable respiration in most children. While ketamine is

Table 44.3 Recommendations for conscious sedation in children

1. Establish protocols, education programmes, and an assessment programme to track efficacy and complications. Efficacy should be judged by patients as well as practitioners.
2. Standardize the choice of drugs and doses for the majority of procedures, so that practitioners are comfortable with a consistent approach.
3. Reduce doses in patients with risk factors for hypoventilation.
4. Observe fasting guidelines for solids and clear liquids to reduce the risk of aspiration.
5. Employ an observer whose only job is to assess level of consciousness and adequacy of respiration.
6. Use pulse oximetry to assess oxygenation.
7. Keep available an oxygen delivery source, suction, a bag and mask, and an airway management cart with a proper range of equipment.
8. Keep available reversal agents, especially naloxone and flumazenil.
9. Recognize that conscious sedation is a continuum, and in some patients, standard doses may produce deep sedation.
10. Recognize that conscious sedation does not permit complete lack of responses to events; it is not general anaesthesia.
11. Refer higher risk patients and more extensive procedures for management by paediatric anaesthesiologists or similar specialists.

useful, it is not risk-free or devoid of adverse reactions. Although respiration is generally well maintained, perhaps better than with opioids dosed to comparable effect, ketamine has the disadvantage of no pharmacologic reversal agent. Respiratory sequelae have been reported (Mitchell et al 1996, Green and Rothrock 1997, Litman 1997, Roelofse and Roelofse 1997). Ketamine should be used primarily in a setting where personnel with advanced airway skills are readily available. The incidence of dysphoria, bad dreams, or prolonged sedation remains in dispute (Valentin and Bech 1996). Coadministration of ketamine with benzodiazepines appears to diminish this risk.

Although many children with cancer have indwelling central venous lines or easy peripheral venous access, others do not. For these children, needle-free routes of administration are helpful. Oral benzodiazepine–opioid or benzodiazepine–ketamine mixtures can be effective, though absorption varies, and oral/parenteral ratios are only approximations (Hollman and Perloff 1995, Qureshi et al 1995). If oral sedation is used, sufficient time should elapse to give peak drug effect. Because of variability in onset and offset, children need to be observed for development of deep sedation or respiratory depression. Some children will become restless or will try to get up and walk, and may injure themselves if unattended. Oral-transmucosal fentanyl has rapid absorption and good efficacy for bone marrow aspiration and lumbar puncture, despite frequent occurrence of nausea and itching.

Nitrous oxide 30–50% in oxygen can be used for sedation (Gamis et al 1989, Bouffet et al 1996) with good safety, rapid onset and offset, no requirement for intravenous access, and good analgesia. Some children will resist the mask, will report bothersome dreams (particularly with concentrations in excess of 50%), or will find nitrous oxide inadequate for portions of more painful procedures. Combination of nitrous oxide with other sedatives or analgesics requires experience; responses vary greatly (Litman et al 1996, 1997). Scavenging of exhaled gas, and high flow turnover of room air is recommended to reduce environmental exposure for health personnel.

The development of shorter duration general anaesthetic agents has greatly facilitated these procedures, both in operating room areas and in remote locations. If intravenous access is available, propofol is widely favoured because of its rapid onset, rapid, pleasant emergence, and antiemetic effects (Van Gerven et al 1992, Frankville et al 1993). If inhalation anaesthesia is required, the vapor anaesthetic sevoflurane has become popular because of its sweet smell and extremely rapid onset and offset. Some children fear the mask or dislike the pungent aroma of volatile anaesthetics, especially halothane and isoflurane (Jay et al 1995).

There is considerable controversy regarding the relative risks and benefits of brief deep sedation or general anaesthesia, provided by anaesthetists (Maunuksela et al 1986), versus conscious sedation provided by non-specialists (Cote 1994, Maxwell and Yaster 1996). Many paediatric centres employ a two-tiered approach, with conscious sedation for certain procedures by oncologists and other non-anaesthetists according to protocol guidelines, and with a 'sedation service' staffed by paediatric anaesthetists for higher risk patients, for more extensive or demanding procedures, or in cases of failed sedation by non-anaesthetists. It is essential that there be close communication and collaboration between paediatricians and anaesthetists, and recognition of each other's practice constraints. We believe that it is important that paediatric residents receive experience and training in use of conscious sedation in preparation for a wide range of subsequent practice settings.

Lumbar puncture

The distress of lumbar puncture is related in part to the required body position and the necessity to remain still, as well as pain due to needle contact with skin, bony spinous processes, or laminae. Topical anaesthesia can facilitate deeper infiltration (Kapelushnik et al 1990). The distress of lumbar puncture may be diminished by using cognitive and behavioural techniques, conscious sedation, or in some cases, general anaesthesia.

Lumbar puncture may produce a sustained cerebrospinal fluid leak, leading to low intracranial pressure headache. The risk of dural-puncture headache can be reduced by use of smaller gauge needles with non-cutting points. Treatment involves simple analgaesics, adequate hydration, and supine position. In adults, caffeine (Camann et al 1990) and sumatriptan have produced mixed results (Carp et al 1994, Choi et al 1996, de las Heras-Rosas et al 1997). In refractory cases, an epidural blood patch (the injection of autologous blood into the epidural space) may be required. Because of the theoretical concern for injecting circulating malignant cells into the neuraxis, we reserve epidural blood patch for prolonged and severe headaches in patients with no evidence of circulating blast cells.

Bone marrow aspiration

Bone marrow aspiration produces pain both with passage of a large needle through periosteum, and with application of suction to the marrow space. The former pain is only partially relieved by local anaesthetic infiltration near periosteum, the latter pain is unrelieved by local anaesthetic. Bone marrow aspiration is a source of severe distress in children (Katz et al 1980, Jay et al 1983). Guided imagery, relaxation, hypnosis, conscious sedation, and general anaesthesia have been shown to be effective modalities for reducing distress in this setting (Jay et al 1987, 1995).

Removal of central venous lines

Tunnelled central venous lines require removal, either electively when treatment courses are completed or more urgently in cases of infection or occlusion. Brief general anaesthesia and conscious sedation are widely used for these procedures.

As noted above, choice among treatments depends on the child's age, temperament, preferences, previous experience with procedures, and on local availability of services. For example, a 12 year old who is an excellent hypnotic subject and who experiences severe nausea or dysphoria with sedation or general anaesthesia may prefer hypnosis to pharmacologic measures. Conversely, a 3 year old who has had severely traumatic experiences with previous procedures may do better with a brief general anaesthetic. Options should be tailored to individual needs (Berde 1995). Pharmacological and psychological approaches should be seen as complementary, not mutually exclusive.

Mucositis

Cancer chemotherapy and radiation therapy attack the rapidly dividing cells of the epithelial lining of the oral cavity and gastrointestinal tract. Mucosal injury and cell death impairs barrier function, and produces pain and inflammation known as mucositis. Topical therapies have been widely used, including diphenhydramine, kaolin, sodium bicarbonate, hydrogen peroxide, sucralfate, clotrimazole, nystatin, lidocaine (lignocaine), and diclonine; efficacy data are limited. Excessive use of topical local anaesthetics can occasionally block protective airway reflexes, resulting in aspiration, or can cause systemic accumulation, with a risk of seizures. When pain persists despite topical therapies, opioids should be used.

Mucositis following bone marrow transplantation is more intense and prolonged than that associated with routine chemotherapy. Mucositis in transplant patients has a continuous component, with sharp exacerbation during mouth care and swallowing. Preventive strategies may reduce the incidence and severity of mucositis (Symonds et al 1996, Larson et al 1998). Opioids are generally partially effective, but for some patients the pain can preclude talking, eating, and on occasions swallowing. Continuous opioid infusions, patient-controlled analgesia (PCA), and nurse-controlled analgesia via a PCA pump are widely used (Hill et al 1991). PCA appears safe and effective for mucositis pain following bone marrow transplantation in children (Mackie et al 1991, Collins et al 1996a). In one comparison, the PCA group required less morphine and had less sedation, less difficulty concentrating, but equivalent analgesia to the group receiving staff-controlled morphine continuous infusion; in other comparisons, PCA groups have lower opioid use and side effects, as well as lower pain scores (Zucker et al 1998). There is a need for further study of optimal methods of management.

Graft versus host disease

Donor-derived immune cells attack host tissues following bone marrow transplantation to create a multiorgan inflammatory process known as graft versus host disease. Abdominal pains and limb pains are common. Abdominal pain may arise from both hepatic and intestinal inflammation and veno-occlusion. Despite pre-emptive anti-T-cell therapies in transplant protocols, this problem remains common, and is a frequent source of pain, which is usually treated with opioids.

Infection

Immunocompromised children are susceptible to painful bacterial, viral, fungal, and protozoal infections in a range of sites, including mouth sores, perirectal abscesses, and skin infection. Analgesics may be required until antimicrobial therapies reduce inflammation.

Acute herpes zoster can be quite painful, and merits use of opioids as needed. Zoster infection in children is less likely to produce prolonged postherpetic neuralgia than that in adults; however, a small subgroup of children may experience long-term postherpetic burning pain, episodic shooting pain, itching, and skin hypersensitivity. Early antiviral therapy should be encouraged (Wood et al 1996). Therapies for postherpetic neuralgia are adapted from those used in adults including tricyclic antidepressants (Bowsher et al 1997, Watson et al 1998a), anticonvulsants (Rowbotham et al 1998), topical, regional, and systemic local anaesthetics, and opioids (Rowbotham et al 1991).

Acute abdominal emergencies

Oncology patients may have any of the causes of an acute abdomen that afflict other patients, such as appendicitis, a perforated ulcer, or a bowel obstruction. Neutropenic patients may present with acute bowel inflammation known as tiflitis. Although they show the signs of an acute surgical abdomen, this condition is usually treated conservatively, and surgical exploration is usually restricted to cases of overt bowel perforation or severe bleeding. Many of these patients are quite ill and require opioids despite their effects on bowel motility.

Pre-emptive treatment of constipation is important in all patients taking opioids, but it is especially important in sick neutropenic patients. Delayed administration of oral laxatives for mild ileus and constipation can lead to a difficult situation with severe abdominal distension, emesis, and a suspicion for tiflitis. Treatment options then become limited, since enemas or rectal laxatives are contraindicated because of their risks of producing bacteraemia or perforation.

Postoperative pain and perioperative care

Postoperative pain management in general is discussed in detail in Chap. 1. It is to be expected that there will be considerable preoperative anxiety and fear for children with cancer and their parents. Heavy premedication may be required, and early anticipation of the need for larger-than-average doses for premedication may prevent unpleasant scenes and distress in the preoperative waiting area.

Children who are or have become opioid tolerant may have a higher risk of intraoperative awareness during anaesthesia, particularly if a nitrous oxide–opioid-relaxant-based anaesthetic technique is used without adjustment for these increased opioid requirements. Unless there is severe haemodynamic instability, we recommend incorporating either volatile anaesthetic agents or adequate doses of hypnotics (e.g., propofol infusions) to ensure unconsciousness.

Postoperatively, patients who have been receiving preoperative opioids should have their daily dose of opioids calculated, and this dose used as a baseline to which additional opioids are added for the purposes of postoperative pain control. This principle is commonly ignored, leading to undermedication of oncology patients postoperatively. Cancer resection can be especially painful postoperatively because of the need to cut across tissues, rather than dividing in natural tissue planes, in order to obtain clear margins.

Epidural analgesia can be used with very good effect for cancer surgery in children (Tobias et al 1992). As with systemic opioids, it is our experience that initial dosing of epidural infusions in children with cancer is often too conservative. Rapid and aggressive bedside titration should be used to relieve their pain. Maximum weight-based local anaesthetic dosing is limited by strict guidelines, as outlined in Chap. 25, while dosing of epidural opioids should be titrated upwards to clinical effect. Placement of the epidural catheter tip at the level of the dermatomes innervating the surgical field permits optimal use of local anaesthetic–opioid synergism. If epidural catheter tips are below the level of surgical dermatomes, or if there is inadequate analgesia with combinations of local anaesthetics with lipid-soluble opioids (e.g., fentanyl), clinicians should not hesitate to switch the opioid component of the epidural mixture to a water-soluble drug such as morphine and hydromorphone to achieve adequate neuraxial spread. Clonidine is being used increasingly as a useful adjunctive medication in epidural infusions. It enhances analgesia from local anaesthetics and opioids, and may provide an improved side effect profile, because it does not produce ileus, itching, or urinary retention.

Postsurgical neuropathic pains

Damage to peripheral nerves is unavoidable in many types of tumour resection, particularly with limb sarcomas, and nerve injury may produce prolonged neuropathic pain. Studies of pre-emptive effects of regional blockade in preventing neuropathic pain are controversial at best. We favour use of perioperative regional blockade whenever feasible for limb sarcoma resections in part because it may provide very good postoperative analgesia, even if the more prolonged benefits are controversial. If a child shows signs and symptoms of neuropathic pain following cancer surgery, early use of tricyclic antidepressants and anticonvulsants should be made. In many cases, they appear beneficial, and are required for several weeks to months. For a tricyclic, we typically begin with nortriptyline in doses of 0.1–0.2 mg/kg at night-time and increase dosing every few days until either there is relief, there are side effects, or full antidepressant levels are achieved, often with addition of a smaller morning dose.

Gabapentin has emerged as the first-line anticonvulsant for treatment of neuropathic pains (Backonja et al 1998). Paediatric experience is limited to case reports or case series (Rusy et al 2001). Our experience with its use has been very favourable, because of both its efficacy and its apparent safety. Occasional children will experience headaches, sedation, abdominal upset, and behavioural disturbances.

Pain due to antineoplastic therapy

Several chemotherapy drugs can produce local necrosis or irritation when a peripheral vein infiltrates. Some forms of chemotherapy are painful when injected via peripheral veins, even when no extravasation occurs. Intrathecal chemotherapy can produce backache, headache, and signs of arachnoiditis or meningeal irritation.

Vincristine commonly produces peripheral nerve dysfunction, with hyporeflexia, sensory abnormalities, paraesthesias, and gastrointestinal hypomotility; in addition, a small subgroup of children report burning or shooting pains and paraesthesias. These are often treated with opioids, tricyclic antidepressants, and anticonvulsants. In the majority of patients, these symptoms improve over several months, but are likely to recur with repeated cycles of chemotherapy.

Granulocyte colony-stimulating factor (GCSF) accelerates neutrophil production, and shortens the duration of neutropenic episodes. It may produce bone marrow pain.

Chronic pains in long-term survivors of childhood cancer

Long-term survivors of childhood cancer occasionally experience chronic pain. Neuropathic pains include peripheral neuralgias of the lower extremity, phantom limb pain, postherpetic neuralgia, and central pain after spinal cord tumour resection. Some patients have chronic lower extremity pain due to a mechanical problem with an internal prosthesis or failure of bony union, or avascular necrosis of multiple joints. Others have longstanding myofascial pains and chronic abdominal pain of uncertain aetiology. Some patients treated with shunts for brain tumours have recurrent headaches that appear unrelated to intracranial pressure or changes in shunt functioning.

Phantom sensations and phantom limb pain are common among children following amputation for cancer in an extremity (Dangel 1998). Phantom pain in children tends to decrease with time. Preamputation pain in the diseased extremity may be a predictor for subsequent phantom pain. Krane

Table 44.4 Dosing recommendations for non-opioid analgesics for children

Drug	Recommended dosing	Comments
Acetaminophen (paracetamol)	Single doses of 15–20 mg/kg. Repeated doses of 10–15 mg/kg every 4 h orally, up to 90 mg/kg/day in children and 60 mg/kg/day in infants.	Generally safe. Does not cause gastric irritation or bleeding.
Choline-magnesium salicylate	10–15 mg/kg every 8–12 h orally	Lower gastric and bleeding risk than most NSAIDs.
Ibuprofen	8–10 mg/kg every 6–8 h orally	Largest paediatric experience among NSAIDs. Potential for bleeding and gastritis limits use in children with cancer.
Naproxen	5–7 mg/kg every 8–12 h orally	Risks similar to ibuprofen. Longer duration permits less frequent dosing.
Amitriptyline or nortriptyline	Begin at 0.1–0.2 mg/kg at bedtime, increase incrementally as limited by side effects and as needed for efficacy up to 2 mg/kg day.	Clearance is variable, so that some patients will benefit from a small morning dose in addition. Plasma concentrations may be a helpful guide at higher dose ranges.
Gabapentin	Begin at 100 mg orally at bedtime, or with 50 mg (1/2 of the smallest capsule's contents) in younger children. If tolerated, advance to twice daily then three times daily over several days. If tolerated, escalate as needed and tolerated up to 60 mg/kg/day, divided in three times daily dosing.	These recommendations are provisional, since current experience is limited.

Table 44.5 General guidelines for opioid use for cancer pain in children

1. Use sufficient doses to keep the patient comfortable and dose frequently enough to prevent most recurrences of pain.
2. Use the oral route first in most circumstances.
3. Use appropriate oral:parenteral conversion ratios.
4. The 'right' dose is whatever it takes to relieve the pain.
5. Treat opioid side effects promptly.
6. Treat constipation pre-emptively.
7. If side effects are bothersome with one opioid, consider opioid switching.

and Heller suggested that phantom pain was quite common in children following cancer resection, and was often under-recognized by physicians (Krane et al 1991). Melzack and coworkers reported that phantom sensation and pain can occur in children with congenital absence of limbs, although the prevalence of pain is less than among children who received amputations (Melzack et al 1997).

Survivors of childhood cancer and their families often worry that pains and other symptoms may imply relapse or a second, treatment-induced malignancy. Care of these children and young adults should be multidisciplinary and should include psychological interventions, physical therapy, and efforts to help these children and young adults return to school and work. A small percentage of long-term survivors take oral opioid analgesics on a daily basis for long-term treatment of pain as part of a multidisciplinary programme.

Pain due to tumour progression

Tumour progression can produce pain, often by infiltration in or pressure on bone, viscera, soft tissues, or nerves. Even where there is no longer curative intent, chemotherapy and radiation therapy may help relieve pain by shrinking the tumour (Stevens et al 1994; Frager 1996; Goldman 1996, 1998; Liben 1996; Dangel 1998).

In Chap. 37, we describe the general difficulties with pain assessment in preverbal children. Several points are worth reiterating here. Behavioural signs of persistent pain may differ from those in the setting of acute medical procedures. Behavioural distress scales developed for acute procedures often under-rate pain in this setting.

Many children with pain due to widespread cancer will lie still, close their eyes, and inhibit body movements. While sometimes this response is due to oversedation, in other cases a withdrawal from their surroundings is a response to undertreated pain. When in doubt, a trial of opioid titration may be diagnostic. If the child becomes more interactive and moves around more freely after opioid dosing, then it is likely that they were previously undermedicated, not oversedated.

Trends in physiologic signs, including heart rate and blood pressure, can provide some information about pain intensity, but should not be used as isolated measures of pain. Many processes unrelated to pain can alter heart rate and blood pressure. Autonomic signs may habituate with persistent pain.

Analgesics for pain due to advanced cancer

The WHO analgesic ladder approach outlined for adults with cancer is in many respects applicable for children as well. General aspects of paediatric analgesic pharmacology are reviewed in Chap. 37. Dosing guidelines for non-opioid and opioid analgesics are summarized in Tables 44.4, 44.5, and 44.6, respectively.

Acetaminophen

Acetaminophen is the most commonly used nonopioid analgesic in children with cancer, particularly because it lacks the antiplatelet and gastric effects of NSAIDs and aspirin. Oral dosing of 10–15 mg/kg every 4 h is recommended, with a daily maximum dose of 90 mg/kg/day in children, 60 mg/kg/day in infants, and 45 mg/kg/day in preterm neonates from 32 weeks to term.

Aspirin and NSAIDs

Aspirin and NSAIDs are frequently contraindicated in paediatric oncology patients because of bleeding concerns. In selected children with adequate platelet number and function, NSAIDs may be very useful, both alone and in combination with opioids. The effectiveness of NSAIDs in cancer is not limited to bone pains (Eisenberg et al 1994).

Choline magnesium salicylate (Trilisate) and related non-acetylated salicylates appear in adult studies to produce less gastric irritation and antiplatelet effects than most NSAIDs. Data are too limited to warrant extrapolating these conclusions to patients with severe thrombocytopenia.

The newer cyclooxygenase-2 (COX2) inhibitors are likely to be enormously beneficial for pain management for children with cancer. If initial studies in adults are replicated, then they should be very safe and effective in many situations, both alone and in combination with opioids.

Weak opioids: codeine, tramadol, and low-dose oxycodone

The WHO ladder distinguishes between weak opioids and strong opioids, although this is a function of dose as well as drug. Codeine is rarely escalated beyond 2 mg/kg because it appears to produce more side effects than comparable doses of other opioids. Recommended pediatric oral dosing is 0.5–1 mg/kg every 4 h. Between 5 and 12% of subjects lack the metabolic enzyme that activates codeine by converting it to morphine; in these subjects, codeine is ineffective. Oxycodone can be regarded as either a 'weak' or a 'strong' opioid depending on the dose used. Dosing of oxycodone can be escalated as long as it is not given in a fixed preparation with acetaminophen (e.g., Percocet) in doses that would risk acetaminophen toxicity.

The practical advantage of the so-called weak opioids is that they can be prescribed in some locations by telephone more easily than many other opioids. In many parts of the United States, there is greater acceptance of telephone prescribing of combinations of acetaminophen with either codeine (e.g., Tylenol #3 or #4) or hydrocodone (e.g., Vicodin). In some countries, such as Germany, tramadol is widely used as an analgesic for pain of moderate severity.

Most available evidence recommends use of standard μ-opioid agonists for cancer pain in preference to mixed agonist–antagonist opioids or opioids acting primarily at κ-receptors. Somnolence and dysphoria are common with the latter drugs, and they may cause withdrawal symptoms in patients receiving μ-opioids. The κ-agonist buprenorphine is widely used for children in countries with limited availability of morphine. It is more properly regarded as a strong opioid, and can have very prolonged duration of action.

Strong opioids: morphine, hydromorphone, fentanyl, meperidine, methadone

For moderate to severe pain, μ-opioid agonists are the cornerstone of treatment. Initial dose recommendations for opioid prescribing for children with cancer are outlined in Table 44.6.

Morphine is the most widely used strong opioid, and is a proper first choice in most circumstances. Age-related differences in morphine conjugation and excretion are summarized in Chap. 24. A typical starting dose for immediate release oral morphine in opioid-naïve subjects is 0.3 mg/kg every 4 h.

Sustained release preparations of morphine and oxycodone are widely available. Dosing sustained release morphine three times, rather than twice, daily may give more constant plasma concentrations (Hunt et al 1999). Crushing sustained release morphine tablets produces immediate release of morphine, which limits their use for children unable to swallow pills.

Hydromorphone is similar in many respects to morphine in its actions, but may be used in settings where there are dose-limiting side effects from morphine. A double-blinded, randomized crossover comparison of morphine to hydromorphone using PCA in children and adolescents with mucositis following bone marrow transplantation showed that hydromorphone was well tolerated, and had an approximate potency ratio of 6:1 relative to morphine in this setting (Collins et al 1996a). Because of its high potency and high aqueous solubility, hydromorphone is convenient for high-

Table 44.6 Starting doses of commonly used opioids in paediatrics

Drug	Usual I.V. starting dose (< 50 kg)	Usual I.V. starting dose (> 50 kg)	Usual P.O. starting dose (< 50 kg)	Usual P.O. starting dose (> 50 kg)
Morphine	0.1 mg/kg q3–4h	5–10 mg q3–4h	0.3 mg/kg q3–4h	30 mg q3–4h
Hydromorphone	0.015 mg/kg q3–4h	1–1.5 mg q3–4h	0.06 mg/kg q3–4h	4 mg q3–4h
Oxycodone	N/A	N/A	0.1–0.2 mg/kg q3–4h[b]	5–10 mg/kg q3–4h
Meperidine[a]	0.75 mg/kg q2–3h	75–100 mg q3h	2–3 mg/kg q3–4h	100–150 mg q3–4h
Fentanyl	0.5–1.5 μg/kg q1–2h	25–75 μg/kg q1–2h	N/A	N/A

N/A = not available; N/R =not recommended. Adapted from Collins and Berde (1997).
[a]Meperidine is not recommended for chronic use because of the accumulation of the toxic metabolite normeperidine.
[b]Smallest tablet size is 5 mg; elixir formulations are available.

dose subcutaneous infusion. Little is known about pharmacokinetics in infants or biologic actions of metabolites.

Fentanyl is about 50–100 times as potent as morphine, depending on whether infusion or I.V. single-dose comparisons are used. It has a rapid onset and offset following intravenous administration, which is convenient for brief painful procedures. With infusions, its duration of action becomes more prolonged. Fentanyl is commonly used for patients who have excessive pruritus from morphine.

Meperidine should be avoided for ongoing use if other opioids are available because its major metabolite normeperidine can cause dysphoria, excitation, and convulsions, particularly in patients with impaired renal function. Meperidine can be used for brief painful procedures, and it has a specific indication in low doses (0.25–0.5 mg/kg I.V.) for treatment of severe shivering or rigors following the infusion of amphotericin and blood components.

Methadone is long acting due to its slow hepatic metabolism. In single parenteral doses, it is equipotent to morphine. Oral absorption is efficient, with an oral:parenteral ratio of approximately 1.5–2:1. Elixir preparations are convenient for prolonged duration in children who are unable to swallow sustained release morphine tablets. Episodic intravenous dosing may be convenient for patients with intravenous access to maintain sustained analgesia without the requirement for an infusion pump (Berde et al 1991).

Methadone requires careful attention in dose titration, both because of variability in its metabolism (Plummer et al 1988) and because of incomplete cross-tolerance with other μ-opioids. Accumulation can produce delayed sedation and hypoventilation several days after a dosing change. Once comfort is achieved, it is often necessary to lower the dose or extend the interval to avoid subsequent oversedation.

Choice among routes of opioid administration The oral route of opioid administration is convenient, inexpensive, and non-technologic, and therefore to be favoured whenever feasible. Some children with advanced cancer either refuse to take oral medications or cannot take them because of nausea, ileus, painful swallowing, or obtundation.

Intravenous administration permits rapid, titrated dosing and complete bioavailability. Where available, indwelling central venous lines obviate the need for repeated intravenous cannulation (Miser et al 1980). Continuous subcutaneous infusions are a useful intermediate technology for parenteral opioid administration for children with poor intravenous access (Miser et al 1983). A small catheter or butterfly needle may be placed under the skin of the thorax, abdomen, or thigh, with sites changed every 3–7 days as needed. Solutions are generally concentrated so that infusion rates do not exceed 1–3 cc/h, although higher rates have been used. Morphine and hydromorphone are commonly used, and are well tolerated; methadone should be avoided because it can produce local irritation and skin necrosis. Needle placement can be made less noxious by prior use of topical local anaesthetic preparations as described above. Pain at the injection site can be diminished by mixing small amounts of lidocaine (lignocaine) in the infusion, as long as cumulative lidocaine dosing does not exceed 1.5 mg/kg/h. Intravenous and subcutaneous infusions can be made more convenient for the home by use of small portable infusion pumps.

Many of the home infusion pumps are equipped with a PCA bolus option as well as a continuous infusion mode. In the United States, there is in general no greater operating cost in adding a PCA option. Most children with cancer have fluctuations in pain intensity and in opioid requirements. A PCA option is a straightforward method for permitting rescue medication via either intravenous or subcutaneous routes (Bruera et al 1988). It is more convenient for patients or parents to push a button than it is to open vials, draw medication into a syringe, and inject medication into the infusion line. General discussion of PCA use in children is given in Chap. 37. In palliative care, pushing the PCA button is often not limited to patients, and parents and nurses frequently participate in dosing.

Transdermal administration of fentanyl via a patch is a convenient method for providing sustained analgesia without the need for intravenous access or infusion pumps (Payne 1992, Patt et al 1993). Initial paediatric studies suggest good efficacy and safety in a small population of paediatric oncology patients. These formulations should be used with caution in opioid-naïve patients or in patients with rapidly changing analgesic requirements. The lowest delivery rate currently available in the United States is 25 μg/h, which may be excessive for some children. There is a considerable delay to obtaining steady-state concentrations, and initial titration to comfort by other routes is required (Zech et al 1992). Absorption may be impaired by severe oedema or impaired circulation, which can be a factor in end-of-life care. For patients with fluctuating pain intensity, another method of opioid administration is required for rescue dosing. These considerations are especially important in treatment of terminal symptoms, such as air hunger.

Oral transmucosal fentanyl produces a rapid onset of effect and bypasses first-pass hepatic clearance. As noted above, OTFC is effective for painful procedures, but it has also been used successfully for adults for breakthrough pain due to tumour (Fine et al 1991).

Management of opioid side effects As with adults, the key to successful use of opioids lies in individualized dosing and treatment of side effects (Table 44.7). Constipation should be prevented and treated with laxatives. Several classes of antiemetics, including 5HT-3 antagonists, phenothiazines, butyrophenones, antihistamines, and cannabinoids have been used effectively for opioid-induced nausea in children.

Opioid dose escalation Opioid dose requirements for children with widespread cancer vary greatly. Opioids are similar in their population

Table 44.7 Management of opioid side effects

Side-effect	Treatment
Constipation	1. Regular use of stimulant and stool softener laxatives (fibre, fruit juices are often insufficient). 2. Ensure adequate water intake.
Sedation	1. If analgesia is adequate, try dose reduction. 2. Unless contraindicated, add non-sedating analgesics, such as acetaminophen or NSAIDs, and reduce opioid dosing as tolerated. 3. If sedation persists, trymethylphenidate or dextroamphetamine 0.05–0.2 mg/kg P.O. b.i.d. in early am and midday. Dosing of methylphenidate can be escalated as tolerated up to at least 0.3 mg/kg at morning and midday, and higher in selected patients. 4. Consider an opioid switch.
Nausea	1. Exclude disease processes (e.g., bowel obstruction, increased intracranial pressure). 2. Antiemetics (phenothiazines, ondansetron, hydroxyzine). 3. Consider an opioid switch.
Urinary retention	1. Exclude disease processes (e.g., bladder neck obstruction by tumour, impending cord compression, hypovolaemia, renal failure, etc.). 2. Avoid other drugs with anticholinergic effects (e.g., tricyclics, antihistamines). 3. Consider short-term use of bethanechol or Crede manoeuvre. 4. Consider short-term catheterization. 5. Consider opioid dose reduction if analgesia adequate or an opioid switch if analgesia inadequate.
Pruritus	1. Exclude other causes (e.g., drug allergy, cholestasis). 2. Antihistamines (e.g., diphenhydramine hydroxyzine). 3. Consider an opioid dose reduction if analgesia adequate, or an opioid switch. Fentanyl causes less histamine release.
Respiratory depression:	
Mild–moderate	1. Awaken, encourage to breathe. 2. Apply oxygen. 3. Withhold opioid dosing until breathing improves, reduce subsequent dosing by at least 25%.
Severe	1. Awaken if possible, apply oxygen, assist respiration by bag, and mask as needed. 2. Titrate small doses of naloxone (0.02 mg/kg increments as needed) stop when respiratory rate increases to 8–10/min in older children or 12–16/min in infants; do not try to awaken fully with naloxone. ****DO NOT GIVE A BOLUS DOSE OF NALOXONE AS SEVERE PAIN AND SYMPTOMS OF OPIOID WITHDRAWAL MAY ENSUE.**** 3. Consider a low-dose naloxone infusion or repeated incremental dosing. 4. Consider short-term intubation in occasional cases where risk of aspiration is high.
Dysphoria/ confusion/ hallucinations	1. Exclude other pathology as a cause for these symptoms before attributing them to opioids. 2. When other causes excluded, change to another opioid. 3. Consider adding a neuroleptic such as haloperidol (0.01–0.1 mg/kg P.O./I.V. every 8 h to a maximum dose of 15 mg/day).
Myoclonus	1. Usually seen in the setting of high-dose opioids, or alternatively, rapid dose escalation. 2. No treatment may be warranted, if this is infrequent and not distressing to the child. 3. Consider an opioid switch or treat with clonezepam (0.01 mg/kg P.O. every 12 h to a maximum dose of 0.5 mg/dose) or a parenteral benzodiazepine (e.g., diazepam) if the oral route is not tolerated.

Adapted from Collins and Berde (1997).

prevalence of side effects, but there may be marked individual variability in these effects. Among opioid-tolerant cancer patients, several studies document incomplete cross-tolerance when switching from one opioid to another, especially when switching from morphine or hydromorphone to methadone. This appears to be a consequence of the NMDA receptor blocking activity of the d-isomer of methadone in the racemic commercial preparations (Ripamonti et al 1998).

If intolerable side effects are found with dose escalation with one opioid, a trial of a second opioid should be considered, beginning at 25–50% of the equianalgesic dose in the case of most opioids, or 15–25% of the equianalgesic dose if the second opioid is methadone. Tolerance to sedation, nausea and vomiting, and pruritus often develops within the first week of commencing opioids.

Patients and parents are often reluctant to increase dosing because of a fear that tolerance will make opioids ineffective at a later date. They should be reassured that tolerance usually can be managed by simple dose escalation, use of adjunctive medications, or opioid switching. There is no justification for withholding opioids to save them for a later time of need. Fears of drug addiction can also be a barrier to opioid use.

Among adults with cancer, rapid opioid dose escalation is most commonly due to tumour spread, rather than rapidly progressive tolerance. We reported on patterns of opioid administration among 199 children who died of malignancy at Boston Children's Hospital and the Dana-Farber Cancer Institute from 1989 to 1993, a time during which the WHO programme was more consistently applied (Collins et al 1995). Over 90% remained comfortable during their terminal course with standard opioid dose escalation and side effect management.

Two subgroups required more intensive management. One group of 6 patients had intolerable side effects before reaching dose escalation more than 100-fold above standard starting rates (i.e., above 3 mg/kg/h I.V. morphine equivalents). All of these patients could be made comfortable by regional anaesthetic approaches (see below). A second group of 12 patients (6% of the overall group) escalated systemic dosing to greater than 3 mg/kg/h I.V. morphine equivalent. Rapid dose escalation was most common in the final weeks of life. Eleven of these 12 patients had solid tumours metastatic to the spine, central nervous system, or major nerve plexus. Maximum opioid dosing ranged from 3.8–518 mg/kg/h I.V. morphine equivalent. Among these 12 patients, 4 were comfortable primarily with opioid escalation, but the rest required either regional anaesthesia or continuous sedation.

Adjunctive medications

Tricyclic antidepressants are widely used for neuropathic pain, as well as to facilitate sleep. Paediatric use of tricyclics for pain is largely extrapolated from adult trials. Reviews of antidepressants in children are given elsewhere (Steingard et al 1995, Birmaher 1998). We begin with single night-time dosing of tricyclics in most patients. If dose escalation is tolerated without sedation, a smaller morning dose can be added. Plasma levels can be useful to guide titration. Electrocardiograms are recommended for screening for rhythm disturbances and to follow changes on therapy, but little is known about their predictive value for risk of severe arrhythmias or cardiac events due to tricyclics. We exercise additional caution with patients who have signs of cardiac dysfunction or ectopy due to anthracyclines. In selected cases where the oral route is not feasible, an injectable preparation of amitriptyline can be used intravenously with slow infusion and careful monitoring (Collins et al 1995).

For children with limiting sedation from opioids, stimulants such as methylphenidate and dextroamphetamine (Bruera et al 1989, Yee and Berde 1994) should be tried. Our impression is that adverse reactions are uncommon, and the improvement in alertness may be impressive. Typically, methylphenidate is started with morning and noontime dosing of 0.1 mg/kg, with dose escalation as needed up to roughly 0.6 mg/kg/day.

Benzodiazepines are useful for sedation for noxious procedures. In our opinion, they are often overused for persistent anxiety. We discourage the prolonged use of benzodiazepines for sleep disturbance, since with chronic use they disrupt sleep cycles, produce tolerance and dependence, and can exacerbate daytime somnolence and confusion.

Corticosteroids are used in adults in a range of settings for cancer pain, including headache due to brain tumours, for nerve compression, for epidural spinal cord compression, and for metastatic bone disease (Watanabe and Bruera 1994). They can be useful for shorter-term pain relief in children as well, although a number of sequelae can arise from prolonged use, including mood disturbances, a Cushingoid body habitus, cataracts, immunosuppression, and fractures.

Anticonvulsants

Anticonvulsants should be considered for pain of neuropathic origin. Gabapentin is commonly chosen because of its safety and tolerability. Carbamazepine, phenytoin, clonezepam, gabapentin, and valproate have all been used, but the evidence is not clear on the relative risks and benefits among these agents in children. Sedation, ataxia, and dysphoria are common symptoms.

Neuroleptics

Phenothiazines and butyrophenones can be used as antiemetics. In general, they are not analgesic, but may reduce reporting of pain. Levomepromazine (methotrimeprazine) has been used as an adjuvant analgesic (Beaver et al 1966), although published experience in children is limited. Levomepromazine (methotrimeprazine) is highly sedating, and may diminish acute agitation.

Interventional approaches to pain management for children with cancer

Epidural and spinal analgesic infusions

A percentage of adults with widespread cancer and a difficulty in controlling pain can be made comfortable by use of spinal analgesic infusions (Plummer et al 1991, Eisenach et al 1995) and neurodestructive procedures (Brown et al 1987, Plancarte et al 1990). Experience with these approaches in children is more limited (Collins et al 1996b), and we approach them with some caution.

It is essential first to optimize pharmacologic and non-pharmacologic approaches and to consider the wishes of the child and his/her parents in the context of a realistic appraisal of their disease and its likely progression.

Our recommendations for use of regional anaesthetic approaches for management of pain due to advanced cancer in children is outlined in Table 44.8.

Spinal infusions can provide excellent analgesia in refractory cases, but they require individualized attention, and should not be undertaken by inexperienced practitioners without guidance. Dose requirements vary dramatically, and the process of converting from systemic to spinal drug is often quite unpredictable, with the potential for either oversedation or withdrawal symptoms. If children with spinal infusions are to be managed at home, it is essential to have resources available to manage new symptoms, such as terminal dyspnoea and air hunger.

Neurodestructive procedures

As with adults (Mercadante 1993), coeliac plexus blockade can provide excellent pain relief for children with severe pain due to massively enlarged upper abdominal viscera due to tumour (Berde et al 1990, Staats and Kost-Byerly 1995). Many children and parents are reluctant to consider procedures with the potential for irreversible loss of somatic function. Decompressive operations on the spine can in occasional cases produce dramatic relief of pain. Treatment algorithms for epidural spinal cord compression depend on a number of issues, and may also involve use of high-dose steroids, chemotherapy, and radiation therapy (Greenberg et al 1980).

Table 44.8 Recommendations for use of epidural and spinal infusions for management of pain due to widespread cancer in children

1. Optimize use of non-pharmacologic approaches, opioids, and adjuvants first.
2. Do not promise perfect pain relief.
3. Be clear with patients and their parents regarding the potential for adverse events and side effects. Where local anaesthetics are used, warn them about the potential for degrees of motor and sensory blockade and impairment of bowel or bladder function.
4. Place catheters under general anaesthesia or deep sedation, not awake.
5. Use fluoroscopic guidance whenever available to ensure proper localization while the child is asleep.
6. We prefer to tunnel catheters with initial placement for improved skin care.
7. The key to success is precise dermatomal application of local anaesthetics; opioids alone are rarely sufficient to achieve an improved therapeutic index. Combine opioids with local anaesthetics, and occasionally add other drugs, such as clonidine.
8. For pain below the umbilicus, we prefer lumbar subarachnoid catheters; for pain in higher dermatomes, we prefer thoracic epidural placement with the catheter tip in the middle of the most important dermatomes innervating the painful area. The subarachnoid route gives the greatest flexibility in escalating local anaesthetic dosing to achieve deafferentation with a margin of safety. With prolonged epidural infusions, local anaesthetic dosing is restricted by concerns for systemic toxicity.
9. Epidural tumour may impede placement, or prevent drug spread to intended sites. Radiographic confirmation of spread of contrast helps ensure a likelihood of access of drug to intended target sites.
10. The optimal combination of drugs must be individualized based on both previous analgesic use, the nature and location of the pain, and the patient's individual preferences in balancing analgesia with side effects. Dose escalation is often needed.

Sedation in end-of-life care

Opioids generally relieve pain with a partial preservation of clarity of sensorium, although many patients require doses of opioids that make them sedated when undisturbed, but rousable when spoken to (Coyle et al 1990). Patients and their families can be told that comfort can be achieved with opioids in most situations (Foley 1997). Providers need to reassure parents that by treating pain with opioids they are not causing their child's death; that the child's disease is the cause of death.

There remains a very small subgroup of patients who have intolerable side effects and/or inadequate analgesia despite extremely aggressive use of analgesics as outlined above. While regional anaesthetic approaches may be chosen by some patients and families, others will chose continuous sedation as a means of relieving suffering.

The choice of sedation generally assumes there is no feasible or acceptable means for providing analgesia with preservation of alertness. We favour continuing high-dose opioid infusions along with sedation to reduce the possibility that a patient might experience unrelieved pain but be too sedated to report on it. The ethical and practical issues around providing sedation in the terminally ill have been discussed (Truog et al 1992, Foley 1997). Sedation for terminally ill patients is widely regarded as providing comfort, not euthanasia, according to the principle of double effect (Foley 1997), although others describe some difficult logical consequences in the use of this ethical justification (Quill et al 1997). Clinicians and ethicists with a range of views regarding assisted suicide and euthanasia agree on the following position: no child or parent should chose death because of our profession's inadequate efforts to relieve pain and suffering, to ameliorate depression, fear, and isolation, or to provide spiritual and emotional support.

HIV and AIDS

Infants now acquire HIV predominantly through transplacental infection from their mothers (Grossman 1988). Transfusion-acquired HIV is declining in prevalence in developed countries, although new cases of transfusion-acquired disease continue in some developing countries. Adolescents become infected through sexual contact and infected needles.

In developed countries, the prognosis for congenitally acquired HIV infection has improved dramatically in recent years due to multidrug therapies. Access to these treatments is severely limited in developing countries, and the majority of infants with AIDS in Africa and Asia continue to suffer cachexia, neurologic devastation, and early death.

Children with HIV infection with access to sophisticated medical treatment undergo an enormous number of painful diagnostic and therapeutic procedures (Hirschfeld et al 1996), which may be treated much like painful oncology procedures as outlined above.

In developing countries and in infants in developed countries with less access to care, HIV-induced neurologic degeneration can produce severe irritability and the appearance of poorly localized pain. Opioids should be considered as first-line agents in preference to sedative hypnotics. This experience differs somewhat from the general impression of treatment of infants with some other neurodegenerative disorders, as outlined below.

Cystic fibrosis

Cystic fibrosis is the most common life-shortening genetic disorder in Caucasian populations. It is a multisystem disorder that arises in different families from one of a series of similar autosomal recessive mutations in a gene encoding a chloride channel. Cystic fibrosis affects a range of organs, including pancreas, intestines, liver, paranasal sinuses, and sweat glands, but the predominant cause of morbidity, mortality, and suffering is due to chronic obstructive lung disease. The ion channel abnormality leads to viscous pulmonary secretions, bronchiectasis, and a particular susceptibility to airways colonization or infection with mucoid strains of *Pseudomonas aeruginosa*.

Longevity has improved dramatically over the past 30 years. Median age at death was less than age 20 in the 1960s. In many centres today, median survival is approaching age 40. There remains a smaller subgroup of patients with rapidly progressive lung disease who are in respiratory failure during their teenage years.

Improved survival has been ascribed to better antibiotics, better nutritional support, or use of chest physiotherapy, although there is little consensus on the relative importance of each of these therapies.

Patients with advanced lung disease suffer several types of distressing symptoms. There can be severe near-constant dyspnoea and air hunger. There is a constant need to cough in an attempt to clear their airways of tenacious sputum, and often the coughing is extremely intense. The high airways resistance and high ratio of alveolar dead space to tidal volume leads to dramatically increased work of breathing and fatigue.

Sleep is often disturbed, and many people with cystic fibrosis develop a fear that they will suffocate during sleep. This may lead them to stay up much of the night and sleep in daytime. Small evening doses of antidepressants may improve sleep. Some tolerate tricyclics, such as nortriptyline. Others are bothered by the peripheral anticholinergic actions in drying their secretions, and instead prefer the tetracyclic, trazodone.

Ravilly and coworkers in our group documented a high prevalence of chronic daily headache and chest pain in patients with advanced cystic fibrosis (Ravilly et al 1996). Headache appears multifactorial, and is usually poorly characterized. Although in many cases, hypoxemia and hypercapnia are present and appear to worsen headache, others experience daily headache before blood gas abnormalities can be demonstrated. Constant violent coughing may contribute to headache, both by associated scalp and neck muscle contraction and possibly because of marked fluctuations in intracranial pressure. Nasal polyposis and sinusitis are ubiquitous, and often contribute to headache.

Chronic chest pain in cystic fibrosis may be due to intercostal muscle fatigue and overuse, both due to the work of breathing and due to coughing. Acute episodes of chest pain with localized rib tenderness may indicate a rib fracture. Acute onset chest pain with dyspnoea may also herald a pneumothorax.

The prevalence of headache and chest pain increases dramatically in the final year of life, and the majority of patients in their final six months of life have chronic daily headache and chest pain.

With a genetic disorder such as cystic fibrosis, the psychological implications for end-of-life and palliative care are different from those for patients with cancer. Most of these patients are aware of their shortened life span from an early age. Conversely, as the natural history of the disease has changed, patients' concepts of their illness have changed.

Patients with cystic fibrosis die predominantly due to respiratory failure, with progressive hypoxaemia, hypercapnia, fatigue, dyspnoea, severe coughing, air hunger, and headache. Opioids can provide some relief of these symptoms, although occasionally opioids may exacerbate headache by worsening hypercapnia. Benzodiazepines are often administered as well for relief of agitation and anxiety associated with terminal dyspnoea.

Patients' concepts of their illness have also been dramatically altered by the development of lung transplantation and heart–lung transplantation, despite the scarcity of available organs. Robinson and coworkers in our group (Robinson et al 1997) documented a dramatic increase in the use of intensive care units for end-of-life care since the beginning of a lung transplant programme at our hospital. Previously, the vast majority of patients died on the adolescent–young adult unit, not in the intensive care unit. In the current era, the majority of patients with advanced disease now die on a waiting list for lung transplantation. Non-invasive assisted ventilation is frequently tried. Home care for end-of-life care is rarely chosen by our patients with cystic fibrosis. Many patients report fear of suffocation; they prefer to be in hospital for end-of-life care, to ensure that they will receive adequate opioids and sedatives to relieve air hunger. This pattern of preference for in-hospital care is not universal; in other centres, a greater proportion of patients with cystic fibrosis die at home (Westwood 1998).

Neurodegenerative disorders

There are a wide range of neurologic or neuromuscular disorders among infants and children that may be associated with suffering (Hunt and Burne 1995) and/or a shortened life span. Although any one of these conditions is relatively rare, taken together, they affect considerable numbers of children who may require symptom management, palliative care, or end-of-life care. These disorders vary greatly in their effects on longevity and quality of life, and on their spectrum of cognitive versus motor impairments. Some disorders, such as Tay–Sachs disease, may cause profound cognitive and motor devastation and death in the first years of life. Conversely, patients with spinal muscular atrophy have intact intelligence and a range of motor impairments according to subtype. At the other end of the spectrum, Duchenne's muscular dystrophy leaves cognition intact and produces slowly progressive weakness, cardiomyopathy, and restrictive lung disease. Depending on its course and on the use of mechanical ventilation, many people with Duchenne's muscular dystrophy are now living well into their 20s.

Decision making in these disorders is complicated by several factors. Making a specific diagnosis in some cases is difficult or delayed. Even when a diagnosis is made, the prognosis can be extremely variable, with the same condition having either a rapidly progressive or slow clinical course (Davies 1996).

Many neurologic and neuromuscular disorders impair cognition and communication abilities. These factors may make it extremely difficult to determine whether the child is experiencing pain, and if so, to determine what is causing the pain.

Some children with neurodegenerative disorders may have persistent screaming or agitation with no apparent cause after extensive medical evaluation to exclude the common treatable causes, such as gastro-oesophageal reflux, hip dislocation, or otitis media. These children can be extraordinarily distressing to their parents, who want physicians to find what is causing the pain and fix it. Experience with drug trials suggests that many of these children remain agitated despite intravenous opioid titration to near-apnoea. Even when an opioid trial is ineffective for relieving pain, it may comfort the parents that an attempt was made to relieve distress. In contrast, some of these children with distress of unknown origin have reduced distress with anticonvulsants (especially those with sodium-channel blocking activity), even when there are no clinical or electroencephalographic signs of seizures. In other cases, the GABA agonist baclofen has appeared effective. There is a need for more systematic study of the roles and risk–benefit ratios of anticonvulsants and sedatives in children with unremitting agitation.

Mechanical ventilation is traditionally regarded as an invasive, painful, extreme, or extraordinary measure for many illnesses. Increasingly, many children with myopathies and other disorders characterized predominantly by motor weakness are now receiving mechanical ventilation both to prolong survival and to improve quality of life. Improvements in nasal or face-mask non-invasive positive pressure devices have made it possible in many cases to support the work of breathing and maintain lung volumes without the need for tracheotomy. Many children use these devices at night-time only, with sustained improvement in their sleep quality and daytime functioning. Non-invasive assisted ventilation may be insufficient for more severely affected children, particularly for those who can no longer control bulbar musculature.

Home, hospice, or hospital care

There is no single 'correct' location for end-of-life care. Children and their families should feel free to chose home, a free-standing hospice, a community hospital, or a paediatric tertiary hospital for end-of-life care (Stevens et al 1994; Frager 1996; Goldman 1996, 1998; Liben 1996; Dangel 1998).

Home has the advantage of a 'natural' and 'safe' environment where the child may feel loved, more in control of his or her surroundings, and less susceptible to the torments of medical intervention. World-wide experience from well-organized paediatric palliative care teams shows that they are able to provide services effectively, and most children and parents appear to feel safe and well-cared-for at home (Goldman 1996, Kopecky et al 1997). Conversely, families should not be 'pushed out the door' against their wishes.

Optimum home care requires planning for contingencies. Support from the local community including clergy can be extremely beneficial. Home care requires local solutions to practical problems, including availability of supplies (e.g., medications, oxygen, special beds). We cannot overemphasize the importance of anticipatory planning for adequate opioid availability. Children in remote areas may use up all their opioid on a weekend day, and be left in pain for extended periods of time. Direct contact with home care pharmacies and nurses can anticipate or fix these problems in many cases. Some pharmacies will accept faxed prescriptions in these situations.

For some children and families, there is a safety and security in continued care by physicians, nurses, psychologists, child life specialists, and others who have guided them through curative therapy. Because of this strong connection between families and their caregivers in paediatric tertiary centres, in many parts of the world a predominant model involves home care with ongoing connection to tertiary hospital specialist physicians and nurses who had previously been involved in curative care (Sirkia et al 1997). Another model involves transfer of care to specific palliative care physicians and nurses (Goldman 1996, 1998). There are few data to recommend one model over another.

Free-standing hospices have been established in many parts of the world, both as a place for children to come to for end-of-life care and as site for coordinating home care (Aquino and Perszyk 1997, Faulkner 1997, Deeley et al 1998, Thompson 1998). Paediatric free-standing hospices face challenges related to size of appropriate populations, staffing, finances, and relationship to paediatric medical centres.

One approach to facilitate staffing and coverage is to have these centres provide two distinct, but complementary services: (1) hospice/end-of-life care and (2) respite care for children with profound disabilities. Caring for a child with serious illness or major disabilities is physically and emotionally exhausting for parents.

Discussions regarding do-not-resuscitate and do-not-intubate orders and no heroic measures must be tailored to the child's particular prognosis, to the child's and parents' views of illness and cure, and to their coping and cognitive styles. Caregivers must be aware of ethnic and cultural differences in how families will respond to these discussions. Truth can be told in many ways (De Trill and Kovalcik 1997).

Deaths in intensive care units and in the operating room

Many neonates, infants, and children die in intensive care units. In some cases, critical illness and death have no warning, as for infants with sudden infant death syndrome or children following motor vehicle accidents. In other cases, death follows prenatal diagnosis (Pearson 1997), long-standing critical illness, or planned surgery with known risks, such as cardiac operations. Even in these technologically oriented settings, efforts can be made to relieve suffering, preserve dignity, and permit parents closeness to their child. Removal of mechanical ventilation need not produce air hunger and distress; terminal sedation and analgesia should be provided as a comfort measure, and parents should be permitted to hold their dying infant or child.

Bereavement programmes provide ongoing support and connection (Carroll and Griffin 1997). Parents respond differently to the loss of a child, and these differences in their patterns of grieving can strain marital relationships (Vance et al 1995).

Siblings of children with terminal illness confront a range of emotions, including sadness and grief, jealousy, and loneliness due to parents' directing more attention towards their sibling's needs, and guilt due to a mistaken fantasy that they may have caused their sibling's illness, and fear that a similar fate could befall them (Lehna 1995, Mahon and Page 1995, Gillance et al 1997).

Conclusions

Children with life-threatening illnesses should receive symptom management, emotional support and spiritual support that is adapted to their needs continuously from the time of diagnosis to end-of-life care. These approaches should be family-centred and should consider developmental and cultural factors. More research is needed on outcomes of different models of delivery of services. There is a need for more attention to supportive care for illnesses other than cancer, particularly neurodegenerative disorders.

References

Abbott K, Fowler-Kerry S 1995 The use of a topical refrigerant anesthetic to reduce injection pain in children. Journal of Pain and Symptom Management 10: 584–590

Anonymous 1993 American Academy of Pediatrics Committee on Hospital Care: child life programs. Pediatrics 91: 671–673

Aquino JY, Perszyk S 1997 Hospice Northeast and Nemours Children's Clinic, Jacksonville, Florida. American Journal of Hospice and Palliative Care 14: 248–250

Backonja M, Beydoun A, Edwards KR, Schwartz SL, Fonseca V, Hes M, LaMoreaux L, Garofalo E 1998 Gabapentin for the symptomatic treatment of painful neuropathy in patients with diabetes mellitus: a randomized controlled trial. Journal of the American Medical Association 280: 1831–1836

Beaver WT, Wallenstein S, Houde RW, Rogers A 1966 A comparison of the analgesic effects of methotrimeprazine and morphine in patients with cancer. Clinical Pharmacology and Therapeutics 7: 436–446

Berde C 1995 Pediatric oncology procedures: to sleep or perchance to dream. Pain 62: 1–2

Berde CB, Sethna NF, Fisher DE, Kahn CH, Chandler P, Grier HE 1990 Celiac plexus blockade for a 3-year-old boy with hepatoblastoma and refractory pain. Pediatrics. 86: 779–781

Berde CB, Beyer JE, Bournaki MC, Levin CR, Sethna NF 1991 Comparison of morphine and methadone for prevention of postoperative pain in 3- to 7-year-old children. Journal of Pediatrics 119: 136–141

Birmaher B 1998 Should we use antidepressant medications for children and adolescents with depressive disorders? Psychopharmacology Bulletin 34: 35–39

Bjerring P, Arendt-Nielsen L 1993 Depth and duration of skin analgesia to needle insertion after topical application of EMLA cream. British Journal of Anaesthesia 64: 173–177

Bouffet E, Douard MC, Annequin D, Castaing MC, Pichard-Leandri E 1996 Pain in lumbar puncture. Results of a 2-year discussion at the French Society of Pediatric Oncology. Archives de Pediatrie 3: 22–27

Bowsher D 1997 The effects of pre-emptive treatment of postherpetic neuralgia with amitriptyline: a randomized, double-blind, placebo-controlled trial. Journal of Pain and Symptom Management 13: 327–331

Brazelton TB, Thompson RH 1988 Child life. Pediatrics 81: 725–726

Brown DL, Bulley CK, Quiel EC 1987 Neurolytic celiac plexus block for pancreatic cancer pain. Anesthesia and Analgesia 66: 869–873

Bruera E, Brenneis C, Michaud M, MacMillan K, Hanson J, MacDonald RN 1988 Patient-controlled subcutaneous hydromorphone versus continuous subcutaneous infusion for the treatment of cancer pain. Journal of the National Cancer Institute 80: 1152–1154

Bruera E, Brenneis C, Paterson A, MacDonald R 1989 Use of methyphenidate as an adjuvant to narcotic analgesics in patients with advanced cancer. Journal of Pain and Symptom Management 4: 3–6

Camann WR, Murray RS, Mushlin PS, Lambert DH 1990 Effects of oral caffeine on postdural puncture headache. A double-blind, placebo-controlled trial. Anesthesia and Analgesia 70: 181–184

Carp H, Singh PJ, Vadhera R, Jayaram A 1994 Effects of the serotonin-receptor agonist sumatriptan on postdural puncture headache: report of six cases. Anesthesia and Analgesia 79: 180–182

Carrie LE 1993 Postdural puncture headache and extradural blood patch. British Journal of Anaesthesia 71: 179–181

Carroll ML, Griffin R 1997 Reframing life's puzzle: support for bereaved children. American Journal of Hospice and Palliative Care 14: 231–235

Choi A, Laurito CE, Cunningham FE 1996 Pharmacologic management of postdural puncture headache. Annals of Pharmacotherapy 30: 831–839

Collins JJ, Berde CB 1997 Pain management. In: Pizzo PA, Poplack DG (eds) Principles and practice of pediatric oncology. Lippincott–Raven, Philadelphia, pp 1183–1199

Collins JJ, Kerner J, Sentivany S, Berde CB 1995 Intravenous amitriptyline in pediatrics. Journal of Pain and Symptom Management 10: 471–475

Collins JJ, Geake J, Grier HE, Houck CS, Thaler HT, Weinstein HJ, Twum-Danso NY, Berde CB 1996a Patient-controlled analgesia for mucositis pain in children: a three-period crossover study comparing morphine and hydromorphone. Journal of Pediatrics 129: 722–728

Collins JJ, Grier HE, Sethna NF, Wilder RT, Berde CB 1996b Regional anesthesia for pain associated with terminal pediatric malignancy. Pain 65: 63–69

Cote CJ 1994 Sedation for the pediatric patient. A review. Pediatric Clinics of North America 41: 31–58

Coyle N, Adelhardt J, Foley KM, Portenoy RK 1990 Character of terminal illness in the advanced cancer patient: pain and other symptoms during the last four weeks of life [see comments]. Journal of Pain and Symptom Management 5: 83–93

Dangel T 1998 Chronic pain management in children. Part I: cancer and phantom pain. Paediatric Anaesthesia 8: 5–10

Davies H 1996 Living with dying: families coping with a child who has a neurodegenerative genetic disorder. Axone 18: 38–44

de las Heras-Rosas MA, Rodriguez-Perez A, Ojeda-Betancor N, Boralla-Rivera G, Gallego-Alonso JI 1997 Failure of sumatripta in post-dural puncture headache. Revista Espanola de Anestesiologia y Reanimacion 44: 378–379

De Trill M, Kovalcik R 1997 The child with cancer. Influence of culture on truth-telling and patient care. Annals of the New York Academy of Sciences 809: 197–210

Deeley L, Stallard P, Lewis M, Lenton S 1998 Palliative care services for children must adopt a family centred approach. British Medical Journal 317: 284

Doyle E, Freeman J, Im NT, Morton NS 1993 An evaluation of a new self-adhesive patch preparation of amethocaine for topical anaesthesia prior to venous cannulation in children. Anaesthesia 48: 1050–1052

Eisenach JC, DuPen S, Dubois M, Miguel R, Allin D 1995 Epidural clonidine analgesia for intractable cancer pain. The Epidural Clonidine Study Group. Pain 61: 391–399

Eisenberg E, Berkey CS, Carr DB et al 1994 Efficacy and safety of nonsteroidal antiinflammatory drugs for cancer pain: a meta-analysis. Journal of Clinical Oncology 12: 2756–2765

Faulkner KW 1997 Pediatric hospice reference library. American Journal of Hospice and Palliative Care 14: 228–230

Fine P, Marcus M, De Boer A, Van der Oord B 1991 An open label study of oral transmucosal fentanyl citrate (OTFC) for the treatment of breakthrough cancer pain. Pain 45: 149–153

Foley KM 1997 Competent care for the dying instead of physician-assisted suicide. New England Journal of Medicine 336: 54–58

Frager G 1996 Pediatric palliative care: building the model, bridging the gaps. Journal of Palliative Care 12: 9–12

Frankville DD, Spear RM, Dyck JB 1993 The dose of propofol required to prevent children from moving during magnetic resonance imaging. Anesthesiology 79: 953–958

Gamis AS, Knapp JF, Glenski JA 1989 Nitrous oxide analgesia in a pediatric emergency department. Annals of Emergency Medicine 18: 177–181

Gauvain-Piquard A, Rodary C, Rezvani A, Lemerle J 1984 Development of a new rating scale for the evaluation of pain in young children (2–6 years) with cancer. In: Rizzi R, Visentin M (eds) Pain. Piccin/Butterworths, Padua, Italy, pp 383–390

Gauvain-Piquard A, Rodary C, Rezvani A, Lemerle J 1987 Pain in children aged 2–6 years: a new observational rating scale elaborated in a pediatric oncology unit—preliminary report. Pain 31: 177–188

Gillance H, Tucker A, Aldridge J, Wright JB 1997 Bereavement: providing support for siblings. Paediatric Nursing 9: 22–24

Gillin S, Sorkin LS 1998 Gabapentin reverses the allodynia produced by the administration of anti-GD2 ganglioside, an immunotherapeutic drug, Anesthesia and Analgesia 86: 111–116

Goldman A 1996 Home care of the dying child. Journal of Palliative Care 12: 16–19

Goldman A 1998 ABC of palliative care. Special problems of children. British Medical Journal 316: 49–52

Green SM, Rothrock SG 1997 Transient apnea with intramuscular ketamine. American Journal of Emergency Medicine 15: 440–441

Greenberg HS, Kim J, Posner JB 1980 Epidural spinal cord compression from metastatic tumor: results with a new treatment protocol. Annals of Neurology 8: 361–366

Grossman M 1988 Children with AIDS. Infectious Disease Clinics of North America 2: 533–541

Hahn YS, McLone DG 1984 Pain in children with spinal chord tumors. Child's Brain 11: 36–46

Halperin DL, Koren G, Attias D, Pellegrini E, Greenberg ML, Wyss M 1989 Topical skin anesthesia for venous, subcutaneous drug reservoir and lumbar punctures in children. Pediatrics 84: 281–284

Hill HF, Mackie AM, Coda BA, Iverson K, Chapman CR 1991 Patient-controlled analgesic administration. A comparison of steady-state morphine infusions with bolus doses. Cancer 67: 873–882

Hirschfeld S, Moss H, Dragisic K, Smith W, Pizzo PA 1996 Pain in pediatric human immunodeficiency virus infection: incidence and characteristics in a single-institution pilot study. Pediatrics 98: 449–452

Hollman GA, Perloff WH 1995 Efficacy of oral ketamine for providing sedation and analgesia to children requiring laceration repair. Pediatric Emergency Care 11: 399

Hunt A, Burne R 1995 Medical and nursing problems of children with neurodegenerative disease. Palliative Medicine 9: 19–26

Hunt A, Joel S, Dick G, Goldman A 1999 Population pharmacokinetics of oral morphine and its glucuronides in children receiving morphine as immediate-release liquid or sustained-release tablets for cancer pain. Journal of Pediatrics 135: 47–55

Jay SM, Ozolins M, Elliot C, Caldwell S 1983 Assessment of children's distress during painful medical procedures. Journal of Health Psychology 2: 133–147

Jay S, Elliot C, Katz E, Siegal S 1987 Cognitive-behavioral and pharmacologic interventions for children's distress during painful medical procedures. Journal of Consulting and Clinical Psychology 55: 860–865

Jay S, Elliott CH, Fitzgibbons I, Woody P, Siegel S 1995 A comparative study of cognitive behavior therapy versus general anesthesia for painful medical procedures in children. Pain 62: 3–9

Joranson DE, Gilson AM 1998 Regulatory barriers to pain management. Seminars in Oncology Nursing 14: 158–63

Kapelushnik V, Koren G, Solh H, Greenberg M, DeVeber L 1990 Evaluating the efficacy of EMLA in alleviating pain associated with lumbar puncture: comparison of open and double-blinded protocols in children. Pain 42: 31–34

Katz ER, Kellerman J, Siegel SE 1980 Behavioral distress in children with cancer undergoing medical procedures: developmental considerations. Journal of Consulting Care 48: 356–365

Kopecky EA, Jacobson S, Joshi P, Martin M, Koren G 1997 Review of a home-based palliative care program for children with malignant and non-malignant diseases. Journal of Palliative Care 13: 28–33

Krane EJ, Heller LB, Pomietto ML 1991 Incidence of phantom sensation and pain in pediatric amputees. Anesthesiology 75: A691

Kuttner L 1989 Management of young children's acute pain and anxiety during invasive medical procedures. Pediatrician 16: 39–44

Larson PJ, Miaskowski C, MacPhail L, Dodd MJ, Greenspan D, Dibble SL, Paul SM, Ignoffo R 1998 The PRO-SELF Mouth Aware program: an effective approach for reducing chemotherapy-induced mucositis. Cancer Nursing 21: 263–268

Lehna CR 1995 Children's descriptions of their feelings and what they found helpful during bereavement. American Journal of Hospice and Palliative Care 12: 24–30

Lewis DW, Packer RJ, Raney B, Rak IW, Belasco J, Lange B 1986 Incidence, presentation, and outcome of spinal cord disease in children with systematic cancer. Pediatrics 78: 438–443

Liben S 1996 Pediatric palliative medicine: obstacles to overcome. Journal of Palliative Care 12: 24–28

Litman RS 1997 Apnea and oxyhemoglobin desaturation after intramuscular ketamine administration in a 2-year-old child. American Journal of Emergency Medicine 15: 547–548

Litman RS, Berkowitz RJ, Ward DS 1996 Levels of consciousness and ventilatory parameters in young children during sedation with oral midazolam and nitrous oxide. Archives of Pediatrics and Adolescent Medicine 150: 671–675

Litman RS, Kottra JA, Berkowitz RJ, Ward DS 1997 Breathing patterns and levels of consciousness in children during administration of nitrous oxide after oral midazolam premedication. Journal of Oral and Maxillofacial Surgery 55: 1372–1377; discussion 1378–1379

Mackie AM, Coda BC, Hill HF 1991 Adolescents use patient-controlled analgesia effectively for relief from prolonged oropharyngeal mucositis pain. Pain 46: 265–269

Mahon MM, Page ML 1995 Childhood bereavement after the death of a sibling. Holistic Nursing Practice 9: 15–26

Marx CM, Stein J, Tyler MK, Nieder ML, Shurin SB, Blumer JL 1997 Ketamine-midazolam versus meperidine-midazolam for painful procedures in pediatric oncology patients. Journal of Clinical Oncology 15: 94–102

Matson DD 1969 Neurosurgery of infancy and childhood, 2nd edn. Thomas, Springfield, IL, pp 847–851

Maunuksela E, Korpela R 1986 Double-blind evaluation of a lignocaine-prilocaine cream (EMLA) in children. Effect on the pain associated with venous cannulation. British Journal of Anaesthesia 58: 1242–1245

Maunuksela EL, Rajantie J, Siimes MA 1986 Flunitrazepam-fentanyl-induced sedation and analgesia for bone marrow aspiration and needle biopsy in children. Acta Anaesthesiologica Scandinavica 30: 409–411

Maxwell LG, Yaster M 1996 The myth of conscious sedation. Archives of Pediatrics and Adolescent Medicine 150: 665–667

Melzack R, Israel R, Lacroix R, Schultz G 1997 Phantom limbs in people with congenital limb deficiency or amputation in early childhood. Brain 120: 1603–1620

Mercadante S 1993 Celiac plexus block versus analgesics in pancreatic cancer pain. Pain 52: 187–192

Miser AW, Miser JS, Clark BS 1980 Continuous intravenous infusion of morphine sulfate for control of severe pain in children with terminal malignancy. Journal of Pediatrics 96: 930–932

Miser AW, Davis DM, Hughes CS, Mulne AF, Miser JS 1983 Continuous subcutaneous infusion of morphine in children with cancer. American Journal of Diseases of Children 137: 383–385

Miser AW, Dothage JA, Wesley M, Miser JS 1987a The prevalence of pain in a pediatric and young adult cancer population. Pain 29: 73–83

Miser AW, McCalla J, Dothage JA, Wesley M, Miser JS 1987b Pain as a presenting symptom in children and young adults with newly diagnosed malignancy. Pain 29: 85–90

Miser AW, Ayash D, Broda E et al 1988 Use of a patient controlled device for nitrous oxide administration to control procedure related pain in children and young adults with cancer. Clinical Journal of Pain 4: 5–10

Miser AW, Goh TS, Dose AM, O'Fallon JR, Niedringhaus RD, Betcher DL, Simmons P, MacKellar DJ, Arnold M, Loprinzi CL 1994 Trial of a topically administered local anesthetic (EMLA cream) for pain relief during central venous port accesses in children with cancer. Journal of Pain and Symptom Management 9: 259–264

Mitchell RK, Koury SI, Stone CK 1996 Respiratory arrest after intramuscular ketamine in a 2-year-old child. American Journal of Emergency Medicine 14: 580–581

Parker RI, Mahan RA, Giugliano D, Parker MM 1997 Efficacy and safety of intravenous midazolam and ketamine as sedation for therapeutic and diagnostic procedures in children. Pediatrics 99: 427–431

Patt R, Lustik S, Litman R 1993 The use of transdermal fentanyl in a six-year-old patient with neuroblastoma and diffuse abdominal pain. Journal of Pain and Symptom Management 8: 317–319

Patt R, Payne R, Farhat G, Reddy S 1995 Subarachnoid neurolytic block under general anesthesia in a 3-year-old with neuroblastoma. Clinical Journal of Pain 11: 143–146

Payne R 1992 Transdermal fentanyl: suggested recommendations for clinical use. Journal of Pain and Symptom Management 7: S40–S44

Pearson L 1997 Family-centered care and the anticipated death of a newborn. Pediatric Nursing 23: 178–182

Peterfreund RA, Datta S, Ostheimer GW 1989 pH adjustment of local anesthetic solutions with sodium bicarbonate: laboratory evaluation of alkalinization and precipitation. Regional Anesthesia 14: 265–270

Plancarte R, Amescua C, Patt RB, Aldrete JA 1990 Superior hypogastric plexus block for pelvic cancer pain. Anesthesiology 73: 236–239

Plummer JL, Gourlay GK, Cherry DA, Cousins MJ 1988 Estimation of methadone clearance: application in the management of cancer pain. Pain 33: 313–322

Plummer JL, Cherry DA, Cousins MJ, Gourlay GK, Onley MM, Evans KH 1991 Long-term spinal administration of morphine in cancer and non-cancer pain: a retrospective study. Pain 44: 215–220

Quill TE, Dresser R, Brock DW 1997 The rule of double effect—a critique of its role in end-of-life decision making. New England Journal of Medicine 337: 1768–1771

Qureshi FA, Mellis PT, McFadden MA 1995 Efficacy of oral ketamine for providing sedation and analgesia to children requiring laceration repair. Pediatric Emergency Care 11: 93–97

Ravilly S, Robinson W, Suresh S, Wohl ME, Berde CB 1996 Chronic pain in cystic fibrosis. Pediatrics 98: 741–747

Ripamonti C, Groff L, Brunelli C, Polastri D, Stavrakis A, De Conno F 1998 Switching from morphine to oral methadone in treating cancer pain: what is the equianalgesic dose ratio. Journal of Clinical Oncology 16: 3216–3221

Robinson WM, Ravilly S, Berde C, Wohl ME 1997 End-of-life care in cystic fibrosis. Pediatrics 100: 205–209

Roelofse JA, Roelofse PG 1997 Oxygen desaturation in a child receiving a combination of ketamine and midazolam for dental extractions. Anesthesia Progress 44: 68–70

Rossitch E, Madsen JR 1993 Neurosurgical procedures for relief of

pain in children and adolescents. In: Schechter NI, Berde CB, Yaster M (eds) Pain in infants, children and adolescents. Williams and Wilkins, Baltimore, pp 237–243
Rowbotham MC, Reisner-Keller LA, Fields HL 1991 Both intravenous lidocaine and morphine reduce the pain of postherpetic neuralgia. Neurology 41: 1024–1028
Rowbotham M, Harden N, Stacey B, Bernstein P, Magnus-Miller L 1998 Gabapentin for the treatment of postherpetic neuralgia: a randomized controlled trial. Journal of the American Medical Association 280: 1837–1842
Ruffin JE, Creed JM, Jarvis C 1997 A retreat for families of children recently diagnosed with cancer. Cancer Practice 5: 99–104
Rusy LM, Troshynski TJ, Weisman SJ 2001 Gabapentin in phantom limb pain management in children and young adults: report of seven cases. Journal of Pain and Symptom Management 21: 78–82
Schechter N, Weisman S, Rosenblum M, Bernstein B, Conard P 1995 The use of oral transmucosal fentanyl citrate for painful procedures in children. Pediatrics 95: 335–339
Schechter NL, Blankson V, Pachter LM, Sullivan CM, Costa L 1997 The ouchless place: no pain, children's gain. Pediatrics 99: 890–894
Sievers TD, Yee JD, Foley ME, Blanding PJ, Berde CB 1991 Midazolam for conscious sedation during pediatric oncology procedures: safety and recovery parameters. Pediatrics 88: 1172–1179
Sirkia K, Saarinen UM, Ahlgren B, Hovi L 1997 Terminal care of the child with cancer at home. Acta Paediatrica 86: 1125–1130
Staats PS, Kost-Byerly S 1995 Celiac plexus blockade in a 7-year-old child with neuroblastoma. Journal of Pain and Symptom Management 10: 321–324
Steggles S, Damore-Petingola S, Maxwell J, Lightfool N 1997 Hypnosis for children and adolescents with cancer: an annotated bibliography, 1985–1995. Journal of Pediatric Oncology Nursing 14: 27–32
Steingard RJ, DeMaso DR, Goldman SJ, Shorrock KL, Bucci JP 1995 Current perspectives on the pharmacotherapy of depressive disorders in children and adolescents. Harvard Review of Psychiatry 2: 313–326
Stevens M, Dalla Pozza L, Cavalletto B, Cooper M, Kilham H 1994 Pain and symptom control in paediatric palliative care. Cancer Surveys 21: 211–231
Symonds RP 1998 Treatment-induced mucositis: an old problem with new remedies. British Journal of Cancer 77: 1689–1695
Thompson M 1998 Children's hospices: 15 years on. Paediatric Nursing 10: 24
Tobias JD, Oakes L, Rao B 1992 Continuous epidural anesthesia for postoperative analgesia in the pediatric oncology patient. American Journal of Pediatric Hematology and Oncology 14: 216–221
Truog RD, Berde CB, Mitchell C, Grier HE 1992 Barbiturates in the care of the terminally ill. New England Journal of Medicine 327: 1678–1682
Valentin N, Bech B 1996 Ketamine anaesthesia for electrocochleography in children. Are psychic side effects really rare? Scandinavian Audiology 25: 39–43
Van Gerven M, Van Hemelrijck J, Wouters P, Vandermeersch E, Van Aken H 1992 Light anaesthesia with propofol for paediatric MRI. Anaesthesia 47: 706–707
Vance JC, Boyle FM, Najman JM, Thearle MJ 1995 Gender differences in parental psychological distress following perinatal death or sudden infant death syndrome. British Journal of Psychiatry 167: 806–811
Watanabe S, Bruera E 1994 Corticosteroids as adjuvant analgesics. Journal of Pain and Symptom Management 9: 442–445
Watson CP, Babul N 1998 Efficacy of oxycodone in neuropathic pain: a randomized trial in postherpetic neuralgia. Neurology 50: 1837–1841
Watson CP, Vernich L, Chipman M, Reed K 1998 Nortriptyline versus amitriptyline in postherpetic neuralgia: a randomized trial. Neurology 51: 1166–1171
Weisman SJ, Bernstein B, Schechter NL 1998 Consequences of inadequate analgesia during painful procedures in children. Archives of Pediatrics and Adolescent Medicine 152: 147–149
Westwood AT 1998 Terminal care in cystic fibrosis: hospital versus home. Pediatrics 102: 436; discussion 436–437
Wolfe J, Grier HE, Klar N, Levin SB, Ellenbogen JM, Salem-Schatz S, Emanuel EJ, Weeks JC 2000 Symptoms and suffering at the end of life in children with cancer. New England Journal of Medicine 342 326–333
Wood MJ, Kay R, Dworkin RH, Soong SJ, Whitley RJ 1996 Oral acyclovir therapy accelerates pain resolution in patients with herpes zoster: a meta-analysis of placebo-controlled trials. Clinical Infectious Diseases 22: 341–347
Yee JD, Berde CB 1994 Dextroamphetamine or methylphenidate as adjuvants to opioid analgesia for adolescents with cancer. Journal of Pain and Symptom Management 9: 122–125
Zech D, Grond S, Lynch J, Dauer H, Stollenwerk B, Lehmann K 1992 Transdermal fentanyl and initial dose-finding with patient-controlled analgesia in cancer pain. A pilot study with 20 terminally ill cancer patients. Pain 50: 293–301
Zeltzer L, Jay S, Fisher D 1989 The management of pain associated with pediatric procedures. Pediatric Clinics of North America 36: 941–964
Zeltzer L, Regalado M, Nichter LS, Barton D, Jennings S, Pitt L 1991 Iontophoresis versus subcutaneous injection: a comparison of two methods of local anesthesia delivery in children. Pain 44: 73–78
Zucker TP, Flesche CW, Germing U, Schroter S, Willers R, Wolf HH, Heyll A 1998 Patient-controlled versus staff-controlled analgesia with pethidine after allogeneic bone marrow transplantation. Pain 75: 305–312

Chapter 45

Cancer pain and AIDS-related pain: psychiatric and ethical issues

William Breitbart, Steven D Passik, and Barry D Rosenfeld

Introduction

The cancer patient faces a wide range of psychological and physical stressors throughout the course of illness. These stressors include fears of a painful death, physical disability, disfigurement, and growing dependency on others. Although such fears exist in most, if not all cancer patients, the degree of psychological distress experienced varies greatly between individuals and depends in part on the patient's personality style, coping abilities, available social supports, and medical factors (Holland and Rowland 1989). One of the most feared consequences of cancer, however, is the potential for pain. Pain has a profound impact on a patient's level of emotional distress, and psychological factors such as mood, anxiety, and the meaning attributed to pain can intensify a patient's experience of cancer pain (Ahles et al 1983). Because of the relationship between psychological factors and pain experience, clinicians who treat patients with cancer pain face complex diagnostic and therapeutic challenges. The appropriate management of cancer pain therefore requires a multidisciplinary approach, recognizing the importance of accurate diagnosis and treatment of concurrent psychological symptoms and psychiatric syndromes (Breitbart 1989a). This chapter reviews the common psychological issues and psychiatric complications (e.g., anxiety, depression, delirium) seen in cancer pain patients and provides guidelines for their assessment and management. Finally, the problem of pain in AIDS is addressed with special focus on psychiatric issues in pain assessment and management.

Psychological impact of cancer and the role of pain

A cancer diagnosis is typically followed by a series of emotional responses that appear quite consistent across many studies, settings, and patient populations (Massie and Holland 1987, Breitbart and Holland 1988, Breitbart 1989a). The initial responses usually consist of shock, denial, and disbelief, which typically evolve into a period of anxiety and/or depression. Disturbed sleep, diminished appetite and impaired concentration, irritability, pervasive thoughts about cancer, and fears about the future often interfere with normal daily activities. These 'stress responses' generally occur at specific points in the course of cancer and its treatment: after diagnosis, with relapse, prior to diagnostic tests, surgery, radiation, and chemotherapy, as well as after treatment has concluded and patients enter the phase of survivorship. Distress usually resolves slowly over a period of several weeks, and patients gradually return to their prior level of homeostasis once the patient's emotional resources have been marshalled and supports have been rallied, although many patients require clinical intervention (e.g., anxiolytic or sedative medications, relaxation techniques) in order to regain their previous level of functioning. For most patients, the support of family and friends, social workers, clergy, and hospital staff are sufficient to cope with these brief crisis periods.

The degree of psychological distress observed in cancer patients also varies considerably between individuals. Some patients experience persistently high levels of anxiety and depression for weeks or months, which significantly impede their ability to function, or at times, even comply with cancer treatment. Others experience only mild or transient symptoms that remit rapidly even without intervention. A number of factors influence this variability, including the presence and degree of pain, stage of disease, pre-existing psychiatric disorders, coping abilities, and level of social support. When significant levels of distress do occur in response to cancer diagnosis or treatment, these reactions often require mental health intervention. For the most part, however, physicians treating cancer patients are confronted with psychologically healthy individuals who are reacting to the stresses imposed by cancer and its treatment. Nearly 90% of the psychiatric disorders observed in cancer patients are thought to represent reactions to or manifestations of the disease or treatments rather than an extension of a pre-existing mental disorder (Derogatis et al 1983, Massie and Holland 1987). One of the most distressing elements of a cancer diagnosis is the anticipation of pain, and the lay public typically believes that pain is a common, if not inevitable, consequence of cancer (Levin et al 1985). Yet only about 15% of cancer patients without metastatic disease report significant pain (Kanner and Foley 1981, Daut and Cleeland 1982), although this proportion climbs dramatically in the presence of advanced disease, with between 60 and 90% of all patients with metastatic disease reporting debilitating pain and as many as 25% of all cancer patients die while still experiencing considerable pain (Foley 1975, 1985; Twycross and Lack 1983; Cleeland 1984).

Not only does pain have a profound impact on psychological distress in cancer patients, psychological factors appear to influence the experience and intensity of cancer pain. Psychological factors such as perceived control, meaning attributed to the pain experience, fear of death, hopelessness, and anxious or depressed mood all appear to contribute to the experience of cancer pain and suffering (Bond 1979, Spiegel and Bloom 1983a, Ahles et al 1983). For example, in a study of women with metastatic breast cancer, Spiegel and Bloom (1983a) found that although the site of metastasis did not predict the intensity of pain report, greater depression and the belief that pain represented the spread of disease (e.g., the meaning attributed to the pain) corresponded to greater levels of pain experienced. Daut and Cleeland (1982) also found that cancer patients who believed that their pain represented disease progression reported significantly more interference with their ability to function and enjoy daily activities than did patients who attributed their pain to a benign cause. Other research has demonstrated that patients with advanced disease who report high levels of emotional distress also report more pain (Bond and Pearson 1969, Bond 1973, McKegney et al 1981).

Current models of cancer pain emphasize the multidimensional nature of the pain experience, incorporating the contributions of cognitive, motivational, behavioural, and affective components in addition to sensory (nociceptive) phenomena. This multidimensional formulation of cancer pain has opened the door to psychiatric and psychological participation in pain research, assessment, and treatment (Melzack and Wall 1983, Lindblom et al 1986). Pain is no longer considered simply a nociceptive event, but is recognized as a psychological process involving nociception, perception, and expression. Because of the important role played by psychological factors in the experience of cancer pain, appropriate and effective management of cancer pain requires a multidisciplinary approach that incorporates neurology, neurosurgery, anaesthesiology, and rehabilitative medicine in addition to psychiatrists and/or psychologists (Foley 1975, 1985; Breitbart 1989a). The challenge of untangling and addressing both the physical and psychological issues involved in cancer pain is essential to developing a rational and effective management strategy. Psychosocial therapies directed primarily at psychological variables have a profound impact on nociception, while somatic therapies directed at nociception have beneficial effects on psychological sequelae of cancer pain. Ideally such somatic and psychosocial therapies are used simultaneously in a multidisciplinary approach to cancer pain management (Breitbart 1989a, Breitbart and Holland 1990, Ahles and Martin 1992).

Unfortunately, psychological variables are too often proposed as the sole explanation for continued pain reports or lack of response to conventional therapies, when in fact medical factors have not been adequately appreciated or examined. The psychiatrist or psychologist is often the last member of the treatment team to be asked to consult on a cancer patient with unrelieved pain and, in that role, must be vigilant that an accurate pain diagnosis is made. They also must be capable of assessing the adequacy of the medical analgesic management provided. In this context, psychological distress in patients with cancer pain should be initially assumed to be the consequence of uncontrolled pain since personality traits may appear distorted or exaggerated by the presence of pain and the pain relief often results in the disappearance of a perceived psychiatric disorder (Marks and Sachar 1973, Cleeland 1984).

Psychiatric disorders in cancer pain patients: assessment and management

A number of psychiatric disorders are common among patients with cancer and the frequency of most of these disorders increases in the context of pain (e.g., Woodforde and Fielding 1970, Ahles et al 1983). The Psychosocial Collaborative Oncology Group, which described the prevalence of psychiatric disorders in cancer patients (Table 45.1), noted that 39% of patients with a psychiatric diagnosis also reported experiencing significant pain, while only 19% of patients without a psychiatric diagnosis reported significant pain (Derogatis et al 1983). The most frequent diagnoses included adjustment disorder with depressed or anxious mood, major depression, and delirium.

However, assessing the mental state of a cancer patient is greatly confounded by the presence of pain. Because of the potentially confounding influence of pain on a patient's psychological state, it is imperative that the patient be reassessed after pain has been adequately controlled in order to determine whether a psychiatric disorder is indeed present. When present, the management of psychiatric complications of cancer pain is essential to maintaining an optimal quality of life. For cancer pain patients, interventions that help decrease mood disturbance also help to reduce pain. A multidisciplinary approach, incorporating psychotherapeutic, behavioural, and psychopharmacological interventions, is the optimal method for treating psychiatric complications in cancer pain patients. Treatment decisions, however, are predicated on the assumption that a thorough medical and psychiatric assessment has led to an accurate diagnosis, thus allowing specific and effective intervention. The management of specific psychiatric disorders such as depression, delirium, and anxiety in cancer patients (including those with pain) has been reviewed in detail in *Handbook of Psychiatry in Palliative Medicine* edited by Breitbart and Chochinov (2000), *Handbook of Psychooncology* edited by Holland and Rowland (1989), *Psychooncology* edited by Holland et al (1998), and other sources (Massie and Holland 1987, 1990; Breitbart

Table 45.1 Rates of DSM-III psychiatric disorders and prevalence of pain observed in 215 cancer patients from three cancer centres[a]

Diagnostic category	Number in diagnostic class	Psychiatric diagnoses (%)	Number with significant pain[b]
Adjustment disorders	69 (32%)	68	
Major affective disorders	13 (6%)	13	
Organic mental disorders	8 (4%)	8	
Personality disorders	7 (3%)	7	
Anxiety disorders	4 (2%)	4	
Total with DSM-III psychiatric disorder diagnosis	101 (47%)		39 (39%)
Total without DSM-III psychiatric disorder diagnosis	114 (53%)		21 (19%)
Total patient population	215 (100%)		60 (28%)

[a]Adapted from Derogatis et al (1983).
[b]Score greater than 50 mm on a 100-mm VAS for pain severity.

and Holland 1988, Holland 1989). A brief guide to the diagnosis and management of these disorders is presented below.

Depression in cancer pain patients

Depression occurs in roughly 20–25% of all cancer patients and the prevalence increases with higher levels of disability, advanced illness, and pain (Plumb and Holland 1977, Bukberg et al 1984, Massie and Holland 1990). Because somatic symptoms of depression (e.g., anorexia, insomnia, fatigue, and weight loss) are often present in cancer patients, these symptoms are less reliable as indicators of depression, and cognitive/affective symptoms (e.g., dysphoric mood, hopelessness, worthlessness, guilt, suicidal ideation) are given greater weight (Plumb and Holland 1977, Endicott 1983, Bukberg et al 1984, Massie and Holland 1990). In addition, patients with a history of previous depressive episodes, or a family history of depression, are at greater risk for depression in response to cancer or cancer-related pain. Once the presence of depressive symptomatology has been established, evaluation of potential 'organic' etiologies is prudent and, if present, would require treatment before addressing the depression per se. Among the possible causes of an organic depression include treatment with corticosteroids (Stiefel et al 1989), chemotherapeutic agents (vincristine, vinblastine, asparaginase, intrathecal methotrexate, interferon, interleukin) (Holland et al 1974, Young 1982, Adams et al 1984, Denicoff et al 1987), amphotericin (Weddington 1982), whole-brain radiation (DeAngelis et al 1989), central nervous system metabolic–endocrinological complications (Breitbart 1989b), and paraneoplastic syndromes (Posner 1988, Patchell and Posner 1989).

Treatment of depression

Depressed cancer pain patients are usually treated with a combination of antidepressant medications, supportive psychotherapy, and cognitive-behavioural techniques (Massie and Holland 1990, Massie and Popkin 1998). Many of these techniques are useful in the management of psychological distress in cancer patients and have been applied to the treatment of depressive and anxious symptoms related to cancer and cancer pain. Psychotherapeutic interventions, in the form of either individual or group therapy, have been shown to effectively reduce psychological distress and depressive symptoms in cancer pain patients (Spiegel et al 1981; Spiegel and Bloom 1983a, b; Massie et al 1989). Cognitive-behavioural interventions, such as relaxation, distraction with pleasant imagery, and cognitive restructuring, also appear to be effective in reducing symptomatology in patients with mild to moderate levels of depression (Holland et al 1991). Psychopharmacological interventions (i.e., antidepressant medications), however, are the mainstay of symptom management in cancer patients with severe depressive symptoms (Massie and Popkin 1998). The efficacy of antidepressants in the treatment of depression in cancer patients, including those with or without pain, has been well established in case observations and clinical trials (Purohit et al 1978; Costa et al 1985; Popkin et al 1985; Rifkin et al 1985; Massie and Holland 1987, 1990; Breitbart and Holland 1988; Breitbart 1989a). Antidepressant medications used in cancer pain patients are listed in Table 45.2.

Tricyclic antidepressants

Although long considered the gold standard for treatment of depression, tricyclic antidepressants (TCAs) have gradually lost their preferred status for most patients with cancer. When used, TCAs are often selected because of their side effect profile (e.g., when sedation or weight gain is desired), although, as always when implementing pharmacological interventions with cancer patients, concerns regarding potential drug interactions must be addressed. For example, because some TCAs are highly anticholinergic, patients receiving multiple drugs with anticholinergic properties (e.g., meperidine, atropine, diphenhydramine, phenothiazines) are at risk for developing an anticholinergic delirium. When used with cancer patients, treatment is typically initiated at low dose (10–25 mg at bedtime) and slowly increased by 10–25 mg every 1–2 days until a therapeutic effect has been achieved. Depressed cancer patients often respond to doses considerably lower (25–125 mg orally) than those typically required by the physically healthy (150–300 mg o.d.).

Selective serotonin reuptake inhibitors

Since breaking into the antidepressant market in the 1980s, the SSRIs have gradually emerged as the first-line treatment for most patients with depression, whether or not they are also diagnosed with cancer. In fact, the SSRIs have a number of advantages that often make them a preferred choice for the first-line treatment in cancer settings. Not only have SSRIs consistently been demonstrated to

Table 45.2 Antidepressant medications used in cancer pain patients[a]

Generic name	Approximate daily dosage range (mg)[b]	Route[b]
Tricyclic antidepressants		
Amitriptyline	10–150	PO, IM, PR
Doxepin	12.5–150	PO, IM
Imipramine	12.5–150	PO, IM
Desipramine	12.5–150	PO, IM
Nortriptyline	10–125	PO
Clomipramine	10–150	PO
Second-generation antidepressants		
Buproprion	200–450	PO
Buproprion SR	150-300	PO
Trazodone	25–300	PO
Serotonin specific reuptake inhibitors		
Fluoxetine	20–60	PO
Sertraline	50–200	PO
Paroxetine	10–40	PO
Citalopram	10-60	PO
Fluvoxamine	50-300	PO
Nefazodone	50–500	PO
Serotonin/noradrenaline reuptake inhibitors		
Venlafaxine	37.5–450	PO
Heterocyclic antidepressants		
Maprotiline	50–75	PO
Amoxapine	100–150	PO
Monoamine oxidase inhibitors		
Isocarboxazid	20–40	PO
Phenelzine	30–60	PO
Tranylcypromine	20–40	PO
Psychostimulants		
Dextroamphetamine	2.5–20 b.i.d.	PO
Methylphenidate	2.5–20 b.i.d.	PO
Pemoline	37.5–75 b.i.d.	PO, SL[c]
Modafinil	100-400	PO
Benzodiazepines		
Alprazolam	0.25–2.0 t.i.d.	PO
Lithium carbonate	600–1200	PO

[a]Adapted from Massie and Holland (1990).
[b]PO = peroral; IM = intramuscular; PR = per rectum; SL = sublingual; SR = sustained release; b.i.d. = two times a day; t.i.d. = three times a day; intravenous infusions of a number of tricyclic antidepressants are utilized outside of the USA; this route is, however, not FDA approved.
[c]Available in chewable tablet form that can be absorbed without swallowing.

be as effective in the treatment of depression as TCAs (e.g., Mendels 1987) but their side effect profile is often advantageous for those patients with advanced disease. For example, SSRIs have a low affinity for adrenergic, cholinergic, and histamine receptors, thus accounting for negligible orthostatic hypotension, urinary retention, memory impairment, sedation, or reduced awareness (Popkin et al 1985). They have not been found to cause clinically significant alterations in cardiac conduction and are generally favourably tolerated along with a wider margin of safety than the TCAs in the event of an overdose. While not without possible side effects (e.g., loose stools, nausea, vomiting, insomnia, headaches, and sexual dysfunction), these side effects tend to be dose related and may be problematical for patients with advanced disease. Moreover, of the available SSRSs, only fluoxetine has a potent active metabolite—norfluoxetine—whose elimination half-life is 7–14 days, leading many clinicians to try alternative SSRIs first. Fluoxetine and norfluoxetine do not reach a steady state for 5–6 weeks, compared with 4–14 days for paroxetine, fluvoxamine, and sertraline. These differences are important, especially for the terminally ill patient in whom a switch from an SSRI to another antidepressant is being considered. All the SSRIs have the ability to inhibit the hepatic isoenzyme P450 11D6, with sertraline (and citalopram) being least potent in this regard. This is important with respect to dose/plasma level ratios and drug interactions, because the SSRIs are dependent on hepatic metabolism. For the elderly patient with advanced disease, the dose–response curve for sertraline appears to be relatively linear. On the other hand, particularly for paroxetine (which appears to most potently inhibit cytochrome P450 11D6), small dosage increases can result in dramatic elevations in plasma levels. Paroxetine, and to a somewhat lesser extent fluoxetine, appear to inhibit the hepatic enzymes responsible for their own clearance (Preskorn 1993). The coadministration of these medications with other drugs that are dependent on this enzyme system for their catabolism (e.g., tricyclics, phenothiazines, type IC antiarrhythmics, and quinidine) should be carried out cautiously. Luvox has been shown in some instances to elevate the blood levels with propranolol and warfarin by as much as twofold, and should thus not be prescribed together with these agents. If patients experience activating effects on SSRIs, they should not be given at bedtime but rather moved earlier into the day. Gastrointestinal upset can be reduced by ensuring the patient does not take medication on an empty stomach.

Psychostimulants

Psychostimulants (dextroamphetamine, methylphenidate, and pemoline) have recently emerged as yet another alternative in the treatment of depression in patients with cancer (Katon and Raskind 1980, Kaufmann et al 1982, Fisch 1985, Chiarillo and Cole 1987, Fernandez et al 1987). Even at relatively low dosage levels, psychostimulants can increase appetite, promote a sense of well-being, and decrease weakness and fatigue in cancer pain patients. These effects can be particularly beneficial in patients with cancer pain, who may feel somewhat sedated from their analgesic regimen. More importantly, particularly when treating terminally ill patients, psychostimulants are often effective quite rapidly, with most patients experiencing some benefit within the first few days (although often longer for a more full antidepressent effect). Treatment is usually initiated at a low dose (e.g., 2.5 mg of methylphenidate at 8.00 a.m. and noon) and gradually increased over several days until a desired effect is achieved or side effects (overstimulation, anxiety, insomnia, paranoia, confusion) intervene. Although patients who respond to psychostimulants can be maintained on these drugs for extended periods of time, eventually patients will develop a tolerance that may require periodic dose increases. Pemoline, another psychostimulant that was initially preferred over methylphenidate because of its decreased abuse potential (Chiarillo and Cole 1987, Breitbart and Mermelstein 1992) and governmental regulation (in the USA), has recently been questioned in cancer patients because of a number of reports of liver toxicity. Thus, although often effective and with a milder side effect profile, pemoline requires careful oversight to monitor liver function (Nehra et al 1990, Pizzuti 1999). Several case reports of irreversible liver failure have resulted in a FDA advisory to obtain written formal consent from patients when pemoline is prescribed. Modafinil, a novel psychostimulant that has shown efficacy in treating excessive daytime sleepiness associated with narcolepsy, has recently demonstrated potential for the adjuvant treatment of depression, fatigue, and opioid-induced sedation (Menza et al 2000).

Alternative antidepressants

If a patient does not respond to an SSRI, TCA, or psychostimulant, or cannot tolerate the side effects of these agents, a number of alternative antidepressants exist. These include 'second-generation' antidepressants (buproprion, trazodone), heterocyclic (maprotiline, amoxapine), and serotonin–noradrenaline reuptake inhibitors (SNRIs; venlafaxine). The selection of one of these antidepressants, like any pharmacological intervention under consideration, should be made with careful consideration of the possible side effects and/or drug interactions. For example, trazodone is highly sedating and, in low doses (100 mg at bedtime), is particularly helpful for treating depressed cancer patients with insomnia. Higher doses of trazodone (up to 300 mg/day) are also useful, but can be associated with orthostatic hypotension and its problematic sequelae (e.g., falls, fractures). Trazodone also has been associated with priapism and should therefore be used with caution in male patients (Sher et al 1983). Venlafaxine (effexor, a serotonin–noradrenaline reuptake inhibitor), although often useful in treating depression, has been associated with elevated blood pressure, especially at doses above the recommended initiating dose, and also therefore requires careful monitoring. However, compared with the SSRIs, effexor has lower protein binding (< 35%) and therefore may have fewer protein binding-induced drug interactions than the SSRIs. Other drugs, such as buproprion, have been used occasionally but with caution, particularly in patients with seizure disorders or brain tumours and in those who are malnourished (Peck et al 1983). Monamine oxidase inhibitors (MAOI), once popular in the treatment of depression, are rarely recommended for use in patients with cancer because of the potentially dangerous side effects. Use of MAOIs entails necessary dietary restrictions (avoidance of tyramine-containing foods), which are often bothersome to cancer patients who often already have diminished appetite. Use of MAOIs in conjunction with narcotics may also be problematic (or even dangerous) because of the possibility of myoclonus or delirium (Breitbart and Holland 1988). Thus, these agents are rarely used and virtually never recommended in treating cancer patients with depression. Finally, some depressed patients with cancer are successfully treated with lithium carbonate, although this is typically only utilized when the patient had utilized this medication sucessfully prior to the diagnosis of cancer illness. Although lithium can be prescribed (and taken) throughout cancer treatment, close monitoring is nevertheless necessary (especially in preoperative and postoperative periods when fluids and salt may be restricted and fluid balance shifts can occur). Maintenance doses of lithium may also need reduction in seriously ill patients, particularly in patients receiving *cis*-platinum and other nephrotoxic agents, since lithium carbonate is primarily eliminated through renal excretion.

Electroconvulsive therapy

Occasionally, it is necessary to consider electroconvulsive therapy (ECT) for severely depressed cancer pain patients such as those whose depression includes psychotic features or patients for whom treatment with antidepressants pose unacceptable side effects. The safe, effective use of ECT in depressed cancer patients has been reviewed by others (Massie et al 1994) and will not be elaborated here, although this alternative may yield secondary analgesic benefits for the depressed patient with otherwise unrelieved pain.

Anxiety in cancer pain patients

A number of different types of anxiety syndrome commonly appear in cancer patients with and without pain, including:

1. Reactive anxiety related to the stresses of cancer and its treatment,
2. Anxiety that is a manifestation of a medical or physiological problem related to cancer, such as uncontrolled pain, and
3. Phobias, panic, and chronic anxiety disorders that predate the cancer diagnosis but are exacerbated during illness (Massie and Holland 1987, Holland 1989).

Reactive anxiety

Although many, if not all, patients experience some anxiety at critical moments during the evaluation and treatment of cancer (e.g., while waiting to hear of diagnosis or possible recurrence, before procedures, diagnostic tests, surgery, or while awaiting test results), intense anxiety may disrupt a patient's ability to function normally, interfere with interpersonal relationships and even impact upon the ability to understand or comply with cancer treatments. In such cases, anxiety can be effectively treated pharmacologically with benzodiazepines such as alprazolam, oxazepam, or lorazepam. In patients whose level of anxiety is relatively mild, and when sufficient time exists for the patient to learn a behavioural technique, relaxation and imagery exercises or cognitive restructuring can be useful in reducing levels of distress (Holland et al 1991). The optimal treatment of anxiety generally incorporates both a benzodiazepine and relaxation exercises or other behavioural interventions.

'Organic' anxiety

The diagnosis of organic anxiety disorder (renamed anxiety disorder due to a general medical condition in DSM-IV) assumes that a medical factor is the aetiological agent in the production of anxious symptoms. Cancer patients with pain are exposed to multiple potential organic causes of anxiety, including medications, uncontrolled pain, infection, and metabolic derangements. Patients in acute pain and those with acute or chronic respiratory distress often appear anxious. The anxiety that accompanies acute pain is best treated with analgesics; the anxiety that accompanies severe respiratory distress is usually relieved by oxygen and the judicious use of morphine and/or antihistamines. Many patients receiving corticosteroids experience insomnia and anxiety symptoms that vary from mild to severe. Because steroids prescribed as part of cancer therapy usually cannot be discontinued, anxiety symptoms are often relieved with benzodiazepines or low-dose antipsychotics (Stiefel et al 1989). Patients developing an encephalopathy (delirium) or who are in the early stages of dementia can also appear restless or anxious. Symptoms of anxiety are also frequent sequelae of a withdrawal from narcotics, alcohol, benzodiazepines, and barbiturates. Because patients who abuse alcohol often inaccurately report alcohol intake before admission, the physician needs to consider alcohol withdrawal in all patients who develop otherwise unexplained anxiety symptoms during early days of admission to the hospital. Other medical conditions that may have anxiety as a prominent or presenting symptom include hyperthyroidism, phaeochromocytoma, carcinoid, primary, and metastatic brain tumour, and mitral valve prolapse (Breitbart 1989b, Holland 1989).

Phobias and panic

Occasionally, patients have their first episode of panic or phobia while in the cancer setting. In one study, approximately 20% of patients scheduled to have an MRI developed anxiety (typically claustrophobia) of such intensity that they were unable to complete the procedure (Brennan et al 1988). Other anxiety symptoms such as panic attacks, needle phobia, and claustrophobia can complicate treatment and necessitate mental health intervention. The techniques available to treat these disorders include both behavioural interventions (relaxation training, systematic desensitization and exposure for specific phobias) and pharmacological approaches (described below). If there is the luxury of time (days to weeks) and the patient will have to face the stress (venipunctures, bone marrow aspirations) repeatedly, behavioural interventions may be advisable in order to enable the patient to gain some control over such fear. Often, however, the need for anxiety relief is immediate because of the urgency of many medical procedures and benzodiazepines (e.g., alprazolam 0.25–1.0 mg P.O.), in addition to providing emotional support, are used to help the phobic patient undergo necessary procedures.

Pharmacological treatment of anxiety symptoms and disorders

The most commonly used drugs for the treatment of anxiety are the benzodiazepines (Massie and Holland 1987, Holland 1989). Other medications used to alleviate anxiety include buspirone, antipsychotics, antihistamines, beta-blockers, and antidepressants (Table 45.3).

Benzodiazepines

For cancer pain patients, the preferred benzodiazepines are those with shorter half-lives (i.e., alprazolam, lorazepam, and oxazepam). These medications are better tolerated and are complicated less frequently by toxic accumulation of active metabolites when combined with other sedating medications (e.g., analgesics, diphenhydramine). Determining the optimal starting dose depends on a number of factors, including the severity of the anxiety, the patient's physical state (respiratory and hepatic impairment), estimated tolerance to benzodiazepines, and the concurrent use of other medications (antidepressants, analgesics, antiemetics). The dose schedule also depends on the half-life of the drug; shorter-acting benzodiazepines must be given three to four times a day, while longer-acting diazepam can be used on a twice-daily schedule. Anxiolytic medications are often prescribed only on an as-needed basis for patients whose anxiety is limited to specific events such as medical procedures or chemotherapy treatments. However, patients with chronic anxiety should be treated with anxiolytics on an around-the-clock schedule as with analgesics for chronic pain. The most common side effects of the benzodiazepines are drowsiness and motor incoordination, but possible synergistic effects when they are used with other CNS depressants exist and the result may be an acute confusional state. In patients taking benzodiazepines chronically (for periods of several weeks), abrupt discontinuation

Table 45.3 Anxiolytic medications used in cancer pain patients

Generic name	Approximate daily dosage range (mg)	Route[a]
	Benzodiazepines	
Very short acting		
Midazolam	10–60 per 24 h	IV, SC
Short acting		
Alprazolam	0.25–2.0 t.i.d.–q.i.d.	PO, SL
Oxazepam	10–15 t.i.d.–q.i.d.	PO
Lorazepam	0.5–2.0 t.i.d.–q.i.d.	PO, SL, IV, IM
Intermediate acting		
Chlordiazepoxide	10–50 t.i.d.–q.i.d.	PO, IM
Long acting		
Diazepam	5–10 b.i.d.–b.i.d.	PO, IM, IV, PR
Clorazepate	7.5–15 b.i.d.–q.i.d.	PO
Clonazepam	0.5–2 b.i.d.–q.i.d.	PO
	Non-benzodiazepines	
Buspirone	5–20 t.i.d.	PO
	Neuroleptics	
Haloperidol	0.5–5q 2–12 h	PO, IV, SC, IM
Levomepromazine (methotrimeprazine)	10–20q 4–8 h	PO, IV, SC
Thioridazine	10–75 t.i.d.–q.i.d.	PO
Chlorpromazine	12.5–50q 4–12 h	PO, IM, IV
Molindone	10–50q 8–12 h	PO
Oroperidal	0.625–2.5q 4–8 h	IV, IM
	Atypical neuroleptics	
Olanzapine	2.5–20q 12–24 h	PO
Risperidone	1–3q 12–24 h	PO
Quetiapine	25–200q 12–24 h	PO
	Antihistamine	
Hydroxyzine	25–50q 4–6 h	PO, IV, SC
	Tricyclic antidepressants	
Imipramine	12.5–150 h	PO, IM
Clomipramine	10–150 h	PO

[a]PO = per oral; IM = intramuscular; PR = per rectum; IV = intravenous; SC = subcutaneous; SL = sublingual; b.i.d. = two times a day; t.i.d. = three times a day; q.i.d. = four times a day; q (2–12)h, every (2–12) h.
Parenteral doses are generally twice as potent as oral doses; intravenous bolus injections or infusions should be administered slowly.

can lead to a serious withdrawal syndrome similar to alcohol withdrawal.

Non-benzodiazepine anxiolytics

Buspirone is a non-benzodiazepine anxiolytic that is useful, along with psychotherapy, in patients with chronic anxiety or anxiety related to adjustment disorders. The onset of anxiolytic action is delayed relative to a benzodiazepine, taking 5–10 days for the relief of anxiety to begin. Because buspirone is not a benzodiazepine, it is not useful in preventing benzodiazepine withdrawal, and so one must be cautious when switching from a benzodiazepine to buspirone. Antipsychotic agents are also potentially useful in treating severe anxiety unresponsive to high doses of benzodiazepines, particularly when cognitive impairment (e.g., dementia) puts the patient at risk of worsening confusion due to benzodiazepines. Antihistamines are infrequently prescribed for anxiety because of their low efficacy but hydroxyzine can be useful for anxious patients with respiratory impairment in whom benzodiazepines are relatively contraindicated. Propranolol can also be a helpful adjunct in blocking the physiological manifestations of anxiety in patients with panic disorders (Holland 1989).

Delirium (cognitive disorders)

Delirium and other cognitive disorders occur in roughly 15–20% of hospitalized cancer patients (Levine et al 1978, Posner 1979) and are the second most common group of psychiatric diagnoses ascribed to cancer patients. Delirium and other cognitive disorders are an even more common occurrence in patients with advanced illness. Massie et al (1983) found delirium in more than 75% of terminally ill cancer patients they studied. Initially termed 'organic mental disorders', the *Diagnostic and Statistical Manual of Mental Disorders*, 4th edn (DSM-IV) (American Psychiatric Association 1994), renamed this class of disorders 'cognitive' disorders and, like its predecessors, divided the various syndromes into the subcategories of delirium, dementia, amnestic disorder, and other cognitive disorders. Lipowski (1987) has grouped these different disorders into those characterized by general cognitive impairment (i.e., delirium and dementia), and those in which cognitive impairment is selective, limited, or non-existent (e.g., amnestic disorder).

Delirium has been described as an aetiologically non-specific, global cerebral dysfunction characterized by concurrent disturbances in any of a number of different functions, including level of consciousness, attention, thinking, perception, emotion, memory, psychomotor behaviour, and sleep–wake cycle. Disorientation, fluctuation, or waxing and waning of the above symptoms, as well as acute or abrupt onset of such disturbances, are critical features of a delirium. Delirium is also conceptualized as a reversible process (e.g., as compared to dementia), even in patients with advanced illness. Delirium, however, may not be reversible in the last 24–48 h of life. This is most likely to be due to the influence of irreversible processes such as multiple-organ failure occurring in the final hours of life. Delirium in these last days of life is often referred to as 'terminal restlessness' or 'terminal agitation' in the palliative care literature. Aside from the complications for patient care and management that result from delirium, patients, family members, and nursing staff typically find this experience to be extremely distressing.

Early symptoms of delirium or other 'organic' disorders are often misdiagnosed as anxiety, anger, depression, or psychosis. Because of the potential for diagnostic error, the possibility of an aetiology should be considered in *any* medically ill patient demonstrating an acute onset of agitation or uncooperative behaviour, impaired cognitive function, altered attention span, a fluctuating level of consciousness, or intense, uncharacteristic anxiety or depression (Lipowski 1987). A common error among medical and nursing staff is to conclude that a new psychological symptom represents a functional psychiatric disorder without adequately considering, evaluating, and/or eliminating possible organic aetiologies. For example, the patient with mood disturbance meeting DSM-IV criteria for major depression, who is severely hypothyroid or on high-dose corticosteroids, may be more accurately diagnosed as having an organic mood disorder (e.g., mood disorder secondary to thyroid dysfunction) rather than a major depressive episode. Differentiating between delirium and dementia can also be extremely difficult, both because they commonly occur in elderly, medically ill individuals and because they share a number of clinical features (e.g., impaired memory and judgement, disorientation). Dementia, however, typically appears in relatively alert individuals with little or no clouding of consciousness. The temporal onset of symptoms in dementia is also less acute (i.e., chronically progressive) and the sleep–wake cycle appears less impaired. Most prominent in dementia are difficulties in short- and long-term memory, impaired judgement, and abstract thinking as well as disturbed higher cortical functions (e.g., aphasia, apraxia). Occasionally one will encounter delirium superimposed on an underlying dementia, particularly in elderly patients or patients with AIDS or a paraneoplastic syndrome.

Organic mental disorders can be caused by either the direct effects of cancer on the central nervous system (CNS) or the indirect CNS effects of the disease or treatments (medications, electrolyte imbalance, failure of a vital organ or system, infection, vascular complications, and pre-existing cognitive impairment or dementia). Given the large numbers of medications cancer pain patients require, and their fragile physiological state, even routinely ordered hypnotics may engender an episode of delirium. Perhaps most relevant to cancer pain management is the role that narcotic analgesics play in the development of delirium. Many opioid analgesics have been reported to cause confusional states, particularly in the elderly cancer patient and in the terminally ill patient (Bruera et al 1989, 1990b). For example, the toxic accumulation of meperidine's metabolite, normeperidine, is associated with florid delirium accompanied by myoclonus and possible seizures. Despite this risk, the routine use of stable regimens of oral narcotic analgesics for the control of cancer pain is rarely complicated by overt delirium or confusional states (Liepzig et al 1987). On the other hand, delirium and other forms of cognitive impairment are more likely to occur during periods of rapid dosage escalation, especially in older patients receiving intravenous infusions of opioids (Portenoy 1987, Bruera et al 1989, Eller et al 1992).

Chemotherapeutic agents known to cause delirium (Table 45.4) include methotrexate, fluorouracil, vincristine, vinblastine, bleomycin, BCNU, *cis*-platinum, asparaginase, procarbazine, and the glucocorticosteroids (Holland et al 1974, Weddington 1982, Young 1982, Adams et al 1984, Denicoff et al 1987, Stiefel et al 1989). With the exception of steroids, however, most patients receiving chemotherapeutic agents do not develop prominent CNS effects. The spectrum of mental disturbances caused by corticosteroids ranges from minor mood lability to mania or depression, cognitive impairment (reversible dementia) to delirium (steroid psychosis). Although these disturbances are most common with higher doses and usually develop within the first 2 weeks of steroid use, they can occur at any time, on any dose, even during the tapering phase (Stiefel et al 1989). Prior psychiatric illness or prior mental disturbance due to steroid use does not predict susceptibility to, or the nature of, subsequent mental disturbance with steroids. These disorders often reverse rapidly upon dose reduction or discontinuation (Stiefel et al 1989).

Table 45.4 Neuropsychiatric side effects of chemotherapeutic drugs

Drug	Neuropsychiatric symptoms
Methotrexate (intrathecal)	Delirium, dementia, lethargy, personality change
Vincristine, vinblastine	Delirium, hallucinations, lethargy, depression
Asparaginase	Delirium, hallucinations, lethargy, cognitive dysfunction
BCNU	Delirium, dementia
Bleomycin	Delirium
Fluorouracil	Delirium
cis-Platinum	Delirium
Hydroxyurea	Hallucinations
Procarbazine	Depression, mania, delirium, dementia
Cytosine arabinoside	Delirium, lethargy, cognitive dysfunction
Hexylmethylamine	Hallucinations
Isophosphamide	Delirium, lethargy, hallucinations
Prednisone	Depression, mania, delirium, psychoses
Interferon	Flu-like syndrome, delirium, hallucinations, depression
Interleukin	Cognitive dysfunction, hallucinations

Management of delirium

The appropriate approach in the management of delirium in the cancer pain patient includes interventions directed at both the underlying causes and symptoms of delirium. Identification and correction of the underlying cause(s) for delirium must take place while symptomatic and supportive therapies are initiated (Lipowski 1987, Fleishman and Lesko 1989). In the case of the cancer patient in pain who develops delirium while on a high-dose opioid infusion, often the mere reduction of dose or infusion rate (if pain is controlled) will begin to resolve symptoms of delirium within hours. Other strategies include switching from one opioid to another. Symptomatic treatment measures include support for and communication with the patient and family, reassurance, manipulation of the environment to provide a reorienting, safe milieu, and then appropriate use of pharmacotherapies. Measures to help reduce anxiety and disorientation (i.e., increased structure and familiarity) may include a quiet, well-lit room with familiar objects, a visible clock or calendar, and the presence of family. Judicious use of one-to-one nursing observation, or even at times physical restraints, may also be necessary and useful. Often, these supportive techniques alone are not adequate and symptomatic treatment with neuroleptic or sedative medications is necessary (Table 45.5).

Table 45.5 Medications useful in managing delirium in cancer pain patients

Generic name	Approximate daily dosage range (mg)	Route[a]
	Neuroleptics	
Haloperidol	0.5–q2–12 h	PO, IV, SC, IM
Thioridazine	10–75q 4–8 h	PO
Chlorpromazine	12.5–50q 4–12 h	PO, IV, IM
Levomepromazine (methotrimeprazine)	12.5–50q 4–8 h	PO, IV, SC
Molindone	10–50q 8–12 h	PO
Droperidol	0.5–5q 12 h	IV, IM
	Novel antipsychotics	
Risperidone	1–3q 12–24 h	PO
Olanzapine	2.5–20q 12–24 h	PO
Quetiapine	25–200q 12–24 h	PO
	Benzodiazepines	
Lorazepam	0.5–20q 1–4 h	PO, IV, IM
	Anaesthetics	
Propofol	10–50q 1 h	IV
Midazolam	30–100 per 24 h	IV, SC

[a]Parenteral doses are generally twice as potent as oral doses; IV = intravenous infusions or bolus injections should be administered slowly; IM = intramuscular injections should be avoided if repeated use becomes necessary; PO = oral forms of medication are preferred; SC = subcutaneous infusions are generally accepted modes of drug administration in the terminally ill; q (2–12)h = every (2–12) h.

Pharmacological management of delirium

Neuroleptic medications vary in their sedating properties and in their potential for producing orthostatic hypotension, neurological side effects (acute dystonia, extrapyramidal symptoms), and anticholinergic effects. The acutely agitated cancer patient requires a sedating medication; the patient with hypotension requires a drug with the least effect on blood pressure; the delirious post-operative patient who has an ileus or urinary retention should receive an antipsychotic with the least anticholinergic effects. For many years, haloperidol, a neuroleptic agent that is a potent dopamine blocker, was considered the drug of choice for the treatment of delirium in the cancer pain patient because of its useful sedating effects and low incidence of cardiovascular and anticholinergic effects (Adams et al 1986, Lipowski 1987, Murray 1987). This medication can be given intramuscularly or subcutanously, if necessary (and, although not yet FDA-approved, through intravenous injection), and is usually effective in targeting agitation, paranoia, and fear. More recently, however, newer 'atypical' antipsychotic medications have become increasingly utilized in managing delirium, including olanzapine and risperidone. Unfortunately, as of yet, these medications are only available for oral administration. These atypical antipsychotic medications appear to be equally effective in managing the symptoms of delirium but with somewhat lower rates of extrapyramidal side effects and movement disorders (Singh 1996, Sipahimalani and Masand 1998, Breitbart et al 2002). When extrapyramidal side effects do occur, these symptoms can usually be controlled by the use of antiparkinsonian medications (e.g., diphenhydramine, benztropine, trihexyphenidyl); akathisia, another common side effect from neuroleptic medications, often responds to low doses of propranolol, lorazepam, or benztropine. A rare but at times fatal complication of antipsychotics is the neuroleptic malignant syndrome (NMS). NMS usually occurs after prolonged high-dose administration of neuroleptics and is characterized by hyperthermia, increased mental confusion, leucocytosis, muscular rigidity, myoglobinuria, and high serum creatine phosphokinase (CPK). Treatment consists of discontinuing the neuroleptic and use of dantrolene sodium or bromocriptine mesylate (Fleishman and Lesko 1989).

Another common strategy in the management of agitated delirium is to add parenteral lorazepam to a regimen of haloperidol (Adams et al 1986, Murray 1987, Fernandez et al 1989). Although lorazepam is often effective in rapidly sedating the agitated delirious patient, its use should be restricted to that of an adjuvant medication as benzodiazepines alone have limited benefit in the treatment of delirium. In a double-blind, randomized comparison trial of haloperidol versus chlorpromazine versus lorazepam, it was demonstrated that lorazepam alone was ineffective in the treatment of delirium and in fact contributed to worsening delirium and cognitive impairment (Breitbart et al 1996c). Both neuroleptic drugs, however, in low doses were highly effective in controlling the symptoms of delirium and improving cognitive function. In addition, haloperidol and chlorpromazine have both been found effective in improving the symptoms of both hypoactive and hyperactive delirium (Platt et al 1994). Perhaps the only setting in which benzodiazepines alone have an established role is in the management of delirium in the dying patient.

Complications in the context of pain and terminal illness

The treatment of delirium in the dying cancer pain patient is unique for the following reasons:

1. Most often, the aetiology of terminal delirium is multifactorial or may not be found; Bruera et al (1990b) reported that an aetiology was discovered in less than 50% of terminally ill patients with cognitive dysfunction.
2. When a distinct cause is found, it is often irreversible (such as hepatic failure or brain metastases).
3. Work-up may be limited by the setting (home, hospice).
4. The consultant's focus is usually on the patient's comfort and ordinarily helpful diagnostic procedures that are unpleasant or painful (i.e., CT scan, lumbar puncture) may be avoided.

When confronted with a delirium in the terminally ill or dying cancer patient, a differential diagnosis should always be formulated; however, studies should be pursued only when a suspected factor can be identified easily and treated effectively. The use of medications in the management of delirium in the dying patient remains controversial in some circles. Some have argued that pharmacological interventions with neuroleptics or benzodiazepines are inappropriate in the dying patient. This approach argues that delirium is a natural part of the dying process that should not be altered. Another rationale often raised is that these patients are so close to death that aggressive treatment is unnecessary. Parenteral neuroleptics or sedatives may be mistakenly avoided because of exaggerated fears that they might hasten death through hypotension or respiratory depression. Many clinicians are unnecessarily pessimistic about the possible results of neuroleptic treatment for delirium. They argue that because the underlying pathophysiological process often continues unabated (such as hepatic or renal failure), no improvement can be expected in the patient's mental status. There is concern that neuroleptics or sedatives may worsen a delirium by making the patient more confused or sedated. Clinical experience in managing delirium in dying cancer patients suggests that the use of neuroleptics in the management of agitation, paranoia, hallucinations, and altered sensorium is safe, effective, and quite appropriate. Management of delirium on a case-by-case basis is always the most logical course of action. The agitated, delirious dying patient should probably be given neuroleptics to help restore calm. A 'wait-and-see' approach, prior to using neuroleptics, may be most appropriate with patients who have a lethargic or somnolent presentation of delirium. The consultant must educate staff and patients and weigh each of these issues in making the decision about whether to use pharmacological interventions for the dying patient who presents with delirium. Among the most commonly used medications for dying cancer patients are levomepromazine (methotrimeprazine) (IV or SC), which is often utilized to control confusion and agitation in terminal delirium (Oliver 1985) but can lead to hypotension and excessive sedation. Midazolam (IV or SC) is also used to control agitation related to delirium in the terminal stages (de Sousa and Jepson 1988, Bottomley and Hanks 1990) and propofol (IV), a short-acting anaesthetic agent, has also begun to be utilized primarily as a sedating agent for the control of agitated patients with 'terminal' delirium (de Sousa and Jepson 1988, Mercandante et al 1995, Moyle 1995). All of these drugs primarily serve to sedate the patient, as opposed to neuroleptic drugs which may help clear a delirious patient's sensorium or improve cognition. These clinical differences may be caused by the underlying pathophysiology of delirium. One hypothesis postulates that an imbalance of central cholinergic and adrenergic mechanisms underlies delirium and so a dopamine blocking drug may initiate a rebalancing of these systems (Itil and Fink 1966). While neuroleptic drugs such as haloperidol are most effective in achieving the goals of diminishing agitation, clearing the sensorium, and improving cognition in the delirious patient, this is not always possible in the last days of life. Processes causing delirium may be ongoing and irreversible during the active dying phase. Ventafridda et al (1990) and Fainsinger et al (1991) have reported that a significant group (10–20%) of terminally ill patients experience delirium that can be controlled only by sedation to the point of a significantly decreased level of consciousness.

Cancer, pain, suicide, and assisted suicide

Uncontrolled pain is a major factor in cancer suicide (Breitbart 1987, 1990). Cancer is perceived by the public as an extremely painful disease compared to other medical conditions. In Wisconsin, a study revealed that 69% of the public agreed that cancer pain could cause a person to consider suicide (Levin et al 1985). The majority of suicides were observed among patients with cancer who had severe pain, which was often inadequately controlled or tolerated poorly (Bolund 1985). Although relatively few cancer patients commit suicide, they are at increased risk (Farberow et al 1963, Breitbart 1987). Factors associated with an increased risk of suicide in cancer patients are listed in Box 45.1. Patients with advanced illness are at highest risk and are the most likely to have the complications of pain, depression, delirium, and deficit symptoms. Psychiatric disorders are frequently present in hospitalized cancer patients who attempt suicide. A review of the psychiatric consultation data at Memorial Sloan-Kettering Cancer Center (MSKCC) showed that one-third of cancer patients who were seen for evaluation of suicide risk received a diagnosis of major depression; approximately 20% met criteria for delirium and more than 50% were diagnosed with an adjustment disorder (Breitbart 1987).

Thoughts of suicide occur quite frequently in patients with advanced cancer, although there is some dispute as to whether these 'thoughts' of suicide reflect genuine suicidal ideation or serve as a 'steam valve' for patient distress more generally. Patients may comment that 'If things get too bad, I always have a way out' as a way of coping with their illness and failing health. More importantly, these passing thoughts of suicide which may occur so often appear to be quite different from the active, overwhelming suicidal thoughts that preoccuppy some depressed patients with cancer. A study conducted at St Boniface Hospice in Winnipeg, Canada, found that 10 of 44 terminally ill cancer patients expressed an interest in suicide or an early death and all 10 were diagnosed with clinical depression (Brown et al 1986). In fact, although the lay public often cite pain as a primary reason for thoughts of suicide or requests for assisted suicide or euthanasia, the scientific literature has not always supported this perception (Breitbart et al 1996d). Chochinov et al (1995) found that of 200 terminally ill patients in a palliative care facility, 44.5% acknowledged at least a fleeting desire to die. However 17 patients (8.5%) reported an unequivocal desire for death to come soon and indicated that they held this desire consistently over time. Among this group, 10 (58.8%) met criteria for a diagnosis of depression, compared to a prevalence of depression of only 7.7% in patients who did not endorse a genuine, consistent desire for death. Patients with a desire for death were also more likely to report severe pain and lower levels of social support than those patients without a desire for death. More recent studies, however, have failed to observe even these weak associations between pain and desire for hastened death (e.g., Breitbart et al 2000), suggesting that the role of pain may be more indirect (e.g., through its influence on mood and hopelessness). In our own research with terminally ill cancer patients (Breitbart et al 2000), we have found depression and hopelessness to be the strongest factors driving desire for hastened death with little apparent impact of pain or symptom distress. Among patients who were both depressed and hopeless, more than ½ indicated a high desire for hastened death, whereas only ¼ of patients who were depressed but not hopeless or hopeless but not depressed had a high desire for hastened death.

BOX 45.1
Cancer pain suicide vulnerability factors

Pain; suffering aspects
Multiple physical symptoms
Advanced illness; poor prognosis
Depression; hopelessness
Delirium; disinhibition
Control; helplessness
Preexisting psychopathology
Suicide history; family history
Inadequate social support

Among patients who were neither depressed nor hopeless, none had a high desire for hastened death.

Perhaps the most relevant data for U.S. physicians is the rapidly growing literature from Oregon, where legalization of physician-assisted suicide was officially approved by ballot referendum in 1994 and ultimately legalized by state statute in 1997. This statute, the Oregon Death with Dignity Act (ODDA), has received considerable attention in both the medical and legal literature since its passage. Like the Dutch law, the ODDA specifies a number of conditions that must be met in order for a request for assisted suicide to be considered valid: the patient must be terminally ill (less than 6 months to live), the physician must seek a second opinion regarding the patient's medical condition and prognosis, the patient must be capable of making a competent decision (i.e., without gross impairment in his or her decision making ability), and there must be a 2-week waiting period between the initial written request for assisted suicide and the provision of a prescription. Contrary to the opinions of some writers, mandatory mental health consultation was not included in this process although the law recommends that consultation be sought whenever concerns regarding the patient's ability to make rational decisions exists. Although challenges to this law have thus far been unsuccessful, many writers have expressed concerns that legalization of assisted suicide would lead to widespread abuses, including the possibility that terminally ill individuals from around the country would flock to Oregon to receive their fatal prescriptions. These fears, however, have not been generally realized as several early studies of the frequency of PAS requests and actions have been far lower than the rates observed in the Netherlands (Meier et al 1998, Sullivan et al 2000). Regardless of the frequency with which cancer patients request assisted suicide or euthanasia, these requests certainly pose many ethical and practical dilemmas for the clinician who receives them. Whether one approves of assisted suicide or opposes it, there is little doubt that such requests should be met with a discussion of the patients' reasons for making the request and a thorough assessment of any inadequately managed symptoms that might be influencing the patient's request.

Assessment issues in the treatment of cancer pain: obstacles to adequate pain control

Cancer pain is often inadequately managed. Cleeland and colleagues (1994) estimate that roughly 40% of cancer pain patients receive inadequate analgesic therapy. A survey of 1177 oncologists who participate in the Eastern Cooperative Oncology Group (ECOG) was undertaken to assess cancer pain management (von Roenn et al 1993). Over 85% reported that they felt the majority of cancer patients are undermedicated for pain. Only 51.4% believed that pain control in their own setting was good or very good. We found even more striking rates of undertreatment in a study of patients with AIDS, with 84% being classified as undertreated based on a comparison of their pain severity and prescribed analgesic medications. A number of barriers to adequate pain management have been recognized, based on the results of several recent surveys (Ward et al 1993, Breitbart et al 1999). These factors include:

1. Patient reluctance to report pain,
2. Patient reluctance to take medications,
3. Physician reluctance to prescribe pain medication (including fears of addiction), and
4. Most importantly, poor pain assessment knowledge and skills.

Inadequate management of cancer pain is also hindered by the frequent unfamiliarity with techniques to properly assess pain (Marks and Sachar 1973, Foley 1985, Breitbart 1989a). All too frequently, psychological variables are proposed to explain continued pain or lack of response to therapy, when in fact medical factors have not been adequately appreciated. Other causes of inadequate cancer pain management include:

1. Lack of knowledge of current therapeutic approaches,
2. Focus on prolonging life and cure versus alleviating suffering,
3. Inadequate physician–patient relationship,
4. Limited expectations of patients,
5. Unavailability of narcotics,
6. Fear of respiratory depression, and
7. Most important, fear of addiction.

Fear of addiction affects both patient compliance and physician management of narcotic analgesics, leading to undermedication of cancer pain (Marks and Sachar 1973, Macaluso et al 1988, Passik et al 2000). Yet studies of the patterns of chronic narcotic analgesic use in patients with cancer have demonstrated that, although tolerance and physical dependence commonly occur, addiction (psychological dependence) is rare and almost never occurs in an individual without a history of drug abuse prior to cancer illness (Kanner and Foley 1981). Passik (1992) reviewed the requests for psychiatric consultation at Memorial Sloan-Kettering Cancer Center for a 1-year period. In only 36 of 1200 (3%) requests for psychiatric consultation was substance abuse cited as the primary reason for the request. Interestingly, in one-third of these cases the psychiatry service consultant did not go on to concur with the labelling of the patient as a substance abuser (usually citing uncontrolled pain as the reason for the supposedly aberrant behaviour on the part of the patient). Fears of iatrogenic addiction result largely from the erroneous assumption that the opioids are highly addictive drugs and that the problem of addiction resides in the drugs themselves. Cancer patients allowed to self-administer morphine for several weeks during an episode of painful mucositis do not demonstrate escalating use (Chapman 1989). Of 11 882 inpatients surveyed in the Boston Collaborative Drug Surveillance Project, who had no prior history of addiction and were administered opioids, only four cases of psychological dependence could be documented (Porter and Jick 1980). A survey of burn centres identified no cases of iatrogenic addiction in a sample of over 10 000 patients without prior drug abuse history, who were administered opioids for pain (Perry and Heidrich 1982). A study of opioid use in headache patients identified opioid abuse in only 3 of 2369 patients prescribed opioids (Medina and Diamond 1977). These data suggest that patients without a prior history of substance abuse are highly unlikely to become addicted following the administration of opioid drugs as part of their medical treatment.

Escalation of narcotic analgesic use by cancer pain patients is usually a result of the progression of cancer or the development of tolerance. Tolerance means that a larger dose of narcotic analgesic is required to maintain an original analgesic effect. Physical dependence is characterized by the onset of signs and symptoms of withdrawal if the narcotic is suddenly stopped or a narcotic antagonist is administered. Tolerance usually occurs in association with physical dependence, but does not imply psychological dependence or addiction, which is not equivalent to physical dependence or tolerance and is a behavioural pattern of compulsive drug abuse characterized by a craving for the drug and overwhelming involvement in obtaining and using it for effects other than pain relief. The cancer pain patient with a history of intravenous opioid abuse presents an often unnecessarily difficult management problem. Macaluso et al (1988) reported on their experience in managing cancer pain in such a population. Of 468 inpatient cancer pain consultations, only 8 (1.7%) had a history of intravenous drug abuse, but none had been actively abusing drugs in the previous year. All 8 of these patients had inadequate pain control and more than half were intentionally undermedicated because of concern by staff that drug abuse was active or would recur. Adequate pain control was ultimately achieved in these patients by using appropriate analgesic dosages and intensive staff education. Refer to the section below on 'Psychotherapy and cancer pain' for a more extensive review of the management of substance abuse problems in cancer pain patients.

The risk of inducing respiratory depression is too often overestimated and can limit the appropriate use of narcotic analgesics for pain and symptom control. Bruera et al (1990a) demonstrated that, in a population of terminally ill cancer patients with respiratory failure and dyspnoea, administration of subcutaneous morphine actually improved dyspnoea without causing a significant deterioration in respiratory function. The adequacy of cancer pain management can be influenced by the lack of concordance between patient ratings or complaints of their pain and those made by caregivers. Persistent cancer pain is often ascribed to a psychological cause when it does not respond to treatment attempts. In our clinical experience we have noted that patients who report their pain as 'severe' are quite likely to be viewed as having a psychological contribution to their complaints. Staff members' ability to empathize with a patient's pain complaint may be limited by the intensity of the pain complaint. Grossman et al (1991) found that while there is a high degree of concordance between patient and caregiver ratings of patient pain intensity at the low and moderate levels, this concordance breaks down at high levels. Thus, a clinician's ability to assess a patient's level of pain becomes unreliable once a patient's report of pain intensity rises above 7 on a visual analogue rating scale of 0–10. Physicians must be educated as to the limitations of their ability objectively to assess the severity of a subjective pain experience. Additionally, patient education is often a useful intervention in such cases. Patients are more likely to be believed and adequately treated if they are taught to request pain relief in a non-hysterical business-like fashion.

The optimal treatment of cancer pain is multimodal and includes pharmacological, psychotherapeutic, cognitive-behavioural, anaesthetic, stimulatory, and rehabilitative approaches. Psychiatric participation in cancer pain management involves the use of psychotherapeutic, cognitive-behavioural, and psychopharmacological interventions, which are described below.

Psychotherapy and cancer pain

The goals of psychotherapy with cancer pain patients are to provide support, knowledge, and skills. Utilizing short-term supportive psychotherapy based on a crisis intervention model, the therapist can provide emotional support, continuity of care, and information and assist in overall adaptation to the crisis. The therapist has a role in emphasizing past strengths, supporting previously successful coping strategies, and teaching new coping skills such as relaxation, cognitive restructuring, use of analgesics, self-observation, assertiveness, and communication skills. Communication skills are of paramount importance for both patient and family, particularly around pain and analgesic issues. The patient and family are the unit of concern, and often require a more general long-term, supportive relationship within the health care system, in addition to specific psychological approaches dealing with pain that a psychiatrist, psychologist, social worker, or nurse can provide.

Group interventions with individual patients, spouses, couples, and families are a powerful means of sharing experiences and identifying successful coping strategies. Utilizing psychotherapy to decrease symptoms of anxiety and depression, factors that can intensify pain, has been empirically demonstrated to have beneficial effects on cancer pain and overall quality of life. Spiegel and Bloom (1983b) demonstrated, in a controlled randomized prospective study, the effect of both supportive group therapy for metastatic breast cancer patients in general and, in particular, the effect of hypnotic pain control exercises. Patients were divided into either a support group focused on the practical and existential problems of living with cancer, a self-hypnosis exercise group, or a control group. Results indicated that the patients receiving treatment experienced significantly less pain than the control patients.

While psychotherapy in the cancer pain setting typically focuses on more current issues around illness and treatment (rather than psychoanalytic or insight-oriented approaches), the exploration of reactions to cancer often facilitates insight into more pervasive life issues. Theoretical constructs derived from psychotherapy with chronic non-cancer pain patients can be helpful in guiding psychotherapy with the cancer pain patient. Alexithymia and pain-induced dissociative symptoms (remnants of early life trauma) have proven to be relevant constructs for the psychotherapeutic treatment of many cancer pain patients and are discussed in more detail below. Psychiatric observations of chronic non-cancer pain patients may have relevance to a subset of cancer pain patients, although the degree of overlap between these two populations has received little empirical investigation.

Alexithymia, or the inability to express and articulate emotional experiences, is thought to be a trait associated with chronic pain and somatization. Research has demonstrated the utility of this construct in understanding the cancer pain patient as well. Dalton and Feuerstein (1989), for example, demonstrated that patients who reported more prolonged and severe pain also scored higher on a measure of alexithymia than did patients experiencing sporadic or less intense pain. Given the range of emotionally charged issues revolving around loss, disability, disfigurement, and death that arise in the context of cancer (Massie and Holland 1987), many patients are faced with intense emotions that can be threatening or difficult to articulate. Therapists can be quite helpful to alexithymic patients by acknowledging such feelings and allowing for their verbalization. In many instances, the therapist must actually provide the patient with a lexicon for their expression (Passik and Wilson 1987). Analogously, the meaning patients attribute to their pain can influence the amount of pain they report. Therapists can help to correct misperceptions about pain when appropriate and allow for the open discussion of issues and fears that might prolong or intensify a pain experience.

Increased awareness of the impact of traumatic events on psychological functioning and, in particular, on the development of dissociative states and disorders (psychogenic amnesia, fugue states, multiple personality disorder, conversion, post-traumatic stress disorder), has led to a growing acknowledgement of the traumatic impact of pain. Patients with dissociative disorders suffer from a wide variety of transient physical problems such as dysaesthesias, anaesthesias, and pain (Terr 1991). In the chronic non-malignant pain population there has also been growing empirical support for the existence of such sequelae of chronic pain. Patients with chronic pelvic pain and premenstrual syndrome, for example (Walker et al 1988, Paddison et al 1990), were found to have an unusually high prevalence of early sexual abuse. The prevalence of such phenomena in the cancer pain population is unknown. However, the cancer setting, with its life-threatening backdrop, toxic and disfiguring treatments, and invasive procedures, can reawaken long-dormant traumata in even high-functioning patients with abuse histories. Inquiry into such issues can be essential to the evaluation and treatment of such patients. Although not generally a part of a routine psychiatric assessment in the medical setting, the recognition of the need to inquire into these areas requires attentive listening with the 'third ear' (Reik 1948).

The substance-abusing patient

Substance abuse is increasingly prevalent in the population at large and is inevitably encountered in the treatment of cancer pain patients. The management of cancer pain in the active abuser and in the patient with a history of substance abuse is a particularly difficult and challenging problem (Payne 1989, McCaffery and Vourakis 1992). Portenoy and Payne (1992) have outlined a range of aberrant drug-taking behaviours that help to identify the substance-abusing cancer pain patient. When patients obtain and use street drugs, purchase opioids from non-medical sources, or engage in illegal behaviours such as forging prescriptions or selling their prescription medications, a diagnosis of substance abuse is clear. More subtle and difficult to interpret are behaviours such as dose escalation without contact with the physician, contacting multiple physicians to obtain opioids, making frequent visits to emergency rooms, hoarding medications and using medications to relieve symptoms other than pain. What renders these behaviours difficult to interpret (though many physicians might feel that they are uniformly aberrant regardless of mitigating circumstances) is that such behaviours usually arise in the setting of an evolving pain complaint with fluctuating intensity and degree of relief. Many behaviours used to define addiction in the physically healthy have limited utility when assessing the cancer pain patient. Relapse after withdrawal from a substance is a common feature in definitions of addiction (Jaffe 1985). However, relapse of pain complaints after decrease or withdrawal from a particular medication in a cancer pain patient may simply signal the return to the baseline level of the underlying pain and may reflect the need for continued treatment with opioids. Furthermore, the need for chronic use of an opioid presupposes that the patient will become tolerant and physiologically dependent. The fact that the patient develops an abstinence syndrome upon abrupt discontinuation of the drug, or requires higher doses for continued pain control, has little bearing upon the diagnosis of drug abuse.

Psychological dependence is generally accepted as central to the definition of addiction and can be inferred from such behaviours as loss of control over the drug, compulsive use, or use despite harm. Patients may directly state that they have lost control over their pain medicines or have become overly concerned with acquisition of these drugs. They may even be aware that their behaviour in seeking pain medicines has alienated their health care team and jeopardized their cancer treatment. Pain, psychological distress, the adequacy and duration of pain relief, and the patient's prior cancer pain experience must be taken into account when assessing the 'drug-seeking' patient. What appears to be highly aberrant drug-seeking behaviour (obsessive preoccupation with the availability of opioids) may simply be a reflection of inadequate pain control. The term 'pseudoaddiction' (Weissman and Haddox 1989) has been coined to describe the phenomenon in which the highly preoccupied and apparently out-of-control patient ceases to act in an aberrant fashion upon the provision of adequate pain control. Drug-taking behaviours unsanctioned by the physician and that fall in the less severe end of the range of these behaviours should be given the benefit of the doubt and seen as reflections of inadequate pain control, especially if the physician's expectations about the patient's responsibility for communication about dose escalation has not been made explicit. Some patients, such as those with a prior history of drug abuse (but not actively abusing), may require more explicit discussions of the rules for treatment than that given to other patients being started on opioid therapy. Paradoxically, such an explicit outline of the parameters of opioid therapy will provide structure as well as comfort to patients who are concerned about relapsing into active abuse.

The psychiatrist or psychologist in the oncology setting who consults in the care of the active substance-abusing patient is faced with many obstacles. Foremost among them is the limited access patients with serious medical illnesses have to traditional modes of treatment for drug and alcohol problems. The demands of cancer treatment are not generally accommodated by inpatient drug treatment centers. Twelve-step and methadone maintenance programmes can be rigid in their approach to the cancer patient's use of opioids and psychiatric medications for symptom control. Hospital staff members are often resentful and frightened of the substance-abusing patient and this can detract from the psychiatrist's or psychologist's ability to create a caretaking environment and alliance with the patient. The addict, frightened and regressed in the face of potentially life-threatening illness, can be tremendously distrustful of the staff and may attempt to cope through drug use, guile, and manipulation rather than trusting in the staff's competence and goodwill. Through our clinical experience working with substance-abusing patients, we have developed a multifaceted approach to minimize the potential problems caused by these individuals. This approach, which is usually agreed upon in advance, includes early admission to allow stabilization of withdrawal symptoms if necessary, restricted access to visitors and possessions (e.g., only allowing drug-free visitors and limiting the patient's access to the outside environment), and frequent urine toxicology screens. In exchange for these limitations, the patient is provided frequent pain assessments to ensure adequacy of pain control (often complicated by the patient's tolerance to opioids) and usually managed with around-the-clock dosing to minimize staff involvement in PRN dosing. With these steps, patients are typically managed with a minimum of staff anger and mistrust that might otherwise become a self-fulfilling prophecy in which the undertreated substance-abusing cancer pain patient acts in an aberrant fashion that compromises treatment. Despite the seeming simplicity of these management guidelines, there is little doubt that active substance abuse can present a significant obstacle to both adequate pain management and cancer treatment more generally.

The dying cancer pain patient

For many years, psychotherapy with the dying patient in pain consisted solely of active listening with supportive verbal interventions (Cassem 1987). More recently, however, active interventions have emerged to help patients cope with their rapidly approaching death. Greenstein and Breitbart (2000) described a Meaning-Centered Group Psychotherapy designed to help patients with advanced cancer explore their sense of meaning and purpose in life, in hopes of decreasing feelings of despair, isolation, and depression. Although only preliminary research has been conducted using this approach, their early results suggest that this and perhaps other spirituality-based interventions might be useful in helping patients deal with issues specifically related to death and dying. However, regardless of the specific approach utilized by the therapist, a number of structural aspects of psychotherapy also warrant note. For example, the therapist's demeanor in dealing with dying patients is of great importance in helping the patients themselves feel comfortable discussing their thoughts and feelings. Often, it is only the psychotherapist, of all the patient's caregivers, who is comfortable enough to converse lightheartedly and allow the patient to talk about his life and experiences, rather than focus solely on impending death. The dying patient who wishes to talk or ask questions about death and pain and suffering should be allowed to do so freely, with the therapist maintaining an interested interactive stance. In addition, it is not uncommon for the dying patient to benefit from pastoral counselling. If a chaplaincy service is available, it should be offered to the patient and family. As the dying process progresses, psychotherapy with the individual patient may become limited by cognitive and speech deficits. It is at this point that the focus of supportive psychotherapeutic interventions shifts primarily to the family. In our experience, a very common issue for family members at this point is the level of alertness of the patient. Attempts to control pain are often accompanied by sedation that can limit communication between patient and family. This can sometimes become a source of conflict, with some family members disagreeing among themselves or with the patient about what constitutes an appropriate balance between comfort and alertness. It can be helpful for the physician to clarify the patient's preferences as they relate to these issues early, so that conflict can be avoided and work related to bereavement can begin.

Cancer pain and the family

The many stressors faced by the families of cancer patients have prompted mental health professionals who work with such patients to refer to them as 'second-order patients' (Rait and Lederberg 1990). Family members face a difficult and ongoing process of adjustment throughout the stages of the cancer patient's illness. They are called upon to perform the sometimes onerous tasks of providing emotional support, meeting basic caretaking needs, sharing the responsibility for medical decision making, weathering financial and social costs, and maintaining stability in the midst of the changes caused by cancer. Cancer pain can impact upon the performance of each of these tasks and the presence of pain has been found to be associated with increased emotional and financial burden in the family (Mor et al 1987). Pain is viewed as a major concern by family members of cancer patients and, perhaps more than other physical symptoms, it is perceived as a powerful threat to the ongoing ability to manage the disease (Ferrell 1991). Many studies have documented the concern family members have about cancer pain and the priority families place upon patient comfort (Hinds 1985,

Rowat 1985, Kristjanson 1986, Blank et al 1989, Hull 1989). Hence, the adequate management of cancer pain should include educating family members regarding pain management issues (i.e., the assessment of pain, proper administration and scheduling of medications, addiction), as well as emotional support and stress management skills and structured opportunities for respite from caregiving responsibilities (Warner 1992).

As was noted above, cancer patients with pain are more likely to develop psychiatric disorders than are patients without pain. The presence of serious depression or organic mental syndromes can seriously disrupt family–patient relationships and further hinder the ability of family members to provide emotional support for their ill relative. Family members too are vulnerable to developing stress-related emotional disorders that can further break down the support they can afford the patient. Ferrell et al (1991) examined the functioning of caregivers who cared for patients in pain, finding that caregivers consistently described the patient's pain as highly distressing to themselves. Pain appeared to heighten the burden of caregiving, especially impacting sleep, physical strain, and overall emotional adjustment. In the advanced cancer patient, whose pain may be difficult to relieve without some sacrifice of mental clarity, family members and patients may disagree about the goals of pain treatment (mental clarity with residual pain versus greater comfort even if accompanied by sedation). Thus, discussions of the patient's and family members' goals for treatment should be held early in the disease course, so that conflicts can be resolved with the full participation of the patient. Another issue that can impede family support is family misconceptions about drug tolerance, dependence, and addiction. Family members often become alarmed at the patient's increasing need for opioids and may withold treatment or limit their advocacy for the patient for fear that the patient will become addicted to their medication or 'use up' the drug's ability to relieve pain. Education about addiction, tolerance, and the meaning of physiological dependence is crucial in avoiding such unnecessary conflicts.

Finally, the family's ability to provide the patient with continuity in the midst of change can be seriously threatened by the development of or changes in cancer pain. To provide for such continuity, family members need to feel as if they are able to predict or exert some control over the disease course. Cancer pain is often viewed as a harbinger of disease progression and as such can be a signal for the patient and family that they are about to enter a new phase of the disease. When cancer pain is continually unrelieved, it can confuse such signals and sacrifice family members' sense of control. The ability to maintain stability and provide the patient with a safe and supportive family environment can thus be disrupted.

Cancer pain and staff stress

Those of us who work intensively with cancer patients have chosen a rewarding but stressful occupation. The painful nature of cancer and its treatment, difficult ethical dilemmas in treatment decision making, emotional reactions of patients and staff to cancer pain, and poor staff communication or conflict all contribute to the stressful cancer work environment. Intense medical involvement with cancer pain patients tends to elicit common reactions that are well known to health care workers in the field. The first is the need to try to 'save' patients from their cancer illness or death. The health care worker may wish to rescue patients from their dreadful plight. Unfortunately, disease often progresses and failure to save patients often leads to feelings of helplessness and a sense of futility. Low self-esteem and depression may result and sometimes engender resentment towards the patient. In an attempt to deal with these feelings of helplessness and futility, the physician or nurse may become overinvolved in the patient's medical care, encouraging or demanding inappropriately aggressive or unrealistic interventions. Staff members often find the transition from active treatment to palliative care difficult. Accepting altered treatment goals and relinquishing the hope of survival for a special patient can be very painful (Spikes and Holland 1975). The inability to recognize that such a transition in care is necessary can lead to a delay in dealing with issues such as DNR orders or other practical issues. Unaware of such reactions, a nurse or physician with a cancer patient may develop an adversarial relationship with other health professionals involved in that individual's care. A grandiose or self-serving attitude may develop in which the nurse or physician feels that only he or she understands the patient and knows how best to care for him medically. Such attitudes often reflect an exaggerated sense of responsibility for the patient's fate, which can result in enormous guilt once the patient's condition ultimately worsens.

Another common staff reaction is the need to 'protect' the patient. This often takes the form of an avoidance to confront or bring up for discussion, even when appropriate, topics that may be painful or emotionally distressing to the patient. Consequently, important issues may go unaddressed, such as the patient's feelings about pain, suffering, and death, practical issues such as a will, DNR status, and tying up financial loose ends. It is also important for the health professional to confront extreme denial and other maladaptive defenses on the part of the patient, especially when they interfere with treatment compliance. Recognition of our human limitations and personal vulnerabilities to loss are as important as being aware of these common countertransference reactions. Hopefully such awareness can benefit our patients, colleagues, and ourselves.

A third common reaction is the tendency to blame the patients for their continued complaints of pain and discomfort. Ignoring the fact that cancer pain management is complex, this reaction takes the form of interpreting the patients' failure to respond to efforts at pain and symptom control as a desire on their part to perpetuate their symptomatology. Patients who have failed to respond to efforts at pain control are seen as 'needing their pain', 'communicating through pain', or drug seeking. In an effort to protect oneself from feelings of inadequacy, health care workers can displace their anger upon patients and withhold appropriate diagnostic tests or interventions.

The consequences of stress in the cancer work environment are many, including the development of physical and/or psychological symptoms, 'burnout', or even more serious difficulties such as substance abuse or depression. Common physical symptoms of chronic stress include tension headache, exhaustion, fatigue, insomnia, and gastrointestinal disturbances with no apparent medical cause. Psychological symptoms of stress in cancer staff include loss of enthusiasm for work, depression, irritability and frustration, and a cynical view of medicine and colleagues (Hall et al 1979, Maslach 1979, Holland and Holland 1985, Mount 1986). Physicians and nurses can become overinvolved in their work, with excessive dedication and commitment, spend longer hours with less productivity, and show decreased sensitivity to the emotional needs of patients and others; conversely, they may become detached and disinterested in medical practice. These two presentations of burnout in oncologists and oncology nurses have been described as the 'I must do everything' syndrome and the 'I hate medicine' syndrome. Potential outcomes of both of these syndromes, if allowed to progress, include substance abuse, depression, and even suicide (Hall et al 1979, Holland and Holland 1985, Mount 1986).

A variety of coping methods can be introduced at both the personal and organizational levels and can be useful in the prevention and management of burnout (Hartl 1979, Koocher 1979, Mount 1986). One of the most important strategies is to be able to recognize the physical and psychological symptoms of stress in oneself. It is additionally important to identify them in colleagues and point out that such symptoms are common, transient, and reversible when dealt with early. Discomfort in pointing out emotional distress in a colleague should not be any greater than suggesting a consultation for a medical symptom. In the cancer centre, having the support of one's peers helps to decrease feelings of demoralization (Kash and Holland 1990). Providing ongoing staff education in pain management can help reduce stress and feelings of inadequacy for staff members. Mental health professionals can also provide invaluable staff support in oncology settings including providing support and backup to unit leaders, and faciliting staff communication (Lederberg 1989). Providing support to colleagues, helping identify and deal with troubled staff, leading groups and conferences, or participating in daily rounds are all useful methods of bolstering staff morale and helping avoid burnout. Ideally, an active role on the unit makes the liaison psychiatrist most familiar with the problems of the unit but even outside mental health consultants can be useful in providing staff support, albeit often somewhat less effective than mental health professionals who are fully integrated into the mileau.

Cognitive-behavioural interventions in cancer pain

Cognitive-behavioural techniques useful in cancer pain (Box 45.2) include passive relaxation with mental imagery, cognitive distraction or focusing, cognitive restructuring, progressive muscle relaxation, biofeedback, hypnosis, systematic desensitization, and music therapy (Cleeland and Tearnan 1986, Cleeland 1987, Fishman and Loscalzo 1987). Some techniques are primarily cognitive in nature, focusing on perceptual and thought processes, and others are directed at modifying patterns of behaviour that help cancer patients cope with pain. Behavioural techniques include methods of modifying physiological pain reactions, respondent pain behaviours, and operant pain behaviours. The most fundamental technique is self-monitoring. The development of the ability to monitor one's behaviours allows a person to notice dysfunctional reactions and learn to control them. Systematic

BOX 45.2
Cognitive-behavioural techniques used for cancer pain patients

Psychoeducation
Preparatory information
Relaxation
Passive breathing
Progressive muscle relaxation
Distraction
Focusing
Controlled mental imagery
Cognitive distraction
Behavioural distraction
Combined relaxation and distraction techniques
Passive relaxation with mental imagery
Progressive muscle relaxation with imagery
Systematic desensitization
Meditation
Hypnosis
Biofeedback
Music therapy
Cognitive therapies
Cognitive restructuring
Behavioural therapies
Self-monitoring
Modelling
Behavioural rehearsal
Graded task management
Contingency management

desensitization is useful in extinguishing anticipatory anxiety that leads to avoidant behaviours and in remobilizing inactive patients. Graded task assignment is analogous to *in vivo* systematic desensitization, in which patients are encouraged to delineate and then execute a series of small steps towards an ultimate goal. Contingency management, a behavioural intervention in which healthy or adaptive behaviours are reinforced, has also been applied to the management of chronic pain as a method for modifying dysfunctional operant pain behaviours associated with secondary gain (Cleeland 1987, Loscalzo and Jacobsen 1990). Primarily cognitive techniques for coping with pain are aimed at increasing relaxation and reducing the intensity and emotional distress that accompany the pain experience. Cognitive restructuring, a technique often used in the treatment of depression or anxiety, is an effective method of altering a patient's interpretation of events and bodily sensations. Because many patients are plagued by disturbing and maladaptive thoughts or beliefs, identifying and modifying these beliefs can allow for more accurate assessment of the situation and thereby decrease subjective distress (Fishman and Loscalzo 1987).

Most cancer patients with pain are appropriate candidates for useful application of cognitive and behavioural techniques; the clinician, however, should take into account the intensity of pain and the mental clarity of the patient. Ideal candidates have mild to moderate pain and can benefit from these interventions, whereas patients with severe pain can expect limited benefit from psychological interventions unless somatic therapies can lower the level of pain to some degree. Confusional states also interfere dramatically with a patient's ability to focus attention and thus limit the usefulness of these techniques (Loscalzo and Jacobsen 1990). Occasionally these techniques can be modified to enable patients with mild cognitive impairments to benefit. This often involves the therapist taking a more active role by orienting the patient, creating a safe and secure environment, and evoking a conditioned response to the therapist's voice or presence.

Cancer patients are usually highly motivated to learn and practice cognitive-behavioural techniques because they are often effective not only in symptom control, but in restoring a sense of self control, personal efficacy, and active participation in their care. It is important to note that these techniques must not be used as a substitute for apropriate analgesic management of cancer pain but rather as part of a comprehensive multimodal approach. The lack of side effects associated with psychological interventions makes them particularly attractive in the oncology setting as a supplement to already complicated medication regimens. The successful use of these techniques should never lead to the erroneous conclusion that the pain was of psychogenic origin and therefore not 'real'. Although the specific mechanisms by which these cognitive and behavioural techniques relieve pain vary, most share the elements of relaxation and distraction. Distraction or redirection of attention helps reduce awareness of pain and relaxation reduces muscle tension and sympathetic arousal (Cleeland 1987).

Other behavioural interventions

Several techniques are used to achieve a mental and physical state of relaxation. Muscular tension, autonomic arousal, and mental distress exacerbate pain (Cleeland 1987, Loscalzo and Jacobsen 1990). Some specific relaxation techniques include: (i) passive relaxation, (ii) progressive muscle relaxation, and (iii) meditation. Passive relaxation, focused breathing, and passive muscle relaxation exercises involve the focusing of attention systematically on one's breathing, on sensations of warmth and relaxation, or on release of muscular tension in various body parts. Verbal suggestions and imagery are used to help promote relaxation. Muscle relaxation is an important component of the relaxation response and can augment the benefits of simple focused breathing exercises, leading to a deeper experience of relaxation and self-control. Progressive or active muscle relaxation involves the active tensing and relaxing of various muscle groups in the body, focusing attention on the sensations of tension, and relaxation. Clinically, in the hospital setting, relaxation is most commonly achieved through the use of a combination of focused breathing and progressive muscle relaxation exercises. Once patients are in a relaxed state, imagery techniques can then be used to induce deeper relaxation and facilitate distraction from or manipulation of a variety of cancer-related symptoms. Scripts that can be utilized by therapists to aid in teaching patients passive and/or active relaxation techniques are available in the literature (McCaffery and Beebe 1989, Loscalzo and Jacobsen 1990, Horowitz and Breitbart 1993). Hypnosis has also been used in the treatment of some cancer pain (Barber and Gitelson 1980, Redd et al 1982, Spiegel and Bloom 1983b, Spiegel 1985), although the specific efficacy of hypnosis (rather than expectancy effects) has increasingly been questioned.

Psychotropic adjuvant analgesics for cancer pain

While the mainstay of pharmacological management of cancer pain is the aggressive use of narcotic analgesics, there is a growing appreciation for the role of adjuvant analgesic drugs in providing maximal comfort (Breitbart 1989a, Breitbart and Holland 1990, Walsh 1990). Psychotropic drugs, particularly antidepressants, psychostimulants, neuroleptics, and anxiolytics, are useful as adjuvant analgesics in the pharmacological management of cancer pain. Psychiatrists are often the most experienced in the clinical use of these drugs and so can play an important role in assisting pain control. Table 45.6 lists the various psychotropic medications with their analgesic properties, routes of administration, and approximate daily doses. These medications have been shown earlier (see Tables 45.2, 45.3) to be effective in managing symptoms of depression, anxiety, or delirium that commonly complicate the course of cancer patients with pain. They also potentiate the analgesic effects of opioid drugs and often have analgesic properties of their own. The most widely studied, and most empirically supported adjuvant analgesics are the tricyclic antidepressants (Walsh 1983, 1990; Butler 1986; France 1987; Getto et al 1987; Magni et al 1987; Ventafridda et al 1987). Amitriptyline is the tricyclic antidepressant most studied, and proven effective as an analgesic, in a large number of clinical trials, addressing a wide variety of chronic pain syndromes (Pilowsky et al 1982; Watson et al 1982; Max et al 1987, 1988; Sharav et al 1987). Other tricyclic antidepressants that have been shown to have efficacy as analgesics include imipramine (Kvindesal et al 1984, Young and Clarke 1985, Sindrup et al 1989), desipramine (Kishore-Kumar et al 1990, Max et al 1991), nortriptyline (Gomez-Perez et al 1985), clomipramine (Langohr et al 1982, Tiengo et al 1987), and doxepin (Hammeroff et al 1982). Other antidepressents (e.g., heterocyclic, SSRIs), while possibly effective, have not been as clearly supported by empirical research and are not necessarily first-line choices for adjuvant analgesic therapy.

Psychiatric aspects of pain in AIDS

Studies conducted between 1990 and 1995 have documented that pain in individuals with HIV infection or AIDS is highly prevalent, diverse, and varied in syndromal presentation; associated with significant psychological and functional morbidity; and alarmingly undertreated (Lebovits et al 1989; McCormack et al 1993; O'Neill and Sherrard 1993; Singer et al 1993; Breitbart 1996, 1997; Breitbart et al 1996a, b; Rosenfeld et al 1996; Hewitt et al 1997). With the introduction of highly active antiretroviral therapies (i.e., combination therapies including protease inhibitors), the face of the AIDS epidemic, particularly for those who can avail themselves of and/or tolerate these new therapies, is indeed changing. Death rates from AIDS in the USA have dropped dramatically in the past 5 years, and rates of serious opportunistic infections and cancers are declining. Despite these hopeful developments, the future is still unclear, and millions of patients with HIV disease worldwide will continue to die of AIDS and suffer from the enormous burden of physical and psychological symptoms. Even with the advances in AIDS therapies, pain continues to be an issue in the care of patients with HIV disease. As the epidemiology of the AIDS epidemic changes in the USA, managing pain in AIDS patients with a

Table 45.6 Psychotropic adjuvant analgesic drugs for cancer pain

Generic name	Trade name	Approximate daily dosage range (mg)	Route
		Tricyclic antidepressants	
Amitriptyline	Elavil	10–150	PO, IM, PR
Nortriptyline	Pamelor, Aventyl	10–150	PO
Imipramine	Tofranil	12.5–150	PO, IM
Desipramine	Norpramin	10–150	PO
Clomipramine	Anafranil	10–150	PO
Doxepin	Sinequan	12.5–150	PO, IM
		Heterocyclic and non-cyclic antidepressants	
Trazodone	Desyrel	25–300	PO
Maprotiline	Ludiomil	50–300	PO
		Serotonin specific reuptake inhibitors	
Fluoxetine	Prozac	20–60	PO
Paroxetine	Paxil	10–40	PO
		Amine precursors	
L-Tryptophan		500–3000	PO
		Psychostimulants	
Methylphenidate	Ritalin	2.5–20 b.i.d.	PO
Dextroamphetamine	Dexedrine	2.5–20 b.i.d.	PO
		Phenothiazines	
Fluphenazine	Prolixin	1–3	PO, IM
Methotrimeprazine	Levoprome	10–20q 6 h	IM, IV
		Butyrophenones	
Haloperidol	Haldol	1–3	PO, IM, IV
Pimozide	Orap	2–6 b.i.d.	PO
		Antihistamines	
Hydroxyzine	Vistaril	50q 4–6 h	PO, IM, IV
		Steroids	
Dexamethasone	Decadron	4–16	PO, IV
		Benzodiazepines	
Alprazolam	Xanax	0.25–2.0 t.i.d.	PO
Clonazepam	Klonopin	0.5–4 b.i.d.	PO

PO = per oral; IM = intramuscular; PR = parenteral; IV = intravenous; q 6 h = every 6 h; b.i.d. = two times a day, t.i.d. = three times a day.

history of substance abuse is becoming an ever-growing challenge. Pain management needs to be more integrated into the total care of patients with HIV disease.

Prevalence of pain in HIV disease

Estimates of the prevalence of pain in HIV-infected individuals have been reported to range from 30 to over 90%, with the prevalence of pain increasing as disease progresses (Lebovits et al 1989; Schofferman and Brody 1990; Breitbart et al 1991, 1996a, b; Singer et al 1993; Kimball and McCormick 1996; Larue et al 1997), particularly in the latest stages of illness.

Studies suggest that approximately 30% of ambulatory HIV-infected patients in the early stages of HIV disease (pre-AIDS; Category A or B disease) experience clinically significant pain, and as many as 56% have had episodic painful symptoms of less clear clinical significance (Singer et al 1993, Breitbart et al 1996b, Larue et al 1997). In a prospective cross-sectional survey of 438 ambulatory AIDS patients in New York City, 63% reported 'frequent or persistent pain of at least two weeks duration' at the time of assessment (Breitbart et al 1996b). The prevalence of pain in this large sample increased significantly as HIV disease progressed, with 45% of AIDS patients with Category A3 disease reporting pain, 55% of those with Category B3 reporting pain, and 67% of those with Category C1, 2, or 3 disease reporting pain. Patients in this sample of ambulatory AIDS patients also were more likely to report pain if they had other concurrent HIV-related symptoms (e.g., fatigue, wasting), had received treatment for an AIDS-related opportunistic infection, or had not been receiving antiretroviral medications (e.g., AZT, ddl, ddC, d4t).

In a study of pain in hospitalized patients with AIDS in a public hospital in New York City, over 50% of patients required treatment for pain, with pain being the presenting complaint in 30% and the second most common presenting problem after fever (Lebovits et al 1989). In a French multicentre study, 62% of hospitalized patients with HIV disease had clinically significant pain (Larue et al 1997). Schofferman and Brody (1990) reported that 53% of patients with far-advanced AIDS cared for in a hospice setting had pain, while Kimball and McCormack (1996) reported that up to 93% of AIDS patients in their hospice experienced at least one 48-h period of pain during the last 2 weeks of life.

Larue and colleagues (1994) demonstrated that patients with AIDS being cared for in a hospice or at home had prevalence rates and intensity ratings for pain comparable to and even exceeded those of cancer patients. Breitbart and colleagues (1996a) reported that ambulatory AIDS patients in their New York City sample reported a mean pain intensity 'on average' of 5.4 (on the 0–10 numerical rating scale of the Brief Pain Inventory) and a mean pain 'at its worst' of 7.4. In addition, as with pain prevalence, the intensity of pain experienced by patients with HIV disease increases significantly as disease progresses. AIDS patients with pain, like their counterparts with cancer pain, typically describe an average of 2.5 to 3 concurrent pains at a time (Breitbart et al 1996a, Hewitt et al 1997).

Pain syndromes in HIV/AIDS: aetiologies and classification

Pain syndromes encountered in AIDS are diverse in nature and aetiology. The most common pain syndromes reported in studies to date include painful sensory peripheral neuropathy, pain due to extensive Karposi's sarcoma, headache, oral and pharyngeal pain, abdominal pain, chest pain, arthralgias and myalgias, and painful dermatological conditions (Lebovits et al 1989; Schofferman and Brody 1990; Breitbart et al 1991, 1996b; Penfold and Clark 1992; O'Neill and Sherrard 1993; Singer et al 1993; Larue et al 1994; Hewitt et al 1997). In a sample of 151 ambulatory AIDS patients who underwent a research assessment that included a clinical interview, neurological examination, and review of medical records (Hewitt et al 1997), the most common pain diagnoses included headaches (46% of patients; 17% of all pains), joint pains (arthritis, arthralgias, etc.—31% of patients; 12% of pains), painful polyneuropathy (distal symmetrical polyneuropathy—28% of patients; 10% of pains), and muscle pains (myalgia, myositis—27% of patients; 12% of pains). Other common pain diagnoses included skin pain (Kaposi's sarcoma, infections—25% of patients; 30% of homosexual males in the sample had pain from extensive KS lesions), bone pain (20% of patients), abdominal pain (17% of patients), chest pain (13%), and painful radiculopathy (12%). Patients in this sample had a total of 405 pains (averaging 3 concurrent pains), with 46% of patients diagnosed with neuropathic-type pain, 71% with somatic pain, 29% with visceral pain, and 46% with headache (classified separately because of controversy as to pathophysiology). When pain type was classified by pains (as opposed to patients) 25% were neuropathic pains, 44% were nociceptive-somatic, 14% were nociceptive-visceral, and 17% were idiopathic-type pains. Patients in this study with lower CD4+ cell counts were significantly more likely to be diagnosed with polyneuropathy and headache. Hewitt and colleagues (1997) demonstrated that while pains of a neuropathic nature (e.g., polyneuropathies, radiculopathies) certainly compose a large proportion of pain syndromes encountered in AIDS patients, pains of a somatic and/or visceral nature are also extremely common clinical problems.

BOX 45.3
Pain syndromes of HIV/AIDS

Pain related to HIV/AIDS infection or consequences of infection
HIV neuropathy
HIV myelopathy
Kaposi's sarcoma
Secondary infections (intestines, skin)
Organomegaly
Arthritis/vasculitis
Myopathy/myositis
Pain related to HIV/AIDS therapy
Antiretrovirals, antivirals
Antimycobacterials, pneumocystis carinii
Pneumonia prophylaxis
Chemotherapy (vincristine)
Radiation
Surgery
Procedures (bronchoscopy, biopsies)
Pain unrelated to AIDS or AIDS therapy
Disc disease
Diabetic neuropathy

Pain syndromes seen in HIV disease can be categorized into three types (Box 45.3):

1. Those directly related to HIV infection or consequences of immunosuppression,
2. Those due to AIDS therapies, and
3. Those unrelated to AIDS or AIDS therapies (Breitbart 1997, Hewitt et al 1997).

In studies to date, approximately 45% of pain syndromes encountered are directly related to HIV infection or consequences of immunosuppression; 15–30% are caused by therapies for HIV- or AIDS-related conditions, as well as diagnostic procedures; and the remaining 25–40% are unrelated to HIV or its therapies (Hewitt et al 1997).

Our group at Memorial has reported on the experience of pain in women with AIDS (Breitbart et al 1995, Hewitt et al 1997). Our studies suggest that women with HIV disease experience pain more frequently than men with HIV disease and report somewhat higher levels of pain intensity. This may in part be a reflection of the fact that women with AIDS-related pain are twice as likely to be undertreated for their pain compared to men (Breitbart et al 1996a). Women with HIV disease have unique pain syndromes of a gynaecological nature specifically related to opportunistic infectious processes and cancers of the pelvis and genitourinary tract (Marte and Allen 1991). Women with AIDS were significantly more likely to be diagnosed with radiculopathy and headache in one survey (Hewitt et al 1997).

Children with HIV infection also experience pain (Strafford et al 1991). HIV-related conditions in children observed to cause pain include meningitis and sinusitis (headaches); otitis media; shingles; cellulitis and abscesses; severe candida dermatitis; dental caries; intestinal infections, such as *Mycobacterium avium intracellulare* (MAI) and cryptosporidium; hepatosplenomegaly; oral and oesophageal candidiasis; and spasticity associated with encephalopathy that causes painful muscle spasms.

Impact of pain: psychological distress

Pain in patients with HIV disease has a profound negative impact on physical and psychological functioning, as well as overall quality of life (Rosenfeld et al 1996, Larue et al 1997). In a study of the impact of pain on psychological functioning and quality of life in ambulatory AIDS patients (Rosenfeld et al 1996), depression was significantly correlated with the presence of pain. In addition to being significantly more distressed, depressed, and hopeless, those with pain were twice as likely to have suicidal ideation (40%) as those without pain (20%). HIV-infected patients with pain were more functionally impaired (Rosenfeld et al 1996). Such functional interference was highly correlated to levels of pain intensity and depression. Patients with pain were more likely to be unemployed or disabled and reported less social support. Larue and colleagues (1997) reported that HIV-infected patients with pain intensities greater than 5 (on a 0–10 numerical rating scale (NRS)) reported significantly poorer quality of life during the week preceding their survey than patients without pain. Pain intensity had an independent negative impact on HIV patients' quality of life, even after adjustment for treatment setting, stage of disease, fatigue, sadness, and depression. Singer and colleagues (1993) also reported an association between the frequency of multiple pains, increased disability, and higher levels of depression. Psychological variables, such as the amount of control people believe they have over pain, emotional associations and memories of pain, fears of death, depression, anxiety, and hopelessness, contribute to the experience of pain in people with AIDS and can increase suffering (Breitbart 1993, Rosenfeld et al 1996). Our group also reported (Payne et al 1994) that negative thoughts related to pain were associated with greater pain intensity, psychological distress, and disability in ambulatory patients with AIDS. Those AIDS patients who felt that pain represented a progression of their HIV disease reported more intense pain than those who did not see pain as a threat.

Undertreatment of pain in AIDS

Reports of dramatic undertreatment of pain in AIDS patients have appeared in the literature (Lebovits et al 1989, McCormack et al 1993, Breitbart et al 1996a, Larue et al 1997). These studies suggest that all classes of analgesics, particularly opioid analgesics, are underutilized in the treatment of pain in AIDS. Our group has reported (Breitbart et al 1996b) that less than 8% of individuals in our cohort of ambulatory AIDS patients reporting pain in the severe range (8–10 on a NRS of pain intensity) received a strong opioid, such as morphine, as recommended by published guidelines (i.e., the WHO Analgesic Ladder). In addition, 18% of patients with 'severe' pain were prescribed no analgesics whatsoever, 40% were prescribed a non-opioid analgesic (e.g., NSAID), and only 22% were prescribed a 'weak' opioid' (e.g., acetaminophen in combination with oxycodone). Utilizing the Pain Management Index (PMI) (Zelman et al 1987), a measure of adequacy of analgesic therapy derived from the Brief Pain Inventory's (BPI) record of pain intensity and strength of analgesia prescribed, we further examined adequacy of pain treatment. Only 15% of our sample received adequate analgesic therapy based on the PMI. This degree of undermedication of pain in AIDS (85%) far exceeds published reports of undermedication of pain (using the PMI) in cancer populations of 40% (Cleeland et al 1994). Larue and colleagues (1997) report that in France, 57% of patients with HIV disease reporting moderate to severe pain did not receive any analgesic treatment at all, and only 22% received a 'weak' opioid.

While opioid analgesics are underutilized, it is also clear that adjuvant analgesic agents, such as antidepressants, are also dramatically underutilized (Lebovits et al 1989, McCormack et al 1993, Breitbart et al 1996a, Larue et al 1997). Breitbart and colleagues (1996a) report that less than 10% of AIDS patients reporting pain received an adjuvant analgesic drug (e.g., antidepressants, anticonvulsants), despite the fact that approximately 40% of the sample had neuropathic-type pain. This class of analgesic agents is a critical component of the WHO Analgesic Ladder, particularly in managing neuropathic pain, and is vastly underutilized in the management of HIV-related pain.

A number of different factors have been proposed as potential influences on the widespread undertreatment of pain in AIDS, including patient, clinician, and health care system-related barriers (Passik et al 1994; Breitbart et al 1996a, 1998, 1999). Sociodemographic factors that have been reported to be associated with undertreatment of pain in AIDS include gender, education, and substance abuse history (Breitbart et al 1996b). Women, less educated patients, and patients who reported injection drug use as their HIV risk transmission factor are significantly more likely to receive inadequate analgesic therapy for HIV-related pain.

Psychiatric management of pain in AIDS

The psychiatric management of HIV-related pain involves the use of psychotherapeutic, cognitive-behavioural, and psychopharmacological techniques. Psychotherapists can offer short-term supportive psychotherapy, based on a crisis–intervention model, and provide emotional support, continuity of care, information about pain management, and assistance to patients in adapting to their crises. This often involves working with 'families' that are not typical and that may consist of gay partners, estranged spouses or parents, and fragmented or extended families. People with HIV disease may also require treatment for substance abuse.

Cognitive-behavioural techniques for pain control, such as relaxation, imagery, hypnosis, and biofeedback, are effective as part of a comprehensive multimodal approach, particularly among patients with HIV disease who may have an increased sensitivity to the side effects of medications. Non-pharmacological interventions, however, must never be used as a substitute for the appropriate analgesic management of pain. The mechanisms by which these non-pharmacological techniques work are not known; however, they all seem to share the elements of relaxation and distraction. Additionally, patients often feel a sense of increased control over their pain and their bodies. Ideal candidates for the application of these techniques are mentally alert and have mild to moderate pain. Confusion interferes significantly with a patient's ability to focus attention and so limits the usefulness of cognitive-behavioural interventions.

Psychiatric disorders, particularly organic mental disorders such as AIDS–dementia complex, can occasionally interfere with adequate pain management in patients with HIV disease. Opiate analgesics, the mainstay of treatment for moderate to severe pain, may worsen dementia or cause treatment-limiting sedation, confusion, or hallucinations in patients with neurological complications of AIDS. The judicious use of psychostimulants to diminish sedation and neuroleptics to clear confusion can be quite helpful.

Psychotropic drugs, particularly the TCAs and the psychostimulants, are useful in enhancing the pain-blocking properties of analgesics in pharmacological management of HIV-related pain. The tricyclic antidepressants (amitriptyline, nortriptyline, imipramine, desipramine, doxepin) and some of the newer non-cyclic antidepressants (trazodone and fluoxetine) have potent analgesic properties and are widely used to treat a variety of chronic pain syndromes. They may have their most beneficial effect in the treatment of neuropathic pain, that is, pain due to nerve damage, such as the peripheral neuropathies seen commonly in people with HIV infection. Antidepressants have direct analgesic effects and the capacity to enhance the analgesic effects of morphine.

Psychostimulants such as dextroamphetamine or methylphenidate are useful antidepressants in people with HIV disease who are cognitively impaired and are also helpful in diminishing sedation secondary to narcotic analgesics. Psychostimulants also enhance the analgesic effects of opiate analgesics.

The inadequate management of pain is often caused by the inability to properly assess pain in all its dimensions. All too frequently, physicians presume that psychological variables are the cause of continued pain or lack of response to medical treatment, when in fact they have not adequately appreciated the role of medical factors. Other causes of inadequate pain management include lack of knowledge of current pharmaco- or psychotherapeutic approaches, a focus on prolonging life rather than alleviating suffering, lack of communication or unsuccessful communication between doctors and patients, limited expectations of patients to achieve pain relief, limited capacity of patients impaired by organic mental disorders to communicate, unavailability of narcotics, doctors' fear of causing respiratory depression, and, most importantly, doctors' fear of amplifying addiction and drug abuse.

References

Adams F, Quesada JR, Gutterman JU 1984 Neuropsychiatric manifestations of human leukocyte interferon therapy in patients with cancer. Journal of the American Medical Association 252: 938–941

Adams F, Fernandez F, Andersson BS 1986 Emergency pharmacotherapy of delirium in the critically ill cancer patient. Psychosomatics 27: 36–37

Ahles TA, Martin JB 1992 Cancer pain: a multidimensional perspective. Hospice Journal 8: 25–48

Ahles TA, Blanchard EB, Ruckdeschel JC 1983 The multidimensional nature of cancer related pain. Pain 17: 277–288

American Psychiatric Association 1994 Diagnostic and statistical manual of mental disorders, 4th edn (DSM-IV). American Psychiatric Association, Washington, DC

Barber J, Gitelson J 1980 Cancer pain: psychological management using hypnosis. CA: A Cancer Journal for Clinicians 3: 130–136

Blank SS, Clark L, Longman AJ, Atwood JR 1989 Perceived home care needs of cancer patients and their caregivers. Cancer Nursing 12: 78–84

Bolund C 1985 Suicide and cancer: II. Medical and care factors in suicide by cancer patients in Sweden, 1973–1976. Journal of Psychosocial Oncology 3: 17–30

Bond MR 1973 Personality studies in patients with pain secondary to organic disease. Journal of Psychosomatic Research 17: 257–263

Bond MR 1979 Psychological and emotional aspects of cancer pain. In: Bonica JJ, Ventafridda V (eds) Advances in pain research and therapy, vol 2. Raven, New York, pp 81–88

Bond MR, Pearson IB 1969 Psychological aspects of pain in women with advanced cancer of the cervix. Journal of Psychosomatic Research 13: 13–19

Bottomley DM, Hanks GW 1990 Subcutaneous midazolam infusion in palliative care. Journal of Pain Symptom Management 5: 259–261

Breitbart W 1987 Suicide in cancer patients. Oncology 1: 49–53

Breitbart W 1989a Psychiatric management of cancer pain. Cancer 63: 2336–2342

Breitbart WB 1989b Endocrine-related psychiatric disorder. In: Holland J, Rowland J (eds) The handbook of psychooncology: the psychological care of the cancer patient. Oxford University Press, New York, pp 356–366

Breitbart W 1990 Cancer pain and suicide. In: Foley KM et al (eds) Advances in pain research and therapy, vol 16. Raven, New York, pp 399–412

Breitbart W 1993 Suicide risk and pain in cancer and AIDS patients. In: Chapman R, Foley KM (eds) Current emerging issues in cancer pain: research and practice. Raven, New York, pp 49–65

Breitbart W 1996 Pharmacotherapy of pain in AIDS. In: Wormser G (ed) A clinical guide to AIDS and HIV. Lippencott-Raven, Philadelphia, pp 359–378

Breitbart W 1997 Pain in AIDS. In: Jensen J, Turner J, Wiesenfeld-Hallin Z (eds) Proceedings of the 8th world congress on pain, progress in pain research and management, vol. 8. IASP Press, Seattle, pp 63–100

Breitbart W, Chochinov H (eds) 2000 Handbook of psychiatry in palliative medicine. Oxford University Press, New York

Breitbart W, Holland JC 1988 Psychiatric complications of cancer. In: Brain MC, Carbone PP (eds) Current therapy in hematology oncology, vol 3. BC Decker, Toronto, pp 268–274

Breitbart W, Holland J 1990 Psychiatric aspects of cancer pain. In: Foley KM et al (eds) Advances in pain research and therapy, vol 16. Raven, New York, pp 73–87

Breitbart W, Mermelstein H 1992 Pemoline: an alternative psychostimulation in the management of depressive disorders in cancer patients. Psychosomatics 33: 352–356

Breitbart W, Passik S, Bronaugh T et al 1991 Pain in the ambulatory AIDS patient: prevalence and psychosocial correlates. 38th annual meeting, Academy of Psychosomatic Medicine, October 17–20, Atlanta, GA (abstract)

Breitbart W, McDonald M, Rosenfeld B et al 1995 Pain in women with AIDS. Proceedings of the 14th annual meeting of the American Pain Society, Los Angeles, CA (abstract)

Breitbart W, Rosenfeld B, Passik S, McDonald M, Thaler H, Portenoy R 1996a The undertreatment of pain in ambulatory AIDS patients. Pain 65: 239–245

Breitbart W, McDonald MV, Rosenfeld B et al 1996b Pain in ambulatory AIDS patients—I: Pain characteristics and medical correlates. Pain 68: 315–321

Breitbart W, Marotta R, Platt M et al 1996c A double blind trial of haloperidol, chlorpromazine and lorazepam in the treatment of delirium in hospitalized AIDS patients. American Journal of Psychiatry 153: 231–237

Breitbart W, Rosenfeld BD, Passik SD 1996d Interest in physician-assisted suicide in ambulatory HIV-infected patients. American Journal of Psychiatry 153: 238–242

Breitbart W, Passik S, McDonald M et al 1998 Patient-related barriers to pain management in ambulatory AIDS patients. Pain 76: 9–16

Breitbart W, Kaim M, Rosenfeld B 1999 Clinician's perceptions of barriers to pain management in AIDS. Journal of Pain and Symptom Management 18: 203–212

Breitbart W, Rosenfeld B, Pessin H, Kaim M, Funesti Esch J, Galietta M, Nelson C, Brescia R 2000 Depression, hopelessness, and desire for death in terminally ill cancer patients. Journal of the American Medical Association 284: 2907–2911

Breitbart W, Tremblay A, Gibson C 2002 An open trial of olanzapine for the treatment of delirium in hospitalized cancer patients. Psychosomatics 43: 175–182

Brennan SC, Redd WH, Jacobsen PB et al 1988 Anxiety and panic during magnetic resonance scans. Lancet ii: 512

Brown JH, Henteleff P, Barakat S, Rowe JR 1986 Is it normal for terminally ill patients to desire death? American Journal of Psychiatry 143: 208–211

Bruera E, MacMillan K, Kuehn N et al 1989 The cognitive effects of the administration of narcotics. Pain 39: 13–16

Bruera E, MacMillan K, Pither J, MacDonald RN 1990a Effects of morphine on the dyspnea of terminal cancer patients. Journal of Pain and Symptom Management 5: 341–344

Bruera E, Miller L, McCalion S 1990b Cognitive failure in patients with terminal cancer: a prospective longitudinal study. Psychosocial Aspects of Cancer 9: 308–310

Bukberg J, Penman D, Holland J 1984 Depression in hospitalized cancer patients. Psychosomatic Medicine 43: 122–199

Butler S 1986 Present status of tricyclic antidepressants in chronic pain therapy. In: Benedetti C et al (eds) Advances in pain research and therapy, vol 7. Raven, New York, pp 173–196

Cassem NH 1987 The dying patient. In: Hacket TP, Cassem NH (eds) Massachusetts General Hospital handbook of general hospital psychiatry, 2nd edn. PSG Publishing, Littleton, MA, pp 332–352

Chapman CR 1989 Giving the patient control of opioid analgesic administration. In: Hill CS, Fields WS (eds) Advances in pain research and therapy, vol 11. Raven, New York, pp 339–352

Chiarillo RJ, Cole JO 1987 The use of psychostimulants in general psychiatry. A reconsideration. Archives of General Psychiatry 44: 286–295

Chochinov HM, Wilson LG, Enns M 1995 Desire for death in the terminally ill. American Journal of Psychiatry 152: 1185–1191

Cleeland CS 1984 The impact of pain on the patient with cancer. Cancer 54: 2635–2641

Cleeland CS 1987 Nonpharmacologic management of cancer pain. Journal of Pain and Symptom Control 2: 523–528

Cleeland CS, Tearnan BH 1986 Behavioral control of cancer pain. In: Holzman D, Turk DC (eds) Pain management. Pergamon, New York, pp 193–212

Cleeland CS, Gonin R, Hatfield AK et al 1994 Pain and its treatment in outpatients with metastatic cancer: the Eastern Cooperative Oncology Group's outpatients study. New England Journal of Medicine 330: 592–596

Costa D, Mogos I, Toma T 1985 Efficacy and safety of mianserin in the treatment of depression of women with cancer. Acta Psychiatrica Scandinavica 72: 85–92

Dalton JA, Feuerstein M 1989 Fear, alexithymia and cancer pain. Pain 38: 159–170

Daut RL, Cleeland CS 1982 The prevalence and severity of pain in cancer. Cancer 50: 1913–1918

DeAngelis LM, Delattre J, Posner JB 1989 Radiation-induced dementia in patients cured of brain metastases. Neurology 39: 789–796

Denicoff KD, Rubinow DR, Papa MZ et al 1987 The neuropsychiatric effects of treatment with interleukin-w and lymphokine-activated killer cells. Annals of Internal Medicine 107: 293–300

Derogatis LR, Morrow GR, Fetting J et al 1983 The prevalence of psychiatric disorders among cancer patients. Journal of the American Medical Association 249: 751–757

de Sousa E, Jepson A 1988 Midazolam in terminal care. Lancet i: 67–68

Eller KC, Sison AC, Breitbart W, Passik S 1992 Morphine-induced acute confusional states: a retrospective analysis (abstract). Academy of Psychosomatic Medicine 39th annual meeting, San Diego, CA

Endicott J 1983 Measurement of depression in patients with cancer. Cancer 53: 2243–2248

Fainsinger R, MacEachern T, Hanson J et al 1991 Symptom control during the last week of life in a palliative care unit. Journal of Palliative Care 7: 5–11

Farberow NL, Schneidman ES, Leonard CV 1963 Suicide among general medical and surgical hospital patients with malignant neoplasms. Medical Bulletin 9, US Veterans Administration, Washington, DC

Fernandez F, Adams F, Holmes VF et al 1987 Methylphenidate for depressive disorders in cancer patients. Psychosomatics 28: 455–461

Fernandez F, Levy JK, Mansell PWA 1989 Management of delirium in terminally ill AIDS patients. International Journal of Psychiatry in Medicine 19: 165–172

Ferrell B 1991 Pain as a metaphor for illness: impact of cancer pain on family caregiver. Oncology Nursing Forum 18: 1303–1308

Fisch R 1985–1986 Methylphenidate for medical inpatients. International Journal of Psychiatry in Medicine 15: 75–79

Fishman B, Loscalzo M 1987 Cognitive-behavioral interventions in the management of cancer pain: principles and applications. Medical Clinics of North America 71: 271–287

Fleishman SB, Lesko LM 1989 Delirium and dementia. In: Holland J, Rowland J (eds) The handbook of psychooncology: psychological care of the cancer patient. Oxford University Press, New York, pp 342–355

Foley KM 1975 Pain syndromes in patients with cancer. In: Bonica JJ, Ventafridda V, Fink RB, Jones LE, Loeser JD (eds) Advances in pain research and therapy, vol 2. Raven, New York, pp 59–75

Foley KM 1985 The treatment of cancer pain. New England Journal of Medicine 313: 845

France RD 1987 The future for antidepressants: treatment of pain. Psychopathology 20: 99–113

Getto CJ, Sorkness CA, Howell T 1987 Antidepressants and chronic nonmalignant pain: a review. Journal of Pain Symptom Control 2: 9–18

Gomez-Perez FJ, Rull JA, Dies H et al 1985 Nortriptyline and fluphenazine in the symptomatic treatment of diabetic neuropathy. A double-blind cross-over study. Pain 23: 395–400

Greenstein MG, Breitbart W 2000 Cancer and the experience of meaning: a group psychotherapy program for people with cancer. American Journal of Psychotherapy 54: 486–500

Grossman SA, Sheidler VR, Swedeon K et al 1991 Correlations of patient and caregiver ratings of cancer pain. Journal of Pain and Symptom Management 6: 53–57

Hall RCW, Gardner ER, Perl M, Stickney SK, Pfefferbaum B 1979 The professional burnout syndrome. Psychiatric Opinion 16: 12–17

Hammeroff SR, Cork RC, Scherer K et al 1982 Doxepin effects on chronic pain, depression and plasma opioids. Journal of Clinical Psychiatry 2: 22–26

Hartl DE 1979 Stress management and the nurse. In: Sutterley DC, Donnelly GF (eds) Stress management. Aspen, Germantown, MD, pp 163–172

Hewitt D, McDonald M, Portenoy R, Rosenfeld B, Passik S, Breitbart W 1997 Pain syndromes and etiologies in ambulatory AIDS patients. Pain 70: 117–123

Hinds C 1985 The needs of families who care for patients with cancer at home: are we meeting them? Journal of Advanced Nursing 10: 575–585

Holland JC 1989 Anxiety and cancer: the patient and family. Journal of Clinical Psychiatry 50: 20–25

Holland JC, Holland JF 1985 A neglected problem: the stresses of cancer care on physicians. Primary Care and Cancer 5: 16–22

Holland JC, Rowland J (eds) 1989 Handbook of psychooncology. Psychological care of the patient with cancer. Oxford University Press, New York

Holland JC, Fassanellos, Ohnuma T 1974 Psychiatric symptoms associated with L-asparaginase administration. Journal of Psychiatric Research 10: 165

Holland JC, Morrow G, Schmale A et al 1991 A randomized clinical trial of alprazolam versus progressive muscle relaxation in cancer patients with anxiety and depressive symptoms. Journal of Clinical Oncology 9: 1004–1011

Holland JC, Breitbart W, Jacobsen PB, Lederberg MS, Loscalzo M, Massie MJ and McCorkle R (eds) 1998 Psycho-oncology. Oxford University Press, New York

Horowitz SA, Breitbart W 1993 Relaxation and imagery for symptom control in cancer patients. In: Breibart W, Holland JC (eds) Psychiatric aspects of symptom management in cancer patients. American Psychiatric Press, Washington, DC, pp 147–172

Hull MM 1989 Family needs and supportive nursing behaviors during terminal cancer: a review. Oncology Nursing Forum 16: 787–792

Itil T, Fink M 1966 Anticholinergic drug-induced delirium: experimental modification, quantitative EEG and behavioral correlations. Journal of Nervous and Mental Disease 143: 492–507

Jaffe JH 1985 Drug addition and drug abuse. In: Gilman AG, Goodman LS, Rall TW, Murad F (eds) The pharmacological basis of therapeutics, 7th edn. Macmillan, New York, pp 532–581

Kanner RM, Foley KM 1981 Patterns of narcotic use in a cancer pain clinic. Annals of the New York Academy of Sciences 362: 161–172

Kash KM, Holland JC 1990 Reducing stress in medical oncology house officers: a preliminary report of a prospective intervention study. In: Hendrie HC, Lloyd C (eds) Educating competent and humane physicians. Indiana University Press, Bloomington, pp 183–195

Katon W, Raskind M 1980 Treatment of depression in the medically ill elderly with methylphenidate. American Journal of Psychiatry 137: 963–965

Kaufmann MW, Murray GB, Cassem NH 1982 Use of psychostimulants in medically ill depressive patients. Psychosomatics 23: 817–819

Kimball LR, McCormick WC 1996 The pharmacologic management of pain and discomfort in persons with AIDS near the end of life: use of opioid analgesia in the hospice setting. Journal of Pain and Symptom Management 11: 88–94

Kishore-Kumar R, Max MB, Schafer SC et al 1990 Desipramine relieves postherpetic neuralgia. Clinical Pharmacology and Therapeutics 47: 305–312

Koocher GP 1979 Adjustment and coping strategies among the caretakers of cancer patients. Social Work in Health Care 5: 145–150

Kristjanson LJ 1986 Indications of quality of palliative care from a family perspective. Journal of Palliative Care 1: 8–17

Kvindesal B, Molin J, Froland A, Gram LF 1984 Imipramine treatment of painful diabetic neuropathy. Journal of the American Medical Association 251: 1727–1730

Langohr HD, Stohr M, Petruch F 1982 An open and double-blind crossover study on the efficacy of clomipramine (anafranil) in patients with painful mono- and polyneuropathies. European Neurology 21: 309–315

Larue F, Brasseur L, Musseault P, Demeulemeester R, Bonifassi L, Bez G 1994 Pain and HIV infection: a French national survey [abstract]. Journal of Palliative Care 10: 95

Larue F, Fontaine A, Colleau S 1997 Underestimation and undertreatment of pain in HIV disease: multicentre study. British Medical Journal 314: 23–28

Lebovits AK, Lefkowitz M, McCarthy D et al 1989 The prevalence and management of pain in patients with AIDS. A review of 134 cases. Clinical Journal of Pain 5: 245–248

Lederberg M 1989 Psychological problems of staff and their management. In: Holland JC, Rowland J (eds) Handbook of psychooncology: psychological care of the patient with cancer. Oxford University Press, New York, pp 678–682

Levin DN, Cleeland CS, Dan R 1985 Public attitudes toward cancer pain. Cancer 56: 2337–2339

Levine PM, Silverfarb PM, Lipowski ZJ 1978 Mental disorders in cancer patients: a study of 100 psychiatric referrals. Cancer 42: 1385–1391

Liepzig RM, Goodman H, Gray P et al 1987 Reversible narcotic-associated mental status impairment in patients with metastatic cancer. Pharmacology 53: 47–57

Lindblom U, Merskey H, Mumford JM et al 1986 Pain terms: a current list with definitions and notes on usage. Pain 3: 5215–5221

Lipowski ZJ 1987 Delirium (acute confusional states). Journal of the American Medical Association 285: 1789–1792

Loscalzo M, Jacobsen PB 1990 Practical behavioral approaches to the effective management of pain and distress. Journal of Psychosocial Oncology 8: 139–169

Macaluso C, Weinberg D, Foley KM 1988 Opiod abuse and misuse in a cancer pain population. Second international congress on cancer pain, July 14–17, Rye, NY (abstract)

Magni G, Arsie D, DeLeo D 1987 Antidepressants in the treatment of cancer pain. A survey in Italy. Pain 29: 347–353

Marks RM, Sachar EJ 1973 Undertreatment of medical inpatients with narcotic analgesics. Annals of Internal Medicine 78: 173–181

Marte C, Allen M 1991 HIV-related gynecologic conditions: overlooked complications. Focus: A Guide to AIDS Research and Counseling 7: 1–3

Maslach C 1979 The burnout syndrome and patient care. In: Garfield CA (ed) Stress and survival, the emotional realities of life-threatening illness. Mosby, St Louis, pp 89–96

Massie MJ, Gagnon P, Holland JC et al 1994 Depression and suicide in patients with cancer. Journal of Pain and Symptom Management 9(5): 325–340

Massie MJ, Holland JC 1987 The cancer patient with pain: psychiatric complications and their management. Medical Clinics of North America 71: 243–258

Massie MJ, Holland JC 1990 Depression and the cancer patient. Journal of Clinical Psychiatry 51: 12–17

Massie MJ, Popkin MK 1998 Depression. In: Holland JC et al (eds), Psycho-oncology. Oxford University Press, New York, pp 518–541
Massie MJ, Holland JC, Glass E 1983 Delirium in terminally ill cancer patients. American Journal of Psychiatry 140: 1048–1050
Massie MJ, Holland JC, Straker N 1989 Psychotherapeutic interventions. In: Holland JC, Rowland J (eds) Handbook of psychooncology: psychological care of the patient with cancer. Oxford University Press, New York, pp 455–469
Max MB, Culnane M, Schafer SC et al 1987 Amitriptyline relieves diabetic-neuropathy pain in patients with normal and depressed mood. Neurology 37: 589–596
Max MB, Schafer SC, Culnane M, Smollen B, Dubner R, Gracely RH 1988 Amitriptyline, but not lorazepam, relieves postherpetic neuralgia. Neurology 38: 1427–1432
Max MB, Kishore-Kumar R, Schafer SC et al 1991 Efficacy of desipramine in painful diabetic neuropathy: a placebo-controlled trial. Pain 45: 3–10
McCaffrey M, Beebe A 1989 Pain: clinical manual for nursing practice. Mosby, Philadelphia, pp 353–360
McCaffrey M, Vourakis C 1992 Assessment and relief of pain in chemically dependent patients. Orthopaedic Nursing 11: 13–27
McCormack JP, Li R, Zarowny D, Singer J 1993 Inadequate treatment of pain in ambulatory HIV patients. Clinical Journal of Pain 9: 247–283
McKegney FP, Bailey CR, Yates JW 1981 Prediction and management of pain in patients with advanced cancer. General Hospital Psychiatry 3: 95–101
Medina JL, Diamond S 1977 Drug dependency in patients with chronic headaches. Headache 17(1): 12–74
Meier DE, Emmons C, Wallenstein S, Quill T, Morrison RS, Cassel CK 1998 A national survey of physician-assisted suicide and euthanasia in the United States. New England Journal of Medicine 338: 1193–1201
Melzack R, Wall PD 1983 The challenge of pain. Basic Books, New York
Mendels J 1987 Clinical experience with serotonin reuptake inhibiting antidepressants. Journal of Clinical Psychiatry 48(suppl): 26–30
Menza MA, Kaufman KR, Castellanos AM 2000 Modafanil augmentation of antidepressant treatment in depression. Journal of Clinical Psychiatry 61(5): 378–381
Mercadante S, DeConno F, Ripamonti 1995 Propofol in terminal care. Journal of Pain and Symptom Management 10: 639–642
Mor V, Guadagnoli E, Wool M 1987 An examination of the concrete service needs of advanced cancer patients. Journal of Psychosocial Oncology 5: 1–17
Mount BM 1986 Dealing with our losses. Journal of Clinical Oncology 4: 1127–1134
Moyle J 1995 The use of propofol in palliative medicine. Journal of Pain and Symptom Management 10: 643–646
Murray GB 1987 Confusion, delirium, and dementia. In: Hackett TP, Cassem NH (eds) Massachusetts General Hospital handbook of general hospital psychiatry, 2nd edn. PSG Publishing, Littleton, MA, pp 84–115
Nehra A, Mullick F, Ishak KG, Zimmerman AJ 1990 Pemoline associated hepatic injury. Gastroenterology 99: 1517–1519
Oliver OJ 1985 The use of methotrimeprazine in terminal care. British Journal of Clinical Practice 39: 339–340
O'Neill WM, Sherrard JS 1993 Pain in human immunodeficiency virus disease: a review. Pain 54: 3–14
Paddison PL, Gise LH, Lebovits A et al 1990 Sexual abuse and premenstrual syndrome: comparison between a lower and higher socioeconomic group. Psychosomatics 31: 265–272
Passik S 1992 Psychotherapy of the substance abusing cancer patient. American Psychiatric Association annual meeting, 4–10 May, Washington, DC (abstract)
Passik S, Wilson A 1987 Technical considerations of the frontier of supportive and expressive modes in psychotherapy. Dynamic Psychotherapy 5: 51–62
Passik S, Breitbart W, Rosenfeld B et al 1994 AIDS specific patient-related barriers to pain management. American Pain Society, 13th annual meeting, Miami, FL, 10–13 November (abstract)
Passik SD, Schreiber J, Kirsh KL, Portenoy RK 2000 A chart review of the ordering and documentation of urine toxicology screens in a cancer center: do they influence patient management? Journal of Pain and Symptom Management 19: 40–44
Patchell RA, Posner JB 1989 Cancer and the nervous system. In: Holland J, Rowland J (eds) The handbook of psychooncology: the psychological care of the cancer patient. Oxford University Press, New York, pp 327–341
Payne RM 1989 Pain in the drug abuser. In: Foley KM, Payne RM (eds) Current therapy of pain. BC Decker, Philadelphia, pp 46–54
Payne D, Jacobsen P, Breitbart W, Passik S, Rosenfeld B, McDonald M 1994 Negative thoughts related to pain are associated with greater pain, distress and disability in AIDS pain. American Pain Society, 13th scientific meeting, Miami, FL, November (abstract)
Peck AW, Stern WC, Watkinson C 1983 Incidence of seizures during treatment with tricyclic antidepressant drugs and buproprion. Journal of Clinical Psychiatry 44: 197–201
Penfold R, Clark AJM 1992 Pain syndromes in HIV infection. Canadian Journal of Anesthesia 39: 724–730
Perry S, Heidrich G 1982 Management of pain during debridement: a survey of US burn units. Pain 13: 267–280
Pilowsky I, Hallett EC, Bassett DL, Thomas PG, Penhall RK 1982 A controlled study of amitriptyline in the treatment of chronic pain. Pain 14: 169–179
Pizzuti D, Abbott Laboratories 1999 Cylert (pemoline) FDA Medwatch safety information and package labeling changes. Available at www.fda.gov/medwatch/safety/1999/Cylert.htm
Platt M, Breitbart W, Smith M, Marotta R, Weisman H, Jacobsen P 1994 Efficacy of neuroleptics for hypoactive delirium [letter]. Journal of Neuropsychiatry and Clinical Neurosciences 6: 66–67
Plumb MM, Holland JC 1977 Comparative studies of psychological function in patients with advanced cancer. Psychosomatic Medicine 39: 264–276
Popkin MK, Callies AL, Mackenzie TB 1985 The outcome of antidepressant use in the medically ill. Archives of General Psychiatry 42: 1160–1163
Portenoy RK 1987 Continuous intravenous infusion of opioid drugs. Medical Clinics of North America 71: 233–241
Portenoy RK, Payne R 1992 Acute and chronic pain. In: Lowinson JH, Ruiz P, Millman RB (eds) Comprehensive textbook of substance abuse. Williams & Wilkins, Baltimore, pp 691–721
Porter J, Jick H 1980 Addiction rate in patients treated with narcotics. New England Journal of Medicine 302: 123
Posner JB 1979 Delirium and exogenous metabolic brain disease. In: Beeson PB et al (eds) Cecil's textbook of medicine. Saunders, Philadelphia, pp 644–651
Posner JB 1988 Nonmetastatic effects of cancer on the nervous system. In: Wyngaarden JB et al (eds) Cecil's textbook of medicine. Saunders, Philadelphia, pp 1104–1107
Preskorn SH 1993 Recent pharmacologic advances in antidepressant therapy for the elderly. American Journal of Medicine 94(suppl 5A): 2S–12S
Purohit DR, Navlakha PL, Modi RS et al 1978 The role of antidepressants in hospitalized cancer patients. Journal of the Association of Physicians of India 26: 245–248
Rait D, Lederberg M 1989 The family of the cancer patient. In: Holland J, Rowland J (eds) The handbook of psychooncology: the psychological care of the cancer patient. Oxford University Press, New York, pp 585–598

Redd WB, Reeves JL, Storm FK, Minagawa RY 1982 Hypnosis in the control of pain during hyperthermia treatment of cancer. In: Bonica JJ et al (eds) Advances in pain research and theory, vol 5. Raven, New York, pp 857–861

Reik T 1948 Listening with a third ear. Farrar Straus, New York

Rifkin A, Reardon G, Siris S et al 1985 Trimipramine in physical illness with depression. Journal of Clinical Psychiatry 46: 4–8

Rosenfeld B, Breitbart W, McDonald MV, Passik SD, Thaler H, Portenoy RK 1996 Pain in ambulatory AIDS patients—II: Impact of pain on psychological functioning and quality of life. Pain 68: 323–328

Rowat K 1985 Chronic pain: a family affair. In: King K (ed) Recent advances in nursing long term care. Churchill Livingstone, Edinburgh, pp 259–271

Schofferman J, Brody R 1990 Pain in far advanced AIDS. In: Foley KM et al (eds) Advances in pain research and therapy, vol 16, Raven Press, New York, pp 379–386

Sharav Y, Singer E, Schmidt E, Dione RA, Dubner R 1987 The analgesic effect of amitriptyline on chronic facial pain. Pain 31: 199–209

Sher M, Krieger JN, Juergen S 1983 Trazodone and priapism. American Journal of Psychiatry 140: 1362–1364

Sindrup SH, Ejlertsen B, Froland A et al 1989 Imipramine treatment in diabetic neuropathy: relief of subjective symptoms without changes in peripheral and autonomic nerve function. European Journal of Clinical Pharmacology 37: 151–153

Singer EJ, Zorilla C, Fahy-Chandon B et al 1993 Painful symptoms reported for ambulatory HIV-infected men in a longitudinal study. Pain 54: 15–19

Singh A 1996 Safety of risperidone in patients with HIV and AIDS. In: Proceedings of the 149th annual meeting, American Psychiatric Association, 4–9 May, p 126 (abstract)

Sipahimalani A, Masand PS 1998 Olanzapine in the treatment of delirium. Psychosomatics 39: 422–430

Spiegel D 1985 The use of hypnosis in controlling cancer pain. CA: A Cancer Journal for Clinicians 4: 221–231

Spiegel D, Bloom JR 1983a Pain in metastatic breast cancer. Cancer 52: 341–345

Spiegel D, Bloom JR 1983b Group therapy and hypnosis reduce metastatic breast carcinoma pain. Psychosomatic Medicine 4: 333–339

Spiegel D, Bloom JR, Yalom ID 1981 Group support for patients with metastatic cancer: a randomized prospective outcome study. Archives of General Psychiatry 38: 527–533

Spikes J, Holland J 1975 The physician's response to the dying patient. In: Strain JJ, Grossman S (eds) Psychological care of the medically ill. Appleton–Century–Crofts, New York, pp 138–148

Stiefel FC, Breitbart W, Holland JC 1989 Corticosteroids in cancer: neuropsychiatric complications. Cancer Investigation 7: 479–491

Strafford M, Cahill C, Schwartz T et al 1991 Recognition and treatment of pain in pediatric patients with AIDS. Journal of Pain and Symptom Management 6: 146 (abstract)

Sullivan AD, Hedberg K, Fleming DA 2000 Legalized physician-assisted suicide in Oregon—the second year. New England Journal of Medicine 342: 598–604

Terr L 1991 Childhood traumas: an outline and overview. American Journal of Psychiatry 148: 10–20

Tiengo M, Pagnoni B, Calmi A, Rigoli M, Braga PC, Panerai AE 1987 Chlorimipramine compared to pentazocine as a unique treatment in post-operative pain. International Journal of Clinical Pharmacology Research 7: 141–143

Twycross RG, Lack SA 1983 Symptom control in far advanced cancer: pain relief. Pitman Books, London

Ventafridda V, Bonezzi C, Caraceni A et al 1987 Antidepressants for cancer pain and other painful syndromes with deafferentation component: comparison of amitriptyline and trazodone. Italian Journal of Neurological Sciences 8: 579–587

Ventafridda V, Ripamonti C, DeConno F et al 1990 Symptom prevalence and control during cancer patients' last days of life. Journal of Palliative Care 6: 7–11

von Roenn JH, Cleeland CS, Gonin R et al 1993 Physicians' attitudes toward cancer pain management survey: results of the Eastern Cooperative Oncology Group survey. Annals of Internal Medicine 119: 121–126

Walker E, Katon W, Griffins JH et al 1988 Relationship of chronic pelvic pain to psychiatric diagnosis and childhood sexual abuse. American Journal of Psychiatry 145: 75–80

Walsh TD 1983 Antidepressants and chronic pain. Clinical Neuropharmacology 6: 271–295

Walsh TD 1990 Adjuvant analgesic therapy in cancer pain. In: Foley KM et al (eds) Advances in pain research and therapy, vol 16. Second international congress on cancer pain. Raven Press, New York, pp 155–166

Ward SE, Goldberg N, Miller-McCauley C, Mueller C et al 1993 Patient-related barriers to management of cancer pain. Pain 52: 319–324

Warner MM 1992 Involvement of families in pain control of terminally ill patients. Hospice Journal 8: 155–170

Watson CP, Evans RJ, Reed K, Merskey H, Goldsmith L, Warsh J 1982 Amitriptyline versus placebo in postherpetic neuralgia. Neurology 32: 671–673

Weddington WW 1982 Delirium and depression associated with amphotericin B. Psychosomatics 23: 1076–1078

Weissman DE, Haddox JD 1989 Opioid pseudoaddiction—an iatrogenic syndrome. Pain 36: 363–366

Woodforde JM, Fielding JR 1970 Pain and cancer. Journal of Psychosomatic Research 4: 365–370

Young DF 1982 Neurological complications of cancer chemotherapy. In: Silverstein A (ed) Neurological complications of therapy: selected topics. Futura, New York, pp 57–113

Young RJ, Clarke BF 1985 Pain relief in diabetic neuropathy: the effectiveness of imipramine and related drugs. Diabetic Medicine 2: 363–366

Zelman D, Cleeland C, Howland EB 1987 Factors in appropriate pharmacological management of cancer pain: a cross-institutional investigation. Pain (suppl): S136

Chapter 46

Pain and impending death

Cicely Saunders and Michael Platt

Introduction

Fear of pain in dying is still common and was the reason for the majority of requests for euthanasia in one study from a hospice in the Netherlands that not only cares for inpatients but also consults with a large number of family doctors. However, once reassured by effective consultation and/or treatment, few requests were repeated and the patients died peacefully from their illness (Zylicz 1997). It is commonly thought that heavy sedation is required for such an outcome but a recent survey revealed that only a small percentage of '61 palliative care experts' questioned had to induce sedation for intractable distress in the dying (Chater et al 1998).

Pain at the end of life can usually be controlled, without such sedation by teams experienced in the multiprofessional practice of palliative medicine presented in detail in the *Oxford Textbook of Palliative Medicine* (Doyle et al 1998). However, it is sadly true that not all patients benefit from this experience. In some developing countries, this is due to lack of resources, but it is not only in such deprived conditions that patients suffer relievable terminal distress. Myths concerning the use of narcotics still abound (Wall 1997). Furthermore, some patients fail to obtain satisfactory pain relief even from large doses of narcotics.

The SUPPORT Study (SUPPORT Principal Investigators 1995) is the most extensive report published, with a total of 9105 adults hospitalized with one or more of nine life-threatening diagnoses and an overall six-month mortality rate of 47%. The study documented the results of the intervention of specially trained nurses in an attempt to improve communication and care and found that there was no overall improvement, including the level of reported pain. Half of the patients who died had moderate or severe pain during most of their final three days of life in the intervention group of 2652 patients, and there was no difference in their experience compared with the control group. Communication between physicians and patients remained poor; for example, the former failed to implement patients' refusal of cardiopulmonary resuscitation (CPR) intervention, while they misunderstood patients' preferences regarding CPR in 80% of cases. A regional study in the UK revealed stories of similar distress. These results have led to a number of calls to address education, leading to better practice in decision making and the control of distress (Addington-Hall and McCarthy 1995).

The efficacy of the World Health Organization Guidelines for Cancer Pain Relief (WHO 1990), which has been translated into many languages, was examined in 401 dying patients by Grond et al

(1991). They report that at the time of death, only 3% of patients experienced severe or very severe pain, whereas 52% had no pain at all, 24% only mild or moderate pain, and 20% were unable to rate pain intensity. Forty-four percent of patients required parenteral drugs. Additional adjuvant drugs were used in 90% of patients. This study was carried out by a department of anaesthesiology and a pain clinic with 45% of the patients treated in a general ward.

The research summarized by the United Kingdom's National Council for Hospice and Specialist Palliative Care Services is available from the address given at the end of this chapter, and is the basis of their booklet *Changing Gear—Guidelines for Managing the Last Days of Life* (National Council for Hospice and Specialist Palliative Care Services 1997), which gives clear guidance for recognition, assessment, and treatment. It recognizes relatives' needs and calls for the collaborative multi-professional approach that is needed, especially for the rare intractable situation. Rehydration with intravenous or subcutaneous fluids has been shown not to be of benefit at this stage and may cause peripheral and pulmonary oedema in patients with severe hypoalbuminaemia (Ellershaw et al 1995), but this remains a subject of debate and calls for further work (Sarhill et al 2001).

There is mounting evidence of the way in which a palliative care consultancy team can alter hospital practice. Their availability makes an impact on prescribing, taking shared responsibility in an area where the usual team is often unsure about opioid and other drug use. They can raise the awareness of the importance of psychosocial care for patients whose problems can seem overwhelming. They can institute and maintain contact with the referring primary care physician who may later have to offer bereavement support to the family. They can also help staff face patients in spiritual need and help in making important contacts. Some teams are developing an integrated care pathway for the dying patient as part of their impact on overall hospital policy (Ellershaw et al 1997). Many countries are establishing education programmes in a previously neglected area, underpinned by a growing body of research and specialist publications.

Therapy in intensive care units

The problem

The intensive care environment is a place where aggressive long-term life-saving techniques are used with the latest high-technology medicine and pharmacology. It is inevitable that pain and death occur frequently, neither of which are handled well in such an environment (Hall et al 1994, Hanson et al 1997). Advanced surgical techniques, improved resuscitation, and trauma life support, together with greater media and public expectations, result in ever-increasing demands for intensive care beds. The general ageing of the population at one end and the increasing survival of premature neonates at the other are also driving this demand.

Deciding on the futility of continuing interventions

Perhaps the most difficult decisions are involved in triaging patients for intensive therapy. This may include deciding on the 'futility of further medical management' in patients during assessment for possible admission to intensive care, or during intensive care management, when it is realized that further therapy is indeed futile (Sanders and Raffin 1993, Campbell and McHaffie 1995, Robb 1997, Yu 1997). Adequate management of pain and suffering is mandatory in any case. This encompasses a large age range of patients, from the 20-week-old premature neonate to the very elderly.

Problems associated with sedation and analgesia in the ITU patient

The patient in intensive care usually requires artificial ventilation, requiring sedation and sometimes paralysis. However, they may be aware, particularly to pain and discomfort, and may also be very distressed about family, finances, and other worries (Cherny et al 1994). The normal indications of pain and distress in a patient who is sedated, anaesthetized, or paralysed consist of increased sympathetic activity such as sweating, lacrimation, increased blood pressure, and tachycardia. However, in the critically ill patient, cardiac support drugs, sedative and anaesthetic drugs, and pathophysiological states such as septic shock and cerebral injury may mask or confuse these signs. Additionally, use of pharmacological paralysing agents prevent the patient from moving in response to pain. Paediatric and neonatal patients present particular problems (Chambliss and Anand 1997).

Sources of pain and suffering

Sources of pain are often multiple, with combinations of chronic neuropathic, inflammatory, chemical, mechanical, ischaemic, or acute pain.

These may be from the primary pathology, from treatment modalities such as radiation, from bedsores and skin ulcers, from pre-existing concurrent disease such as chronic arthritis, or simply from the discomfort of an endotracheal tube or intravenous line. Pain may be considered as contributing significantly to an overall sense of suffering. Cherny devised a model of suffering that incorporated pain and the various factors that affect quality of life (Cherny et al 1994). This model also includes the importance of family and social stresses, emphasizing the importance of adequate communication and counselling with close family and friends—especially once a decision of futility of further treatment has been made (Jones 1997). Psychosocial and spiritual processes strongly influence the impact and expression of pain, and these need to be taken into account in the assessment and treatment of pain in intensive care. This needs a holistic approach to the patient (Kolcaba and Fisher 1996) as well as some novel approaches to the treatment of pain.

How to assess suffering in ITU

The data used by critical care nurses in assessing pain appear to be a combination of facial appearances (grimacing, etc), movements of the patient, and the sympathetic activity mentioned above. Studies assessing the use of pain measurement scores using this sort of data (behavioural and physiological) suggest that pain is better managed this way (Puntillo et al 1997). Many units are now using pain and sedation scores to assess the adequacy of pain control in patients on life support in intensive care. The intensive care unit at St. Mary's Hospital in London uses a scoring system for pain and sedation (appended to the Glasgow coma scale) with an action flow chart (Fig. 46.1).

On withdrawal of active medical management

Once a decision, on the grounds of futility, is made to withdraw active treatment from a clinically ill patient (which should be seen as a positive one), adequate pain control and sedation continue to be of paramount importance. The close relatives of the patient also need to be properly consulted and counselled as necessary and in many cases involved in the decision making process. It should be noted that a withdrawal of active treatment is not the same as euthanásia, and patients die of the disease processes for which they were being treated. The use of adequate analgesia does not of itself cause death, which should be as pain free and dignified as possible, with the wishes of the patient, who should be as informed as possible (Horton 1996), and the relatives being respected.

Withdrawal of artificial ventilation

When life support for a ventilator-dependent patient is to be withdrawn, rather than having to cease artificial ventilation prior to death, the reduction of inspired oxygen concentration to that of room air, together with the removal of adjunctive ventilatory support such as PEEP (positive end-expiratory pressure), is usually sufficient before death ensues. At all stages, adequate analgesia and sedation for the patient must be provided (Edwards and Ueno 1991). A recent study showed that 10% of relatives of patients who died in hospital felt that pain could have been better managed (Hanson et al 1997). The relatives and close friends must not be forgotten, and they should be fully informed on the decisions that are made and the reasons for them.

Harvesting organs for transplantation after brain death

The diagnosis of brain death and the harvesting of organs for transplantation are no excuse for inadequate sedation and analgesia. Ultra-short-acting drugs such as the opioid remifentanil and intravenous anaesthetic agents such as propofol can be used to prevent accumulation of sedative drugs to allow for the diagnosis of brainstem death. The patient should always be appropriately anaesthetized for organ harvest, and good analgesia and sedation must always be assured. There are many modern potent opioids that can be used to provide profound analgesia without affecting cardiac output and help maintain adequate tissue perfusion.

Conclusion

Whatever the situation, even at life's end on a 'life support machine,' we have the pharmacology and the technology to treat pain and distress (although not always the means to treat spiritual distress), without recourse to euthanasia. Patients and their relatives should be confident that we as practitioners are always acting in the patient's best interests, including the relief of suffering. Patients should never have to fear that pain will not be treated or that their lives will end in undignified pain and terror.

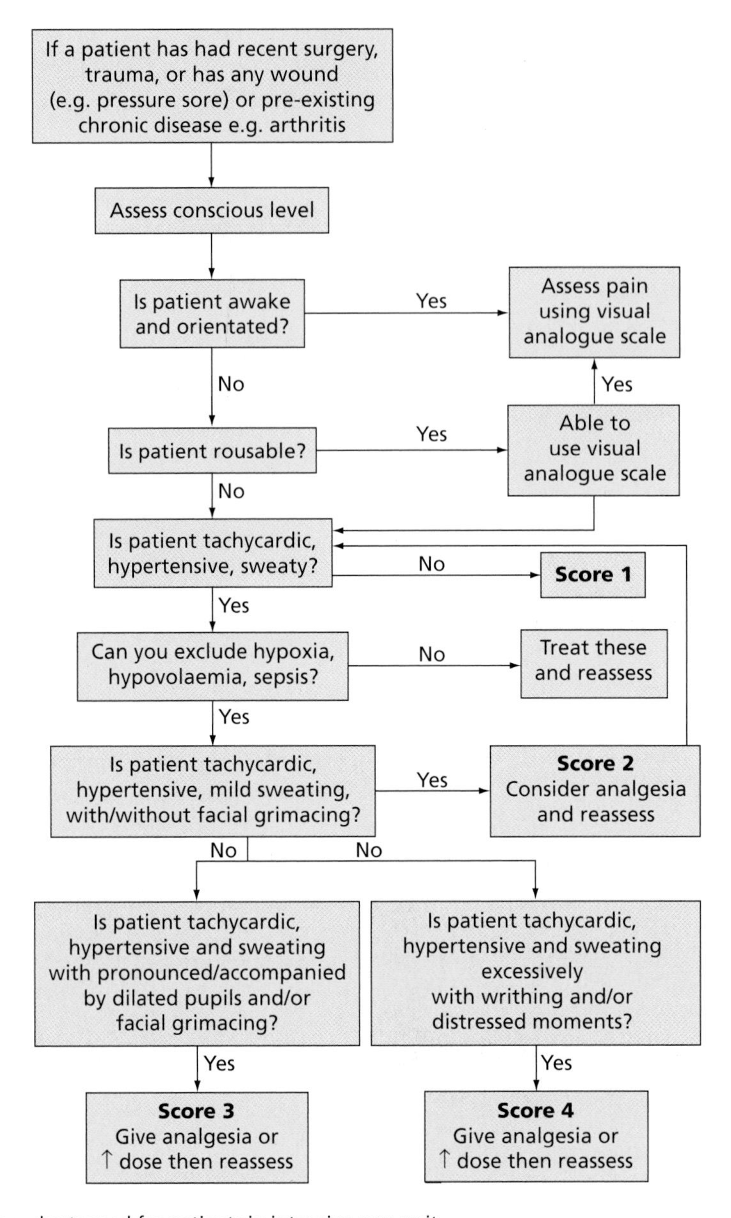

Fig. 46.1 Action flow charts used for patients in intensive care unit.

Guidelines for managing the last days of life

The Appendix to the National Council's booklet *Changing Gear—Guidelines for Managing the Last Days of Life in Adults* gives help in the control of all likely symptoms. The following suggestions are clear and direct:

1. Pain

   Pain (non-neuropathic)

   NSAIDs

- Indicated for superficial or deep somatic pain and pain of bone secondaries should be continued in patients already taking NSAIDs.
- Suppositories, e.g., diclofenac 100 mg b.d.
- Injections, e.g., ketorolac 30 mg per 24 h.
- Gel, e.g., diclofenac, may be used for painful decubitus ulcers.

Opioids

- Diamorphine is the drug of choice for parenteral administration (other opioids of high solubility may be used).

- Regular 4 hourly injections.
- Continuous subcutaneous infusion by syringe driver.

2. Dose conversion from oral morphine to parenteral diamorphine

1. Calculate total daily dose or oral morphine.
2. Divide total oral dose by 3 to give equivalent daily dose of parenteral diamorphine.
3. Increase diamorphine dose by 50% if pain is not controlled.
4. Infuse total daily dose in 24 h by syringe driver.

OR

Divide total daily dose by 6 to calculate dose for 4 hourly injection.

3. Use of portable infusion devices

Portable infusion devices, commonly known as syringe drivers, allow continuous infusions of medications to be given subcutaneously. This prevents the need for multiple injections and maintains a smooth delivery of medication. There are a number of such devices currently available. It is always important to follow the manufacturers instructions for safe administration of drugs.

Drugs commonly given by this method include:

Diamorphine
Midazolam
Hyoscine hydrobromide or butylbromide
Glycopyrronium
Haloperidol
Cyclizine (may precipitate in combination with other drugs)
Metoclopramide
Levomepromazine (methotrimeprazine)

Only one of these may be combined with diamorphine at one time.

4. Management of specific symptoms

Pain (neuropathic)

Anticonvulsants

- Indicated for treatment of burning or shooting pains when patient unable to take oral anticonvulsants.
- Midazolam 5–10 mg 4 hourly SC
- Clonazepam 0.25–1 mg 4 hourly SC
- Phenothiazines
- Levomepromazine (methotrimeprazine)
- Also has sedative and antiemetic properties.
- Indicated for pain when sedation is also required.
- 20–25 mg t.d.s. by SC injection.
- Local reaction can occur at the injection site.

Breathlessness

- May be more distressing than pain.
- Some patients have a fast respiratory rate but are not distressed by this.

Opioids

- Diamorphine is the opioid of choice (or another opioid of high solubility may be used).
- 2.5–5 mg 4 hourly by SC injection for opioid-naïve patients.

Benzodiazepines

- Indicated for breathlessness associated with anxiety.
- Lorazepam 0.5–1 mg sublingually.
- Midazolam 2.5–5 mg by SC injection 4 hourly or via syringe driver.

Phenothiazines

- Indicated for breathlessness associated with anxiety or extreme agitation.
- Less commonly used since introduction of water-soluble benzodiazepines.
- Levomepromazine (methotrimeprazine) 25–50 mg 6–8 hourly.

Oxygen therapy

- Several studies have shown that oxygen is more effective than air at relieving dyspnoea when given acutely, even in patients with normal oxygen saturation.
- Should be administered in least obtrusive way, via nasal prongs.
- Humidification is needed to minimize drying out mucous membranes.
- Often not needed if dyspnoea is relieved by other measures.

Cough/noisy respirations

- Cough and 'rattly' breathing usually herald tracheo-bronchitis or bronchopneumonia as a terminal event because the patient is too weak to clear secretions.
- Antibiotics are rarely appropriate.
- Appropriate positioning of patient by nurse.

Anticholinergics reduce the volume of secretions.

- Hyoscine hydrobromide 0.2–0.4 mg hourly SC.
- Indicated if sedation is also required.
- Compatible with diamorphine in syringe driver.

This may cause agitated confusion in the elderly, in which case change to:

- Glycopyrronium 0.2 mg 4 hourly.
- Less likely to cause confusion/agitation.

Local anaesthetics suppress distressing cough when patient is too weak to clear secretions:

- Bupivacaine 2.5 ml 0.25% via nebulizer 6 hourly.

Terminal restlessness

Exclude correctable causes such as urinary retention (catheterize) or steroid therapy (discontinue).

Benzodiazepines

- Midazolam 5–20 mg 4 hourly SC or via syringe driver has become the treatment of choice.

Agitation/delirium

Major tranquillizers

- Levomepromazine (methotrimeprazine) 25–50 mg 6–8 hourly by SC injection.
- Haloperidol 5–20 mg 4–6 hourly by SC injection.

Benzodiazepines

- Midazolam 5–20 mg 4 hourly SC as an adjunct to major tranquillizer.

Myoclonic jerking

Usually due to rapid escalation of opioid dose.

Benzodiazepines

- Midazolam 5–10 mg SC.

From *Changing Gear—Guidelines for Managing the Last Days of Life in Adults*, published by the National Council for Hospice and Specialist Palliative Care Services, First Floor, Hospice House, 34–44 Britannia Street, London WC1X 9JG.

The selection of these drugs needs to be individualized. A blanket ordering of what may be an overdose for a particular patient would hardly seem to be the way to end a long-term commitment to a patient's care on the part of his or her doctors and nurses. Drugs are used as fine instruments and to turn to their use as a blunderbuss at the end would intimate a final attitude tantamount to 'writing off the patient'. Clinical assessment and response to the needs of the patient cease only at death and support for the family afterwards depends on the doctor's presence and interest throughout the illness he has committed himself to manage.

References

Addington-Hall JM, McCarthy M 1995 Dying from cancer: results of a population based investigation. Palliative Medicine 9(4): 295–305

Campbell, AGM, McHaffie HE 1995 Prolonging life and allowing death: infants. Journal of Medical Ethics 21(6): 339–344

Chambliss CR, Anand KJ 1997 Pain management in the pediatric intensive care unit. Current Opinion in Pediatrics 9(3): 246–253

Chater S, Viola R, Paterson J, Jarvis V 1998 Sedation for intractable distress in the dying – a survey of experts. Palliative Medicine 12(4): 255–269

Cherny NI, Coyle N, Foley KM 1994 Sufferirng in the advanced cancer patient: a definition and taxonomy. Journal of Palliative Care 10(2): 57–70

Doyle D, Hanks GWC, MacDonald N 1998 Oxford textbook of palliative medicine, 2nd edn. Oxford University Press, London

Edwards BS, Ueno WM 1991 Sedation before ventilator withdrawal (Case presentation). Journal of Clinical Ethics 2(2): 118–122

Ellershaw JE, Sutcliffe JM, Saunders CM 1995 Dehydration and the dying patient. Journal of Pain and Symptom Management 10(3): 192–197

Ellershaw J, Foster A, Murphy D et al 1997 Developing an integrated care pathway for the dying patient. European Journal of Palliative Care 4(6): 203–208

Grond S, Zech D, Schug A et al 1991 Validation of World Health Organization guidelines for cancer pain relief during the last days and hours of life. Journal of Pain and Symptom Management 6(7): 411–422

Hall Lord ML, Larsson G, Bostrom I 1994 Elderly patients' experiences of pain and distress in intensive care: a grounded theory study. Intensive Critical Care Nursing 10(2): 133–141

Hanson LC, Danis M, Garrett J 1997 What is wrong with end-of-life care? Opinions of bereaved family members. Journal of the American Geriatric Society 45: 1339–1344

Horton S 1996 Imparting the knowledge of impending death to the intensive care patient who is unable to respond. Nursing Critical Care 1(5): 250–253

Jones A 1997 Family therapy in a critical care unit. Nursing Standard 11(21): 40–42

Kolcaba KY, Fisher EM 1996 A holistic perspective on comfort care as an advance directive. Critical Care in Nursing Quarterly 18(4): 66–76

National Council for Hospice and Specialist Palliative Care Services 1997 Changing gear—guidelines for managing the last days of life in adults. Proceedings of working party on clinical guidelines in palliative care. National Council for Hospice and Specialist Palliative Care Services, London

Puntillo KA, Miaskowski C, Kehrle K et al 1997 Relationship between behavioural and physiological indicators of pain, critical care patients' self-reports of pain, and opioid administration. Critical Care Medicine 25(7): 1159–1166

Robb YA 1997 Ethical considerations relating to terminal weaning in intensive care. Intensive Critical Care Nursing 13(3): 156–162

Sanders LM, Raffin TA 1993 The ethics of withholding and withdrawing critical care. Cambridge Quarterly of Healthcare Ethics 2(2): 175–184

Sarhill N, Walsh D, Nelson K, Davis M 2001 Evaluation and treatment of cancer-related fluid deficits: volume depletion and dehydration. Support Cancer 9: 408–419

'SUPPORT' Principal Investigators 1995 A controlled trial to improve care for seriously ill hospitalized patients. The study to understand prognoses and preferences for outcomes and risks of treatments (SUPPORT). Journal of the American Medical Association 274(20): 1591–1598

Wall PD 1997 The generation of yet another myth on the use of narcotics. Pain 73: 121–122

World Health Organization (WHO) 1990 Cancer pain relief. World Health Organization, Geneva

Yu VY 1997 Ethical decision-making in newborn infants. Acta Medica Portuguesa 10(2–3): 197–204

Zylicz Z 1997 Dealing with people who want to die. Palliative Care Today 6(3): 38

Index

C

D

E

G

H

I

J

K

L

M

O

Q

R

S

U

V

W

X

Y

Z